Essentials of Pathophysiology

Essentials of Pathophysiology

Edited by

Chris E. Kaufman, M.D.
Professor and Chief, Section of Nephrology,
University of Oklahoma College of Medicine;
Staff Physician, University Hospital, Oklahoma City

Patrick A. McKee, M.D.
George Lynn Cross Professor of Medicine and Scientific Director,
William K. Warren Medical Research Institute,
University of Oklahoma College of Medicine, Oklahoma City

Little, Brown and Company
Boston   New York   Toronto   London

To all our teachers, that this may represent
a spark of their torch passed on

Library of Congress Cataloging-in-Publication Data

Essentials of pathophysiology / edited by Chris E. Kaufman,
   Patrick A. McKee.
      p.   cm.
    Includes bibliographical references and index.
    ISBN 0-316-48405-9
    1. Physiology, Pathological.   I. Kaufman, Chris E.
  II. McKee, Patrick A.
    [DNLM: 1. Disease.   2. Physiology.   QZ 140 E78 1996]
  RB113.E87   1996
  616.07 — dc20
  DNLM/DLC
  for Library of Congress   95-26499
                         CIP

Printed in the United States of America
MV-NY

Editorial: Evan R. Schnittman, Rebecca Marnhout
Production Services: Textbook Writers Associates, Inc.
Copyeditor: Lawrence Feinberg
Indexer: Michael Loo
Cover Design: Hannus Design Associates
Cover Illustration: Kristen Wienandt

Contents

Plate Legends

Plate 1. Peripheral blood smear in acute lymphocytic leukemia. The lymphoblast (arrow) is of the L3 histologic subtype. Note the enormity of this cell in comparison to normal erythrocytes in the field. The blast cell has the characteristic high nuclear : cytoplasmic ratio, dark blue cytoplasm, and vacuoles seen in L3 lymphoblasts. In addition, immature neutrophils and a nucleated red blood cell are characteristic of the myelophthisic blood picture.

Plate 2. Peripheral blood smear in chronic lymphocytic leukemia. The malignant cells appear histologically like normal lymphocytes. The size approximates that of an erythrocyte and is markedly smaller and quite distinct from the appearance of the lymphoblast in Plate 1. Also shown is the typical smudge cell seen in chronic lymphocytic leukemia. Some variability of the size and shape of the malignant cells is not uncommon, but the majority of the lymphocytes are rather bland.

Plate 3. Bone marrow aspirate in multiple myeloma. The marrow shows a large number of plasma cells (PC). These cells may be morphologically normal or abnormal, such as the binucleate plasma cell (BN). The erythroid (E) and myeloid (M) cells in the background appear normal, because they are unaffected by the malignant clone.

Plate 4. Monosodium urate monohydrate crystals aspirated from a tophus of a patient with gout. Numerous needle-shaped crystals are seen, without inflammatory cells. A. Under polarized light with a red compensator, urate crystals show negative birefringence; thus, all crystals whose long axis is parallel to the slow axis of vibration of the

red compensator (arrow) appear yellow (white in these photographs), while those lying perpendicular appear blue. Some crystals lying obliquely are seen to extinguish (appear dark). B. When the same field is viewed so the axis of the compensator (arrow) is turned 90 degrees from that in A, each individual crystal that appeared yellow becomes blue, and those appearing blue become yellow. (Courtesy of Jan Pitha, M.D.)

Plate 5. Immunofluorescence of a glomerulus showing linear staining for IgG typical of anti–glomerular basement membrane glomerulonephritis. (Courtesy of Fred Silva, M.D.)

Plate 6. Immunofluorescence of a glomerulus showing granular staining of the peripheral capillary loops and mesangial areas. (Courtesy of Zoltan Laszik, M.D.)

Plate 7. Red cell cast, unstained (original magnification 400×).

Plate 8. Acute tubulointerstitial nephritis. Marked inflammatory cell infiltrate in the interstitium along with edema causing tubular separation (hematoxylin-eosin stain, original magnification 250×). (Courtesy of K. Min, M.D.)

Plate 9. Photomicrograph of Cowdry type A intranuclear inclusions.

Plate 10. Photomicrograph of cerebral toxoplasmosis shows three cysts (arrows) and free multiple organisms (tiny spots near bottom arrows).

Preface

Essentials of Pathophysiology emphasizes the relationships between abnormal function and clinical manifestations of disease. It was created according to four pedagogic principles. First, throughout the text, the reader will review the language of physiology and, to a certain extent, pathology from the standpoint of *words* and *symbols* that depict normal and abnormal function. Second, factual knowledge about disease is laid out in an economical way to facilitate retention of key information. Third, the reader is guided to recall and arrange this information in logical ways that lead to the correct interpretation and understanding of signs and symptoms of illness. Fourth, frequent repetition of facts and concepts throughout the text, and their presentation in different formats and relationships, augment the ability to recall information and construct a conceptual framework for its application.

The text does not provide detailed descriptions of cellular and molecular aberrations that lead to disease, it does not address all diseases known, and it cannot substitute for more comprehensive textbooks. Instead, the text primarily discusses how deranged function becomes manifest in frequently encountered and illustrative human diseases.

Essentials of Pathophysiology was written primarily to help medical students and residents make the transition from the basic science–oriented years of learning to the patient's bedside, by explaining structure-function relationships for each organ system and the resultant signs and symptoms of common illnesses. Each chapter begins with a list of learning objectives and concludes with one or more case histories that exemplify how the history, physical examination, and laboratory findings can be explained if one comprehends the underlying pathophysiology.

The book contains numerous tables and illustrations selected to enhance understanding. Board examination–type questions are provided at the end of each part to test whether facts can be logically integrated and applied to clinical problems. In short, the overarching goal is to draw the reader toward an enhanced ability for clinical problem solving through orderly arrangements and interpretations of factual knowledge.

The book should be a powerful complement to most medical school pathophysiology courses. We expect that physicians-in-training and practicing physicians will find the book useful for review of the basic science concepts underlying clinical practice. The book should also facilitate preparation for medical board examinations as well as those required for certification by the osteopathic, dental, nursing, and physician assistant professions.

We are most appreciative of the hard work and caring attention that Beverly Clarke, our administrative assistant, provided in assembling and editing this book.

C. E. K.
P. A. M.

Contributing Authors

Mary Zoe Baker, M.D.
Assistant Professor of Medicine, University of Oklahoma College of Medicine; Staff Physician, University Hospital, Oklahoma City

Karen J. Beckman, M.D.
Associate Professor of Medicine, University of Oklahoma College of Medicine; Staff Physician, University Hospital, Oklahoma City

Marie A. Bernard, M.D.
Associate Professor of Medicine, University of Oklahoma College of Medicine; Associate Chief of Staff, Department of Geriatrics and Extended Care, Veterans Affairs Medical Center, Oklahoma City

Brian G. Birdwell, M.D.
Instructor and National Institutes of Health Research Fellow, Department of Medicine, University of Oklahoma College of Medicine; Staff Physician, University Hospital, Oklahoma City

Gary B. Bobele, M.D.
Director, Section of Pediatric Neurology, Driscoll Children's Hospital, Corpus Christi, Texas

Sylvia S. Bottomley, M.D.
Professor of Medicine, University of Oklahoma College of Medicine; Staff Physician, University Hospital and Veterans Affairs Medical Center, Oklahoma City

James E. Bourdeau, M.D., Ph.D.
Nephrology Associates of Waukesha, S.C., Waukesha, Wisconsin

Brent R. Brown, M.D.
Assistant Professor of Medicine, University of Oklahoma College of Medicine; Staff Physician, University Hospital, Oklahoma City

Roger A. Brumback, M.D.
Professor of Pathology, University of Oklahoma College of Medicine; Staff Pathologist, University Hospital, Oklahoma City

Vikki A. Canfield, M.D.
Assistant Professor of Medicine, University of Oklahoma College of Medicine; Staff Physician, University Hospital, Oklahoma City

Paul V. Carlile, M.D.
Associate Professor of Medicine, University of Oklahoma College of Medicine; Staff Physician, University Hospital, Oklahoma City

L. Philip Carter, M.D.
Professor and Chairman, Department of Neurosurgery, University of Oklahoma College of Medicine; Chief, Department of Neurosurgery, University Hospital, Oklahoma City

Thomas H. Carter, M.D., Ph.D.
Assistant Professor of Medicine, University of Oklahoma College of Medicine; Staff Physician, University Hospital, Oklahoma City

Keith F. Clark, M.D.
Associate Professor of Otorhinolaryngology, University of Oklahoma College of Medicine; Staff Physician, University Hospital, Oklahoma City

Dennis L. Confer, M.D.
Associate Professor of Medicine, University of Oklahoma College of Medicine; Director, Bone Marrow Transplant Unit, University Hospital, Oklahoma City

James R. Couch, Jr., M.D., Ph.D.
Professor and Chairman, Department of Neurology, University of Oklahoma College of Medicine; Staff Physician, University Hospital, Oklahoma City

Matthew T. Draelos, M.D.
Assistant Professor of Medicine, University of Oklahoma College of Medicine; Staff Physician, University Hospital and Veterans Affairs Medical Center, Oklahoma City

E. Randy Eichner, M.D.
Professor of Medicine, University of Oklahoma College of Medicine; Staff Physician, University Hospital, Oklahoma City

Bradley K. Farris, M.D.
Associate Professor of Ophthalmology, University of Oklahoma College of Medicine; Staff Physician, University Hospital, Oklahoma City

Douglas P. Fine, M.D.
Professor and Chairman, Department of Medicine, University of Oklahoma College of Medicine; Staff Physician, University Hospital and Veterans Affairs Medical Center, Oklahoma City

Dale A. Freeman, M.D.
Associate Professor of Medicine, University of Oklahoma College of Medicine; Staff Physician, University Hospital, Oklahoma City

James N. George, M.D.
Professor and Chief, Section of Hematology-Oncology, University of Oklahoma College of Medicine; Staff Physician, University Hospital and Veterans Affairs Medical Center, Oklahoma City

Barry A. Gray, M.D., Ph.D.
Professor of Medicine, University of Oklahoma College of Medicine; Staff Physician, University Hospital and Veterans Affairs Medical Center, Oklahoma City

Ralph T. Guild III, M.D.
Associate Professor of Medicine, University of Oklahoma College of Medicine; Chief, Section of Digestive Diseases/Nutrition, Veterans Affairs Medical Center, Oklahoma City

Mary K. Gumerlock, M.D.
Associate Professor of Neurosurgery, University of Oklahoma College of Medicine; Surgeon, Veterans Affairs Medical Center, Oklahoma City

Michael R. Hahn, M.D.
Resident, Department of Neurosurgery, University of Oklahoma College of Medicine, Oklahoma City

Karen K. Hamilton, M.D.
Associate Professor of Medicine, University of Oklahoma College of Medicine; Staff Physician, University Hospital and Veterans Affairs Medical Center, Oklahoma City

John B. Harley, M.D., Ph.D.
Professor and James R. McEldowney Chair in Immunology, University of Oklahoma College of Medicine; Associate Member, Arthritis and Immunology Program, Oklahoma Medical Research Foundation, Oklahoma City

Gary W. Harris, M.D.
Clinical Assistant Professor of Ophthalmology, University of Oklahoma College of Medicine, Staff Physician, University Hospital and Veterans Affairs Medical Center, Oklahoma City

Richard F. Harty, M.D.
Professor and Chief, Section of Digestive Disease and Nutrition, University of Oklahoma College of Medicine; Staff Physician, University Hospital, Oklahoma City

Farhat Husain, M.B.B.S.
Assistant Professor of Neurology, University of Oklahoma College of Medicine; Staff Physician, University Hospital, Oklahoma City

Donald J. Kastens, M.D.
Associate Professor of Medicine, University of Oklahoma College of Medicine; Staff Physician, University Hospital, Oklahoma City

Chris E. Kaufman, M.D.
Professor and Chief, Section of Nephrology, University of Oklahoma College of Medicine; Staff Physician, University Hospital, Oklahoma City

David C. Kem, M.D.
Professor and Chief, Section of Endocrinology, Metabolism, and Hypertension, University of Oklahoma College of Medicine; Staff Physician, University Hospital, Oklahoma City

Sudhir K. Khanna, M.D., M.R.C.P., F.R.C.P.C.
Staff Nephrologist, Baptist Medical Center,
Oklahoma City

Gary T. Kinasewitz, M.D.
Professor and Chief, Section of Pulmonary
Diseases, University of Oklahoma College of
Medicine; Staff Physician, University Hospital,
Oklahoma City

Jeanne A. King, M.D.
Assistant Professor of Neurology, University of
Oklahoma College of Medicine; Staff Physician,
University Hospital, Oklahoma City

Michael A. Kolodziej, M.D.
Assistant Professor of Medicine, University of
Oklahoma College of Medicine; Staff Physician,
University Hospital, Oklahoma City

Satish Kumar, M.D.
Assistant Professor of Medicine, University of
Oklahoma College of Medicine; Staff Physician,
University Hospital and Veterans Affairs Medical
Center, Oklahoma City

Ralph Lazzara, M.D.
Professor and Chief, Section of Cardiology,
University of Oklahoma College of Medicine; Staff
Physician, University Hospital, Oklahoma City

Richard W. Leech, M.D.
Professor and Vice-Chairman for Administrative
Affairs, Department of Pathology, University of
Oklahoma College of Medicine; Staff Pathologist,
University Hospital, Oklahoma City

David C. Levin, M.D.
Professor of Medicine, University of Oklahoma
College of Medicine; Staff Physician, University
Hospital and Veterans Affairs Medical Center,
Oklahoma City

D. Robert McCaffree, M.D.
Professor of Medicine, University of Oklahoma
College of Medicine; Chief of Staff, Veterans Affairs
Medical Center; Staff Physician, University
Hospital, Oklahoma City

Paul N. Maton, M.D.
Director, Oklahoma Foundation for Digestive
Research; Staff Physician, Presbyterian Hospital,
Oklahoma City

Anil Minocha, M.D.
Associate Professor of Medicine, University of
Oklahoma College of Medicine; Staff Physician,
University Hospital and Veterans Affairs Medical
Center, Oklahoma City

Harry S. Ojeas, M.D.
Fellow, Section of Digestive Diseases and Nutrition,
University of Oklahoma College of Medicine,
Oklahoma City

Leann Olansky, M.D.
Associate Professor of Medicine, University of
Oklahoma College of Medicine; Staff Physician,
University Hospital, Oklahoma City

Samuel R. Oleinick, M.D., Ph.D.
Professor of Medicine, University of Oklahoma College of Medicine; Staff Physician, University Hospital
and Veterans Affairs Medical Center, Oklahoma City

Edwin G. Olson, M.D.
Attending Physician, Section of Cardiology,
Methodist Medical Center, Dallas

Edward Overholt, M.D.
Associate Professor of Pediatrics, University of
Oklahoma College of Medicine; Staff Physician,
Children's Hospital of Oklahoma, Oklahoma City

Julie T. Parke, M.D.
Clinical Associate Professor of Neurology, University
of Oklahoma College of Medicine; Staff Physician,
Children's Hospital of Oklahoma, Oklahoma City

James A. Pederson, M.D.
Professor of Medicine, University of Oklahoma College of Medicine; Staff Physician, University Hospital
and Veterans Affairs Medical Center, Oklahoma City

Osvaldo H. Perurena, M.D.
Assistant Professor of Neurology, University of
Oklahoma College of Medicine; Staff Physician,
University Hospital, Oklahoma City

Laura I. Rankin, M.D.
Adjunct Professor of Medicine, University of Oklahoma College of Medicine; Staff Nephrologist, Baptist Medical Center, Oklahoma City

Robert A. Rankin, M.D.
Staff Gastroenterologist, University Hospital, Oklahoma City

Morris Reichlin, M.D.
Professor and Chief, Section of Immunology, University of Oklahoma College of Medicine; Staff Physician, University Hospital, Oklahoma City

Regina Resta, M.D.
Assistant Professor of Medicine, University of Oklahoma College of Medicine; Staff Physician, University Hospital, Oklahoma City

Eliot Schechter, M.D.
Professor of Medicine, University of Oklahoma College of Medicine; Director, Cardiac Catheterization Laboratory, Veterans Affairs Medical Center, Oklahoma City

Sanford Schneider, M.D.
Presbyterian Health Foundation Professor of Neurology, University of Oklahoma College of Medicine; Chief, Section of Child Neurology, Children's Hospital of Oklahoma, Oklahoma City

R. Hal Scofield, M.D.
Assistant Professor of Medicine, University of Oklahoma College of Medicine; Staff Physician, University Hospital and Veterans Affairs Medical Center, Oklahoma City

Chittur A. Sivaram, M.D.
Associate Professor of Medicine, University of Oklahoma College of Medicine; Chief, Section of Cardiology, Veterans Affairs Medical Center, Oklahoma City

Haraldine A. Stafford, M.D., Ph.D.
Assistant Professor of Medicine, University of Oklahoma College of Medicine; Staff Physician, University Hospital, Oklahoma City

Leslie S. Staudt, M.D.
Assistant Professor of Medicine, University of Oklahoma College of Medicine; Staff Physician, University Hospital, Oklahoma City

Ira N. Targoff, M.D.
Associate Professor of Medicine, University of Oklahoma College of Medicine; Staff Physician, University Hospital, Oklahoma City

Udho Thadani, M.B.B.S., M.R.C.P., F.R.C.P.C.
Professor and Vice-Chief and Director of Clinical Research, University of Oklahoma College of Medicine; Staff Physician, University Hospital, Oklahoma City

Martin H. Welch, M.D.
Professor of Medicine, University of Oklahoma College of Medicine; Director, Pulmonary Function Laboratory, University Hospital, Oklahoma City

James H. Wells, M.D.
Professor of Medicine, University of Oklahoma College of Medicine; Staff Physician, University Hospital, Oklahoma City

Thomas L. Whitsett, M.D.
Professor of Medicine and Pharmacology, University of Oklahoma College of Medicine; Director, Vascular Medicine Program, University Hospital, Oklahoma City

Peggy J. Wisdom, M.D.
Associate Professor of Neurology, University of Oklahoma College of Medicine; Staff Physician, University Hospital, Oklahoma City

I Cardiovascular Diseases

Part Editor
Udho Thadani

Notice

The indications and dosages of all drugs in this book have been recommended in the medical literature and conform to the practices of the general medical community. The medications described do not necessarily have specific approval by the Food and Drug Administration for use in the diseases and dosages for which they are recommended. The package insert for each drug should be consulted for use and dosage as approved by the FDA. Because standards for usage change, it is advisable to keep abreast of revised recommendations, particularly those concerning new drugs.

1 Cardiac Arrhythmias and Conduction Disturbances

Karen J. Beckman and Ralph Lazzara

Objectives

After completing this chapter, you should be able to

Understand the three mechanisms of tachyarrhythmias

Understand the mechanisms of bradyarrhythmias

Understand the types of clinical arrhythmias

Understand the treatment of clinical arrhythmias

Normal Cardiac Electrophysiology

Resting State

The movement of ions across cardiac cellular membranes can be measured as voltage changes over time, which are represented by the action potential (Fig. 1-1). The transmembrane voltage potentials of cardiac cells are determined by the permeability of the membrane to specific ions and by the differences in concentrations of those ions in the interior and exterior of the cell. In the resting state, the membrane is highly permeable to potassium in comparison with the other major ion species (sodium, calcium, chloride, bicarbonate, and magnesium). The concentration of potassium is much greater inside the cell than outside, resulting in a chemical gradient across the membrane which serves to drive potassium out of the cell and generates a counteracting electrical potential gradient to retain potassium in the cell. Since potassium is a positively charged ion, the electrical potential required to retain it in the cell is a negative potential. Thus, during the resting state, the intracellular compartment has a negative voltage (approximately –90 mV) in comparison to the extracellular compartment — the so-called resting potential. The cell is at its resting potential during phase 4 of the action potential (see Fig. 1-1).

Depolarization (Excitation) and Propagation

When a cell is excited, a marked change in permeability occurs: the membrane becomes transiently more permeable to sodium due to opening of ion channels, called fast channels, that are relatively selective for sodium. Since sodium is in relatively high concentration outside the cell and is a positively charged ion, the increase in sodium permeability results in an intense transient flow of sodium ions into the cell (inward current) and a shift in membrane potential toward the positive direction, resulting in an upstroke and overshoot to +30 mV (phase 0 of the action potential). The process of excitation occurs when the transmembrane potential in the resting state is shifted to approximately –60 mV, a level called the threshold potential. The shift can also occur because of the passage of electrical current through the membrane or with mechanical deformation of the membrane. During natural propagation, the shift from resting to threshold potential occurs because of current flow generated by the difference in internal potential between a cell that has been excited to a level of +30 mV and a cell that is in the resting state at a level of –90 mV. Current flows through the interior of the cell and across the membranes because of this potential

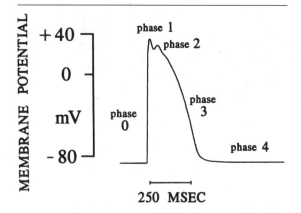

VENTRICULAR MUSCLE

Fig. 1-1. Action potential of a myocardial cell. The action potential is divided into five phases. Phase 0 is the upstroke/overshoot and corresponds to excitation of the cell. Phases 1, 2, and 3 are all phases of repolarization. Phase 4 is the resting stage.

gradient. Thus, the process of propagation depends on the passage of current between the excited cells and the resting cells and the excitation of the cells in the resting state by this current. In addition, all cardiac cells are connected together in a syncytium and linked by low resistance junctions called intercalated discs through which current passes more readily. There are more intercalated discs on the ends of myocardial fibers than on the sides; therefore, conduction proceeds more readily in the longitudinal direction than the transverse direction (uniform anisotropy).

Repolarization

After a cell has been excited, a series of changes in ionic permeabilities occurs. An increase in permeability to calcium results from the opening of channels called slow channels that are relatively selective for calcium. The opening of the slow channels causes an inflow of calcium ions because calcium is in higher concentration in the exterior than the interior of the cell. The slow inward flow of calcium begins near the end of the upstroke, peaks just after the overshoot (phase 1 of the action potential), and persists at low intensity during the plateau phase (phase 2 of the action potential). During the plateau, there is a gradual increase in permeability to potassium due to the open-

ing of a potassium selective channel, which reaches sufficient intensity to initiate rapid repolarization (phase 3). The outward flow of positive potassium ions is largely responsible for restoring the membrane to the negative resting potential (phase 4).

The myocardial cells are refractory to excitation for a period of time after being depolarized. The refractory period corresponds approximately to the duration of the action potential. The absolute refractory period occurs from the upstroke to the time when the membrane potential has repolarized to the level of the threshold potential; the relative refractory period corresponds to the time that the membrane potential is repolarizing from the level of the threshold potential to the level of the resting potential. During the absolute refractory period, no stimulus can excite cardiac cells. During the relative refractory period, a larger than usual stimulus is required and the upstroke velocity and amplitude are reduced, resulting in a poorly conducted action potential. After its return to resting state, the ordinary working myocardial cell will remain stable until an excitatory current is generated by a cell connected to it. In certain cardiac cells, such as the atrioventricular (AV) nodal cells, the refractory period outlasts the action potential duration and the cell is refractory during diastole. It is advantageous for the AV node to have a long refractory period in order to protect the ventricles in the event of excessively rapid atrial rates. In such a circumstance, not all of the atrial impulses would be able to traverse the AV node because of refractoriness.

Specialized Conduction System

In addition to working myocardial cells in the atria and ventricles, there exist specialized cells which together comprise the conduction system: the sinoatrial (SA) node, the AV node, the His bundle, the bundle branches, and the Purkinje network (Fig. 1-2). The cells in this system have the ability to generate an action potential de novo, that is, to generate action potentials without the stimulus of excitatory current from another cell. This property is called automaticity and is the result of a slow, gradual depolarization of the membrane potential during phase 4 of the action potential. The basis for this depolarization is not completely understood but appears to be due to the opening of nonselective cation channels that conduct an inward depolarizing current of positive ions. Other inward currents, such as calcium current, have been implicated as well. When the membrane potential drifts to the threshold potential (–60 mV), the potential at which fast channels open, depolarization of the cell will occur. The rate of dia-

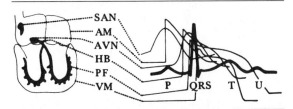

Fig. 1-2. The specialized conduction system. The figure on the left is a schematic drawing of the heart showing the anatomic location of the sinoatrial node (SAN), the atrial myocardium (AM), the AV node (AVN), the His bundle (HB), the Purkinje fibers (PF), and the ventricular muscle (VM). On the right are the action potentials that would be recorded at each of the sites. Note that they are all different, reflecting the different electrophysiologic functions of the different cell types. The heavy line shows a schematic drawing of an ECG recorded from the skin. The P wave, QRS complex, and T and U waves correspond respectively to atrial depolarization, ventricular depolarization, and ventricular repolarization. (Reprinted with permission from: Kaufman CE and Papper S. (eds.) *Review of Pathophysiology*. Boston: Little, Brown, 1983, p. 17.)

stolic depolarization is the primary determinant of the rate of firing of pacemaker cells. Thus the SA node is the pacemaker of the heart because it has the fastest rate of diastolic depolarization and therefore the most intrinsic automaticity. After the SA node, the AV node has the most automaticity, followed by the bundle branches, His bundle, and the Purkinje network.

In addition to the pacemaker function, the specialized conducting cells have other special properties depending on their location. In most people, there are two inputs (pathways) from the atrium into the AV node: the fast pathway enters the AV node anteriorly and has fast conduction properties but a longer refractory period than the slow pathway which enters the AV node posteriorly and has slower conduction properties and a shorter refractory period. The AV nodal cells are specialized for slow conduction. Several factors contribute to this property. The AV nodal cells are small in diameter and circuitously arranged. Depolarization of AV nodal cells occurs due to opening of channels that slowly transport calcium ions inward. The slow conduction of calcium inward results in the action potential having a slow upstroke velocity. In contrast, the bundle branches and subendocardial Purkinje network are specialized for rapid conduction and rapid dispersal of the impulse through the ventricular myocardium. They have large diameters and are aligned in parallel-like cables.

These cells are depolarized by opening of rapid sodium channels, which results in rapid upstroke velocities and high overshoots. Normally the only electrical connection of the atria to the ventricles is through the AV node, His bundle, and bundle branches. The His bundle and upper portions of the bundle branches are not directly connected to the adjacent myocardial cells but are surrounded by a fibrous sheath that does not conduct electrical impulses. Thus interruption of the AV node or His bundle will prevent the impulse from entering the ventricular myocardium. Once the impulse enters the Purkinje network, there are many connections between Purkinje cells and myocardial cells.

Surface Electrocardiography

Assessments of normal and abnormal heart rhythms can be made by recording the changes in voltage across the whole heart over time from the body surface. This recording is called the electrocardiogram (ECG). The relationship of the electrocardiographic patterns to electrophysiologic events is shown in Fig. 1-2. The P wave is the potential generated by depolarization of the left and right atria. The current generated by the sinus node is too small to be seen on the surface ECG but the sinus node would have been depolarized just before the onset of the P wave. The flat segment between the P wave and the onset of QRS complex is called the PR interval and represents the conduction time through the AV node, the His bundle, and the bundle branches. Again the current generated from these structures is too small to be seen on the ECG. The QRS complex reflects depolarization of the ventricles. The T wave corresponds to repolarization of the ventricles. The U wave is also probably a phenomenon of repolarization. The appearance and timing of the various components of the ECG (especially the relationship between the P wave and the QRS complex) can be used to diagnose various kinds of arrhythmias.

Abnormalities of Electrophysiology (Arrhythmias)

Abnormalities of excitable cardiac tissue can lead to abnormalities of heart rhythm which are called arrhythmias or dysrhythmias. Arrhythmias can cause the heart to beat either too quickly (tachycardia) or too slowly (bradycardia), either of which may cause hemodynamic embarrassment or death (Tables 1-1 and 1-2). Tachycardia which is completely contained within the ventricles is called ven-

Table 1-1. Types of Bradycardia

SINUS NODE DYSFUNCTION

Sinus bradycardia
Sinus arrest

HEART BLOCK

1° AV block
2nd° AV block Type I
2nd° AV block Type II
3rd° AV block (complete heart block)
Bundle branch block

Table 1-2. Types of Tachycardia

SINUS TACHYCARDIA

SUPRAVENTRICULAR TACHYCARDIA

Paroxysmal supraventricular tachycardia
   Sinoatrial reentry
   Atrial reentry
   AV nodal reentry
   AV reentry
Ectopic atrial tachycardia
Atrial flutter
Atrial fibrillation

VENTRICULAR TACHYCARDIA

Monomorphic ventricular tachycardia
   Bundle branch reentry
   Idiopathic ventricular tachycardia
Polymorphic ventricular tachycardia
   Torsade de pointes
Bidirectional ventricular tachycardia

VENTRICULAR FIBRILLATION

---

tricular tachycardia. Tachycardias which originate entirely or in part above the ventricles are called supraventricular tachycardias. All arrhythmias (both fast and slow) stem from one of two causes: abnormalities of impulse generation or abnormalities of impulse propagation.

Bradycardia

Pacemaker Failure

Pacemaker failure is an abnormality of impulse generation. Age, disease, or drugs can lead to depression in the rate of diastolic depolarization of the SA node which in turn causes the normal heart rate to slow (sinus bradycardia) or to become absent (sinus arrest). In the event of the latter circumstance, subsidiary pacemakers in the atrium,

AV node, or Purkinje network usually assume the pacemaking responsibilities in the heart. If no latent pacemakers emerge, the heart will not be electrically excited (asystole) and cardiac function will cease.

Heart Block

If the sinus impulse is generated but fails to be conducted to the ventricles, the result is heart block. Heart block is caused by the failure of the electrical impulse to be propagated normally through the conduction system. Heart block can occur at the level of the AV node, His bundle, or distal conduction system (see Table 1-1). Subsidiary pacemakers below the level of block may emerge to provide an escape rhythm. As is the case with pacemaker failure, heart block can be caused by disease, drugs, and age.

Treatment

If a reversible cause of the bradycardia (such as drugs) cannot be identified, the treatment for symptomatic bradycardia (due either to pacemaker failure or heart block) is implantation of an artificial electronic pacemaker to electrically stimulate the heart.

Tachycardia

Automaticity

Enhanced Automaticity. Enhanced automaticity is caused by partial depolarization of the pacemaker cell which allows it to reach the threshold for depolarization sooner than it would ordinarily. Enhancement of normal automaticity may be produced by increased catecholamines.

Abnormal Automaticity. Under certain conditions, nonpacemaker cardiac cells may acquire abnormal automaticity that allows them to fire more rapidly and usurp the normal pacemaker of the heart (the sinus node). Abnormal automaticity is also caused by partial depolarization of the cell which allows it to reach the threshold for depolarization sooner than it would ordinarily (Fig. 1-3). Abnormal automaticity can be seen after ischemic injury to the cell (which partially depolarizes the cell by damaging the sodium-potassium ATP pump).

Treatment. It is unclear to what extent abnormal automaticity plays a role in clinical arrhythmias, but many of the rhythms thought to be from abnormal automaticity are transient due to a temporary perturbation of the electrophysiologic milieu (such as acute myocardial infarction) and may not require specific treatment. When treatment is required, antiarrhythmic drugs can be used to suppress the

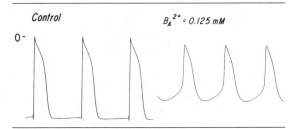

Fig. 1-3. Abnormal automaticity. This figure shows the effects of barium poisoning on the automaticity of a Purkinje cell. The control action potentials on the left are normal. After introduction of barium chloride, the rate of spontaneous depolarization increased. The action potentials on the right can be seen to have an increased rate of spontaneous depolarization caused by the increased slope during phase 4. (From: Dangman KH and Hoffman BF. In vivo and in vitro antiarrhythmic and arrhythmogenic effects of N-acetyl procainamide. Reprinted with permission from: *J Pharmacol Exp Ther,* 217(3): 851–862, 1981.)

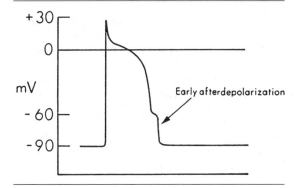

Fig. 1-4. Schematic drawing of an early afterdepolarization. (Reprinted with permission from Cranefield PF and Aronson RS. *Introduction to Cardiac Arrhythmias: The Role of Triggered Activity.* Mt. Kisco, NY: Futura Publishing Co., Inc., 1988, p. 12.)

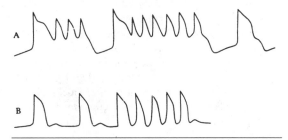

Fig. 1-5. Triggered automaticity. A. Triggered automaticity due to early afterdepolarizations. B. Triggered automaticity due to delayed afterdepolarizations. (Reprinted with permission from Kaufman CE and Papper, S. (eds.) *Review of Pathophysiology.* Boston: Little, Brown, 1983. P. 16.)

abnormal focus or the abnormal focus can be ablated either surgically or by catheter ablation.

Triggered Activity

Triggered activity also stems from an abnormality in impulse generation. Triggered activity is caused by low amplitude potentials called afterdepolarizations. Afterdepolarizations are transient positive shifts in membrane potential that occur after the cell has already been depolarized and an action potential generated. **Early** afterdepolarizations occur during phase 2 and 3 of the action potential and are caused by blockade of the outgoing potassium current and/or an increase in the inward calcium or sodium current (Fig. 1-4). **Delayed** afterpotentials occur in phase 4 after the cell has repolarized and are caused by an increase in intracellular calcium due to release of calcium from an overloaded sarcoplasmic reticulum.

If the afterdepolarization generates enough of a shift in membrane potential to reach the threshold potential for that cell, the cell will be depolarized and excitation will occur. The resulting action potential is said to be "triggered" by the afterdepolarization that initiated it. If the triggered complex also has an afterdepolarization, another triggered complex will ensue and so forth (Fig. 1-5). It is unclear to what extent triggered activity accounts for arrhythmias in man. Triggered activity due to early afterdepolarizations is thought to be the mechanism for torsade de pointes (a form of polymorphic ventricular tachycardia),

which may be congenital (the long QT syndrome) or acquired. The acquired (pause-dependent) form of torsade de pointes is most commonly caused by drugs which prolong repolarization (by blocking potassium channels) or by electrolyte abnormalities (hypokalemia and hypomagnesemia). Triggered activity due to delayed afterdepolarizations is thought to be the mechanism of some of the arrhythmias seen with digitalis intoxication.

Treatment.   The treatment of the congenital form (the long QT syndrome) is beta adrenergic blockade, calcium channel blockade, and pacing. The treatment for acquired forms of torsade de pointes is beta adrenergic stimulation, magnesium, and pacing.

Reentry

The most common mechanism of tachyarrhythmias in man is reentry. Reentry is an abnormality of impulse propagation where an impulse returns to tissue that was already excited and reexcites it, causing the electrical wavefront to become a continuous loop or circuit. The three requirements for a reentrant circuit are (1) a barrier around which the circuit travels, (2) a region of unidirectional block where the impulse can travel in one direction but not the other, and (3) a region of slow conduction to allow the parts of the reentrant loop to recover excitability before the reentrant wavefront passes that way again.

If myocardial fibers all had the same electrophysiologic properties (i.e., identical properties of conduction and refractoriness) and were uniformly connected, any electrical impulses traveling through them would be conducted in a uniform manner. If the impulse met with a barrier to conduction, the impulse would split and go around either side of the barrier at equal speeds only to collide and be extinguished at the other end of the barrier (Fig. 1-6A). If the myocardium on one side of the barrier was still refractory and thus unable to conduct the impulse (Fig. 1-6B, #2), conduction could still proceed down the other side of the barrier (Fig. 1-6B, #1) and then go around the barrier to the area that had been previously refractory (Fig. 1-6B, #3). If the area was still refractory (bidirectional block), the impulse would be extinguished. If conduction around the bar-

rier had been slow enough to allow time for the tissue to recover excitability, the previously refractory area would now be excitable (unidirectional block), and the impulse would be able to return to the area where it first originated (Fig. 1-6B, #4). This is the most common form of reentry.

The rate of the reentrant tachycardia (R, in beats/min) is determined by the length of the reentrant circuit (L, in meters) and the conduction velocity of the impulse that travels around it (V, in meters/sec) R = (V/L)60. The interval between that time when part of the reentrant circuit has recovered excitability and the time when the wavefront actually returns to reexcite that area is called the excitable gap. The obstacle that the impulse travels around may be anatomical (the valve anulus or a scar) or functional. If the barrier is functional (that is, based on abnormal properties of conduction and refractoriness, not a fixed anatomical barrier), the cycle length of the tachycardia will be only just longer than the refractory period, leaving little or no excitable gap. This is called leading circle reentry. Reflection is a rare form of reentry where there is no barrier at all and reentry occurs due to longitudinal electrical dissociation within the myocardial fibers.

Many forms of reentrant tachycardias can occur in the human heart (see Table 1-2). In the Wolff-Parkinson-White syndrome, patients are born with an extra muscular connection between the atrium and the ventricle (in addition to the AV node/bundle of His) called an accessory pathway (Fig. 1-7). The mitral or tricuspid valve anulus serves as an

Fig. 1-6. Schematic drawing of reentry. See text for details. (Reprinted with permission from: Rosen MR. Mechanisms of arrhythmias. In Josephson ME and Wellens JJ (ed.). *Tachycardias: Mechanisms and Management.* Mt. Kisco, NY: Futura Publishing Co., Inc., 1993, p. 2.)

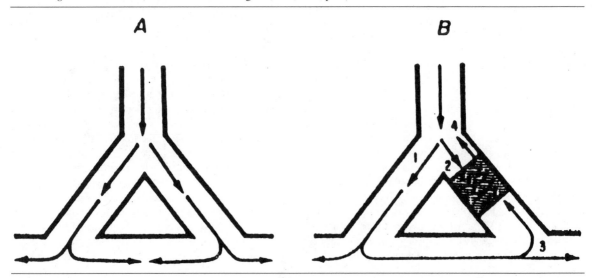

anatomic barrier. (Being composed of fibrous tissue, the anulus is unable to conduct electrical impulses.) When the atrial wavefront arrives at the anulus, if both the accessory pathway and the AV node are excited (left figure), conduction will proceed down both pathways with the two competing wavefronts colliding in the ventricle. However, if, when the atrial wavefront arrives at the anulus the AV node has recovered from the previous impulse, but the accessory pathway is still refractory (second figure), the impulse will travel through just the normal conduction system to excite the ventricle and then try to activate the accessory pathway from the ventricle. If conduction through the AV node was slow enough (that is, slower than the refractory period of the accessory pathway), the accessory pathway will be able to be excited in the retrograde direction and the wavefront will be propagated back to reexcite the atrium (third and fourth figures). This form of supraventricular tachycardia is called atrioventricular (AV) reentrant tachycardia.

Another form of reentrant tachycardia, ventricular tachycardia, can occur in patients who have had a myocardial infarction. In this situation, fibrotic scar in the area of infarction provides a barrier to conduction. In addition myocardium that is damaged may have a prolonged refractory period or only be able to conduct impulses slowly because of partial depolarization of the membrane. This combination of conduction block and slowed conduction can lead to reentry.

Treatment.   Reentrant arrhythmias can be treated by either preventing the reentrant circuit from starting or by causing block within the reentrant circuit once tachycardia has begun. Antiarrhythmic medications and antitachycardia pacing can increase refractoriness in myocardial tissue to turn unidirectional block into bidirectional block. Antiarrhythmic drugs can also directly extinguish excitatory current. Alternatively the critical parts of the reentrant circuit can be ablated either surgically or by catheter ablation. Electrical shocks (cardioversion) can terminate reentrant tachycardias by temporarily imposing uniform electrophysiologic properties on the heart by causing simultaneous depolarization of the myocardium.

Clinical Examples

1. An 83-year-old white male fainted while walking home from the grocery store. He was unconscious for a few minutes. Since that time he had several dizzy spells which occurred without warning and lasted up to two or three minutes. On the day of admission, the patient's wife noticed that while watching television, the patient had lost consciousness, turned pale and then blue. She called the paramedics after trying unsuccessfully to arouse the patient by shaking him. The patient regained consciousness before the paramedics arrived and was taken by ambulance to the hospital. In the emergency room an ECG was recorded (see Fig. 1-8).

Discussion.   The tracing shows recordings made from two ECG channels. The tracings show complete heart block with a junctional escape rhythm. The QRS complexes (which determine the ventricular rate) are occurring at a rate of 33 beats/minute and bear no relation to the P waves which reflect the sinus and atrial rate and are occurring at a rate of 50 beats/minute. The electrical events in the atrium and the ventricle are occurring independently of each other (AV dissociation) because the sinus impulses are not being transmitted through the AV node, resulting in complete heart block. A subsidiary cardiac pacemaker (probably the AV node or His bundle) has taken over, albeit at a slower rate. Unfortunately, pacemakers other than the sinus node are often unreliable (and are slower and more unreliable the lower in the specialized conduction system they originate). When these lower pacemakers fail, patients are prone to syncope due to decreased perfusion from low cardiac output during bradycardia and asystole. The etiology of this patient's heart block is probably fibrosis of the AV node due to age. The most appropriate treatment is implantation of an electronic pacemaker.

Fig. 1-7. Schematic drawing of AV reentrant tachycardia in the Wolff-Parkinson-White syndrome. NSR = normal sinus rhythm, APD = atrial premature depolarization, ECHO = a single reentrant complex, SVT = supraventricular tachycardia. (Reprinted with permission from: Josephson ME. Preexcitation syndromes. In *Clinical Cardiac Electrophysiology,* 2nd ed. Philadelphia: Lea and Febiger, 1993, p. 320.)

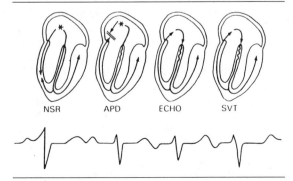

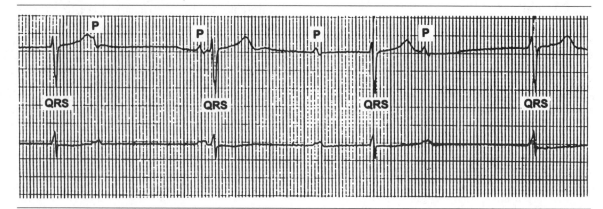

Fig. 1-8. Complete heart block with a junctional escape rhythm.

2. A 28-year-old man had a history of palpitations since he was a teenager. The patient reported his heart would suddenly and without warning start to beat rapidly. The rapid heart beat would be accompanied by chest pain, dyspnea, and dizziness. After about 15–20 minutes, these episodes would stop as abruptly as they had started. Over time he had learned that straining as at stool or coughing sometimes stopped the attacks more quickly. By serendipity, the patient spontaneously developed his usual symptoms while an ECG was being recorded (Fig. 1-9).

Discussion. Figure 1-9 shows three ECG channels. Note that the first four beats show normal sinus rhythm with the delta wave, widened QRS complex, and short PR interval, which are characteristic of conduction through an accessory pathway in the Wolff-Parkinson-White syndrome. A premature atrial complex (X) occurred before the accessory pathway had recovered from refractoriness. The premature atrial beat was conducted through the normal conduction system only (resulting in a normal QRS complex) and initiated AV reentrant tachycardia. During

Fig. 1-9. Initiation of AV reentrant tachycardia in a patient with the Wolff-Parkinson-White syndrome. X = presence of premature atrial complex and initiation of tachycardia. (Reprinted with permission from: Kaufman CE and Papper S. (eds.) *Review of Pathophysiology.* Boston: Little, Brown, 1983, p. 19.)

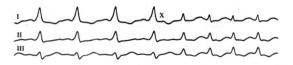

tachycardia, conduction through the accessory pathway is in the retrograde direction and thus not evident on the ECG. Vagal maneuvers (such as straining and coughing) can terminate the tachycardia by causing transient block in the AV node. The patient underwent successful catheter ablation of his accessory pathway and has had no further tachycardia.

3. A 68-year-old woman was admitted to the hospital with new onset of atrial fibrillation (a form of supraventricular tachycardia) for which she was started on the antiarrhythmic drug quinidine. After she had been taking quinidine for a day, her rhythm converted back to normal sinus rhythm. Later that same day the patient had a cardiac arrest due to ventricular tachycardia/ventricular fibrillation (Fig. 1-10) and was resuscitated with electrical defibrillation.

Discussion. This is an example of an iatrogenic (caused by the physician) arrhythmia due to the proarrhythmic effect of an antiarrhythmic medication. Quinidine's antiarrhythmic effect stems in part from its ability to block potassium channels and thus prolong repolarization. The first line of Fig. 1-10 shows normal sinus rhythm; however, the repolarization time (as measured by the time between the beginning of the QRS complex and the end of the T wave, i.e., the QT interval) is markedly prolonged at 600 msec. The second and fourth complexes in the second line are premature ventricular complexes (PVCs) that were caused by triggered activity. The pause after the PVC further exacerbates the repolarization abnormality, and finally polymorphic ventricular tachycardia (torsade de pointes) is initiated with the sixth complex. The ventricular tachycardia quickly degenerated into ventricular fibrillation

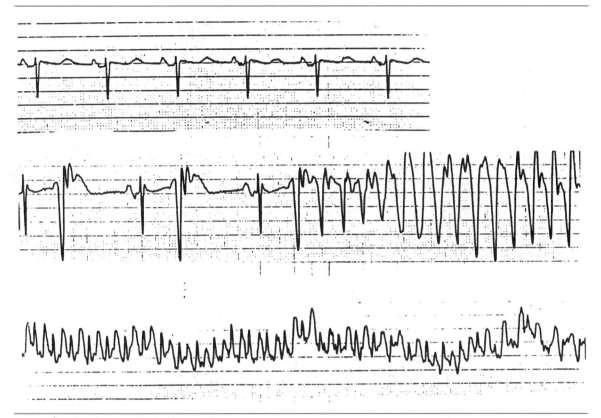

Fig. 1-10. Quinidine-induced torsade de pointes. First line: Sinus rhythm with a prolonged QT interval of 600 msec. Second line: Sinus rhythm with every other complex being a premature ventricular complex (bigeminy) and initiation of torsade de pointes (a particular form of ventricular tachycardia). Third line: Ventricular tachycardia has degenerated into ventricular fibrillation. Note the chaotic rhythm.

(third line). There is no organized electrical or mechanical activity during this rhythm, and ventricular fibrillation is almost always fatal if the patient is not promptly defibrillated with an external electrical shock. After defibrillation, the patient was treated acutely with intravenous magnesium and her quinidine was discontinued. She recovered without incident.

Bibliography

Jackman WM, Friday KJ, Anderson JL, et al. The long QT syndromes: A critical review, new clinical observations and a unifying hypothesis. *Progress Cardiovasc Diseases* 31:115–172, 1988. *A review of ventricular tachycardias thought to be caused by triggered activity.*

Oren JW, Beckman KJ, McClelland JH, et al. A functional approach to the preexcitation syndromes. *Cardiol Clinics* 11:121–149, 1993 *A clinical review of WPW and preexcitation in general.*

Task Force of the Working Group on Arrhythmias of the European Society of Cardiology. The sicilian gambit: A new approach to the classification of antiarrhythmic drugs based on their actions on arrhythmogenic mechanisms. *Circulation* 84:1831–1851, 1991. *A succinct but brilliant review of basic electrophysiology as it relates to mechanism of antiarrhythmic drug action.*

Zipes, DP. Genesis of Cardiac Arrhythmias: Electrophysiological Considerations. In Braunwald E (ed.). *Heart Disease: A Textbook of Cardiovascular Medicine.* Philadelphia: Saunders, 1988, pp. 581–620. *An excellent review of normal and abnormal cardiac electrophysiology.*

2 Myocardial Performance: Systolic and Diastolic Function

Eliot Schechter

Objectives

After completing this chapter, you should be able to

Discuss the conceptual model of the sarcomere and how it relates to changes in pressure and length during contraction

Define *contractility, preload,* and *afterload*

Explain the effects of contractility, preload, and afterload on sarcomere function

Relate the basic physiologic concepts of preload, contractility, and afterload to the function of the heart in situ

Discuss how the pressure-volume loop and end-systolic pressure-volume line describe the function of the heart

Show how the pressure-volume loop and end-systolic pressure-volume line change with preload, afterload, and contractility

Describe the relationship between "forward" and "congestive" or "backward" failure and the implication for therapy

Enumerate the factors that determine the diastolic properties of the heart

Discuss how abnormal diastolic function can mimic the symptoms caused by systolic dysfunction

To the clinician the heart is a pump distributing blood throughout the body. Because of the interaction of heart muscle function, venous return, and neurohumoral factors studying the hearts pump function in the intact organism is difficult. To make this subject more understandable it is helpful to review cardiac muscle function beginning at the simplest level, the isolated muscle cell, expand these concepts to strips of heart muscle, and then to the intact heart.

Cellular Basis of Contraction

Systolic Function

The sarcomere is the fundamental unit of heart muscle and is composed of three conceptual (as opposed to anatomical) elements.

The contractile element contains both of the major contractile proteins, actin (thin filament) and myosin (thick filament) as well as the cross-bridges which link and separate during activation and relaxation. During contraction (systole), the cross-bridges between the actin and myosin filaments interact under the influence of calcium released by the sarcoplasmic reticulum, with the result that the actin filaments are "pulled" by the myosin toward the center of the contractile element. The strength of the contraction depends upon the number of cross-bridges linked, while the velocity depends upon the speed of linking. During relaxation the calcium is pumped back into the sarcoplasmic reticulum and the cross-bridges separate.

Shortening of the contractile element may result in shortening of the sarcomere, development of tension without shortening, or a combination of tension development and shortening. These diverse responses of the sarcomere to shortening of the contractile proteins cannot be entirely

13

explained by the properties of the contractile proteins (which can be thought of as the "power"). Therefore a second component — the series elastic element — is proposed in the model of the sarcomere (Fig. 2-1). The series elastic element stretches to allow shortening of the contractile element without shortening of the sarcomere. In doing so, the shortening of the contractile element is converted to tension at the ends of the sarcomere.

Diastolic Function

In the quiescent state a sarcomere will assume its resting length. An increase in length can only be achieved by the application of force (tension). Although this requirement for force could be attributed to stretching the series elastic element and contractile element, most models of muscle contraction use a separate element, the parallel elastic element (Fig. 2-1), to model the diastolic length-tension relationship.

Fig. 2-1. Schematic representation of the conceptual three-element model of the sarcomere. The contractile proteins and series elastic element produce tension and/or shortening during contraction and the parallel elastic element determines the length and compliance at rest. (Reprinted with permission from: Kaufman CE and Papper S. (eds.) *Review of Pathophysiology.* Boston: Little, Brown, 1983.)

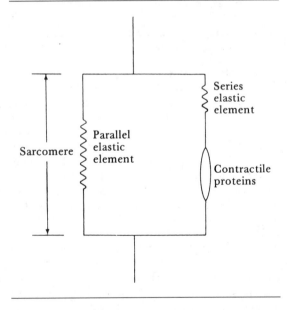

Definitions

To progress from this brief review of muscle contraction at a cellular level to contraction of a muscle strip requires reviewing certain definitions:

Contractility is the fundamental property of muscle that describes its ability to shorten and/or develop tension when stimulated.

Preload is the stretch exerted on the muscle in the resting state. Preload can be thought of as either the resting muscle length or the resting tension. These are related by the diastolic length-tension (compliance) curve.

Afterload is the resistance to shortening that the muscle must overcome during contraction.

Isometric contraction is contraction without shortening; energy is converted to tension by stretch of the series elastic element.

Isotonic contraction is muscle contraction without change in tension; energy is required for shortening of the muscle.

Velocity of shortening (dl/dt) is the rate of change of muscle fiber length, that is, the change in length (dl) during any unit of time (dt). In a more familiar setting, when driving dl/dt would be miles (dl) per hour (dt).

Rate of tension development (dT/dt) is the rate at which a muscle develops tension, that is, the change in tension for any unit of time. Since both this and dl/dt vary from instant to instant during a contraction, they are usually expressed as their maximum value or their value at some arbitrarily defined tension. Both dT/dt and dl/dt are indirect measures of contractility.

Physiology of Contraction in Isolated Muscle Strips

Systolic Function

The systolic function (contraction) of a muscle strip can be studied using a simple "muscle bridge" (Fig. 2-2). Figures 2-3A and Fig. 2-3B show the changes in force and length during a typical contraction using the muscle bridge. When the muscle fibers are stimulated contraction begins. Muscle tension rises, but there is no muscle shortening.

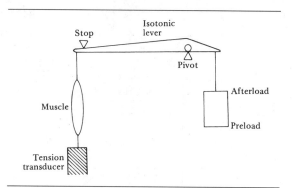

Fig. 2-2. A muscle bridge for studying contractile function. The muscle is attached to one side of a pivoting arm and a weight (afterload) to the other. A stop allows a controlled amount of initial stretch (preload). A tension transducer attached to the muscle measures the tension developed, and the movement of the arm indicates the shortening. (Reprinted with permission from Kaufman CE and Papper S. *Review of Pathophysiology.* Boston: Little, Brown, 1983.)

This is due to stretching of the series elastic element. The rate of tension development is not constant, but is slow at the onset of contraction and more rapid as contraction progresses. The maximum rate of tension development (dT/dt) is at the point where shortening begins. When muscle tension equals afterload, muscle shortening begins while the tension remains constant and equal to the afterload. If the afterload is increased (see Fig. 2-3B), the tension developed is increased, and the velocity and magnitude of shortening is decreased. There is an inverse relationship between the force developed during muscle contraction and the velocity with which the muscle shortens. This force-velocity relationship characterizes the systolic function of muscle. Figure 2-4A shows the velocity of muscle shortening (dl/dt) plotted against afterload. At the maximum developed tension (isometric contraction) the shortening velocity is zero while the maximum shortening velocity (V_{max}) occurs when the tension developed is zero.

In Fig. 2-4B the effect of different preloads is illus-

Fig. 2-3. When the muscle fibers are stimulated, contraction begins. Muscle tension rises (lower portion of diagram), but there is no muscle shortening. This is due to stretching of the series elastic element. The rate of tension development is not constant, but is slow at the onset of contraction and more rapid as contraction progresses. The maximum rate of tension development (dT/dt) occurs at the point where shortening begins. When muscle tension equals afterload, muscle shortening begins (upper portion of diagram) while the tension remains constant and equal to the afterload. The velocity of shortening (dl/dt) is most rapid at the onset of shortening. Panel B shows the effect of increased afterload. Maximum rate or pressure development is higher, and shortening is slower and occurs later. (Reprinted with permission from: Kaufman CE and Papper S. (eds.) *Review of Pathophysiology.* Boston: Little, Brown, 1983.)

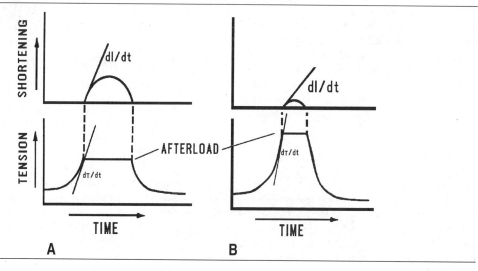

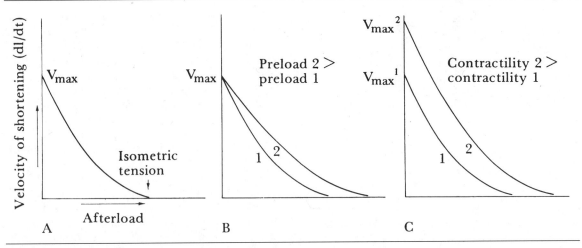

Fig. 2-4. (A) Relationship of force (tension) and velocity. Maximum force is developed at 0 velocity and maximum velocity (V_{max}) at 0 force. (B) Effect of preload on the force-velocity curve. Isometric tension is greater with greater preload. The maximum shortening velocity is unchanged. (C) Effect of increased contractility on the force-velocity curve. With increasing contractility both the maximum tension and the maximum velocity are increased. (Reprinted with permission from: Kaufman CE and Papper S. (eds.) *Review of Pathophysiology.* Boston: Little, Brown, 1983.)

trated. Isometric tension is greater with greater preload. For any given afterload dl/dt is greater with greater preload. The maximum shortening velocity V_{max} is unchanged. Thus preload affects the force of muscle shortening; however, maximum velocity of shortening is independent of preload. Fig. 2-4C shows how changes in contractility shift the force-velocity curve. Increased contractility (curve 2) increases the maximum isometric tension and velocity at any developed tension just as increased preload does. However, with increased contractility, V_{max} is also increased. V_{max} is thus a measure of contractility in isolated muscle strips.

Diastolic Function

The diastolic function of a muscle is described by the relationship between the applied tension (preload) and the resulting muscle length — that is, how much a given amount of tension will stretch the muscle when in a resting state. This relationship is called compliance. A more compliant muscle is one that stretches more for any given tension. In cardiac muscle this relationship is not linear (Fig. 2-5). At short muscle lengths it takes less tension to produce a given increase in muscle length than at longer lengths.

Relationship between Diastolic and Systolic Function

When a muscle contracts from varying resting lengths, varying tension is developed. A family of force-velocity curves exists describing the effect of different preloads on contraction (see Fig. 2-4). This relationship between preload and developed tension is shown in Fig. 2-6, which depicts the tensions developed at a common shortening velocity at different preloads. Up to a point, increases in resting length (increased preload) result in increased tension. This is called the "preload reserve." At some resting length maximum tension is developed. Further increases in length produce no change or a fall in tension. The resting length at which maximum tension is developed is the length at which there is the maximum overlap of the actin and myosin fibers allowing the maximum number of sites for interaction during contraction.

Fig. 2-5. Diastolic length-tension curve. With increasing stretch (length) the amount of tension required for a given increase in length becomes much greater. This increase is not linear, as shown by the right-hand portion of the curve.

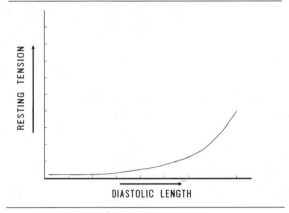

Fig. 2-6. Preload and systolic function. As diastolic tension (and therefore length) is increased the systolic tension developed during contraction increases. At some point the muscle is overstretched and further increases in preload result in no increase or a fall in systolic tension. (Reprinted with permission from: Kaufman CE and Papper S. (eds.) *Review of Pathophysiology.* Boston: Little, Brown, 1983.)

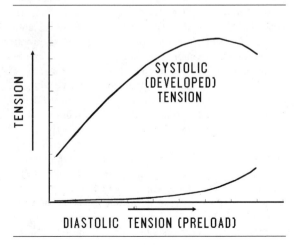

The Intact Heart
Measurements of Function

In the intact heart we cannot eliminate confounding variables such as venous return, coronary blood flow, neurogenic and humoral factors which affect cardiac performance, nor can we measure the basic physiologic variables of muscle length, tension, and velocity. These must be translated into, or approximated from, variables which can be measured, volume and pressure. Volume in a chamber is related to the length of the muscle in the wall. Pressure is related to tension in the wall of that chamber. Velocity is related to the rate of change of pressure and/or volume. Therefore in the intact heart we must modify the previous definitions of muscle mechanics.

Contractility
No satisfactory method exists in the intact, in-situ heart to measure myocardial contractility. Maximum rate of pressure rise (dP/dt) has been used, but it is both preload and afterload dependent. Attempts to extrapolate to V_{max} from pressure and dP/dt measurements during isometric contraction suffer from large errors due to the few points available for extrapolation. The end-systolic pressure-volume point has been suggested as a measure of contractility but has both preload and afterload dependence. The slope of the end-systolic pressure-volume line is independent of both preload and afterload and could be a useful measure of contractility. Its use is, unfortunately, limited by the practical problem of making measurements in several different states (e.g., with different preloads) in order to plot the line.

Preload
In the intact heart diastolic ventricular volume is most directly related to the resting length of the muscle elements in the ventricular wall, that is, preload. Diastole is a dynamic process with continuing filling throughout diastole so volume (and therefore muscle length) are continually increasing. Clinically, preload is the volume just before contraction begins, that is, the end-diastolic volume. Because diastolic volume and pressure are related by the compliance of the ventricle, end-diastolic pressure (EDP) (or mean atrial pressure) is often taken to represent preload, as it is more easily measured.

Afterload
The forces resisting ejection of blood constitute afterload. For practical purposes, arterial pressure, usually peak sys-

tolic or mean pressure, is taken as an estimate of the after-load of the ventricle. This is closely related to the resistance to flow through the arterial vessels. For a true measure of afterload the pressure within the left ventricular cavity must be related to the tension in the wall of the ventricle by geometric formulas that take into account the size, shape, and thickness of the ventricular chamber.

Isovolumic Contraction and Relaxation

Contraction without a change in volume is analogous to isometric contraction in the muscle strip and occurs at the beginning of systole, before the aortic and pulmonic valves open and ejection begins. Isovolumic relaxation is relaxation of the chamber without a change in volume. This occurs in early diastole after the aortic and pulmonic valves close and before the mitral and tricuspid valves open.

Isotonic Contraction

Isotonic contraction does not exist in the intact heart. Even during maximum ejection there are continuing changes in pressure (afterload).

Velocity of Ejection

This corresponds to velocity of shortening. The ejection fraction (that is, the percent of end-diastolic volume that is ejected during the following systole) is commonly measured and is an index of the amount of shortening of the muscle. It is the most commonly used measure of systolic or contractile function.

dP/dt

The rate of pressure development, reported as the maximum rate measured or the rate at a defined pressure, corresponds to the rate of tension development (dT/dt) in the muscle strip.

Ventricular Pressure-Volume Relationship

The ventricle provides a bridge between the low-pressure venous system and the high-pressure arterial tree. During diastole the ventricle fills with blood at low pressure. The diastolic properties of the ventricle are described by its compliance curve, where volume and pressure show the same relationship as length and tension in the isolated muscle strip. However, unlike the muscle strip, the intact heart is stimulated 60 to 180 times a minute; thus the diastolic compliance curve is the result of not just the passive properties of the muscle (the parallel elastic element in our original model), but of the relaxation that takes place at the end of each contraction (Fig. 2-7).

During systole the ventricle generates pressure to produce forward flow. The Frank-Starling curve describes the

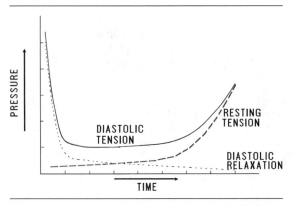

Fig. 2-7. Determinants of diastolic pressure in the intact heart. The pressure at any point in time is the sum of the passive diastolic tension (heavy dashed line) and diastolic relaxation (dotted line), an active process.

basic relationship between the diastolic and systolic functions of the ventricle. It relates filling in diastole (preload) to the volume and pressure output of the ventricle in systole (work). This relationship is similar to the relationship of tension (work) to resting length (preload) noted in the muscle strip (see Fig. 2-6).

Since the work of the intact heart includes both pressure and volume (flow) it is useful to describe cardiac function by plotting the diastolic and systolic pressure and volume changes of the ventricle during a complete cardiac cycle. This produces a pressure-volume or work loop (Fig. 2-8). During diastole the ventricle fills along its diastolic compliance curve. With the onset of systole, pressure builds up in the ventricle until ejection begins. Volume then decreases while pressure increases and then decreases until the end of systole. The volume remaining in the ventricle (the end-systolic volume) and the pressure at the end of systole (the end-systolic pressure) has been suggested as a useful measure of contractility as noted above. With the onset of diastole, pressure falls abruptly to the level determined by the muscle stiffness and the degree of relaxation at that time. The area inside this curve, the pressure-volume loop, represents the work of the ventricle. With increased diastolic filling there is increased stroke volume and more cardiac work as expressed in the Frank-Starling relationship. This preload reserve is a major factor in moment-to-moment regulation of cardiac function, insuring that an increase in filling (preload) is accompanied by an appropriate increase in output (work). The heart thus has a

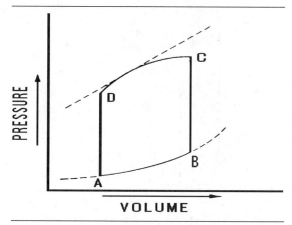

Fig. 2-8. During diastole the ventricle fills along its diastolic compliance curve (A to B). With the onset of systole (point B), pressure builds up in the ventricle until it reaches the level where ejection begins (point C). Volume then decreases while pressure increases and then decreases until the end of systole (point D). With the onset of diastole (isometric relaxation) pressure falls (points D–A) to the level determined by diastolic compliance at the end-systolic volume (point A) and the degree of relaxation at that time. Point D, the end-systolic pressure-volume point, has been suggested as a measure of contractility. (Reprinted with permission from: Kaufman CE and Papper S. (eds.) *Review of Pathophysiology.* Boston: Little, Brown, 1983.)

mechanism that causes input and output to keep pace (more input = more output) on a beat-to-beat basis.

In a ventricle with a stable contractile state the slope of the line relating volume and pressure at end systole is unaffected by differing preloads. It represents the amount of shortening that the myocardium is capable of at any given afterload, that is, its contractility. With increasing preloads the end-systolic pressure and volume both increase as a result of increased output into a constant afterload (Fig. 2-9). With constant preload but increasing afterloads the end-systolic pressure and volumes also increase, but the slope of the end systolic pressure-volume line is increased, an indication of increased contractility. This increase in contractility in response to increased afterload has been termed **homeometric autoregulation.** This enables the heart to maintain its stroke output without increasing its diastolic volume and pressure to compensate for an increased afterload such as high blood pressure.

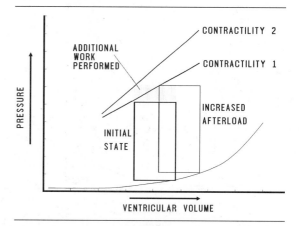

Fig. 2-9. Homeometric autoregulation allows increased work to be performed without an increase in preload by increasing contractility. With an increase in afterload there is initially an increase in end-diastolic pressure and volume shifting the pressure-volume loop to the right. Contractility then increases, allowing return of the loop to its previous position.

Interrelationship of Preload, Afterload, and Contractility in the Intact Heart

The interrelationships of the three determinants of the function of the intact heart are shown in Fig. 2-10. The immediate effect of changes in afterload are shown in panel A. If the afterload is increased (as for example by hypertension), ejection ends sooner, the stroke volume is reduced, and the end-diastolic volume increased. Subsequently there is an increase in contractility due to homeometric autoregulation that restores the initial EDP and stroke volume. If afterload is reduced (as might occur with the vasodilatation induced by a hot environment), there is an increase in stroke volume.

The effect of increased preload is shown in panel B. With an increase in preload (as might occur with the increased venous return induced by elevating the legs or lying down), the stroke volume increases. If preload and afterload remain constant but contractility changes (for example, under the influence of catecholamines), we see the results in panel C. An increase in contractility increases the slope of the end-systolic pressure-volume line, so that at any given afterload there is more shortening and therefore an increase in stroke volume.

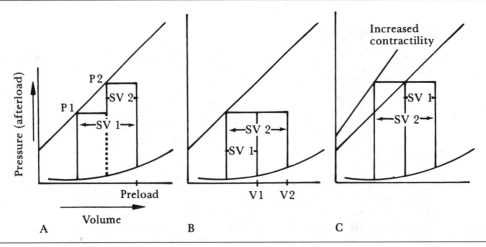

Fig. 2-10. Effect of pathophysiologic changes on the pressure-volume (work) loop. Panel A shows the effect of changes in afterload. With afterload of P1 the heart ejects a stroke volume of SV1. If the afterload is increased to P2, as for example by hypertension, ejection ends sooner and the stroke volume is reduced to SV2. Panel B shows the effect of changes in preload. A preload of V1 results in ejection of stroke volume SV1. With an increase in preload to V2, as might occur with the increased venous return induced by elevating the legs or lying down, the stroke volume increases to SV2. Panel C shows the effect of a change in contractility. If contractility increases, as for example under the influence of cathecholamines, the slope of the end-systolic pressure-volume line increases so that at any given afterload there is more shortening and therefore an increase in stroke volume. (Reprinted with permission from: Kaufman CE and Papper S. (eds.) *Review of Pathophysiology.* Boston: Little, Brown, 1983.)

Changes in Function with Myocardial Disease

Systolic Dysfunction

During systole the ventricle must develop sufficient pressure to equal the pressure in the great vessels (aorta or pulmonary artery) so that flow may begin, and enough shortening of the muscle fibers so that sufficient blood for the needs of the body is pumped. Both pressure development (isovolumic contraction) and stroke volume are affected by many factors, but the primary determinant is the contractile state of the myocardium. Systolic dysfunction implies impairment of this contractile ability. A number of diseases primarily affect the ability of the myocardium to contract. These include myocarditis (usually viral), alcoholism, toxins (including some drugs), ischemia, and a large group of patients with myocardial failure of un-

known cause, the idiopathic congestive cardiomyopathies. In each of these cases of systolic dysfunction the pump function of the heart is inadequate for the needs of the tissues. This activates a number of compensatory mechanisms which themselves may be deleterious. These mechanisms are discussed further in Chapter 10. Figure 2-11 shows the changes in the pressure-volume curve as a result of impaired ventricular contractile function. With impaired contractility the end-systolic pressure-volume line has a flatter slope (at any pressure [afterload] the ventricle empties less well), and therefore a smaller stroke volume and higher end-systolic volume results. Also, for any increase in afterload there is a larger decrease in the ejected volume, so the ventricle is unable to handle stress as well. The clinical picture is that of inadequate cardiac output — poor tissue perfusion (cold, clammy skin), poor renal perfusion (oliguria), and poor cerebral perfusion (confusion). The reduced stroke volume can be partially compensated by an

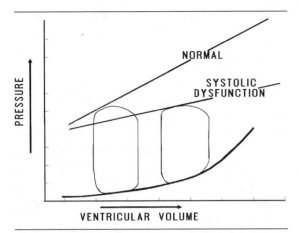

Fig. 2-11. Effect of systolic dysfunction on cardiac work. The left-hand curve demonstrates the normal pressure-volume loop. With impaired contractility the end-systolic pressure-volume line has a flatter slope (at any pressure [afterload] the ventricle empties less well). A smaller stroke volume, higher end-systolic volume, and higher diastolic volume and pressure results.

increased heart rate (cardiac output = stroke volume times beats/minute), so tachycardia is a frequent clinical manifestation of systolic myocardial failure. This picture has been called "forward cardiac failure." However, the forward cardiac output can be maintained by increasing the preload. This results in increased venous pressure in the lungs (if dealing with the left ventricle) or systemic veins (if dealing with the right ventricle), a condition referred to as "congestive" or "backward failure."

It is clear from the inter-relationships of preload and cardiac output that forward and backward failure are simply different manifestations of the same pathologic physiology. If the filling pressure is high we have congestion with adequate forward cardiac output; if the filling pressure is normal or low we have no congestion but the forward cardiac output is inadequate. By evaluating preload (ventricular EDP), afterload (arterial pressure), and contractility (stroke volume and ejection fraction), the pathophysiology in any given patient can be characterized and therapy can be designed physiologically. We can increase preload (volume expansion) as much as possible without causing congestion, decrease afterload (vasodilators) as much as possible without causing hypotension, and increase contractility (inotropic agents such as digitalis and amrinone) without causing side effects such as arrhythmias.

Diastolic Dysfunction

The diastolic properties of the ventricle are defined by its compliance curve and its state of relaxation at the time. A less compliant ventricle may be due to alterations in the myocardium itself as seen in patients with restrictive myocardial diseases including amyloidosis (deposition of amyloid material in the myocardium), hypertrophy, and scarring from myocardial infarction. Impaired relaxation may be due to inadequate energy supply. Relaxation is not passive, but rather is an energy-requiring activity. ATP is needed to return Ca^{++} to the sarcoplasmic reticulum against a concentration gradient and allow decoupling of the actin-myosin cross-bridges. Reduced compliance, especially in ischemic heart disease, often is due to delayed relaxation secondary to decreased energy stores. It is now becoming evident that endothelial cells, both in the myocardial vascular system and in the endocardium, play a role in diastolic function. Endothelium-derived relaxing factor (EDRF) shortens contraction and promotes myocardial relaxation while an as yet uncharacterized agent "endocardin" appears to have the opposite effect.

Increasingly, diastolic dysfunction is being recognized as a cause of symptoms (pulmonary congestion — with dyspnea and orthopnea) often attributed incorrectly to congestive heart failure due to systolic dysfunction. The compliance curve is not linear but rises more steeply as the ventricle is stretched (Fig. 2-12). The normal left ventricle has an end-diastolic volume (preload) of about 135 cc at a distending pressure of 12 mm Hg. A patient with restric-

Fig. 2-12. Effect of diastolic dysfunction. For the same stroke volume and end-systolic volume a higher end-diastolic pressure (EDP) is needed to fill the ventricle to the same end-diastolic volume (same preload).

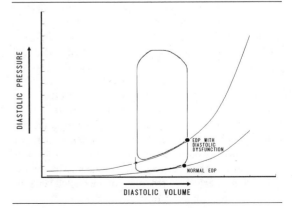

tive myocardial disease may require a pressure of 30 mm Hg to achieve the same volume. This places the patient on the steep portion of the compliance curve so additional venous return, for example with exercise, results in very high levels of pressure and congestive symptoms.

Alternatively, the inability to elevate the filling pressure to these high levels will markedly restrict cardiac output. Note that, although the pathophysiology of systolic and diastolic dysfunction is different, the effects on the pump function of the heart and therefore on the patient are the same, elevated filling pressures with congestive symptoms or reduced forward flow with symptoms of inadequate perfusion. Further, the elevation of diastolic pressure in the ventricle reduces the gradient between aortic diastolic pressure and the left ventricle that serves as the driving force for coronary perfusion. The resultant ischemia further impairs myocardial function.

Clinical Examples

1. A 12-year-old girl came to the hospital because of difficulty breathing. She had a sore throat two weeks earlier followed by fever and transient swelling of first one, then her other knee 3 days earlier. For the past 24 hours she had difficulty breathing when lying flat or with any activity. Examination showed a regular pulse of 112, and blood pressure of 100/80. Jugular venous pressure was elevated. There were rales over the lower half of both lung fields. The apex impulse was displaced leftward and downward, the first sound was soft, there was a ventricular (S3) gallop and soft systolic murmur at the apex.

Discussion.   This girl presented with the typical picture of acute rheumatic fever. Rheumatic myocarditis is an inflammatory condition of the myocardium which primarily impairs its systolic function. As a result of this impaired systolic emptying, her diastolic filling pressure rose to compensate. This elevated filling pressure was reflected back into the lungs, producing symptoms of left-sided congestive failure, difficulty breathing. On examination she had a tachycardia, as is common in patients with impaired systolic function. The reduced pulse pressure (100/80) is evidence of her reduced stroke volume. The reduced emptying of the heart produces dilatation reflected in the displacement of the apex impulse to the left and downward. The soft first sound reflects the impaired rate of pressure buildup (dP/dt) by the damaged myocardium. The ventricular gallop reflects impaired filling of the dilated ventricle and the systolic murmur reflects stretching of the mitral

annulus by the ventricular dilatation with resultant mitral regurgitation.

2. A 45-year-old male was seen in consultation because of "heart failure." The day after an uncomplicated gastric resection he complained of shortness of breath. On examination his neck veins were distended when lying with his head elevated 45 degrees and there were rales at the bases of both lungs. His apex impulse was hyperactive. The first and second sounds were accentuated. A medium-pitched systolic ejection murmur of grade 2 intensity was heard at the left sternal border. There was no edema.

He had no past history of heart disease. His ECG was normal except for sinus tachycardia. A chest x-ray showed pulmonary congestion.

Review of the postoperative records revealed that he had inadvertently received 6 liters of intravenous fluid in the first day since his surgery.

Discussion.   This patient presented with signs of high filling pressures on both the right side (dilated neck veins) and left side (pulmonary rales and congestion on the chest x-ray). While this usually is the result of impaired myocardial function producing heart failure, in this case there was no evidence of impaired pumping ability of the heart. In fact the hyperdynamic cardiac action suggested a high cardiac output. The answer lies in the inadvertent fluid overload. As a result of the increased filling, the diastolic pressure rose, producing venous congestion. In response to the increased diastolic filling, the cardiac output increased (the Frank-Starling mechanism or preload reserve), but until the kidneys excrete the extra intravascular volume, the venous congestion will persist — a normal response to a volume load.

3. A 55-year-old man was under care because of multiple myeloma. On a routine followup visit he complained of trouble breathing and was noted to have venous distention and rales over both lung fields. He had no chest pain. Examination showed an enlarged heart with normal first and second heart sounds. An early diastolic sound was heard. At diagnostic catheterization his diastolic pressures were markedly elevated and endomyocardial biopsy revealed amyloidosis.

Discussion.   Amyloid (and other infiltrative cardiomyopathies) markedly reduce diastolic compliance. These patients require high venous pressures to adequately fill their hearts and achieve an adequate cardiac output. Although this type of myocardial failure mimics systolic dysfunction, the problem is really quite different with impairment to filling rather than inadequate emptying being the cause of the venous congestion. It is important to recognize diastolic dysfunction since the usual treatments for heart failure (vasodilators, inotropic agents) are ineffective or detrimental.

Bibliography

Baan J, van der Velde ET, and Steendijk P. Ventricular pressure-volume relations in vivo. *European Heart J* 1992;13(suppl E):2–6. *A review of the physiology of pressure and volume in the heart.*

Pouleur H. Diastolic dysfunction and myocardial energetics. *European Heart J* 1990;11(suppl C):30–34. *A simple review of the energetics of myocardial relaxation and the diseases that affect it.*

Pasipoularides A. Cardiac mechanics: Basic and clinical contemporary research. *Ann Biomed Eng* 1992;20:3–17. *A very sophisticated review of the mechanics of myocardial function and a good overview of the whole area.*

Shah AM and Lewis MJ. Endothelial modulation of myocardial contraction: mechanisms and potential relevance in cardiac disease. *Basic Res Cardiol* 1992;87 (suppl 2):59–67. *A review of some new findings with insights into how this may be of importance in myocardial diseases.*

3 Common Forms of Volume and Pressure Overload: Valvular Heart Disease

Eliot Schechter

Objectives

After completing this chapter, you should be able to

Explain the relationships between the cardiac cycle, valve function, and heart sounds

List the common causes of volume overload

Describe the response of the heart to an acute volume load

Contrast the response of the heart to chronic volume overload with the response to acute volume loading

List the common causes of pressure overload

Describe the initial and long-term response of the ventricle to pressure overload

Explain the hemodynamic changes produced by the common valvular diseases:

mitral stenosis

mitral regurgitation

aortic stenosis

aortic regurgitation

List the normal values for cardiac chamber pressures, cardiac output, and ejection fraction

---

Review of Normal Physiology

Valve Function

The normal cardiac valves are wonders of engineering. They open with minimal pressure. They allow flow without obstruction over a wide range of flow rates during systole. They close rapidly and completely, preventing regurgitation of blood.

Normal Heart Sounds

Examination of the heart provides bedside clues to the pathophysiology of valvular function and dysfunction. The closure of the atrioventricular valves (mitral valve and tricuspid valve) produces the first heart sound; closure of the semilunar valves (aortic valve and pulmonic valve) produces the second heart sound. Because right-sided pressures are far lower than those on the left side, the sounds produced by the tricuspid and pulmonary valves are softer than those produced by the mitral and aortic valves. Closure of the atrioventricular and semilunar valves on the right side of the heart is not synchronous with the closure of the corresponding valves on the left. This asynchronous closure gives rise to splitting of the first and second heart sounds. The left-sided valves close before the right, so the mitral first sound precedes the tricuspid and the aortic second sound precedes the pulmonic.

Atrioventricular Valves

The tricuspid and mitral valves separate the right atrium and ventricle and the left atrium and ventricle respectively. The cardiac cycle begins with contraction of the atrium. The resulting rise in pressure, the a-wave in the atrial pressure tracing (Fig. 3-1), provides the final 10% of filling of the ventricle and the last bit of preload. At the onset of systole the rising pressure in the ventricles closes the atrioventricular valves, producing the first heart sound and a small wave in the atrial pressure tracing, the c-wave. The first heart sound reflects the physiology of valve closure. Its loudness reflects the separation of the leaflets at the time of closure (wide separation = loud sound) and the rate of pressure change in the ventricle (high rate of pressure change = loud sound) as well as the structure of the leaflets (thickened immobile leaflets = soft sound). During systole the high pressure in the ventricles keeps the atrioventricular valves closed and atrial pressure falls as the atrium relaxes (the x-descent). As venous inflow to the atrium gradually fills this chamber its pressure rises (the v-wave). When ventricular pressure falls at the onset of diastole it becomes lower than atrial pressure. The AV valves open. This valve opening is normally silent. The pressure in the atrium falls rapidly as blood fills the ventricles (the y-descent). The atrioventricular valves are thus closed during systole, preventing regurgitation of blood from the ventricles to the atria and open during diastole to allow ventricular filling.

Semilunar Valves

The pulmonic and aortic valves lie between the right ventricle and pulmonary artery and the left ventricle and aorta respectively. At the beginning of the cardiac cycle atrial contraction produces an abrupt rise in ventricular pressure as described above. The contraction of the ventricle begins from this point, the end-diastolic pressure which is a measure of its preload (Fig. 3-2). As ventricular pressure rises it exceeds the atrial pressure and the atrioventricular valves close. The subsequent phase of isovolumic contraction continues until ventricular pressure exceeds that in the great vessels (pulmonary artery and aorta), at which point the semilunar valves open and the ejection phase of systole begins. The pressure continues to rise and then falls as systole ends. When the pressure drops below that in the great vessels the semilunar valves close, preventing regurgitation of blood back into the ventricles. The period of isovolumic relaxation extends from this point until opening of the AV valves.

Ventricles

The left and right sides of the circulation normally differ markedly in their pressure levels. While systemic (left-sided) arterial pressure is in the range of 120/60, pulmonary

Fig. 3-2. Pressure recordings of the normal left ventricular and aortic pressures. EDP = end-diastolic pressure.

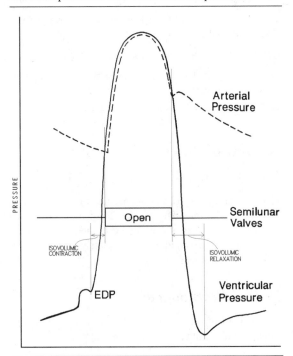

Fig. 3-1. Pressure recordings of the normal left atrial and left ventricular pressures.

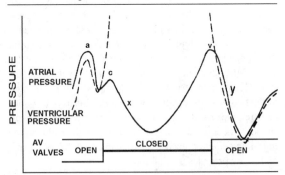

(right-sided) pressure is much lower, 20/12. The shape of the ventricles is adapted for these pressures. The left ventricle is conical shaped and thick walled, suitable for pressure development. The right ventricle is bellows shaped and thin walled, suitable for handling a large volume when necessary, but ill equipped to maintain high pressures.

Pathophysiology of Volume Overload

Failure of an atrioventricular valve to close properly (incompetence) produces volume overload of the atrium because of the regurgitation of blood during systole and of the ventricle because of the increased filling during diastole owing to the volume regurgitated being returned in addition to the normal volume. Incompetence of a semilunar valve causes volume overload of the respective ventricle due to regurgitation of blood during diastole. In the clinical setting the common causes of volume overload are mitral regurgitation, aortic regurgitation, and atrial septal defect (see Chapter 4). The pathophysiologic changes due to volume overload progress through three stages.

Acute volume loading increases the preload by increasing end-diastolic volume (Fig. 3-3, V_1 to V_2), with the re-

Fig. 3-3. Pressure-volume loops in volume overload. P_1, P_2, and P_3 are the pressures at the corresponding volumes V_1 and V_2.

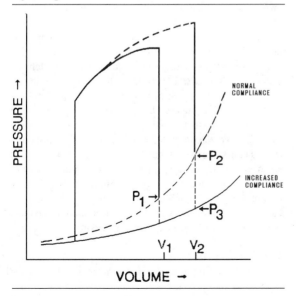

sultant increase in end-diastolic pressure (P_1 to P_2) because of the shape of the diastolic compliance curve. If the volume load is large, the increase in pressure may be marked and will be reflected into the lungs (pulmonary edema) or systemic vein (venous congestion). This increased diastolic stretch, by utilizing the Frank-Starling mechanism, results in increased stroke volume and maintains a normal end-systolic volume. There are increases in the peak rate of diastolic filling, ejection fraction, and peak rate of systolic ejection. Because of the increase in the size of the pressure-volume loop there is an increase in cardiac work.

If the volume load is maintained, cardiac dilation due to rearrangement (remodeling) of the myocardial fibers occurs. In this way the myocardial fiber length returns to normal but slippage of fibers in relation to each other allows diastolic compliance to increase so this larger end-diastolic volume is accommodated at a normal end-diastolic pressure (Fig. 3-3, P_3). Systolic function remains normal — that is, stroke volume and ejection fraction remain high and end-systolic volume is not increased.

After prolonged existence of volume overload, systolic function deteriorates. Patients with mitral regurgitation eject a significant proportion of their left ventricular volume into the low-pressure left atrium. This ejection begins early in systole before the aortic valve opens and continues later in systole after the aortic valve closes because of the low pressure in the left atrium. This decrease in afterload allows the ventricle to maintain its systolic function longer in patients with mitral regurgitation than in those with aortic regurgitation, where afterload is maintained. In both cases, however, deterioration of systolic and diastolic function invariably occurs. There are many manifestations of this dysfunction. Ventricular systolic volume at any pressure is greater and ejection fraction is lower, indicating poorer emptying. Increasing diastolic volumes are associated with increased wall tension and decreased coronary flow. There is endocardial ischemia as a result of the decreased coronary flow with buildup of fibrous tissue. An increased level of intracellular calcium prevents normal ATP-dependent relaxation of the myocardium. Thus diastolic compliance is reduced (the ventricle is stiffer) in addition to systolic dysfunction.

Pathophysiology of Pressure Overload

Pressure overload (increased afterload) increases the systolic work of the ventricle. Common diseases resulting in pressure overload include obstruction of the semilunar valves (aortic stenosis or pulmonic stenosis), coarctation of the aorta, and systemic or pulmonary hypertension. Faced with increased resistance to outflow the ventricle progresses through several pathophysiologic states.

Acutely the ventricle empties less completely as a result of the increased afterload, resulting in a higher end-systolic and, therefore, early diastolic ventricular volume (Fig. 3-4, point ESV_2 vs ESV_1). Since venous return is unchanged the result is increased diastolic stretch of the ventricle (increased preload, dilatation) because filling starts from a larger volume (see Fig. 3-4, point ESV_2) and therefore ends at a larger volume (see Fig. 3-4, point EDV_2). The initial compensation for a pressure load thus utilizes the Frank-Starling mechanism to increase cardiac work.

If the afterload is maintained for some time the contractility of the myocardium alters so that increased pressure can be generated from a lower preload, a phenomenon termed homeometric autoregulation. This shifts the ventricular end systolic pressure-volume line upward and left. The ventricle is now able to develop more pressure from the same end-diastolic volume and to empty to a normal end-systolic volume. The work curve is larger and, if pressure overload is maintained, hypertrophy develops.

Ventricular hypertrophy is an adaptive response to a sustained increase in afterload, allowing normalization of systolic wall stress despite increased pressure in the chamber by increasing wall thickness. This hypertrophy is due both

to the addition of more sarcomeres and to an increase in the size of the sarcomeres and, unlike the hypertrophy in volume overload, is concentric, resulting in a marked increase in wall thickness. Despite its benefits, the presence of left ventricular hypertrophy in conditions of pressure overload affecting the left ventricle indicates a poorer prognosis. Whether this is due to the left ventricular hypertrophy itself or occurs because the presence of LVH indicates more severe disease is uncertain.

While ventricular hypertrophy is beneficial in maintaining systolic function the hypertrophied ventricle becomes less compliant (stiffer). Eventually the ventricle is unable to fill adequately without systemic or pulmonary congestion. Intuitively, systolic dysfunction might be expected in patients with pressure overload, but diastolic dysfunction is actually more common.

Valvular Heart Disease

Mitral Stenosis

Hemodynamic Changes

Until a critical degree of narrowing occurs, no disturbance of function results from stenosis of the mitral valve. The reserve is so great that the area of the valve orifice has to be at least halved before the obstruction causes any compensatory pressure changes. Even when the obstruction is not hemodynamically important, the increased rate of flow across the narrowed area produces a murmur, facilitating early diagnosis. With progressive narrowing of the valve orifice, a pressure gradient develops between the left atrium and the left ventricle (Fig. 3-5) and the left atrial pressure rises, causing the left atrium to hypertrophy. This pressure is reflected back into the pulmonary veins, capillaries, and arteries with eventual pulmonary hypertension and right ventricular hypertrophy. Increasing pulmonary capillary pressure can lead to the development of pulmonary edema if it occurs suddenly. Since atrial systole is crucially important to the filling of the ventricle across the stenotic valve, the onset of atrial fibrillation (the most common disturbance of rhythm seen in patients with mitral stenosis) is often a turning point in the natural history of this condition. Patients deteriorate rapidly because of the loss of the atrial component of ventricular filling and because the rapid heart rate results in a decreased filling time, both resulting in an acute rise in pressure in the left atrium.

Clinical Picture

The symptoms in patients with mitral stenosis are related to the increased pressure in the pulmonary capillaries (difficulty breathing), reduced cardiac output (fatigue), and

Fig. 3-4. Pressure-volume loops in pressure overload. P_1, P_2, and P_3 = increasing pressures (afterloads). ESV = end-systolic volume. EDV = end-diastolic volume.

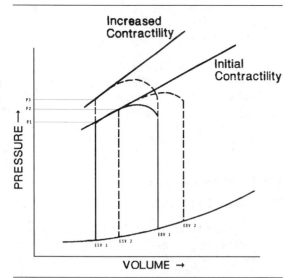

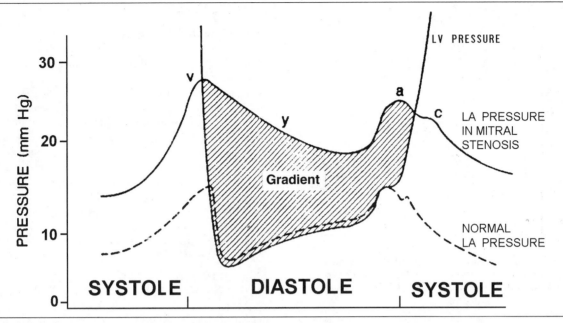

Fig. 3-5. Left atrial and left ventricular pressure tracings in a patient with mitral stenosis. Note the differences between the normal y-descent and the slowed y-descent in mitral stenosis, the larger a-wave in mitral stenosis, and the gradient (pressure difference) between the atrium and ventricle in mitral stenosis due to the obstruction.

the rapid irregular heart rate when atrial fibrillation develops (palpitations). Hemoptysis is relatively common. The patient may also complain of chest pain. Emboli occur secondary to thrombi forming within the enlarged left atrium as a result of stasis of blood. The physical examination reflects the altered physiology. The peripheral pulse is reduced in volume due to the low stroke volume. Precordial examination usually reveals the apex to be normal in position. There is a parasternal lift due to right ventricular hypertrophy. The first sound is accentuated since the mitral valve leaflets are widely separated and since the rate of pressure change is high at the time of valve closure. There is an opening snap following the second heart sound, as the abnormally thickened mitral leaflets are opened by a high atrial pressure. The higher the atrial pressure the sooner the mitral leaflets open, so the interval from the second sound to the opening snap provides a bedside estimate of left atrial pressure, a short interval indicating more severe stenosis. A mid-diastolic rumbling murmur and, in patients who are in sinus rhythm, a presystolic murmur are bedside evidence of the turbulent flow through the stenotic valve.

Mitral Regurgitation

Hemodynamic Changes

The blood regurgitated from the left ventricle into the left atrium produces left atrial distention. This blood, along with the normal venous return, fills the left atrium rapidly, resulting in a large c-v wave (Fig. 3-6). The subsequent increased diastolic filling of the left ventricle results in increased stroke volume utilizing the Frank-Starling mechanism. The total volume of blood pumped by the left ventricle is thus increased to maintain forward output, resulting in volume overload of the left ventricle as well as atrium. Since regurgitation usually develops slowly, rearrangement of myocardial fibers can occur, allowing the chambers to become more compliant and minimizing the pressure rise due to this increased volume.

Clinical Picture

The left ventricle can tolerate mitral regurgitation for many years but when heart failure develops it usually progresses steadily and relentlessly. Symptoms are predominantly related to the rise in filling pressures when

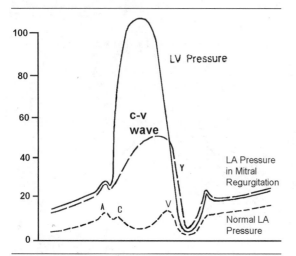

Fig. 3-6. Left atrial and left ventricular pressure tracings in a patient with mitral regurgitation. Note the large systolic c-v wave and the rapid y-descent as well as the exaggerated filling in early diastole.

compensatory mechanisms fail. As in mitral stenosis, these pressures are reflected into the lungs, resulting in effort dyspnea, orthopnea, nocturnal dyspnea, and acute pulmonary edema. Embolism is less frequent than in mitral stenosis as there is no stasis in the left atrium. Patients may complain of palpitations due to the hyperdynamic left ventricle or the development of atrial fibrillation. Fatigue is a common complaint. Physical examination usually reveals an enlarged left ventricle with a hyperdynamic apex beat due to the increased left ventricular stroke volume. The first sound may be reduced as the overfilling of the left ventricle in diastole allows the mitral leaflets to float together so there is less separation at the time of closure and the incompetent mitral valve eliminates the isovolumic phase of contraction with its rapid buildup of pressure. There is invariably an apical pansystolic murmur. The murmur commences with the first heart sound, which it may obscure, and runs through to aortic second sound. It is maximum at the apex, medium pitched, blowing in quality, and usually radiates to the axilla. The severity of the incompetence cannot be assessed from the intensity of the murmur. A third heart sound is frequently present at the apex and this may be followed by a mid-diastolic flow murmur, both reflecting the increased diastolic filling of the left ventricle and indicating severe regurgitation.

Aortic Stenosis

Hemodynamic Changes

Aortic stenosis results in obstruction of flow from the left ventricle to the aorta and therefore a systolic pressure gradient exists between these chambers (Fig. 3-7). To overcome this increase in afterload the left ventricle generates a higher systolic pressure to maintain normal forward flow. This increased pressure load results in concentric hypertrophy. The hypertrophied ventricle is less compliant and therefore requires higher filling pressures to maintain a normal volume. When heart failure occurs, cardiac output drops and left ventricular filling pressure increases further. Inadequate coronary flow to the hypertrophied muscle may occur, producing myocardial ischemia. This results both from the increased oxygen demand of the afterloaded myocardium and the failure of the coronary bed to hypertrophy along with the muscle.

Clinical Picture

The patient with aortic stenosis has a long asymptomatic period during which the left ventricular myocardium is able to compensate for the increased afterload by homeometric autoregulation and then by hypertrophy. Eventually symptoms of dyspnea result from increased left ventricular

Fig. 3-7. Pressure tracings from a patient with aortic stenosis showing the gradient between the left ventricle (LV) and aorta.

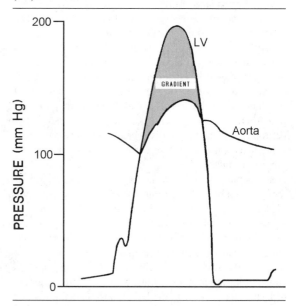

stiffness and then from systolic dysfunction. Both of these result in a rise in filling pressure (preload) which is reflected back into the lungs. Angina pectoris may occur as a result of ischemia from increased demand and increased muscle mass which may outstrip its capillary supply. This is often aggravated by coexisting coronary disease since both are common in older males. Syncope was thought to reflect low cardiac output but is now known to often result from ventricular tachycardia. The onset of symptoms in aortic stenosis is associated with a poor prognosis since they occur only after compensatory mechanisms have failed. On physical examination the pulse is characteristically slow rising since the rate of ejection through the stenotic valve is slow. The apex impulse is displaced downward and outward, reflecting left ventricular enlargement, and is sustained since the rate of ventricular emptying is slow. A harsh loud systolic ejection murmur is characteristic. It starts after the first sound (at the onset of ejection) and may be preceded by an ejection click. It increases in amplitude as systolic pressure increases, and then tapers off as pressure drops and ejection slows. The aortic second sound is often soft and delayed.

Aortic Regurgitation

Hemodynamic Changes

Insufficiency of the aortic valve allows regurgitation of blood from the aorta into the left ventricle during diastole. Most of the leak occurs during early diastole when the pressure difference is greatest (Fig. 3-8). The increased volume of blood results in diastolic distention of the left ventricle (increased preload) and the Frank-Starling mechanism produces increased stroke volume. This leads to ventricular dilatation as the ventricular myocardium is rearranged to increase its compliance and eventually results in hypertrophy.

Clinical Picture

As with mitral regurgitation and aortic stenosis, the natural history of aortic insufficiency includes a prolonged asymptomatic period during which compensatory mechanisms maintain an adequate forward output at a filling pressure which can be tolerated by the patient. The onset of shortness of breath, orthopnea, paroxysmal nocturnal dyspnea, or pulmonary edema signal the onset of decompensation when adequate cardiac output can only be achieved by an unacceptably high filling pressure. Palpitations and awareness of arterial throbbing in the neck due to the large stroke volume are sometime troublesome. Characteristically, the pulse is collapsing due to the rapid diastolic

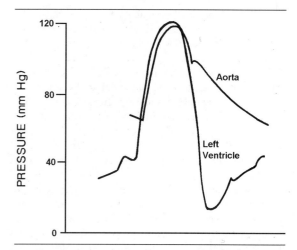

Fig. 3-8. Pressure tracings from a patient with aortic insufficiency. Note the rapid fall in the aortic pressure and rise in the left ventricular pressure in diastole as well as the rapid pressure rise and large pulse pressure in systole.

runoff from the aorta into the left ventricle. Examination of the precordium usually reveals an apex impulse that is displaced laterally and downward due to left ventricular dilatation and is hyperdynamic due to the increased left ventricular stroke volume. The characteristic auscultatory finding is an early diastolic murmur, which commences with A-2 and is usually high pitched and soft. The murmur is decrescendo, reflecting the rapid decrease in the pressure gradient between the aorta and left ventricle.

Lesions of the Right-Sided Valves

Tricuspid stenosis, tricuspid insufficiency, pulmonic stenosis, and pulmonic insufficiency have hemodynamics similar to the corresponding left-sided lesions. While left-sided lesions cause changes in the arterial waveform that can be appreciated by examination of the carotid pulse, changes in the venous pulse with left-sided lesions cannot be detected by physical examination since the pulmonary veins are deep in the chest. Conversely, the changes in the pulmonary arterial pulse from the right-sided lesions are inaccessible by physical examination while venous changes are easily seen in the jugular veins. Only the key differences between right- and left-sided lesions will be discussed below.

Tricuspid stenosis is characterized by an increased a-wave on the jugular venous pulse as a result of atrial hypertrophy and increased strength of contraction due to the afterload imposed by the stenotic tricuspid valve. Also as a result of the tricuspid obstruction the y-descent is slowed since blood flow into the right ventricle is slowed.

Tricuspid regurgitation most commonly occurs secondary to right heart failure and is due to disturbance of the architecture of the tricuspid valve apparatus rather than disease of the leaflets. The physical examination is characterized by a large v- or c-v wave in the jugular venous pulse and systolic expansion of the liver. Auscultation reveals a systolic murmur that increases with inspiration, and is heard best along the left sternal border.

Pulmonic stenosis results in right ventricular hypertrophy due to the increased afterload which can be appreciated as a systolic impulse along the left sternal border. As the right atrium hypertrophies in response to the decreased diastolic compliance of the hypertrophied right ventricle, the size of the a-wave in the jugular venous pulse increases. Wide splitting of the second sound due to marked delay in right ventricular emptying is characteristic, with the pulmonic component of the second sound delayed and soft.

Pulmonic regurgitation is characterized by an early to mid-diastolic murmur occurring along the left sternal border similar to that of aortic regurgitation. The murmur increases with inspiration. Because of the ability of the right ventricle to handle large volumes of blood, pulmonic insufficiency is well tolerated and only occasionally produces other signs or any symptoms.

Clinical Examples

Normal Values

Right atrial mean pressure	3–6 mm Hg
Left atrial mean pressure	6–12 mm Hg
Stroke volume	50–80 cc/beat
Heart rate	60–100 beats/min
Cardiac output	4–6 L/min
LV end-diastolic volume	60–100 cc/m^2 BSA
Ejection fraction	55–65%

1. The patient, a 65-year-old man, had no cardiac history. He came to the emergency room with acute pulmonary edema. The patient's pulse was 92 and regular, his blood pressure 110/70. Jugular pulse was normal. The carotid pulse volume was reduced and the upstroke was slow. A sustained left ventricular impulse was palpable. The first sound was normal, the aortic component of the second sound was soft, and a fourth sound was heard at the apex. A loud, rough systolic ejection murmur was heard at the upper right and left sternal borders and in the neck. Moist rales were heard over the entire extent of both lung fields. Cardiac catheterization was performed.

Hemodynamics

Left atrial pressure	30 mm Hg
Left ventricular systolic pressure	200 mm Hg
Aortic systolic pressure	120 mm Hg
Aortic valve gradient	75 mm Hg
Cardiac output	3.5 L/min
Ejection fraction	40%

Discussion.   This patient with aortic stenosis has developed severe left ventricular hypertrophy. In the face of continuing afterload, compensatory mechanisms in the ventricle have failed, and at the present time, despite a high filling pressure, the ejection fraction and cardiac output have fallen, representing loss of compensation. Increasing cardiac output by the Frank-Starling mechanism is impossible because the high filling pressure is already producing pulmonary symptoms. The stiff ventricle and high diastolic pressure result in the generation of a fourth sound at the apex. Following surgical aortic valve replacement the patient's symptoms improved. His hemodynamic measurements were then:

Left atrial pressure	15 mm Hg
LV systolic pressure	120 mm Hg
Aortic systolic pressure	120 mm Hg
Cardiac output	4 L/min
Ejection fraction	50%

Reduction of ventricular afterload has now allowed a return to more normal function. The severe hypertrophy, however, will not regress completely and still results in some decreased compliance (elevated left ventricular filling pressure) and reduced function (somewhat reduced ejection fraction and cardiac output).

2. A 38-year-old woman gave a history of a constitutional illness with joint pains at the age of 15. The doctor told her that she had a heart murmur. She recovered uneventfully and remained totally asymptomatic until her first pregnancy seven years later, when she noticed that she had become short of breath when she exerted herself. She delivered a second child five years later and again noticed some deterioration in her effort tolerance. She had pneumonia, requiring hospitalization and treatment with antibiotics, six years later. She noticed that her effort tolerance had diminished even further, and she began for the first

time to have some difficulty doing her housework. She also complained of being tired and at times coughed up blood-stained sputum. About 4 years after that, she noticed some irregularity of her heartbeat and consulted her doctor. On physical examination her rhythm was totally irregular with a pulse rate of 144. Her blood pressure was 105/80. The cardiac apex was normal. She had a parasternal heave. The first heart sound was accentuated. She had an opening snap which followed closely upon the second heart sound, and a low-pitched diastolic rumble.

Cardiac catheterization showed a loss of A-wave in the left atrial pressure tracing due to atrial fibrillation.

Left atrial mean pressure	20 mm Hg
Mitral gradient	15 mm Hg
PA pressure (mean)	50 mm Hg

The y-descent of the atrial pressure was slowed.

Discussion. This woman developed progressive obstruction of her mitral valve over many years. The mitral stenosis produced afterloading of the left atrium, which hypertrophied. The increased left atrial pressure owing to increased residual volume from obstructed emptying was transmitted to the lungs, producing pulmonary symptoms which were worst at times of volume loading such as pregnancy and exertion. Eventually the pressure was reflected back into the right ventricle, which subsequently hypertrophied. As the stenosis became more severe her symptoms (which initially were only present during times of increased volume loading) were present with normal exertion. The enlarged left atrium provided a substrate for atrial fibrillation and the loss of atrial contraction further impaired atrial emptying. The atrial fibrillation was evident on physical examination as irregular rhythm. The right ventricular enlargement could be felt as an impulse along the left sternal border. The loud first sound was indicative of mitral leaflets that were widely separated at the time of closure, and were closed briskly by the normally contracting left ventricle. The pulmonic component of the second sound was accentuated because of the high pulmonary artery pressure. The opening snap of the abnormally thickened mitral leaflets could be heard, and was close to the second sound because of the high left atrial pressure. The turbulent flow across the obstructed mitral valve in diastole produced the characteristic rumbling murmur.

Bibliography

Corin WJ, Murakami T, Monrad ES, et al. Left ventricular passive diastolic properties in chronic mitral regurgitation. *Circulation* 83:797–807, 1991. *This clinical study compares diastolic function in normals and in two groups of patients with mitral regurgitation — those with normal and those with impaired systolic function.*

Holt W, Auffermann W, Wu ST, et al. Mechanism for depressed cardiac function in left-ventricular volume overload. *Am Heart J* 121:534–537, 1991. *An experimental study of the effect of progressive volume loading on coronary flow and cellular calcium ions.*

Lorell BH, Apstein CS, Weinberg EO, and Cunningham MJ. Diastolic function in left ventricular hypertrophy: Clinical and experimental relationships. *European Heart J* 11(suppl G):54–64, 1990. *A comprehensive review of changes in diastolic function in the presence of left ventricular hypertrophy. Well written, complete with 55 references.*

Rumberger JA and Reed JE. Quantitative dynamics of left ventricular emptying and filling as a function of heart size and stroke volume in pure aortic regurgitation and in normal subjects. *Am J Cardiol* 70:1045–1050, 1992. *Presents a study of the response of a normally functioning heart to aortic regurgitation.*

Villari B, Campbell SE, Hess O, et al. Influence of collagen network on left ventricular systolic and diastolic function in aortic valve disease. *J Am Cell Cardiol* 22:1477–84, 1993. *Pathologic study of changes in the myocardium with hypertrophy that sheds light on the ensuing physiologic changes.*

Villari B, Hess OM, Kaufmann P, et al. Effect of aortic valve stenosis (pressure overload) and regurgitation (volume overload) on left ventricular systolic and diastolic function. *Am J Cardiol* 69:927–934, 1992. *A study comparing left ventricular function in 28 patients with aortic stenosis and 30 with aortic regurgitation to each other and to 11 control subjects.*

Yun KL, Rayhill SC, Niczporuk MA, et al. Left ventricular mechanics and energetics in the dilated canine heart: Acute versus chronic mitral regurgitation. *J Thorac Cardiovasc Surg* 104:26–39, 1992. *An experimental study of mitral regurgitation induced in dogs studied early (1 week) and late (3 months), looking at progressive changes in left ventricular function.*

4 Congenital Heart Disease and Intracardiac Shunts

Edward Overholt

Objectives

After completing this chapter, you should be able to

Describe fetal circulation, including the location of the major anatomic shunts

Outline the circulatory changes that normally occur following birth

List the four major categories of congenital heart defects and give at least two examples of each

Describe the typical features and characteristic pathophysiologic disturbances for each of the major types of congenital heart disease

Explain the pathophysiologic basis for the typical signs and symptoms of each of the major categories of congenital heart disease

Basic Concepts of Intracardiac Shunting

An understanding of several basic concepts is critical to comprehension of the principle of intracardiac shunting and the clinical effects of the variety of congenital heart defects. The following terms are selected as those particularly important to the concepts presented later in this chapter and are supplemental to other basic concepts such as preload, afterload, and contractility, which are covered in Chap. 2.

Pressure

Pressure is the force, either actual or potential, generated within a cavity. In a fluid-filled system, it is analogous to voltage (potential electromotive force) in an electrical system. It should not be confused with resistance, since in many cases pressure may be elevated, e.g., pulmonary hypertension, but resistance is actually low.

Resistance

Resistance is the opposition to passage of a material through a system. In the vascular system, resistance can be defined as either **alteriolar resistance** (opposition to flow through the arteriolar bed) or **total resistance** (arteriolar resistance plus the resistance of the column of fluid downstream).

Flow

Flow is the amount of fluid which moves through the system within a specified amount of time. It is analogous to current in an electrical system. In the vasculature, flow can be defined as **effective blood flow** (the flow entering the system which actually exits) or **total blood flow** (effective blood flow plus any flow which is shunted into or out of the system).

Cyanosis

Cyanosis is a clinical description of the bluish color seen in the presence of desaturated hemoglobin. Approximately

5 grams per deciliter desaturated hemoglobin must be present before it is detectable by physical exam. **Peripheral cyanosis or acrocyanosis** (detected in distal capillary beds such as the fingers, toes, circumoral area) may be due to sluggish capillary blood flow and is *not* necessarily an indication of arterial hypoxemia. However, **central cyanosis** (detected in central capillary beds such as the mucosae or trunk) is thought to be a more reliable indication of "arterial" hypoxemia.

Fetal Circulation

The majority of information regarding the fetal and neonatal circulation is derived from animal studies, particularly in the fetal lamb, and the results are then used for extrapolations to the human. These extrapolations are useful but may not always be entirely accurate, considering differences between species and the instrumentation required for many of the measurements. However, with more recent studies of cardiac hemodynamics made possible by improvements in echocardiography and Doppler flow measurements, much of the original work in fetal lambs has been validated in the human fetus and newborn.

The Immature Myocardium

The ability of the myocardium to contract against a load improves with maturation. This inability to contract in the immature appears to be primarily due to decreased availability of intracellular calcium. The Frank-Starling relationship appears to be intact in the developing heart; the effects of changes in cardiac rate, volume loading, and inotropic stimulation on fetal cardiac output are similar to those seen in the adult. Myocardial oxygen consumption is higher in the fetus due to increased demands by the mitochondria. The metabolic substrates used by the fetal myocardium (glucose, lactate, and pyruvate) change to more utilization of long chain fatty acids in the neonate and adult. Due to this fact and differences in utilization of high-energy phosphates, the fetal and neonatal myocardium is more resistant to hypoxemia and ischemia than the adult myocardium.

Pattern of Fetal Blood Flow

The general course of fetal blood flow is shown in Fig. 4-1. The major difference between the fetal and the adult circulation is the different site of gas exchange (the placenta vs. the lungs). The effects of this difference on variations

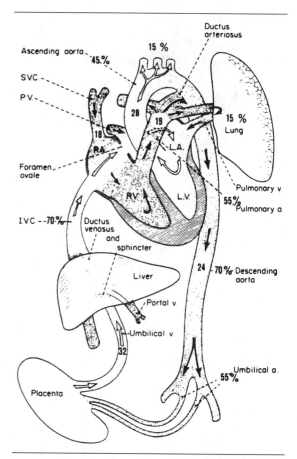

Fig. 4-1. Diagram of the fetal circulation showing the four sites of shunt. The intravascular shading is in proportion to oxygen saturation. The intravascular numbers represent the pO_2, the number outside the vascular structures represent the relative flows in the major tributaries. (From Guntheroth WG, et al. Physiology of the circulation: Fetus, neonate and child. In Kelley VC (ed.). *Practice of Pediatrics.* Philadelphia: Harper & Row, 1983. With permission from J. B. Lippincott and the author.)

in flow, pressure, and resistance are summarized as follows:

1. The placenta represents a large low-resistance system of blood vessels designed for optimal exchange of gases and nutrients. As such, it receives the largest proportion of combined ventricular output (55%) with relatively low oxygen content.
2. The inferior vena cava carries approximately 70% of the total venous return to the heart, receiving oxy-

genated (pO_2 = 32 mm Hg) blood from the placenta via the ductus venosus, which connects to the umbilical vein through the hepatic/portal circulation. Two-thirds of this flow is directed through the foramen ovale into the left atrium. The remainder mixes with the majority of the superior vena caval flow and is directed through the tricuspid valve into the right ventricle.

3. The right ventricular output (55% of the combined ventricular output) is directed primarily through the ductus arteriosus due to the high pulmonary vascular resistance (only 15% traverses the pulmonary capillary bed). This results in relatively poorly oxygenated blood (pO_2 = 24 mm Hg) entering the descending aorta, which returns to the low-resistance placenta via the umbilical arteries.

4. The left ventricle pumps the remaining 45% of the combined output into the ascending aorta, where the more highly oxygenated blood (pO_2 = 28 mm Hg) enters the coronary and cerebral circulations.

Postnatal Circulatory Changes

The primary alteration in the circulation following birth is related to redirection of blood flow into the lungs for gas exchange.

Interruption of Umbilical Circulation

Removal of the low-resistance capillary bed of the placenta from the circulation occurs with interruption of the umbilical cord flow, usually within the first minute after birth. Later the umbilical arteries constrict and eventually fibrose and the ductus venosus closes due to loss of flow from the placenta. These changes result in an increase in systemic vascular resistance.

Pulmonary Circulation

The pulmonary vascular resistance is essentially equal to systemic resistance before birth and is maintained at this high level by a combination of a thick muscular layer in the arteriolar walls, relative hypoxia in the pulmonary arteries, and the response to factors such as pH, pO_2, pCO_2, and vasoactive substances. Following birth, the pulmonary arteriolar bed undergoes a rapid fall in resistance in response to several factors: (1) expansion of alveoli with gas, (2) increases in arterial oxygenation and pH, (3) decreases in arterial CO_2 levels, and (4) related changes in the levels of vasoactive substances such as prostaglandins. This re-

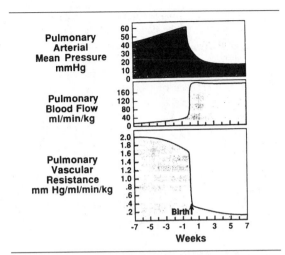

Fig. 4-2. Graphic representation of the changes in pulmonary artery pressure, blood flow, and vascular resistance in the perinatal period. (Reproduced with permission from: Rudolph AM. The pre- and postnatal pulmonary circulation. In *Congenital Diseases of the Heart.* Chicago: Year Book Medical, 1974, p. 31.)

sistance fall is quite dramatic within the first few minutes to hours following birth and continues on particularly within the first 6 to 8 weeks of life (Fig. 4-2). This relative change in resistance to pulmonary blood is a critical factor affecting the degree of intracardiac shunting in various congenital defects and the appearance of various clinical signs and symptoms (tachypnea, tachycardia, poor feeding) of congestive heart failure in infants with these lesions.

Closure of Ductus Arteriosus and Foramen Ovale

Functional closure of the ductus arteriosus occurs in response to an increase in arterial oxygen tension and changes in local prostaglandin levels. This closure usually occurs within the first 12 to 24 hours after birth, but may be delayed in response to conditions such as hypoxemia and prematurity. Timing of ductal closure is an important predictor of the appearance of clinical signs such as cyanosis or cardiogenic shock seen in defects which require the ductus for maintenance of pulmonary or systemic blood flow. Final anatomic closure of the ductus arteriosus usually occurs with the first few months of life.

Because of increased pulmonary blood flow after birth

and thus increased flow and pressure in the left atrium, functional closure of the flap valve of the foramen ovale occurs within minutes after birth. However, the foramen ovale continues to allow interatrial shunting for weeks to months following birth, with anatomical closure of the foramen often not occurring for years.

Congenital Heart Disease

To simplify understanding, we will consider four major categories of congenital heart defects. While some infants exhibit several anomalies, this "simple" approach can explain fundamental concepts of pathophysiology and helps predict the clinical consequences of the dominant lesion.

Left Heart Obstructive Lesions

Left heart obstructive lesions (aortic stenosis, coarctation of the aorta, hypoplastic left heart syndrome, mitral stenosis, and total anomalous pulmonary venous return with obstruction) make up an important group of defects in children. They are the **most common** cause of **congestive heart failure** in infants in the first 2 weeks of life. The severity of symptoms and timing of their presentation depends on the degree of obstruction and the timing of closure of the ductus arteriosus. Since the fetal ductus primarily supplies the systemic circulation, loss of this supply sometime after birth leads to a marked increase in left heart afterload with secondary elevation of left ventricular pressure. This elevation results in increased pulmonary capillary pressures and subsequent development of transudation of fluid into alveoli (pulmonary edema). Pulmonary edema causes a lack of compliance of the lungs and results in tachypnea and eventual respiratory distress. Eventually, elevated left heart pressures cause right-sided pressure increases and development of right heart failure. In infancy, elevated central venous pressures are clinically evident as hepatomegaly and central edema (not peripheral edema, seen in adults). Finally, increased sympathetic activity (seen as tachycardia, diaphoresis) with its increased myocardial oxygen demand combines with decreased myocardial perfusion (reduced due to elevated ventricular diastolic and lowered aortic pressures) to cause a reduction in myocardial contractility. In infants less than 2 weeks of age with severe symptoms, marked improvement can be accomplished by redilation of the ductus arteriosus using an infusion of prostaglandins. This results in improved systemic perfusion due to a "right-to-left" shunt of blood from the pulmonary arteries. This circulation is demonstrated in Fig. 4-3.

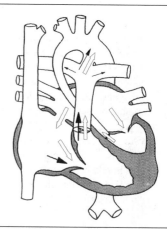

Fig. 4-3. Diagram of the circulation in mitral stenosis, hypoplastic left ventricle, severe aortic stenosis, and persistent patent ductus arteriosus. In this and subsequent diagrams, the arrows indicate direction and proportionate volume of blood flow. Filled arrows indicate poorly oxygenated blood and open arrows designate well-oxygenated blood. In this circulation, the patent ductus arteriosus is the primary source of blood supply to the body.

Milder degrees of obstruction do not cause the picture of congestive heart failure and generally present at an older age with a cardiac murmur or rarely symptoms of reduced cardiac output.

Right Heart Obstructive Lesions

Right heart obstructive lesions (tetralogy of Fallot, pulmonary stenosis, tricuspid atresia, pulmonary atresia) are a frequent cause of **severe cyanosis** in newborn infants. Obstruction of the flow of poorly oxygenated blood returning from the body causes "right-to-left" shunting through any existing communications such as ventricular septal defects or the foramen ovale (tetralogy of Fallot represents a combination of pulmonic stenosis and ventricular septal defect). This shunted blood combines with the reduction in pulmonary blood flow to cause severe cyanosis often evident immediately at birth or upon loss of the supplemental pulmonary blood flow through the ductus arteriosus. Signs of congestive heart failure are not present in these infants since there is actually a reduction in combined ventricular flow. Re-establishment of a patent ductus arteriosus using prostaglandins causes a significant improvement in arterial oxygen tension due to "left-to-right" shunting from the aorta into the pulmonary circulation (Fig. 4-4).

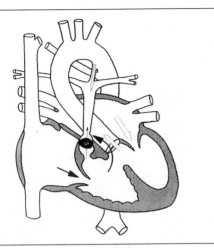

Fig. 4-4. Diagram of the circulation in severe tetralogy of Fallot and persistent patent ductus arteriosus (PDA). Note the primary source of pulmonary blood flow is due to left-to-right shunting through the PDA; closure of the PDA would therefore lead to severe hypoxemia.

Intuitively, it follows that the degree of cyanosis would parallel the severity of obstruction to pulmonary blood flow. In older children, right heart obstructive lesions typically present as a cardiac murmur with a milder degree of cyanosis. A special exception to this principle is the development of **hypercyanotic episodes** in children with two basic defects — tetralogy of Fallot or tricuspid atresia with pulmonary blood flow dependent solely on shunting through a ventricular septal defect. In these circumstances, the child is susceptible to episodes of dramatic reduction in pulmonary blood flow caused by a variety of triggering factors (dehydration, tachycardia, emotional stress, exercise) which result in lowered systemic vascular resistance, increased contractility, and increased pulmonary outflow obstruction. This combination of changes produces severe hypoxemia which can be life threatening if not treated promptly.

Left-to-Right Shunt Lesions

Left-to-right shunt lesions (ventricular septal defect, atrial septal defect, patent ductus arteriosus, total anomalous pulmonary venous return without obstruction, arteriovenous malformation, atrioventricular canal) represent several of the most common congenital heart defects. The amount of left-to-right shunting is dependent on several factors including (1) size of the communication, (2) com-

pliance of the cardiac chambers, (3) anatomic location of the communication, and (4) the relative pulmonary-systemic vascular resistances. Of these factors, location of the defect is the least important in determining the shunt amount except in the case of a direct left ventricle-right atrial communication. An understanding of the changes in vascular resistance (especially pulmonary) following birth is necessary when studying these lesions. As previously noted, the high fetal pulmonary vascular resistance drops rapidly after birth and continues to decrease relatively rapidly within the first 6 to 8 weeks of life. This decline in resistance in the right heart leads to a progressive increase in left-to-right shunting over the same time period. For this reason, the clinical signs of a large left-to-right lesion (Fig. 4-5) are usually not evident in the first few days or even weeks after birth. Subsequently, congestive heart failure and growth failure become apparent.

Not all lesions in this category lead to the clinical picture of congestive heart failure. In general, defects which cause shunting before flowing through the tricuspid valve are less likely to cause early congestive heart failure. Also, the persistence or development of elevated pulmonary vascular resistance can lessen the degree of intracardiac shunting and actually cause an improvement of cardiac symptoms. This apparent "golden period" is in reality an

Fig. 4-5. Diagram of the circulation in complete atrioventricular canal defect (one of the endocardial cushion defects commonly seen in patients with Down's syndrome). Relatively low pulmonary arteriolar resistance leads to a large left-to-right shunt through the atrial and ventricular septal defects.

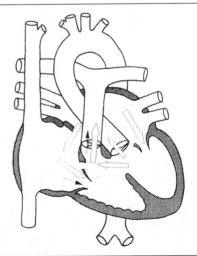

ominous sign of the development of anatomic changes in the pulmonary vascular bed. These changes begin with medial hypertrophy of the pulmonary arterioles, followed by fibrous intimal hyperplasia, plexiform and angiomatoid lesions of the small arteries, and finally necrotizing arteritis. This process becomes irreversible and causes so-called Eisenmenger's syndrome (described in patients with septal defects and elevated pulmonary resistance who first develop a balanced circulation and then progressively increasing right-to-left shunting as pulmonary vascular obstructive disease ensues). The elements which predispose toward the development of these vascular changes include (1) increased pulmonary blood flow, (2) pulmonary hypertension, (3) arterial hypoxemia, and (4) elevated blood viscosity. Congenital defects are therefore assessed with respect to these factors and the possibility of early development of pulmonary vascular disease when making plans for therapeutic interventions such as surgical repair.

Admixture Lesions

Admixture is a term used to define a circulation which includes both left-to-right and right-to-left shunting. This circulation therefore leads to a combination of signs and symptoms of both problems, namely congestive heart failure and cyanosis. Lesions in this group include transposition of the great arteries, truncus arteriosus, double outlet right ventricle, and many of the so-called "single-ventricle" defects. The primary presentation of children with these lesions depends on the predominant shunt, i.e., children with predominant right-to-left shunting (e.g., transposition of the great arteries) exhibit cyanosis; children with predominant left-to-right shunting (e.g., truncus arteriosus) show more obvious congestive symptoms than cyanosis.

Figure 4-6 demonstrates the circulation seen in transposition of the great arteries. In this lesion, the pulmonary and systemic circulations are in parallel rather than in series as seen in normal hearts. Loss of the fetal communications (the foramen ovale or ductus arteriosus) which allow mixing of well and poorly oxygenated blood in the parallel circuits results in marked hypoxemia. This results in death within hours unless one or both of these communications can be re-established. The foramen ovale can be "permanently" opened by the Rashkind procedure, in which a balloon-tipped catheter is guided into the left atrium by a transvenous approach. The catheter is then rapidly withdrawn across the flap valve over the foramen, creating an opening which allows interatrial mixing. Alternatively, the ductus arteriosus can be reopened using a prostaglandin

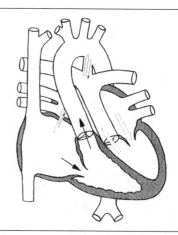

Fig. 4-6. Diagram of the circulation in D-transposition of the great arteries and persistent patent ductus arteriosus (PDA). Note the bidirectional shunting at the level of the PDA and the interatrial septum: This shunting provides the only route for poorly oxygenated blood to return to the pulmonary circuit and for well-oxygenated blood to exit to the body.

infusion, as previously described. These maneuvers are not necessary to achieve adequate mixing if "permanent" communications are present such as septal defects or surgically created shunts.

Clinical Examples

1. A one-day-old male infant has developed cyanosis. This infant is the product of a term, uncomplicated gestation and delivery. The child was first noted to have cyanosis at 6 hours of age. At that time, rapid respirations but no distress was noted. Supplemental oxygen administration resulted in little or no improvement in the child's level of cyanosis.

Physical Examination

Temperature	37.5°C
Heart rate	140/minute
Respiratory rate	60/minute
Blood pressure	70/50 in right arm

General examination reveals a cyanotic, well-nourished infant in no acute respiratory distress. There is a mildly prominent cardiac impulse at the left sternal border but no thrills are palpable. Cardiac auscultation reveals a regular rate and rhythm with a normal first heart sound and mildly accentuated second heart sound which is closely split. A grade 2/6 systolic ejection murmur is heard best at the upper left sternal border. No diastolic murmurs or other abnormal cardiac sounds are heard. Abdominal examination shows mild hepatomegaly without other abnormalities. The pulse examination is normal in the upper and lower extremities.

A chest x-ray demonstrates normal heart size, narrow superior mediastinum, and increased pulmonary vascular markings. The electrocardiogram shows sinus rhythm, right axis deviation, and right ventricular hypertrophy. Arterial blood gases on room air: pH 7.37, pCO_2 35, pO_2 22. Arterial blood gases during administration of high flow supplemental oxygen: pH 7.35, pCO_2 38, pO_2 28.

Discussion. Several points are important to note from the history and physical examination: (1) the primary sign of cardiac disease (cyanosis, which appeared within the first few hours of life) suggests a predominant right-to-left shunt lesion related to closure of the ductus arteriosus, (2) the lack of prominent heart failure symptoms points toward either a right heart obstructive lesion or an admixture lesion with predominant right-to-left shunting, and (3) a normal pulse exam points away from a left heart obstructive lesion.

The chest x-ray showed increased pulmonary vascular markings, suggesting significant left-to-right shunting. The electrocardiogram suggests significant right heart volume or pressure loading. The arterial blood gas results indicate a large right-to-left intracardiac shunt (failure of hypoxemia to improve with high-flow O_2 is characteristic of a shunt). This constellation of findings suggests a cardiac lesion with both right-to-left and left-to-right shunting (i.e., an admixture lesion), predominantly right-to-left.

An echocardiogram was performed and showed transposition of the great arteries without septal defects and a closing patent ductus arteriosus. A prostaglandin infusion was started and resulted in prompt improvement in arterial oxygenation. The child was maintained on this infusion until surgical repair was performed at 3 days of age. The child was discharged one week later in good condition with normal oxygenation.

2. A 10-month-old female infant was brought to a family physician by her mother with a history of "pale spells" which had been noted for the past 3 to 4 weeks. She was the product of a term, uncomplicated gestation and delivery. She grew and developed normally since birth. Her family "did not believe in doctors" therefore, she had not received routine immunizations or examinations in the past. Her mother stated these episodes usually occurred in the early morning and were often precipitated by crying. After crying for several minutes, the child would develop rapid breathing and "poor color." She would then become lethargic, pale, and diaphoretic with occasional "twitching spells." The episodes gradually ended within 30 to 60 minutes when the child was held and comforted.

Physical Examination

Temperature	37°C
Heart rate	100/minute
Respiratory rate	30/minute
Blood pressure	100/75 in right arm

General examination demonstrated a well-nourished infant who appeared developmentally normal. A prominent impulse was felt near the left sternal border, but no thrills were palpable. Auscultation showed a regular rate and rhythm with normal first and second heart sounds. A grade 2–3/6 high-pitched systolic ejection-type murmur was best heard at the mid to upper left sternal border. No diastolic murmurs were heard. The lung and abdominal exams were normal. The pulses were normal in the upper and lower extremities. The capillary refill was normal but mild cyanosis of the nail beds and oral mucosae was noted. No clubbing of the fingers or toes was noted.

A chest x-ray demonstrated a normal heart size with upturned apex and concave left upper border, mildly decreased pulmonary vascular markings, and possible right aortic arch. The electrocardiogram showed sinus rhythm, right axis deviation, and right ventricular hypertrophy.

After several attempts were made to obtain arterial blood, the child began breathing quite deeply and rapidly. Her general color changed to deep cyanosis and she developed a lethargic, disoriented appearance. The mother stated that this episode was similar to those noted at home. Cardiac auscultation during this period showed no murmur but a heart rate of 180/minute.

Discussion. Of interest in the history was the relatively recent onset of symptoms, which does not suggest a ductal-dependent lesion. The child had grown normally, which indicates absence of any significant element of congestive heart failure. The physical examination showed mild cyanosis and a heart murmur of pulmonary outflow obstruction. The chest x-ray and electrocardiogram both suggest right ventricular enlargement and decreased pulmonary blood flow. These findings indicate the presence of a right-to-left shunt lesion (non-ductal dependent) such as severe pulmonary stenosis (with a patent foramen ovale allowing the right-to-left shunt) or tetralogy of Fallot. The timing of the onset of these episodes at 9–10 months of age suggests the progressive development of obstruction to pulmonary blood flow. The episode of severe cyanosis witnessed was compatible with a "hypercyanotic episode" owing to transient worsening of a right-to-left shunt. The loss of the murmur during the episode suggests loss of significant pulmonary blood flow secondary to critical obstruction.

The hypercyanotic episode was initially treated with supplemental oxygen and by placing the child in her mother's arms with its knees close to her chest. (This maneuver increases systemic vascular resistance and reduces right-to-left shunting.) Following stabilization, an echocardiogram showed tetralogy of Fallot with severe pulmonary outflow obstruction. Urgent surgical repair was performed and the child was discharged home 8 days after surgery in good condition.

3. A six-week-old infant was the product of an uncomplicated, term gestation and delivery. No cardiac murmur or other neonatal problems were noted. At routine exams, the child was noted to have a slow weight gain since birth. Over the past two weeks, the parents noted the child was feeding very slowly and was quite irritable. They also noted the infant became very diaphoretic with feedings.

Physical Examination

Temperature	37.0°C
Heart rate	165/minute
Respiratory rate	65–70/minute
Blood pressure	65/40

General exam reveals a thin, ill-appearing infant with mild respiratory distress and acrocyanosis. Cardiac examination shows a hyperactive precordium with a thrill palpable at the left lower sternal border. First and second heart sounds are accentuated and a grade 4/6 harsh, low-pitched holosystolic murmur is heard at the left sternal border. A third heart sound, and a mid-diastolic flow rumble are heard at the apex. The abdominal examination reveals an enlarged, nontender liver. Mildly decreased pulse amplitudes are noted in the upper and lower extremities. Chest x-ray shows an enlarged cardiac silhouette and increased pulmonary vascular markings. Sinus tachycardia, biventricular hypertrophy, and left atrial enlargement are noted on the electrocardiogram.

Discussion.   This infant's history suggests the onset of congestive heart failure as the natural decline in pul-

monary vascular resistance occurred. The absence of a murmur at birth is very typical since pulmonary resistance is quite high at that point, and therefore little flow is present across any communication which may exist. This picture can change dramatically over the first few weeks of life with the natural decline in pulmonary vascular resistance. A child who initially has no murmur at birth can later develop prominent signs of a large left-to-right shunt. The development of tachycardia, tachypnea, and evidence of high-output congestive heart failure in this infant are suggestive of a large left-to-right shunt lesion. The absence of central cyanosis suggests the lack of any significant right-to-left shunt. If this child had Down's syndrome, the possibility of an atrioventricular canal defect would be increased since this is the most common lesion seen among these patients. Otherwise a large ventricular septal defect is the most likely defect.

This child underwent an echocardiogram and was diagnosed with a large perimembranous VSD and also a secundum-type atrial septal defect. The child responded moderately well to administration of digoxin and furosemide (diuretic), but continued to show signs of chronic congestive heart failure and growth failure. Surgical repair of the septal defects was therefore performed when the child reached three months of age.

Bibliography

Garson A Jr., Bricker JT, and McNamara DG (eds.). *The Science and Practice of Pediatric Cardiology.* Philadelphia: Lea and Febiger, 1990. *A comprehensive pediatric cardiology textbook with chapters on fetal physiology, the pulmonary circulation, and the physiology of different types of lesions.*

Moller JH and Neal WA (eds.). *Fetal, Neonatal, and Infant Cardiac Disease.* Englewood Cliffs, NJ: Prentice Hall, 1990. *A comprehensive textbook on most aspects of cardiac physiology of the fetus and infant.*

Park MK. *Pediatric Cardiology for Practitioners.* Chicago: Year Book Medical, 1984. *A general textbook which displays the physiology of different congenital defects, their clinical presentation and management in outline form.*

Rudolph AM. *Congenital Diseases of the Heart.* Chicago: Year Book Medical, 1974. *An older textbook with a classic section on the circulation of the fetus and newborn.*

5 Myocardial Ischemia and Infarction

Udho Thadani

Objectives

After completing this chapter, you should be able to

Define the terms *myocardial ischemia* and *infarction*

State the factors that determine myocardial oxygen demand

State the factors that determine coronary blood flow

Understand the mechanisms and causes of myocardial ischemia

Understand the pathophysiologic differences between stable angina pectoris and acute ischemic syndromes (unstable angina and myocardial infarction)

State the consequences of ischemia

Understand the clinical manifestation of various forms of ischemic syndromes

Understand the rationale of treatment in different ischemic syndromes

---

The term "myocardial ischemia" implies deprivation of oxygen to the myocardium accompanied by inadequate removal of metabolites secondary to decreased perfusion. Ischemia may be reversible or irreversible with different functional, pathologic, and clinical consequences. In this chapter, factors that determine normal coronary blood flow and myocardial oxygen supply are described and the alterations in coronary blood flow or myocardial oxygen demand in different clinical ischemic syndromes are discussed.

Normal Physiology

The heart is an aerobic organ and can develop only a small oxygen debt without undergoing irreversible damage. Under physiologic conditions, myocardial oxygen supply equals myocardial oxygen consumption (Fig. 5-1). In a steady state, determination of the heart's oxygen consumption provides an accurate measure of its metabolism. Factors determining myocardial oxygen consumption are (1) the tension time index (the area under the left ventricular pressure curve), tension being directly related to the radius and the intraventricular pressure and inversely related to ventricular wall thickness; (2) contractile state of the myo-

cardium (contractility); and (3) heart rate. Acceleration of heart rate increases the frequency of tension development per unit time and also augments myocardial contractility. Oxygen supply is determined by the coronary blood flow.

The heart is supplied by the left and right coronary arteries, which course across the epicardial surface of the heart and then give rise to arteries which turn at right angles and penetrate the myocardium and branch into smaller arteries and finally to arterioles and capillaries. Myocardial blood flow is determined by the driving pressure and resistance offered to flow at the level of arterioles and precapillary sphincters (Fig. 5-2).

Resistance in the vessels is variable due to the compressive effect of the contractile myocardium and it is also influenced by neural, metabolic, myogenic, and humoral factors. In the normal heart, there are over 2000 capillaries per cubic millimeter of which only between 60–80% are usually open. When myocardial oxygen tension falls, more capillaries are recruited. This capillary recruitment is very important in meeting the increased myocardial oxygen requirement. Effective driving or perfusion pressure is the pressure gradient between the aorta and the intramyocardial capillaries. During systole, coronary ostia are partly occluded by the open aortic valve leaflets. However, during diastole when the aortic valve is closed, aortic diastolic

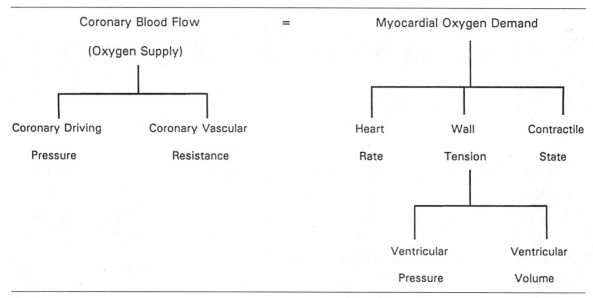

Fig. 5-1. Determinants of myocardial oxygen demand and coronary blood flow. Under normal circumstances, coronary blood flow matches myocardial oxygen demand. For autoregulation of coronary blood flow, downward or upward adjustment of coronary vascular resistance plays the dominant role at wide ranges of coronary driving pressure in normal subjects.

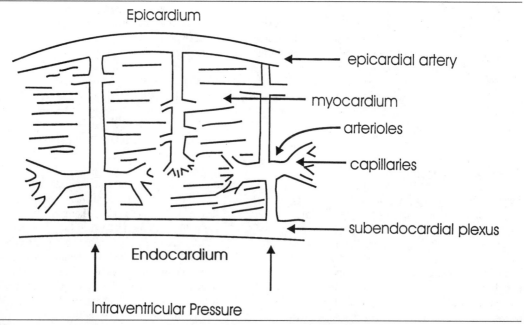

Fig. 5-2. Coronary artery and its branches. Metabolic, neurogenic, myogenic, and hormonal factors regulate the caliber of the resistance vessels and hence regulate coronary blood flow.

pressure is transmitted directly to the coronary ostia. The intramyocardial portions of the branches of the coronary arteries supplying the left ventricle are compressed during systole in the contracting thick left ventricle and coronary blood flow, therefore, occurs primarily during diastole. In the right coronary artery, which supplies both the right and left ventricle, flow occurs both in systole and diastole, since right ventricular pressure is lower than aortic pressure in both systole and diastole. Intramyocardial pressure is higher in the subendocardial region compared to the subepicardial region, but diastolic flow is preferentially shunted to the subendocardial region because of reduced coronary resistance in this region secondary to the relative ischemia during systole.

Accordingly, overall flow to the subendocardial region equals or is greater than subepicardial flow when coronary perfusion pressure is normal. If coronary perfusion pressure is reduced, as occurs with hypotension or with partial obstruction of epicardial coronary arteries by atheroma, blood can be shunted away from subendocardial regions. Therefore, subendocardial regions are more vulnerable to diminished flow than are subepicardial regions.

Normal coronary blood flow is 60–90 ml/minute per 100 g of myocardium, but can decrease by 50% when metabolic requirements decrease as during total-body hypothermia or cardiac arrest and can increase four- to fivefold during exercise.

Even under basal conditions, myocardial oxygen extraction is near maximum as indicated by very low coronary sinus oxygen saturation. Therefore, the increase in myocardial oxygen supply is achieved primarily by an increase in coronary blood flow. The myocardium communicates its oxygen requirements to the coronary arteries by the rate of production of adenosine which in turn produces vasodilation and hence an increase in coronary blood flow. Other proposed mechanisms of coronary dilation are prostaglandins and other vasoactive compounds such as potassium and lactate.

Coronary collateral vessels (connections between coronary arteries) are abundant in the canine heart but are highly variable in human hearts. Under physiologic conditions, they are of little consequence but play an important role when coronary blood flow is compromised by obstruction of a major vessel.

Mechanisms of Myocardial Ischemia

Myocardial ischemia is a state of myocardial oxygen deprivation accompanied by inadequate removal of metabolites secondary to decreased perfusion. Myocardial ischemia results when myocardial oxygen demand outstrips supply. This is brought about either by a reduction or cessation of coronary blood flow or by an increase in oxygen demand during stress that cannot be met by an increase in coronary blood flow (Fig. 5-3).

The cross-sectional area of a coronary artery may be reduced by 70–80% without inducing ischemia at rest. With this degree of narrowing in the proximal position of a coronary artery, ischemia can often be induced by any stimulus (e.g., exercise, atrial pacing, or psychologic stress) that increases myocardial oxygen demand.

Myocardial ischemia is most commonly caused by organic narrowing or obstruction of coronary arteries, but it may result from coronary artery spasm or from increased oxygen demand in the presence of normal coronary arteries, as in aortic stenosis and subaortic muscular stenosis.

Atherosclerosis

Atherosclerosis is by far the most common pathologic process for organic narrowing of the coronary arteries. Atherosclerotic plaques typically develop in the proximal segments of coronary arteries. However, in some patients there is diffuse involvement of coronary arteries with atherosclerosis. Coronary narrowing increases resistance to blood flow. The resistance increases by a power of 4 as the radius decreases. When the lumen diameter decreases to 50% or lower (cross-sectional area narrowing of 75% or more), manifestations of myocardial ischemia invariably occur during stresslike exercise and with higher grades of stenosis myocardial ischemia may also occur during rest. The severity and extent of ischemia varies with the number of vessels involved in the atherosclerotic process, the severity of the lesions, the length of the stenosis, and the amount of myocardium supplied by the vessel distal to the stenosis.

Nonatherosclerotic Coronary Artery Disease

Coronary arteries may be narrowed due to inflammatory and autoimmune processes. The vessels involved are usually small branches of coronary arteries, in contrast to the larger epicardial coronary arteries affected by atherosclerosis. Small-vessel coronary disease occurs in polyartertis nodosa, systemic lupus erythematosus, rheumatoid arthritis, scleroderma, and diabetes; it may be an important cause of myocardial ischemia in this group of patients.

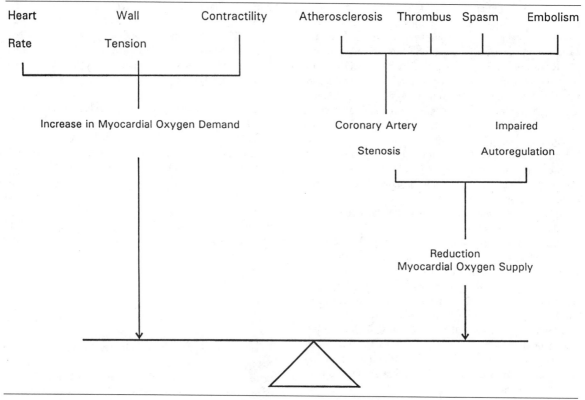

Fig. 5-3. Mechanisms of myocardial ischemia. Myocardial ischemia may become manifest when there is an increase in myocardial oxygen demand in relation to myocardial oxygen supply or when there is a primary reduction in coronary blood flow without a change in myocardial oxygen demand.

Coronary Thrombosis and Platelet Aggregation

Partial occlusion of a coronary artery due to platelet deposition is an important cause of prolonged myocardial ischemia (unstable angina) and thrombotic occlusion of an atherosclerotic vessel is found in as many as 80–90% of cases at the time of an acute myocardial infarction. What initiates the thrombotic process remains speculative. Both coronary spasm and platelet aggregation have been implicated. Fissuring, rupture, or ulceration of an atheromatous plaque is invariably present at the site of platelet deposition or thrombotic occlusion. Exposure of subendothelial tissue is a potent stimulus for platelet aggregation. This increased platelet aggregation is the most likely factor initiating the thrombotic process in a diseased coronary artery,

leading to myocardial infarction. The extent of myocardial injury from sudden disruption of coronary blood flow is determined by the presence or absence of collateral circulation in the ischemic area, the site of occlusion, and the status of the remaining coronary arteries. In the absence of collateral blood flow, ischemic myocardium invariably becomes necrotic, but the severity and extent of necrosis varies with the site of occlusion and the size and number of vessels involved.

Coronary Artery Spasm

Spasm of a normal or previously diseased coronary artery is an important cause of myocardial ischemia. The exact mechanism which triggers coronary artery spasm remains speculative. Coronary artery spasm and platelet aggregation may be interrelated. Platelet aggregation releases thromboxane A$_2$, which is a potent vasoconstrictor and which may be a mechanism of spasm, especially in coronary arteries with obstructive organic narrowing because platelets often adhere to these lesions and under appropriate stimuli might release thromboxane A$_2$. There may be a local coronary supersensitivity to vasoconstrictive stimuli in some patients. The end result of coronary arterial spasm is a profound reduction in myocardial blood flow with resultant ischemia. Although coronary artery spasm is not a common cause of prolonged myocardial ischemia, it may lead to irreversible myocardial damage (myocardial infarction) and serious, often fatal, arrhythmias, even in the absence of myocardial infarction.

Coronary Embolism

This is a rare cause of a sudden reduction in coronary blood flow but can produce severe myocardial ischemia and even myocardial necrosis. The source of emboli is usually thrombi in the left atrium or left ventricle. Atrial fibrillation, valvular heart disease, cardiomyopathy, and endocarditis predisposes to coronary embolism.

Diminished Coronary Flow Reserve

Coronary flow reserve is the ratio of maximum coronary flow to resting flow. It represents the maximum increase in oxygen that can be mustered in response to stress. Myocardial ischemia may occur due to an abnormally high resistance at the level of small coronary arteries or arterioles with a reduction in maximum coronary vascular flow reserve. This leads to the impairment of an increase in coronary blood flow during stress as seen in some patients with severe hypertension. This mechanism is also operative in patients with syndrome X (normal coronary arteries and exercise-induced chest pain and myocardial ischemia).

Increased Myocardial Oxygen Demand

The important determinants of myocardial oxygen demand are heart rate, contractile state of the ventricle, and the tension time index. In the presence of moderate to severe organic narrowing of coronary arteries, any stimulus that increases myocardial oxygen demand may induce myocardial ischemia.

The stress may be exercise, which increases heart rate, myocardial contractility and tension time index or anxiety, which augments heart rate and blood pressure. Anemia,

thyrotoxicosis, and infection also increase myocardial oxygen demand and may induce myocardial ischemia in a patient who has obstructive narrowing of one or more coronary arteries. However, these conditions rarely precipitate myocardial ischemia in the presence of normal coronary arteries. Increased myocardial oxygen demand in the presence of normal coronary arteries is rarely a cause of myocardial ischemia but it can lead to ischemia in patients with severe aortic stenosis and in those with subaortic muscular stenosis. In these two conditions, myocardial oxygen demand is greatly augmented due to a thickened, hypertrophied ventricle and due to a marked elevation of intraventricular pressure.

Functional Consequences of Ischemia

Contractile Dysfunction

Contractile dysfunction is one of the earliest consequences of myocardial ischemia (Fig. 5-4). Contractile force and myocardial segment shortening are reduced within 6–10 seconds after abrupt coronary occlusion in animal experiments. Two explanations for such abrupt changes in contractility are (1) reduced high-energy phosphate supplies and (2) rapidly developing cellular acidosis. Both consequences of ischemia result in alterations in membrane ion flux and myofibrilar Ca^{++} binding. Abnormalities of excitation-contraction coupling and contractile dysfunction result. Acute coronary artery occlusion leads to paradoxical motion in the central ischemic zone and reduced contractility in the adjacent area. There is increased contractility of the uninvolved normal myocardium through the Frank-Starling mechanism. Patients with obstructed but not occluded coronary arteries usually do not show impaired myocardial function at rest, but the increase in myocardial oxygen demand during stress often precipitates myocardial dysfunction. Regional areas of impaired myocardial contractility, whether sustained or transient, may depress overall left ventricular function, producing reductions of left ventricular systolic function (cardiac output, stroke volume, ejection fraction, and stroke work). Myocardial ischemia also impairs diastolic relaxation, leading to increased resistance to ventricular filling. Through its direct effect on contractility, ischemia causes incomplete ventricular emptying and elevation of left ventricular end-diastolic pressure, which may lead to left ventricular failure. Cardiogenic shock may ensue when myocardial damage is extensive (>40%).

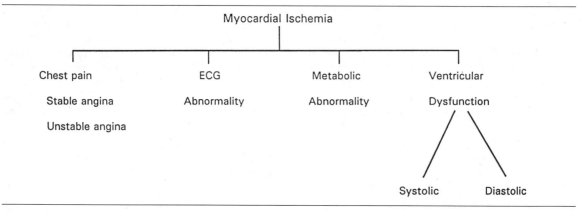

Fig. 5-4. Consequences of myocardial ischemia. Depending upon the severity and duration of ischemia, one may observe metabolic or electrocardiographic or ventricular functional abnormalities and/or the patient may experience chest pain.

Electrolyte and Electrophysiologic Changes

Another early consequence of myocardial ischemia is a net loss of total cellular K^+ due to an increased rate of efflux from the cell. The cause of increased K^+ efflux is unknown. K^+ loss occurs concurrently with the onset of anaerobic glycolysis and contractile failure. Maintenance of electrolyte gradients across cell membrane is energy dependent, and K^+ loss may be the result of decreased high-energy phosphates. Microelectrode studies during ischemia show T-Q depression (resulting from a reduced K^+ gradient) and ST segment elevation. These changes summate to produce ST segment elevation on surface electrocardiograms within 15–30 seconds after the onset of ischemia. In general, ST segment elevation is a reasonable index of the extent of myocardial ischemia. However, changes in temperature, drugs, and pericardial injury also influence ST segments.

Myocardial Infarction

When myocardial ischemia is transient, biochemical and physiologic changes are often reversible, and near complete function recovery occurs. However, during prolonged ischemia, irreversible myocardial damage or myocardial infarction occurs. Location and extent of the infarction depend on a number of factors: (1) location and severity of coronary arterial narrowing, (2) the extent of collateral circulation to the ischemic area, (3) the size of the vascular bed perfused by the narrowed vessel, and (4) the oxygen needs of the jeopardized myocardium.

If the myocardial damage is irreversible, the affected region appears pale, bluish, and slightly swollen; 18–36 hours later the myocardium appears tan or reddish purple. These changes persist for 48 hours, when the infarct turns gray. By 8–10 days following infarction, the infarcted muscle is removed by mononuclear cells. Over the next 2 or 3 months, the infarcted area is converted to a shrunken, thin scar, which whitens and firms with time. The endocardium below the infarct becomes thickened and opaque. In man, myocardial infarction may occur after occlusion of one or more arteries. However, it may be due to coronary arterial spasm without occlusive coronary artery disease. If the coronary artery becomes completely occluded and there is poor collateral blood flow to the ischemic area, the infarct is often transmural (whole thickness of myocardium). Occlusion of the left anterior descending coronary artery results in involvement of the areas supplied by this artery (septum, apical area, and anterior wall). Occlusion of the left circumflex artery may lead to infarction of the lateral and inferoposterior wall of the left ventricle. Occlusion of the right coronary artery results in infarction of the inferoposterior wall of the left ventricle, the inferior portions of the septum, and the posteromedial papillary muscle. Nontransmural myocardial infarction often occurs in the presence of severely narrowed coronary arteries which are not completely occluded. Myocardial infarction usually involves the left ventricle, but right ventricular infarction occurs in some 20% of cases of inferior myocardial infarction.

Myocardial infarction may be complicated by myocardial rupture. If this rupture involves the free wall, it may lead to hemopericardium and immediate death from cardiac tamponade. Rupture of the infarcted septum may lead to a communication between the two ventricles (ventricular septal defect). Rupture of the papillary muscle may lead to severe mitral regurgitation and acute pulmonary edema. Many patients die suddenly due to ventricular arrhythmias following an acute myocardial infarction. Of those who survive the first few hours and are hospitalized, 10–25% die due to various complications (pump failure, arrhythmias, cardiac rupture, mitral regurgitation, or ventricular septal defect).

Pericarditis is a frequent complication of myocardial infarction but is usually transient and is secondary to the involvement of the epicardial layer of the myocardium. A late complication of myocardial infarction is left ventricular aneurysm, which develops in 12–15% of patients who survive. The aneurysm predisposes to clot formation, with resultant increased risk of systemic embolization.

Clinical Manifestations of Myocardial Ischemia and Infarction

Depending upon the severity, duration, and extent of ischemic periods, there may be reversible or irreversible myocardial damage with resultant clinical consequences (see Fig. 5-4).

The clinical manifestations of transient reversible ischemia are (a) stable angina pectoris, (b) unstable angina pectoris, (c) variant angina, (d) mixed angina, and (e) silent myocardial ischemia. The pathophysiology is somewhat different for each syndrome.

Stable Angina Pectoris

The term "stable angina pectoris" is used to describe ischemic myocardial pain which is usually substernal in location and may radiate to neck or left arm and sometimes to the back. The pain is usually precipitated by activity or emotional upset and is relieved after discontinuation of activity or ingestion of a sublingual nitroglycerin. By definition, "stable" implies that the frequency of angina episodes has been unchanged for at least a period of 2–3 months.

The underlying cause of stable angina is usually severe

atherosclerotic coronary artery disease. Because of coronary artery narrowing, coronary blood flow is restricted and cannot increase in proportion to increase in myocardial oxygen demand. In a majority of patients, angina can be reproduced by exercise at identical workloads and rate pressure product. As the severity of disease worsens, effort tolerance decreases progressively and it may be difficult to avoid precipitation of angina even with minimal effort like brushing the teeth, toweling, etc. Thus, the major pathogenetic factor for stable angina is an increase in myocardial oxygen demand in the presence of relatively fixed coronary blood supply. In addition, there is an impairment of release of endothelial-derived relaxation factor (NO) and stimuli which normally produce vasodilation produce vasoconstriction. Thus, further narrowing of a stenotic site during exercise may reduce coronary blood flow.

The mechanism by which anginal pain is produced is not known but may be related to stretching of the ischemic myocardium or to stimulation of the nerve endings due to accumulation of metabolites. During an episode of angina pectoris, there is usually ECG evidence of subendocardial ischemia manifested by ST segment depression. When the territory of ischemia is large, one may observe changes in systolic and diastolic function which can be assessed by an echocardiogram or a nuclear ventriculogram. Depending upon the extent of ischemia, global ventricular function (ejection fraction) may or may not decrease but regional function often shows some abnormality.

Some patients with classical exertional angina do not have underlying coronary artery disease. In these patients, there may be impairment in maximum coronary flow reserve due to an abnormally high tone in the arterioles or precapillary sphincters. Some of these patients may have small vessel disease which cannot be visualized by conventional angiography. In a minority of patients with stable angina, a superimposed coronary artery spasm may compromise flow.

Some patients with severe aortic regurgitation and normal coronary arteries may experience angina. This can be explained on the basis of raised left ventricular end-diastolic pressure and lowered aortic diastolic pressure, which reduces coronary flow in diastole.

Unstable Angina Pectoris

The term "unstable angina" has been used to describe four different entities: (1) progressive or crescendo angina in a patient with a previous history of stable angina; (2) angina of recent onset precipitated by minimal exertion; (3) angina at rest during which pain lasts more than 15 minutes; this form has also been called pre-infarction angina or intermediate coronary syndrome; and (4) angina occurring within 4 weeks of acute myocardial infarction.

In some patients with unstable angina, especially in those with progressive or recent onset angina, increase in myocardial oxygen demand via increase in heart rate, blood pressure, or myocardial contractility may precipitate ischemic episodes. However, a primary reduction in myocardial oxygen supply due to a reduction in coronary flow plays a more important role in the majority of patients, especially in those with rest angina. The reduction in coronary blood flow is brought about by platelet aggregation or thrombus formation and alterations in coronary vasomotor tone at the site of plaque fissuring (complicated atherosclerotic plaque). The waxing and waning nature of the partial platelet occlusion, or thrombus formation, accounts for variable prognosis in this group of patients. Antiplatelet agent (aspirin) and heparin both reduce mortality and incidence of myocardial infarction in unstable angina. Thrombolytic treatment, however, is not indicated and is no more effective than treatment with heparin and aspirin.

Variant Angina Pectoris

This syndrome was first described by Prinzmetal and is also referred to as vasospastic angina or Prinzmetal angina. The syndrome is usually characterized by pain at rest with associated ST elevation due to transmural ischemia but at times only ST segment depression occurs. The pain typically occurs at night and may wake the patient from sleep. Pain may last several minutes. In some patients, pain may be brought on by exertion, but in many patients exercise performance may be normal.

Painful episodes may recur for several weeks and months and then may disappear spontaneously. In 85% of patients, there is evidence of underlying atherosclerosis while the remainder may have normal-looking coronary arteries.

This syndrome is produced by focal spasm of an epicardial coronary artery or arteries. The mechanism which triggers spasm still remains speculative. Local hypersensitivity of a segment of a coronary artery to various stimuli in a nonspecific nature could be responsible for spasm. It is rare for these patients to have a myocardial infarction, although occasional cases have been reported.

Mixed Angina Pectoris

Some patients with angina pectoris do not fit into any of the above categories. They may have classical exertional angina but at times also experience resting chest pain or

the exercise tolerance may vary on the same day or on different days. These variations in angina threshold may be due to coronary artery spasm, intermittent platelet aggregation, or thrombosis at the atherosclerotic plaque site.

Silent Myocardial Ischemia

This term implies electrocardiographic ST segment depression or elevation during ambulatory monitoring in the absence of symptoms. Some patients with silent ischemia never experience chest pain but more often patients who have angina also experience episodes of silent ischemia. The term has been further extended to include a fall in ejection fraction or abnormal thallium myocardial uptake during exercise in asymptomatic patients.

Why patients with silent ischemia do not experience pain remains speculative. It has been explained on the basis of elevated pain threshold in comparison to patients who experience symptoms during myocardial ischemia. The role of high endorphin levels to explain silent ischemia remains controversial at the present time. Another postulation is that the extent of territory involved in silent ischemia is smaller than in the painful ischemia.

Acute Myocardial Infarction (Irreversible Myocardial Ischemia)

An abrupt cessation of coronary blood flow due to coronary artery thrombosis is the usual cause of acute myocardial infarction. The occluded artery is almost always narrowed by a pre-existing atherosclerotic lesion.

Plaque fissuring in an area with subcritical narrowing (< 50% diameter narrowing) is probably the initial factor which leads to formation of a thrombus due to an adhesion of platelets, liberation of vasoactive substances, and an increase in coronary vasomotor tone. However, spontaneous reperfusion occurs in 20–40% of patients and may occasionally cause reperfusion necrosis and arrhythmias. Arrhythmias are common and may be due to reentry, secondary to slow conduction in the area of the infarction, increased automaticity, or late triggered activity (see Chap. 1 for discussion of these mechanisms).

Myocardial infarction is usually accompanied by chest pain and characteristic electrocardiographic changes (Fig. 5-5). Some patients (15–20%) may experience myocardial infarction without pain — silent myocardial infarction.

Infarct expansion, rupture of the myocardium, and aneurysm formation are all complications of a transmural infarction and are not seen in patients with subendocardial or nontransmural infarction. Left ventricular aneurysm

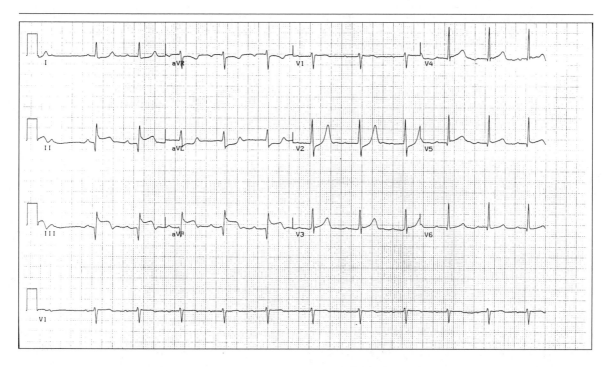

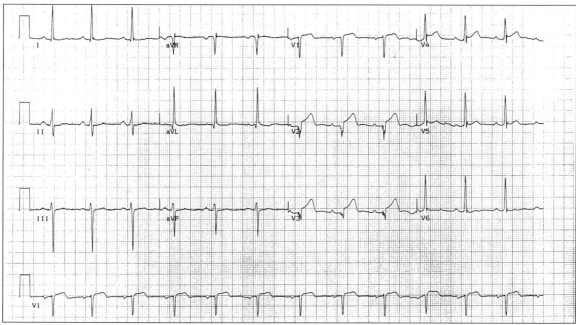

Fig. 5-5. Top: Acute inferior myocardial infarction. The electrocardiogram shows ST elevation (acute injury pattern) in limb leads II, III, and aVF with reciprocal changes in leads I and aVL. Bottom: Acute anterior myocardial infarction. The electrocardiogram shows ST elevation in leads V_1–V_3 (acute anteroseptal injury pattern) associated with ST–T changes in leads V_1–V_6 and leads I and aVL.

often develops at the apex or lateral wall and some 50% of these are complicated by intramural thrombus — which may predispose the patient to systemic embolization. Patients with aneurysms are more prone to ventricular arrhythmias. Remodeling after a myocardial infarction produces ventricular dilation and eventual ventricular failure, especially in patients with large infarcts.

Sudden Cardiac Death

Sudden death is a very common presentation of ischemic heart disease. Ventricular fibrillation is the most common cause of death within 1 hour of an acute myocardial infarction. Patients resuscitated from sudden death and myocardial infarction are also at a risk of sudden death in subsequent years.

Earlier studies suggested that coronary thrombosis accounted for only a minority of patients with sudden death. Recent careful pathologic studies have, however, shown that intraluminal thrombi occur in 74% of patients in whom sudden cardiac ischemic death occurred compared with none of those dying suddenly from other causes. Platelet aggregates have been found in small intramyocardial vessels in about 30% of the patients. Platelet aggregates are often confined to the segment of the myocardium downstream to a major epicardial coronary artery containing an atherosclerotic plaque which has undergone fissuring and on which thrombus has developed. Thus platelet aggregation in the myocardium probably represents an embolic phenomenon. The association of myocardial necrosis with such emboli could precipitate ventricular fibrillation and sudden death.

In hospital survivors of sudden death associated with myocardial infarction, the pathogenesis of ventricular fibrillation is different. In this group of patients, there is usually a preceding episode of ventricular tachycardia which degenerates into ventricular fibrillation. Arrhythmias in this group of patients probably occur by reentrant excitation of relatively discrete circuits that form during the healing of acute infarction.

Clinical Examples

1. A 50-year-old man came to the hospital with severe chest pain of 4 hours duration. On examination, he was in sinus rhythm with a heart rate of 120 beats/minute and blood pressure of 70/50 mm Hg. He was mentally confused and acutely dyspneic.

An electrocardiogram showed evidence of a recent anterior myocardial infarction (ST segment elevation in anterior chest leads V_1–V_6). Chest x-ray showed gross pulmonary edema. He was given intravenous furosemide (diuretic) and tissue plasminogen activator (thrombolytic agent). However, he remained hypotensive. He was taken to the catheterization laboratory. The left main coronary artery was found to be completely occluded and was opened by balloon angioplasty. This resulted in marked improvement in blood pressure and breathlessness.

Discussion.   This patient's chest pain was secondary to severe myocardial ischemia. (The mechanism by which pain occurs during myocardial ischemia is poorly understood.) His mental confusion and severe hypotension indicate very poor ventricular function secondary to extensive myocardial damage. His dyspnea was due to marked elevation of left ventricular end-diastolic pressure owing to a failing left ventricle. Radiologic evidence of pulmonary edema supports this hypothesis. Intravenous furosemide was given to induce diuresis and tissue plasminogen activator (tPA) to dissolve the coronary occlusion which is invariably responsible for acute infarction. In some 20–30% of patients, tPA fails to recanalize the occlusion as in this patient and opening of the artery with a balloon catheter may be life-saving.

2. A 64-year-old patient reported having recurrent episodes of chest pain during exertion for the past 3 years. Physical examination did not reveal any abnormality. A resting electrocardiogram was normal. During exercise, the patient complained of breathlessness and developed ST segment depression in the anterior chest leads. His heart rate increased from 50 to 120 beats/per minute and blood pressure increased from 110/80 to 170/90 mm Hg. Electrocardiograms returned to normal within 5 minutes of stopping exercise. Patient was treated with long-acting nitrates (veno and arterial dilator) and atenolol (beta blocker), with marked improvement in symptoms.

Discussion.   Myocardial ischemia was precipitated during exercise, which increases myocardial oxygen demand due to increases in heart rate, systolic blood pressure, and myocardial contractility. Breathlessness was due to a transient increase in left ventricular end-diastolic pressure secondary to myocardial ischemia. Electrocardiographic ST depression represents subendocardial ischemia. With the cessation of exercise, myocardial oxygen demand decreased and manifestations of myocardial ischemia (ST changes, chest pain, breathlessness) subsided. Drugs which reduce myocardial oxygen demand (nitrates which reduce venous return, beta blockers which reduce heart rate and contractility, or calcium channel blockers which reduce afterload and dilate coronary arteries) are often effective. Patients who do not adequately respond to medication often improve with revascularization procedures which increase blood flow to ischemic areas.

Bibliography

Braunwald E (ed). *Heart Disease.* Philadelphia: Saunders, 1992. *A comprehensive textbook of cardiology with five chapters on ischemic heart disease.*

Davies MJ and Thomas AC. Plaque fissuring — the cause of acute myocardial infarction, sudden ischemic death, and crescendo angina. *Br Heart J* 53:363–368, 1985. *An original description of pathophysiology of acute ischemic syndromes.*

Fuster V and Chesebro JH. Mechanisms of unstable angina. *N Eng J Med* 315:1023–1026, 1986. *An excellent review of the subject.*

Thadani U. Pathophysiology of myocardial ischemia: Major clinical syndromes. In Abrams J, Pepine CJ, and Thadani U (eds). *Medical Therapy of Ischemic Heart Disease.* Boston: Little, Brown, 1992. *A good review, easy to read and extensively referenced.*

Angina pectoris in Cardiology Clinics 9:1–189, 1991. *A multiauthor volume devoted to pathophysiology and treatment of stable and unstable angina.*

6 Cardiomyopathies

Chittur A. Sivaram

Objectives

After completing this chapter, you should be able to

Understand the classification of cardiomyopathy

Understand the morphological description of the subtypes of cardiomyopathy

Describe the pathophysiological mechanisms involved in the symptomatology of cardiomyopathy

Understand the differences in the manifestation of the subtypes of cardiomyopathy

Describe the principles of treatment of cardiomyopathy

The term "cardiomyopathies" applies to diseases of the cardiac muscle excluding myocardial disorders secondary to ischemic, hypertensive, congenital, or valvular heart disease. A commonly used scheme of classification divides cardiomyopathy into primary (i.e., cause unknown) and secondary (i.e., associated with a known cause or systemic disease, e.g., alcoholism, pregnancy, amyloidosis, sarcoidosis, etc.).

Classification of Primary Myocardial Diseases

Based on anatomic and pathophysiological considerations, cardiomyopathies can be of three types; dilated, hypertrophic, and restrictive (Table 6-1; Fig. 6-1).

Dilated Cardiomyopathy

Dilated cardiomyopathy was previously known as congestive cardiomyopathy. The characteristic feature is dilatation of the ventricles (left more than right) owing to ventricular systolic dysfunction (Fig. 6-2). The ventricular end-diastolic volumes and diastolic pressures are invariably elevated, giving rise to varying degrees of pulmonary and systemic vascular congestion. Often the involvement is equally severe on both right and left ventricles, causing biventricular

failure. The weight of the heart is increased at autopsy. Patches of subendocardial fibrosis are seen in the ventricles even in the presence of normal epicardial coronary arteries. Overall the prognosis of patients with dilated cardiomyopathy is poor, with 5-year mortality ranging from 40 to 80%. Spontaneous improvement occurs in a small proportion of patients with dilated cardiomyopathy. Dilated cardiomyopathy has been found in association with alcoholism, pregnancy, and familial clustering (Table 6-2).

An association between viral myocarditis and dilated cardiomyopathy has been known for many years. It is proposed that some patients with viral myocarditis proceed to develop biventricular dilatation resulting from chronic myocardial damage due to immunological injury. However, no viral isolates have been recovered from the myocardium.

Clinical Presentation

The most common symptoms of dilated cardiomyopathy are symptoms of congestive heart failure such as dyspnea on exertion, orthopnea, paroxysmal nocturnal dyspnea, and edema. Patients occasionally present with arrhythmias, particularly malignant ventricular tachycardia leading to syncope. Atrial fibrillation is common in patients with advanced dilated cardiomyopathy. Ventricular thrombi lead to embolic phenomena as the presenting symptom in some patients. Chest pain occurs occasionally in dilated cardiomyopathy despite normal epicardial coronary arteries.

Table 6-1. Features of Primary Cardiomyopathies

Feature	Dilated Cardiomyopathy	Hypertrophic Cardiomyopathy	Restrictive Cardiomyopathy
LV size	dilated	normal or small	normal
Systolic function	decreased	supernormal	normal
LV hypertrophy	absent	present	absent
Diastolic dysfunction	absent	present	present
LV outflow obstruction	absent	present	absent

Physical Examination

The pulse volume is decreased due to low stroke volume. Peripheral cyanosis and cold clammy extremities may be present. The venous pressure is frequently elevated owing to right-sided heart failure. The apical impulse is displaced laterally and may be diffuse. A right ventricular heave may be palpable. The intensity of first sound is decreased and P2 may be accentuated. Third and fourth sound gallops may be present. Murmurs of mitral and tricuspid regurgitation may be also present secondary to ventricular and annulus dilatation. In patients with advanced heart failure, secondary to dilated cardiomyopathy hepatomegaly, ascites, bibasilar crackles, marked peripheral and sacral edema are present.

Investigations

Abnormalities in the electrocardiogram are frequent and include atrial enlargement, atrial fibrillation, varying de-grees of ventricular ectopy, bundle branch block, and ventricular hypertrophy. Chest x-ray reveals enlargement of the cardiac silhouette, evidence for left-sided failure with upper lobe venous prominence and pleural effusions.

Echocardiogram can confirm the enlargement of the ventricular chambers and the diffusely abnormal wall mo-

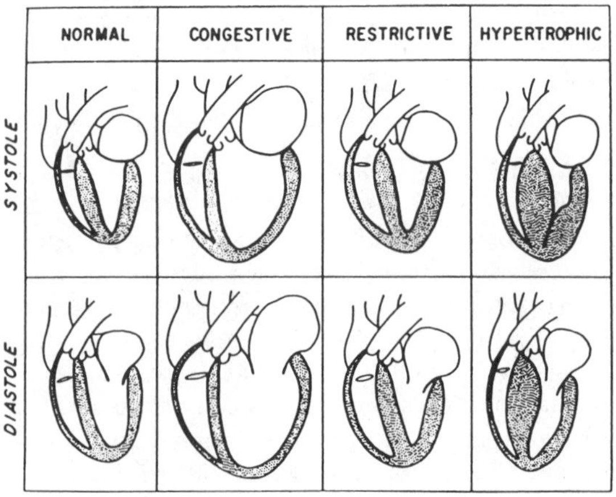

Fig. 6-2. Gross postmortem heart of a patient with dilated cardiomyopathy. The ventricles are dilated without proportional increase in wall thickness. (Reprinted with permission from: Fang KS, Dec W, and Lilly LS. The Cardiomyopathies. In Lilly LS (ed). *Pathophysiology of Heart Disease.* Philadelphia: Lea & Febiger, 1993, p. 169.)

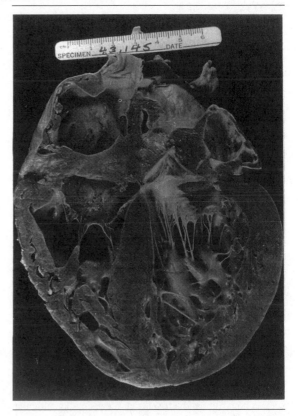

Fig. 6-1. Diagram of the 50° left anterior oblique view of the heart in the different types of cardiomyopathy at end-systole and end-diastole. (Reprinted with permission from: *American Journal Cardiology:* Vol. 46; 1980, p. 1232.)

Table 6-2. Some Examples of Dilated Cardiomyopathy

IDIOPATHIC

INFLAMMATORY

Infectious (especially viral)
Noninfectious
    Connective tissue diseases
    Peripartum cardiomyopathy
    Sarcoidosis

TOXIC

Chronic alcohol ingestion
Chemotherapeutic agents (e.g., adriamycin)

METABOLIC

Hypothyroidism
Chronic hypocalcemia or hypophosphatemia

NEUROMUSCULAR

Muscular or myotonic dystrophy

Reprinted with permission from: Fang KS, Dec W, and Lilly LS. The Cardiomyopathies. In Lilly LS (ed). *Pathophysiology of Heart Disease*. Philadelphia: Lea & Febiger, 1993, p. 169.

tion. The presence of diffuse biventricular wall motion abnormalities is helpful in the differentiation of dilated cardiomyopathy from advanced ischemic heart disease where regional rather than global wall motion abnormalities are typically found.

Radionuclear ventriculogram shows findings that are very similar to those found on echocardiogram but estimation of LV ejection fraction is more accurate with the radionuclide technique. It is advisable that the same noninvasive test (echocardiography or nuclear ventriculography) be used serially to follow ventricular function.

Cardiac catheterization may be required in patients with dilated cardiomyopathy over the age of 40 years in order to rule out ischemic heart disease as the underlying cause. Since coronary bypass grafting prolongs survival in patients with three-vessel coronary disease and modest depression of ventricular function (ejection fraction around 35%), the exclusion of coronary disease is important. During cardiac catheterization, the ventricular end-diastolic pressures, ejection fraction, pulmonary artery pressures, and pulmonary vascular resistance can be determined. Myocardial biopsy is sometimes required if inflammatory myocarditis is considered in the differential diagnosis.

Special Types of Dilated Cardiomyopathy

Alcoholic Cardiomyopathy. Chronic heavy alcohol use can lead to biventricular dilatation and systolic dysfunction. Patients with this entity have a history of heavy alcohol use for many years. In some patients with a history of heavy alcohol use, asymptomatic ventricular dilatation might be present. Periods of atrial fibrillation may punctuate the preclinical stages of the cardiomyopathic process. These patients have a reasonable chance of recovery of ventricular function if they stop alcohol abuse. In addition to the direct toxic effects of alcohol on the myocardium, the myocardial dysfunction may also be precipitated by thiamine deficiency which occurs in some alcoholics. Classically heart failure due to alcoholic cardiomyopathy is a low output state with high peripheral vascular resistance, whereas thiamine deficiency produces a state of elevated cardiac output and decreased peripheral vascular resistance (wet Beriberi).

Peripartum Cardiomyopathy. Peripartum cardiomyopathy may occur in the late stages of pregnancy or following delivery. A clear cause-and-effect relationship between heart failure and pregnancy exists in this condition but the pathogenesis is unknown. The typical patient at risk for developing peripartum cardiomyopathy is of lower socioeconomic status, multiparous state, and age over 40. A history of hypertension is frequently present. In some patients with peripartum cardiomyopathy, recovery of ventricular function occurs within the first 6 months following delivery. Ventricular dysfunction present more than 6 months after delivery is likely to progress. Subsequent pregnancies are contraindicated for women who have had peripartum cardiomyopathy.

Treatment

The treatment of dilated cardiomyopathy follows the standard lines of treatment for congestive heart failure and includes restriction of activity, salt restriction, diuretics, afterload reducing agents, digitalis, and occasionally long-term anticoagulation. Diuretics decrease the high left ventricular filling pressures and decrease the symptoms of dyspnea. Afterload reducing agents improve cardiac output and ameliorate symptoms such as fatigue and dyspnea. Long-term therapy with afterload-reducing agents such as ACE inhibitors and hydralazine-isosorbide combination have been shown to improve survival in patients with heart failure. Markers for poor prognosis in dilated cardiomyopathy include severe symptomatic status, severe depression of ejection fraction, presence of left ventricular conduction delay on electrocardiogram, complex ventricular ectopy, and marked activation of the neuroendocrine system with elevation of plasma catecholamine and vasopressin levels. Causes of death in dilated cardiomyopathy include ventricular arrhythmias, heart failure, and thromboembolism.

Hypertrophic Cardiomyopathy

Hypertrophic cardiomyopathy is characterized by left ventricular hypertrophy (Fig. 6-3) in the absence of an appropriate stimulus such as aortic stenosis or systemic hypertension. This condition has been previously called hypertrophic obstructive cardiomyopathy and idiopathic hypertrophic subaortic stenosis. The characteristic distribution of hypertrophy in this condition is asymmetric septal hypertrophy (hypertrophy of the interventricular septum disproportionate to the hypertrophy of the left ventricular free wall) but symmetric hypertrophy can also occur. Left ventricular systolic function is normal or supernormal in hypertrophic cardiomyopathy, with the left ventricular cavity being normal or smaller than normal in size.

Fig. 6-3. Severe hypertrophic cardiomyopathy, with marked left ventricular hypertrophy, especially of the intraventricular septum. (Reprinted with permission from: Fang KS, Dec W, and Lilly LS. The cardiomyopathies. In Lilly LS (ed). *Pathophysiology of Heart Disease.* Philadelphia: Lea & Febiger, 1993, p. 170.)

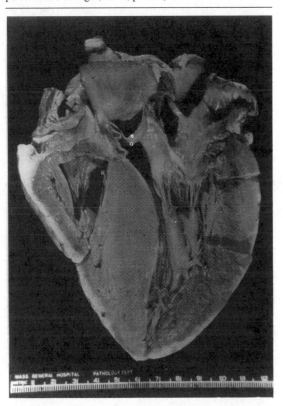

However, the marked hypertrophy leads to impaired left ventricular relaxation. Other abnormalities include larger size of the mitral valve with enlargement and elongation of the valve leaflets as well as anterior displacement of the mitral valve and papillary muscles. The left atrium is frequently dilated. The histology of the myocardium is characteristic with disorganization of the muscle fibers and a pattern of whorl-like arrangement. Abnormalities of the intramural coronary arteries have also been described with thickening of the wall due to proliferation of smooth muscles, collagen, and elastic fibers. Hypertrophic cardiomyopathy is familial in some patients.

A characteristic feature of hypertrophic cardiomyopathy is the occurrence of left ventricular outflow obstruction. However, this phenomenon is not universally present. The narrowing of the outflow tract during systole in hypertrophic cardiomyopathy is due to the anterior migration of the anterior leaflet of the mitral valve due to a Venturi effect produced by hyperdynamic left ventricular ejection. This high-velocity jet combined with hypertrophy of the basal part of the intraventricular septum produces left ventricular outflow obstruction, which may result in syncope or presyncope due to reduced cerebral perfusion. (Fig. 6-4).

Fig. 6-4. Two-dimensional echocardiogram with four-chamber view of patient with hypertrophic cardiomyopathy; arrow demonstrates systolic anterior motion of mitral valve. LV = left ventricle; LA = left atrium; RV = right ventricle; RA = right atrium; S = septum.

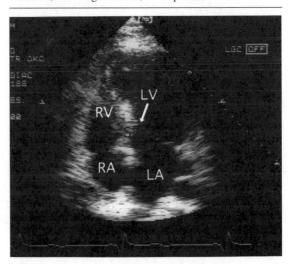

Clinical Presentation

Patients with hypertrophic cardiomyopathy may present with symptoms of dyspnea on exertion, syncope, or chest pain suggestive of angina pectoris. The dyspnea is due to raised pulmonary capillary wedge pressure resulting from poor ventricular compliance. Syncope is often exercise induced and is the result of left ventricular outflow tract obstruction due to apposition of anterior mitral leaflet to the intraventricular septum. Chest pain suggestive of myocardial ischemia occurs due to increased myocardial oxygen demands even in absence of coronary atherosclerosis. In the later stages of the disease atrial dilatation leads to atrial fibrillation, which can produce significant hemodynamic compromise as the hypertrophied ventricle is dependent on the atrial transport mechanism. Embolic phenomena can also occur.

Physical Examination

The pulse upstroke is rapid as the left ventricular ejection is supernormal during early systole. In some patients the characteristic bifid carotid pulse (pulses bisferiens) can be felt. The apical impulse is not displaced but has characteristic heaving quality secondary to left ventricular hypertrophy. A fourth heart sound is often present consistent with powerful atrial contraction owing to left ventricular hypertrophy. The second heart sound may be paradoxically split. The most characteristic feature of hypertrophic cardiomyopathy is a midsystolic murmur heard in the left parasternal area as well as the aortic area and occasionally at the apex with radiation to the neck. This murmur is due to turbulent flow across the left ventricular outflow tract due to the systolic anterior motion of the mitral valve. This murmur characteristically undergoes variations in loudness with various bedside maneuvers depending on the effect of the maneuver on left ventricular cavity size. Typically the strain phase of the Valsalva maneuver, standing, and amyl nitrite inhalation decrease venous return and left ventricular filling and the smaller LV cavity worsens outflow obstruction and accentuates the murmur. On the other hand, squatting, isometric hand grip, and intravenous beta-blockade increase left ventricular cavity size, which in turn produces a decrease in the intensity of the murmur.

Investigations

The electrocardiogram shows evidence of left ventricular hypertrophy and left atrial enlargement. Frequently, abnormal Q-waves may be seen in the lateral precordial leads due to septal hypertrophy. This may lead to the false diagnosis of myocardial infarction. On chest x-ray the cardiac silhouette is within normal limits but some suggestion of pulmonary venous congestion may be present.

The characteristic echocardiographic feature is left ventricular hypertrophy along with asymmetric septal hypertrophy. The ratio of septal to posterior wall thickness exceeds 1.3. Abnormal anterior motion of the mitral valve producing outflow obstruction during systole may also be present. Varying degrees of mitral regurgitation may be seen, depending upon the degree of distortion of mitral valve coaptation induced by anterior motion of the mitral leaflet. The left atrium is frequently dilated in patients with left ventricular outflow tract obstruction. The Doppler signal demonstrates increase in the left ventricular velocities during systole. The gradient across the outflow tract may be present either at rest or with provocation using Valsalva maneuver or amyl nitrite inhalation.

Differential Diagnosis

The symptomatology of hypertrophic cardiomyopathy could mimic aortic stenosis and other types of fixed left ventricular outflow tract obstruction. The condition may also be confused with coronary artery disease based on history of chest pain. The auscultatory findings of systolic murmur might be confused with the mitral regurgitation or ventricular septal defect. The characteristic changes in the murmur produced by the various bedside maneuvers will be useful in clarifying the diagnosis. However, many patients require investigations for establishing or excluding the diagnosis of hypertrophic cardiomyopathy.

Treatment

Therapeutic approaches to hypertrophic cardiomyopathy includes medication, surgery, and cardiac pacing.

Medical Therapy.   The two classes of drugs used are beta-blockers and calcium channel blockers. Beta-blockers produce a negative inotropic effect which leads to an increase in the ventricular cavity size. This leads to a decrease in left ventricular outflow tract obstruction and relief of symptoms. Calcium channel blockers improve the diastolic properties of the hypertrophied ventricle. Both beta-blockers and calcium channel blockers (e.g., verapamil) slow heart rate, which may also improve ventricular filling. Both classes of drugs improve symptomatology in hypertrophic cardiomyopathy even though calcium channel blockers are superior to beta-blockers. The risk of sudden cardiac death is not significantly altered by either therapy.

Surgery.   Ventricular septal myectomy can be employed in patients not responding to medical therapy and manifesting significant outflow tract obstruction.

Pacing.   Dual-chamber pacing is effective because right ventricular pacing causes the septum to contract with the right ventricle and move away from the left ventricular freewall and anterior mitral leaflet during systole.

Restrictive Cardiomyopathy

Restrictive cardiomyopathy denotes a group of conditions characterized by normal ventricular cavity size, and impairment/restriction to diastolic filling. Systolic function is usually normal. Restrictive cardiomyopathy may be idiopathic or may be associated with an infiltrative disease of the myocardium such as amyloidosis. Other systemic diseases that produce restrictive abnormalities of diastolic function include hemochromatosis, sarcoidosis, and endomyocardial fibrosis (hypereosinophilic syndrome).

Impaired ventricular filling is the hallmark of restrictive cardiomyopathy. The cardiac size and systolic function are near normal or normal. The restriction to diastolic filling leads to a rise in end-diastolic pressures, left atrial and pulmonary capillary pressures, and congestion in the lungs. The atria are commonly dilated. In cardiac involvement due to amyloidosis, significant thickening of the ventricular walls due to infiltration of amyloid is seen. Thickening of the mitral and tricuspid valves, atrial septum, and pericardium are also commonly present. Abnormal restriction to diastolic filling also occurs in constrictive pericarditis which is due to fibrous thickening of the pericardium as a result of an infectious or fibrotic process. The differentiation between constrictive pericarditis and restrictive cardiomyopathy is important as constrictive pericarditis is surgically resectable with a reasonable chance of cure.

Physical Examination

Findings related to the underlying systemic disease may be present in amyloidosis, hemochromatosis, and sarcoidosis. The cardiac findings include elevated venous pressure with prominent x- and y-descents, dependent edema, ascites, and enlargement of the liver. A third heart sound due to abrupt termination of rapid filling and holosystolic murmurs due to mitral and/or tricuspid regurgitation may be present. A paradoxical rise in jugular venous pressure with inspiration (Kussmaul's sign) may occasionally be elicited.

Investigations

The electrocardiogram often shows evidence of left or right bundle branch block. This finding is very helpful in differentiating restrictive cardiomyopathy from constrictive pericarditis. In spite of increase in wall thickness owing to an infiltrative process, the electrocardiogram typically shows normal or low voltages.

Cardiac catheterization is used to establish the diagnosis of restrictive cardiomyopathy, differentiate it from constrictive pericarditis, and to perform myocardial biopsy if a systemic disease such as amyloidosis, hemochromatosis, or sarcoidosis are suspected. The atrial pressures are typically increased and a steep x- and y-descent are seen in the right atrium. Right ventricular systolic pressure is usually elevated and a characteristic dip and plateau pattern is seen during diastole due to rapid rise in ventricular diastolic pressure during the rapid filling phase. Pulmonary artery pressures are modestly elevated. When the left atrial pressure is significantly higher than right atrial pressure, the diagnosis of restrictive cardiomyopathy can be confirmed and the possibility of constrictive pericarditis excluded. However, when both pressures are elevated and equal, the differential diagnosis is difficult.

Differential Diagnosis

Restrictive cardiomyopathy must be distinguished from constrictive pericarditis while the clinical features may be identical. CT of the chest or magnetic resonance imaging may demonstrate pericardial thickening and calcification and indirectly provide clues to the diagnosis of constrictive pericarditis. Occasionally cardiac catheterization is required to demonstrate dissimilar filling pressures on the left and right side of the heart and obtain an endomyocardial biopsy. Some patients require thoracotomy to exclude constrictive pericarditis after extensive investigations prove inconclusive as constrictive pericarditis is a surgically treatable condition.

Treatment

Diuretics may be used cautiously to relieve congestive symptoms. However, aggressive diuretic therapy is contraindicated as the diastolic filling abnormalities require higher filling pressures and over-diuresis will decrease cardiac output. Afterload reducing agents are of limited value and may precipitate hypotension. Digoxin is of little help and should be used with caution in patients with amyloid heart disease since the chance of digitalis intoxication is increased.

Specific therapy aimed at an underlying disease is occasionally undertaken (e.g., Melfalan therapy for amyloidosis, phlebotomy and/or chelation for hemochromatosis, and steroid therapy for sarcoidosis).

Clinical Examples

1. A 45-year-old male complained of dyspnea on exertion and occasional episodes of shortness of breath at

night. Ten years earlier, when he was evaluated for mild dyspnea, a chest x-ray revealed enlargement of cardiac silhouette and an electrocardiogram revealed left bundle branch block. At that time he was using alcohol heavily. He quit drinking but he remained minimally symptomatic until 6 months prior to the current evaluation, when his symptoms worsened. His family history is negative for cardiac disease. He had no history of myocardial infarction, hypertension, or diabetes. Examination revealed pulse 80, blood pressure 110/70, respiration 22/minute. Venous pressure was elevated by 7 cm, mild pitting ankle edema was present, and bilateral basal crackles were audible. Apical impulse was displaced to the left sixth intercostal space and diffuse. S1 and S2 were normal, with a clearly audible S3 at the apex. Electrocardiogram revealed left axis deviation and left bundle branch block. Chest x-ray showed enlargement of cardiac silhouette, a left atrial double shadow, and prominent upper pulmonary veins. An echocardiogram revealed dilatation of the left and right ventricles with diffuse hypokinesis, mild mitral and tricuspid regurgitation. He was treated with furosemide, captopril, and digoxin with improvement. One year later the patient became extremely limited with dyspnea and was unable to perform his day-to-day activities. He underwent successful orthotopic cardiac transplantation after appropriate evaluation.

Discussion.   This patient's history is typical for dilated cardiomyopathy. Even though he had a history of excessive intake of alcohol, the etiology of heart failure is unlikely to be alcoholic cardiomyopathy since he discontinued alcohol for over 10 years. The presence of biventricular enlargement, abnormal left axis deviation, and left bundle branch block on EKG would be consistent with dilated cardiomyopathy. His symptomatology suggests both right and left ventricular dysfunction. Absence of regional wall motion abnormalities on echocardiography is more consistent with dilated cardiomyopathy than coronary artery disease. Many patients with dilated cardiomyopathy initially improve with medical therapy as did this patient. When symptoms continue to become severe in spite of medical therapy, particularly when normal day-to-day activities are interfered with, cardiac transplantation is a viable option.

2. A 25-year-old male was referred for investigation of a cardiac murmur. He had minimal fatigue but denied chest pain, palpitations, lightheadedness, or dyspnea. His family history included hypertrophic cardiomyopathy in his 50-year-old mother. There was no history of cardiac disease in any other member of the family. No family history of sudden cardiac death was noted. Examination revealed brisk

carotid pulse upstroke, blood pressure 110/70 mm Hg, heaving apical impulse, normal S1 and S2, and a grade 2/6 systolic ejection murmur in the left parasternal area. The murmur intensified during the strain phase of the Valsalva maneuver and with standing. EKG showed sinus rhythm and left ventricular hypertrophy with deep T inversions in leads V4–V6. Chest x-ray was within normal limits. An echocardiogram showed asymmetric septal hypertrophy with ratio of septal to posterior wall thickness of 1.9, systolic anterior motion of the mitral valve, and moderate mitral regurgitation. The outflow tract gradient at rest was estimated at 60 mm Hg and increased to 80 mm Hg with the strain phase of the Valsalva maneuver. A diagnosis of hypertrophic cardiomyopathy, probably familial in type, was made. In spite of the minimal symptomatology, the patient was treated with propranolol (a beta adrenergic blocker), and was advised to have regular followup.

Discussion.   This young male has classic hypertrophic cardiomyopathy. In view of the family history of hypertrophic cardiomyopathy, his risk of developing symptoms including sudden cardiac death is higher than average. The outflow tract gradient of 60 mm Hg at rest is markedly abnormal. The gradient increases to 80 mm Hg with provocation. This would suggest that the risk of syncope with exercise is significant in this particular patient. Even though most patients with similar findings will be expected to have symptoms, occasionally patients are asymptomatic despite outflow tract obstruction. Treatment of such patients is somewhat controversial as neither calcium channel blocker or beta-blocker therapy have been proven to either regress left ventricular hypertrophy or decrease the chance of sudden cardiac death.

3. An 80-year-old man was admitted to the hospital for progressively increasing dyspnea on exertion, lower extremity swelling, and frequent episodes of lightheadedness on standing. He had no history of hypertension or myocardial infarction. He denied use of alcohol. An electrocardiogram done 10 years ago was reportedly normal. Examination revealed a chronically ill-appearing elderly male. Blood pressure was 100/70 supine and 70/50 mm Hg upon standing. His heart rate was 100/minute, and irregular supine and standing. Jugular venous pressure was markedly elevated and a prominent y-descent was noted. Edema of the lower extremities was present up to the knees. His extremities were cool and peripheral cyanosis was present. There were no palpable precordial impulses and heart sounds were faint. A third heart sound was noted. Bilateral crackles were noted in the lung bases. The liver was enlarged with a span of 15 cm and the spleen tip was palpable.

There was free fluid in the abdomen. Electrocardiogram revealed atrial fibrillation with rapid ventricular response, left axis deviation, low voltage and nonspecific T changes in the precordial leads. Chest x-ray showed bilateral pleural effusions, prominent upper lobe veins, and absence of any calcification in the region of the pericardium. Urinalysis showed 2+ proteinuria, but the urine sediment was within normal limits. CBC revealed a hemoglobin of 11 gm/dl with normal white count and platelet count. Sedimentation rate was 40 mm/hour. Liver enzymes were abnormal with elevation of transaminases to 1.5 times normal. An echocardiogram revealed normal size of the LV cavity, markedly increased thickness of the septum and posterior wall (16 mm each), with thickening of the mitral and tricuspid valves and atrial septum. Mild mitral and tricuspid regurgitation were seen on colorflow Doppler echocardiography. Granular sparkling was seen in the septum as well as the posterior wall. The patient was treated with intravenous furosemide with improvement of his dyspnea and leg swelling. However, postural hypotension initially worsened, then stabilized after he began using elastic support hose.

Discussion.   The above patient represents a classical example of a restrictive cardiomyopathy due to amyloidosis. Amyloid heart disease typically presents in the elderly with symptoms of biventricular failure. Postural hypotension is frequently seen due to autonomic neuropathy, which is also secondary to amyloidosis. Elevation of the venous pressure is consistent with abnormal diastolic filling. The third heart sound implies restriction to rapid filling phase. The EKG findings of low voltage and atrial fibrillation are also consistent with the diagnosis of amyloidosis. Proteinuria is also suggestive of amyloid involvement of the kidneys even though mild proteinuria can result from severe heart failure. The echocardiographic findings are classical for amyloidosis with thickening of the walls of the ventricle and granular sparkling. The nondilated ventricle with well-preserved systolic function would not be consistent with dilated cardiomyopathy. The diagnosis of amyloidosis could be confirmed by a biopsy obtained from myocardium, rectum, gingivum, or subcutaneous fat. The treatment of patients with amyloid heart disease is difficult because the dose of diuretic needed to relieve congestive symptoms reduces preload sufficiently to further reduce cardiac output. The result is often worsening fatigue and hypotension.

Bibliography

Goodwin JF and Oakley CM. The cardiomyopathies. *Br Heart J* 34:545–552, 1972. *A classic article dealing with the classification and pathogenesis of cardiomyopathies.*

Johnson RA and Palacios I. Dilated cardiomyopathies of the adult. *N Eng J Med* 307:1051–1058, 1119–1126, 1982. *A two-part article describing the pathophysiology and pathogenesis of dilated cardiomyopathy including peripartum and alcoholic cardiomyopathies.*

Maron BJ, Bonow RO, Cannon RO, et al. Hypertrophic cardiomyopathy: Interrelation of clinical manifestations, pathophysiology, and therapy. *N Eng J Med* 316:780–789, 844–852, 1987. *An excellent two-part article with comprehensive account of the pathophysiology and discussion of the treatment modalities of hypertrophic cardiomyopathy.*

Wynne J and Braunwald E. The cardiomyopathies and myocarditides: toxic, chemical, and physical damage to the heart. In Braunwald, E (ed). *Heart Disease* (4th ed). Philadelphia: Saunders, 1992. *A comprehensive, contemporary review of the subject.*

7 Pulmonary Heart Disease

Karen K. Hamilton

Objectives

After completing this chapter, you should be able to

Understand the pressure-volume relationships in the normal right ventricle

Understand the normal physiology of the pulmonary circulation

Know the definition of cor pulmonale and recognize that there are other causes of right ventricular dysfunction

Describe the mechanisms by which chronic lung diseases result in right heart dysfunction

Know the common physical findings and methods of diagnosing pulmonary heart disease

Understand the common causes of both acute and chronic cor pulmonale

Normal Physiology of the Right Ventricle and Pulmonary Circulation

Right Ventricular Function

The left ventricle (LV) is an ellipsoid chamber which contracts concentrically. The normal right ventricle (RV) is a thin-walled, crescent-shaped chamber whose pumping function has been likened to a bellows. The RV volume is larger than that of the LV and its ejection fraction is lower (0.45–0.55). Pulmonary artery (PA) pressures are in the range of 15–30 mm Hg systolic and 3–12 end-diastolic. In contrast to the normal mean aortic pressure (80–100 mm Hg or more), the mean PA pressure is normally 9–16 mm Hg and rarely exceeds 20–25 mm Hg. Because the RV outflow impedance ("afterload") is low, the RV stroke work for generating the same cardiac output is about 25% of that of the LV. Like the LV, the RV has the capacity to dilate in response to an increase in volume load and to hypertrophy in response to an increase in pressure work. The RV is more compliant than the LV, that is, the RV is able to accept large increases in volume with relatively little increase in pressure (Fig. 7-1). By contrast, acute increases in ejection pressure are relatively well tolerated by the LV, but may cause decompensation of RV pump function. An acute increase in mean aortic pressure of 5–15 mm Hg would go unnoticed by the left ventricle, whereas a similar increase in mean PA pressure to 20–25 mm Hg may result in significant fall in RV stroke volume.

Ventricular Interdependence

It must also be recognized that the RV and LV do not function independently, but share a common wall (the septum) and a maximal diastolic filling volume that is limited by the pericardium. Acute increases in RV filling volume result in shifting of the septum toward the LV, which decreases LV compliance and end-diastolic volume; this may result in a fall in cardiac output.

Effects of Intrathoracic Pressure on Cardiac Function

Intrathoracic pressure falls during normal inspiration, which increases venous return to the right ventricle, shifts the septum toward the LV, and decreases the LV end-diastolic volume. Intrapleural pressure also affects LV "af-

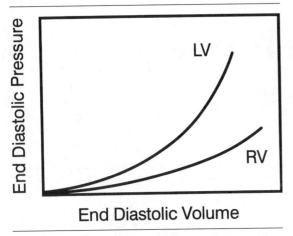

Fig. 7-1. Compliance curves for the left and right ventricle. The relationship of end-diastolic pressure to end-diastolic volume is shown for the left and right ventricles. The right ventricle is more compliant (accepts larger increases in volume with small changes in pressure).

terload." Although it is common to consider systemic arterial systolic pressure as the LV "afterload," the systolic arterial pressure relative to intrapleural pressure is a better estimate of LV afterload. Thus a decrease in intrathoracic pressure increases the effective LV ejection pressure (the difference between the extrathoracic arterial pressure and the intrathoracic LV end-diastolic pressure). This decrease in LV preload and increase in afterload results in an inspiratory decrease in stroke volume and an inspiratory fall in blood pressure referred to as pulsus paradoxus. Pulsus paradoxus is normally less than 10 mm Hg but may increase in patients with exaggerated respiratory effort and large negative intrapleural pressure, such as patients with obstructive lung disease.

Pulmonary Circulation

Compliance
The normal pulmonary vascular bed is a highly compliant system able to accommodate the large increases in cardiac output with little increase in pressure. The individual pulmonary vessels are not more compliant than systemic vessels; however, in the normal lung, a significant proportion of vessels are not perfused. Increases in flow are accommodated predominantly by recruitment of these previously unperfused vessels and to a lesser extent by vasodilation of already perfused vessels. Flow in the normal

pulmonary circulation can increase 2.5–3-fold before a significant increase in pulmonary artery pressure occurs (Fig. 7-2).

Resistance
Vascular resistance is defined as the pressure drop across a vascular bed (P in mm Hg) divided by the flow through the bed (Q in liters/min) (Fig. 7-3). Pulmonary vascular resistance (PVR) may be expressed in Woods units (mm Hg/liters/min) or in dynes-sec-cm^{-5}. The normal range for PVR is 20–120 dynes-sec-cm^{-5}, whereas the normal range for systemic vascular resistance is 800–1500 dynes-sec-cm^{-5}. The small muscular arteries and arterioles are the primary determinants of pulmonary vascular resistance. Normally, PVR decreases slightly as flow increases because of the increase in cross-sectional area of the pulmonary vascular bed as vessels open or dilate. In addition to the cross-sectional area, other important determinants of PVR include alveolar gas and lung volumes. Because resistance vessels are exposed to alveolar gas, hypoxia results in vasoconstriction initially and eventually in smooth

Fig. 7-2. Relationship between cardiac output and pulmonary artery pressure. In normal subjects, the cardiac output may increase 2.5–3-fold before pulmonary artery (PA) pressures will increase. In patients with a mild reduction in the cross-sectional area or distensibility of the pulmonary vascular bed, the PA pressure is normal at rest but will increase with increased flow as during exercise. In patients with a severe reduction in the pulmonary bed (e.g., a patient with chronic bronchitis and resting pO$_2$ < 60), PA pressures will be elevated even at rest and will increase further with increased flow.

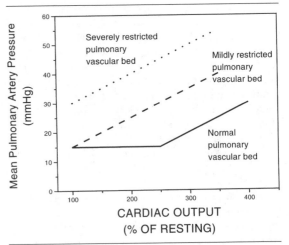

$$PVR(mmHg/L/min \text{ or Wood units}) =$$
$$\frac{\text{mean PA pressure (mmHg) - mean LA pressure (mmHg)}}{Q \text{ (L/min)}}$$

or

$$PVR \text{ (dynes-sec-cm}^{-5}\text{) } =$$
$$\frac{\text{mean PA pressure (mmHg) - mean LA pressure (mmHg)}}{Q \text{ (L/min)}} \times 80$$

Fig. 7-3. Calculation of pulmonary vascular resistance. Q is pulmonary blood flow in liters/min. In the absence of a significant shunt, the pulmonary blood flow is equal to cardiac output. Left atrial pressure can be estimated by pulmonary artery occlusion pressure (PAOP), also called the pulmonary capillary wedge pressure (PCW).

muscle hypertrophy and muscularization of previously nonmuscular arterioles. PVR is also increased by both high and low lung volumes: At high lung volumes or during positive pressure ventilation, alveolar arterioles may be compressed, which increases resistance; at very low lung volumes, the extra-alveolar vessels, which depend on lung inflation to maintain patency, will collapse, thus increasing resistance.

Ventilation-Perfusion Matching

Normally, hydrostatic pressure in the upright position results in a gradient of pulmonary arterial and venous pressures from highest in the lung bases to lowest in the apices. At rest, the lung bases receive more perfusion and apical vessels are relatively less distended than those in the base; this normal distribution of pulmonary vessel caliber can be confirmed on chest radiograph. Ventilation is distributed more homogeneously, with only slightly more ventilation to the dependent portions of the lung. Regions of the lung which are ventilated but relatively underperfused (wasted ventilation) are termed "physiologic dead space." On the other hand, regions of the lung which are perfused but poorly ventilated are equivalent to shunting of venous blood into the systemic circulation and result in hypoxemia. The vasoconstriction which occurs in pulmonary ar-

terioles exposed to alveolar hypoxia serves to direct blood flow away from poorly ventilated regions of the lung and maintain normal ventilation-perfusion matching.

Cor Pulmonale

Pulmonary heart disease or cor pulmonale refers to right ventricular dysfunction which is secondary to alteration in structure or function of the lungs or pulmonary vasculature. Right ventricular dysfunction includes RV hypertrophy and/or dilatation; cor pulmonale does not necessarily imply frank RV failure. Other causes of right ventricular dysfunction include (1) chronic increases in LV filling pressures (e.g., LV failure or mitral stenosis), (2) large left-to-right shunts, (3) obstruction to RV outflow (e.g., pulmonic stenosis or infundibular stenosis as seen in tetralogy of Fallot), (4) RV infarction, or (5) intrinsic RV cardiomyopathy (e.g., arrhythmogenic RV dysplasia). This discussion will be limited to RV dysfunction secondary to abnormalities of lung structure or function or pulmonary vascular diseases. In patients over the age of 50, cor pulmonale is the third most common form of heart disease. The most common etiologies of cor pulmonale are listed in Table 7-l.

Table 7-1. Causes of Cor Pulmonale

DISEASES OF THE LUNG

Chronic obstructive lung disease
Chronic suppurative lung diseases (e.g., cystic fibrosis)
Restrictive lung diseases/pulmonary fibrosis

IMPAIRED VENTILATION

Chronic hypoventilation syndromes (e.g., central sleep
   apnea, extreme obesity)
Obstructive sleep apnea

ABNORMALITIES OF THORACIC CAGE FUNCTION

Thoracic cage deformity (e.g., kyphoscoliosis)
Neuromuscular disorders resulting in impairment of respi-
   ratory muscle function (e.g., myasthenia gravis,
   Guillain-Barré syndrome, multiple sclerosis)

PULMONARY THROMBOEMBOLIC DISORDERS

Pulmonary emboli
   Acute massive
   Chronic recurrent
Small-vessel pulmonary thrombosis

DISEASES OF THE PULMONARY VASCULATURE

Primary pulmonary hypertension
Toxin-induced pulmonary hypertension
Vasculitis/autoimmune diseases involving the pulmonary
   vessels (e.g., systemic lupus erythematosus, sclero-
   derma)
Pulmonary venoocclusive disease
Surgical loss of vascular bed (e.g., lobectomy, pneu-
   monectomy)

Pathogenesis

Pulmonary hypertension invariably precedes RV dysfunction. Poiseuille's law relates the intraluminal pressure generated by flow in a tube to its length and cross-sectional
area (Pressure difference = 8 (fluid viscosity)(vessel
length)(flow) / π (radius)^4). Clearly, pressure will increase
with increases in blood flow and viscosity, and pressure
will decrease with increases in cross-sectional area of
the vascular bed. Thus, changes in cross-sectional area of
the pulmonary vascular bed, pulmonary blood flow, and
viscosity may each contribute to the development of pulmonary hypertension.

Reduction of the Pulmonary Vascular Bed

Loss of cross-sectional area of the pulmonary vascular bed
may occur through a variety of mechanisms including, for
example, resection of lung tissue. However, even with loss
of up to 50–60% of the pulmonary vascular bed, as may

occur after pneumonectomy, pulmonary artery pressures at
rest remain normal. When flow increases with exercise, the
reserve capacity for vasodilation to accommodate additional blood flow is limited and PA pressures increase (Fig.
7-2). Other mechanisms for reduction of the pulmonary
vascular bed include:

1. Destruction of small arteries and arterioles by inflammation and fibrosis
2. Obstruction of vessels by thromboemboli, tumor metastasis, or parasites.
3. Fixed structural narrowing of the pulmonary vessels,
   including plexogenic lesions in patients with primary
   pulmonary hypertension, intimal fibrosis in patients
   with recurrent thromboemboli, and medial hypertrophy
   in response to chronic hypoxia.
4. Vasoconstriction, most commonly in response to alveolar hypoxia or acidosis. Vessel diameter may also be
   dynamically altered by neurogenic input and by circulating hormones and cytokines. For example, beta
   adrenergic agonists such as epinephrine result in pulmonary vasodilation. Probably the most potent pulmonary vasoconstrictor is low alveolar oxygen tension,
   as may occur at high altitudes and in patients with
   chronic obstructive lung disease or generalized hypoventilation syndromes.
5. Compression of vessels by hyperinflated alveoli at high
   lung volumes and high intrathoracic pressures.

Increased Pulmonary Blood Flow

A compensatory increase in cardiac output is seen in response to chronic hypoxemia in many disorders associated
with cor pulmonale, and increased flow may further aggravate pulmonary hypertension.

Increased Viscosity

Increases in blood viscosity may occur in patients with
lung disease when hematocrit rises above 55% as a compensatory response to chronic hypoxemia.

Clinical Presentation

Symptoms and Signs

No symptom is specific for cor pulmonale. Prior to the
onset of frank RV failure, the patient's complaints are
often related to the underlying respiratory disorder. Dyspnea and cough are common. Chest pain may occur in patients with acute pulmonary emboli or primary pulmonary
hypertension. Lower-extremity edema is common once
RV failure develops.

The physical examination in patients with cor pulmonale will vary with the severity of RV dysfunction. Early findings may include a prominent A-wave of the jugular venous pulse and a fourth heart sound of RV origin, both of which result from decreased RV compliance during atrial contraction. The pulmonic component of the second heart sound (P2) will become louder than the aortic component, due to the increased PA pressures. Later, as RV hypertrophy and dilatation develop, a heave may be palpable in the left parasternal area, and the patient may develop an S3 of RV origin. As RV failure progresses, systemic venous pressure rises and jugular venous distension and lower-extremity edema appear. The increased RV systolic pressure results in a very high-pitched murmur of tricuspid regurgitation. A murmur of pulmonic regurgitation may be found in severe pulmonary hypertension.

Diagnosis

Diagnosis of cor pulmonale requires confirmation of the presence of pulmonary hypertension and assessment of RV size and function. Chest x-ray may suggest pulmonary hypertension when the main and proximal pulmonary arteries are enlarged. Pulmonary artery pressures may be measured directly by right heart catheterization, or may be estimated noninvasively using Doppler echocardiography in most patients. Cardiac catheterization may be required to exclude intracardiac shunting and elevation of left-sided filling pressure as the etiology for pulmonary hypertension. RV size and function may also be assessed qualitatively by 2D echocardiography. In addition, first-pass or gated equilibrium nuclear blood pool scans can measure RV volume and ejection fraction.

Common Etiologies

Acute Cor Pulmonale

Acute cor pulmonale is usually due to a sudden increase in pulmonary pressure secondary to acute pulmonary emboli. The presenting symptoms in these patients are quite variable and include sudden onset of dyspnea, wheezing, chest pain, cough and hemoptysis, hypotension, syncope, and the sense of impending doom. The increase in PA pressure which occurs in patients with acute pulmonary emboli is in part due to obstruction of a segment of the pulmonary vascular bed by thrombus (loss of cross-sectional area) and in part due to continued generation of activated clotting factors and release of vasoconstrictors from activated platelets. Heparin is an essential tool in current therapy because of its ability to inhibit both coagulation and thrombin-

initiated platelet activation. Acute right heart failure may also occasionally occur in association with acute respiratory failure in a patient with chronic obstructive pulmonary disease (COPD) with previously compensated RV function.

Chronic Cor Pulmonale

Chronic Obstructive Pulmonary Disease

The most common cause of chronic cor pulmonale is chronic obstructive lung disease due to emphysema, chronic bronchitis, or both, usually in patients with a long history of cigarette smoking. Emphysema, a pathologic diagnosis, is associated with the destruction, coalescence, and enlargement of alveolar sacs and/or respiratory bronchioles, which results in loss of intra-alveolar arterioles and capillaries, loss of support for small bronchioles, and airflow obstruction. Chronic bronchitis is a clinical diagnosis given to patients with cough and sputum production on most days. Pathological changes include inflammation and narrowing of the terminal bronchioles, metaplasia of the bronchial epithelium, enlargement of mucous glands in the bronchi, and hypersecretion of mucus. Emphysema and chronic bronchitis occur together to some degree on most patients with COPD. Mild hypoxemia may be the only gas exchange abnormality initially, and exacerbation of hypoxemia and pulmonary hypertension may occur only during acute respiratory infections. As the disease progresses, some patients will develop progressive dyspnea and hyperinflated lungs, but will not have chronic sputum production. These patients, often referred to as "pink puffers," have only mild to moderate hypoxemia ($pO_2 > 65$) and are not likely to develop cor pulmonale. By contrast, other patients ("blue bloaters") will develop chronic sputum production, marked hypoxemia, carbon dioxide retention, pulmonary hypertension, and right heart failure.

Factors which contribute to the pulmonary hypertension in these disorders include alveolar hypoxia (which results in vasoconstriction of adjacent vessels) and acidosis (which acts synergistically with hypoxemia to exacerbate vasoconstriction). Emphysema is associated with loss of pulmonary capillary bed and perhaps compression of microvessels by hyperinflated alveoli. When systemic hypoxemia ensues, patients develop compensatory polycythemia and increased cardiac output in order to maintain oxygen delivery, but the increase in flow and red cell mass (which increases viscosity) further increase pulmonary artery pressures. Initially, patients may have normal PA pressures at rest, but develop pulmonary hypertension during exercise due to the limited ability of the reduced pulmonary vascular bed to accommodate increases in flow during exercise (see Fig. 7-2). This increase in RV afterload during exercise may result in RV dilatation and failure to increase RV ejection fraction with exercise and may limit the increase in cardiac output. The development of resting hypoxemia ($PaO_2 < 60$) in patients with COPD, rather than the severity of airflow obstruction, appears to be the most important factor in the development of pulmonary hypertension.

It should be noted that cardiac output may be normal or high in patients with cor pulmonale, especially early in the course of the disease. Nevertheless, a low mixed venous oxygen saturation after exercise or at rest will indicate poor tissue oxygenation. Whereas the cardiac output may appear to be in the "normal" range, it is inadequate for oxygen delivery because of the low arterial oxygen content.

Restrictive Lung Diseases

A group of interstitial or restrictive lung diseases associated with alveolar and interstitial inflammation and progressive fibrosis may result in pulmonary hypertension and cor pulmonale. These disorders include sarcoidosis, radiation pneumonitis, pulmonary fibrosis secondary to collagen vascular disorders, and idiopathic pulmonary fibrosis. The inflammatory process may destroy small septal arterioles and fibrosis may encase the remaining vessels and limit their ability to dilate. The inflammatory process also results in arterial hypoxemia, which exacerbates pulmonary hypertension. The disorders have in common a restrictive abnormality on pulmonary function testing with low lung volumes, a decreased lung diffusing capacity, and no evidence of airflow obstruction.

Hypoventilation Syndromes

Alveolar hypoventilation in patients with normal lungs may result from inadequate central ventilatory drive, upper airway obstruction (obstructive sleep apnea), and limitation of chest wall function due to deformity or neuromuscular disorder. These patients develop severe alveolar hypoxia, hypercapnia, hypoxemia, and respiratory acidosis. The alveolar hypoxia and acidosis lead to pulmonary vasoconstriction, pulmonary hypertension, and RV dysfunction. Therapy is directed toward reversing the hypoxemia and hypercapnia and varies with the underlying disorder. Mechanical ventilation may be required in patients with neuromuscular weakness. Tracheostomy or continuous positive airway pressure masks may be of benefit in patients with obstructive sleep apnea.

Primary Pulmonary Hypertension

Primary pulmonary hypertension may be diagnosed when pulmonary hypertension is discovered in a patient with no identifiable abnormality of the lung or ventilatory function, normal left heart function, and no evidence of pulmonary emboli or intracardiac shunting. Pulmonary function testing, right heart catheterization, and pulmonary angiography may be required to exclude other diagnoses. Pulmonary angiography carries a significant risk in these patients, however, and should not be undertaken unless other evidence suggests major pulmonary emboli. Idiopathic pulmonary hypertension occurs most frequently in young adults, women more often than men, and occasionally appears to be familial. Patients present with insidious and progressive dyspnea on exertion, and pulmonary hypertension is often quite severe by the time of diagnosis. Other symptoms include chest pain and syncope. Many patients also experience other vasospastic disorders such as Raynaud's phenomenon and migraine.

Prognosis in this disease is generally poor. Survival is limited to 1–2 years after the development of heart failure. Many patients are treated with vasodilator drugs but none has been shown to be consistently effective or to alter prognosis.

Chronic Recurrent Pulmonary Thromboembolism

Pulmonary hypertension may result from multiple proximal pulmonary emboli which fail to lyse. Pathologic studies have also shown a subset of patients with unexplained pulmonary hypertension who have thrombosis and recanalization of small pulmonary arteries; these patients have no source for embolization and are believed to have thrombosis in situ.

Management of Cor Pulmonale

The primary goal of management of cor pulmonale is the reduction of pulmonary hypertension. In patients with obstructive lung disease, specific therapy should be directed toward improving respiratory function and oxygenation. This would include bronchodilators, antibiotics for associated bronchitis, steroids to reduce inflammation, and supplementary oxygen. If the patient's arterial pO_2 is below 60, continuous oxygen should be prescribed for home use. Continuous oxygen therapy has been shown to decrease mortality and to improve quality of life. Many vasodilator drugs have been used to treat pulmonary hypertension.

Only oxygen has shown consistent benefit. In patients with marked polycythemia (hematocrit > 60%), phlebotomy has been shown to reduce pulmonary artery pressure and to improve exercise performance.

Digoxin has been utilized for inotropic support of the right ventricle but benefit has not been demonstrated unless the patient also has LV failure. This drug is utilized in patients with atrial fibrillation to control ventricular rate. Patients with lung disease are believed to be more sensitive to the toxic effects of digoxin (arrhythmias), probably because of hypoxemia, and the drug should be used with caution.

Patients with RV failure will often have peripheral edema. Although this may worry the patient, it is usually well tolerated. Use of diuretics in such patients may result in a significant fall in cardiac output. Nevertheless, careful diuresis may be required to alleviate severe edema and ascites.

Trials of vasodilator drugs in both primary pulmonary hypertension and COPD have been in general disappointing. Unfortunately, there is no drug which specifically dilates only the pulmonary vascular bed (except perhaps oxygen in the patient with alveolar hypoxia). Thus, administration of vasodilator drugs frequently results in systemic hypotension and may impair coronary perfusion and thus depress both RV and LV performance. In addition, pulmonary vasodilators may worsen hypoxemia by dilating the vascular beds of poorly ventilated regions of the lung, thus worsening ventilation-perfusion mismatch.

Heart-lung transplantation may be an option for selected patients with severe pulmonary hypertension. Right ventricular function has even been shown to improve significantly after single lung transplantation.

In patients with pulmonary thromboembolic disease, acute and chronic anticoagulation is indicated. Patients with acute pulmonary emboli with hemodynamic compromise may be candidates for pulmonary embolectomy or for thrombolytic therapy. Patients with chronic recurrent pulmonary thromboemboli often present with severe pulmonary hypertension and have a poor prognosis. These patients may benefit from pulmonary thromboendarterectomy, although mortality remains high.

Clinical Examples

1. A 64-year-old man complained to his physician of increasing shortness of breath with exertion and swelling in his feet over the past 6 months. For 2 days, he also noted shortness of breath even at rest. He admitted to a chronic cough with daily production of whitish sputum, but now noted that his sputum was yellowish. His physician made the diagnosis of heart failure and bronchitis. He was treated with digoxin, a potent diuretic, an angiotensin converting enzyme (ACE) inhibitor, and an antibiotic. His cough improved but he remained very short of breath and became so weak and lightheaded that he went to the hospital emergency room.

On examination there, his BP was 88/60, HR 110, respirations 24. There was no jugular venous distension and no edema remaining in the lower extremities. Lung exam revealed diffuse end-inspiratory crackles and occasional wheezes. A high-pitched 2/6 holosystolic murmur was present at the left sternal border which increased slightly with inspiration.

Chest radiograph showed hyperinflated lungs without pulmonary vascular congestion. Arterial blood gas while the patient was breathing room air revealed pH 7.32, pCO_2 47, pO_2 55. An echocardiogram was performed to assess ventricular function. The left atrium and ventricle were normal in size and function, whereas the right atrium and ventricle were mildly enlarged and the right ventricle appeared hypokinetic. The systolic PA pressure was estimated to be 40 mm Hg.

Discussion. This patient was told he had heart failure on the basis of his complaints of exertional dyspnea and lower-extremity edema. He was managed as if he had LV failure. However, diuresis and reduction of systemic vascular resistance with an ACE inhibitor resulted in systemic hypotension, weakness, and lightheadedness. His exacerbation of chronic bronchitis was treated with an antibiotic, but the other underlying problems of airflow obstruction, chronic hypoxemia, and pulmonary hypertension were not addressed by his initial therapy.

At this point, the patient was admitted to the hospital to receive IV fluids and bronchodilator therapy. Diuretics were held, and the ACE inhibitor and digoxin, given to treat presumed LV failure, were discontinued. The patient's blood pressure and pulse returned to normal, and he no longer complained of weakness and lightheadedness. Although his shortness of breath improved some with bronchodilator therapy, his pO_2 on room air never increased above 58. He was discharged on home oxygen, bronchodilators, and a small dose of diuretic.

2. A 26-year-old woman presented to the emergency room complaining of the sudden onset of right-sided chest

pain and shortness of breath. She was 5 weeks postpartum, and she and her husband had been driving most of the day to visit her parents.

On exam, the patient was anxious and in obvious respiratory distress. BP was 125/80, pulse 110, respiratory rate 30. Her lungs were clear. On cardiac exam, the pulmonic component of the second heart sound was increased, and a fourth heart sound of right ventricular origin was heard. Her right lower extremity was noted to be slightly swollen when compared to the left.

The chest radiograph was normal. EKG showed evidence of possible acute RV "strain" or ischemia (T-wave inversion in the right precordial leads). Arterial blood gas on room air showed a pH 7.48, pCO_2 30, pO_2 70.

Discussion.   The patient's symptoms were highly suggestive of acute pulmonary embolus. In addition, pregnancy and the postpartum period are associated with an increased risk of thromboembolism. Prolonged sitting would further increase the likelihood of venous stasis. The patient was started immediately on supplemental oxygen and intravenous heparin. Doppler studies of the right lower extremity showed evidence of deep-vein thrombosis and a lung perfusion scan showed a segmental defect which was felt to be highly suggestive of pulmonary embolus.

Bibliography

Matthay RA, Niederman MS, and Wiedemann HP. Cardiovascular-pulmonary interactions in chronic obstructive pulmonary disease with special reference to the pathogenesis and management of cor pulmonale. *Med Clin N Am* 74:571–618, 1990. *Comprehensive discussion of the effects of chronic lung disease on right and left ventricular function at rest and during exercise.*

Palevsky HI and Fishman AP. Chronic cor pulmonale. *JAMA* 263:2347–2353, 1990. *Excellent brief clinical review of the pathophysiology and management of cor pulmonale.*

Timms RM, Khaja FU, and Williams GW. The nocturnal oxygen therapy trial: Hemodynamic response to oxygen therapy in chronic obstructive pulmonary disease. *Ann Intern Med* 102:29–36, 1985. *Report of one of the large trials demonstrating the benefit of continuous oxygen therapy in patients with COPD.*

Wiedemann HP and Matthay RA. Cor pulmonale in chronic obstructive pulmonary disease. *Clin Chest Med* 11:523–545, 1990. *Discussion of the circulatory pathophysiology of cor pulmonale and the rationale and effectiveness of a wide range of management options.*

8 Pericardial Disease

Edwin G. Olson

Objectives

After completing this chapter, you should be able to

Understand the normal physiology of the pericardium

Understand the meaning of the terms *pericardial constraint, intrapericardial and transmural distending pressure*

Recognize the different clinical signs, symptoms, and hemodynamic characteristics between cardiac tamponade and constriction

Comprehend the pathophysiology of symptoms and signs of acute, subacute, and chronic tamponade

Understand the pathophysiology of symptoms and signs of constrictive pericarditis

Comprehend the importance of early recognition of tamponade

Understand the diagnostic procedures needed to differentiate constriction from tamponade

Know general treatment guidelines for pericardial disorders

Physiology of the Normal Pericardium

The normal pericardium is composed of two layers. The inner layer, called the visceral pericardium, is a thin serous membrane, composed of a single layer of mesothelial cells. It is attached to the epicardial fat on the surface of the heart and forms the epicardium. The outer layer, called the parietal pericardium, is a fibrous sac composed of collagen and elastin fibers. It has attachments to the sternum, vertebral column, and diaphragm. The two layers are separated by pericardial fluid. Normal pericardial fluid is an ultrafiltrate of plasma. It is clear yellow and has a volume of less than 50 ml.

The normal pericardium serves several functions. It positions the heart within the chest cavity and prevents displacement of the heart during changes in body position. It may also prevent sudden dilatation of the heart. The pericardium reduces friction between the heart and surrounding organs. It potentially functions as a barrier, limiting the spread of infections and malignancies.

The normal pericardium is relatively stiff and nondisten-

sible. The compliance characteristics of the pericardium can be studied by plotting the intrapericardial pressure against the intrapericardial volume (Fig. 8-1). The intrapericardial volume consists of the volume occupied by the heart plus the pericardial fluid. At low volumes the pericardial pressure is negligible and rises very slowly. However, once the intrapericardial volume increases to the point where the pericardium is being distended, the pericardial pressure rises very steeply.

The normal pericardium is able to slowly stretch to accommodate chronic dilatation of the heart. However, sudden increases in intrapericardial volume may elevate intrapericardial pressure dramatically and may prevent adequate cardiac filling, as in acute cardiac tamponade. Similarly, a diseased pericardium which is thickened and fibrosed may not be able to stretch and may cause pericardial constriction.

Relationship of Pericardium to Cardiac Function

In the past, most authorities believed that the normal pericardium did not affect cardiac function. The pericardium

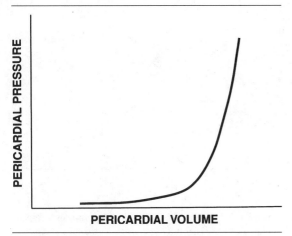

Fig. 8-1. Pressure-volume curve for the normal pericardium. Pericardial volume, plotted along the abscissa, includes both the volume of pericardial fluid and the volume of the heart. Pericardial pressure, plotted along the ordinate, is measured in the pericardial space. The curve is initially flat, but then becomes extremely steep after it reaches a critical volume. The normal pericardium is relatively stiff and noncompliant.

was not felt to restrain ventricular filling. The pericardial pressure was felt to be very low and to reflect the intrathoracic pressure. These beliefs were based on measurements of pericardial pressure using fluid-filled catheters. However, the normal pericardial space has little fluid and acts more like a potential space. Recently, investigators have measured pericardial pressures with flat, fluid-filled balloons instead of catheters. Using these new techniques, they have found that even the normal pericardium can restrain ventricular filling. This restraint of filling is referred to as "pericardial constraint."

In order to understand the concept of "pericardial constraint," one must understand the concept of "transmural distending pressure." Simply stated, the transmural distending pressure of a chamber is the difference between the pressure within the chamber and the pressure outside the chamber. Since the pericardium usually transmits pressure equally to all the cardiac chambers, the transmural distending pressure is the pressure within either ventricle minus the intrapericardial pressure.

Using the new balloon technique, investigators have measured intrapericardial pressure in experimental animals and in patients undergoing open-heart surgery. In subjects with normal pericardiums and normal heart sizes, the pericardial pressure is almost identical to the right

atrial and right ventricular diastolic pressures (Fig. 8-2). This near equalization between the RV diastolic pressure and the pericardial pressure indicates that the transmural distending pressure of the right ventricle is close to zero. Furthermore, the transmural distending pressure of the left ventricle can be estimated by subtracting the right ventricular diastolic pressure from the left ventricular diastolic pressure, since the right ventricular diastolic pressure and the pericardial pressures are almost equal.

In patients with chronically dilated hearts, the relationship between pericardial pressure and right ventricular pressure has not been well studied. Chronic dilatation may stretch the pericardium enough so that pericardial pressure is no longer as high as right ventricular diastolic pressure.

The concept of pericardial constraint has important implications for understanding normal cardiac physiology. Since the pericardium "constrains" both ventricles equally, there must be an interdependence of filling of both ventricles. If one ventricle has increased filling within the pericardial space, then the other ventricle will require higher pressure to maintain its filling. In other words, the increased filling will cause increased intrapericardial pressure, which will increase diastolic pressure of the other ventricle. The other ventricle will have an *apparent* change in its diastolic pressure-volume relationship. Although the filling pressure within the other ventricle appears increased,

Fig. 8-2. Right atrial pressure versus pericardial pressure in dogs. A wide range of right atrial pressures was obtained by volume loading, administering nitroglycerine and phenylephrine, and inducing ischemia. Right atrial pressure and pericardial pressure were almost identical over a wide range. (Modified with permission from: Smithseth OA et al. Pericardial pressure assessed by right atrial pressure. *Am Heart J* 108:603, 1984.)

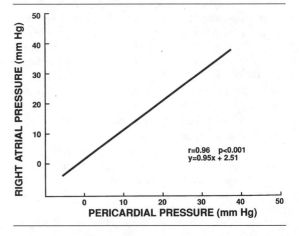

the transmural distending pressure is not increased. Similarly, medications which reduce filling of one ventricle by vasodilation and venous pooling may allow filling of the other ventricle to be maintained at a lower filling pressure.

Pericardial Tamponade

Pericarditis of any etiology may produce pericardial effusion. When the effusion is large enough to limit filling of the ventricles, cardiac tamponade results. The develop-

ment of tamponade is dependent on three factors: (1) the volume of the effusion, (2) the rate of growth of the effusion, and (3) the compliance of the pericardium. In a normal patient, the pericardium is relatively small and noncompliant. As little as 150–200 ml of fluid can cause tamponade, if accumulated rapidly. In a patient with a slowly developing pericardial effusion, the pericardium can stretch to accommodate 1500–2000 ml of fluid without hemodynamic compromise.

Generally, tamponade is produced by effusions large enough to raise the intrapericardial pressure to the same level as the diastolic pressures of both ventricles (Fig. 8-3).

Fig. 8-3. Cardiac tamponade. In (A), the pericardial effusion is small and the pericardial pressure is low. Equalization is not present. The transmural distending pressure (TDP) of the RV is close to zero, but the TDP of the LV is 8. In (B), the effusion is large and the pericardial pressure is high. Equalization of the diastolic pressures in the pericardium, RV, and LV is present. The transmural distending pressure of both ventricles is close to zero and tamponade is present. (Modified from: Cosio FG, et al. Abnormal septal motion in cardiac tamponade with pulsus paradoxus. *Chest* 71:787, 1977.)

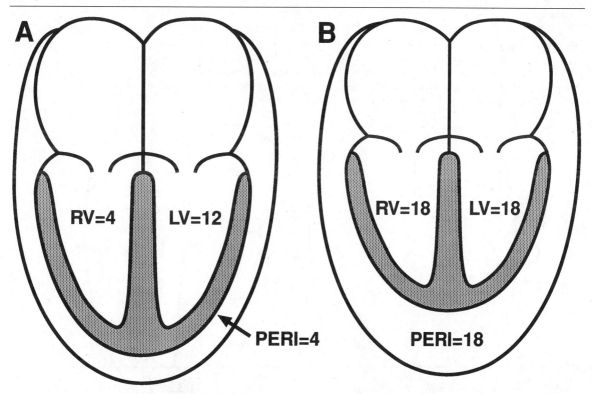

TRANSMURAL DISTENDING PRESSURES
RVTDP   = 4 - 4 = 0
LVTDP   = 12 - 4 = 8

TRANSMURAL DISTENDING PRESSURES
RVTDP   = 18 - 18 = 0
LVTDP   = 18 - 18 = 0

When the diastolic pressures are equal in the pericardial space, the right ventricle, and the left ventricle, then all three spaces are filling against a common compliance — the pericardium. The ventricles are no longer filling against the compliance of their individual muscle walls. In fact, the transmural distending pressure of both ventricles is close to zero. Thus all three spaces are competing for volume against the other two spaces. Increased filling of one ventricle can occur only at the expense of the other. Thus the hallmark of cardiac tamponade is equalization of the intrapericardial, right ventricular, and left ventricular diastolic pressures.

The decrease in transmural distending pressures (approaching zero) of both ventricles produces a decrease in filling of both ventricles. The decrease in filling produces a decrease in stroke volume and cardiac output. Ultimately, blood pressure is decreased. Thus tamponade produces high filling pressure, but the filling volume remains low because the transmural distending pressure is low.

Pulsus Paradoxus

The three clinical features of tamponade are (1) elevated filling pressures (elevated jugular venous pressure), (2) hypotension, and (3) pulsus paradoxus, defined as a fall in systolic blood pressure greater than 10 mm Hg during inspiration. Pulsus paradoxus is an exaggeration of the normal fall in left ventricular stroke volume and systolic pressure, which occurs during inspiration. The mechanism of pulsus paradoxus is related to the competition between the ventricles for filling. As previously stated, both ventricles are filling against the common compliance of the pericardium. One ventricle fills at the expense of the other. During inspiration, the decrease of intrathoracic pressure results in increased filling of the right ventricle. The increased size of the RV results in decreased filling of the LV. The ventricular septum is actually displaced toward the LV (Fig. 8-4).

The increased filling of the right ventricle during inspi-

Fig. 8-4. Mechanism of pulsus paradoxus. During inspiration, decreased intrathoracic pressure causes increased filling of the RV and decreased filling of the LV. This produces a decrease of aortic pressure. During expiration, increased intrathoracic pressure causes decreased filling of the RV and increased filling of the LV. This produces an increase of aortic pressure. (Modified from: Cosio FG, et al. Abnormal septal motion in cardiac tamponade with pulsus paradoxus. *Chest* 71:787, 1977.)

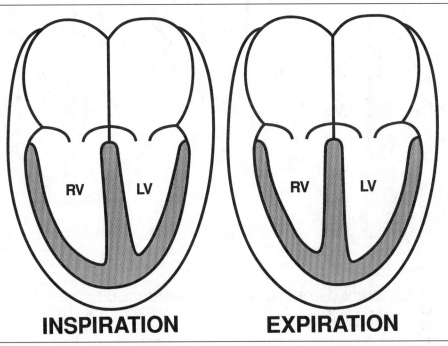

INSPIRATION　　　**EXPIRATION**

ration produces an increase in right ventricular stroke volume and a subsequent increase in RV and PA systolic pressure. The simultaneous decreased filling of the left ventricle during inspiration produces a decrease in left ventricular stroke volume and a subsequent decrease in left ventricle and aortic systolic pressure. During expiration, the situation is reversed. Thus, there is a phasic shift in filling which produces phasic variations in pressures. The pulmonary artery pressure increases while the aortic pressure decreases during inspiration, and the PA pressure decreases while the aortic pressure increases during expiration (Fig. 8-5).

Of note, there are several situations in which pulsus paradoxus is absent during the cardiac tamponade: (1) atrial septal defect prevents the cyclic shifting of ventricular filling with respiration, (2) aortic regurgitation produces a major component of left ventricular filling independent of respiratory variation, and (3) marked cardiac hypertrophy produces elevated left ventricular diastolic pressure, such that tamponade occurs before equalization of diastolic pressures in both ventricles.

Also, pulsus paradoxus can be seen in conditions other than cardiac tamponade. It can be seen with chronic obstructive lung disease, acute asthma, and pulmonary embolism.

Clinical Manifestations

Acute Cardiac Tamponade

The classic description of acute cardiac tamponade includes three elements: (1) elevated jugular venous pressure, (2) hypotension, and (3) a small, quiet heart. This presentation of tamponade is often seen in the surgical emergency department and is produced by sudden hemorrhage into the pericardium. The etiology may include trauma, stab wounds of the heart, rupture of the heart, aortic dissection, and hemorrhage following cardiac surgery. The effusion develops rapidly before the pericardium can stretch. Severe hypotension develops quickly after as little as 150–200 ml of fluid accumulates in the pericardial space. Pulsus paradoxus is present. In fact, the pulse may not be palpable during inspiration. The neck veins are markedly elevated. The precordial impulse is quiet and the heart sounds faint. The situation is emergent and tamponade must be relieved immediately for the patient to survive.

Subacute and Chronic Cardiac Tamponade

Most cases of tamponade seen in the medical wards have developed more slowly from chronic pericardial effusions. The effusions are much larger, up to 1500–2000 ml of fluid, because the pericardium has had time to stretch. The etiologies include idiopathic pericarditis, malignancies, uremia, radiation, infection, and connective tissue diseases.

The most common symptoms of chronic tamponade are dyspnea and tachycardia. The cardinal signs on physical exam include (1) jugular venous distension, (2) pulsus paradoxus, and (3) hypotension. It is extremely important to note that many patients with chronic tamponade do *not* have significant hypotension or only have hypotension during fluid shifts such as occur with dialysis. For this reason, it is extremely important to search for pulsus paradoxus as an early clue to tamponade.

Patients with tamponade have elevated jugular venous pressure. The wave form is important: x-descents are preserved and may be prominent; however, y-descents are usually absent (Fig. 8-6).

Laboratory studies may be useful in confirming cardiac tamponade. The chest x-ray is nonspecific. However, a pericardial effusion is suggested by a large heart shadow with a globular or "water bottle" shape. The EKG is also nonspecific. However, electrical alternans is very suggestive of tamponade. In electrical alternans, the magnitude of the QRS complex varies with every other or every third beat as the heart "swings" within the large pericardial space.

Fig. 8-5. Respiration, aortic (Ao) pressure, right ventricular (RV) pressure, and electrocardiogram (LG) in patient with cardiac tamponade and hypovolemia. Pulsus paradoxus is a fall in systolic aortic pressure greater than 10 mm Hg during inspiration. The right ventricular systolic pressure also varies with respiration. Note that the right ventricular and aortic systolic pressures are out of phase with each other. (From Shabetai R et al. The hemodynamics of cardiac tamponade and constrictive pericarditis. *Am J Cardiol* 26:480, 1970. Reprinted with permission from *American Journal of Cardiology*.)

Pulsus Paradoxus

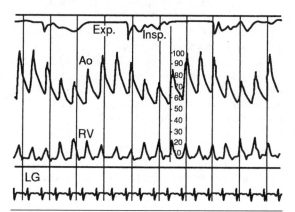

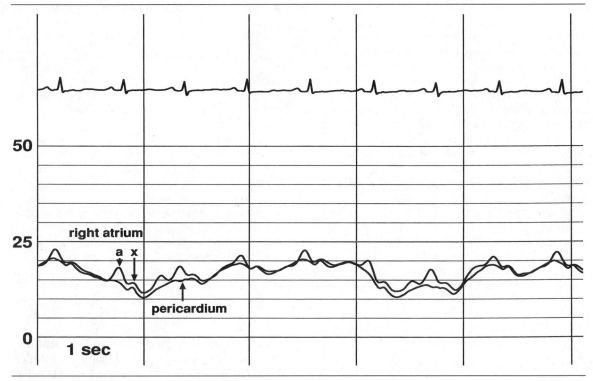

Fig. 8-6. Right atrial and pericardial pressures in cardiac tamponade. The RA pressure is elevated and almost identical to the pericardial pressure (note the slight separation during inspiration). The x-descent is still evident, but the y-descent is absent.

The echocardiogram is essential to document the presence of an effusion. In most cases of subacute and chronic tamponade, there is time to obtain an echocardiogram prior to pericardiocentesis.

The conclusive diagnosis of cardiac tamponade is made by combined cardiac catheterization and pericardiocentesis. The diastolic pressures in the right atrium, right ventricle, left atrium, left ventricle, and intrapericardial space are all equal (Fig. 8-7). Finally, the hemodynamics should improve after drainage of the fluid.

Constrictive Pericarditis

Constrictive pericarditis may develop from months to years after an episode of pericarditis. The pericardium becomes markedly thickened and scarred with fibrous tissue. Usually, pericardial fluid is absent, and the visceral and pari-

etal layers are fused together. In rare cases, a pericardial effusion may exist with selective thickening of the visceral pericardium. Constrictive pericarditis may be caused by any form of pericarditis: idiopathic, infectious, malignant, uremic, radiation-induced, and postpericardiotomy. Prior to effective chemotherapy, the most common cause was tuberculosis. Often the pericardium was heavily calcified and visible on routine chest x-rays.

The pathophysiology of classic constrictive pericarditis can be understood by visualizing the heart surrounded by a rigid shell. The rigid shell restricts filling of both ventricles and results in marked elevations of filling pressure. Since the shell effects both ventricles equally, there is equalization of the RV and LV diastolic pressures (Fig. 8-8).

The pattern of diastolic filling of the ventricles is characteristic for constrictive pericarditis. In early diastole, the rigid shell does not restrict filling, so filling occurs more rapidly than normal due to elevated filling pressures. How-

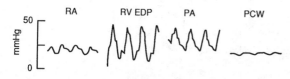

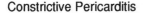

Fig. 8-7. The "pressure plateau" in cardiac tamponade. Equalization of right arterial, right ventricular end-diastolic, pulmonary artery diastolic, and pulmonary capillary wedge pressures. RA = right atrial pressure, RV EDP = right ventricular end-diastolic pressure, PA = pulmonary artery pressure, PCW, pulmonary capillary wedge pressure. (Reproduced with permission from: Weeks KR, et al. Bedside hemodynamic monitoring. *J Thorac Cardiovasc Surg* 71:250, 1976.)

Constrictive Pericarditis

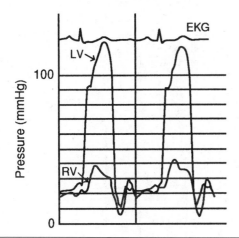

Fig. 8-8. Equalization of the right ventricular and left ventricular diastolic pressures in constrictive pericarditis. Note the waveform has a "dip-and-plateau" or "square-root" configuration. (Reproduced with permission from: Shabetai R and Grossman W. Profiles in constrictive pericarditis, restrictive cardiomyopathy, and cardiac tamponade. In Grossman W (ed), *Cardiac Catheterization and Angiography,* 2nd ed. Philadelphia: Lea & Febiger, 1980, pp. 358–376.)

ever, the ventricular volumes quickly increase to the limits imposed by the surrounding rigid shell. Further filling in late diastole is markedly decreased or even absent. Thus, almost all ventricular filling occurs in early diastole. This situation is in marked contrast to cardiac tamponade, where filling is restricted throughout diastole.

The characteristic pattern of ventricular filling is also reflected in diastolic filling pressures. At the onset of diastole, there is no constraint on filling. Therefore, early diastolic pressures are low. However, the diastolic pressures rapidly rise once the ventricles have expanded to the limits of the rigid pericardial shell. Further filling is extremely limited, so the pressures tend to plateau throughout late diastole. This cardiac pressure pattern has been referred to as "dip and plateau" or "square root sign" (Fig. 8-9).

The atrial pressure patterns are also characteristic for constrictive pericarditis. During diastole, the atrioventricular valves are open and the pressures in the atria and ventricles are equal (Fig. 8-10). The early dip in the ventricular pressures is reflected as a prominent y-descent in the atrial pressures. The atrial pressures also have a prominent x-descent, as in tamponade. The combination of prominent x- and y-descents results in a characteristic appearance referred to as the M or W configuration (Fig. 8-11). This pattern can often be discerned in the examination of the jugular veins at the bedside.

Another characteristic of the atrial and jugular venous pressures is the lack of respiratory variation. Apparently the rigid pericardium prevents transmission of changes in intrathoracic pressure to the heart. Normally, inspiration results in a reduction of intrathoracic pressure and a similar reduction of right atrial pressure. In constrictive pericarditis, the right atrial pressure remains the same or even increases — the so-called Kussmaul's sign.

Thus, the classic features of constrictive pericarditis are (1) elevation of diastolic filling pressures (including the jugular venous and pulmonary capillary wedge pressures), (2) equalization of RV and LV diastolic pressures, (3) dip-and-plateau configuration of ventricular diastolic pressures, (4) prominent x- and y-descents of atrial and jugular venous pressures, and (5) lack of respiratory variation of the right atrial and jugular venous pressure. Of particular note: These features can be mimicked by several other conditions, including restrictive cardiomyopathy and right ventricular infarction.

Clinical Features

The clinical features of constrictive pericarditis are predominantly caused by elevations of the ventricular filling pressures. The elevation of right atrial pressure produces symptoms of venous congestion: edema, ascites, and hepatic congestion. For unknown reasons, ascites is usually more prominent than edema. Some patients may be mistakenly diagnosed as having cirrhosis of the liver.

The elevation of the left atrial pressure produces symp-

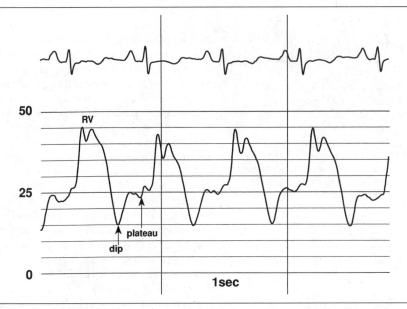

Fig. 8-9. Ventricular pressure in constrictive pericarditis. In constrictive pericarditis the diastolic pressures of both ventricles usually display a characteristic "dip-and-plateau" configuration. Ventricular filling is rapid during early diastole and very limited during late diastole.

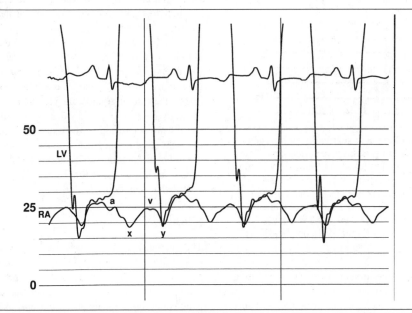

Fig. 8-10. Atrial pressures in constrictive pericarditis. The right atrial pressure is equal to the right ventricular pressure during diastole, since the tricuspid valve is open. The prominent y-descent in the atrial pressure corresponds to the prominent dip in the ventricular pressure.

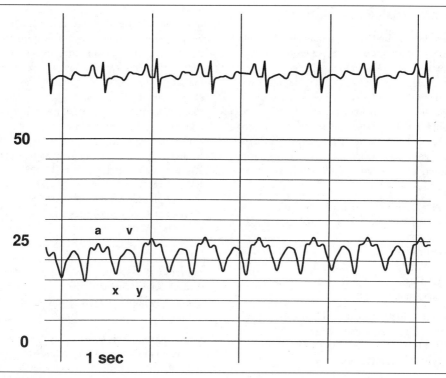

Fig. 8-11. Right atrial pressure in constrictive pericarditis. In constrictive pericarditis, the right atrial pressure usually has prominent x- and y-descents, producing the characteristic M or W configuration.

toms of pulmonary congestion, mainly exertional dyspnea. Orthopnea may occur. Frank pulmonary edema is extremely rare.

Although the cardiac output is usually normal, reduced cardiac output can result in symptoms of fatigue, weight loss, and muscle wasting. The physical exam invariably reveals an elevated jugular venous pressure with prominent x- and y-descents. The Kussmaul's sign (increase of jugular venous pressure during inspiration) may be present. Blood pressure is usually normal and pulsus paradoxus is rare. Auscultation of the heart is usually marked by a diastolic pericardial knock, an early diastolic heart sound similar to an S3, but occurring slightly earlier and having slightly higher pitch. The liver is usually enlarged and ascites may be massive. Edema is a variable feature, but may be quite marked.

The chest x-ray is often normal. However, many patients with tubercular pericarditis have dense calcification of the pericardium. The EKG is nonspecific, but atrial fibrillation is common. The echocardiogram is generally nonspecific, but may reveal thickening of the pericardium. Both the CT scan and magnetic resonance imaging have been found to be very useful in defining thickening of the pericardium.

The diagnosis of constrictive pericarditis is usually made by cardiac catheterization. If the characteristic hemodynamic findings are present and if pericardial involvement is documented by thickening on CT scan or calcification on chest x-ray, then the diagnosis is certain. Occasionally, constrictive pericarditis cannot be distinguished from restrictive cardiomyopathy on clinical grounds. A percutaneous biopsy of the right ventricle may suggest restrictive cardiomyopathy by revealing myocardial fibrosis, amyloidosis, or hemochromatosis. Rarely, surgical exploration of the pericardium is required to distinguish constrictive pericarditis from restrictive cardiomyopathy.

Clinical Examples

1. A 53-year-old man, undergoing hemodialysis for end-stage renal disease, develops severe hypotension with systolic blood pressures as low as 60 mm Hg. The patient is resuscitated with elevation of the feet and rapid infusion of 500 ml of normal saline. Following saline infusion the BP increases to 90/60 with a paradox of 20 mm Hg. The neck veins are distended with an estimated central venous pressure of 15 cm H_2O. Chest x-ray reveals a massively enlarged heart with a "water bottle" shape. An echocardiogram reveals a large anterior and posterior pericardial effusion.

Hemodynamics

BP   95/60 mm Hg with paradox of 20 mm Hg
RA   16 mm Hg with prominent x-descents, no
            y-descents
RV   30/16 mm Hg
PA   30/16 mm Hg
PCW   17 mm Hg
CO   3.8 liters/min

Pericardiocentesis is performed in the cardiac catheterization laboratory. The pericardial pressure is 16 mm Hg (equal to RA and PCW pressure). Approximately 1400 ml of serosanguinous fluid is removed.

Follow-Up Hemodynamics

BP   105/70 mm Hg with paradox of 8 mm Hg
RA   8 mm Hg with normal a- and v-waves and
            normal x- and y-descents
RV   30/9 mm Hg
PA   30/12 mm Hg
PCW   16 mm Hg
CO   4.85 liters/min

Discussion.   This case reveals all the features of chronic pericardial effusion with tamponade: (1) large pericardial effusion, (2) pulsus paradoxus, (3) elevated CVP with absent y-descents, (4) mild hypotension, (5) equalization of RA, RV diastolic, PCW and pericardial pressure, and (6) most significantly, resolution of abnormalities following pericardiocentesis. Note that the PCW pressure remained elevated, probably secondary to left ventricular hypertrophy and/or fluid overload secondary to renal failure. Also note that if LV filling pressures are extremely high, tamponade can occur **before** complete equalization of LV and RV filling pressures. In that situation, pulsus paradoxus will **not** be observed.

2. A 46-year-old man was referred to the gastroenterology service for evaluation of cirrhosis and ascites. He had a one-year history of progressive abdominal swelling and mild ankle edema. On physical examination, he had elevated jugular venous pressure with prominent x- and y-descents. Cardiac exam revealed a third heart sound, suspected to be a pericardial knock. The abdomen was massively distended with a fluid wave and marked hepatomegaly. The chest x-ray and EKG were unremarkable. The echocardiogram revealed normal ventricular function and possible thickening of the pericardium.

Cardiac catheterization was performed and revealed hemodynamics typical of constrictive pericarditis. Both RA and PCW pressures were elevated to 18 mm Hg. The RV and LV diastolic pressures were equal and revealed a dip-and-plateau configuration. The RA pressure had prominent x- and y-descents and increased during inspiration. The LV had a normal ejection fraction. Fluoroscopy revealed mild calcification of the pericardium.

Thoracotomy revealed a thickened pericardium. Following removal of the pericardium, the patient gradually improved. After 6 months, the patient's physical exam was completely normal, and his exercise capacity had returned to normal.

Discussion.   This case reveals the importance of careful examination of the jugular venous pulsations in **any** patient presenting with ascites or edema. Constrictive pericarditis is a potentially curable cause of hepatomegaly, massive ascites, or edema. Of note, the hemodynamics of constriction may take several months to resolve. In some cases, complete resolution will not occur due to either incomplete pericardial resection or extension of fibrosis into the myocardium.

Bibliography

Corey GR, Campbell PT, Van Trigt P, et al. Etiology of large pericardial effusions. *Am J Med* 95:209–213, 1993. *This study examined the usefulness of pericardial fluid and pericardial tissue in diagnosing the etiology of large pericardial effusions.*

Kern MJ and Aguirre F. Interpretation of cardiac pathophysiology from pressure waveform analysis: pericardial compressive hemodynamics, Part I, II, and III. *Cathet Cardiovasc Diagn* 25:336–342, 1992, 26:34–40, 1992, and 26:152–158, 1992. *This series of articles analyzes pressure waveforms in patients with cardiac tamponade and constrictive pericarditis.*

Spodick DH. Macrophysiology, microphysiology, and anatomy of the pericardium: a synopsis. *Am Heart J*

124:1046–1051, 1992. *A concise review of the anatomy and physiology of the normal pericardium.*

Trabouls M, Scott-Douglas NW, Smith ER, et al. The right and left ventricular intracavitary and transmural pressure-strain relationships. *Am Heart J* 123:1279–1287, 1992. *Examines the effects of the normal pericardium on ventricular function, referred to as pericardial constraint.*

Vaitkus PT and Kussmaul WG: Constrictive pericarditis versus restrictive cardiomyopathy: a reappraisal and up-date of diagnostic criteria. *Am Heart J* 122:1431–1441, 1991. *An excellent review of the clinical and hemodynamic criteria used to distinguish constrictive pericarditis and restrictive cardiomyopathy.*

Watkins MW and LeWinter MM. Physiologic role of the normal pericardium. *Ann Rev Med* 44:171–180, 1993. *A concise review of the physiology of the normal pericardium in normal conditions and several selected disease states.*

9 Infective Endocarditis

Chittur A. Sivaram and Douglas P. Fine

Objectives

After completing this chapter, you should be able to

Have a basic understanding of the types of endocarditis

Know the differences in the microbiology of acute, subacute, and prosthetic valve endocarditis

Understand the characteristic clinical features in infective endocarditis and their pathogenesis

Know the nature of the complications of infective endocarditis

Identify the appropriate tests for the confirmation of the diagnosis of infective endocarditis

---

Infective endocarditis is the general term for bacterial or fungal infection of the endocardial surface, and particularly cardiac valves; more specific terms for subcategories of infective endocarditis include subacute or acute bacterial endocarditis, fungal endocarditis, etc. (see below). Many of the general principles regarding infective endocarditis could also be applied to infections of other endothelial surfaces (e.g., aortic aneurysms, arteriovenous shunts); however, this discussion will confine itself to endocardial infections.

Acute and subacute infective endocarditis are two different clinical syndromes. Subacute endocarditis is of weeks' or months' duration and is associated with a relatively indolent course and rather more subtle or mild symptoms. As a general rule, subacute endocarditis requires a predisposing abnormality of the valve and is caused by organisms of lesser virulence. In contrast, acute endocarditis may involve previously normal valves, is caused by organisms of greater virulence, and has a more fulminant, rapidly progressive course with a poorer prognosis. Historically, subacute was the most common form of infective endocarditis, but in recent decades acute endocarditis has been commonly encountered.

In addition to native valves, bacteria and fungi may also infect prosthetic valves. Organisms causing prosthetic endocarditis differ, depending on whether the infection occurs early or late after valve replacement.

Bacteria or fungi circulating in the bloodstream from any peripheral site initiate endocarditis by attaching to the heart valve (particularly at a previously damaged site with a fibrin and platelet nidus) and then proliferating locally. Eventually macrocolonies of organisms enmeshed in platelets and fibrin form the hallmark of endocarditis, the "vegetation." Not only does the vegetation continuously seed the bloodstream with bacteria and sometimes with larger fragments of the mass (emboli), but the underlying inflammation and valve injury can lead to dysfunction and destruction of the valve (Fig. 9-1).

Infections of heart valves (and other intravascular structures) are unique in one very important way. Valves are fibrous structures without the soft-tissue matrix and vascular supply of most other tissues, and they exist within the rapidly flowing environment of the bloodstream. Therefore, polymorphonuclear neutrophilic leukocytes cannot protect against or combat infection. Defenses against endocarditis are the bactericidal activity of serum (complement and antibody), which can kill circulating microorganisms, the continuous flowing of the bloodstream,

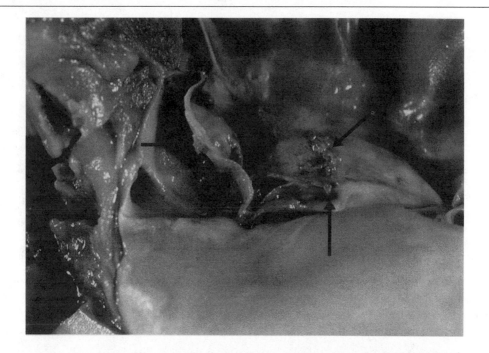

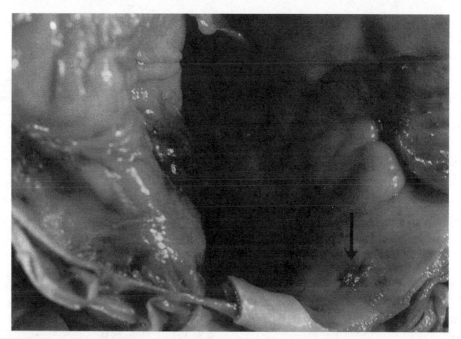

Fig. 9-1. Vegetations in a patient with *Staphylococcus aureus* aortic valve endocarditis. (Top) Arrows point to vegetations at three separate sites on the aortic valve. (Bottom) Endocardial surface lesions on the cardiac wall away from the valve. (Figure provided courtesy of Leonard N. Slater, M.D.)

which inhibits initial attachment, and the ability of endothelial cells to resist attachment of bacteria. Cure of endocarditis can probably only rarely be accomplished by the host without antimicrobial chemotherapy, which must be executed so that microbicidal concentrations of the antimicrobial agent bathe the valve almost continuously for prolonged periods.

Pathophysiology

Susceptible Cardiac Lesions

Development of infective endocarditis is favored by a susceptible cardiac lesion on which microorganisms may adhere and infection progress. Endocarditis can develop on anatomically normal valves, but does so usually in intravenous drug addicts or in association with specific highly virulent organisms. In addition to native valves, prosthetic valves and occasionally endocardium may develop infection. The most susceptible cardiac lesions are prosthetic valve, bicuspid aortic valve, mitral valve prolapse with mitral regurgitation, ventricular septal defect, patent ductus arteriosus, and coarctation of aorta. History of previous endocarditis is also thought to be a risk factor. Lesions with intermediate risk for endocarditis are mitral stenosis, tricuspid valve disease, hypertrophic cardiomyopathy, sclerotic aortic valve of the elderly, and nonvalvular intracardiac implants such as pacemakers. Certain lesion such as atrial septal defect (secundum type), mitral valve prolapse without mitral regurgitation, coronary artery disease, and surgically corrected cardiac lesions (without prosthetic implants 6 months after surgery) have low risk for development of endocarditis.

Historically, the most common cause of valvular lesions was rheumatic carditis. That disease has been uncommon in developed countries in recent decades; however, recent localized epidemics in the United States and elsewhere may presage a resurgence.

Microbiology

The organisms which cause infective endocarditis vary, depending upon the clinical syndrome, the underlying state of the valve, and, in the case of prosthetic valve endocarditis, the length of time since valve replacement (Table 9-1).

Subacute Endocarditis, Native Valve

Viridans streptococci (e.g., *Streptococcus mutans, Streptococcus sanguis*), normal inhabitants of the oral and intestinal cavities, are the most common causes of the syndrome

Table 9-1. Organisms Causing Endocarditis Under Known Conditions

SUBACUTE ENDOCARDITIS, NATIVE VALVE

Viridans streptococci
Enterococci
Haemophilus species
Streptococcus bovis

ACUTE ENDOCARDITIS, NATIVE VALVE

Staphylococcus aureus
Neisseria gonorrhoeae
Streptococcus pyogenes
Streptococcus pneumoniae
Pseudomonas aeruginosa
Candida albicans

PROSTHETIC VALVE ENDOCARDITIS, WITHIN 2 MONTHS

Staphylococcus aureus
Staphylococcus epidermidis
Gram-negative enteric bacilli
Pseudomonas aeruginosa
Haemophilus species
Enterococci

PROSTHETIC VALVE, GREATER THAN 2 MONTHS

Staphylococcus epidermidis
Viridans streptococci
Gram-negative enteric bacilli
Pseudomonas aeruginosa
Acinetobacter calcoaceticus
Haemophilus species
Staphylococcus aureus
Enterococci
Corynebacteria
Propionibacteria
Candida species

of subacute endocarditis and generally infect previously damaged valves. Enterococci (*Enterococcus faecalis* and *Enterococcus faecium*) and *Streptococcus bovis* may cause subacute disease. Less commonly encountered are *Haemophilus* species such as *H. aphrophilus* and *H. parainfluenzae*.

Acute Endocarditis, Native Valve

Staphylococcus aureus is the major cause of acute endocarditis. Organisms which can do so but have been uncommonly encountered in recent years include *Neisseria gonorrhoeae, Streptococcus pyogenes,* and *Streptococcus pneumoniae*. Among intravenous drug users, *Pseudomonas aeruginosa* may cause this syndrome, particularly affecting the tricuspid valve. More recently, *Candida albicans* and occasionally other fungi have been encountered.

Prosthetic Valve Endocarditis, Within 2 Months of Surgery

Staphylococci, particularly *S. aureus* but also including *Staphylococcus epidermidis,* are predominant organisms causing prosthetic valve infection early after surgery. Gram-negative enteric bacteria (e.g., *Klebsiella pneumoniae, Serratia marcescens*) and *Haemophilus* species are important pathogens. Enterococci may be encountered as well. These infections tend to be associated with a syndrome similar to acute endocarditis.

Prosthetic Valve Endocarditis, After 2 Months

Later infections are more likely to resemble subacute endocarditis and the organisms encountered include viridans streptococci, corynebacteria, propionibacteria, and *S. epidermidis,* as well as *S. aureus* and a variety of gram-negative bacteria.

Consequences of Lesions of Endocarditis

The development of progressive valvular destruction and valvular regurgitation is the most serious consequence in infective endocarditis. Uncontrolled infection leads to erosion of valve cusps, rupture of chordae tendineae, and in the most severe instances total disappearance of the valve tissue. The consequence is varying degrees of valvular regurgitation. Effective compensatory mechanisms cannot be generated in the acute valvular regurgitation of infective endocarditis, and symptoms of heart failure develop precipitously. The onset of acute heart failure in a patient with infective endocarditis strongly suggests progressive valve destruction and acute regurgitant lesions. Aortic and mitral valve endocarditis may be complicated by severe pulmonary edema, which may be very rapid in onset and progression. The inability of the ventricles and atria to dilate and accommodate the regurgitant volume results in marked elevation of ventricular end-diastolic and left atrial pressures.

Vegetations in infective endocarditis tend to be friable and capable of embolism. Occasionally, embolic phenomena may be the presenting symptom. The size of the vegetation (larger than 1.0–1.5 cm^2 by echocardiography) and fungal etiology have been found to increase chances of embolism. The consequences of embolism depend on the circulation involved in the process. Cerebrovascular accidents, ischemia of an extremity leading to gangrene, splenic infarction, renal infarction, and mesenteric infarction leading to acute abdomen may result. In the daily evaluation of a patient with infective endocarditis, careful examination of the peripheral pulses and cardiac auscultation are important. In endocarditis of the tricuspid valve, the embolic phenomena lead to pulmonary embolism and pulmonary infarction.

Occasionally abscesses extend from the vegetation into the perivalvular area (valve ring abscess) or myocardium. These abscesses may compress or destroy the cardiac conduction tissue and produce heart block. A rare complication of aortic valve endocarditis is weakening of the region between aortic and mitral annuli with formation of an aneurysmal pouch (aneurysm of the intervalvular fibrosa). Such an aneurysm may occasionally rupture into the left atrium, causing mitral regurgitation.

Clinical Presentation

Fever and Constitutional Symptoms

Fever is a hallmark of endocarditis, and it is a rare patient who will not manifest it at some point. In acute endocarditis, fever is usually high and associated with systemic symptoms, including chills, myalgia, arthralgia, malaise, all of which may be severe. Headaches and gastrointestinal symptoms (e.g., nausea, vomiting, diarrhea) may be present. Patients appear very ill and may be confused. In contrast, subacute endocarditis is usually a much more subtle disease. Fever is often low grade, and systemic symptoms mild. Night sweats may be the only clue to fever. Malaise, fatigue, and weight loss are more likely to dominate the clinical picture. Myalgia, arthralgia, and headache may be present.

Stigmata of Endocarditis

Extracardiac physical findings, if present, include pallor as a manifestation of the anemia common in endocarditis, wasting, splenomegaly, and certain cutaneous lesions characteristic (but not diagnostic) of endocarditis. Osler nodes are small (1–2 mm), tender erythematous nodules particularly noted on the finger or toe pads. Janeway lesions are flatter subcutaneous macular purplish or reddish lesions on the palms or soles. They are painless. Nail beds may show splinter hemorrhages, small subungual flamelike hemorrhagic streaks near the base of the nail. Petechiae are common and may be seen on skin, conjunctivae, or soft palate. Roth spots, 1–3 mm hemorrhages with a whitish center, may be seen on the retinal surface. These lesions reflect end-arteritis due to infected microemboli from the vegetation or immune-complex disposition. In general, all the stigmata are more likely to be present in subacute endocarditis or in endocarditis due to *S. aureus,* but even in these circumstances they are uncommon.

Cardiac Findings

Sinus tachycardia is frequently present as a result of infection. Pulse pressure may be increased in aortic valve endocarditis due to regurgitation, even though in acute aortic regurgitation the pulse pressure may remain normal. Clinical evidence for left ventricular failure may be present if hemodynamically severe left-sided regurgitant lesions exist. In tricuspid valve endocarditis with regurgitation, jugular venous pressure may be elevated, with venous pulse showing large v-waves and sharp y-descent. In acute endocarditis, no significant displacement of PMI is present. The murmurs of acute mitral and aortic regurgitation tend to be quite different from the murmurs of chronic mitral and aortic regurgitation. The murmurs of hemodynamically severe acute mitral and aortic regurgitation may be brief and soft because the rapid rise of pressures in the chamber receiving the regurgitant jet stop the turbulent flow earlier than in chronic lesions. In acute mitral regurgitation, a loud fourth heart sound is often heard. Third heart sound is common. The murmurs may be particularly difficult to auscultate in patients with pulmonary edema due to interference from lung sounds. Changing heart murmurs have been thought to be characteristic of infective endocarditis, even though the value of the finding is not clearly known. However the appearance of a new diastolic murmur always suggests progressive valve disruption in endocarditis. Rarely obstruction to flow and resultant murmur may be produced by a very large vegetation. A pericardial friction rub is rare in infective endocarditis and may suggest aortic valve ring abscess.

Complications

Complication of infective endocarditis can be divided into cardiac and noncardiac. Cardiac complications include progressive valvular regurgitation, progressive heart failure, pericarditis, heart blocks and other conduction disturbances due to development of abscesses, and mycotic aneurysms (weakening of a vessel wall due to embolization into the vessel wall). Noncardiac complications are renal failure, systemic embolism (leading to cerebrovascular accidents, ischemia of various organs, and gangrene), intracranial hemorrhage due to ruptured cerebral mycotic aneurysms, and meningoencephalitis.

Diagnosis
Clinical Laboratory

The only way to establish the diagnosis of infective endocarditis (short of surgery or autopsy) is to culture mi-croorganisms from blood. Even then, a logical, analytical approach is necessary to be able to diagnose endocarditis. Endovascular infections such as endocarditis are characterized by nearly continuous bacteremia, whereas with other infections (e.g., urinary tract infection, pneumonia, meningitis, soft-tissue abscess) if bacteremia occurs it is intermittent or transient. Therefore, the diagnosis of endocarditis requires multiple (three is usually sufficient) blood cultures obtained over a period of time (1–2 hours for acute endocarditis in which therapy cannot be delayed, 12–48 hours for subacute endocarditis). If only one is positive, endocarditis is less likely, whereas two or more positive cultures strongly indicate endovascular infection.

Culturing the organism also, of course, permits in vitro susceptibility testing to identify the most effective and safe antimicrobials for the prolonged (4–8 weeks) intravenous therapy necessary. Effectiveness of therapy may be monitored by serum bactericidal titer (serum-killing power) which documents bactericidal concentrations of antimicrobials in the blood; use of these tests is complicated and of debated benefit.

Other laboratory tests are primarily important to identify complications. Patients are typically mildly to moderately anemic. Leukocyte counts are elevated with a left shift. Platelet counts may be decreased (acute toxicity) or increased (chronic infection) or normal. In the event of renal involvement by emboli or immune-complex mediated glomerulonephritis, hematuria may be noted. In immune-complex disease, the urine sediment may demonstrate pyuria, hematuria, proteinuria, and the presence of erythrocyte casts. Creatinine clearance may be reduced. Other laboratory studies are of limited value. In the presence of neurological symptoms, cerebrospinal fluid pleocytosis and protein elevation may indicate parameningeal microabscesses secondary to bacteremia, or even purulent meningitis, in which case the spinal fluid glucose would be decreased and organisms may be identified by culture or stain.

Following institution of appropriate therapy, serial blood cultures should be obtained to document microbiological cure. A reasonable plan would be one culture daily or every other day until negative.

Echocardiography

The role of echocardiography in the diagnosis of infective endocarditis has been well validated. The diagnosis of endocarditis by echo is based on the demonstration of vegetations (Fig. 9-2). Typically vegetations appear as echogenic masses on valves with irregular and shaggy edges. Vegetations also exhibit excessive mobility — unlike

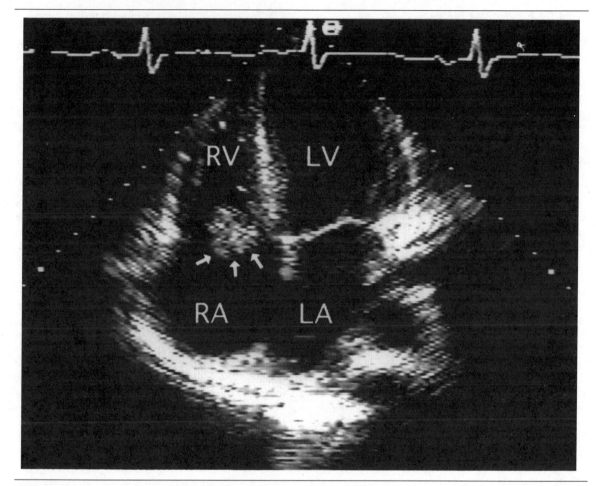

Fig. 9-2. Transthoracic echocardiogram (four-chamber view) showing a large vegetation on the tricuspid valve in a drug addict with *Staph. aureus* endocarditis. LV = left ventricle; LA = left atrium; RV = right ventricle; RA = right atrium. Arrows indicate the vegetation.

fibrosis or calcification of the valves, with which they may be confused. The presence of varying degrees of valvular regurgitation will be an additional echocardiographic finding consistent with endocarditis. Echocardiography can also reveal the presence of an underlying valve lesion susceptible to endocarditis. Since the resolution of echocardiography is about 2 mm, only vegetations larger than 2 mm will be demonstrated. When complications such as severe valvular regurgitation or valve ring abscess are present in infective endocarditis, echocardiography may be highly valuable for demonstration and localization of lesions. Colorflow Doppler can assess the severity of regur-

gitant lesions. Diagnosis of prosthetic valve endocarditis by echocardiography is more difficult due to multiple artefacts from reverberation and shadowing originating in the mechanical components of the prosthesis.

For evaluation of infective endocarditis, often transesophageal rather than transthoracic echocardiography is required. The sensitivity of transthoracic echo in endocarditis is only 40–50%, whereas the sensitivity of transesophageal echo is 80%. The diagnostic accuracy of transesophageal echocardiography is higher than transthoracic echo in detection of valve ring abscess as well. Information from the echocardiogram should always be used in conjunction with clinical and microbiologic data. Occasionally, serial echocardiograms may be required for the confirmation of endocarditis. The size of the vegetations can indicate high risk for embolism.

Treatment

Antimicrobial Therapy

In the case of acute infective endocarditis, the severity of illness usually demands empiric therapy based on likely organisms. The most commonly employed empiric regimen is vancomycin and an aminoglycoside (e.g., gentamicin, tobramycin, amikacin). Vancomycin is effective for staphylococci (including methicillin-resistant *S. aureus* and *S. epidermidis*), most enterococci, and other gram-positive bacteria. The aminoglycoside adds synergy for enterococci and treatment for gram-negative bacteria. An alternative regimen would combine nafcillin (or oxacillin) plus an aminoglycoside. Unless the clinical situation mandates, therapy for subacute endocarditis can usually be deferred until cultures are positive.

In either case, antimicrobial choices should be tailored to the organism(s) isolated from blood, guided by in vitro susceptibility tests. Antimicrobials chosen should be microbicidal if possible. Therapy should be continued a minimum of 4 weeks and often longer.

Surgery

Surgical therapy is reserved for patients with infective endocarditis who develop complications. Progressive valvular regurgitation due to destruction of the valve by infection is the most common indication for surgery. Depending on the degree of hemodynamic instability, decision for elective or emergency surgery is made. Risk of valve replacement in the face of ongoing infection should be balanced with risk of intractable heart failure from severe valvular regurgitation, but surgery during acute infective endocarditis can usually be undertaken with acceptable risk. The presence of abscess (myocardial or valve ring) is another indication for surgery. Occasionally surgery is required due to recurrent embolism. Even though valve replacement is the commonest surgical procedure done in endocarditis, excision of the tricuspid valve is occasionally performed in tricuspid valve endocarditis in drug addicts and vegetations have sometimes been excised from otherwise functional valves. Allografts (homografts) are the ideal prosthesis in endocarditis as they resist infection the best. Antibiotic therapy is invariably continued in the postoperative period.

Clinical Examples

1. A 65-year-old man presents with progressive malaise, weakness, low-grade fever, and joint pains of 3 weeks' duration. He was hospitalized 3 weeks ago for Crohn's disease. In preparation for elective bowel surgery in a couple of weeks, he has been receiving parenteral hyperalimentation through a central line. He denies prior history of cardiac disease. He has no chest pain, dyspnea, or paroxysmal nocturnal dyspnea. Examination reveals an ill-appearing male, with temperature 100 degrees, pulse 100 beats/minute with brisk upstroke, blood pressure 150/60 mm Hg. He has no clubbing, Osler nodes, or splinter hemorrhages. A few conjunctival petechiae are present. Jugular venous pressure is normal. PMI is impalpable, S1 and S2 are normal. A grade 3/6 ejection systolic murmur and a soft early diastolic decrescendo murmur are heard along the left sternal border. Abdomen and respiratory system are normal. Fundi are normal. There is erythema and tenderness of the insertion site of the central venous catheter. Investigations reveal hemoglobin of 10 g%, hematocrit of 30%, leukocyte count of 21,000 cells/μl with left shift. Urinalysis shows 10–15 red blood cells per high-powered field. Blood urea nitrogen is 20 dl and creatinine 0.9 dl. EKG shows sinus rhythm, PR interval of 0.26 sec, nonspecific T inversions. Chest x-ray shows normal-sized cardiac silhouette, no signs of failure and no lung abnormalities. A transthoracic echocardiogram (technically difficult study) shows thickening of the aortic valve and aortic regurgitation of uncertain severity. Within 6 hours of admission the patient develops acute dyspnea followed by syncope. During cardiopulmonary resuscitation, it is noted that the patient is in severe respiratory distress and complete heart block. The patient is intubated and temporary transvenous pacing is started. In an hour the patient stabilizes. An emergency transesophageal echocardiogram shows large vegetations on the aortic valve, severe aortic regurgitation, and an abscess in the region of the left cusp. Blood cultures show growth of gram-positive cocci. The presumptive diagnosis is staphylococcal endocarditis of the aortic valve (portal of entry being the central line) with severe aortic regurgitation, valve ring abscess, and complete heart block. Antibiotic therapy is initiated with vancomycin and gentamicin. Patient undergoes emergency surgery to drain a valve ring abscess and replace the aortic valve with an allograft.

Discussion.   This patient, whose valves were apparently previously normal, developed a syndrome of acute endocarditis, characterized by onset over a few days of high fever, malaise, weakness, and arthralgia. The diagnosis of endocarditis was suggested by the syndrome, the physical examination findings (murmur of aortic insufficiency, conjunctival petechiae), and an obvious portal of entry (the visibly inflamed central venous catheter). Diagnosis was confirmed by positive blood cultures. However, shortly after his arrival at the hospital, he developed rapidly progressing valve failure, heart block, and congestive failure. The occurrence of complete heart block as well as the pre-existing first degree AV block are consistent with the development of aortic valve ring abscess. He required emergent surgery to debride the valve ring abscess and replace the now-destroyed valve. Surgery was followed by prolonged antimicrobial therapy. This course is entirely compatible with *S. aureus* acute endocarditis: nondamaged valve, rapid progression of valve destruction, severe clinical syndrome.

2. A 62-year-old man was in good health until 3 months ago, when he developed low-back pain consequent to heavy lifting. A diagnosis of degenerative joint disease was made; roentgenograms of the lumbar spine were consistent. At that time, his physician noted a low-grade fever (38.0°C orally), of which the patient was unaware. No further workup or therapy was done at that time. However, over the next two months the patient has become aware of almost daily fever, usually low grade, but occasionally as high as 39.2°C. With fever, he feels fatigued and "yucky." He notes anorexia and a 20-lb. weight loss. He has received several courses of oral antibiotics without obvious benefit. He continues to note moderately severe low-back pain. Physical examination is normal except for marked tenderness over the lumbosacral spine. Careful auscultation by several observers reveals no murmur. Laboratory studies are remarkable for a persistent mild leukocytosis (12–16,000 cells/μl over the previous 2 months) with a persistent left shift, progressive anemia (hemoglobin now 9.9 g/dl), persistent thrombocytosis (542,000–659,000 cells/μl). Repeat lumbosacral spine films suggest osteomyelitis of L4–5. EKG and chest roentgenograms are normal. Three separate blood cultures obtained over a 48-hour span grow *Enterococcus faecalis*. Therapy is initiated with vancomycin and gentamicin, which is followed by rapid defervescence, improved sense of well-being, and

gradually decreasing low-back pain. His course, however, is stormy and complicated: severe allergic reactions to vancomycin and penicillins, progressive valve dysfunction and aortic insufficiency, eventual surgical replacement of the aortic valve, and postoperative *S. aureus* sternal wound infection. Eventually, after prolonged parenteral and then oral antibiotic therapy for the sternal wound and (presumed) enterococcal vertebral osteomyelitis, he recovers completely.

Discussion. This man had an illness lasting over 2 months before diagnosis. The vertebral osteomyelitis may have been the primary site of infection (seeded from urinary or gastrointestinal tract) or secondary to the endocarditis. At any rate, by time of presentation, he had sustained bacteremia and then gradually developed clinically evident endocarditis. His syndrome was characteristic of subacute endocarditis.

Bibliography

Baddour LM, Christensen GD, Lowrance JH, and Simpson WA. Pathogenesis of experimental endocarditis. *Rev Infect Dis* 11:452–463, 1989. *Relatively recent review of experimental endocarditis and information gained relevant to human disease.*

Bayer AS. Infective endocarditis. *Clin Infect Dis* 17:313–322, 1993. *Excellent recent review.*

Fang G, Keys TF, Gentry LO, et al. Prosthetic valve endocarditis resulting from nosocomial bacteremia. *Ann Intern Med* 119:560–567, 1993. *A multicenter prospective evaluation. Thorough and informative.*

Freedman LR. The pathogenesis of infective endocarditis. *J Antimicrob Chemother* 20 (suppl A):1–6, 1987. *Reflective article principally focused on experimental endocarditis and unanswered questions.*

Von Reyn CF, Levy BS, Arbeit RD, et al. Infective endocarditis: An analysis based on strict case definitions. *Ann Intern Med* 94:505–518, 1981. *Standard reference in the field and a source for strict criteria for diagnosis.*

Wilson WR, Jaumin PM, Danielson GK, et al. Prosthetic valve endocarditis. *Ann Intern Med* 82:751–756, 1975. *An early and excellent review.*

10 Congestive Heart Failure

Udho Thadani

Objectives

After completing this chapter, you should be able to

List the types of heart failure

Understand systolic versus diastolic left ventricular dysfunction

Distinguish differences between volume and pressure overload

List the common causes of heart failure

Understand the importance of neurohormonal activation in perpetuating heart failure

Recognize symptoms and signs of failure

State general treatment guidelines for heart failrue

Congestive heart failure is a constellation of symptoms and signs due to the impaired function of the heart. Clinical heart failure manifests when normal physiologic compensatory mechanisms fail. Activation of the neuroendocrine factors that are initially compensatory may perpetuate heart failure with deleterious consequences.

This chapter focuses on the pathophysiological aspects of heart failure and lays the foundation for understanding the mechanisms responsible for the symptoms and signs of heart failure and how these can be appropriately treated.

General Description

Congestive heart failure is a syndrome in which an abnormality of cardiac function is responsible for the failure of the heart to pump blood at a rate adequate for the metabolic demand of peripheral tissues (organs). It is characterized by an abnormal relationship between left ventricular filling pressure and cardiac output. Clinical presentations result from the combination of depressed myocardial performance (Fig. 10-1), inadequate peripheral organ function, greater ventricular filling pressure due to decreased inotropic state or decreased ventricular compliance leading to increased venous pressure, neurohu-

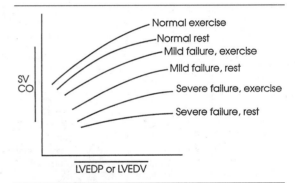

Fig. 10-1. Frank-Starling function curves in normal and in mild and severe heart failure. SV = stroke volume; CO = cardiac output; LVEDP = left ventricular end-diastolic pressure; LVEDV = left ventricular end-diastolic volume. (Reprinted with permission from: Kaufman CE and Papper S. (eds.). *Review of Pathophysiology.* Boston: Little, Brown, 1983, p. 66.)

moral changes, fluid retention, peripheral congestion, and edema.

Although heart (pump) failure is usually due to myocardial (muscle) failure, it may occur from impaired ventricular filling, as in restrictive cardiomyopathy and in constrictive pericarditis. In the early stages of heart failure, various compensatory mechanisms come into play in order to maintain the cardiac output. However, with time these compensatory mechanisms often are exhausted or overshoot and may produce detrimental effects and perpetuate further heart failure (Fig. 10-2).

Heart failure may develop acutely or be of insidious onset. In acute heart failure, attributable either to sudden increase in afterload to the heart (for example, acute hypertensive crisis) or to a sudden volume overload (for example, mitral regurgitation due to papillary muscle rupture), the heart does not have adequate time to develop

Fig. 10-2. The pathophysiology of heart failure involves the interaction of intrinsic cardiac function with neurohormonal activation, peripheral vasoconstriction, and volume expansion. Neurohormonal activation may increase vasoconstriction and lead to a vicious cycle of worsening cardiac function. Natriuretic peptides and other hormones with vasodilating properties may have potentially beneficial effects on vasoconstriction and volume expansion. This complex model is influenced by numerous factors, including age of patient, drugs, presence of coronary artery disease, and the constant feedback of the various regulatory systems. → Demonstrated effect; - - - → Possible effect; + Positive feedback; – Negative feedback; ↓ Decrease; ↑ Increase; Ca^{2+} Intracellular calcium concentrations. (From: Johnstone DE et al. Diagnosis and management of heart failure. *Can J Cardiol* 10:614, 1994. Reproduced with permission of *Canadian Journal of Cardiology,* 1994; 10:614.)

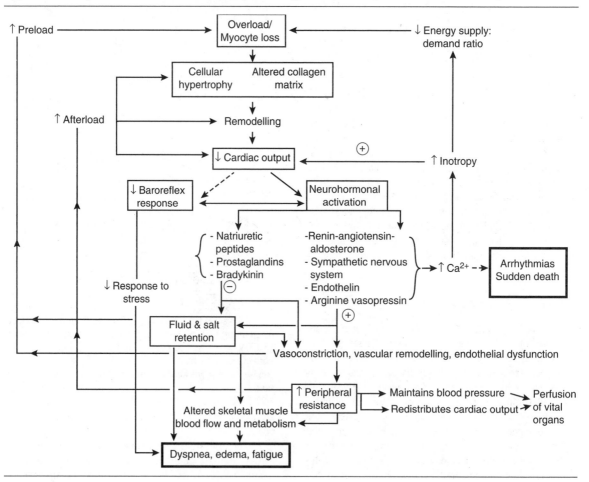

compensatory mechanisms. Therefore, heart failure is abrupt and more severe.

Compensatory Mechanisms

Four principal compensatory mechanisms are available to maintain adequate cardiac output and organ perfusion in the early stages of heart failure:

1. Use of the Frank-Starling mechanism (preload reserve) is achieved by increasing ventricular end-diastolic volume (increasing preload). This leads to increased muscle fiber length with resultant increase in contractile force and cardiac output.
2. Increased catecholamine release from adrenergic nerves and adrenal medulla results in increased heart rate and myocardial contractility.
3. Activation of the renin-angiotensin system leads to fluid retention and therefore an increase in preload. Both this system and the increased catecholamine levels produce vasoconstriction in an effort to maintain blood pressure.
4. Cardiac hypertrophy leads to augmentation of the heart pump function due to an increased myocardial muscle mass. However, myocardial contractility per unit muscle mass is usually depressed, although it may occasionally be normal.

All these compensatory mechanisms are of limited and finite potential and take place at the expense of increased myocardial metabolic (oxygen) consumption. Heart rate, myocardial contractility, and myocardial tension developed are the major determinants of myocardial oxygen consumption. Myocardial tension (wall tension, T) is directly related to the ventricular pressure (P) and the radius (R) of the ventricular cavity ($T = PR$). Myocardial dilation leads to increased radius with resultant increase in myocardial oxygen consumption. In early stages of heart failure, cardiac compensatory mechanisms may be adequate to maintain ventricular performance but ultimately ventricular function deteriorates and clinical heart failure becomes manifest (see Fig. 10-2). In severe heart failure, there is a marked increase in circulating catecholamines and depletion of myocardial catecholamines, resulting in decreased myocardial contractility and increased afterload. Cardiac dilation may increase until the heart exhausts the preload reserve and functions on the plateau limb of the Frank-Starling curve, where stroke volume does not increase with further increases of end-diastolic volume.

Pathophysiologic Mechanisms of Heart Failure

Pressure Overload

Pressure overload of the left ventricle is commonly caused by systemic hypertension or by outflow tract obstruction, such as valvular aortic stenosis (Table 10-1). Pressure overload of the right ventricle is commonly secondary to back pressure from a failing left heart but may also occur due to severe pulmonary stenosis, or pulmonary hypertension secondary to pulmonary emboli, or parenchymal lung disease. The initial response to increased afterload (pressure overload) is a decrease in cardiac emptying. There is, therefore, an increased amount of blood in the ventricle during diastole. This increased diastolic stretch (increased preload) causes increased myocardial contraction (Frank-Starling mechanism), so that more pressure can be generated and emptying (stroke volume) remains normal. Contractility increases with time (hemometric autoregulation), so that increased pressure and ejection can be achieved from a smaller end-diastolic volume. These changes provoke cardiac hypertrophy as the primary compensatory changes. Because of the thickened, hypertrophied ventricle, diastolic compliance decreases. The ratio of ventricular diastolic volume (V) change per unit pressure (P) change (V/P) decreases (Fig. 10-3), i.e., there is an increase in ventricular stiffness. This leads to an elevation of ventricular end-diastolic pressure with resultant elevation of pulmonary or systemic venous pressure.

Volume Overload

Volume overload may result from various causes. On the left side of the heart, the most common are mitral or aortic regurgitation. High cardiac output states secondary to hyperthyroidism, anemia, Paget's disease, arteriovenous fistula, and hepatic cirrhosis may also be responsible for volume loading of the ventricles. An intracardiac shunt such as an atrial septal defect may produce right ventricular volume overload.

Due to a chronic volume load, ventricular diastolic volume increases and the ventricle dilates. Dilation of the ventricle (or atria) causes slippage of myocardial fibers, so the wall becomes thinner. This increases compliance, so that with any increase in volume there is less increase in pressure (see Fig. 10-3). However, with time continued stretch causes intrinsic changes in the heart muscle which are essentially irreversible and result in reduction in cardiac contractility and development of heart failure.

Table 10-1. Pathologic and Physiologic Correlations in Various Forms of Heart Failure*

Pathologic State	HR	SV	CO	LVEDV	LVEDP	LAP	RAP	Cardiac Contractility	Heart Size
Increased pressure load (aortic stenosis)	↑	NL or ↓	NL or ↓	NL or ↑	↑↑	↑↑	↑	NL ↑ or ↓	NL or ↑
Increased volume load (aortic and mitral regurgitation)	↑	NL or ↑	NL or ↑	↑↑↑	↑	↑	↑	↓	↑↑
Impaired contractility	↑	↓	↓	↑↑	↑↑	↑↑	↑	↓↓	↑
Diminished LV filling									
LV hypertrophy	↑	NL or ↓	NL or ↓	NL or ↓	↑↑	↑	NL	↑↑	NL or ↑
Mitral stenosis	↑	↓	↓	NL or ↓	↓	↑	↑ or NL	NL	NL or ↑ (LA ↑)
Pericardial constriction or restrictive cardiomyopathy	↑↑	↓↓	↓	NL or ↓	↑↑↑	↑↑↑	↑↑↑	↓ or NL	↑ or NL

*HR = heart rate; SV = stroke volume; CO = cardiac output; LVEDV = left ventricular end-diastolic volume; LVEDP = left ventricular end-diastolic pressure; LAP = left atrial pressure; RAP = right atrial pressure; NL = normal; LV = left ventricular; ↑ = increased; ↓ = decrease; → = no change.
Adapted from Kaufman CE and Papper S (eds). *Review of Pathophysiology.* Boston: Little, Brown, 1983, p. 71.

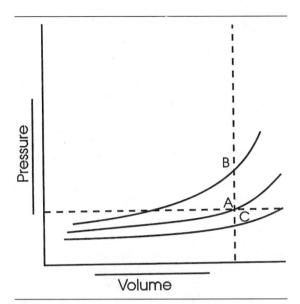

Fig. 10-3. Ventricular compliance curves. A = curve of normal left ventricle; B= curve of less compliant ventricle; C = curve of more compliant ventricle. (Reprinted with permission from: Kaufman CE and Papper S. (eds.) *Review of Pathophysiology.* Boston: Little, Brown, 1983, p. 28.)

On the other hand, when volume loading is acute (as in cases of aortic regurgitation secondary to rupture of the aortic valve due to endocarditis or mitral regurgitation due to papillary muscle rupture), the ventricle or atrium does not have time to dilate. Because of the small chamber size and normal compliance, regurgitation of blood leads to marked elevation of diastolic pressure which is passively transmitted to the pulmonary veins and leads to acute pulmonary edema.

Decreased Contractility

Myocardial disease (loss of muscle) secondary to myocardial infarction or muscle damage secondary to inflammation results in decreased pumping capability of the heart. Initially, the remaining normal myocardium tries to compensate by increasing its contractility; but with time even the normal myocardium may undergo irreversible changes, leading to a further reduction in pumping capacity and hence heart failure. Because of reduction in myocardial contractility, the end-systolic volume of the left ventricle increases. Depending upon the amount of loss of muscle, cardiac output may or may not be impaired at rest but is in-

variably diminished during exercise due to impaired myocardial performance.

In acute myocardial infarction, when more than 40% of the myocardium is damaged, cardiogenic shock occurs which carries a very high mortality. Primary abnormality of cardiac muscle (cardiomyopathy) is also associated with decreased cardiac contractility and hence reduced cardiac output. This eventually leads to heart failure due to cardiac dilation and elevated ventricular volumes.

Impaired or Restricted Filling

Impaired or restricted filling of the ventricles may be due to extrinsic factors such as cardiac tamponade or constrictive pericarditis, or intrinsic factors such as increased stiffness of the ventricular chamber in hypertrophic cardiomyopathy or hypertensive heart disease or infiltration of the myocardium, for example, with amyloid. Both intrinsic stiffness and external constraints on the heart lead to restriction of ventricular filling, with resultant decrease in end-diastolic volume and preload. Paradoxically, however, end-diastolic pressure increases considerably due to reduced compliance of the ventricle or the pericardium or of both the ventricle and the pericardium (see Fig. 10-3).

In mitral stenosis, left ventricular filling is reduced due to the reduced flow across the mitral valve. The primary burden falls on the left atrium, where pressure is elevated behind the obstruction. As mitral stenosis worsens, elevated left atrial pressure is transmitted to the pulmonary veins and this leads to pulmonary venous hypertension and eventually to pulmonary arterial hypertension and right heart failure. Left ventricular contractility and systolic function are usually not impaired. However, left ventricular stroke volume is decreased because of decreased left ventricular end-diastolic volume. The heart responds to these conditions by increasing heart rate in order to maintain cardiac output. However, increased heart rate has a deleterious effect by shortening the left ventricular filling time and thus diminishing ventricular filling and ventricular diastolic volume, with resultant further decrease in cardiac output.

Common Causes of Heart Failure

Heart failure is a symptom of underlying heart disease. Common etiologies of heart disease are coronary artery disease, systemic hypertension, valvular heart disease, pulmonary hypertension, cardiomyopathy, and congenital heart disease. Coronary artery disease is the most frequent cause of heart failure since it is the most common cause of heart disease in the United States. In addition to the loss of muscle due to myocardial infarction, ischemia impairs both the systolic and diastolic function of the left ventricle with impairment of cardiac contractility and compliance and elevation of ventricular end-diastolic pressure. Also, cardiac dilation increases wall stress and thus further increases the myocardial oxygen demand of the compromised ischemic ventricle.

Consequences of Heart Failure

Heart Rate

Heart rate is usually increased in congestive heart failure presumably due to elevated circulating catecholamines and enhanced sympathetic tone. This increase in heart rate tends to maintain cardiac output in the face of low stroke volume. However, there is failure to increase the heart rate in response to normal stimuli and in response to vasoconstriction. The normal decrease of parasympathetic tone during exercise does not occur in congestive heart failure.

Myocardial Changes in Heart Failure

Both the length-tension and force-velocity relationships of failing myocardium are depressed. These findings are the opposite of those evoked by an increased inotropic state such as that resulting from catecholamine stimulation. There is decreased velocity of shortening at any given tension, decreased force development at any given length, and decreased maximum rate of force development.

Defects in oxidative phosphorylation, high-energy phosphate metabolism, calcium ion movements, contractile proteins, protein synthesis and breakdown, and catecholamines have all been reported in heart failure. However, there is no unifying hypothesis to explain these divergent findings.

Neurohumoral Activation

In response to low cardiac output, there is an increase in catecholamine secretion from the adrenal medulla and sympathetic nerve endings and activation of the renin-angiotensin system (see Fig. 10-2). Both the elevated catecholamines and elevated angiotensin initially tend to maintain blood pressure by producing vasoconstriction. However, excessive vasoconstriction increases afterload and produces an extra burden on the already failing heart. This perpetuates heart failure. Elevated levels of angiotensin II may contribute to troublesome hyponatremia, by causing water retention secondary to stimulation of the thirst center and release of antidiuretic hormone. Angiotensin II also leads to an increased release of aldosterone, which promotes further retention of salt and water. Much of the congestion in advanced heart failure is due to these neurohumoral mechanisms rather than the inability of the heart to empty adequately. Increased arteriolar vascular stiffness, possibly related to sodium and water retention, also increases peripheral vascular resistance. Although these compensatory neurohumoral mechanisms may be helpful in maintaining cardiac function, they have the potential for overshooting and producing deleterious effects. Excessive retention of salt and water can lead to an excessive increase in preload. Initially, an increase in preload is effective in increasing cardiac output through the Frank-Starling mechanism. With further increase in preload, cardiac performance does not increase and symptoms become manifest (see Fig. 10-2).

In addition to the neurohumoral changes which produce vasoconstriction and water retention, there are increased levels of atrial natruretic peptide which produce diuresis and local increases in prostaglandins which tend to produce vasodilation (see Fig. 10-2). The secretion of endothelial-derived relaxation factor (NO) is impaired, while the level of endothelial-derived constricting factor (endothelin) is increased in heart failure. The vasodilatory mechanisms are less potent and do not completely offset those that produce vasoconstriction and fluid retention (see Fig. 10-2).

These neuroendocrine alterations also produce redistribution of blood in various tissues. Thus, blood flow to exercising muscles increases while flow to the skin and splanchnic areas decreases.

Myocardial Catecholamines and Receptors

Myocardial norepinephrine levels are low in heart failure due to decreased synthesis. There is a block of normal conversion of dopamine to norepinephrine. There is also decreased uptake of synthesized catecholamines by nerve terminals in the myocardium which results in spill of catecholamines into the circulation. In severe heart failure, the beta-receptor density in the myocardium is very low. This limits the response of myocardium to stimulation by circulating catecholamines.

Ventricular Function Curve (Starling Curve) in Heart Failure

Regardless of the mechanism, cardiac failure is associated with a depressed ventricular function curve. In the normal heart, the ventricle functions on the ascending limb of the ventricular function curve (see Fig. 10-1). Stroke volume and cardiac output vary directly with the end-diastolic ventricular volume (preload). During exercise, cardiac output may increase five- to tenfold over the resting state. This is brought about by increased myocardial contractility, heart rate and venous return, and decreased peripheral resistance. The ventricular function curve shifts upward to the left side. In heart failure, the curve is depressed and shifted downward to the right of the normal curve. There is still a direct relationship between ventricular filling (preload) and cardiac output, but it is flatter than normal. In severe heart failure the function curve is markedly depressed, shifted downward and to the right; the heart exhausts the compensatory mechanisms afforded by the Starling mechanism and functions on the plateau part of the ventricular function curve (maximum preload reserve). Thus, for a given change in end-diastolic volume, the change in stroke volume is markedly depressed or absent in severe heart failure. During exercise, the heart responds poorly, with minimal or no increase in stroke volume.

Signs and Symptoms in Heart Failure

Various signs and symptoms of heart failure can be explained easily on the basis of hemodynamic alterations that occur in myocardial failure. The depressed left ventricular function curve explains the symptoms of low cardiac output (weakness, fatigue) while the increased end-diastolic ventricular pressure produces the symptoms due to pulmonary and systemic venous congestion. In early stages of heart failure, the only symptoms may be fatigue on exertion due to low cardiac output and dyspnea on exertion.

In left ventricular failure, the raised left ventricular pressure is transmitted to the left atrium, pulmonary veins, and capillaries and results in pulmonary congestion and pulmonary edema. The latter becomes clinically manifest as dyspnea (shortness of breath) during exertion and at rest, orthopnea (dyspnea when supine), and bilateral pulmonary crepitations on physical exam.

A third heart sound (ventricular filling gallop) is a common physical finding in heart failure. Filling of the diseased, flabby left ventricle occurs rapidly in early diastole, and then abruptly stops as the stiffness of the ventricle increases steeply at large volumes. This abrupt checking of inflow causes a low-pitched filling sound, the S3 or ventricular gallop. The fourth heart sound is often audible and is due to the forceful contraction of the atrium in order to boost the ventricular filling at high end-diastolic pressures. This sound is not pathognomonic of heart failure but is usually audible in moderate and severe heart failure.

Right heart failure is usually secondary to left heart failure; the signs and symptoms of right heart failure therefore develop quite late in the disease process. However, patients with severe pulmonary parenchymal or occlusive pulmonary vascular disease may present primarily with signs and symptoms of right heart failure. In these patients, symptoms of low cardiac output are secondary to low right ventricular output, with resultant decrease in pulmonary blood flow and decrease in left ventricular filling.

In right ventricular failure, the increased right atrial pressure is eventually transmitted to the systemic veins and leads to systemic congestion. Engorgement of neck veins, congestion of liver (which is often tender due to stretching of the liver capsule), accumulation of fluid in tissues (pitting ankle and leg edema), and increase in body weight are the clinical manifestations.

Prognosis

Prognosis of patients with congestive heart failure is influenced by the underlying left ventricular systolic function; the lower the left ventricular ejection fraction (EF), the worse the prognosis. Three years after the initial presentation, nearly 50% of patients with moderate and severe heart failure (EF < 30–35%) die either due to progressive failure or with sudden death owing to cardiac arrhythmias. In addition to the severity of systolic left ventricular dysfunction, severity of symptoms, presence of complex ventricular arrhythmias, low serum sodium level, and markedly elevated plasma norepinephrine levels are associated with a poor prognosis. Paradoxically, treatment with positive inotropic agents (with the exception of digoxin, which has only a mild inotropic effect) increases mortality. Treatment with angiotensin converting enzyme (ACE) inhibitors improves survival.

Treatment

The principles of treatment of heart failure are to increase cardiac output and to reduce elevated ventricular filling pressures (Fig. 10-4). Diuretics (by reducing intravascular

Algorithm for Management of Heart Failure

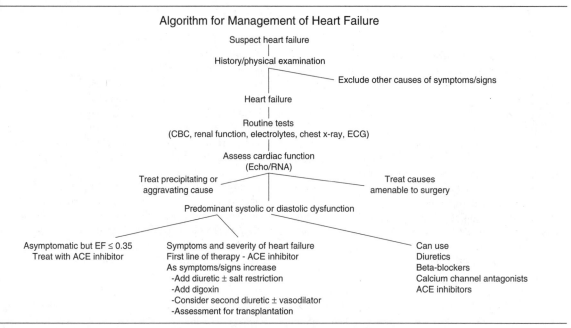

Fig. 10-4. Critical pathway recommended to manage patients with known or suspected heart failure. Once the diagnosis is made, cardiac function should be assessed and the relative contribution of systolic and diastolic dysfunction to the syndrome of heart failure determined. Guidelines have been recommended for choice of therapeutic agents based on the clinical findings and the results of noninvasive tests. ACE angiotensin-converting enzyme; CBC complete blood count; ECG electrocardiogram; Echo echocardiography; EF ejection fraction; HF heart failure; RNA radionuclide angiography. (From Johnstone DE, et al. Diagnosis and management of heart failure. *Can J Cardiol* 10:614, 1994. Reproduced with permission of *Canadian Journal of Cardiology,* 1994; 10:613–631.)

volume) and nitrates (by reducing venous return) lower ventricular filling pressure but have little effect on cardiac output. The arterial vasodilator hydralazine reduces peripheral resistance and improves ventricular emptying and thus increases cardiac output and lowers filling pressures. Treatment with nitrates plus hydralazine improves survival. Treatment with potent inotropic agents and antiarrhythmic agents adversely affects prognosis. ACE inhibitors, by blocking the effects of the activated renin-angiotensin system, reduce impedance to left ventricular emptying and have been consistently shown to improve quality of life and survival of patients with heart failure.

Clinical Examples

1. A 60-year-old man sustained an extensive acute myocardial infarction 4 years before his recent admission. Since that time, he has become progressively more breathless on exertion. During the past 6 months, he developed swelling of his abdomen and feet despite vigorous diuretic and digoxin therapy. Examination revealed an emaciated man who was breathless even at rest. Cardiac rhythm was regular and blood pressure was 90/60 mm Hg. Jugular venous pressure was elevated and there was ankle edema, hepatomegaly, and ascites. Heart sounds were faint but a loud third sound was audible. Chest x-ray revealed marked cardiac enlargement, bilateral pleural effusions, and pulmonary venous congestion. Cardiac catheterization revealed severe inoperable three-vessel coronary artery disease, poor left ventricular function with marked elevation of left ventricular end-diastolic pressure, and low cardiac output.

Discussion. In this patient, myocardial infarction was responsible for extensive damage to the left ventricular muscle, which resulted in chronic elevation of left ventricular end-diastolic pressure. This accounted initially for breathlessness on exertion and, with time, exudation of fluid into the alveoli (pulmonary edema). Subsequently, the right heart also started to fail, manifested by venous congestion (elevated jugular venous pressure, ascites, ankle edema, and liver enlargement).

The final outcome in this kind of patient remains grave. Afterload-reducing agents such as hydralazine often lead to some improvement in left ventricular performance by reducing the impedance to left ventricular outflow. The nitrate group of drugs are also useful; their venodilator effects reduce venous return to the heart, which leads in turn to a reduction in ventricular volumes and end-diastolic pressures.

Angiotensin converting enzyme inhibitors are one of the most effective treatments in patients with congestive heart failure due to myocardial disease. By blocking the effects of excessive activation of the renin-angiotensin system, these agents not only reduce impedance to left ventricular emptying but also limit the influence of angiotensin II on thirst, renal vasoconstriction, and aldosterone secretion. Both symptoms and patient survival improve by treatment with these agents. In contrast, long-term treatment with potent inotropic agents is not useful and increases mortality.

2. A 35-year-old man presented with a complaint of increasing shortness of breath. This initially occurred with exertion, but now occurred at rest as well. He had no previous cardiac symptoms. His father suffers from chest pain and heart failure. Examination revealed a normal upstroke and bifid systolic impulse on palpation of the carotid artery. Presystolic and forceful sustained systolic apical impulses were palpable. The first and second sounds were normal. A loud fourth sound was heard. A systolic ejection murmur that increased with valsalva was heard along the left sternal border. Echocardiogram revealed a markedly hypertrophied left ventricle with disproportionate thickening of the septum and a small left ventricular cavity.

Discussion. The thick ventricular walls with disproportionate septal thickening are characteristic of hypertrophic cardiomyopathy. The small chamber is stiff (fourth sound is heard and presystolic impulse is palpable due to vigorous atrial contraction) and requires high pressures to fill (dyspnea reflects pulmonary congestion due to high left ventricular filling pressures). Because the obstruction to left ventricular ejection is dynamic and develops during systolic emptying, the carotid upstroke is initially normal but a second, slower impulse is evident after obstruction develops. The valsalva maneuver reduces left ventricular filling and makes the outflow obstruction more severe; hence the increase in the intensity of the murmur. Treatment should be directed at decreasing stiffness (calcium channel blockers, beta-blockers) rather than increasing contractility.

Bibliography

Braunwald E (ed). *Heart Disease.* Philadelphia: Saunders, 1992. *A classic textbook of cardiology with four chapters on heart failure (pp. 393–519) and extensive references.*

Heart failure. Management of patients with systolic dysfunction. Prevention, initial evaluation, patient counseling and education, pharmacologic management, role of myocardial revascularization and algorithm. U.S. Department of Health and Human Services. AHCPR Publication No. 94–0613. June 1994. *A concise overview makes this easy bedtime reading for the busy student.*

Johnstone DE et al. Diagnosis and management of heart failure. Canadian Cardiovascular Society's Consensus Conference. *Can J Cardiol* 10:613–631, 1994. *A timely and extremely useful concise review.*

Packer M. Pathophysiology of chronic heart failure. *Lancet* 340:88–92, 1992. *An authoritative but concise review.*

11 Shock Syndrome

Karen K. Hamilton

Objectives

After completing this chapter, you should be able to

Define shock syndrome and describe its common physical findings and the associated biochemical abnormalities

List the three types of shock syndrome and describe the underlying pathophysiology and common causes of each type

Understand the consequences of shock, e.g., the effect on organ function

Explain the utility of hemodynamic monitoring in differentiating types of shock and in guiding therapy

Explain the therapeutic modalities available to correct the pathophysiology in each form of shock

Types of Shock Syndrome

Definition

The terms "shock syndrome" or "hypoperfusion syndrome" refer to the consequences of inadequate oxygen delivery to tissues. Common causes of shock are listed in Table 11-1. The multiple manifestations of the syndrome are results of tissue ischemia and failure to clear products of metabolism, with subsequent organ dysfunction.

Classification of Shock

Hypovolemic Shock

This form of shock results from loss of intravascular volume (inadequate preload). The Frank-Starling curve relating preload or end-diastolic volume to ventricular output is shown in Fig. 11-1, and the effect of a decrease in preload on cardiac output is illustrated. Such volume loss may occur through hemorrhage, loss of fluid through the urinary or gastrointestinal (GI) tracts or skin, or loss of fluid into the extravascular space (e.g., ascites). Rapid loss of 20–30% of intravascular volume may result in shock.

Cardiogenic Shock

Cardiogenic shock is present when preload is adequate and yet cardiac output is inadequate to achieve effective tissue perfusion (inadequate pump function). This form of shock may occur in patients with large myocardial infarction, in patients with primary myocardial disease and severe pump failure, and in patients with sudden and severe valvular dysfunction, such as aortic or mitral insufficiency. A subtype of cardiogenic shock has been termed "obstructive shock." In this form of shock, generation of adequate cardiac output is impaired by obstruction to filling or forward flow. Examples include severe mitral and aortic stenosis, massive pulmonary embolus, and pericardial tamponade. The most common form of cardiogenic shock (pump failure due to impaired contractility as occurs in acute myocardial infarction) is illustrated in Fig. 11-2.

Distributive Shock

This form of shock results from inappropriate vasodilatation of selected vascular beds (inadequate afterload) resulting in maldistribution of intravascular volume. It has also been designated hyperdynamic, vasodilatory, or vasogenic shock. Examples of such vasodilatation include sepsis, anaphylaxis, and neurologic disorders such as spinal cord injury. The typical hemodynamics of vasodilatory

Table 11-1. Common Etiologies of Shock

HYPOVOLEMIC SHOCK

Hemorrhage

Fluid loss

    Gastrointestinal (e.g., vomiting, diarrhea)

    Urinary (e.g., hyperglycemia, diabetes insipidus, diuretic therapy, postobstructive diuresis)

    Skin (e.g., burns)

    Internal sequestration (e.g., ascites)

CARDIOGENIC SHOCK

Myocardial failure

    Left ventricular (e.g., ischemia, infarction, cardiomyopathy)

    Right ventricular (e.g., infarction, pulmonary hypertension, cor pulmonale)

Arrhythmias

Valvular regurgitation or stenosis

Ventricular septal rupture or free-wall rupture

Obstructive lesions

    Myxoma

    Pulmonary embolus

    Pericardial tamponade

DISTRIBUTIVE SHOCK

Septic shock

Neurogenic shock (e.g., severe central nervous system depression, spinal cord injury)

Anaphylaxis

Adrenal cortical failure

Fig. 11-1. The effects of hypovolemia on cardiac output. The Frank-Starling curve relating preload or end-diastolic volume to ventricular output is shown. The fall from normal intravascular volume (●) to hypovolemia (■) is accompanied by a marked fall in cardiac output, which is likely to be accompanied by hypoperfusion and shock syndrome. Administration of fluids (△) may restore normal cardiac output.

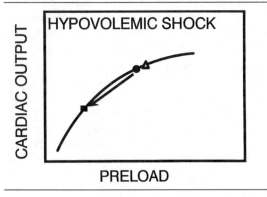

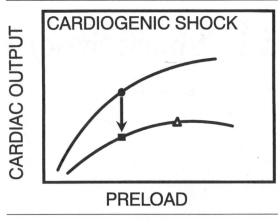

Fig. 11-2. The effects of depressed cardiac contractility on cardiac output. The upper Frank-Starling curve represents the relationship between preload and cardiac output when ventricular function is normal, as shown in Fig. 11-1. The fall from normal contractility (●) to impaired contractility (lower curve, ■) as might occur at the time of large acute myocardial infarction is accompanied by a marked fall in cardiac output, which is likely to be accompanied by hypoperfusion and shock syndrome. Administration of fluids (△) may improve cardiac output. However, an inotropic agent to improve contractile function may also be required to reverse the shock state.

shock are illustrated in Fig. 11-3. Vasodilation often results in a variable fall in preload and a compensatory increase in contractility (hyperdynamic circulatory state). Thus cardiac output may be high, normal, or low.

Clinical Overview

The clinical manifestations of shock are those of impaired organ perfusion, including decreased urine output, confusion, agitation, obtundation or other forms of altered mental status, peripheral cyanosis, and metabolic acidosis. The skin is frequently cool and clammy but may be warm in distributive shock. Blood pressure (BP) may be low or may initially be maintained in the normal range by compensatory tachycardia, vasoconstriction, or increased stroke volume. Patients may subsequently develop a syndrome of multiorgan system failure (often including respiratory, hepatic, and renal failure) which ultimately becomes irreversible even when adequate tissue perfusion is restored. Reticuloendothelial function and gastrointestinal barrier function may deteriorate and predispose to overwhelming infection.

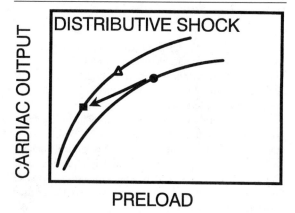

Fig. 11-3. The effects of vasodilation (reduced afterload) on cardiac output. The lower Frank-Starling curve represents the normal relationship between preload and ventricular output (●). A decrease in afterload (■) typically results in a decrease in preload (due to peripheral pooling of volume) and a compensatory increase in cardiac contractility (shift to the upper Frank-Starling curve). Cardiac output may initially be high, normal, or low, depending on the severity of vasodilation and the patient's ability to respond by increasing cardiac contractility and heart rate. Administration of fluids (△) may increase cardiac output. However, the hypoperfusion syndrome in these patients results from maldistribution of cardiac output and impaired oxygen utilization and often persists when cardiac output is normal or high.

Pathophysiology

Hypovolemic Shock

These patients have low right- and left-sided filling pressures due to external or internal fluid losses.

Hemorrhage

Hemorrhage is probably the most frequent cause of the syndrome of hypovolemic shock. Blood loss may occur secondary to trauma, surgery, or aneurysm rupture. Blood may be lost externally or sequestered in tissues or body cavities (e.g., fracture with hematoma, hemothorax, or hemoperitoneum). Bleeding may also occur spontaneously in patients who have received anticoagulants or thrombolytic drugs, or who have coagulation disorders such as hemophilia. Treatment requires prompt localization of the bleeding site and surgical repair if appropriate, correction of any coagulopathy, volume replacement, and frequently transfusion.

Excessive Fluid Loss from the GI Tract

Vomiting or prolonged bouts of diarrheal illnesses may result in hypovolemic shock, especially in infants and children.

Urinary Tract Fluid Losses

Excessive diuresis may occur in patients with uncontrolled diabetes mellitus, diabetes insipidus, after relief of urinary tract obstruction, in salt-wasting disorders such as adrenocortical insufficiency, or following administration of diuretic agents.

Fluid Loss from the Skin

Sufficient fluid loss from the skin to cause shock may occur in patients with extensive burns or skin inflammation (e.g., generalized exfoliative dermatitis).

Internal Sequestration of Fluid

Loss of volume into the interstitial spaces or body cavities, frequently referred to as "third-spacing," may be seen in patients with disorders resulting in low plasma oncotic pressure (e.g., chronic liver disease), inflammation (e.g., acute pancreatitis), or abnormal capillary leakiness (e.g., angioedema).

Cardiogenic Shock

When the heart is unable to generate cardiac output adequate to maintain tissue perfusion, the syndrome is referred to as cardiogenic shock. Cardiogenic shock may result from abnormalities in the myocardium itself, from valvular dysfunction, and from lesions that impair filling or obstruct outflow.

Impaired Pump Function

Left Ventricular Failure.   Cardiogenic shock is seen most commonly in the setting of acute myocardial infarction. The syndrome is more common with large infarcts involving more than 40% of the left ventricle (LV) and in patients who have had previous infarctions. Diagnosis and management usually require invasive hemodynamic monitoring. The diagnosis of cardiogenic shock requires the demonstration that preload is adequate and yet cardiac output remains low. Treatment often includes inotropic support (e.g., dobutamine). If peripheral vasoconstriction is present, vasodilator therapy may improve perfusion. If pulmonary congestion is present and LV filling pressure is high, diuretics or intravenous (IV) nitroglycerin may be useful to decrease preload.

Right Ventricular Failure.   Failure of the right ventricle (RV) may develop in patients with severe pulmonary hypertension from any cause (e.g., recurrent pulmonary emboli, obstructive lung disease, or primary pulmonary hypertension). Low cardiac output may also follow acute RV infarction, which is usually recognized in association with inferior wall infarction. Dilatation of the RV in these circumstances also results in shift of the ventricular septum toward the LV with impairment of LV filling, resulting in a further drop in cardiac output.

Arrhythmia

Incessant or prolonged tachyarrhythmia, either ventricular or supraventricular, will compromise cardiac output and may result in shock. Patients may also develop shock secondary to bradyarrhythmias such as severe sinus bradycardia or sinus arrest with a slow junctional or ventricular escape rhythm, and high grade or complete atrioventricular block. Sinus bradycardia may respond transiently to a vagolytic drug such as atropine. Slow sinus rates may also be increased with beta adrenergic drugs such as isoproterenol or dobutamine. Temporary pacing may also be used to treat shock resulting from heart block or other bradyarrhythmia.

Obstructive Valvular Disease

Both severe mitral and aortic stenosis can contribute to the development of cardiogenic shock, especially when compensatory mechanisms fail. In a patient with severe aortic stenosis, an increase in metabolic demand, a decrease in preload, or a negative inotropic drug may precipitate shock. Vasodilatation may impair coronary perfusion during diastole, resulting in ischemia of the hypertrophied LV and inability to maintain cardiac output. In severe mitral stenosis, tachycardia, which compromises diastolic filling time, is a common precipitant of pulmonary congestion and shock.

Severe Acute Valvular Regurgitation, Ventricular Septal Defect, or Ventricular Rupture

Rupture of a papillary muscle, the interventricular septum, or the free wall of either ventricle may occur in the setting of acute myocardial infarction and lead to shock. Acute severe mitral or aortic regurgitation may also occur in patients with endocarditis or myxomatous valvular degeneration.

Massive Pulmonary Emboli

Obstruction of the main pulmonary artery with thrombus will result in acute RV failure and shock.

Impairment to Filling

Filling of cardiac chambers may be impaired by pericardial tamponade and constriction, intracavitary masses such as myxoma, and external cardiac compression, e.g., by tumor or hematoma.

Distributive Shock

Sepsis

Bacterial sepsis is the most common cause of vasodilatory shock. In these patients, peripheral vascular resistance is low, and cardiac output is frequently high. A myocardial depressant factor of sepsis has been invoked to explain the inappropriately decreased cardiac contractility which may be seen in patients with previously normal cardiac function, especially in the later stages of sepsis. While cardiac output may be high in these patients, metabolic demand is also increased and oxygen utilization is often impaired. This finding is believed to be due to maldistribution of flow, possibly due to arteriovenous shunting or to impaired tissue utilization of oxygen.

Anaphylaxis

Systemic anaphylaxis may result when a sensitized individual is exposed to an antigen which triggers an IgE-mediated activation of mast cells. Anaphylactic reactions are most commonly seen in response to drugs (e.g., penicillin), foods (e.g., egg white, nuts, and seafood), and Hymenoptera venom (e.g., wasp stings). Mast cells release a variety of potent mediators, including histamine, leukotrienes, and platelet-activating factor; these mediators alter vascular tone and permeability and recruit other inflammatory cells. Manifestations of anaphylaxis include urticaria, diffuse erythema of the skin, respiratory distress (tachypnea, stridor, and wheezing), and hypotension. Patients may also complain of nausea, vomiting, or abdominal cramping.

Neurogenic Shock

Severe central nervous system depression of any cause and spinal cord injury may result in dysfunction of the autonomic nervous system and inability to maintain normal peripheral vascular resistance.

Hemodynamic Interactions in Shock States

Shock is classified by its inciting event (preload failure, pump failure, or afterload failure). Nevertheless, combination syndromes are common and must be recognized for appropriate treatment. For example, a patient with severe hypotension due to sepsis or hemorrhage may also develop myocardial ischemia secondary to inadequate diastolic coronary perfusion pressure. Patients with acute myocardial ischemia often have not only pump failure but inadequate preload for the damaged ventricle. And patients with cardiogenic shock may develop bowel ischemia and cytokine-induced vasodilation or frank sepsis. Patients with adrenocortical insufficiency have both intravascular volume depletion (due to mineralocorticoid deficiency and failure of sodium retention) and inadequate cardiac contractility and vascular tone (due to impaired ability to secrete and respond to catecholamines).

Additional Consequences of Shock

The metabolic consequences of prolonged organ hypoperfusion are the same regardless of the etiology of shock.

Tissue Hypoxia and Accumulation of End-Products of Anaerobic Metabolism

In the presence of oxygen, cells metabolize glucose to carbon dioxide, which is excreted by the lungs, and water. In states of tissue ischemia, pyruvate is metabolized to lactic acid. Lactate is removed by the liver and, to a lesser extent, the kidney. Normally, lactate is effectively metabolized at rates up to 320 mEq/hour (e.g., during strenuous exercise). However, in shock, lactic acid accumulates due not only to increased production but also to impaired metabolism, probably because of decreased hepatic and renal perfusion.

Sympathetic Overactivity

Shock results in release of norepinephrine from adrenergic nerve terminals and epinephrine from the adrenal medulla. High catecholamine levels usually result in tachycardia, increased cardiac contractility, and vasoconstriction. These alterations may increase cardiac output and partially restore tissue perfusion, particularly perfusion of the brain and heart. Catecholamine stimulation may result in cardiac ischemia in patients with underlying coronary artery disease, and intense vasoconstriction may result in decreased perfusion of some vascular beds (e.g., renal, hepatic, and splanchnic ischemia). Even transient severe hypoperfusion in these territories may result in prolonged organ dysfunction (e.g., renal failure due to acute tubular necrosis). Renal insufficiency worsens metabolic acidosis. Epinephrine release also results in hypokalemia due to movement of potassium into cells and may predispose to arrhythmias.

Circulation of Vasoactive Toxins and Cytokines

Bacterial toxins such as the lipopolysaccharide endotoxin from gram-negative organisms and the exotoxin from *Staphylococcus aureus* which induces toxic shock syndrome are known to contribute to the syndrome of septic shock. However, septic shock may be seen with infections by organisms which do not produce known bacterial toxins. Release of cytokines and other mediators which alter vascular tone probably plays a role in both septic shock and shock syndromes which are not initiated by infection. Tumor necrosis factor (TNF) is released from macrophages in response to endotoxin and causes a fall in blood pressure and vascular resistance, and antibodies against TNF appear to be protective in animal models of septic shock. Several interleukins have also been shown to decrease blood pressure, vascular resistance, or cardiac contractility. Shock states may also result in disseminated intravascular coagulation and activation of the complement system, both of which produce additional vasoactive substances.

Management
Clinical Assessment in Shock

Basic clinical assessment of patients in shock must include vital signs, mental status, hematocrit, and urine output. Evidence for decreased intravascular volume may include orthostatic changes in blood pressure and pulse, thready pulses, poor skin turgor, and dry mucous membranes. Evidence for cardiac dysfunction should also be sought on examination, including pulmonary rales, distended neck veins, third heart sound of left or right ventricular origin, and murmurs compatible with valvular stenosis or regurgitation. Peripheral vasoconstriction may be manifest as cool, mottled skin and even peripheral cyanosis.

Hemodynamic Monitoring

Invasive hemodynamic monitoring is invaluable in the optimal management of shock. An indwelling arterial catheter is frequently used to monitor arterial pressure and to provide blood for assessment of arterial oxygenation. Central venous pressure (CVP) may be measured using a catheter inserted into a large central vein (internal jugular or subclavian). CVP may be used as an indicator of intravascular volume in patients who are very unlikely to have any form of cardiac dysfunction. However, it must be recognized that in many circumstances the CVP may be considerably higher or lower than the LV filling pressure. The CVP will often be higher than LV filling pressure in RV infarction and in pulmonary hypertension of any cause (e.g., pulmonary embolus or cor pulmonale). By contrast, CVP will be lower than LV filling pressure in patients with LV systolic failure (e.g., acute ischemia) or diastolic dysfunction (e.g., hypertensive heart disease or hypertrophic cardiomyopathy).

Bedside monitoring of left-sided filling pressures via a balloon flotation catheter in the pulmonary artery was first reported by Swan and Ganz in 1970. One year later, this group of investigators reported measurement of cardiac output at the bedside by the thermodilution method. The flow-directed balloon-tipped thermodilution pulmonary artery (PA) catheter has revolutionized management of shock. This catheter allows the measurement of cardiac output (CO) and pressures in the right atrium (RA), RV, and PA. In addition, the small balloon at the tip is briefly inflated in a pulmonary artery branch. The pressure measured distal to this occluding balloon is referred to as the pulmonary artery occlusion pressure (PAOP) or pulmonary capillary wedge pressure (PCWP). In the absence of obstruction between the PA and the LV (e.g., pulmonary veno-occlusive disease or mitral stenosis), the PAOP closely approximates LV filling pressure. Systemic vascular resistance (SVR) can then be calculated using an invasively measured or noninvasively estimated mean arterial pressure (MAP).

$$SVR = \left(\frac{[MAP - PAOP]}{CO}\right) \times 80 \ (\text{normal}: \ 800 - 1500 \ \text{dynes} \cdot \text{sec} \cdot \text{cm}^{-5}$$

These data may suggest an unsuspected etiology for the shock state, and also help guide therapy and assess its efficacy. The hemodynamic alterations which are typical for various forms of shock are presented in Table 11-2. Hemodynamic abnormalities (low cardiac output, volume depletion, or vasodilatation) should be identified and corrected as rapidly as possible. When tissue hypoperfusion becomes prolonged, the patient is much more likely to develop prolonged or irreversible organ failure.

Patients are generally considered to have been successfully resuscitated from shock when heart rate is less than

Table 11-2. Hemodynamic Alterations in Shock

| Type of Shock | End-Diastolic Pressure | | CO | SVR |
	RV	LV		
Hypovolemic	↓↓	↓↓	↓	↑↑
Cardiogenic				
RV dysfunction	↑	0,↓,↑	↓↓	↑↑
LV dysfunction	0,↑,↓	↑↑	↓↓	↑↑
Distributive	0 or ↓	0 or ↑	↑,0, or ↓	↓↓

90, mean blood pressure is greater than 80 (in previously normotensive patients), cardiac output is close to normal, arterial oxygen saturation is greater than 90%, and systemic acidosis has resolved. Some patients who appear by these parameters to have been adequately resuscitated nevertheless progress to multiorgan system failure. Increasing evidence suggests that inadequate oxygen delivery and acidosis may persist in some tissues, particularly the gastrointestinal mucosa, even after apparently successful resuscitation. This is especially likely in cases where metabolic demand is high, such as in severe trauma or postsurgical patients. Deterioration of gastrointestinal barrier function may then result in entry of endotoxins or bacteria into the circulation, contributing to poor outcome. Recognition of these complications has led to the search for new methods to assess adequacy of oxygen delivery in tissues at high risk (such as GI mucosal pH monitoring) and trials of new interventions (monoclonal antibodies to endotoxin) which may be available in clinical practice in the future.

Correction of Hemodynamic Derangements

Hypovolemic Shock

Attention must be given to maintaining adequate intravascular volume, which can be assessed by measuring CVP and PAOP. A CVP of 5–12 mm Hg and a PAOP of 14–18 mm Hg usually represent adequate preload. Where possible, ongoing fluid loss should be identified and treated (e.g., surgical repair or cauterization of a source of bleeding). Optimizing preload is essential for all forms of shock, regardless of etiology.

Cardiogenic Shock

In some cases, the acute precipitating event will be readily identifiable and correctable. For example, a tachyarrhythmia may be controlled with an antiarrhythmic drug or a bradyarrhythmia with a pacemaker. The severity of LV dysfunction secondary to acute myocardial infarction (MI) may be ameliorated by reperfusion using a thrombolytic agent or emergency angioplasty. Acute severe aortic insufficiency may require emergency valve replacement, and pericardial tamponade may be relieved by pericardiocentesis.

Management of pump failure causing shock usually requires invasive hemodynamic monitoring to determine cardiac output, right and left ventricular filling pressures, and systemic vascular resistance. These data will confirm the suspected low cardiac output. If preload is determined to be inappropriately low for the clinical setting, intravenous fluids may be administered to optimize cardiac output. An ischemic or failing ventricle requires a higher than normal filling pressure. In patients with significant LV dysfunction or acute LV infarction, a PAOP of 18 mm Hg will usually represent adequate preload. In patients with RV ischemia or dysfunction, a CVP, obtained via a catheter in the superior vena cava or RA, greater than 12 mm Hg should be adequate. Inotropic drugs are the mainstay of therapy for primary LV or RV pump failure as occurs with acute myocardial infarction or severe cardiomyopathy. These drugs which increase cardiac contractility include catecholamines such as dobutamine, phosphodiesterase inhibitors such as amrinone or milrinone, and digoxin. If the systemic vascular resistance is high, vasodilator drugs may actually improve tissue perfusion without significantly decreasing blood pressure. The intra-aortic balloon pump may be used in patients with severe LV failure who do not have significant dysrhythmia or aortic regurgitation. The balloon inflates in the proximal descending aorta during diastole (which augments perfusion of the coronary arteries) and deflates during systole (which decreases afterload).

Distributive or Vasodilatory Shock

Initial resuscitation is directed toward increasing intravascular volume and reversing inappropriate vasodilatation. This is achieved by intravenous administration of colloid or crystalloid and a vasopressor agent. Wedge pressure (PAOP) should be used as an indicator of the adequacy of intravascular volume. Volume may be infused as long as cardiac output continues to increase or until the PAOP of 18 mm Hg is reached. It should be noted that while vasopressor drugs may return mean arterial pressure toward normal and improve flow to the brain, they increase central venous pressures and often decrease perfusion to other vital organs and worsen lactic acidosis. Specific therapy of the underlying disorder must also be considered. Broad spectrum antibiotic coverage is initiated for suspected sepsis. For anaphylaxis, intravenous epinephrine is administered, along with oxygen and bronchodilators as needed. Antihistamines and corticosteroids are also frequently utilized, although there is little evidence in support of their effectiveness.

Clinical Examples

1. An 82-year-old man was brought to the emergency room by his grandson, who reported that the man had been eating poorly for 2 days and had been difficult to arouse that morning. The patient had no specific complaints.

On exam, the patient would open his eyes and mumble incoherently in response to pain. His temperature was 38.6°C, BP 75/40, HR 124 regular, respirations 26. His lungs were clear. No murmurs or extra sounds were appreciated on cardiac exam. His skin was warm, with bounding peripheral pulses.

His chest radiograph and EKG were normal.

Laboratory data: white blood cell count 19,500 (normal less than 10,000). A bladder catheter was inserted (with difficulty) and yielded cloudy urine, which was noted to contain many white cells and bacteria. Urine was sent for culture.

Discussion.   Initial evaluation suggests that this patient has septic shock probably originating from a urinary tract infection. Altered mental status and poor appetite are often the only presenting symptoms of infection in elderly patients. Prostatic hypertrophy is a likely predisposing factor for urinary tract infection in an elderly man. Blood and cerebrospinal fluid samples were obtained and sent for culture, and the patient was immediately started on intravenous antibiotic coverage for common gram-negative urinary tract pathogens. He also received intravenous fluids which resulted in an increase in his blood pressure to 110/80 over the next 4 hours and marked improvement in his mental status. Vasopressor drugs were not required in this patient.

2. A 35-year-old woman presented to an emergency room complaining of a headache present since a myelogram which had been performed 4 days before. Her past medical history was unremarkable and her physical examination was normal. She was given an injection of meperidine for her pain. After the injection she began to complain of numbness and tingling in her fingertips, lightheadedness, shortness of breath, and diffuse itching. Her pulse was noted to be 140 and blood pressure was palpable at 70/0 mm Hg. Faint wheezes were noted throughout the lungs. Although she had initially denied drug allergies, she now remembered similar symptoms which had followed an injection of "pain medicine" 2 years before.

Discussion.   The physician must now treat this patient based on a presumptive diagnosis of anaphylactic shock. She received IV fluids, IV diphenhydramine (an antihistamine), and subcutaneous epinephrine. Her blood pressure and pulse returned to normal over the next 45 minutes.

3. A 67-year-old female arrived in the emergency room complaining of chest pain and severe weakness present for 12 hours. These symptoms had been preceded by several

days of nausea and vomiting, poor appetite, and subjective fever.

On examination, she had a pulse rate of 110 and BP 85/50. There was no jugular venous distension. Her lungs were clear and no murmur or gallop were heard on auscultation of the heart. There was no extremity edema.

EKG showed new ST elevation in the inferior leads, suggesting an evolving inferior myocardial infarction. Right precordial leads did not show evidence of RV infarction at that time.

The patient was given sublingual nitroglycerin and within minutes became confused and unable to respond to questions. Systolic blood pressure dropped to 60 and pulse slowed to 70. Her legs were elevated and rapid infusion of intravenous fluids was begun. Her mental status improved but she remained hypotensive. The decision was made to place a pulmonary artery catheter to help with management of cardiogenic shock.

Initial Hemodynamic Data

BP	80/50, mean 60
RA	4 mm Hg, RV 22/3, PA 22/10, PAOP 6
Cardiac output	1.9 liters/min
SVR	2350 dynes-cm^{-5}-sec (normal 400–1900)

Discussion.   This patient's pain and EKG changes allow the presumptive diagnosis of acute inferior myocardial infarction. Although this patient's cardiac output is low, the diagnosis of cardiogenic shock can be made only in the presence of adequate intravascular volume. Both right- and left-sided filling pressures are low. Her left ventricular filling pressure, as estimated by pulmonary artery occlusion pressure, is particularly low, as patients with acute or chronic ischemia in general require higher filling pressures to maintain adequate cardiac output than patients with normal ventricular function. It appears likely that this patient became mildly volume depleted during the preceding viral

syndrome when her intake was poor. When her compensatory increase in stroke volume was then compromised by the myocardial ischemia, she developed hypotension. It should also be noted that patients with volume depletion and patients with inferior ischemia are particularly susceptible to developing a hypotensive response to nitroglycerin. This drug is a venodilator, and further reduces preload. When this patient received additional fluids to increase her PAOP to 12, her cardiac index increased to 3.1 liters/minute/m^2 and her blood pressure increased to 115/70. The remainder of her hospital course was uncomplicated.

Bibliography

Fiddian-Green RG, Haglund U, Gutierrez G, et al. Goals for the resuscitation of shock. *Crit Care Med* 21(2):S21–S31, 1993. *Excellent summary of the limitations of current techniques for monitoring successful resuscitation and a look at what may be available for clinical use in the future.*

Ganz W, Donoso R, Marcus HS, Forrester JS, and Swan HJ. A new technique for measurement of cardiac output by thermodilution in man. *Am J Cardiol* 27:392–396, 1971. *First report of bedside measurement of cardiac output using the pulmonary artery balloon floatation catheter.*

Mouchawar A and Rosenthal M. A pathophysiological approach to the patient in shock. *Internat Anesthesiol Clinics* 31:1–20, 1993. *Comprehensive review of the pathophysiology and management of shock.*

Swan HJ, Ganz W, Forrester J, Marcus H, Diamond G, and Chonette D. Catheterization of the heart in man with use of a flow-directed balloon-tipped catheter. *N Engl J Med* 283:447–451, 1970. *First report of the use of a flow-directed pulmonary artery catheter for bedside hemodynamic monitoring.*

12 Hypertension

David C. Kem

Objectives

After completing this chapter, you should be able to

Understand the basic dependency of the systemic blood pressure upon changes in peripheral resistance and cardiac output

Recognize the contribution that each of these components may have in the hypertension associated with several disease states

Learn that renovascular stenosis can sustain hypertension through a spectrum ranging from volume- to pressor-dependent mechanisms depending on sodium intake and diuretic status

Recognize several hypotheses which serve as models for the etiology of essential hypertension

Identify several diseases which are recognized as secondary causes of hypertension

Recognize how this knowledge can assist in the management of patients with hypertensive diseases

Introduction and General Concepts

Hypertension is estimated to affect 20% of the American population, increases with age, and occurs more frequently in susceptible populations. It is a major risk factor for most cardiovascular diseases.

An elevated blood pressure (BP) relative to the age of the patient (> 140/90 or 160/95 after age 60) should be considered a sign of an underlying pathological condition rather than a disease in itself. A large number of diseases are associated with an elevated BP. To understand the pathophysiology of hypertension, therefore, requires knowledge of a wide variety of conditions that may interact with or alter the blood pressure response.

It is essential to know how BP is normally maintained in order to understand hypertension. In its simplest form, the mean arterial pressure (MAP) is directly proportional to the product of the cardiac output (CO) and the total peripheral resistance (TPR) (Ohm's law).

$$MAP = CO \times TPR$$

The peripheral resistance is frequently described by a modification of Poiseuille's law:

$$TPR = k \frac{VL}{r^4}$$
where V = viscosity
      L = length of vessels
    TPR = total peripheral resistance
      r = average radius of resistance vessels

indicating that the resistance is exquisitely sensitive to small changes in the radius, but also proportional to the length of the vessels and the blood viscosity. However, alterations in the latter two parameters are rarely associated with hypertension.

Changes in the cardiac output are an early component of some forms of hypertension and are important in modulating BP control. Cardiac output is determined by the stroke volume (SV) and the heart rate (r) (CO = SV × r). The SV, in turn, is altered by a complex interaction of blood volume (venous return) and myocardial integrity. Changes in the TPR will alter the SV as increased afterload (TPR) tends to decrease stroke volume. A diminished volume or pressure of blood returning to the heart, which leads to a decreased volume of blood in the ventricle at the end of diastole (preload), also will decrease stroke volume.

Several neural and humoral mechanisms modulate changes in the TPR and CO. Autonomic efferent innervation of the heart and peripheral vasculature is controlled by a complex interaction of high- and low-pressure baroreceptors located in the carotid artery, the aorta, great veins, and the atria. Afferent signals from these receptors are carried via the vagus or by sympathetic afferents to the central nervous system where the signals are integrated and subsequently modify adrenergic and parasympathetic outflow to the heart and peripheral vessels.

Blood volume is regulated through central nervous system, hormonal, and renal mechanisms. Thirst and salt appetite are altered by changes in osmolality, angiotensin levels, and neurogenic input from the atria. The kidney is the effector organ for regulation of blood volume in response to blood pressure (an increase in perfusion pressure leads to increased filtration and excretion of sodium and water), and hormonal and neural control mechanisms.

Perturbation of these complex systems may be observed in several types of secondary hypertension (caused by a known etiology). These secondary forms of hypertension comprise at most 5% of all patients with high blood pressure (Table 12-1). Their importance is greater than this figure might suggest since the study of these diseases has led to a better understanding and a more rational therapy of the remaining 95%, which are defined as "primary" or "essential" hypertension.

It is useful to look upon the major types of hypertension as encompassing a spectrum ranging from those characterized by "volume dependency" to those with a predominantly pressor (vasoconstriction) mechanism. In the following schema (Fig. 12-1), the various types of secondary hypertension have been placed in relative position delineating the degree of volume overload as compared to the pressor component contributing to elevation of the blood pressure. This judgment is an approximation based on both clinical and laboratory studies. Several factors influence where a given type of patient might be placed in this scheme, including dietary salt intake, medications, age, duration of disease, and coexistent diseases. This

Table 12-1. Secondary Causes of Hypertension

Chronic end-stage renal disease
Renovascular stenosis
1° aldosteronism
    Aldosterone-producing adenoma
    Idiopathic adrenal hyperplasia
    Glucocorticoid suppressible hyperplasia
Pheochromocytoma
Hypercalcemia
Cushing's syndrome
Hyper- and hypothyroidism
Acromegaly
Renin-producing JG cell tumor of kidney
Hypertension of pregnancy
Hypertension associated with drug use
    Oral contraceptives
    Cocaine abuse
    Cyclosporin
Hypertension associated with insulin resistance
Isolated systolic hypertension in the elderly

Fig. 12-1. The mechanisms of secondary hypertension depending on the degree of volume overload and/or pressor factors.

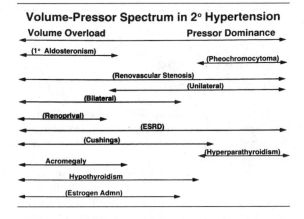

chapter will examine a predominantly volume-dependent hypertension (primary hyperaldosteronism), a pressor-dependent form (pheochromocytoma), as well as a type of hypertension that may appear anywhere in this spectrum depending on sodium intake and renal function (renovascular hypertension). Then several hypotheses directed toward essential hypertension will be examined, utilizing these same concepts to explain the pathophysiology.

Three Types of Secondary Hypertension

Primary Hyperaldosteronism

Primary hyperaldosteronism is characterized by overproduction of the mineralocorticoids aldosterone, corticosterone, 18-hydroxycortisol, and 18-oxocortisol which lead to renal retention of sodium and water, resulting in expansion of extracellular fluid volume. The overproduction of these mineralocorticoids is usually due to a benign adrenal cortical adenoma (Fig. 12-2) or to bilateral hyperplasia of the glomerulosa cells. (See Chap. 23 for additional discussion of primary hyperaldosteronism.)

Several features of mineralocorticoid hypertension support a major role for abnormal volume retention in elevating blood pressure. (1) Animals given excess mineralocorticoid do not become hypertensive unless volume overload is allowed to occur (e.g., concurrent salt-loading). (2) Suppression of the volume-sensitive renin-angiotensin system is a constant feature of mineralocorticoid hypertension. (3) An increase in atrial natriuretic peptide (ANP) has been found and is consistent with volume expansion. ANP levels return to normal following effective therapy. (4) Blood pressure can usually be normalized early in the disease by measures which reduce extracellular volume, such as diuresis and/or blockade of mineralocorticoid activity.

These patients may demonstrate an increased cardiac

Fig. 12-2. An aldosterone producing adrenal-cortical tumor which produced hyperaldosteronism, hypertension, and a hypokalemic alkalosis. Resection of the tumor led to a normalization of these abnormalities.

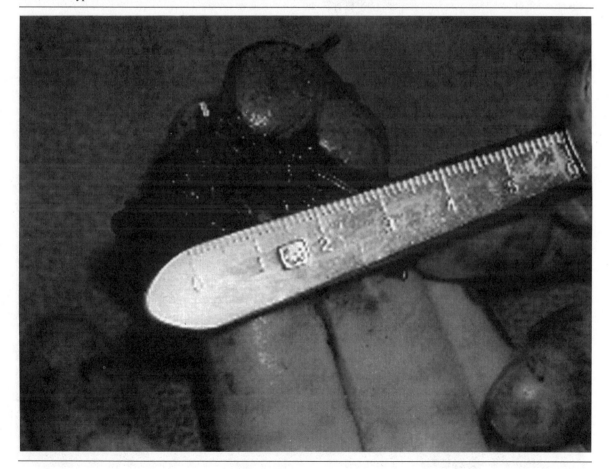

output and/or peripheral vascular resistance. These changes result from volume-loading and may also reflect increased sympathetic activity following activation of CNS mineralocorticoid receptors. In addition, long-standing renal damage may lead to a mild increase in the renin-angiotensin system. However, the initial pathophysiological abnormality is abnormal salt and water retention.

Pheochromocytoma

Patients with a pheochromocytoma, a tumor of the adrenal medulla (Fig. 12-3), are characterized by increased levels of norepinephrine and epinephrine, hormones excreted by the tumor. Norepinephrine predominates, causing periph-

eral vasoconstriction, pressure natriuresis, and elevated BP in the face of volume reduction. In addition, there is an alteration in the baroreceptor responsivity and mild elevation in heart rate. This condition, present in 0.1–0.5% of hypertensive patients, represents the purest form of predominantly "pressor" hypertension. Effective blockade of adrenergic hormone receptors alone frequently normalizes the blood pressure in these patients.

Renovascular Hypertension

This is the most interesting model for demonstrating how pathophysiological mechanisms can vary, depending on factors such as dietary sodium intake and renal function.

Fig. 12-3. A CT scan showing a left adrenal medullary pheochromocytoma (arrow). Resection led to normalization of blood pressure and disappearance of episodic adrenergic symptoms.

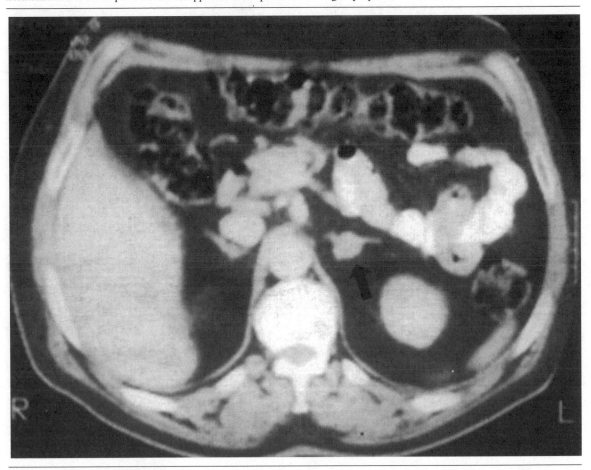

Hemodynamically significant unilateral stenosis of the renal artery (Fig. 12-4) leads to a lower renal perfusion pressure in the affected kidney. The renin-angiotensin system is activated, thereby increasing production of the potent vasoconstrictor angiotensin II (Ang II) which causes pressor hypertension. Under these conditions, acute blockade of Ang II production by an angiotensin converting enzyme inhibitor (CEI) or use of an Ang II receptor antagonist will lower the elevated BP. In contrast, bilateral renal artery stenosis is generally characterized by suppressed renin and angiotensin caused by volume overload. In this setting, blockade of the renin-angiotensin (R-A) system has little effect on the BP. However, diuretic therapy, by returning extracellular volume to normal, will temporarily lower blood pressure until or unless the volume reduction activates the R-A system and restores the blood pressure to its elevated level.

Patients with renovascular hypertension may occupy either extreme in this pathophysiological spectrum at different times, depending on circumstances. Using animal models and clinical human studies, it has been demonstrated that salt-loading the individual with a unilateral stenosis will transform the hypertension into a "volume-dependent" type. Conversely, volume depletion activates the R-A system in the bilaterally stenotic model and it becomes "pressor-dependent." Knowledge of the underlying pathophysiology has permitted development of clinical tests which utilize converting enzyme inhibitors to identify renin-dependent changes in these patients and to select a rational surgical or drug therapy based on these concepts.

Patients with advanced renal failure can also be made to change from a volume-overload status to a renin-dependent pressor mechanism with the use of potent diuretics or dialysis techniques. In this situation there is often an interplay between loss of renal vasodilator hormones (prostaglandins), volume-overload status, and the presence of pressor agents (norepinephrine and angiotensin II). Renoprival hypertension (resection of both kidneys) eliminates the role of renal pressor substances and usually converts the hypertension to a volume-dependent type.

Response to Therapy as an Indicator of Secondary Hypertension

Therapy of hypertension generally involves use of potent drugs which diminish the effectiveness of one or more of the physiological mechanisms which are responsible for the blood pressure elevation. The absence of a beneficial effect with a given agent can be used as an indicator that the blood pressure in that patient is not primarily dependent upon an abnormality targeted by the drug. An exam-

Fig. 12-4. Arteriogram showing narrowing of the proximal left renal artery. Poststenotic dilatation is present. Renal artery graft bypass normalized the blood pressure.

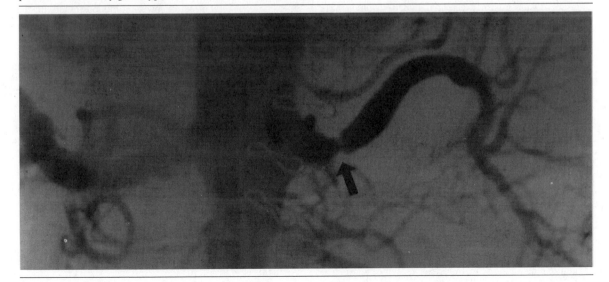

ple would be the absence of a beneficial effect of a diuretic on hypertension caused by a norepinephrine-secreting adrenal medullary tumor (pheochromocytoma).

Some authorities advocate careful testing of most patients with hypertension for secondary causes prior to beginning pharmacological therapy. A more prevalent practice, in view of the great predominance of patients with essential hypertension, is to treat them initially after using information from their history, physical examination, a urinalysis, and serum chemistry screen. If they have a poor therapeutic response or demonstrate clues to an underlying cause, then more extensive testing for one of the secondary forms of hypertension listed in Table 12-1 might be indicated.

Essential Hypertension

Mechanisms

Several hypotheses have been formulated to characterize the pathophysiology of essential (idiopathic) hypertension. Data can be marshalled to support each hypothesis probably because more than one component is operative either sequentially or concurrently in most patients. Early essential hypertension is frequently characterized as having increased CO with a normal (rather than suppressed) TPR. Over time, secondary changes in the vasculature lead to an increase in TPR, a normalization of the CO, and eventually to a markedly increased TPR and suppressed CO.

The hypotheses formulated to account for the increased CO during early essential hypertension include the following:

1. Central nervous system abnormalities increase the CO through direct cardiac effects but do not alter the peripheral resistance.
2. An increased retention of dietary sodium leads to mild volume retention and secondary changes in CO. Support for this hypothesis has been generated by studies indicating that hypertensive African-Americans tend to be more salt-sensitive (BP rises disproportionally following sodium-loading) than other hypertensives. This trait is shared to a smaller extent by many non-black hypertensives and may be present in up to 35% of patients with idiopathic hypertension. Most hypertensives, however, excrete an acute intravenous sodium load more rapidly compared to normotensives.
3. Alterations in Ca^{2+} and Na^+ transport occur across the cellular membranes in hypertensive subjects. Such a

defect would alter both volume and peripheral resistance.
4. The association of type II diabetes mellitus, obesity, and hypertension has been recognized for some time. Recent studies have supported the concept that elevated insulin concentrations, associated with insulin resistance, may contribute to sodium retention and result in the elevated arterial pressure.
5. Other hypotheses include overactivity of the adrenergic system or the renin-angiotensin system.

People with hypertension of long duration have been shown to "reset" their baroreceptors to a higher BP. When vasodilator medications are used, the CNS interprets the lowered BP as "abnormal" and increases autonomic tone to bring the lowered systemic pressure up to the previously elevated BP that was misinterpreted as "normal." If the BP is lowered for a long period of time, the opposite resetting may occur.

Clinical Consequences

Hypertension is one of the most important reversible risk factors for development of cardiovascular diseases. When hypertension coexists with obesity, smoking, and lipid disorders, there is a 20-fold increased likelihood for death from coronary heart disease. Hypertension is also strongly linked to development of stroke, end-stage renal disease, peripheral vascular occlusive diseases, and congestive heart failure.

The beneficial effect of lowering blood pressure on the occurrence of these complications constitutes one of the major advances in medicine during the 1960–1980s. Data clearly indicate that the risk of stroke, end-stage renal disease, and congestive heart failure is markedly diminished with effective control of blood pressure.

The effect of therapy on coronary artery occlusive disease and sudden cardiac death is more complicated. Many investigators currently believe the lack of a clear-cut improvement for these cardiac events is due to the complex etiology and long duration of antecedent coronary artery disease, the concurrence of other factors including cardiac hypertrophy, and the possibility that some pharmacologic agents may have deleterious secondary effects on atherosclerosis and intracellular ionic composition or may fail to prevent or reverse cardiac hypertrophy despite control of the blood pressure. These considerations have led to a searching re-evaluation of treatment goals and methods in patients at high risk for cardiac events.

Clinical Examples

1. A 52-year-old woman was found to have a BP of 186/104. She was tried on various drugs with indifferent success. Subsequently, she was admitted to the hospital because of the sudden onset of right-sided weakness.

Physical exam showed a BP of 165/100 while on three antihypertensive medications, and a right upper quadrant bruit. Mild weakness was noted in the right arm and leg. Her serum Na was 134 mEq/liter, K = 3.6 mEq/liter, creatinine = 1.4 mg/dl, and Hgb = 12.2 g/dl. Following a period of rehabilitation for her stroke, a renal angiogram was done. It showed a right renal artery stenosis that was asymmetrical, suggestive of atherosclerotic disease. Plasma renin activity (PRA) measured in samples obtained from each renal vein following acute administration of a converting enzyme inhibitor was 26 ng/ml/hour on the right and 10 ng/ml/hour on the left. A peripheral venous PRA was 11.5 ng/ml/hour. Surgical bypass of the right renal artery lowered her BP to normal for 18 months, after which it rose again into the hypertensive range.

Discussion.   This patient had a rather typical presentation of renovascular hypertension. She demonstrated increasingly severe hypertension, mild hypokalemia with a slightly low serum Na, and an upper quadrant abdominal bruit. An arteriogram demonstrated a stenosis in the right renal artery, and the selective renal vein determination confirmed the significance of this lesion. The patient initially had an excellent response to surgical bypass of the stenotic right renal artery. After her BP rose again, a repeat renal vein renin study demonstrated an elevated left renal venous value with a ratio 1.8 times that of the right and to the peripheral PRA. A repeat arteriogram with oblique views demonstrated a significant narrowing of the left renal artery that had been obscured on the previous standard views. The right renal artery bypass graft was widely patent. Surgical bypass of the left side led to long-standing improvement in her BP.

This patient demonstrates how clinical procedures built upon an understanding of the underlying pathophysiology can be of great assistance.

2. A 38-year-old male took an insurance exam and had a BP of 150/98 mm Hg. His urinalysis showed a trace of albumin. A repeat exam 2 months later showed the BP to be 145/94 and a normal urinalysis, but his application for insurance coverage was denied. He was asymptomatic. Physical examination revealed a 15% overweight male with minimal A/V nicking of the retinal vessels. The rest of the exam was normal. No abdominal bruit was heard. Serum electrolytes, BUN and creatinine, and a repeat urinalysis were normal. Twenty-four hour urinary protein excretion was 78 mg (normal < 150 mg/24 hours). A fasting serum glucose was 108 mg/dl. The patient was advised to lose 15 lb. In 2 months, he lost 7 lb. and his BP was 144/94. Eventually he lost 12 lb., his BP was 140/88, and his fasting plasma sugar was 92 mg/dl. Two months later, he passed his insurance exam. He missed two subsequent appointments and switched to a different health maintenance organization. Two years later, he returned weighing 15% over ideal body weight; his BP was 148/98 and a fasting plasma glucose was 134 mg/dl.

Discussion.   This patient with essential hypertension had associated obesity and mild elevation of his fasting blood sugar. Loss of weight was effective in lowering both his BP and his fasting plasma glucose values. Once the stimulus of obtaining life insurance was removed, he returned to his usual overweight condition, and again demonstrated hypertension and insulin resistance.

Bibliography

Guyton AC, ed. The circulation: Overview. In *Textbook of Medical Physiology* (8th ed). Philadelphia: W.B. Saunders, 1991, pp. 150–158. *A simplified physiologic view of hypertension.*

Kaplan NM, ed. Primary hypertension: pathogenesis. In *Clinical Hypertension* (6th ed). Baltimore: Williams & Wilkins, 1995. *An easily understood compilation of various aspects of hypertension. Easily the best text to use.*

Neaton JD and Wentworth D. Multiple Risk Factor Intervention Trial Group. Serum cholesterol, blood pressure, cigarette smoking, and death from coronary heart disease: Overall findings and differences by age for 316,099 white men. *Arch Int Med* 152:56–63, 1992. *The MRFIT research study has generated a great deal of useful information on mortality and risk in a very large sampling of the male population. If reasons are needed to stop smoking, lose weight, and accomplish control of blood pressure, here they are!*

The Fifth Joint National Committee Report on the detection, evaluation and treatment of high blood pressure. *Arch Int Med* 153:154–183, 1993. *This is a "working paper" with consensus recommendations from a broad range of experts on the diagnosis and management of the hypertensive patient. It is very useful as a reference guide to management of the average patient.*

13 Peripheral Vascular Disease

Brian G. Birdwell and Thomas L. Whitsett

Objectives

After completing this chapter, you should be able to

Understand the factors that determine and regulate organ/tissue blood flow

Differentiate between arterial insufficiency and other factors that cause claudication-type symptoms

Realize how an occlusive lesion that is not flow-limiting can become hemodynamically significant

Recognize when altered blood components can affect viscosity and reduce blood flow

Differentiate between normal and abnormal Doppler blood flow signals

Know the named deep and superficial veins of the lower extremities

Understand the functional differences among the deep, superficial, and communicating veins.

Explain the basic pathophysiology of the "post-phlebitic syndrome"

Know Virchow's Triad: Explain the significance of these factors, and give an example of each

Explain the role of objective testing in the diagnosis of deep-vein thrombosis (DVT)

Principles of Blood Flow (in Health and Disease)

Flow Regulation

Blood flow is described by the expression

$$Q = \frac{P_1 - P_2}{R}$$

where $P_1 - P_2$ is the arterial pressure differences between the respective ends of the vessels and R is vascular resistance. Under normal conditions P_2, being venous pressure, is relatively insignificant compared to P_1 and can be ignored. However, during low perfusion pressure and elevated venous pressure (e.g., arterial occlusive disease and heart failure), increases in P_2 may further impair tissue perfusion. Resistance to flow is in large part a function of the geometric aspects of the arterioles (resistance vessels)

and is controlled by autoregulation and neuronal (sympathic and cholinergic) effects. Vascular smooth-muscle contractility is controlled by intracellular Ca^{++} concentration as it lacks fast sodium channels; thus contractions are slow, prolonged, and associated with a low degree of ATP utilization.

Autoregulation

Autoregulatory factors predominate control of flow to the brain, heart, and skeletal muscles, while neuronal factors control flow to the skin and splanchnic regions. Humoral factors (hormones and drugs, e.g., catecholamines, histamine, acetylcholine, serotonin, angiotensin, adenosine, and prostaglandins) have varying sensitivities for different vascular beds. Autoregulation due to local or intrinsic factors seek to maintain blood pressure and flow adequate to maintain tissue metabolic needs. For most tissues an arteriolar/capillary pressure of 35–50 mm Hg is necessary for normal resting perfusion. Under conditions of stress (e.g., exercise, trauma, infection, or postsurgical healing), higher levels of perfusion and hence pressure are necessary to prevent ischemic conditions. The mediators of autoregulation include lactic acid, CO_2, hydrogen and potassium ions, and possibly adenosine and prostaglandins. Arterial oxygen concentration has little influence on vascular smooth-muscle tension. In the cerebral circulation autoregulation maintains constant blood flow to pressures of approximately 60 mm Hg assuming there are no hemodynamically significant occlusive lesions. Hydrogen ion and arterial pCO_2 produce vasodilatation and increase cerebral blood flow. That is why respiratory depressants (narcotics) are dangerous in people with head injuries, since hypoventilation results in cerebral vasodilatation and increased flow that worsens cerebral edema.

Endothelial Factors

Vascular endothelium, besides providing a nonthrombogenic barrier between soluble coagulation factors and the vessel wall, is a source of numerous substances that modulate smooth-muscle activity. Prostacyclin and endothelium-derived relaxing factor (EDRF) are vasodilators and also suppress vascular smooth-muscle growth. Prostacyclin also inhibits platelet aggregation. Endothelin and angiotensin II are vasoconstrictors, both of which have a mitogenic vascular smooth-muscle effect. Angiotensin II and vasopressin produce vasoconstriction acting through endothelial receptors, while atrial natriuretic factors vasodilate. There is a local tissue renin-angiotensin system that is active irrespective of circulating hormones.

Endothelium-Derived Relaxing Factors

Nitric oxide is thought to be the potent substance called EDRF that causes vasodilation by stimulating guanylate cyclase to increase cyclic GMP activity. EDRF is released by acetylcholine, ATP, serotonin, thrombin, shear stress, increased flow, vasopressin, and norepinephrine. When EDRF response is impaired (denuded endothelium, diabetes mellitus, atherosclerosis, hypercholesterolemia, and hypertension) vasoconstrictor stimuli predominate or have exaggerated effect that can further affect flow and possibly lead to thrombosis.

Endothelins

The endothelins are a family of peptides that are synthesized as a propeptide, cleaved to form big endothelin and then further cleaved by endothelin-converting enzyme to form the active peptide. Endothelin I is formed in vascular endothelium, and endothelin III in neural tissue. They are potent, long-acting vasoconstrictors which act by stimulating voltage-sensitive calcium channels. Endothelins are activated by thrombin, angiotensin II, vasopressin, and decreased blood flow.

Characteristics of Flow

Arterial flow is normally laminar with migration of cellular elements to the center (axial streaming) and a thin cell-free zone at the vessel wall. Flow velocity is maximum in the axial stream and zero at the wall. Movement between the adjacent fluid layers (shear rate) is thus maximum at the wall and least at the center of the vessel. Velocity (cm/sec) refers to the rate of displacement per unit time. Volume flow (cm^3/sec) refers to volume per unit time and is represented by the equation

$$Q = VA$$

where Q is volume flow, V is velocity of flow, and A is cross-sectional area. Radial mixing of fluid is referred to as turbulence and a greater pressure is required to maintain turbulent flow. The Reynolds number is the ratio of inertial to viscous forces and is expressed as

$$N_R = \frac{pDv}{n}$$

where p is the fluid density, D is the tube or vessel diameter, v is the mean velocity, and n is the fluid viscosity. For $N_R < 2000$ flow is laminar when $N_R > 3000$ turbulence develops. Thus, large-diameter vessels with high velocity and low viscosity will predispose to turbulence. Also, abrupt variations in vessel dimensions or surface irregularity will predispose to turbulence. This usually causes vibrations that can be detected by stethoscope (bruit) in anemia (reduced viscosity) in close proximity to a stenotic lesion or tortuous vessel and with increased cardiac output (increased velocity). Blood clots are more likely to occur with turbulent flow, thus explaining the tendency of thrombi to form in aneurysms, at sites of stenotic lesions, and with prosthetic valves.

The resistance to flow is represented functionally by **resistance = vascular hindrance** (geometry of vessel) × **blood viscosity** (flow properties of blood), or specifically:

$$R = \frac{1}{r^4} \times n$$

where r is the radius of the vessel, l is the length of the conduit involved, and n is viscosity of blood. Clearly the caliber of a vessel is the major factor determining resistance and, with the arteriolar/capillary bed being the smallest, it is the principal determinant. Since capillaries lack smooth muscle, vasoreactivity in the arterioles is the major factor influencing peripheral vascular resistance under normal conditions. However, with hyperviscosity syndromes or during hypotensive perfusion, blood fluidity becomes important.

Hemorrheologic Aspects of Flow

Viscosity, the internal friction of a fluid, exerts a direct effect on the resistance equation, but under normal circumstances does not change dramatically nor influence flow as long as shear stress (the force that produces a relative motion of fluid layers) is adequate to counteract effects created by viscosity. Under conditions of low shear stress, deformability of erythrocytes and leukocytes and their movement through capillaries are important determinants of resistance to flow and adequacy of perfusion. Ischemia, diabetes, endotoxemia, and sickle cell disease are conditions that may reduce erythrocyte and leukocyte deformability and thereby increase resistance to flow through the capillaries. Narrow capillary diameters due to basement membrane thickening in diabetes would further increase the "cellular" aspects of blood viscosity and favor flow through larger-diameter, thoroughfare-type capillaries that lack adequate exchange of oxygen and other metabolic products. Plasma is about 1.5 times as viscous as water and its viscosity depends on the concentration of high molecular weight asymmetric proteins, e.g., fibrinogen, alpha-2 macroglobulins, and immunoglobulins M and G. Plasma viscosity increases acutely with dehydration. Blood (which exhibits a viscosity about 2–15 times that of water) is a non-Newtonian fluid, so that viscosity is a function of shear rate and hematocrit (Fig. 13-1).

Under conditions of normal shear stress, hematocrit must be above 60% to exert a significant influence on viscosity. However, when a bed is perfused by low shear stress (e.g., distal to a stenotic lesion), when a vessel is occluded and dependent on collateral flow, or during a hypotensive disorder, then even normal hematocrits have a negative effect on blood fluidity and consequently oxygen delivery. An optimal hematocrit for oxygen delivery in low shear stress perfusion is in the range of 30–35%.

Rouleaux or erythrocyte aggregation is an important aspect to the loss of fluidity of sluggish or low shear blood flow. This occurs in capillaries, veins, and other sites where low flow exists. It is correlated with plasma fibrinogen concentration, which creates a charge that causes erythrocytes to aggregate like stacked coins when shear stress

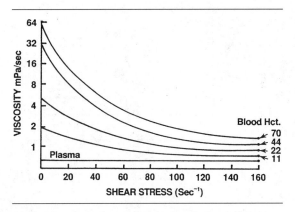

Fig. 13-1. Erythrocyte aggregation causes blood to behave as a non-Newtonian fluid. As hematocrit increases blood becomes more viscous and this tendency is exaggerated under conditions of low shear rate (flow).

is low and particularly at normal or higher hematocrits. Rouleaux formation has been shown in vivo by capillary microscopy; how important it is in patients is uncertain, but is likely significant.

Patterns of Flow in Lower Extremities

Resting blood flow at the common femoral region and below is triphasic. This is easily discerned by a handheld Doppler instrument which detects erythrocyte velocity by the Doppler-shift effect (Fig. 13-2). Initial forward flow follows cardiac systole and is associated with dilation of the conducting arteries. This is followed by elastic recoil and the direction of flow is towards vascular beds with lower resistance. Since the lower extremities have relatively high resistance and the renal and spanchnic beds are of low resistance, a brief reversal of flow occurs during early diastole. In the remainder of diastole, flow is in a forward direction. In the presence of infection, trauma, or following exercise, the resistance in the legs may be less than in the splanchnic region and the reversal phase of flow is attenuated or absent. Hence the waveform may normally be biphasic under these conditions.

Flow Obstruction

Stenotic lesions (under stable resting conditions) that compromise the diameter of an artery in a mild to moderate degree are usually not hemodynamically significant. This can be attributed to the Bernoulli effect, which describes the reduction of pressure distal to a site of stenosis, accompanied by an increase in velocity of fluid flow to maintain a constant flow volume. The flow is often laminar at the site

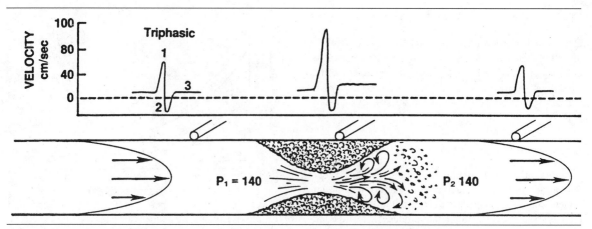

Fig. 13-2. Flow through a nonhemodynamically significant stenosis with corresponding Doppler flow velocity waveforms. Note higher velocity within the stenosis and poststenotic turbulence with reconstitution of laminar flow. P_1 and P_2 represent peak systolic pressure in mm Hg.

of maximum stenosis, but in the poststenotic areas it becomes turbulent (a bruit may be heard) with eddy current formation and recirculation near the vessel wall producing boundary-layer separation. There is also an increased lateral pressure directed toward the vessel wall that may lead to "poststenotic" dilatation which may predispose to thromboembolism. Note: Volume flow is maintained (under stable resting conditions) until there is an approximate 70–80% stenosis (diameter narrowing).

As luminal area becomes critical, i.e., exceeds the ability to maintain volume flow by increasing velocity within the stenosis, the lesion is said to be hemodynamically significant and is associated with a pressure drop with an equivalent decrease in volume flow (Fig. 13-3). Initially, systolic pressure decreases while diastolic values remain unchanged. As the degree of stenosis increases, pressure and flow are decreased exponentially.

When a vessel becomes occluded or contains a tight stenosis (> 80% diameter narrowing), flow in the distal vessels is dependent upon reconstitution by collaterals which are relatively high-resistance conduits. This results in a monophasic waveform.

It is important to understand that as peripheral resistance distal to a stenotic lesion decreases (due to exercise or some other metabolic demand), the degree of stenosis that produces hemodynamic significance is reduced; thus a subcritical stenosis is transformed to a functionally critical one during exercise.

When these conditions exist in a lower extremity, modest exercise produces ischemia, resulting in ankle pressures of less than 60 mm Hg and inadequate flow to the foot. On physical examination, the patient will have blanching of the affected foot after exercise with no palpable pulses or detectable Doppler flow. Obviously, patients with ischemic foot ulcers who require an increase in skin blood flow to achieve healing would experience greater ischemic ulcer problems during ambulation as blood is diverted to exercising muscles.

Flow Assessment

Patients with arterial occlusive disease are usually asymptomatic at rest but develop claudication with exercise when the demand for skeletal muscle blood flow exceeds supply. The symptoms of intermittent claudication vary from person to person but usually include pain (often starting in the calf) and often numbness or weakness during exercise (10 yards to 1 mile) that is relieved by a short rest. On physical examination there is a pallor with elevation of the feet and a dependent rubor. Trophic skin changes are present as disease progresses and consist of digital atrophy, thickened nails, loss of hair on the dorsum of the toes, and thinning of the skin. Gangrene is a reflection of severe disease. The femoral pulses reflect inflow (aorto-iliac) disease. As severity of disease increases, resting pulses become difficult to palpate. In milder forms of disease, pulses may only be diminished or absent after a brisk walk. Palpating

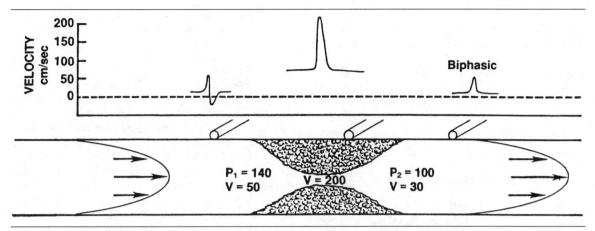

Fig. 13-3. Flow through a hemodynamically significant stenosis with a 40 mm Hg pressure drop and a corresponding decrease in volume flow. V represents flow velocity in cm/sec. Note higher Doppler waveform velocities and poststenotic biphasic waveforms.

pulses is sometimes difficult and imprecise. Elevating the legs to approximately 45° and observing the plantar surface of the feet and toes for pallor is also a good technique for assessing the adequacy of circulation. The more severe the disease the quicker pallor develops. If no blanching develops, supine ankle pressure is likely greater than 80 mm Hg. Compressing the nail bed and then assessing capillary refill of the toes with the legs elevated provides further information in patients who do not blanch spontaneously.

Measurement of ankle arterial pressure is a common technique for evaluating patients with claudication symptoms. A Doppler probe is placed over the posterior tibial or dorsalis pedis artery to detect flow. A cuff placed on the ankle is inflated and, when pressure is released, the first Doppler flow sounds represent the systolic pressure at the cuff site. A common parameter is the ankle/arm index (AAI), which is the ankle systolic pressure divided by the brachial artery systolic pressure. Normally, this value is one or higher. If it is higher than 1.3, suspect calcific medial sclerosis (often seen in diabetics) or interference with arterial compression by the blood pressure cuff. AAI values less than 0.9–1.0 reflect occlusive disease. Values less than 0.8 are consistent with moderate disease and values less than 0.5 severe disease. Patients may have a normal AAI at rest yet have a significant stenotic lesion that becomes flow limiting with exercise, producing an abnormal AAI. However, ankle pressures of less than 60 mm Hg (irrespective of the AAI) immediately after exercise is required to confirm that arterial insufficiency is the cause of the symptoms.

A common scenario is a patient with known peripheral artery disease (PAD) and an AAI around 0.8 who develops symptoms suggesting claudication but immediately after exercise has an ankle pressure that is not in the ischemic range. When this occurs, one should suspect some other cause for the exercise symptoms, e.g., spinal stenosis, degenerative disc disease, or other musculoskeletal abnormality.

There are other techniques available in the noninvasive vascular laboratory to assess the adequacy of flow. These include (1) pulse volume recordings (a plethysmographic cuff that assesses the sum total of all pulsatile phenomena beneath the cuff) (2) photoplethysmography (PPG) that measures microvascular skin flow in the digits or adjacent to skin lesions, (3) transcutaneous pO_2 ($tcpO_2$), which measures the partial pressure of oxygen within the skin; this is a function of skin perfusion as well as hemoglobin O_2 saturation, and is used to detect ischemic rest pain and predict successful amputation sites, and (4) duplex scan (ultrasound with Doppler flow) to observe lesions and assess hemodynamic significance.

Compartment Syndrome
Following reperfusion of an ischemic limb (after thrombolytic therapy or surgical revascularization), swelling may occur within an anatomically confined area (e.g., the

anterior compartment of the lower leg). This is the result of capillary leak in ischemic tissue that increases compartmental pressure. If excessive, this pressure (which can be measured at the bedside) causes muscle paralysis from both damage to the nerves within the compartment and impaired arterial flow. Treatment is by fasciotomy, which is either performed prophylactically in certain postischemic revascularization procedures, or as clinically indicated employing direct measurement of compartmental pressures.

Aneurysmal Disease

A vessel is considered aneurysmal when the diameter is twice the size of its more proximal segment. A weakness within the wall permits expansion of the lumen and thinning of the wall itself. Atherosclerosis is a major risk factor, but defects in type III collagen and elastin likely play a major role. Wall tension is described by the law of Laplace:

$$T = Pr$$

where T is tension in the vessel wall (a force that is tangential to the vessel wall, tending to pull apart a theoretical longitudinal slit in the vessel), P is transmural pressure, and r is the vessel radius. Thus, as aneurysmal diameter increases, there is a proportional elevation in wall tension, and as thinning occurs, wall stress is further increased. Thus an expanding aneurysm has two factors at work that predispose to rupture, an increase in diameter and wall thinning. Another complication is that laminated thrombi may form in the aneurysm that can be the source of emboli or progress to total vessel occlusion.

In the clinical setting, an abdominal aortic aneurysm that is 4–5 cm in diameter (normal aorta being approximately 1–2 cm) should be considered for surgical repair. A 6-cm aneurysm has such a high incidence of rupture that surgery should be considered even in the high-risk patient.

Venous Disorders

Anatomy of Lower-Extremity Venous System

Venous drainage of the lower extremities is accomplished via three systems: (1) the deep system, which carries approximately 85% of the blood from the legs to the central circulation; (2) the superficial system, which includes the visible and sometimes palpable veins familiar to patients

and clinicians; and (3) the perforator (or communicating) venous system, small veins which connect the superficial and deep systems (Fig. 13-4).

Deep System

In the lower leg the deep system consists of the deep plantar veins of the foot and six paired veins (not featured in the figure) in the calf which converge in the upper third of the calf to form three veins: **posterior tibial, peroneal, anterior tibial.** The posterior tibial and peroneal veins converge to form the tibioperoneal trunk in the proximal calf. The anterior tibial vein joins the tibioperoneal trunk, usually at the distal popliteal fossa, to form the **popliteal vein.** At the level of the obturator canal in the distal thigh the popliteal vein is renamed the **superficial femoral vein** (note: still very much a "deep vein"). In the upper thigh, the deep femoral vein, which drains the muscles of the thigh, joins the superficial femoral vein to form the **common femoral vein.** At the level of the inguinal ligament this vein is renamed the **external iliac,** which when joined by the internal iliac becomes the **common iliac vein.** The right and left common iliac veins converge to form the **inferior vena cava.**

Superficial System

Lying within the subcutaneous tissues, the superficial veins of the leg are familiar structures: Varicose veins are dilated superficial veins, and many normal superficial veins may be visible and/or palpable. The superficial system consists of two major veins, the greater (or long) saphenous vein and the lesser (or short) saphenous vein. The **greater saphenous vein,** formed by the confluence of veins from the medial sole of the foot and the medial marginal vein, courses upward anterior to the medial malleolus and along the anteromedial surface of the leg and thigh, finally emptying into the common femoral vein just distal to the inguinal ligament. The **lesser saphenous vein** drains the lateral aspect of the heel and calf. It ascends along the lateral border of the Achilles tendon until it reaches the middle third of the calf. Typically it empties into the popliteal vein in the popliteal fossa, but it may instead join the greater saphenous vein in the calf, the popliteal vein high in the popliteal fossa, or join the femoral vein in the upper thigh.

Communicating Veins

Blood from the superficial system flows into the deep system via the communicating veins. The largest communicating veins are the terminal portions of the greater and lesser saphenous veins; they drain into the femoral and popliteal veins, respectively.

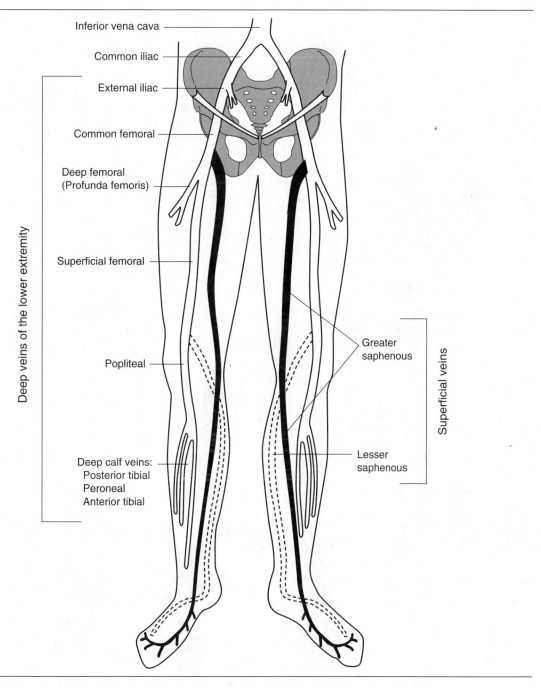

Fig. 13-4. The deep and superficial veins of the lower extremities. The communicating veins, which connect the deep and superficial veins, are represented by the terminal greater and lesser saphenous veins as they empty into the common femoral and popliteal veins, respectively. (Many other important communicating veins, particularly in the calf, are not featured here.)

Normal Venous Physiology

The deep veins of the calf function as reservoirs from which the venous blood is propelled when squeezed by the calf muscles. (This anatomical arrangement is called "the calf muscle pump.") (Fig. 13-5) This action is analogous to the cardiac ventricles, with a systolic and diastolic phase. During the "diastolic phase," the relaxed calf muscles allow the deep calf veins to fill with venous blood — in part by flow from the superficial system via the communicating veins. During the "systolic phase," calf muscle contraction pushes the blood into more proximal deep veins. Pressures in the deep veins are actually lower than in the superficial system during the diastolic phase, but greatly exceed superficial venous pressure during muscle contraction, as depicted in Fig. 13-5. The communicating veins have valves which allow flow from the superficial system into the deep veins during "diastole" (when the differential

Fig. 13-5. The calf muscle pump in normal and abnormal legs. A. During calf muscle relaxation ("diastolic phase") in both normal legs or legs with insufficient valves, the pressure differential favors the flow of venous blood from the superficial to the deep veins, and the communicating vein valves allow flow in that direction. B. When the calf muscle pump contracts ("systolic phase") in the normal leg, pressure in the deep veins rises far above that in the superficial veins, but intact valves in the communicating veins prevent flow back into the superficial system and preserves the low-pressure environment. Venous flow is exclusively proximal, toward the heart. C. Calf muscle contraction in the leg with insufficient communicating valves allows the venous blood to flow back into the superficial veins, exposing them to abnormally high pressures.

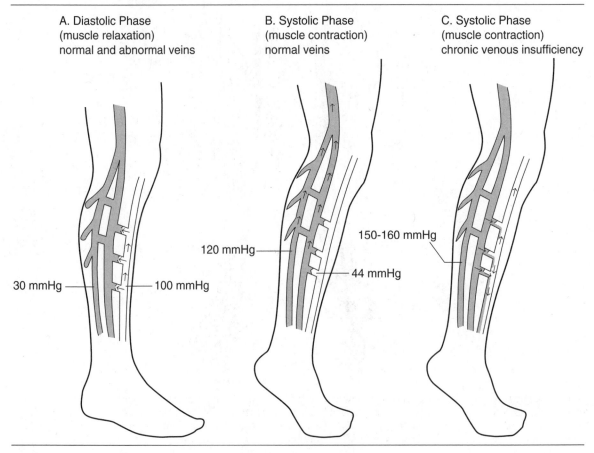

A. Diastolic Phase
(muscle relaxation)
normal and abnormal veins

B. Systolic Phase
(muscle contraction)
normal veins

C. Systolic Phase
(muscle contraction)
chronic venous insufficiency

30 mmHg — — 100 mmHg

120 mmHg —

— 44 mmHg

150-160 mmHg

pressures favor superficial-to-deep flow), but prevent re-fluxing of high-pressure venous blood from the deep-vein system back into the superficial veins during the "systolic phase." Therefore these one-way valves have two important functions during the contraction of the calf muscle pump: (1) promote exclusively forward deep venous blood flow toward the heart and (2) protect the superficial system from the high venous pressures generated during the "systolic phase." The deep veins themselves also have one-way valves which perform the same two functions: prevent retrograde flow and help to limit the peak tissue or venous calf pressures during muscle contraction to approximately 120 mm Hg.

Chronic Venous Insufficiency and Postphlebitic Syndrome

If lower-extremity venous valves don't function properly, the pathophysiological state is termed **chronic venous insufficiency.** It is believed that the most common cause of this problem is damage or destruction of venous valves from deep-vein thrombosis (see below). But many patients present to physicians with insufficient venous valves and neither past symptoms nor any objective signs of recent or remote venous thrombosis. While many of these patients may have had an asymptomatic episode of deep-vein thrombosis which left no "tracks," most authorities now acknowledge that some individuals acquire chronic venous insufficiency for unknown reasons. Whatever the cause, improperly functioning valves have the same pathophysiological consequences (Fig. 13-6). The malfunctioning valves of the communicating veins fail to shield the superficial system from the high venous pressure generated during the "systolic phase" of the calf muscle pump. (Those "systolic phase" pressures are especially high in persons whose deep veins also have insufficient valves: When the patient is upright, significant hydrostatic pressure is created by the effect of gravity upon the uninterrupted column of blood.) In patients with chronic venous insufficiency, **the most potent pathophysiological factor is the exposure of the superficial venous system to high venous pressures.** In response to these high pressures, the subcutaneous venous capillaries then develop increased permeability, allowing fibrin- and protein-rich serum to leak into the interstitial tissues. The proteins attract water and trap it in the interstitial space, producing edema, while the fibrin impairs the normal exchange of oxygen and nutrients across the capillaries, causing subsequent disruption of cellular metabolism and cell death. In advanced cases of chronic venous insufficiency, these forces lead to chronic

edema, fibrosis, skin breakdown and chronic ulceration, and typical pigmentary changes due to hemosiderin deposition from leaked erythrocytes (see Fig. 13-6). Although chronic venous insufficiency causes 85% of lower-extremity skin ulcers, these nonhealing ulcers must be distinguished from other causes (Table 13-1). These physical findings, along with swelling and pain, constitute a clinical picture known as the postphlebitic syndrome. Early detection of chronic venous insufficiency is key: Correct diagnosis in a patient with unexplained leg edema saves further workup for other potential causes and allows the application of treatment (compression stockings) that prevents progression to the postphlebitic syndrome. Diagnosis may be formally accomplished at a noninvasive vascular laboratory; there are, however, two easily applied bedside maneuvers which may provide useful information about venous valvular function.

Trendelenburg's Test

This test evaluates for incompetence of the valves in the long saphenous vein (a common, inherited defect with primarily cosmetic implications) and is useful in those patients who have associated varicosities of this vein. The patient lies on an examining table and raises the involved leg above heart level to empty the veins. A rubber tourniquet is applied to the upper thigh and the patient is asked to stand up quickly for about 15 seconds. If the valves of the long saphenous vein are incompetent, when the tourniquet is released the veins will immediately fill with blood.

Perthes' Test

It detects incompetence of the perforating (communicating) veins at the ankle. Patients are asked to exercise the calf by rapidly raising and lowering themselves on their toes. A tourniquet is applied to the upper leg just below the knee to prevent additional filling from an incompetent long or short saphenous system. The patient begins the exercise again. If the veins at the ankle become less prominent, the results suggest that the valves of the perforating veins are competent. If the veins become more prominent, the results suggest that the high pressure of the deep system is being transmitted through incompetent perforating (communicating) veins at the superficial ankle veins.

The aim of treatment of patients with chronic venous insufficiency or more advanced postphlebitic disease is the same: reducing the accumulation of edema due to lower-extremity venous hypertension. This is accomplished in a simple way by elevating the leg, thereby employing gravity to reduce venous pressure in the lower leg. For ambulatory or wheelchair-bound patients, maintaining externally

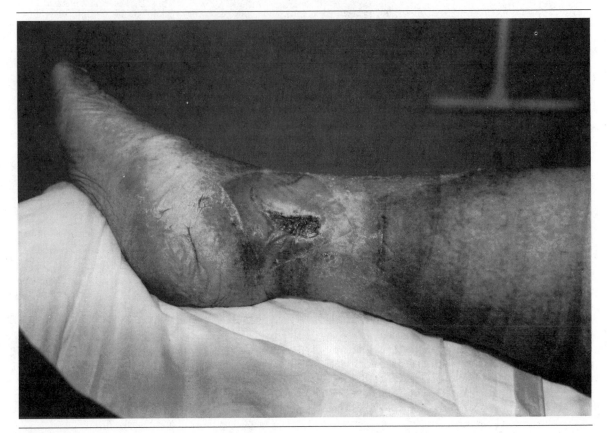

Fig. 13-6. Longstanding chronic venous insufficiency and postphlebitic syndrome. Note pigmentary change, which demarcates the level distal to which communicating vein valves are insufficient. Even with meticulous care, ulceration may take many months to heal.

Table 13-1. Causes of Chronic Lower-Extremity Ulceration

VASCULAR	MALIGNANT	MISCELLANEOUS
Venous stasis	Squamous cell	Blood dyscrasias
Ischemic	carcinoma	Mechanical
Vasculitic	Kaposi's carcinoma	Chemical
	Malignant melanoma	Thermal
INFECTIOUS	Malignant breast	Neuropathic
Bacterial	carcinoma	Insect bite
Fungal	Basal cell carcinoma	Radiation
Syphilitic		Frostbite
		Factitial
	METABOLIC	
	Diabetes mellitus	

applied pressure of 30–40 mm Hg via custom-fitted gradient compression hose is remarkably effective in preventing the leakage of serum and formed blood elements from the venous capillaries into the subcutaneous tissues.

Deep-Vein Thrombosis

The topic of **venous thromboembolism,** which is comprised of deep-vein thrombosis (DVT) and pulmonary embolism (PE) is also covered in Chapter 50.

Venous thrombosis represents a collection of fibrin, erythrocytes, leukocytes, and platelets which occurs as a result of an imbalance between the forces of thrombogenesis and thrombolysis. This disequilibrium may result from an inborn abnormality of the blood itself leading to a proclivity to clot, as seen in inherited deficiencies of anticlotting proteins such as Protein C and Protein S. Much more commonly, the balance is tipped by injury to vein endothelium, stasis of venous blood flow (e.g., prolonged bed rest; congestive heart failure), and/or an acquired state of hypercoagulability such as pregnancy, surgery, or certain malignancies. These three factors — endothelial injury, venostasis, and hypercoagulability — were identified by Virchow over a century ago, but Virchow's Triad remains a valid conceptualization of the factors which promote abnormal clot formation in the deep veins of the leg.

It is postulated that deep-vein thrombus begins at side branches or behind valve cusps, sites of turbulent currents and eddy flow. These sites may facilitate the deposition of platelets and fibrin on the endothelium, because turbulent flow may cause endothelial injury, and the geometry of branching veins and valve cusps creates small pockets of sluggish flow. Undoubtedly, tiny thrombi frequently form in normal individuals, but whether this nidus propagates into a substantial thrombus or is harmlessly dissolved is largely due to other factors such as immobility, recent surgery, bed rest — in other words, factors which fit into the categories of Virchow's Triad.

Patients with DVT may have no leg symptoms. Indeed some patients present only with pulmonary symptoms due to embolized thrombus. In symptomatic patients pain and swelling occur most often, but anatomic sites of the symptoms are **not** a guide to location of disease: calf vein clot can present with thigh symptoms and thrombus in thigh veins may manifest as pain or swelling in the calf only. Pain in this setting is caused by associated inflammation but may be negligible or absent, in contrast to thrombosis in the superficial veins, which is usually quite painful, exquisitely tender, and palpably inflamed. Edema reflects the extravasation of capillary and lymphatic fluid due to vein inflammation and increased venous and lymphatic pressures. Acute iliofemoral thrombosis may present with massive swelling, pain, tenderness, and cyanosis of the affected extremity, a clinical picture termed "phlegmasia cerulea dolens." (The cyanotic hue comes from the accumulation of reduced hemoglobin due to sluggish venous outflow.) Even more ominous is "phlegmasia alba dolens" where the leg is pallid, a sign of embarrassment of arterial inflow caused by venous pressures approaching or exceeding systemic blood pressure.

DVT, then, manifests a broad spectrum of symptomatic severity and may be mimicked by a number of other conditions (Table 13-2). Consequently, objective testing for DVT is essential to confirm its presence or absence.

Table 13-2. Conditions That Can Mimic Symptomatic DVT

CONDITIONS THAT LEAD TO PAIN

Ruptured popliteal (Baker's) cyst
Subfascial or intramuscular hematoma
Ruptured plantaris muscle
Nerve entrapment

CONDITIONS THAT CAUSE EDEMA

Postphlebitic syndrome
Congestive heart failure
Lymphedema
Extrinsic venous compression by trauma, hematoma, malignancy
Prolonged dependency (paralysis, ischemic rest pain)
Hypothyroidism

CONDITIONS THAT CAUSE LEG INFLAMMATION

Cellulitis
Lymphangitis
Subcutaneous fat necrosis

Clinical Examples

1. A 61-year-old man describes left calf cramping and fatigue which manifests at one-half block of ambulation, and is relieved with 5 minutes of rest. A recent serum cholesterol was 274 mg% at a screening health check. His father died from an acute myocardial infarction at age 50. The patient has smoked for 45 years. His blood pressure was 140/80. Both common femoral pulses were readily palpable (2/2), while the right posterior tibialis pulse was diminished (1/2) and the left posterior tibialis pulse was undetected (0/2). Noninvasive vascular examination revealed triphasic Doppler waveforms at the common femoral arteries bilaterally, biphasic Doppler waveforms at the right popliteal artery, monophasic Doppler waveforms at the left popliteal artery, a right ankle systolic pressure of 102 mm Hg, and a left ankle systolic pressure of 46 mm Hg.

Discussion.   Peripheral arterial disease often manifests in the lower extremities as intermittent claudication provoked by exertion and relieved with rest. Modifiable risk factors for the development of atherosclerotic disease include smoking, hypercholesterolemia, and hypertension. This patient exhibited signs of bilateral occlusive vascular disease which was more severe on the left. This was confirmed by the deterioration in Doppler waveforms between the common femoral artery and the popliteal artery and the diminished ankle/arm indices (left 0.33; right 0.73). An abdominal aortogram with aortofemoral runoff revealed a discrete 75% stenosis in the left superficial femoral artery which was dilated successfully with an angioplasty catheter, followed by a resolution of his symptoms.

2. A 45-year-old insulin-dependent diabetic man purchased a new pair of workshoes and broke them in on a weekend walk. The following morning, he noted blisters on the right first toe and on the bottom of his left foot. On examination, he had normal femoral pulses, difficult-to-feel popliteal pulses, and weak to normal posterior tibial pulses. There were no skin changes other than the blisters and large callouses over the metatarsal heads on both feet. The feet did not blanch with elevation to 45°. Bilateral ankle/arm indices were 0.9. Sensation was markedly diminished in both feet.

Discussion.   Diabetic neuropathic lower-extremity ulcerations occur as a result of unrecognized trauma since pain is often not perceived in the setting of diabetic neuropathy. A callous acts as a foreign body and requires prompt, aggressive treatment when discovered on the foot of a diabetic. Progression to limb-threatening and life-threatening infection may ensue if not interrupted with appropriate wound debridement and dressing changes, antibiotic administration, and revascularization as possible. The patient developed a potentially lethal lower-extremity lesion as a complication of purchasing a pair of new shoes. (All diabetic patients should be instructed on proper foot care and should examine their feet on a daily basis. The physician should also examine their feet at each clinic visit.) The findings on examination and the ankle/arm index of 0.9 suggest only minimal macrovascular disease.

3. A 69-year-old woman had a total knee replacement one month before appearing at the emergency room. She complained of left lower-extremity pain and swelling, which 2 days previously involved the calf but had spread to involve the thigh as well. Earlier in the day she experienced the acute onset of pleuritic chest pain accompanied by dyspnea, tachypnea, and cough, and she has a low-grade fever. Hemoptysis and sputum production are absent.

Discussion.   Venous thromboembolism is the most common disease of the vascular system. It may present with symptoms of either deep-vein thrombosis (DVT), pulmonary embolism (PE), or both, as in this case. DVT is common after surgeries or trauma to the lower extremities; prophylaxis against such events is very helpful but by no means eliminates them all. The diagnosis of DVT and PE is suggested by this patient's presentation but must be confirmed with objective testing. Once the diagnosis is secure, treatment — intravenous heparin — should be instituted immediately, followed by at least 3 months of warfarin. Chronic venous insufficiency in the wake of this DVT is likely. It may be treated prophylactically by fitting the patient with compression stockings prior to discharge from the hospital, thereby lessening the chances of the morbidity of the postphlebitic syndrome.

Bibliography

European Working Group on Chronic Critical Leg Ischemia. Second European consensus document on chronic critical leg ischemia. *Circulation* 84(suppl.):IV 1–26, 1991. *A comprehensive statement endorsed by the American Heart Association detailing problems related to leg ischemia.*

Kilo C. Vascular complications of diabetes. *CVR&R* 6:18, 21–23, 1987. *A review of peripheral vascular problems associated with diabetes.*

Localzo J, Creager MA, and Dzau VJ (eds). *Vascular Medicine.* Boston: Little, Brown, 1992. *A textbook covering all aspects of vascular disease.*

Moser K. Venous thromboembolism. *Am Rev Respir Dis* 141:235–249, 1990. *A comprehensive review of all aspects by an internationally recognized authority.*

O'Donnell TF. Chronic venous insufficiency and varicose veins. In Young JR, Graor RA, Olin JW, and Bartholomew JR (eds). *Peripheral Vascular Diseases.* New York: Mosby, 1991. *A lucid review of a common but poorly understood disorder which generally receives little attention in textbooks of medicine. Features a thorough rendering of pathophysiology, and reviews surgical aspects as well.*

14 Cardiovascular Wellness, Exercise, and Prevention of Heart Disease

E. Randy Eichner

Objectives

After completing this chapter, you should be able to

Distinguish the "healthful physiology" of athlete's heart from the pathophysiology of heart disease

Differentiate 12 risk factors or lifestyle factors that may contribute to coronary heart disease

Identify eight "nondrug" or lifestyle measures that can help prevent or treat hypertension

Explain how "body shape" — where excess fat is deposited — interacts with physiology and metabolism to shape the risk of heart disease

Understand about gender and coronary risk factors key for men; for women

Heart disease is our nation's leading killer. Despite the declining death rate from acute myocardial infarction (AMI) over the past two decades, coronary heart disease (CHD) — mainly AMI — still causes about one death in three, nearly 600,000 deaths a year. The pathophysiology of AMI — essentially coronary atherosclerosis and thrombosis — is covered in Chap. 5. Stroke, our third leading killer, is covered in Chap. 68. Accordingly, this chapter, on cardiovascular wellness, covers prevention of AMI. For each risk factor and/or lifestyle considered, physiology is covered where relevant; pathophysiology is detailed as known. In this chapter, clinical epidemiology and clinical trials are also key.

Exercise

Hippocrates said "To keep well, avoid too much food, too little toil." Cicero added "Exercise and temperance can

preserve something of our strength in old age." William Osler declared "A man is only as old as his arteries." Despite this sage advice, many Americans are sedentary. Recent surveys find that only 20% of adults exercise enough to reap maximal cardiovascular benefit. Another 40% may be active enough to gain some cardiovascular benefit. The final 40%, alas, are sedentary, which doubles their risk of CHD and AMI.

In the past 40 years, many epidemiological studies have related exercise habits to risk of AMI. A recent meta-analysis of 35 studies finds a relative risk of death from CHD of 1.9 for sedentary compared with active people. To be sure, selection bias and other confounding occurs in such studies, which are observational, not randomized. This begs the question: Do active people stay healthy; do healthy people stay active; or is it both?

Because we lack a randomized, controlled trial, a minority of experts holds that "The hypothesis that regular exercise can prevent CHD and prolong life is not yet proved." But the majority holds that we know sloth causes AMI in the same way we know smoking causes cancer. The link between sloth and AMI is consistent, supported by many studies using different methods, biologically plausible, fairly strong, "dose-related," and apparently independent of other CHD risk factors, such as hypercholesterolemia, smoking, hypertension, and overweight. Both the American Heart Association and the U.S. Public Health Service declare physical inactivity a key risk factor for CHD.

Many recent studies support the "exercise hypothesis." Former elite Finnish athletes stay more active lifelong and outlive peers who were equally healthy when young. In a 16-year followup of initially healthy, middle-aged Norwegian men, physical fitness predicted CHD death: The most fit men were only 40% as apt to die as the least fit. In a long-term followup of over 10,000 Harvard men, those who began playing sports in mid-life cut their risk of death 23%. And in a five-year study of nearly 1,200 initially healthy Finnish men, those most active and most fit had the lowest risk of first AMI.

Of course, sudden exertion can trigger AMI and/or sudden cardiac death. Yet remaining sedentary is unwise. In a Seattle community study, for sedentary men, the relative risk of cardiac arrest during exercise (compared with the rest of the day) was 56. For active men, the risk during exercise was also elevated over baseline, but only by a factor of 5, and the overall risk of cardiac arrest — at any time — was only 40% that for sedentary men.

Similarly, in a recent study of over 1,200 heart-attack victims, the relative risk of AMI in the hour after heavy physical exertion, compared with lighter exertion or none, was about 6. But this risk was borne mainly by the sedentary: risk was 45 times greater for sedentary people than for those who exercised five or more times a week. Sudden, heavy exertion can trigger AMI, but mainly in sedentary people.

In other words, although the risk of cardiac arrest or AMI is higher during intense exertion than at rest, this risk is small enough — and the benefit of regular exercise great enough — that it pays to stay active and fit. In the long run, exercisers fare better than couch potatoes.

How does habitual exercise help prevent AMI? Physiologically, regular exercise improves functional work capacity and lowers heart rate and blood pressure, two major determinants of myocardial oxygen demand. Specifically, the heart adapts to chronic overload: "athlete's heart."

With pressure overload, as in weightlifting, the heart increases in septal and free-wall thickness to normalize myocardial-wall stress even at high afterload (LaPlace's law). With volume overload, as in jogging, the heart increases in left ventricular end-diastolic diameter, with a proportional rise in septal and free-wall thickness to normalize wall stress. This increase in left ventricular volume increases the stroke volume. Ejection fraction and myocardial contractility seem not to change, but the greater stroke volume, along with the thickened ventricular wall and a bradycardia in the trained exerciser, make the heart a better pump.

Bradycardia in exercisers correlates with fitness, and owes to increased vagal tone, decreased sympathetic tone, and an intrinsic cardiac component. Vagally-mediated arrhythmias and physiologic changes in electrocardiographic configurations can also occur in athletes.

Relevant to risk of AMI is that regular, strenuous exercise may enlarge the coronary arteries. Autopsy studies suggest that active men have enlarged epicardial coronaries. And in a recent cross-sectional study, in response to nitroglycerin, the coronary arteries of highly-trained, middle-aged endurance runners dilated more than those of inactive men.

The degree of athlete's heart varies greatly by type, intensity, and duration of training, and by age, sex, and genetic makeup. Most exercisers, however, have at least some features of athlete's heart (Table 14-1).

During submaximal exertion, heart rate, blood pressure, and adrenergic activity increase less in fit people than in unfit. This protects the fit from exercise-induced disruption ("cracking") of coronary atherosclerotic plaques. Also, research finds that exercise-induced platelet activation is less likely in fit people than unfit, thus protecting the fit against coronary thrombosis should plaque-cracking occur.

Besides conferring athlete's heart, exercise fends off AMI by reducing weight, improving lipoprotein profile, decreasing blood viscosity, mitigating platelet hyperreactivity, enhancing fibrinolysis, curbing adrenergic response to stress, and improving mental outlook (see below).

Just as exercise confers these many benefits, sloth confers the opposing detriments. Therein lies the pathophysiology.

Table 14-1. Features of Athlete's Heart

Resting bradycardia
Enlarged left ventricle
Increased stroke volume
Systolic flow murmur
3rd or 4th heart sound
Increased EKG voltage
Altered EKG repolarization
Vagally-mediated arrhythmias
Enlarged coronary arteries

Smoking

Epidemiologists estimate that smoking accounts for about 20% of all mortality from heart disease. Even "passive smoking" has been tied to AMI; a recent review of 10 epidemiological studies concludes that, each year in the U.S., heart disease from environmental tobacco smoke kills 37,000 people.

Smoking is a key risk factor for AMI in women, partly because, compared with the risk for AMI in men, women have more favorable hormonal, behavioral, and cholesterol profiles. A prospective cohort study of nearly 120,000 female nurses suggests that smoking is the leading cause of CHD in middle-aged women, accounting for about half of all AMIs in women under 55.

Sadly, young women today are smoking more, although the rest of society is smoking less. For example, over the past few years, more high school senior girls than boys have smoked. This gender trend continues into adulthood.

Epidemiologic studies record the CHD toll that smoking takes. Smoking compounds other risks: obesity, hypertension, diabetes, and high cholesterol. Women who have diabetes and smoke, compared with the general population, have a 20-fold increased risk of fatal CHD. Women on oral contraceptives who smoke increase their risk of AMI up to 23-fold. Women who smoke 25 cigarettes a day have five times the CHD risk of nonsmokers. Even the lightest smokers (1 to 4 cigarettes a day) have at least twice the CHD risk of nonsmokers.

Smoking is rich in pathophysiology: it can accelerate atherosclerosis and CHD by injuring vascular endothelium, oxidizing low-density lipoprotein, activating platelets, inhibiting fibrinolysis, and promoting upper-body fat. Smoking saps a woman's natural protection from CHD by enhancing breakdown of estrogen and raising plasma levels of adrenal androgens. Acutely, nicotine and smoking-generated carbon monoxide tax the heart by constricting blood vessels, raising heart rate and blood pressure, and displacing oxygen from hemoglobin.

Fortunately, recent research finds that in women who smoke, as in men, the increase in risk of first AMI declines soon after they stop smoking and disappears after two or three years.

Cholesterol

Population studies in the U.S. agree there is a positive, curvilinear relationship between plasma cholesterol level and relative risk of CHD. As cholesterol level rises, especially above 200 mg/dl, risk of CHD rises ever more steeply. At 250 mg/dl, risk is double that at 200 mg/dl; at 300 mg/dl, risk is triple or quadruple that at 200 mg/dl (Fig. 14-1).

Some studies suggest a link between plasma triglyceride level and risk of CHD, but debated is whether risk from hypertriglyceridemia is independent of that from cholesterol profile. Of course, plasma levels of cholesterol and triglyceride just reflect the lipoproteins that carry them.

The lipoproteins are key in atherogenesis, because they transport lipids into and out of arterial walls. Increasingly, the CHD risk of individuals will be defined by analyzing lipoprotein profiles.

The five major lipoprotein classes, in order of decreasing size and lipid content and increasing density, are: chylomicrons, large, triglyceride-rich particles secreted by the gut after meals; very-low-density lipoprotein (VLDL), secreted by the liver and a key triglyceride-transporter; intermediate density lipoprotein (IDL), a transient lipolytic product of VLDL; low-density lipoprotein (LDL), which derives from IDL or VLDL remnants and carries most of the plasma cholesterol to cells; and high-density lipoprotein (HDL).

Atherogenicity varies considerably among lipoproteins. Chylomicrons may not be atherogenic, whereas VLDL remnants are. LDL is the most atherogenic of all lipoproteins, but HDL is not atherogenic. In fact, many good epidemiologic studies agree that high plasma levels of HDL protect against CHD.

In simple terms, then, LDL is the "bad" cholesterol, HDL the "good." Exactly how HDL wards off CHD is unclear. One hypothesis is that HDL enters arterial walls, scavenges excess cholesterol there, and takes it to the liver for excretion: "reverse cholesterol transport." Another hy-

Fig. 14-1. Curvilinear relationship between plasma cholesterol and risk of CHD. (Reprinted with permission from: Grundy SM. Disorders of lipids and lipoproteins. In Stein JH, ed. *Internal Medicine* (2nd ed). Boston: Little, Brown, 1987, pp. 2035–2052.)

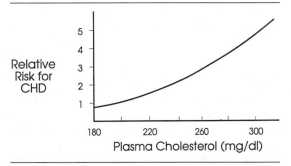

pothesis is that a high HDL level is but a marker of a "healthy" plasma transport system: a cart, not a horse.

As for pathophysiology, genetic errors in lipoprotein metabolism can increase the risk of CHD. One person in 500 is heterozygous for familial hypercholesterolemia, having one defective gene for the hepatic LDL receptor, which delays clearance of LDL from plasma. About 85% of such people suffer AMI by age 60. Other people are born with low plasma HDL from defects in apoprotein A and/or C; some of these defects are atherogenic, some not. Lipoprotein (a), a genetic variant of LDL that binds to a plasminogenlike molecule, is atherogenic and thrombogenic. Two other genetically influenced LDL variants that are atherogenic are: an increase in apoprotein B; and an increase in small, dense LDL particles, which are easily oxidized.

Oxidation of LDL is in vogue to explain pathophysiology in CHD. The emerging hypothesis is that oxygen free radicals, either from toxins or as normal byproducts of mitochondrial respiration, oxidize LDL in the artery wall, making it more atherogenic. Oxidized LDL, it seems, is atherogenic in four ways: (1) it recruits monocytes; (2) it inhibits migration of macrophages from artery wall to plasma; (3) it boosts uptake of LDL by macrophages via an acetyl LDL receptor, creating foam cells; and (4) it is "cytotoxic," somehow damaging arterial endothelium.

The oxidation hypothesis explains the fad of taking antioxidants (beta carotene, vitamins C and E) to prevent CHD. Two recent studies suggest that vitamin E supplements, for example, may ward off AMI. Followed for 4 to 8 years were over 87,000 female nurses and nearly 40,000 male health professionals. People who took at least 100 units of vitamin E a day for two years or longer had about a 40% lower risk of CHD. Such observational studies, however, cannot prove cause and effect. In both studies, for example, vitamin takers were more apt to exercise, eat right, and not smoke.

Antioxidant-vitamin supplements, then, are unproven in preventing CHD. In fact, disappointing is the first randomized, placebo-controlled trial of antioxidants in a Western population. When over 29,000 middle-aged Finnish men — overweight smokers with high cholesterols — took supplements of beta carotene, vitamin E, both, or neither for 5 to 8 years, the vitamins failed to prevent either lung cancer or CHD. Similar trials are ongoing in American men and women. For now, it seems prudent to get antioxidants mainly from food — fruits and vegetables — not from pills.

Studies of twins raised together or apart find that both genetics and diet shape plasma lipoprotein levels. In most people, a high-cholesterol diet increases plasma LDL levels. The likely mechanism is as follows: The dietary cholesterol reaches the liver in chylomicron remnants, suppresses synthesis of cholesterol and LDL receptors by the liver, and thus impairs clearance of LDL from plasma. Some people, however, do not respond to a high-cholesterol diet with an increase in plasma LDL levels, owing to differences in absorption of cholesterol, synthesis of bile salts, and metabolism of LDL.

Like cholesterol, some saturated fatty acids (especially those with 14, 16, and perhaps 12 carbons) tend to raise plasma LDL, probably by suppressing synthesis of hepatic LDL receptors. Saturated fatty acids come from animal meat, dairy products, the hard fat of plants (coconut oil, palm oil), and baked goods. *Trans* fatty acids, the "unnatural" fatty acids created by the partial hydrogenation that converts vegetable oils to solid fats (like stick margarine), also boost plasma LDL. Conversely, polyunsaturates like linoleic acid and mono-unsaturates like oleic acid (in olive oil) lower plasma LDL level when exchanged for saturated fatty acids.

Diet, then, is key to CHD risk. In the past 20 years, many randomized, clinical end-point trials have found that diet and/or drug therapy that lowers blood cholesterol (especially LDL), 10–20% can reduce CHD. The longer the trial, the greater the CHD risk of those studied, and the greater the fall in LDL, the greater the benefit in preventing AMI.

Lowering blood cholesterol can even reverse CHD, as in a recent review of 10 controlled clinical trials using coronary arteriography. Three trials used no drugs, just a low-fat diet alone or with other lifestyle measures. The mean fall in LDL was 20%; this cut the odds of CHD progression (gauged by arteriography) or increased the odds of regression by 20–40%.

Studies agree that vegetarians — white or African-American — have lower LDL levels and lower CHD risk. To cut CHD risk, one should cut dietary fat to below 30% of calories, saturated fat below 10%. In general, each 1% reduction in a person's cholesterol level (or 1% increase in HDL) yields a 2–3% reduction in CHD risk.

Hypertension

Many prospective observational studies show that high blood pressure is positively and independently related to risk of AMI. Systolic pressure may predict CHD risk better than diastolic, perhaps because systolic has a larger range and can be gauged more precisely. In a recent report from the Framingham Heart Study, even borderline isolated systolic hypertension (systolic pressure 140–159 mm Hg; diastolic, below 90 mm Hg) increased the risk of CHD. Blood pressure, systolic or diastolic, is a continuous variable, and its associated CHD risks increase from lowest to highest values.

Pathophysiologically, hypertensive heart disease results from afterload imposed on the left ventricle by the progressive increase in arterial pressure and total peripheral resistance caused by hypertensive vascular disease. This hemodynamic overload causes left ventricular hypertrophy (LVH). Over time, LVH may increase myocardial oxygen demand by inducing microvascular disease that cuts coronary blood flow and flow reserve. Hypertension also boosts CHD risk by accelerating the progression of coronary atherosclerosis.

LVH, an ominous sign, is an independent risk factor for CHD and sudden cardiac death. Hypertension is the leading cause of LVH, but the correlation between height of blood pressure and degree of LVH is poor. Recent studies find that many people with LVH have no hypertension, or at least have systolic blood pressures under 140 mm Hg.

Indeed, LVH is shaped by genetic and humoral factors, and by age, race, and gender. For example, LVH tends to be more severe in men with DD genotype for angiotensin-converting enzyme, in people who get hypertension when young rather than old, in blacks more than whites, and in men more than women.

Obesity, too, influences LVH. Any increase in body mass — be it fat or muscle — requires a higher cardiac output and expanded blood volume to meet the higher metabolic demands. Obesity increases cardiac output and contributes to LVH by increasing left ventricular filling pressure and stroke volume. In other words, when obesity and hypertension coexist, the heart has to carry the high preload of obesity and strain against the high afterload of hypertension. In such patients, losing weight reduces LVH more than would be expected from the fall in blood pressure alone.

Essential hypertension, which accounts for 90% of high blood pressure, is the upper quintile of blood-pressure distribution in the general population. Probably, several genes interact with environmental stimuli to raise blood pressure in susceptible persons. For example, variants of the angiotensinogen (renin substrate) gene may predispose to hypertension, and lifetime salt intake is key.

"Intersalt," a recent observational study of over 10,000 people in 52 populations worldwide, ties salt intake to blood pressure, both within and across populations. About 25% of normotensive people and 50% of hypertensive patients are "sodium-sensitive," meaning that excess dietary salt increases their blood pressure. In general, most apt to be salt-sensitive are older people, African-Americans, those with low plasma renin levels, and those with a family history of hypertension. In such people, cutting salt can

reduce blood pressure, but only if sodium intake is cut sharply — to 90 mmol or less a day — which means not adding salt in cooking or at the table and not eating processed foods high in salt.

Reversing hypertension reduces CHD risk. In prospective observational studies, a long-term decrease of 5–6 mm Hg in usual diastolic blood pressure is associated with about 20–25% less CHD. A recent meta-analysis of 14 randomized trials of antihypertensive drugs, with a mean treatment duration of 5 years, reports about a 15% reduction in AMI.

The first step for mild hypertension is "nondrug" or lifestyle therapy. Studies agree that weight loss, exercise, and cutting salt and alcohol can help control mild hypertension. Other helpful measures: increasing potassium and calcium intake, curbing caffeine, eating more fish, and learning to relax. The most practical way to cut sodium and increase potassium is to eat lots of fruits and vegetables. Foods "straight from the ground" are high in potassium and low in sodium; processed foods are the reverse.

Lifestyle measures can also prevent hypertension. For example, 200 men and women with high-normal blood pressure were randomized: half (controls) had no intervention; half ("lifestyle group") cut calories, salt, and alcohol, and began to exercise regularly. After 5 years, hypertension had developed in one in five of the controls, but in only one of 11 of the lifestyle group.

Obesity

Obesity, especially upper-body obesity (the "apple" shape), increases risk of CHD by contributing to hypertension and LVH and by causing diabetes mellitus and lipid abnormalities.

Unfortunately, America is the fattest nation on earth. Food is abundant and — rich in sugar and fat — tasteful and energy dense. Alcohol, also energy dense, is consumed liberally, accounting for 5–7% of caloric intake among men. As we eat more calories, we burn fewer. We use labor-saving devices at work and play, and at leisure we favor passive pleasures — TV or computer games — over active sports. Genetic and cultural traits — and the difficulty of permanently losing excess weight — complete the recipe for the "fattening of America."

One-third of American adults are now overweight, up from one-quarter a decade ago. This means that 32 million women and 26 million men weigh at least 20% more than they should. Men and women are eight pounds heavier, on average, than a decade ago. Even young adults are heavier than ever.

Recent epidemiologic studies probe aspects of body weight and CHD risk. A long-term followup of 508 Boston people finds that men who were overweight as teenagers — even if they lose weight as adults — are twice as apt as lean cohorts to die of CHD. The Framingham Heart Study, from 32 years of data on nearly 3,200 men and women, suggests that "yo-yo" dieting increases CHD risk. That is, compared with people who gain "normally" over time (nearly one pound every two years), those who repeatedly gain and lose lots of weight are nearly twice as apt to die of CHD. Also, results of the Nurses' Health Study suggest that 40% of CHD in women owes to obesity.

Controversy on body weight and CHD stems from epidemiologic studies that differ on whether the relationship is positive and linear or J-shaped, with more CHD in both leanest and fattest people. "J-shaped studies," however, are confounded by (1) not adjusting for lower weight because of cigarette smoking or antecedent disease and (2) inappropriately adjusting for biological effects of obesity — hypertension, dyslipidemia, hyperglycemia — that cause CHD. When such flaws are avoided, as in a recent 27-year followup of more than 19,000 middle-aged men, Harvard alumni, the relationship between body weight and CHD mortality is positive and linear: The lowest CHD death rate is among men who weigh 20% below the current U.S. average (Fig. 14-2).

Pathophysiology of obesity and CHD involves "Syndrome X," also called the insulin-resistance syndrome or the "Deadly Quartet": upper-body obesity, glucose intolerance, hypertriglyceridemia, and hypertension. Other CHD risk factors in this "metabolic cluster" tied to insulin resistance are low level of HDL; high level of plasminogen activator inhibitor; small, dense particles of LDL; and enhanced postprandial lipemia.

How this pathophysiology interrelates is yet unclear, but it may go roughly as follows: Upper-body fat ("apple-shape") — in men and women — is driven by androgen, lower-body fat ("pear-shape") by estrogen. Upper-body fat is "busy" or metabolically active; lower-body fat is "lazy," locked-in energy for pregnancy and lactation. Upper-body fat that accrues from sloth, gluttony, and/or alcohol causes insulin resistance and glucose intolerance.

The pancreas compensates with hyperinsulinemia; this can prevent frank diabetes mellitus, but at a cost that promotes CHD. The upper-body fat floods the liver with fatty acids that, in the face of hyperinsulinemia, increase the output of VLDL and cause hypertriglyceridemia. Muscle and fat cells, resistant to insulin and deficient in lipoprotein lipase, process VLDL poorly, promoting hypertriglyceridemia and lowering HDL. Hyperinsulinemia, the hypothesis goes, may contribute to hypertension by upping renal sodium resorption, activating sympathetic nerves, and inducing smooth-muscle hypertrophy in arterial walls.

The effect of weight reduction on CHD risk is uncertain in prospective studies because few subjects sustain the weight loss. Helping patients lose weight and keep it off is a vexing problem for physicians. The public health imperative is not to reverse obesity, but to prevent it.

Diabetes Mellitus

Diabetes mellitus accelerates atherosclerosis and increases the risk of AMI, especially in women. In population-based studies, age-adjusted CHD death rates are two to three times higher among diabetic men but six to seven times higher among diabetic women than among nondiabetics. Pathophysiology is tied in with Syndrome X. Besides compounding other CHD risk factors, diabetes mellitus seems independently to increase AMI risk, perhaps by a thrombotic tendency, cardiac autonomic neuropathy, or diabetic cardiomyopathy. Strict glycemic control in diabetics should decrease CHD risk, but confirmatory data are sparse.

Hematology of Inactivity

The state of the blood — its viscosity, rheology, tendency to clot, fibrinolytic potential — shapes CHD risk. The

Fig. 14-2. Schematic representations of competing hypotheses for relationship between body weight or obesity and risk of CHD. Best controlled studies find a linear relationship.

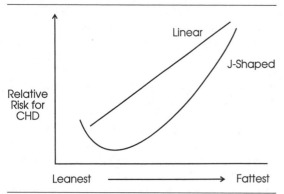

Framingham Heart Study, for example, finds that the higher the hematocrit, the greater the risk of CHD. Many epidemiologic studies agree that baseline fibrinogen concentration is also a CHD risk factor in men and women. Hematocrit and fibrinogen, of course, contribute greatly to blood viscosity, and fibrinogen is key in clotting.

Much evidence implicates platelets in acute coronary events. Autopsy in sudden cardiac death, arteriography in AMI, and angioscopy in unstable angina show that these CHD events begin when platelets adhere to an atherosclerotic plaque and initiate a blood clot. Pilot studies suggest that obesity, sloth, and/or dyslipidemia can make platelets hyperreactive. And a recent study tied platelet hyperreactivity to prognosis in survivors of AMI. During a 5-year followup, those who had "spontaneous platelet aggregation" had five times the rate of cardiac events as those without such aggregation.

Sluggish fibrinolyis, seen with obesity or hypertriglyceridemia, also poses CHD risk. As covered above, the CHD-promoting pathophysiology known as Syndrome X includes inhibited fibrinolysis.

Regular exercise cuts CHD risk partly by reversing the "hematology of inactivity" (Table 14-2). By expanding the baseline plasma volume, exercise lowers the hematocrit, accounting for the "dilutional pseudoanemia" of elite endurance athletes. Perhaps also by dilution exercise lowers fibrinogen, as shown by longitudinal studies of healthy volunteers and CHD patients.

Regular exercise also reverses platelet hyperreactivity, as shown by a randomized clinical trial (3 months of jogging) in men with features of Syndrome X. And exercise spurs fibrinolysis by releasing tissue plasminogen activator (TPA) from the endothelium of blood vessels. Augmented fibrinolysis can last up to 90 minutes after 5 minutes of strenuous exercise. In cross-sectional studies, fibrinolysis correlates with fitness; and in longitudinal studies, exercise programs enhance fibrinolysis even at rest.

Table 14-2. Hematology of Inactivity versus Activity

Inactivity	Activity
High hematocrit	Low hematocrit
High fibrinogen	Low fibrinogen
Overactive platelets	Normal platelets
Sluggish fibrinolysis	Brisk fibrinolysis

Alcohol

There now seems little doubt that alcohol can help prevent CHD in men and women. Most large-scale studies have shown that people who consume one to two drinks a day have fewer CHD events than abstainers. But the relationship between alcohol intake and death rate is J-shaped. More than three drinks a day predicts increased all-cause mortality; five or more drinks a day predicts increased CHD mortality.

The CHD-protecting physiology involves an increase in HDL. As shown most recently in a case-control study of 340 AMI patients, moderate alcohol intake increases HDL2 and HDL3, which cuts AMI risk by about 35%. Alcohol may also cut CHD risk by inhibiting clotting: Pilot evidence suggests that alcohol increases the prostacyclin/thromboxane ratio, reduces platelet aggregability, interacts with aspirin to prolong the bleeding time, and spurs the release of TPA from endothelial cells.

Indeed, a recent survey of more than 600 healthy male physicians finds a positive link between moderate alcohol intake and plasma TPA level, suggesting that alcohol may fend off CHD in part by enhancing fibrinolysis.

Alcohol, of course, is a two-edged sword. At least 100,000 deaths occur yearly from alcohol-related causes. Physicians concerned about public health advise against the wide use of alcohol. Telling nondrinkers to take up alcohol for health benefits would be unwise. Yet some people — those at high risk for CHD but low risk for problem drinking — may benefit from one drink a day.

Fish

Fish fits well in a healthy diet since it replaces red meat, which is rich in saturated fat. But fish confers another benefit: The type of fat in fish oil — omega-3 fatty acids — may reduce the risk of CHD.

Researchers began to explore the health benefits of fish 25 years ago, when they noted that Greenland Eskimos ate lots of fat — from fish — yet had little CHD. Many studies suggest that eating fish helps cut CHD risk. A key study was a 20-year followup of 852 Dutch men initially free of CHD. Men who ate fish at least twice a week had only half the CHD death rate as those who ate no fish. In another study, over 2,000 men, survivors of AMI, were assigned to receive or not receive advice on diet changes, including eating fish. Over the next 2 years, although no differences in rates of second AMI were seen, men who ate fish twice a week were 29% less apt to die of CHD.

The CHD-preventing physiology centers on reducing platelet reactivity and improving blood lipid profile. Fish oil may also reduce blood pressure, fibrinogen level, and blood viscosity.

Eating fish reduces platelet reactivity because the omega-3 fatty acid from fish replaces omega-6 fatty acid (from animal fat) in platelet membranes, reducing production of thromboxane A2 by platelets. Thromboxane A2 is a potent vasoconstrictor and platelet agonist, so anything that curbs its production should be "antithrombotic." Indeed, a recent study in healthy men finds that a salmon-rich, low-fat diet promises to be antithrombotic: It reduces urinary excretion of the metabolite of thromboxane A2.

Fish or fish-oil supplements also cut plasma triglycerides by inhibiting output of VLDL by the liver. Supplements, however, can raise LDL and impair glucose tolerance in diabetics. In contrast, as shown recently in men at risk for CHD, daily fish in a 30% fat diet improves the blood lipid profile: It reduces cholesterol, LDL, and triglycerides, and increases HDL.

Pilot studies suggest that fish oil may reduce blood fibrinogen level and blood viscosity. Fish-oil supplements can lower blood pressure in some patients with moderate hypertension, but so can eating fish. Many controlled trials find little benefit from fish-oil supplements in mild hypertension.

Public-health authorities recommend eating fish — baked or broiled, not fried — at least twice a week. Eating fatty fish makes more sense than adding calorie-rich fish-oil pills to a diet. Fish provides nutrients not in pills, plus a meal low in saturated fat.

Aspirin

It seems likely that daily low-dose aspirin can safely help prevent AMI in people with CHD risk factors. The preventive physiology hinges on the fact that aspirin acetylates and inactivates a platelet enzyme, prostaglandin G/H synthase, thus blocking cyclooxygenase activity and inhibiting production of the platelet agonist and vasoconstrictor thromboxane A2. This "antiplatelet" role of aspirin can be useful clinically because differences in dose-response and duration minimize detrimental or offsetting actions of aspirin on stomach, kidney, and vascular endothelium. See Chapter 34 for details.

Aspirin clearly prevents second heart attacks in AMI victims and first heart attacks in men with unstable angina or even chronic stable angina. As for preventing AMI in healthy people, three studies are key: two in men, one in women.

In a U.S. trial, over 22,000 male physicians took aspirin (325 mg every other day) or placebo. After 5 years, there was a 44% reduction in risk of first AMI in the aspirin group, mostly in men aged 50 and older. In a British trial of over 5,100 male physicians, no such reduction was seen from aspirin. However, an overview of both trials found that aspirin significantly cut first AMI by 33%.

The study in women is observational. In the Nurses' Health Study, women who report taking one to six aspirin per week have a 25% lower risk of first AMI. Women aged 50 and older with CHD risk factors benefit most.

Probably, aspirin can benefit most middle-aged men and women with CHD risk factors. The recommendation of a single loading dose of 200–300 mg followed by a daily dose of 75–100 mg stems from findings that this dose works as well as higher doses and is safer than higher doses, which may boost the risk of hemorrhagic stroke.

Hormone Replacement

In mid-life, the AMI risk for women is one-fourth that for men. Within 30 months after menopause, however, a woman's HDL falls and her LDL rises so that her cholesterol profile resembles a man's. Consequently, within 10 years after menopause, the CHD rate among women approaches that among men.

Estrogen-replacement therapy (ERT) can help prevent AMI in women after menopause. Almost all prospective (but nonrandomized) trials agree that ERT offers benefit in terms of CHD, especially a lower death rate. A recent review of 10 case-control studies and 11 cohort studies finds that ERT cuts CHD risk in postmenopausal women by 40–50%.

The protective physiology centers on the fact that oral estrogen raises HDL and lowers LDL. Oral estrogen also raises triglycerides, but this is not a key detriment. Transdermal estrogen affects HDL little, and only large doses lower LDL. Progesterone tends to attenuate any increase in HDL or decrease in LDL (but it offsets the endometrial-cancer risk from ERT). It is likely that ERT also helps prevent AMI by other poorly understood but beneficial effects on blood rheology, blood pressure, coagulation, and fibrinolysis.

ERT is neither panacea nor elixir of life. It is not risk-free and not all women tolerate it. Decisions to use it are individual, balancing risk of CHD (and stroke and osteoporosis) against, for example, risk of breast cancer. Overall, however, trends are toward wider use of ERT.

Personality Traits

For 40 years, some researchers have pinned a scarlet "A" on people who are hard-driving, competitive, and hostile. Those "Type A" people, mainly men, are said to have an increased risk of CHD. Careful studies, however, tend to refute a broad link between personality and CHD. But recent research suggests that certain personality traits are hard on the heart.

For example, there is "tension" in hypertension. Researchers from the Framingham Heart Study gauged stress in over 1,000 normotensive people and then checked blood pressures every 2 years for 20 years. Among middle-aged men, those scoring highest on anxiety or tension were twice as apt to develop hypertension as calmer men.

Hostility may also harm the heart. Researchers who developed the Type A hypothesis later identified hostility as the "Type A trigger" for high CHD risk. Then followed a slew of studies, most in support, some not. Most of the research was with men; limited data suggest hostility may also boost CHD risk in women, but women tend to be less hostile than men.

The pathophysiology of anxiety and hostility, of course, is the age-old "fight-or-flight" reaction. Researchers find that anger-provoking situations trigger stronger reactions in some than others. "Hot reactors" have sharper increases in heart rate, blood pressure, and stress hormones. Over time, the hypothesis goes, such extreme physiologic reactions can spur pathophysiology: atherosclerosis and CHD.

Anger is "riskier" in the face of CHD. In the most recent report from an ongoing study of immediate triggers of AMI, based on over 1,600 men and women who survived AMI, people with CHD more than double their risk of AMI when they become angry, and the danger lasts 2 hours.

This area of research is "softer" than some, not only because anxiety and hostility are harder to measure than blood pressure and cholesterol, but also because one person's stress is another's joy. Surely, cultural and gender differences also apply. For example, stress in men may come mainly from work, but stress in women may come mainly from men.

Researchers on hostility and CHD offer these practical, self-help tips toward a more trusting heart: acknowledge the problem; reason with yourself; think like the other person; laugh at yourself; practice trust (start small); be assertive, not aggressive; and practice forgiveness. When all else fails, pretend today is your last.

Bibliography

Belchetz PE. Hormonal treatment of postmenopausal women. *N Engl J Med* 330:1062–1071, 1994. *This article provides a comprehensive yet practical review.*

Curfman GD. Is exercise beneficial — or hazardous — to your heart? *N Engl J Med* 329:1730–1731, 1993. *A perceptive, timely editorial.*

Eichner ER: Hematology of inactivity. *Rheum Dis Clin NA* 16:815–825, 1990. *A majestic overview by a pioneering researcher.*

Mannson JE, Tosteson H, Ridker PM, et al. Primary prevention of myocardial infarction. *N Engl J Med* 326:1406–1416, 1992. *A classic, practical review.*

Ridker PM, Vaughan DE, Stampfer MJ, et al. Association of moderate alcohol consumption and plasma concentration of endogenous tissue-type plasminogen activator. *JAMA* 272:929–933, 1994. *New research and concise review of this field.*

Part I Questions: Cardiovascular Diseases

1. Which of the following lesions would result in complete heart block?
   A. Fibrosis of the sinoatrial node
   B. Interruption of the His bundle
   C. Interruption of the left bundle
   D. Interruption of the right bundle
   E. Interruption of an accessory pathway
2. Systolic dysfunction results when
   A. contractility is impaired.
   B. there is volume overload.
   C. compliance is reduced.
   D. preload is reduced.
   E. afterload is reduced.
3. The normal response to acute valvular insufficiency includes all except
   A. Elevated diastolic pressure
   B. Elevated diastolic volume
   C. Elevated stroke volume
   D. Reflex increase in heart rate
   E. Decreased heart rate
4. Which of the following statements are true?
   A. Infants with severe right heart obstructive lesions present with central cyanosis.
   B. An infant with aortic atresia (a severe left heart obstructive lesion) requires ductal patency to allow poorly oxygenated blood to reach the pulmonary circulation.
   C. Hypercyanotic episodes are caused by a variety of factors which raise systemic vascular resistance, lower pulmonary resistance, and therefore cause an increase in right-to-left shunting.
   D. Children with large septal defects almost always have signs and symptoms of congestive heart failure due to the large left-to-right shunt.
   E. The foramen ovale is only necessary during fetal life in children with cyanotic heart defects.
5. A 45-year-old man was admitted to the hospital with severe chest pain of 2 hours' duration. The cardiac rhythm was regular at 90 beats/minute and blood pressure was 150/80 mm Hg. Bilateral basal rales were audible and chest x-ray showed cardiomegaly and pulmonary edema. Which of the following statements is false?
   A. History is compatible with acute myocardial infarction.
   B. Basal rales and pulmonary edema indicate left ventricular failure.
   C. Pulmonary capillary wedge pressure will be high.
   D. Left ventricular end-diastolic pressure will be elevated.
   E. Clinical picture suggests an anginal syndrome.
6. The correct statement about restrictive cardiomyopathy is
   A. Left ventricle is usually dilated.
   B. Amyloidosis causes restrictive cardiomyopathy.
   C. Systolic dysfunction is usually present.
   D. Differential diagnosis includes pericardial effusion.
   E. It may occur after delivery.
7. Which of the following signs, symptoms, or laboratory findings are specific for pulmonary heart disease?
   A. Shortness of breath with exertion
   B. RV hypertrophy and dilation on echocardiogram
   C. Hypoxemia on arterial blood gas
   D. A loud pulmonic component of the second heart sound
   E. None of the above
8. In constrictive pericarditis
   A. equalization of diastolic pressures is relieved by pericardiocentesis.
   B. elevated jugular venous pressure is normalized by pericardiocentesis.
   C. y-descent is not prominent before pericardiocentesis.
   D. y-descents become prominent after pericardiocentesis.
   E. pericardial fluid is not a feature.
9. The single most diagnostic feature of infective endocarditis is

A. Vegetations observed by transesophageal echocardiography

B. Valve dysfunction noted on transthoracic echocardiogram

C. Normochromic normocytic anemia

D. Continuous bacteremia or fungemia

E. Osler's nodes

10. Which of the following statements is true?

A. Cardiac output is always very high in distributive shock.

B. Cardiogenic shock can be diagnosed by obtaining serial creatine kinase MB fraction levels in the patient's blood.

C. Either a central venous pressure or a pulmonary artery occlusion pressure may be used to determine the adequacy of preload in a patient with acute anterior myocardial infarction.

D. Despite high cardiac output, oxygen utilization is frequently abnormal in distributive shock.

E. Pericardial effusion may cause shock by obstructing flow of blood out of the right and left ventricles.

11. Which statement does not apply to congestive heart failure secondary to mitral valvular stenosis?

A. The left atrial pressure is elevated.

B. The pulmonary arterial pressure is elevated.

C. The pulmonary congestion is due to left ventricular failure.

D. A slow heart rate is usually tolerated better than a rapid one.

E. Dyspnea is commonly present.

12. Which of the following conditions does not have a predominantly volume overload contributing to the elevation of blood pressure?

A. Primary aldosteronism

B. Cushing's syndrome

C. Bilateral renal artery stenosis

D. Hypercalcemia

E. Estrogen administration

13. Chronic venous insufficiency

A. is always a result of previous DVT.

B. results in pulmonary embolism.

C. is caused by the exposure of superficial veins to high venous pressure.

D. cannot be treated with compression stockings alone.

E. is due to inflammation in the deep veins.

14. Which dietary change is least likely to increase plasma LDL levels?

A. Lower total fat

B. Lower intake of *trans* fatty acids

C. Lower cholesterol intake

D. Relatively more unsaturated fatty acids

E. Relatively more saturated fatty acids

II Digestive Diseases and Nutrition

Part Editor
Richard F. Harty

15 Esophagus

Donald J. Kastens

Objectives

After completing this chapter, you should be able to

Understand the functional anatomy of the esophagus and the normal physiology of swallowing

Understand the major clinical syndromes of esophageal pathophysiology to include dysphagia, heartburn, and chest pain

Understand the clinical tests for diagnosis of esophageal disorders

Understand the clinical pathophysiology and treatment of esophageal motility disorders

Understand the clinical pathophysiology and treatment of gastroesophageal reflux disease

Normal Esophageal Anatomy and Physiology

Functional Anatomy

The esophagus can be thought of as a hollow muscular tube, composed of striated and smooth muscle, closed at both ends by a sphincter. The cricopharyngeus (upper esophageal sphincter or UES), which is the lowermost segment of the inferior pharyngeal constrictor, guards the proximal end of the esophagus. The body of the esophagus is a 20–22 cm distensible cylinder, potentially about 2.5 cm in diameter, that extends from the UES through the posterior mediastinum and diaphragmatic hiatus to the stomach. The distal end of the esophagus, the lower esophageal sphincter (LES), typically extends approximately 2 cm intra-abdominally. The aortic arch, tracheal carina, and cardiac left atrium are all in close proximity to the esophagus.

The lumen of the esophagus is lined by squamous epithelium throughout. The UES and the muscular layers of the upper 5% of the esophageal body are purely striated muscle and the muscular layers of the lower one-half are entirely smooth muscle, with an intervening transition zone of mixed striated and smooth muscle. The LES consists of a 3–4 cm specialized segment of circular smooth muscle. The esophagus lacks a serosa, and thus a potential containment mechanism for the spread of cancer.

Physiology of Swallowing

The act of swallowing and bolus transport can be divided into voluntary oral and involuntary pharyngeal and esophageal phases. The oral phase includes forming and pushing the bolus to the posterior pharynx with the tongue, an act coupled to the pharyngeal phase, which then consists of a precisely coordinated UES relaxation and pharyngeal contraction. The pharyngeal phase occurs over about 1.5 seconds and also includes airway protection achieved by reflex inhibition of respiration, closure of the glottis and downward deployment of the epiglottis, and elevation and anterior displacement of the larynx. The oral and pharyngeal phases are orchestrated by the swallowing center in the medulla via a number of cranial nerves. The third or esophageal phase results in bolus transport through the esophagus over 7–10 seconds. Bolus transit time is faster with liquids in the upright position and slower with solids in the supine position.

The UES exhibits varying pressure that seems to have two components, an active component of cricopharyngeal contraction and a passive component of tissue elasticity. The active contraction is stimulated by respiration, phonation, esophageal distention, and stress, and typically results in pressures of 50–100 mm Hg. The passive tissue elasticity produces a pressure of approximately 10 mm Hg and is essentially the only pressure present during sleep. The UES transiently relaxes to less than 5 mm Hg during the swallowing process.

The esophageal body has a normal intraluminal resting pressure that is slightly subatmospheric (–5 mm Hg), a reflection of its intrathoracic location. Three patterns of pressure responses can be seen within the body of the esophagus: (1) primary peristalsis is a progressive contraction wave that strips the esophagus from proximal to distal after oropharyngeal initiation of a swallow; (2) secondary peristalsis is a progressive contraction wave initiated by distention of the esophagus (due to remaining food or refluxed material) that is not preceded by a swallow; (3) a tertiary (simultaneous) contraction is a nonperistaltic, nonpropulsive contraction of most or all of the esophagus at the same time. Simultaneous contractions in response to wet swallows are distinctly unusual in normal persons. The LES has a normal resting pressure of 15–35 mm Hg. It relaxes to the level of intraluminal gastric pressure when the UES opens, and remains open until the peristaltic contraction has reached the LES. Esophageal distention, by causing a secondary peristalsis, will initiate similar relaxation of the LES.

Esophageal peristalsis and LES relaxation are controlled extrinsically through vagal innervation and intrinsically by the myenteric plexus of nerves within the muscular layers. Nitric oxide appears to be a major neuromuscular mediator for both of these physiologic events. A peristaltic contraction is coordinated through a latency gradient along the length of the esophagus, such that the latency varies from the shortest time in the proximal esophagus to the longest just above the LES.

Physiology of LES Competence

There are at least several mechanisms for the normal maintenance of the LES resting pressure that limit reflux of gastric contents into the esophagus. Both structural and mechanical factors are important. The phrenoesophageal ligaments help hold the LES in position. The acute angle of entry of the esophagus into the stomach results in a mucosal flap valve that helps prevent reflux of gastric material. The slightly positive intra-abdominal pressure surrounds the subdiaphragmatic portion of the LES and, since thoracic pressure is negative, helps keep the LES closed. However, when other mechanisms fail, this effect can become detrimental in the event of sudden increases in intra-abdominal pressure. The right crus of the diaphragm,

which encircles the LES, also extrinsically augments the LES pressure during inspiration.

Intrinsic myogenic activity of the sphincteric smooth muscle appears to be the most important factor in maintenance of LES pressure. Control of myogenic activity probably represents the interplay between hormonal and neural mechanisms. Agents, including medications and foods, that affect the LES pressure do so primarily by enhancing (Table 15-1) or diminishing (Table 15-2) myogenic tone.

Clinical Syndromes of Esophageal Pathophysiology
Dysphagia

A cardinal manifestation of esophageal disease is difficulty in swallowing or dysphagia. A patient may describe

Table 15-1. Agents Producing *Increased* LES Pressure

Neurotransmitters	Hormones	Other Agents
Alpha-adrenergic agonists (norepinephrine)	Gastrin Motilin Substance P Bombesin	Protein Antacids Metoclopramide Domperidone Cisapride Prostaglandin F2
Cholinergic agonists (bethanechol)		
Anticholinesterase (edrophonium)		

Table 15-2. Agents Producing *Decreased* LES Pressure

Neurotransmitters	Hormones	Other Agents
Beta-adrenergic agonists (isoproterenol)	Progesterone Estrogen Secretin Cholecystokinin Glucagon Vasoactive intestinal polypeptide (VIP) Calcitonin gene-related peptide (CGRP) Somatostatin	Fat Chocolate Ethanol Peppermint Smoking Theophylline Calcium channel blockers Nitrates Diazepam Meperidine Prostaglandin E2
Alpha-adrenergic antagonists (phentolamine)		
Dopamine		
Anticholinergics (atropine)		

trouble initiating a swallow or a sensation that an ingested bolus is stopping or "hanging up" somewhere behind the sternum or at the suprasternal notch. Dysphagia can be divided clinically into two types: oropharyngeal and esophageal.

Oropharyngeal Dysphagia

Oropharyngeal dysphagia or transfer dysphagia is characterized by difficulty in voluntarily transferring a bolus from the mouth into the esophagus when initiating the involuntary phases of swallowing. Any disease affecting the central nervous system, the cranial nerves controlling the oropharynx, or the striated muscles of the oropharynx can cause this symptom through failure of propulsive force. Any mass lesion in the oropharyngeal region may also cause this symptom by obstructing flow in some way. In patients with this type of dysphagia, liquid ingestion often causes more problems than ingestion of solids. Associated symptoms may include nasal regurgitation, coughing or aspiration during swallowing, and change in speech.

Clinical examples where failure of oropharyngeal propulsive force is of primary pathophysiologic importance include cerebrovascular accident or stroke, amyotrophic lateral sclerosis (Lou Gehrig's disease), myasthenia gravis, and polymyositis. Examples where obstruction to oropharyngeal flow is more the problem include retropharyngeal abscess, carcinoma, thyroid enlargement, and abnormalities of UES relaxation or elasticity like those producing a Zenker's diverticulum in the hypopharynx. In Zenker's diverticulum the pouch may fill with food and also obstruct the upper esophagus by compression.

Esophageal Dysphagia

Esophageal dysphagia represents difficulty with the transport of a bolus down the esophagus once it has been successfully transferred from the oropharynx. If the sensation of bolus arrest is localized to the lower sternum, the problem is most likely in the distal esophagus. However, the symptom can be referred to the suprasternal notch area, even though the problem is in the distal esophagus. Esophageal dysphagia may be induced by any disorder causing failure or incoordination of propulsive force, or by mechanical obstruction to flow. Examples of neuromuscular or motility disorders are achalasia, diffuse esophageal spasm, and scleroderma; these disorders usually produce dysphagia equally with solids and liquids. Clinical examples of obstruction to flow such as esophageal carcinoma, reflux peptic stricture, and Schatzki ring generally produce solid dysphagia alone. Esophageal stenosis less than 13 mm in diameter will almost invariably cause solid dysphagia. Rapidly progressive solid dysphagia with weight loss,

in a patient older than age 50, is the most common scenario in esophageal carcinoma. Slowly progressive solid dysphagia associated with chronic heartburn is more typical for a reflux stricture. Intermittent solid dysphagia with a large piece of meat or bread usually characterizes a Schatzki ring, a membranous circular ridge of tissue in the distal esophagus.

Heartburn

Heartburn (pyrosis), the most common manifestation of an esophageal disorder, is classically described as a retrosternal burning sensation which may radiate toward the throat or mouth. It is due to reflux of gastric contents into the esophagus and usually occurs within an hour or two after meals. It is usually made worse when the patient bends over or lies down. A frequent accompanying symptom is regurgitation, usually described by the patient as the spontaneous appearance of an acid or bitter taste in the mouth. Regurgitation may also occur separately from heartburn. These symptoms are usually relieved, or at least improved, by taking some type of antacid preparation.

A number of other symptoms may be associated with heartburn or occur separately on the broad spectrum of gastroesophageal reflux manifestations. Epigastric distress or dyspepsia, nausea, acid belches, and upper abdominal fullness or bloating following meals are all frequently reflux induced. Water brash, or sudden filling of the mouth with slightly salty fluid, is reflex hypersalivation secondary to esophageal acid exposure. Nocturnal cough, hoarseness, nonallergic asthma, chronic hiccoughs, loss of dental enamel, and globus sensation ("lump in the throat") may all be symptoms or presentations of gastroesophageal reflux.

Chest Pain

Chest pain is also a very frequent symptom of esophageal disorders, and may coexist with or occur independently of classical heartburn. The pain may be described as burning or squeezing, substernal in location, and radiating into the back, neck, jaw, or arms, potentially making it very difficult to distinguish from cardiac angina. Two mechanisms proposed for esophageal chest pain are reflux related, the most common, and motility-related. The mechanisms for reflux-related pain are incompletely understood, but some reasonable possibilities are detailed in Fig. 15-1. Exercise may trigger gastroesophageal reflux and induce exertional chest pain, again mimicking cardiac angina. The mechanism for motility-related chest pain is even less well understood. Esophageal motility disorders, frequently seen in

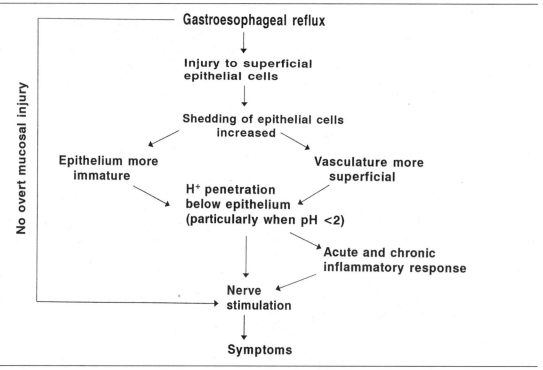

Fig. 15-1. Possible mechanisms for reflux-related symptoms.

patients with noncardiac chest pain, may stimulate mechanoreceptors by producing changes in esophageal wall tension. On the other hand, motility disorders have been frequently associated with altered esophageal visceral nociception, a lowered threshold for afferent visceral pain signals such as described in the irritable-bowel syndrome. Chest pain directly related to swallowing, termed odynophagia, is most commonly due to esophageal infections, drug or reflux-induced esophageal ulcers, or radiation-induced esophageal injury.

Clinical Tests for Esophageal Disorders

Although the history and physical examination are always important basics, specific clinical tests can directly document pathophysiology of the esophagus. Barium contrast radiography and endoscopic esophagoscopy with biopsy can be done to look for esophageal mucosal pathology.

Additionally, esophageal manometry (motility study) and 24-hour intraesophageal pH monitoring can demonstrate disturbances of function. Esophageal manometry utilizes a catheter with pressure transducers to characterize the contractions in the esophageal body (peristaltic versus simultaneous), assess the amplitude and duration of those contraction pressures, quantify the pressure in the LES, assess LES relaxation with swallowing, and evaluate UES function. Twenty-four hour intraesophageal pH monitoring involves placement of an esophageal probe, connected to a portable digital recorder, to measure the frequency and timing of acid reflux events with regard to patient meals, position, and symptom episodes. Finally, an esophageal acid perfusion study (Bernstein test) can help document the esophageal origin of symptoms (heartburn, chest pain). The test is performed by dripping normal saline, alternating with 0.1 N hydrochloric acid into the esophagus. Reproduction of the patient's typical symptoms during the acid perfusion suggests that they are due to acid reflux.

Common Esophageal Disorders

Motility Disorders

Primary Esophageal Motility Disorders

Primary disorders involve a variety of abnormalities of the coordinated neuromuscular apparatus responsible for peristalsis and sphincter function in the esophagus. Some of these abnormalities are manometrically demonstrated in Fig. 15-2.

Achalasia.   It is characterized by low-amplitude simultaneous contractions with complete loss of peristaltic activity (aperistalsis) in the esophageal body and increased LES pressure associated with failure of the LES to relax with swallowing. This is pathophysiologic double trouble

Fig. 15-2. Examples of manometric tracings demonstrating normal and abnormal findings. Upper portion of each tracing: pull-through of catheter from stomach (S), across lower esophageal sphincter (LES), to esophagus (E). Relaxation of LES evaluated during a swallow (Sw). Lower portion of each tracing: catheter positioned in esophageal body to record pressures in proximal (P), middle (M), and distal (D) esophagus. Response to two wet swallows (Sw) is shown. (Reprinted with permission from Geriatrics 40(10):63, 1985. Copyright by Advanstar Communications, Inc. Printed in U.S.A.)

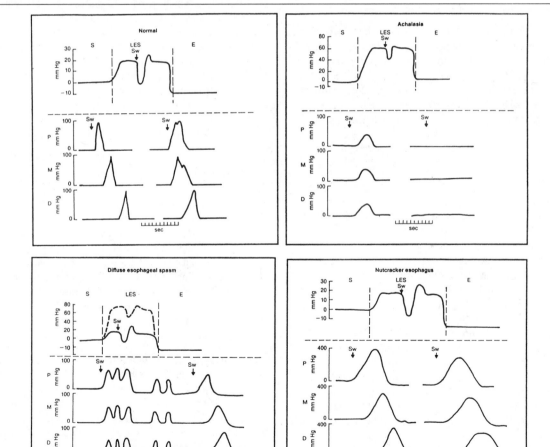

in that there is loss of propulsive force as well as a functional obstruction to flow. The exact etiology of achalasia is unknown, but the mechanism is thought to involve loss of myenteric plexus neurons and vagal denervation of the esophagus. As a result, there may be marked dilatation of the esophagus which can progress to a sigmoid-appearing deformity. Slowly progressive solid and liquid dysphagia is the most common symptom and is mostly related to the inability of the LES to relax with swallowing. Patients may also have chest pain and commonly experience weight loss. Spontaneous regurgitation of food and fluid retained in the esophagus is a fairly common symptom and may occur during and after meals or at night. Nocturnal regurgitation sometimes results in pulmonary aspiration or even pneumonia. The diagnosis is made by a combination of barium studies, endoscopic esophagoscopy, and manometry, the last being of major importance.

Diffuse Esophageal Spasm.   This is characterized by simultaneous (nonperistaltic) contractions, which may be repetitive and/or of increased amplitude, occurring after greater than 10% of wet swallows. Intermixed periods of normal peristalsis must be present. LES pressure is also increased in one-third of patients, and relaxation can be abnormal. Symptoms induced by this disorder include chest pain, solid and liquid dysphagia as the progress of the bolus is interrupted, and occasionally odynophagia. The diagnosis is made by esophageal manometry. This disorder can progress to achalasia over time.

Nutcracker Esophagus.   A more recently described motor disorder, it is defined as peristaltic contractions with markedly increased amplitude (> 180 mm Hg) and usually markedly prolonged duration (> 6.0 seconds). For reference sake, normal contraction amplitudes range from 60 to 140 mm Hg and durations range from 3.5 to 5.5 seconds. In nutcracker esophagus LES pressure and relaxation are normal. This is the most common motility disorder seen in patients with noncardiac chest pain and, likewise, chest pain is the most common symptom. Mild solid and liquid dysphagia is sometimes seen. The symptoms have been difficult to correlate with the contraction abnormalities in nutcracker esophagus, so it may be more of an epiphenomenon or a marker for aberrant esophageal visceral nociception. Reflux-induced pain has also been seen in nutcracker esophagus. The diagnosis can only be made by esophageal manometry.

Secondary Esophageal Motility Disorders

Diseases that affect the striated or smooth muscle of the esophagus can also cause esophageal motor problems and symptoms. Scleroderma is a systemic disease in which the smooth-muscle portion of the esophagus is often involved. Atrophy of the smooth muscle results in loss of LES competence and loss of peristaltic contractions of the lower esophagus. This causes solid and liquid dysphagia as well as severe gastroesophageal reflux, which in turn may progress to esophageal stricture formation. Diseases that affect the striated muscle portion of the esophagus, such as polymyositis, often cause symptoms of oropharyngeal dysphagia as well as loss of peristaltic activity in the upper portion of the esophagus.

Treatment of Esophageal Motility Disorders

Treatment of these disorders can involve pharmacologic agents or more invasive interventions. Treatment approaches for achalasia have been aimed primarily at the poorly relaxing LES. Drugs which decrease LES pressure, like nitrates and calcium channel blockers, given just prior to meals may be of some benefit. Abrupt dilation of the LES by insufflation of a 3–4 cm diameter balloon can frequently produce relief. A surgical myotomy performed on the LES will almost always effect relief. Drugs which modify nociception, such as antidepressants and anxiolytics, have been the most useful for treatment of nutcracker esophagus.

Gastroesophageal Reflux Disease (GERD)

The most common disease of the esophagus, gastroesophageal reflux, is due to reflux of gastric acid and pepsin (or, less commonly, alkaline bile) through the LES and into the esophagus. It is important to recognize that major objective manifestations of reflux, such as esophagitis, are not always present in a patient with chronic reflux. Therefore, it has become more appropriate to use the term GERD to cover the whole spectrum of manifestations of chronic reflux, including the patient who has recurring heartburn without objective mucosal disease and the individual who presents with severe esophageal injury (e.g., stricture with dysphagia), but with no symptoms until this advanced disease develops.

Pathophysiology of GERD

At least four major factors seem important in the pathophysiology of GERD. The first factor is efficiency of the antireflux barrier at the esophagogastric junction, especially the LES. A low resting LES pressure is not required nor is it that helpful at predicting who will develop GERD. In an individual patient it must be quite low (≤ 6 mm Hg) before one can reliably predict significant reflux disease. Of course, drugs, hormones, and dietary elements that decrease LES pressure often promote reflux, as will sudden increases in intra-abdominal pressure. A very common finding in reflux patients is frequent transient complete LES relaxations (not related to swallows) allowing reflux. The mechanism for these transient LES relaxations is incompletely understood, but they may represent a component of the belch reflex. A second factor is the irritant effect of refluxed substances (acid, pepsin, bile) on the esophageal mucosa. Acid hypersecretion is not a usual finding; rather the problem is acid in the wrong place. Mucosal defense factors (mucus production, cell membrane structure and function, blood flow) are important in determining the ability of the mucosa to resist these insults. The third factor is the efficiency of the esophageal clearance mechanism. Effective peristalsis, both primary and secondary, is extremely important in clearing most of the acid after reflux, and then swallowed salivary bicarbonate provides additional neutralizing capability for the remaining small amounts of acid. GERD patients frequently have slower acid clearance, often due to peristaltic dysfunction, and therefore prolonged acid exposure time. This statement correctly implies that normal individuals quickly clear their infrequent reflux events before any problems can arise. Enlisting the aid of gravity can improve esophageal clearance (e.g., elevating the head of the bed). A hiatal hernia (herniation of the proximal stomach up through the diaphragmatic hiatus) may contribute to delayed esophageal clearance by providing a gastric juice reservoir for repeated episodes of reflux, but is by no means required for the development of GERD. A fourth and final factor is the efficiency of gastric emptying. Delayed gastric emptying may contribute to the production of reflux by allowing acid/pepsin mixtures to remain in the stomach for longer periods of time and also by maintaining greater gastric volumes available to reflux.

Through use of 24-hour intraesophageal pH monitoring the concepts of physiologic and pathologic reflux have been defined. Physiologic reflux in normal persons is characterized by infrequent, rapidly cleared postprandial reflux events that result in limited upright esophageal acid exposure, amounting to less than 5% of the 24-hour period. Three types of pathologic reflux patterns involving more numerous and/or more prolonged acid reflux events, and therefore a greater percentage of esophageal acid exposure time, have been documented. Upright refluxers are those patients whose reflux events occur only in the upright position, usually following a meal. Supine refluxers are patients in whom reflux events almost always occur while they are lying down, especially when in bed at night. The third and most common type, combined refluxers, consists of patients who reflux in both the supine and the upright positions. Patients with prolonged supine reflux events seem most prone to develop esophagitis.

Clinical Manifestations of GERD

Patients with GERD most commonly present with heartburn and/or regurgitation. The severity of symptoms does not correlate well with the presence of esophageal mucosal injury and only about half of patients have esophagitis. When esophagitis does occur it may progress to ulcerations, bleeding, stricture formation, and Barrett's metaplastic epithelium. Ulcerations may cause odynophagia or bleeding, and the bleeding can present as hematemesis (bloody emesis), melena (tarry stools), or an iron-deficiency anemia due to chronic occult blood loss. Deep reflux injury stimulates fibrosis with collagen deposition and results in stricture, which manifests as slowly progressive solid dysphagia. Chronic reflux can cause the replacement of normal squamous mucosa with an abnormal columnar mucosa (Barrett's mucosa), which has a predisposition to develop adenocarcinoma. Esophageal carcinoma of this type and the more common squamous-cell carcinoma usually cause rapidly progressive solid dysphagia.

GERD patients may manifest myriad other "atypical" symptoms such as chest pain, hoarseness, sore throat, cough, asthma, and water brash. Patients with extraesophageal symptoms frequently don't have heartburn or esophagitis, further highlighting the large interindividual variability in the perception of reflux. Reflux-induced chest pain can be exertional and/or very severe, simulating cardiac angina or even myocardial infarction. Laryngeal and pharyngeal symptoms appear to be most commonly due to direct contact with refluxed acid. Pulmonary symptoms can be due to aspiration of refluxed acid or in some cases to an "esophagobronchial reflex," a vagally mediated bronchospasm in response to esophageal acid exposure.

Treatment of GERD

Conservative measures are the first step in the treatment of GERD and are aimed at the known pathophysiologic factors. This therapy includes elevation of the head of the bed, avoidance of tight-fitting garments and bending over after meals, restriction of alcohol and smoking, dietary modification, weight loss, avoidance of meals before bedtime, and antacid use. More aggressive treatment includes the use of drugs like H_2-receptor antagonists and proton-pump inhibitors to block gastric acid secretion, and use of prokinetic drugs like metoclopramide and cisapride to enhance esophageal clearance, LES pressure, and gastric emptying. The most aggressive treatment involves surgical augmentation of the antireflux barrier.

Clinical Example

1. A 35-year-old male patient reported a history of dysphagia for 5 years. It had been worse during the past 2 years, and recently he had trouble at each meal. He experienced dysphagia equally with solids and liquids. During meals he typically got a full feeling behind his sternum, frequently experienced regurgitation, and then could slowly finish his meal. The regurgitated matter did not contain any bile, only food and fluid he had just ingested. He had some trouble with regurgitation of undigested food at night when supine, but denied any heartburn or acid/bitter taste. The patient had lost 15 pounds over the past 6 months. He intermittently noted nonexertional squeezing retrosternal chest pain as well.

Physical examination revealed a somewhat thin man in no acute distress. His vital signs were normal and his general physical exam was otherwise unremarkable. Routine laboratory studies were all normal.

A barium esophagram showed a dilated esophagus containing food and a smooth "bird-beak" narrowing of the LES area. Endoscopic esophagoscopy revealed some retained food and fluid and a tightly closed LES area, but no mucosal lesions were seen. Esophageal manometry demonstrated low-pressure simultaneous contractions of the esophageal body with a high LES pressure and failure of LES relaxation with swallowing.

The patient was treated with preprandial sublingual nitrates and a calcium channel blocker with only mild relief of his dysphagia. After an abrupt balloon dilation of the LES, the patient's symptoms resolved and he rapidly regained his lost weight.

Discussion.   The combination of slowly progressive solid and liquid dysphagia and nocturnal regurgitation of undigested food strongly suggests an esophageal motility disorder.

The x-ray and endoscopy findings are consistent with achalasia.

The manometric findings of an elevated pressure in the LES, poor LES relaxation with swallowing, and associated low-pressure simultaneous contractions in the body of the esophagus confirm the diagnosis of achalasia.

Dilation of the hypertensive, poorly relaxing LES was then associated with relief of symptoms.

Bibliography

Castell DO, Richter JE, and Dalton CB, (eds.). *Esophageal Motility Testing.* New York: Elsevier, 1987. *A concise text covering the role of esophageal motility studies in the diagnosis of esophageal diseases.*

DeVault KR and Castell DO. Current diagnosis and treatment of gastroesophageal reflux disease. *Mayo Clin Proc* 69:867–876, 1994. *An excellent overview and assessment of the currently available diagnostic and treatment modalities of GERD.*

Gelfand DW and Richter JE (eds.). *Dysphagia: Diagnosis and Treatment.* New York: Igaku-Shoin Medical Publishers, 1989. *A comprehensive text covering the pathophysiology, disease entities, diagnostic modalities, and treatment of this very important symptom of esophageal disease.*

Richter JE. *Ambulatory Esophageal pH Monitoring: Practical Approach and Clinical Applications.* New York: Igaku-Shoin Medical Publishers, 1991. *A comprehensive text on the important diagnostic role of 24-hour esophageal pH monitoring, with particular attention to the atypical clinical manifestations of GERD.*

Richter JE, Bradley LA, and Castell DO. Esophageal chest pain: Current controversies in pathogenesis, diagnosis, and therapy. *Ann Int Med* 110:66–78, 1989. *An excellent review of all aspects of esophageal chest pain, including the more controversial elements of this symptom of esophageal disease.*

16 Stomach and Duodenum

Paul N. Maton

Objectives

After completing this chapter, you should be able to

Understand the nature of gastroduodenal secretions

Understand the cellular basis of gastric acid secretion

Understand the control of acid secretion

Understand the basic components of mucosal protection

Understand the basic gastric motility

Understand the pathophysiology of peptic ulcer disease

Understand the importance of *H. pylori* to gastroduodenal disease

Normal Physiology

The main secretions produced by the stomach are acid, pepsinogen, lipase, intrinsic factor, mucus, and bicarbonate. Acid is bactericidal, activates the enzyme pepsinogen, and releases vitamin B_{12} (cobalamin) from food. Pepsinogen, when activated to pepsin, initiates protein digestion and lipase initiates fat digestion. Intrinsic factor facilitates absorption of vitamin B_{12}, and mucus and bicarbonate secretion help protect the gastric mucosa. These various functions are distributed in different parts of the stomach (Fig. 16-1). The fundus is responsible for mucus, pepsinogen, and lipase secretion; the body for mucus, acid, pepsinogen, lipase, and intrinsic factor; and the antrum for mucus and gastrin production. The stomach also has important motor functions concerned with the initial storage and processing of meals. In addition to these functions the gastric glands possess other cells that contain peptides and amines whose functions are poorly understood. These include somatostatin-containing cells in the antrum and other endocrine cells in the fundus and body. Furthermore in the gastric submucosal and muscle layers there are many peptides that presumably function as neurotransmitters. Our knowledge of the physiological and pathophysiological role of these chemicals and the cells that contain them is rudimentary.

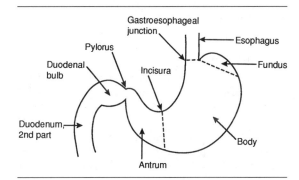

Fig. 16-1. Anatomical aspects of the stomach and duodenum.

The duodenum contains glands that secrete bicarbonate and neutralize gastric acid. In addition the mucosa contains endocrine cells of various types that produce peptides which modulate gastric acid secretion, pancreatic secretion, gallbladder contraction, and other intestinal functions. These will not be discussed in this chapter. The duodenum also possesses motor activity and, as seen in the stomach, numerous motor , sensory, and inter neurons are found whose precise function remains largely unexplored.

Acid Secretion

Acid is secreted by the stomach in an approximately isosmotic concentration, giving rise to pH of around 1, but this is diluted in gastric glands to pH 1–2. Acid is secreted continuously in the basal state at about 4 mmol/hour in women and 7 mmol/hour in men. The initial effect of eating a meal is to reduce gastric acidity because of the buffering effect of food. However, eating stimulates acid secretion in three stages although they can occur simultaneously. The cephalic phase is produced by the sight, smell, and taste of food and is mediated by the vagus. In the gastric phase, food (particularly peptides, beer and wine, coffee, and calcium) within the stomach stimulates secretion through the stimulation of gastrin release and also through intragastric and long vago-vagal reflexes. Gastrin is the major postprandial stimulant of acid secretion. The intestinal phase of secretion is mediated by nutrients reaching the duodenum and the rest of the intestine. In the intestine peptides are more powerful stimuli of acid secretion than carbohydrates, and fats tend to reduce acid secretion. There is a normal diurnal rhythm of acid secretion by the stomach. Acid secretion rises with each meal during the day, and then declines in the early hours of the morning. Maximal acid secretion, as stimulated by exogenously administered gastrin is 30 mmol/hour or more and is higher in males than in females.

Parietal Cell

Parietal cells are situated in the lower half of the gastric glands and are the most numerous cells in gastric body and fundus. The most potent stimulant of parietal cells is histamine acting through H_2 receptors. Histamine is probably released by enterochromaffinlike cells (ECL cells). Parietal cells can be stimulated directly by acetylcholine through occupation of M_3-type muscarinic receptors (Fig. 16-2). Gastrin released from the G cells in the antrum may act directly on gastrin receptors on the parietal cell, but probably acts principally on the ECL cell to release histamine (Fig. 16-2). The intracellular messengers in parietal cells that mediate acid secretion include cyclic AMP, the primary messenger for the histamine H_2 receptor, and calcium released from intracellular stores and entering from the extracellular fluid following occupation of the M_3 receptors.

Proton Pump

Acid secretion by the parietal cell occurs through a final common pathway, that of a proton pump which exchanges hydrogen ions for potassium ions. This enzyme utilizes ATP as an energy source and is therefore termed a hy-

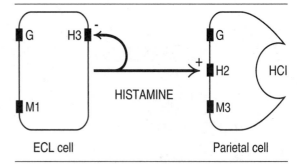

Fig. 16-2. Simplified model of the relationship between ECL cells and parietal cells in relation to acid secretion and occupation of cell surface receptors. G = gastrin receptor; M_1 = muscarinic M_1 receptor; M_3 = muscarinic M_3 receptor; H_2 = histamine H_2 receptor; H_3 = histamine H_3 receptor. (Modified from Lewin MJM. Parietal cell receptors of acid secretion. In Domschke W and Konturek SJ (eds.). *The Stomach.* New York: Springer-Verlag, 1993.)

drogen-ion-potassium, ATPase ($H^+,K^+,$ATPase). This exchanges potassium ions in the lumen for intracellular hydrogen ions (in fact hydronium ions, H_3O^+), resulting in acid secretion. In addition, a potassium channel is necessary to allow hydrogen ion and potassium exchange, and a chloride pathway is also present in order to maintain electroneutrality of the pump. The $H^+,K^+,$ATPase consists of two subunits, a larger alpha subunit with several transmembrane domains and a smaller beta subunit with only a single membrane-spanning domain. In the resting cell, most $H^+,K^+,$ATPase molecules are situated within the cytoplasm in tubulovesicles. However, when the parietal cell is stimulated, these vesicles fuse with the plasma membrane at the apical part of the cell to form a secretory canaliculus. This translocation of the $H^+,K^+,$ATPase is necessary for secretion.

Enterochromaffinlike (ECL) Cell

The ECL cell is situated deep in the gastric glands of the gastric fundus and body. This cell has a typical endocrine cell cuboidal appearance and, like many endocrine cells throughout the body, stains with silver stains. In animals, it is now known that this cell possesses gastrin and muscarinic M_1 receptors, and the ECL cell is the principal source of histamine that stimulates the parietal cell to produce acid. Thus in animals the ECL cell is a central cell in terms of normal physiology (see Fig. 16-2). The data are less complete in humans, but the same situation is thought to pertain.

Pepsinogen Secretion

Pepsinogen, a protease of molecular weight 42,000, is secreted into the gastric juice by four different types of gastric cells: mucus neck cells and chief cells in the proximal stomach, pyloric gland cells in the antrum, and Brunner's gland cells in the duodenum. Most of the pepsinogen is secreted by the chief cells found in the lower part of the gastric glands in the body and fundus of the stomach. Pepsinogen is, in fact, a group of several enzymes that differ on the basis of electronegativity, sensitivity to alkali and heat, and optimal pH activity. Pepsinogens are stored in granules within the cell, and, when the cell is stimulated, these granules fuse with the apical cell membrane and release the pepsinogen into the gastric gland lumen. When pepsinogen is exposed to acid (below pH 4), the active form of the enzyme, pepsin, is released. The optimal pH for pepsin is around 2. Pepsinogen secretion is stimulated intracellularly by both the cyclic AMP and calcium pathways. Stimulation of secretion can be produced by muscarinic agonists, cholecystokinin, and histamine. Vagal activity is responsible for the basal secretion of pepsinogen, and histamine is probably the major physiological stimulant. Gastrin probably stimulates pepsinogen secretion only indirectly through its effect on histamine release.

Lipase Secretion

Gastric chief cells produce an acid lipase that is chemically distinct from pancreatic lipases and does not require a colipase for full activity. Lipolysis in the stomach gives rise to acyl chains and diglyceride. It has been estimated that about 15% of ingested fat is lysed by gastric lipase.

Mucus Secretion

Mucus is a water-insoluble gel consisting of 90–95% water containing a mixture of proteins, glycoproteins, lipids, and electrolytes. Mucins are the major solid in mucus. They are large glycoproteins (500,000 daltons) linked by disulphide bridges into tetramers that are about 15% protein, 85% carbohydrate, and 1% fatty acids. Mucins are continuously synthesized and released by surface mucus cells and degraded and solubilized by enzymatic proteolysis and shear forces. Secretion is stimulated by muscarinic agents, gastrin, cholecystokinin, secretin, and prostaglandins. The mucus layer is 50–400 μm thick, has little buffering capacity, and is quite permeable to acid. However, it constitutes a hydrophobic layer and forms a barrier to physical damage. In addition mucus impedes the back diffusion of acid by creating an unstirred layer of water, electrolytes, and bicarbonate, and can inhibit bacterial proliferation.

Bicarbonate Secretion

There is a passive flux of bicarbonate from blood and the interstitial tissues into the gastric lumen, which is enhanced by mucosal injury. In addition, there is an active secretion of bicarbonate into the lumen by surface-lining cells of the whole stomach through an electroneutral chloride-bicarbonate ion exchanger situated at the apical membrane. The rate of bicarbonate secretion is 5–10% of basal acid secretion, but it can be enhanced by vagal stimulation, luminal acid, cholinergic agents, cholecystokinin, and prostaglandins.

Intrinsic Factor Secretion

Intrinsic factor, a protein of 45,000 daltons, is produced by parietal cells in the gastric body and fundus but is secreted independently of acid. Intrinsic factor is secreted in excess of the requirements for vitamin B_{12} absorption and is resistant to degradation by acid and proteolytic enzymes. Each molecule of intrinsic factor binds one molecule of cobalamin but in the stomach most cobalamin binds to salivary R proteins. When these reach the duodenum, pancreatic proteases cause the release of cobalamin from the R proteins and allow it to bind to intrinsic factor. Intrinsic factor secretion is stimulated by gastrin, histamine, and cholinergic agents, and inhibited by somatostatin, but the physiological significance of these findings is not clear.

Gastrin

Gastrin is produced by antral G cells and by similar cells in the duodenum. These are endocrine-type cells situated at the base of the antral glands. Gastrin release is stimulated by cholinergic and sympathetic pathways and gastrin-releasing peptide. Nutrients (particularly proteins, peptides, and amino acids, especially phenylalanine and tryptophan) also stimulate gastrin release. Gastrin stimulates secretion of acid which (when it reaches the antrum) inhibits further gastrin release. Acid probably inhibits gastrin release through release of somatostatin from antral somatostatin-containing D cells. Thus there is a negative feedback that limits plasma gastrin concentrations.

Duodenal Secretion

The duodenum, and particularly the duodenal bulb, is the first part of the intestine that meets gastric acid and it possesses special protective mechanisms. As in the stomach, passive flux of bicarbonate occurs but here Brunner's glands secrete pepsinogens, bicarbonate, and mucus. Thus the neutralization of gastric acid within the gut begins in the very first part of the duodenum. Subsequent neutralization occurs throughout the duodenum, partly through exchange mechanisms and partly through the addition of the alkaline secretions of the pancreas and biliary tree.

Gastroduodenal Mucosal Protection

With the presence of acid, pepsin, and detergents such as bile salts present in the upper gut, it is important that the mucosa has protective mechanisms to prevent damage. These can be divided into several components, the unstirred layer consisting of mucus and bicarbonate, the epithelial cells, the regenerative capacity of the mucosa including restitution and regeneration, and mucosal blood flow.

The mucosa is a water-repellent hydrophobic layer that contributes to the protection from attack by acid and other water-soluble compounds. Bile salts (which damage the mucosa) reduce hydrophobicity and prostaglandins (which protect the mucosa) can increase hydrophobicity. However, the hydrophobic nature of gastric mucosa is largely dependent on surface mucus. Mucus also provides an unstirred surface layer that can prevent pepsin from digesting underlying epithelial cells. In addition, bicarbonate, when trapped in the mucus gel, can raise the epithelial surface pH of the cell as high as pH 4. Thus the combination of mucus and bicarbonate provides an important defense mechanism.

Following minor mucosal damage, re-epithelialization occurs by the rapid migration of cells along an intact basal lamina to provide a defense against subsequent acid damage. This process is known as restitution. Repair of more severe lesions requires more extensive healing processes involving cell division, an inflammatory response, and angiogenesis.

The gastric mucosa requires generous blood flow partly for metabolic requirements of acid secretion, but also for mucosal protection. Studies in animals suggest that modulation of the gastric microcirculation by nitric oxide, peptides, and prostanoids are all important in regulating gastric mucosal integrity. Endogenous prostanoids in gastric mucosa include prostaglandin E_2 and prostacyclin. Both of these compounds have numerous effects that are protective in addition to their effect on the microcirculation. These include effects on membrane hydrophobicity, mucus secretion, bicarbonate secretion, restitution, and regeneration.

Gastroduodenal Motility

Fasting Gastric Motility

The stomach can be divided into two regions with respect to motility. The proximal stomach (the fundus and upper 1/3 of the body) maintains sustained nonphasic electrical activity. The distal stomach exhibits phasic electrical activity due to the generation of slow waves. These waves of depolarization arise in the pacemaker region, which is situated in the mid-body of the stomach on the greater curve, and travel to the pylorus at a frequency of about three per minute. Slow waves have a prolonged plateau and are only accompanied by muscle contraction if there is a superimposed spike action potential. In fasting, there is a phasic pattern of electrical activity. Phase 1 lasts for about 1 to 1.5 hours, during which slow waves occur without any spike activity, and therefore there are no contractions. In phase 2 (lasting about 30 minutes) there is an increase in spiking associated with slow waves. In phase 3 (which lasts 5–10 minutes) spikes occur with every slow wave, and contractions occur every 15–20 seconds. Then there is a recovery phase (phase 4), which lasts about 10 minutes, followed by the next phase 1. The cyclic activity is called the myoelectric migrating complex and occurs every 90–120 minutes. The muscle contractions also cycle and are termed migrating motor complexes. They begin in the proximal stomach and spread down to the pylorus and then into the duodenum. The proximal stomach shows coordinated contractions associated with the antral contractions. Pyloric activity is closely related to duodenal and antral activity, but is also under control of nerves and circulating agents. The pacemakers for migrating motor complexes either side of the pylorus have a different periodicity. In the stomach, it is about three per minute, whereas in the duodenal bulb it is eleven per minute.

Gastric Motility After Meals

After meals, the stomach motor activity is concerned with storage, grinding of food, and emptying, all of which can occur virtually simultaneously. The storage of food is mainly a proximal gastric function. There are vagal reflexes that mediate a receptive relaxation of the proximal stomach when the resting tonic contractions of the fundus are inhibited. Thus gastric pressure rises very little after a meal. When food is ingested, the cyclical pattern of the fasting activity is disrupted and is replaced by sustained irregular contractions rather like phase 2 of the migrating motor complexes. All solid food is broken down into particles less than 1 mm by mixing and grinding. In addition, the stomach actively controls emptying of the different constituents of the meal, and liquids, digestible solids, and indigestible solids leave the stomach at different rates. Increasing osmolality or acidity slows emptying, while increases in volume accelerates emptying. Warm and cold drinks are emptied more slowly than control drinks, and fat reduces gastric emptying. Cholecystokinin enhances liquid emptying while substance P and neurotensin produce moderate acceleration. Sham feeding inhibits gastric emptying.

Emptying of solids occurs after digestible solids are ground to tiny particles. This occurs mainly in the distal stomach. Solids empty more slowly from the stomach than liquids and this may be due to the time it takes to break down solids into the small particles. Antral contractions, increased viscosity, and fiber content of the meal each reduce gastric emptying. Emptying of both solids and liquids correlates with duodenal phase 3 activity, the migrating motor complex activity resuming soon after completion of gastric emptying. Solids that cannot be broken down to 1–2 mm are emptied from the stomach by a different mechanism. These particles are retained until phase 3 activity of the interdigestive cycle, which empties the stomach.

Control of Gastroduodenal Motility

Humoral factors such as the plasma concentration of the peptide motilin have been shown to be important in the control of myoelectric migrating complexes. Extrinsic nerves are thought to play only a minor role, but atropine does inhibit migrating motor complexes, suggesting that cholinergic nerves are important. Chemical factors also play a role. In the upper intestine fat induces gastric relaxation, proteins have a minor effect, and carbohydrate no effect. However, in the distal intestine carbohydrate and protein reduce gastric tone, whereas fat has no effect. Gastric distention inhibits the interdigestive cycle and duodenal distention inhibits gastric activity. Mild to moderate exercise accelerates, but severe exercise delays, gastric emptying. Excitement, anxiety, fear, fright, and depression inhibit gastric motility, as does cold stress.

Disease States

Gastritis

This inflammation of the mucosal lining of the stomach may be acute or chronic. There are many ways of classifying gastritis but the one used here is the Sydney classification.

Acute Gastritis

These forms of gastritis are characterized by mucosal inflammation associated with acute infiltration by neutrophils. The bacterium *Helicobacter pylori* (*H. pylori*) can cause an acute gastritis that is associated with hypochlorhydria or achlorhydria, and can also lead to a chronic gastritis. Other forms of acute gastritis include phlegmonous (suppurative) gastritis caused by streptococci or staphylococci and the gastritis seen after ingestion of corrosives or after radiation to the stomach.

Special Forms of Gastritis

These are acute or chronic inflammations caused by specific diseases or insults such as Crohn's disease, sarcoidosis, or infections. Reactive gastritis due to nonsteroidal anti-inflammatory drugs (NSAIDs) (typically erosions with little or no inflammatory cell infiltrate) is included in this category as is reactive gastritis caused by other ingested toxins such as alcohol.

Chronic Corpus Gastritis with Atrophy (Type A Gastritis)

Type A gastritis is an autoimmune disease where the mucosa of the gastric body and fundus is attacked by the immune system, leading to chronic inflammation and mucosal atrophy. Plasma markers of this disorder include antibodies to intrinsic factor and parietal cells. There is achlorhydria and failure to secrete pepsinogen and intrinsic factor. Because vitamin B_{12} binds to the receptor in the terminal ileum only when complexed to intrinsic factor, lack of intrinsic factor leads to malabsorption of vitamin B_{12}. These patients usually have few or no gastrointestinal complaints but may develop symptoms of anemia (fatigue, shortness of breath, and pallor) and neurological complaints. In this type of gastritis there is relative sparing of the gastric antrum and thus gastrin is produced normally. As there is no gastric acid to inhibit gastrin secretion, there is marked hypergastrinemia, which over many years can lead to hyperplasia or even tumors of gastric ECL cells.

Chronic Antral Gastritis with Atrophy (Type B Gastritis)

This type of gastritis principally involves the mucosa of the gastric antrum. It is now known that 90% of antral gastritis is caused by chronic infection with *H. pylori* and if the bacterium can be cleared from the stomach the gastritis will heal. This has important implications for peptic ulcer disease. In some cases, particularly those associated with gastric ulcer and gastric cancer, the antral gastritis caused by *H. pylori* spreads to involve the corpus as well as the antrum and is then termed pangastritis (Type AB gastritis).

Hemorrhagic Erosive Gastritis (Stress Gastritis, Stress Ulcers)

This condition (which is principally an endoscopic diagnosis) occurs in severely ill patients such as those with trauma, sepsis, respiratory failure, and intracranial disease. Typically acute erosions are scattered throughout the stomach. The erosions and the ulcers may bleed extensively. There is little or no cellular infiltrate and the appearances are similar to those seen with NSAIDs, but the mechanisms are different. The pathophysiology of hemorrhagic erosive gastritis is poorly understood, but is probably related to changes in the mucosal microcirculation.

Peptic Ulcer Disease

For many decades ulcers were thought to be due to changes in acid secretion, and certainly reduction in acid secretion heals ulcers. Others stressed the importance of mucosal defense mechanisms. However in the last 5–10 years there has been a revolution in the understanding of the pathogenesis of ulcer disease invoking the role of the bacterium *H. pylori*. Although there are some similarities, pathophysiological abnormalities in patients with duodenal ulcer differ from those with gastric ulcer.

Duodenal Ulcer

A duodenal ulcer is a lesion that extends through the mucosa and beyond the muscularis mucosa into the submucosa. About 95% of all duodenal ulcers occur in the duodenal bulb and the rest occur mainly in the immediate postbulbar area. Duodenal ulcers occur more frequently in men, and blood group O and nonsecretors have a slightly increased incidence. Smoking renders ulcers harder to heal and more likely to recur. Typically duodenal ulcers give rise to pain in the epigastrium or right hypochondrium occurring between meals and may wake the patient in the early hours of the morning. The pain is often relieved by eating, by taking antacids, or taking drugs that reduce acid secretion such as histamine H_2 antagonists or H^+,K^+,AT-Pase inhibitors. An ulcer may erode into a blood vessel and cause minor or major bleeding or may erode through the duodenum, causing a perforation. This allows air and fluid from the gut lumen to escape, giving rise to peritonitis, characterized by severe pain and abdominal rigidity with air under the diaphragm seen on abdominal x-ray. An ulcer can penetrate into surrounding tissues and organs such as the pancreas and therefore give rise to pancreatic pain. Rarely ulcers can heal with scarring and cause distortion and obstruction of the duodenal bulb with vomiting and dehydration. After healing, up to 70% of duodenal ulcers recur in the first year.

Abnormalities in Acid Secretion

1. Parietal cell abnormalities. Patients with duodenal ulcers tend to secrete more acid than normal controls. Maximal acid output is higher in patients with duodenal ulcers, and the parietal cell mass is 1.5–2.0 times higher, but there is a considerable overlap with normals. Basal acid output is also elevated in some patients with duodenal ulcers, possibly due to increased vagal tone. Acid secretion from midnight to waking (nocturnal acid secretion) is also increased in ulcer patients. Meal-stimulated acid secretion is increased in some patients with duodenal ulcer. This may be due to an increased sensitivity of parietal cells to gastrin or due to impaired negative feedback on acid secretion through a relative lack of antral somatostatin or other mechanisms.

2. G-cell abnormalities. Meal-stimulated gastrin levels are higher in some duodenal ulcer patients than controls, but most studies have shown normal fasting and postprandial gastrin concentrations in ulcer patients. In the rare Zollinger-Ellison syndrome, where patients have a gastrin-producing tumor, gastrin is not under physiological control, plasma concentrations of gastrin are extremely high, and basal acid secretion is markedly increased. In these patients the huge amounts of acid produced are sufficient to cause ulcers. Furthermore, the hypergastrinemia is trophic to the gastric mucosa and causes an increase in parietal cell mass, and ECL cell hyperplasia.

Because there is such a large overlap of acid secretion in patients with duodenal ulcer and in normals, the role of acid secretion as an etiological factor in most patients with duodenal ulcer has been questioned. This has been particularly so since the discovery of *H. pylori* and recent studies suggest that many of the observed changes in acid and gastrin may be secondary to *H. pylori* infection.

Impaired Mucosal Defenses. There is evidence that in some circumstances mucosal defense mechanisms play an important role in susceptibility to ulceration. This could be due to decreased secretion of bicarbonate or mucus, decreased restitution, decreased blood flow or prostaglandin production, or *H. pylori* infection with or without gastritis. The majority of duodenal ulcers are associated with factors that impair mucosal defenses: the presence of *H. pylori* or the ingestion of such NSAIDs as aspirin. However, these are not the only factors necessary to cause ulcers. Many patients take NSAIDs or have *H. pylori* in their stomach, but do not have peptic ulceration.

It has been suggested that duodenal ulcers occur because the amount of acid reaching the duodenum exceeds the neutralizing capacity within the lumen due to acid hypersecretion, rapid gastric emptying, or impaired duodenal bicarbonate secretion. Others have suggested that the mucus gel formation is impaired in ulcer patients, but the relative functional importance of the mucus bicarbonate layer and surface epithelial cells remains controversial. Nevertheless, one effect of *H. pylori* is to impair the function of mucus. No abnormalities in restitution or mucosal blood flow have been described in patients with duodenal ulcers.

Prostaglandins promote mucosal resistance, possibly by increasing duodenal bicarbonate secretion. Administration of prostaglandin analogues reduces NSAID-induced mucosal injury. NSAIDs block cyclo-oxygenases, reduce mucosal prostaglandins, inhibit bicarbonate and mucus secretion, reduce mucosal blood flow and mucosal cell growth, and may enhance basal and stimulated acid secretion. Because the relative importance of these factors has not been established, the mechanisms whereby prostaglandins prevent NSAID-induced ulceration are not clear.

Gastric Ulcer

Gastric ulcers rather than duodenal ulcers tend to occur in older people. Typically the patients have epigastric pain or discomfort, often with other complaints such as nausea or early satiety. The pain may have no clear relation to meals but may respond to antacids or antisecretory medications. Ulcers often occur at the incisura on the lesser curve of the stomach at the junction of the antrum and the body. Gastric motility may also be impaired. As with duodenal ulcers, gastric ulcers may cause bleeding or perforation or penetrate into other organs. Likewise, they can heal with scarring and cause deformity of the stomach or even gastric outlet obstruction.

Increased acid secretion is not important in gastric ulcer as most patients have a normal or low acid secretion and normal parietal cell mass. Furthermore, there is no evidence of any abnormality of control of acid secretion in patients with gastric ulcer. Gastric emptying studies have provided conflicting results, and it is not clear whether any differences observed are the cause, or the result, of ulcer formation. Some studies have found more duodeno-gastric reflux in patients with gastric ulcers than in healthy controls and duodenal juice is potentially damaging to the gastric mucosa. However, in the typical patient with gastric ulcer, motility disturbances do not play a major role.

As with duodenal ulcer, impaired mucosal defenses have been invoked as a cause of gastric ulcer, but there are no strong data to suggest that abnormalities in gastric bicarbonate secretion or changes in mucus secretion or restitution are important factors in gastric ulcer disease. Nor have abnormalities in mucosal blood flow been shown to be important. Prostaglandins are, however, undoubtedly important in NSAID-associated gastric ulcers as described above for duodenal ulcer. Indeed, the links between mucosal

prostaglandin production and gastric ulcer are stronger than for duodenal ulcer.

Gastritis, Duodenitis, Ulcers, and *H. pylori* Infection

As noted above, 95% of antral (type B) gastritis is caused by *H. pylori* and most patients with a gastric or a duodenal ulcer have chronic gastritis. Patients with a duodenal ulcer usually have gastritis involving only the antrum, but the gastritis may be more extensive, and involve the gastric body, especially in patients with gastric ulcer. Severe gastritis of the body and fundus can result in parietal cell destruction and decreased acid secretion, and may account for the fact that patients with gastric ulcer have lower acid secretion than those with duodenal ulcers. About 90% of patients with duodenal ulcer and about 65% of patients with gastric ulcer have *H. pylori* present in the stomach. However, *H. pylori* is also quite common in the general population who have no ulcers. Although bacteria had been seen in human stomachs for decades, *H. pylori* was only cultured and characterized in 1983. *H. pylori* (called Campylobacter pyloridis at one time) is a curved gram-negative bacillus with 4–6 flagella at the pole. One of its most distinctive characteristics is the production of a urease, which is important in some diagnostic tests for the bacterium. *H. pylori* is found only in gastric mucosa, where it colonizes surface mucus cells. When found in the duodenum it is only in areas of gastric metaplasia. How *H. pylori* damages the mucosa is not yet clear as the bacterium produces several potentially toxic products.

Acid hypersecretion and hypergastrinemia have been found in some patients with *H. pylori* infections and duodenal ulcer; eradication of *H. pylori* reduces basal and meal-stimulated gastrin concentrations and reduces acid output, suggesting that all the abnormalities of acid secretion in patients with duodenal ulcer at one time thought to be causative may be secondary to the infection with *H. pylori*. One finding suggesting that *H. pylori* is of major importance in duodenal ulcer (even though *H. pylori* is common in normals) is that eradication of *H. pylori* in a patient with duodenal ulcer reduces the relapse rate from greater than 50% to less than 10% in a year.

H. pylori is less frequently related to gastric ulcers, possibly because more gastric ulcers than duodenal ulcers are caused by NSAIDs. Treatment of *H. pylori* reduces gastric ulcer recurrence. An outline of current hypotheses for the relationship between *H. pylori* and peptic ulcers is shown in Fig. 16-3.

The reasons for the variability of the effects of *H. pylori* in different individuals are at present unknown. It may be that different strains of *H. pylori* have different effects, or

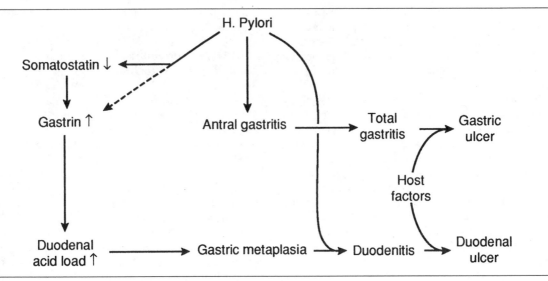

Fig. 16-3. Outline of a hypothesis for the relationship between *H. pylori* and peptic ulceration.

there may be differences in host responses, or both. Certainly there are host factors in ulcer disease that remain unexplained such as the increased frequency in men, the mechanism by which smoking leads to increased ulceration, and the relationship of duodenal ulcers to blood group type O. Thus *H. pylori* is the most important, but not the only factor in non-NSAID ulcer disease.

Disorders of Gastric Motility

Neuropathies

Three patterns of gastric dysrhythmia have been described in association with delayed gastric emptying. These disturbances are evident in the fasting state although postprandial abnormalities are also present. Some patients show reduced numbers or absence of migrating motor complexes, termed bradygastria. Others exhibit an increased frequency of complexes termed tachygastria. Yet other patients have approximately normal rate of generation of migrating complexes, but they occur in an irregular rhythm.

Up to 20% of patients with longstanding insulin-dependent diabetes develop an autonomic neuropathy. Symptoms include early satiety, nausea, vomiting, bloating, and postprandial epigastric pain. These patients show decreased frequency and amplitude of postprandial antral contractions and many also show abnormalities of fasting

motility with reduction or absence of migrating motor complexes.

Other Conditions

Patients who have had a truncal vagotomy and pyloroplasty (a widening of the pylorus), usually for ulcer disease, can develop delayed gastric emptying of solids and, particularly in the early postoperative period, gastric atony. Also, there is sometimes rapid emptying of meals after gastric surgery in part due to lack of distensibility of the stomach after a vagotomy. This may lead to symptoms of faintness due to hypoglycemia, abdominal discomfort, diarrhea, and malabsorption.

Gastric Cancer

Gastric cancer was very common in the USA, but since the 1940s there has been a marked decline in frequency, the cause of which is not clear. Epidemiological studies are consistent with gastric cancer being caused by exposure to an environmental factor early in life. Dietary factors, including salt and nitrates and nitrites that can be converted into carcinogenic nitrosamines, have been considered, but good data have been hard to obtain. Infection with *H. pylori* is associated with an increased risk of gastric adenocarcinoma, probably because the infection can result in a chronic atrophic gastritis. An increase in gastric carcinoma is also seen in patients with pernicious anemia and in patients more than 20 years after a gastric resection.

Typically gastric cancer is asymptomatic early on and only gives rise to symptoms late in the course of the disease. Common symptoms include abdominal pain and weight loss, often with anorexia, weakness, or anemia. The tumor may cause obstruction and give rise to dysphagia or vomiting, or symptoms may be caused by metastases and include abdominal swelling or shortness of breath.

Because of the often late presentation of gastric cancer, treatment is often unrewarding. In the rare patient with local disease, surgical resection is appropriate, but most patients will be candidates only for palliative chemotherapy. Overall the 5-year survival of patients with gastric cancer in the USA is about 15%.

Nonulcer Dyspepsia

This a descriptive term for patients who have dyspeptic symptoms including nausea, upper abdominal pain, burning, and discomfort without any other defined disease. This is a very common disorder and almost certainly patients with this syndrome far outnumber those with peptic ulcers and defined motility disorders. In order to make the diagnosis it is essential to exclude known esophageal, gastric, duodenal, and pancreatic diseases as well as motility disorders and irritable-bowel syndrome. Nevertheless, patients with nonulcer dyspepsia may well consist of several syndromes. Current suggestions as to causation include as yet undefined motility disorders or some response to *H. pylori* infection. However, no current data are available that identify the pathophysiology in these patients.

Clinical Examples

1. A 72-year-old woman with osteoarthritis of hips and hands takes four ibruprofen per day that she buys from the drug store for relief of her symptoms. She recently developed epigastric pain, worse when she was hungry and relieved somewhat by antacids. It also wakes her at night, typically around 2:00 to 3:00 in the morning. She had an endoscopic examination of her stomach which showed she had a duodenal ulcer, and *H. pylori* was present in biopsies taken from the gastric antrum.

Discussion.   This woman has two independent risk factors for the development of duodenal ulcer disease. She has *H. pylori,* which predisposes to ulcer disease and makes recurrence more likely, and she also takes NSAIDs. Appropriate treatment would include an H_2 antagonist

which would allow ulcer healing, but also antimicrobial treatment of the *H. pylori* in order to reduce the chances of recurrence of the ulcer. She should use acetaminophen for her joint pain and avoid NSAIDs. If she must take NSAIDs again, an oral prostaglandin analogue might protect her upper gut from ulceration.

2. A 42-year-old woman presented with shortness of breath on exertion and general fatigue. She was found to be anemic, with a hemoglobin of 7 g/dl and a macrocytosis (MCV 105 fL). She had some epigastric discomfort, and a fasting plasma gastrin was found to be 850 pg/ml (normal <100).

Discussion.   This woman has pernicious anemia. In this condition there is an immune gastritis that involves the body and fundus of the stomach, but not the antrum. The patient does not secrete any intrinsic factor, cannot absorb dietary vitamin B_{12}, and therefore develops the anemia. In addition, she does not make gastric acid, and the negative feedback inhibition of gastrin release is lost. Thus the patient has a high fasting gastrin. In the long term, the hypergastrinemia may prove to be important in that gastrin could cause hyperplasia and even tumors of ECL cells. The anemia, however, can be controlled easily with lifelong vitamin B_{12} injections.

3. A 58-year-old man had a vagotomy and pyloroplasty for a duodenal ulcer 10 years ago. However, since that time, he has been hospitalized once with a bleeding ulcer and has been treated with an H_2 antagonist many times to control his symptoms of epigastric pain, nausea, and heartburn. At endoscopy he is found to have a duodenal ulcer despite taking ranitidine twice per day for the last 6 months. Biopsies show that he does not have *H. pylori* in the stomach.

Discussion.   This man has a history of severe ulcer disease recurring after what should be effective surgical therapy. Furthermore, he has had a complication of an ulcer even after his surgery, and has required numerous courses of medication. This suggests possible Zollinger-Ellison syndrome, a rare condition in which a tumor in the duodenum or pancreas produces gastrin, causing markedly increased acid secretion. The massively increased acid secretion is sufficient to produce ulcers in the absence of *H. pylori* or NSAIDs.

Bibliography

Collen MJ and Benjamin SJ (eds.). *Pharmacology of Peptic Ulcer Disease.* Berlin: Springer-Verlag, 1991. *Essays on drugs and gastric function.*

Domschke W and Konturek SJ (eds.). *The Stomach: Physiology, Pathophysiology and Treatment.* Berlin: Springer, 1993. *Numerous reviews on aspects of the stomach.*

Gustavsson S, Kumar D, and Graham DY (eds.). *The Stomach.* Edinburgh: Churchill Livingstone, 1993. *Collected reviews on all aspects of the stomach.*

Sleisenger MH and Fordtran JS (eds). *Gastrointestinal Disease* (5th Ed). Section IV: Stomach and Duodenum. Philadelphia: Saunders, 1993. *The standard text on gastrointestinal diseases.*

17 Pancreas

Robert A. Rankin

Objectives

After completing this chapter, you should be able to

Review the anatomy and physiology of the pancreas

Define acute pancreatitis and its etiology and pathogenesis

Describe the clinical and biochemical hallmarks of acute pancreatitis

Detail the complications associated with acute pancreatitis

Outline the causes, pathogenesis and consequences of chronic pancreatitis, including abdominal pain, malabsorption and diabetes

Review the complications and treatment options of chronic pancreatitis

---

Anatomy

The pancreas is a relatively small organ weighing 60–110 g and is retroperitoneal in location. It has no capsule but is located close to several vital structures, including the stomach, duodenum, spleen, portal vein, and distal common bile duct. The pancreas receives efferent innervation from the vagus and splanchnic nerves which pass through the hepatic and celiac plexi. Sympathetic efferents supply the blood vessels. Afferent nerves traveling in splanchnic nerves traverse the celiac plexus en route to the spinal cord. Visceral pain originating from the pancreas is transmitted to the central nervous system via these primary sensory afferent nerves. Mechanisms involved in pancreatic pain perception are poorly understood.

Exocrine Pancreas

The exocrine pancreas consists of clusters of microscopic, spherical acini that form lobules. Each acinus consists of a cupped layer of acinar cells that secrete a large variety of proteins into the central lumen. The ductal lumen is partially lined by pale-staining, centroacinar cells that secrete water and sodium bicarbonate.

Endocrine Pancreas

The endocrine pancreas consists of approximately a million islets of Langerhans scattered among the loose tissue between lobules. Their known cell types and secretory products are: beta cells, insulin; alpha cells, glucagon; delta cells, somatostatin, d_1 cells, vasoactive intestinal peptide (VIP); and d_2 cells, pancreatic polypeptide.

Physiology and Biochemistry

The pancreas can secrete up to 4,000 milliliters of fluid per day and produces more protein per gram of tissue than any other organ in the body. It has a tremendous reserve capacity. Steatorrhea occurs only after 80–90% reduction of intraduodenal lipase levels are achieved. The composition of the average daily secretion is described in Table 17-1.

Basal secretion of enzymes is approximately 10% of maximally stimulated secretion, while bicarbonate secretion is only about 2%. As is true with acid secretion of the stomach, postprandial pancreatic enzyme secretion can be divided into cephalic, gastric, and intestinal phases. The sight, smell, and taste of food activate the cephalic phase

Table 17-1. Constituents of Basal Pancreatic Secretion

Constituent	Amount
Water	1,000 ml
Total protein	5–10 g
Na^+	145 mEq
K^+	5 mEq
Ca^{++}	1.6 mEq
Mg^{++}	0.4 mEq
HCO_{3-+Cl-}	155 mEq

of pancreatic secretion (approximately 25% of total) which is mediated by the vagus nerve. The gastric phase is also mediated by the vagus nerve when stimulated by gastric distention and accounts for up to 10% of the total response. The intestinal phase accounts for about 65% of the total meal-related pancreatic secretion. The major stimulants are hydrogen ions entering the duodenum (stimulating secretin release from duodenal cells) and amino acids and fatty acids in the duodenum-releasing cholecystokinin (CCK).

Pancreatic enzymes are made by the acinar cells and are stored intracellularly as zymogen granules until stimulation for release occurs. A large variety of enzymes is found in the pancreatic juice (Table 17-2). Because the proteins produced in the pancreas could destroy it, protective mechanisms are available to prevent autodigestion from occurring. Many enzymes are produced as inactive proenzymes. Secretory granule packaging occurs within the cell to protect the cell as it stores the enzyme. Since trypsin is the major activator for most of the proenzymes, trypsin inhibitors are secreted along with the enzymes into the pancreatic duct. With some exceptions (amylase and lipase, for instance), enzymes are activated only upon reaching the duodenal lumen where enterokinase (released from the duodenum) converts trypsinogen to trypsin, which in turn activates the proenzyme (Fig. 17-1).

Pancreatic enzymes are secreted, in large part, by hormonal stimulation of cholecystokinin. This regulatory peptide is released from endocrine cells in the duodenal wall in response to ingested fatty acids and amino acids in the duodenum (Fig. 17-2). When both secretin and cholecystokinin act on the pancreas simultaneously, the effects are additive. In addition to secretin and cholecystokinin, vagovagal reflexes activate cholinergic postganglionic neurons in the pancreas to stimulate enzyme secretion. Other hormones shown in Fig. 17-2 to have an affect on pancreatic enzyme secretion include gastrin, bombesin, substance P, and neurotensin. Adrenergic stimulation of the pancreas through the sympathetic nervous system is inhibitory and directly related to intense vasoconstriction.

Several peptides are present in nerve cell bodies or fibers in the pancreas. Vasoactive intestinal peptide (VIP) appears to be the most abundant, but it is only a weak agonist for enzyme secretion.

Inhibition of pancreatic secretion is mediated by release of inhibitory hormones. Pancreatic glucagon and somatostatin (both stimulated by hyperaminocidemia) as well as pancreatic polypeptide (PP) and intestinal glucagon all appear to be inhibitory. Their exact role in regulating pancreatic function is yet to be determined.

Table 17-2. Enzymes of Mammalian Pancreatic Secretion

Zymogen	Enzyme	Activator
Trypsinogen	Trypsin	Enterokinase, Ca^{2+}, trypsin
Chymotrypsinogen	Chymotrypsin	Trypsin
Procarboxypeptidase A	Carboxypeptidase A	Trypsin
Procarboxypeptidase B	Carboxypeptidase B	Trypsin
Proelastase	Elastase	Trypsin
Proelastomucase	Elastomucase	Trypsin
	Amylase	Chloride
	Lipase	Emulsifying agents
	Esterase	Bile salts
Prophospholipase A	Phospholipase A	Bile salts
		Trypsin
	Cholesterol esterase	Bile salts

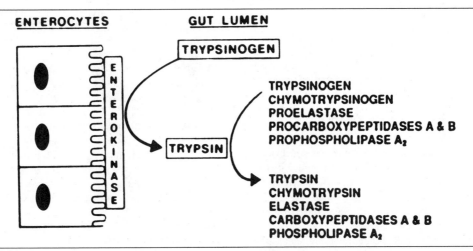

Fig. 17-1. Mechanism of proenzyme activation in the intestinal lumen. (Reprinted with permission from Pandol S. Pancreatic physiology. In Slesinger M and Fordtran J (eds.). *Gastrointestinal Disease* (5th ed.). Philadelphia: W. B. Saunders, 1993, p. 1587.)

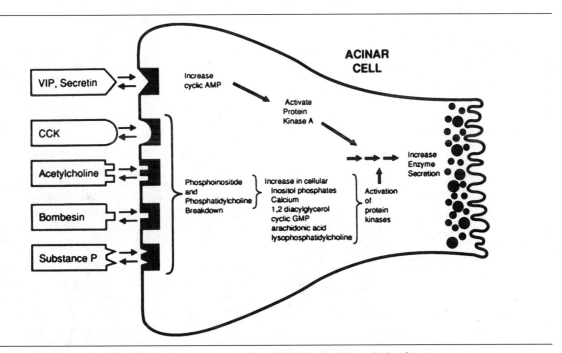

Fig. 17-2. Hormonal control of pancreatic acinar cell secretion. (Reprinted with permission from Pandol S. Pancreatic physiology. In Slesinger M and Fordtran J (eds.). *Gastrointestinal Disease* (5th ed.). Philadelphia: W. B. Saunders, 1993, p. 1589.)

Common Diseases

Acute Pancreatitis

This is defined as acute inflammation with secretory cell damage; complete structural and biological restitution is possible if the cause is eliminated. However, since the pancreas is relatively inaccessible, only clinical resolution of disease can reliably be established. Therefore, acute pancreatitis is defined in clinical terms. The two types of acute pancreatitis that can occur are (1) edematous pancreatitis, which occurs more frequently and is milder in severity (the pancreas becomes swollen, but no major hemorrhage occurs) and (2) hemorrhagic pancreatitis, which is a more severe variety often associated with major retroperitoneal bleeding and relatively high mortality.

Acute pancreatitis is called acute relapsing pancreatitis if more than one episode occurs from the same cause. For instance, this can occur with recurrent passage of gallstones through the common bile duct.

Causes of Acute Pancreatitis

Gallstones are the most common cause of acute pancreatitis. Alcohol is more often associated with chronic pancreatitis (as defined by progressive fibrosis in the pancreas), but alcohol-induced pancreatitis may present acutely and does not always progress to chronic changes. Therefore, alcohol is now felt to be the second most common cause of acute pancreatitis.

Obstructive Causes. Gallstones are the most common obstructive cause of pancreatitis. Pancreatic cancer with partial ductal obstruction can present infrequently (3%) as acute pancreatitis. Also, sphincter of Oddi dysfunction can act as obstruction and account for some cases of acute pancreatitis.

Toxins and Drugs. Ethyl alcohol is the most common toxin, although organophosphorous insecticides, scorpion venom, and methyl alcohol have been associated with pancreatitis. Numerous drugs have also been implicated. Those associated with a high incidence of the disease are azathioprine and 6-mercaptopurine (3–5%), valproic acid (up to 20%), and the antiviral (HIV) agent didanosine (DDI). Other common medications implicated in causing pancreatitis include estrogens, tetracycline, metronidazole, furosemide, sulfonamide, erythromycin, salicylate, H_2 receptor blockers, and acetaminophen.

Trauma. Blunt trauma to the abdomen, endoscopic retrograde cholangiopancreatography (ERCP), and abdominal or thoracic surgery (especially with the use of cardiopulmonary bypass) are all associated with acute pancreatitis.

Metabolic Causes. Hypertriglyceridemia (with triglyceride levels of over 1000 mg/dl) and hypercalcemia can be associated with pancreatitis.

Infection. Viral causes include mumps, coxsackievirus, hepatitis A, B, or C, and cytomegalovirus (CMV). Rarely bacterial agents are implicated. AIDS patients have a very high incidence of pancreatitis with CMV being the most common cause. Numerous other infections as well as the agents used to treat them are associated with pancreatitis.

Miscellaneous. Penetrating ulcers are a rare cause of acute pancreatitis, as is Crohn's disease.

Idiopathic. This is the third most common category of acute pancreatitis.

Pathogenesis

This is still not well understood. The proposed mechanisms of gallstone passage causing pancreatitis include bile reflux, reflux of duodenal content, or extravasation of pancreatic juice into the gland parenchyma. These theories have not held up. Recent studies with experimental pancreatitis suggest that the triggering events may involve derangements in acinar cell function and that activation of digestive enzymes may occur within the acinar cells. Activation of trypsin from trypsinogen in the lysosome vacuoles is believed to be one of the initiating events. Trypsin is then available to activate other enzymes.

Ischemia appears to transform mild, edematous pancreatitis into severe hemorrhagic or necrotizing forms. This, in turn, can lead to the release of toxic factors into the systemic circulation or peritoneal space and ultimately multi-organ compromise and possibly failure.

Activation of phospholipase A2 and release into the circulation is thought to cause acute pulmonary injury by degrading surfactant. Activation of elastase can lead to digestion of the elastic components of blood vessels and thereby contribute to hemorrhage. Since the release of trypsin can activate complement and vasoactive kinins, pancreatitis can lead to shock, renal failure, and disseminated intravascular coagulation. Lipase release can lead to peripancreatic fat necrosis. Tetany may result from rapid calcium or magnesium sequestration following fat necrosis. Jaundice may become evident as swelling of the pancreatic head obstructs the distal common bile duct.

Diagnosis

Pain is usually a major component of the patient's disease at presentation. Nerve involvement, gland swelling, and retroperitoneal hemorrhage may all contribute to the pain. Typically the pain is in the upper abdomen with radiation straight through to the back. Nausea and vomiting usually occur.

The serum amylase and lipase levels are typically elevated. The lipase elevation is more sensitive and specific for acute pancreatitis than is the amylase elevation. Ultrasound or computed tomography (CT) may demonstrate swelling of the pancreas, but these techniques are more useful when looking for causes and complications of pancreatitis.

Complications

Up to 25% of all attacks of acute pancreatitis are associated with complications. The mortality rate can approach 9%, with the most common cause of early death (within one week of admission) being respiratory failure and the most common cause of late death being infection. Obesity is a major risk factor for severe pancreatitis.

Systemic complications can include shock, coagulopathy, respiratory failure, acute renal failure, hyperglycemia, hypocalcemia, subcutaneous fat necrosis, retinopathy, and psychosis. Local complications can include peripancreatic necrosis with or without infection, pseudocysts, abscess formation, gastrointestinal hemorrhage from gastritis, gastric varices from splenic vein obstruction or rupture of a pseudoaneurysm, and splenic rupture or hematoma.

Treatment

This is largely supportive in nature and involves pancreas and bowel rest by eliminating oral intake. Vigorous and appropriate levels of intravenous fluid resuscitation and nutritional support are critical in the more severe forms of pancreatitis. Adequate pain control may require narcotic administration. Treatment of complications should be done as they arise.

Chronic Pancreatitis

With chronic pancreatitis, permanent structural and functional damage already exists at the time of presentation.

Etiology

Alcohol.   It accounts for approximately 70–80% of all cases of chronic pancreatitis. There is a direct relationship between the development of chronic pancreatitis and the amount consumed as well as the duration of alcohol intake. In general, 6–12 years is required to develop symptoms. The risk of alcohol-induced pancreatitis is higher in patients on high-fat, high-protein diets. Higher protein concentrations are found in the pancreatic juice of these individuals.

Tropical (Nutritional) Pancreatitis.   This is the second most common cause of chronic pancreatitis worldwide. It is a prevalent disease among juveniles in Africa and Asia. Diffuse pancreatic calcifications, diabetes, and pain are characteristic of this disease.

Hereditary Pancreatitis.   This disease typically begins in childhood at a mean age of 10–12 years and is inherited through an autosomal dominant gene.

Hyperparathyroidism.   Hypercalcemia is a potent stimulus of human pancreatic enzyme secretion, and this continuous stimulation may lead to chronic pancreatitis. Increased calcium in the pancreatic secretion can precipitate and cause stone formation.

Obstruction.   Obstruction of the main pancreatic duct by tumors, pseudocysts, stricture, or ampullary lesions can lead to a distinct form of chronic pancreatitis. It is characterized by acinar atrophy and fibrosis along with dilation of the pancreatic ductal system. Functional and structural changes may improve when obstruction is relieved.

Trauma.   Although more typically a cause of acute pancreatitis, traumatic damage to the pancreatic duct may lead to localized changes of chronic pancreatitis.

Pancreas Divisum.   Congenital failure of the ducts of the dorsal and ventral pancreas to fuse leads to drainage of most pancreatic exocrine secretions through the duct of Santorini and minor papilla. Relative obstruction of the minor papilla may lead to chronic pancreatitis on an obstructive basis.

Idiopathic.   This is the second most common type of chronic pancreatitis in North America. There appears to be a juvenile type associated with a lot of pain and a "senile" type with little pain but with endocrine and exocrine pancreatic insufficiency.

Pathogenesis

Alcohol can cause an increase in basal secretion of proteases, amylase, and lipase and a decrease in trypsin inhibitor (at least in rats). Alcohol may produce chronic pancreatitis by interfering with intracellular transport of enzymes, thereby initiating localized enzyme activation and local autodigestion. With increased protein in the secretion, localized protein plugs can also occur and cause secondary duct obstruction. These secretions also calcify and can cause intraductal stones.

Although malnutrition is invariably present in tropical (nutritional) pancreatitis, the link with pancreatitis is not known. Toxic products in cassava, which is consumed in large quantities by the majority of the Afro-Asian poor, may be the cause.

Clinical Features

Abdominal pain, malabsorption, and diabetes are the major symptoms and findings in chronic pancreatitis.

Pain.   Possible mechanisms include chronic pancreatic inflammation, increased intraductal pressure, and neural irritation. Many observations suggest that decreased pancreatic secretion (and therefore decreased ductal pressure) may relieve pain. Surgical decompression of the duct seems to decrease pain in a high percentage of patients with dilated ducts and increased ductal pressure. Alterations in the perineural sheath and continuous stimulation of the nerve by inflammation, entrapment, and locally released noxious substances have also been postulated as causes of chronic pain.

Malabsorption.   This occurs only after the capacity for enzyme secretion has decreased by 90%. Lipase secretion decreases more rapidly than protease secretion, so steatorrhea usually occurs before protein malabsorption.

Diabetes.   Destruction of the endocrine pancreas occurs along with the exocrine destruction. With time, diabetes develops in a number of these patients.

Diagnosis

A history of heavy alcohol intake, recurrent or daily pain, and pancreatic calcifications on x-ray are noted in most patients with chronic pancreatitis. Amylase and lipase elevations may or may not be present.

Ultrasound, CT, and endoscopic retrograde cholangiopancreatography (ERCP) have made it possible to routinely assess the gross structure of the pancreas. They all have excellent specificity and good sensitivity. ERCP seems to be the best test, though the most invasive, and CT appears to be more sensitive than ultrasound.

Complications

The most common complication of chronic pancreatitis is pseudocyst formation, which occurs in up to 25% of all cases. Pseudocysts probably result from rupture of a pancreatic duct and subsequent necrosis and phlegmon formation caused by escaping pancreatic juice. Adjacent mesothelium walls off the inflammatory collection. As the core of inflammatory tissue resolves, a pseudocyst is formed. Small pseudocysts (< 4 cm) often resolve spontaneously while larger ones (> 6 cm) rarely do.

Pain is the major symptom of pancreatic pseudocysts. Other more threatening problems include bleeding into the pseudocyst (pseudoaneurysm formation), pseudocyst rupture, infection, and obstruction of the splenic vein leading to gastric varices. If these complications occur or pain persists, surgical drainage is usually necessary.

Pancreatic ascites can occur if there is a persistent leakage of enzyme-rich fluid from a ruptured pancreatic duct or from a pseudocyst. Amylase levels in the ascitic fluid are frequently above 1000 IU/liter and often much higher. After an ERCP is done to define the cause and site of the leak, surgery is usually necessary.

Splenic vein thrombosis with resultant gastric varices formation can occur secondary to pancreatic inflammation or pseudocyst formation. This should be suspected in someone found bleeding from gastric varices who has a previous history of pancreatitis. Splenectomy is curative.

Treatment

Treatment is directed at pain control and correction of maldigestion by pancreatic enzyme replacement, taken with meals. It should be remembered that acid (pH < 4) inactivates pancreatic enzymes, so some patients require reduction of gastric acidity or special acid-resistant coatings for tablets to get adequate amounts of enzymes into the small intestine.

Clinical Example

1. A 54-year-old man was admitted for evaluation of epigastric pain. He had apparently been well until 18 months prior to admission when he experienced several episodes of right upper quadrant pain. An ultrasound study revealed gallstones. Six months later he suffered a severe episode of right upper quadrant and epigastric pain with radiation to the back. He underwent cholecystectomy; at surgery the gallbladder was inflamed but was easily removed. The common bile duct was not explored. Gallstones were seen within the gallbladder. Two months later the patient experienced an episode of periumbilical and epigastric pain which radiated through to his back. He required hospitalization but rapidly improved with intravenous fluids and pain medications. Between that admis-

sion and the present admission, he suffered numerous episodes of similar epigastric pain radiating to his back, but treated himself at home with codeine. Although the codeine would relieve his pain temporarily, he often noted pain again after eating or drinking. The present admission was precipitated by an especially severe episode of pain associated with mild jaundice. He has lost 40 pounds over the past several months. He considered himself a social drinker and had consumed approximately a pint of liquor per day for the last several years.

On physical exam he appeared moderately ill, with a blood pressure of 110/80 and no postural hypotension. General examination was normal except for evidence of muscle wasting and malnutrition. The liver was approximately 15 cm in vertical span in the midclavicular line. There was tenderness to palpation throughout the epigastrium and the periumbilical area. Mild scleral icterus was noted. There was a trace of edema in the lower extremities.

During hospitalization, he was found to have a normal blood count. Urinalysis revealed 1+ glucose and some bilirubin. His serum and urine amylase were normal and his alkaline phosphatase was four times the upper limit of normal. His serum bilirubin was slightly elevated. Examination of his stool showed neutral fat globules and meat fibers. His fasting blood glucose was 200 mg/dl. An endoscopic retrograde cholangiopancreatogram (ERCP) showed alternating stenosis and dilatation of the pancreatic duct, indicating chronic pancreatitis. The common bile duct was slightly dilated except in its distal portion, where it went through the head of the pancreas. At this point it narrowed in a gradual fashion. No stones were seen.

Discussion.   The patient has chronic relapsing pancreatitis, probably secondary to his alcohol intake. Such patients may not have serum amylase elevations late in their disease because much of the pancreas may be destroyed. For this same reason they may develop diabetes (destruction of the islets of Langerhans) and fat, protein, and carbohydrate maldigestion (because of inadequate enzyme production). This patient also developed mild obstructive jaundice because of scarring and inflammation around the common bile duct where it courses through the head of the pancreas.

The diabetes was controlled with insulin and the patient's maldigestion improved with pancreatic enzyme supplementation. He was asked to abstain from alcohol because in some patients abstinence will lessen the painful attacks.

Bibliography

Steinberg W and Tenner S. Acute Pancreatitis. *N Engl J Med* 330;17:1198–1210, 1994. *An excellent review article on acute pancreatitis. Easy to read and understand.*

Yamada T. The Regulatory Peptide Letter: A Quarterly Clinical Review, Vol. I, No. 3. Woodbridge, M.E.D. Communications, 1989. *A review of everything that may or may not be involved in pancreatic secretion including all the known and postulated hormones. This is an indepth review.*

Yamada T. The Regulatory Peptide Letter: A Quarterly Clinical Review, Vol. II, No. 3. Woodbridge, M.E.D. Communications, 1990. *This article reviews the cellular and subcellular mechanisms for pancreatic secretions.*

Yamada T (ed.). Pancreas. In *Textbook of Gastroenterology,* Vol. II. Philadelphia: Lippincott, 1991. *This is basic textbook of gastroenterology with well written chapters on pancreatic physiology as well as all the diseases associated with the pancreas. This is a good starting point for any reading.*

18 Liver and Biliary Tract

Richard F. Harty

Objectives

After completing this chapter, you should be able to

Review briefly pertinent anatomical features of the liver that relate hepatic acinar structure to sinusoidal blood flow and hepatocyte function

Discuss the functional aspects of the liver with regard to hepatocellular uptake, transport metabolism, biotransformation and secretion of exogenous and endogenous substances

Describe the sequence of events involved in bilirubin metabolism and pathophysiological factors that result in hyperbilirubinemias and jaundice

Explain the differential diagnosis of unconjugated versus conjugated hyperbilirubinemia

Provide a basis for interpretation of laboratory tests involving enzyme assays, measures of hepatic synthetic function and immunology tests in liver disease

Outline the clinical and serologic features of viral hepatitis

Detail the causes and complications of cirrhosis including portal hypertension, ascites, hepatic encephalopathy and hepatorenal syndrome

Anatomy

The liver is the largest organ in the body, weighing between 1200 and 1500 g in a healthy adult. It is located in the right upper quadrant and extends across the midline to the left upper quadrant. The right lobe of the liver is predominant over the left lobe in size, weight, and proportion of blood received from its dual blood supply of the portal vein and hepatic artery. Gross anatomical demarcations of the right and left lobes are provided anteriorly by the falciform ligament, a peritoneal reflection on the anterior surface of the liver that extends from the diaphragm to the umbilicus. Functional anatomical divisions of the liver are more accurately defined by the trunks and branches of the hepatic vessels and bile duct. In this perspective the dividing line between right and left hepatic lobes is through the plane passing from the gallbladder bed above and inferior vena cava below. Each hepatic lobe can be further divided into four segments (Figs. 18-1a and 18-1b). These lobular and segmental divisions are particularly important to the

surgeon involved in liver resection. Figure 18-1 illustrates the relative anatomical relationships of hepatic segments to each other and to the four branches of the portal vein and three branches of the hepatic vein. Attention should be paid to the location of the caudate lobe (segment 1) and its blood supply. The caudate lobe receives blood from both the right and left branches of the portal vein and hepatic artery. Of importance in Budd-Chiari syndrome (thrombosis of hepatic veins), this lobe drains directly into the inferior vena cava. Therefore, in states of hepatic venous outflow obstruction, the caudate lobe enlarges dramatically, as reflected by noninvasive imaging, and may be the sole route for hepatic venous outflow.

Normal Function

The liver performs a number of important and complex biological functions that are essential for survival. Biochemical diversity in hepatocytes of the acinus, the functional

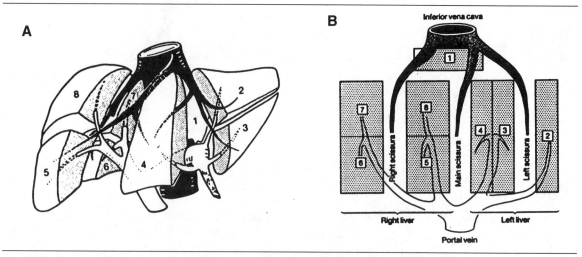

Fig. 18-1. (A) Illustration of the functional divisions of the liver into segments and (B) schematic representation of functional anatomy of the liver noting the three main hepatic veins and four main portal vein branches, thus dividing the liver into four sectors and eight segments. (From: Bismuth H, Aldridge MC, and Kunstlinger F. Macroscopic Anatomy of the Liver. In McIntyre N (ed.). *Oxford Textbook of Clinical Hepatology.* New York: Oxford University Press, 1991, pp. 4–5. By permission of Oxford University Press.)

unit of the liver, accounts for a remarkable number of functions carried out by the liver. Uptake, transport, metabolism and excretion of endogenous and exogenous solutes are principal regulatory functions of the liver. The hepatic acinus is depicted in Fig. 18-2, which shows hepatocytes in relationship to the unidirectional sinusoidal blood flow. Gradients exist between high substrate and oxygen concentrations in the portal area and low concentrations in the region of terminal hepatic venule. The zonal arrangement of hepatocytes described by Rappaport assigns zone 1 to the areas of greatest substrate concentration and zone 3 the least, while zone 2 is intermediate in oxygen and substrate concentrations. The physiological significance of this arrangement is that solutes come in contact with hepatocytes in a sequential manner. Uptake of solutes by hepatocytes in zone 1 means that cells at the periphery of the lobule will be exposed to a different microenvironment. As a consequence of this decreasing substrate concentration within the acinus, there is hepatocyte heterogeneity. Hepatocytes in zone 1 exhibit greater levels of gluconeogenesis and oxidative energy metabolism while liver cells in zone 3 are involved predominantly in glycogenolysis and lipogenesis. Thus, uptake and transport of solutes into hepatocytes determines, in part, phenotypic expression of metabolic activity. Furthermore, the zonal location of hepatocytes within the acinus can preordain its susceptibility to injury in disease states.

Within hepatic cords, the hepatocyte is polarized into basolateral and canalicular or apical domains (Fig. 18-3). The sinusoidal surface (basolateral) is expanded by microvilli that project into the space of Disse, the space between the fenestrated sinusoidal endothelium and hepatocyte. At the apical surface, adjacent hepatocytes are coupled by tight junctions to create the bile canaliculus. Canalicular bile flow is countercurrent to sinusoidal blood flow. Bile flow is directed toward the portal zones and then to coalescing bile ductules and ducts and ultimately reaches the gallbladder and small intestine.

Uptake

In order for the liver to synthesize proteins, carbohydrates, and lipids and to regulate energy homeostasis it must take up the necessary substrate molecules. Amino acids, glucose and fatty acids, triglycerides, and bile acids are examples of such substrates. Uptake of solutes by hepatocytes occurs at its basolateral membrane and is dependent upon specific uptake mechanisms, the affinity of solute for albumin, and hepatocyte location within the acinus. Simple diffusion accounts for the uptake of small molecules such

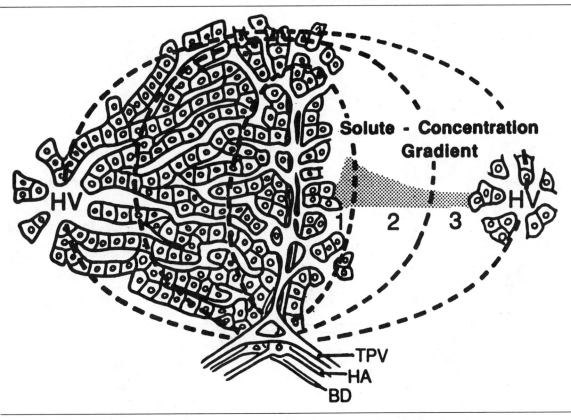

Fig. 18-2. Illustration of the hepatic acinus depicting zones and solute concentration gradient relative to sinusoidal blood flow. TPV terminal hepatic venule, HA terminal hepatic artery, BD bile duct, HV hepatic venule. (Used with permission from: Gumucio JJ. Hepatic transport. In Kelley WN (ed.). *Textbook of Internal Medicine* (2nd ed.). Philadelphia: Lippincott, 1992, p. 422.)

as ammonia which occurs mostly in zone 1. Carrier-mediated transport of solute across the hepatocyte membrane takes place by facilitated diffusion or active transport. Carrier-mediated uptake of substances such as bile acids, an organic anion, is dependent on the distribution of membrane transporters within the acinus. In this instance, bile acid membrane carriers are distributed homogenously in all hepatocytes. Molecules bound tightly to albumin, for example bilirubin, are taken up by ligand:carrier-mediated processes in all acinar zones. The sinusoid membrane transport systems for bile acids and bilirubin are separate. Receptor-mediated endocytosis is another mechanism by which hepatocytes can internalize ligand:receptor complexes. This process of internalization has been described for certain hormones such as insulin and epidermal growth factor.

Transport

Following extraction from admixed portal venous and hepatic arterial blood the hepatocyte must transport substrate to the appropriate intracellular site for metabolism or biotransformation. Thereafter, the resultant biochemical product is transported to a storage locus within the hepatocyte, secreted at the basolateral membrane into sinusoidal blood or excreted via the apical membrane into bile. Macromolecular transport or trafficking within the hepatocyte is also influenced by cytoskeletal structures including microtubules and microfilaments (Fig. 18-3). Membrane-associated transport systems involved in uptake, secretion, and excretion require energy derived from ATP hydrolysis. In turn, these energy-dependent transport processes are susceptible to injury from factors such as hypoxia or ischemia. Reduc-

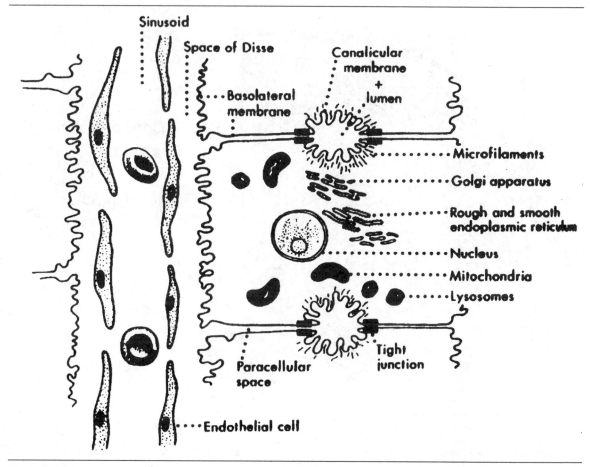

Fig. 18-3. Major structural features of the hepatocyte. (Reprinted with permission from: Traber PG. Hepatic Metabolism. In Kelley WN (ed.). *Textbook of Internal Medicine* (2nd ed.). Philadelphia: Lippincott, 1992, p. 424.)

tion in bile flow as a consequence of impaired canalicular membrane transport may result in cholestasis that is most apparent in zone 3 of the acinus.

Metabolism

Biochemical reactions of the liver involving metabolism of carbohydrates, lipids, and proteins require a cellular infrastructure of organelles. As noted in Fig. 18-3, these include mitochondria, lysosomes, endoplasmic reticulum, and the Golgi apparatus. In the presence of liver disease, these metabolic functions may be impaired and may represent a dominant biochemical feature of underlying organ injury.

Carbohydrates

Carbohydrate metabolism by the liver plays a central role in regulating blood glucose levels. Carbohydrate homeostasis is also closely related to hepatic lipid and protein metabolism. Glucose uptake by the hepatocyte is modulated, in part, by insulin. In the fed state, dietary glucose is either stored as glycogen (glycogenesis) or converted to fatty acids (lipogenesis) which are subsequently incorporated into triglycerides. Fasting, on the other hand, is associated with mobilization of energy stores through the process of glycogenolysis and gluconeogenesis. Glucagon is involved in glycogenolysis and noncarbohydrate substrates (e.g., amino acid) fuel gluconeogenesis. Hypoglycemia or glucose intolerance may be manifestations of liver injury or disease. Severe liver injury due to viral or alcoholic hepatitis may be associated with profound hypoglycemia.

Lipids

Lipid metabolism by the liver involves fatty acid uptake and triglyceride, cholesterol, and phospholipid synthesis (Fig. 18-4). Lipoproteins assembled in the liver are secreted into the circulation. Accumulation of fat, in the form of triglyceride, in the liver can result in a condition termed fatty liver. Fatty liver results from an imbalance between hepatic triglyceride synthesis and secretion. It can be seen in obesity, diabetes mellitus, and protein-calorie malnutrition and can be caused by ingestion of drugs such as ethanol.

Proteins

Protein metabolism and synthesis are important hepatic functions. The majority (50–80%) of total hepatocyte protein synthesis is directed toward proteins which are exported into plasma. Plasma proteins synthesized by the liver include albumin, clotting factors, transferrin, alpha$_1$-antitrypsin, and nonalimentary lipoproteins. Depressed plasma concentrations of proteins such as albumin and prothrombin may reflect severity of acute and chronic liver disease. Amino acids entering the liver via the portal vein are catabolized to urea in the Krebs-Henseleit cycle. In this reaction, amino acids undergo oxidative deamination, whereby the amino group is converted to ammonium ion and, ultimately, to urea. Four amino acids (ornithine, citrulline, arginine, and aspartic acid) are involved in transforming ammonia to urea in this biochemical reaction. Impairment of this important pathway for hepatic detoxification may result in increased levels of circulating ammonia and other bioactive amines which may cause hepatic encephalopathy (see below). Amino acids not catabolized are utilized for protein synthesis or serve as precursors for gluconeogenesis. Transamination of amino acids such as alanine is accomplished by alanine transaminase (ALT), resulting in formation of pyruvate. Pyruvate is then available to act as a substrate for gluconeogenesis.

Biotransformation

The liver, as an excretory organ, performs essential functions in the modification or biotransformation of a wide variety of exogenous (e.g., drugs and toxins) and endogenous substances (e.g., bilirubin and hormones). These excretory functions involve (1) membrane transport of organic substances, (2) intracellular metabolism or biotransformation, and (3) bile secretion. Biotransformation involves the biochemical conversion of lipid-soluble substances into more aqueous-soluble metabolites. As a consequence of the biotransformation process, metabolites are transported by a carrier-mediated mechanism out of the hepatocyte and into the bile or plasma via the canalicular or sinusoidal membrane, respectively. Drug metabolism by the liver involves the cytochrome P-450-dependent microsomal mixed-function oxidase system. There are two sequential phases of drug metabolism: phase 1 reactions are catalyzed by the cytochrome P-450 system and involve oxidation-reduction reactions and phase 2 reactions further the solubility of drugs by conjugating a charged molecule, such as glucuronic acid or glutathione, to the parent compound. As a consequence of these reactions, exogenous and endogenous substances are rendered inactive. However, certain drugs may be activated or made hepatoxic by the biotransformation process. An example of such a drug is acetaminophen, particularly when the drug is taken in large doses. Furthermore, the presence of liver disease and altered biotransformation capability may lead to increased sensitivity to certain drugs (e.g., sedatives and opiates). Depending on the ability of a drug to increase or decrease the activity of enzymes involved in biotransformation, the coadministered drug may have enhanced or diminished biological effectiveness. Alcohol, when ingested acutely or chronically, can cause clinically important drug-drug interactions.

Bile Formation and Secretion

The apical or canalicular membrane portion of the hepatocyte is the site of bile formation. The canalicular membrane contains energy (ATP)-dependent enzymes which transport biotransformed organic substances (e.g., bilirubin and bile acids) by carrier-mediated processes. Bile acid secretion is the driving force for bile formation. Bile acid-dependent bile flow is related to the osmotic activity of bile acids and their associated counter-ions. Electrolyte concentrations in bile closely reflect those in plasma. The majority of osmotic water flow occurs through paracellular pathways. Within bile canaliculi bile acids form aggregates or micelles due to their amphipathic properties. Micelle formation occurs when bile acids are at a critical micellar concentration (CMC) of 3 mmol/liter. Lipid-soluble substances such as cholesterol, steroid hormones, and drugs (e.g., cyclosporine) are incorporated into micelles and transported in the biliary tract and intestine.

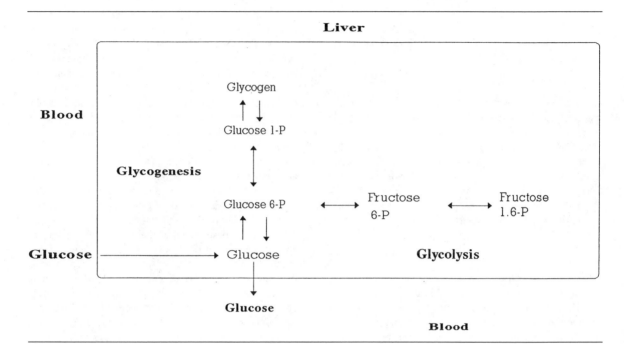

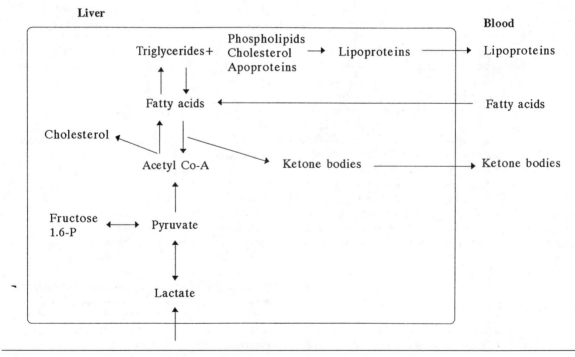

Fig. 18-4. Scheme of carbohydrate and liquid metabolism in the liver. These reversible pathways also include gluconeogenesis and lipolysis. (Reprinted with permission from: Sabesin SM. Hepatic metabolism. In Stein J (ed.). *Internal Medicine* (4th ed.). St. Louis: Mosby-YearBook, 1994, p. 528.)

The liver secretes approximately 1500 ml of bile per day. During fasting, bile is stored and concentrated in the gallbladder. Meal ingestion and cholecystokinin release from the duodenum in response to luminal fat and protein results in gallbladder contraction and delivery of bile to the intestine. Conjugated bile acids entering the intestine are absorbed efficiently in the ileum and returned to the liver via the portal vein for hepatocyte re-uptake to complete their enterohepatic circulation.

Jaundice and Disorders of Bilirubin Metabolism

Jaundice, or icterus, is a clinical condition caused by increased plasma levels of bilirubin. It is manifest as yellowish discolorization of the skin, sclerae, and mucus membranes. Key steps in bilirubin metabolism are shown in Fig. 18-5. Bilirubin is a yellow, tetrapyrrolic pigment

Fig. 18-5. Beginning overview of bilirubin metabolism. Unconjugated bilirubin (UCB) formed from the breakdown of hemoglobin heme and other hemoproteins is transported in plasma reversibly bound to albumin and is converted in the liver to bilirubin monoglucuronide (BMG) and diglucuronide (BDG), the latter being the predominant form secreted in bile. BMG and BDG together normally account for less than 5% of serum bilirubin. In the presence of hepatobiliary disease, BMG and BDG accumulate in plasma and appear in urine. Bilirubin glucuronides in plasma also react nonenzymatically with albumin and possibly other serum proteins to form protein conjugates, which do not appear in urine and have a plasma half-life similar to that of albumin. (Reprinted with permission from: Scharschmidt BF. Bilirubin metabolism and Hyperbilirubinemia. In Wyngaarden JB, Smith LH, and Bennett JC (eds.). *Cecil Textbook of Medicine* (19th ed.). Philadelphia: W.B. Saunders, 1992, p. 756.)

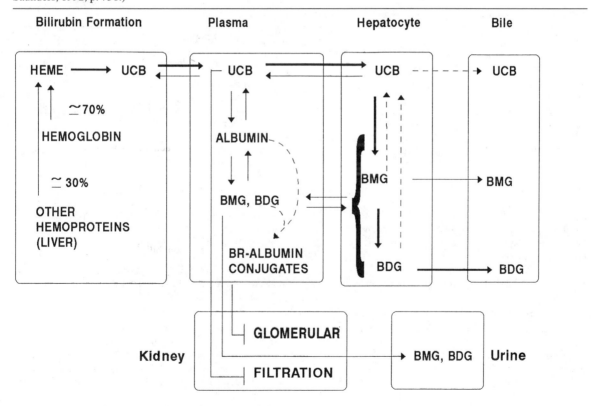

derived principally from heme catabolism. Unconjugated bilirubin is water insoluble and is transported in plasma bound tightly and reversibly to albumin. Unconjugated bilirubin is not excreted in urine. Conjugated bilirubin, which is bound less tightly to albumin, may appear in the urine. Uptake of bilirubin by the hepatocyte from sinusoidal blood is rapid and carrier mediated. After entry into the hepatocyte, bilirubin may be stored temporarily by binding to cytosolic proteins such as ligandin. In order for bilirubin to be excreted into bile it must undergo biotransformation. Conversion of bilirubin from a lipid-soluble to a water-soluble compound is accomplished by conjugation of one or two glucuronic acid molecules to bilirubin. This modification takes place in the smooth endoplasmic reticulum and is catalyzed by uridine diphosphate (UDP) glucuronyl transferase. The bilirubin mono- or di-glucuronide molecules are rendered water soluble because of impairment of hydrogen bonding between pyrrole rings. Transport of conjugated bilirubin from the hepatocyte into bile is accomplished by a carrier-mediated process. Conjugated bilirubin also exits the basolateral membrane of the hepatocyte and enters the circulation. Plasma bilirubin levels range between 0.3 and 1.0 mg/dl. Greater than 90% of circulating bilirubin is normally unconjugated. In the presence of liver or biliary tract disease, circulating bilirubin concentration may be elevated and the proportion of conjugated bilirubin increased.

In the distal small bowel and colon, conjugated bilirubin is hydrolyzed by bacterial enzymes (glucuronidases) to form unconjugated bilirubin and, subsequently, urobilinogen. Urobilinogen is absorbed from the intestine and re-excreted in bile; a small fraction appears in urine. Urobilinogen is absent from the bile and urine of patients with complete biliary obstruction.

The differential diagnosis of hyperbilirubinemia can be divided into three pathophysiologic categories: increased production, reduced hepatic clearance, and extrahepatic obstruction (Table 18-1).

Table 18-1. Causes of Hyperbilirubinemia and Associated Serum Bilirubin Patterns

Disorder	Defect in Bilirubin Physiology
UNCONJUGATED HYPERBILIRUBINEMIA	
Hemolysis and hemolytic anemias	Increased production
Hematomas	Increased production
Ineffective erythropoiesis	1 liter blood = 150 mg hemoglobin = 5 g bilirubin = 20 × normal daily production
Ineffective erythropoiesis (pernicious anemia, thalassemia)	Increased production
Neonatal jaundice (physiologic jaundice)	Increased production; decreased UGT activity; decreased cytosolic ligandin; increased intestinal bilirubin absorption
Breast-milk jaundice	? Inhibition of UGT activity; increased intestinal absorption
Drugs	Reduced hepatic uptake
Crigler-Najjar syndrome type I	Absent bilirubin UGT activity
Crigler-Najjar syndrome type II	Markedly decreased UGT activity
Gilbert's syndrome	Decreased bilirubin UGT activity; ? decreased hepatic uptake; ? hemolysis or dyserythropoiesis
Fasting hyperbilirubinemia (marked response in Gilbert's syndrome)	Increased production; decreased hepatic clearance; ? decreased uptake and conjugation
CONJUGATED HYPERBILIRUBINEMIA	
Intrahepatic cholestasis (hepatocellular, canalicular, or ductular damage)	Decreased biliary secretion; bilirubin deconjugation leads to increased plasma unconjugated bilirubin
Extrahepatic cholestasis (mechanical obstruction)	Decreased biliary secretion; bilirubin deconjugation
Dubin-Johnson syndrome	Impaired biliary secretion (? canalicular membrane defect)
Rotor's syndrome	? decreased hepatic uptake and storage; ? decreased biliary secretion

UGT=uridine-diphosphate glucuronosyltransferase.
Modified from: Crawford JM and Gollan JL. Bilirubin metabolism and the pathophysiology of jaundice. In Schiff L and Schiff ER (eds.). *Diseases of the Liver* (7th ed.) Philadelphia: Lippincott, 1993, p. 58.

Elevated levels of unconjugated bilirubin occur when there is either a marked increase in the rate of formation or a defect in any of the steps involved in the hepatic clearance of unconjugated bilirubin (i.e., hepatic uptake, intracellular binding, and conjugation). On the other hand, conjugated hyperbilirubinemia reflects impaired hepatic clearance of conjugated bilirubin due to either decreased biliary excretion or reduced bile flow at the level of the canaliculus or more distally. Often, liver diseases (e.g., hepatitis, cirrhosis) disrupt both hepatic conjugation and biliary excretion. Thus, in certain instances, the relative amounts of unconjugated and conjugated bilirubin may not be helpful in determining the etiology of jaundice.

Unconjugated Hyperbilirubinemia

Increased Production of Bilirubin

Bilirubin production in adults is 250 mg/day. When the rate of bilirubin formation is increased and the capacity of the liver to clear this load is exceeded, then unconjugated hyperbilirubinemia results. Red-cell hemolysis and ineffective erythropoiesis result in increased heme degradation and bilirubin formation. Plasma levels of unconjugated bilirubin in hemolysis are modest and rarely exceed 4–5 mg/dl. Hemolytic anemia, hematoma, pulmonary infarction, transfusion reaction, or transfusion of stored blood can cause unconjugated hyperbilirubinemia.

Impaired Uptake and Clearance of Bilirubin

Neonatal jaundice is associated with impaired conjugation of bilirubin due, in part, to decreased glucuronyl transferase activity. This condition is also called physiologic jaundice of the newborn and occurs in the first week of life. Kernicterus may develop if plasma bilirubin levels exceed 10 mg/dl. In this condition bilirubin is deposited in brain tissue, resulting in permanent neurologic injury. Neonatal infants fed breast milk may also develop jaundice. The cause of breast-milk jaundice is not completely understood, but may be due to maternal steroid hormones. Drugs may also cause elevations in unconjugated bilirubin secondary to decreased hepatocyte uptake and binding to cytosolic proteins.

Inherited disorders of bilirubin metabolism (see Table 18-1) can cause a spectrum of chronic unconjugated hyperbilirubinemias. Gilbert's syndrome is a relatively frequent (7% of the population) cause of jaundice due to mild unconjugated hyperbilirubinemia (< 3 mg/dl). It is inherited as an autosomal dominant trait and is usually recognized clinically as asymptomatic icterus during the second and third decades. Decreased hepatic glucuronyl trans-

ferase activity and impaired uptake of unconjugated bilirubin are thought to be factors accounting for the pathogenesis of Gilbert's syndrome. Crigler-Najjar syndrome type I (autosomal recessive inheritance) is a rare and fatal condition due to virtual absence of glucuronyl transferase. Type II Crigler-Najjar syndrome is associated with less severe jaundice and survival into adulthood without neurologic damage.

Combined Conjugated and Unconjugated Hyperbilirubinemia

In many clinical situations, jaundice and hyperbilirubinemia are a consequence of cholestasis. Cholestasis refers to impairment of bile formation and/or bile flow secondary to hepatic parenchymal disease or extrahepatic biliary tract obstruction. Unconjugated and conjugated hyperbilirubinemia often coexist in cholestasis.

The differential diagnosis of conjugated hyperbilirubinemia is extensive and includes congenital defects of conjugated bilirubin transport. Rare hereditary defects in transport include Dubin-Johnson syndrome and Rotor's syndrome. Both entities are inherited as autosomal recessive traits. More commonly, disorders such as acute viral hepatitis, chronic hepatitis, alcoholic hepatitis, cirrhosis, and drug-induced hepatotoxicity impair canalicular secretion of conjugated bilirubin.

Extrahepatic Obstruction

Although the above definition of cholestasis includes extrahepatic obstruction, it is helpful to consider this cause of jaundice separately. The pathophysiology of obstructive jaundice is straightforward; however, clinical and biochemical presentations may be confusing. Alternatively, certain hepatic disorders may present with severe cholestasis (e.g., viral and alcoholic hepatitis and primary biliary cirrhosis), suggestive of extrahepatic obstruction. With the availability of abdominal ultrasound, CT scan, and endoscopic techniques to directly visualize the biliary tree, uncertainties in diagnosis can be resolved. Furthermore, the presence of biliary tract obstruction provides clear direction for surgical, endoscopic, or radiologic intervention to define the cause and decompress the biliary system. Choledocholithiasis or gallstones in the biliary tract and tumors account for the majority of cases of extrahepatic biliary obstruction. Obstruction of the distal common bile duct by pancreatic cancer causes painless and progressive jaundice. Absence of bile in the intestinal tract results in clay-colored acholic stools. The presence of positive fecal hemoccult testing in the setting of obstructive jaundice suggests carcinoma of the ampulla of Vater. Inflammatory and postoperative strictures of the common bile duct due to acute cholecystitis and its surgical treatment may also cause biliary obstruction.

Interpretation of Laboratory Tests in Liver Disease

Clinical history, physical examination, and routine laboratory tests are sufficient to diagnose the cause of jaundice in the majority of cases. Exposure to infectious agents through sexual contact, intravenous drug use, or blood transfusions suggest possible viral hepatitis. Alcohol, drugs, organic solvents, or oral contraceptive agents can cause cholestatic jaundice or hepatocellular damage. History of previous biliary tract surgery, gallstones, prior bouts of jaundice, or inflammatory bowel disease suggest extrahepatic cholestasis. Family history of jaundice and chronic liver disease should prompt consideration of inheritable liver diseases such as hemochromatosis, Wilson's disease, or alpha$_1$-antitrypsin deficiency.

In addition to measuring plasma concentrations of bilirubin and the proportion of unconjugated:conjugated bilirubin, enzyme assays, test of hepatic synthetic functions, and immunologic tests can aid in diagnosing and monitoring liver disease (Table 18-2).

Enzyme Assays

Aspartate transaminase (AST, formerly SGOT) and alanine transferase (ALT, formerly SGPT) are hepatic enzymes involved in amino-acid metabolism, namely, the transfer of the alpha-amino groups of alanine and aspartic acid to the alpha-keto groups of ketoglutaric acid. Both enzymes are found in other tissues (e.g., cardiac and skeletal muscle) containing aminotransferases. Serum levels of transaminases (normally < 40 IU/liter) are elevated in most hepatic diseases and reflect hepatocyte injury or death. The highest elevations (> 1000 IU/liter) are observed in extensive hepatocellular injury seen in viral and drug-induced hepatitis and hepatic ischemia and hypoxia. Acute biliary obstruction due to gallstone passage can cause transient elevation in transaminases above 1000 IU/liter. Alcoholic hepatitis is associated with modest transaminase elevations in the range of 200–300 IU/liter. Interestingly, in this condition AST is usually at least twice the ALT value. Identification of an altered AST/ALT ratio may be helpful in etiologic considerations of abnormal transaminase levels. Serum transaminase values do not accurately predict severity of liver disease or prognosis.

Alkaline phosphatase represents a group of isoenzymes found in a number of tissues including liver, bile duct, bone, placenta, intestine, and kidney. Elevated serum alkaline phosphatase in the presence of liver disease (> 4 × normal) usually indicates cholestasis either originating at an intrahepatic site or due to extrahepatic obstruction. It is believed that increased pressure within the biliary system is transmitted to the canicular membrane where synthesis of alkaline phosphatase is stimulated. Bile acids appear to play a role in increased alkaline phosphatase synthesis and release into the circulation. Hepatic origin of alkaline phosphate can be confirmed by demonstrating parallel elevations in one or more of the following enzymes: gamma-glutamyl transpeptidase, leucine aminopeptidase, or 5′ nucleotidase. These enzymes are not increased in bone disease (e.g., Paget's disease) associated with elevation of alkaline phosphatase. Increases in serum alkaline phosphatase may also be seen in infiltrative liver diseases such

Table 18-2. Representative Biochemical Tests in the Patient with Hepatobiliary Disease

Test	Hepatocellular Necrosis	Cholestasis	Infiltrative Process
Aminotransferase	++/+++	0/+	0/+
Alkaline phosphatase	0/+	++/+++	++/+++
Total/direct bilirubin	0/+++	0/+++	0/+
Prothrombin time	Normal or prolonged	Normal or prolonged; responsive to vit. K	Normal
Albumin	Decreased in chronic disorders	Normal	Normal

0 = normal; + to +++ = degrees of abnormality.
Modified with permission from: Moseley RH. Approach to the patient with abnormal liver chemistries. In Yamada T (ed.). *Textbook of Gastroenterology.* Philadelphia: Lippincott, 1991, p. 839.

as lymphoma, leukemia, sarcoidosis, and primary or metastatic cancer.

Hepatic Synthetic Function

Albumin, prothrombin, fibrinogen and factors V, VII, IX, X, XI, and XII are synthesized by the liver. Acute or chronic liver disease may disrupt hepatic protein synthesis sufficiently to depress circulating levels of these proteins.

Prothrombin synthesis depends on an adequate supply of the fat-soluble vitamin K. Thus abnormal prothrombin activity may be caused by vitamin K deficiency, liver disease, or both. Failure to correct prolongation of the prothrombin time with parenteral vitamin K administration indicates severe hepatocellular disease and rules out deficiency of vitamin K due to malabsorption associated with cholestasis. Because the serum half-life of albumin (3 weeks) is long, hypoalbuminemia may not be seen uniformly in acute liver disease; however, serum albumin levels may be an important indicator of chronic liver disease.

Prolonged cholestasis is associated with increased serum levels of cholesterol and phospholipids. Xanthoma and xanthelasma are examples of cutaneous lipid deposition seen in chronic cholestatic syndromes such as primary biliary cirrhosis.

Immunologic Tests

Immunologic abnormalities occur in a variety of liver diseases. Autoimmune hepatitis is associated with antinuclear (ANA) and smooth-muscle antibodies. Antibodies to liver/kidney microsomes (anti-LKM) are present in a subset of cases of autoimmune hepatitis: young females with an aggressive clinical course of hepatitis. Antimitochondrial antibodies (AMA) are present in over 90% of patients with primary biliary cirrhosis and in about 25% of patients with autoimmune chronic active hepatitis. Hypergammaglobulinemia is commonly observed in patients with chronic liver disease and may reflect impairment of reticuloendothelial cells of the hepatic sinusoids. Globulin levels above 3.0 g/dl are frequently seen in autoimmune liver disease. Elevation of IgM is a feature of primary biliary cirrhosis.

Acute Hepatitis

In the United States, acute viral hepatitis is due most commonly to four hepatitis viruses: A, B, C, and D. Hepatitis E is a cause of acute viral hepatitis in Asia, Africa, and Mexico. Characteristics of these agents are summarized in Table 18-3. In the majority of cases hepatocellular necrosis

Table 18-3. Differentiation of the Etiologic Forms of Viral Hepatitis

Feature	Hepatitis A	Hepatitis B	Hepatitis C	Hepatitis D	Hepatitis E
Viral characteristic					
Size of the virus (nm)	27	42	30–60	35–37	32
Nucleic acid	RNA	DNA	RNA	RNA	RNA
Incubation period (days)					
Range	15–49	28–160	15–160	21–140	15–65
Mean	30	70–80	50	?35	42
Patterns of immunity					
Heterologous immunity	No	No	No	No	No
Homologous immunity	Yes	Yes	Second attacks may indicate another distinct agent or weak immunity	Yes	Unknown
EPIDEMIOLOGIC AND CLINICAL FEATURES					
Fecal-oral transmission	Yes	No	No	No	Yes
Percutaneous transmission	Rare	Yes	Yes	Yes	?No
Carrier state	No	Yes	Yes	Yes	No
Risk of chronic hepatitis and cirrhosis	No	Yes	Yes	Yes	No
Risk of hepatocellular carcinoma	No	Yes	Yes	?No	No

Modified with permission from: Koff RS. Viral hepatitis. In Schiff L and Schiff ER (eds.). *Diseases of the Liver* (7th ed.). Philadelphia: Lippincott, 1993, p. 494.

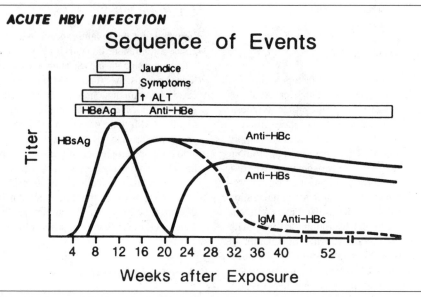

Fig. 18-6. Acute HBV infection-sequence of events. Terminology for serological events and viral agents is included in Table 18-5. (Reprinted with permission from: Koff RS et al. *AGA Clinical Teaching Project, Unit 3. Viral Hepatitis.* Thorofare, N.J.: Slack, 1988, p. 15.)

Table 18-4. Serologic Tests in Viral Hepatitis

Agent	Terminology	Definition	Significance
Hepatitis A (HAV)	Anti-HAV IgM type IgG type	Antibody to HAV	Current or recent infection or convalescence Current or previous infection; indicates immunity
Hepatitis B (HBV)	HBsAg HBeAg	HBV surface antigen e antigen; HBV core component	Positive in most cases of acute or chronic infection Transiently positive during active virus replication, acute hepatitis, and in some chronic cases; reflects Dane particle concentration and infectivity
	Anti-Hbc (IgM or IgG)	Antibody to HBV core antigen	Positive in all acute and chronic cases and in carriers; thus, marker of HBV infection; not protective; IgM anti-HBc may reflect active virus replication
	Anti-HBe	Antibody to e antigen	Transiently positive during convalescence and in some chronic cases and carriers; not protective; reflects low infectivity
	Anti-HBs	Antibody to surface antigen	Becomes positive late in convalescence in most acute cases; protective
Hepatitis C (HCV)	Anti-HCV	Antibody to cloned C100-3 polypeptide	Becomes positive on average 15 weeks after clinical onset; not protective; may be infectious
Hepatitis D (HDV)	Anti-HDV (IgM or IgG)	Antibody to HDV antigen	Similar to anti-HBc in indicating infection; not protective

Reprinted with permission from: Ockner RK. Acute viral hepatitis. In Wyngaarden JB, Smith LH, and Bennett JC (eds.). *Cecil Textbook of Medicine* (19th ed.). Philadelphia: W.B. Saunders, 1992, p. 766.

is self-limited and uncomplicated. Malaise, poor appetite, right upper quadrant pain, and jaundice may be clinical presentations, but frequently the infection is asymptomatic and anicteric. This is particularly true with hepatitis A and hepatitis C. Rarely, acute viral hepatitis leads to acute liver failure and death. Serologic tests and terminology in viral hepatitis are listed in Table 18-4. Hepatitis B virus infection is associated with a complex series of serologic events in response to different antigenic and genetic components of the virus. The clinical and laboratory findings in acute hepatitis B are illustrated in Fig. 18-6. Causes of acute hepatitis in individuals who are HBsAg positive include reactivation of chronic HBV infection and superinfection by other hepatitis viruses. Hepatitis D virus occurs in the presence of HBV infection and is acquired as a coinfection or superinfection. Persistence of abnormal laboratory tests in hepatitis B, C, or D beyond 6–12 months suggests development of chronic hepatitis which does not occur with hepatitis A.

Chronic Hepatitis

Chronic hepatitis is defined as liver cell necrosis and inflammation lasting for more than 6–12 months. Chronic hepatitis may develop in up to 10% of individuals following hepatitis B infection and in up to 50% of cases infected with hepatitis C virus. The clinical and laboratory features of chronic hepatitis are nonspecific and the diagnosis is established by liver biopsy. Histologic classification of chronic hepatitis is based upon the extent of inflammation and liver injury. Chronic persistent hepatitis refers to inflammation confined primarily to the portal areas. Chronic active hepatitis is a more severe form of liver injury which extends beyond the portal tract into the parenchyma with varying degrees of piecemeal necrosis and fibrosis. Ongoing liver cell injury is reflected by elevated levels of aminotransferase enzymes. In general, prognosis is thought to be more favorable with chronic persistent hepatitis and worse with chronic active hepatitis. Experience indicates, however, that these assurances are not absolute. Apparent benign histology at one point in time may change and progress to irreversible liver injury. Progression to cirrhosis may take years to develop. In chronic hepatitis C infection, 10–20 years may pass before cirrhosis is established. Hepatocellular carcinoma is a potential complication of chronic hepatitis B, C, and D.

A number of drugs may induce chronic hepatic inflammation. Histologically, drug-induced chronic hepatitis can be indistinguishable from chronic viral hepatitis or metabolic forms of chronic liver injury (e.g., hemochromatosis,

Wilson's disease). A careful drug history is essential to identifying potential drug or toxin-mediated causes of chronic liver disease.

Alcoholic liver disease results from chronic abuse of ethanol. Alcohol is the most common cause of liver disease in the Western hemisphere. Daily ethanol consumption of 40–80 g (36–72 oz. of beer, 4.5–9.0 oz. of liquor, 15–30 oz. of wine) for 10–15 years are associated with an increase in the incidence of cirrhosis. The hepotoxic effects of ethanol on the liver are manifest pathologically as fatty liver, alcoholic hepatitis, and cirrhosis. These lesions may appear separately in a sequential manner or they may be present together in a mixed picture. Fatty liver is caused by the accumulation of triglycerides in the liver. Hepatomegaly, elevated transaminases ($AST > 2 \times ALT$), and mild jaundice are frequently observed. Fatty liver is a reversible lesion with abstinence from alcohol. Alcoholic hepatitis is a serious consequence of alcoholism because it may lead to hepatic failure and cirrhosis. A spectrum of clinical features may be seen in alcoholic hepatitis. Typically, the patient is ill with abdominal pain, nausea, vomiting, and weight loss. Ascites, jaundice, fever, hepatosplenomegaly, and encephalopathy are common findings. Complete resolution may occur in some patients; however, other individuals experience progression to diffuse fibrosis and cirrhosis. Mortality in alcoholic hepatitis is between 10 and 40%. The toxic effects of ethanol are not restricted to the liver and may effect the central and peripheral nervous system, heart, bone marrow, and pancreas.

Cirrhosis and Complications of Liver Failure

Cirrhosis

Cirrhosis is the end result of sustained or repeated injury to hepatocytes and/or bile ducts that lead to hepatic fibrosis, nodular regeneration of remaining hepatocytes, and interruption of normal sinusoidal blood flow. The causes of cirrhosis are multiple and a representative list is provided in Table 18-5.

Physical examination is frequently helpful in providing evidence of chronic liver disease and cirrhosis. Jaundice, hepatomegaly, splenomegaly, and ascites suggest hepatic functional compromise and portal hypertension. Spider angiomas of the face and upper trunk, palmar erythema, Dupuytren's contracture (fibrous thickening and contraction of the palmar fascia), parotid gland enlargement, gynecomastia, and testicular atrophy are additional findings in cirrhosis.

Table 18-5. Causes of Cirrhosis

DRUGS AND TOXINS	METABOLIC
Alcohol	Wilson's disease
Methyldopa	Hemochromatosis
Methotrexate	Erythropoietic protoporphyria
Isoniazid	Pediatric: alpha$_1$-antitrypsin
Perhexiline maleate	deficiency, galactosemia,
Amiodarone	hereditary fructose intoler-
Oxyphenisatin	ance, glycogen storage dis-
Vitamin A	ease type IV, tyrosinosis
Carbon tetrachloride	
	CARDIOVASCULAR
INFECTIONS	Chronic right heart failure
Hepatitis B and C	Budd-Chiari syndrome
Syphilis (tertiary)	Veno-occlusive disease
Schistosoma japonicum	
	MISCELLANEOUS
BILIARY OBSTRUCTION	Chronic active hepatitis
Carcinoma (pancreatic	Primary biliary cirrhosis
or bile duct)	Sarcoidosis
Chronic pancreatitis	Jejunoileal bypass
Common duct stones	Neonatal hepatitis
Strictures	Indian childhood cirrhosis
Cystic fibrosis	Hereditary hemorrhagic
Biliary atresia	telangiectasia
Sclerosing cholangitis	CRYPTOGENIC

Reprinted with permission from: Boyer TD. Cirrhosis of the liver and its major sequelae. In Wyngaarden JB, Smith LH, and Bennett JC (eds.). *Cecil Textbook of Medicine* (19th ed.). Philadelphia: W.B. Saunders, 1992, p. 786.

Complications

Complications of cirrhosis relate directly to progressive hepatic fibrosis and parenchymal dysfunction. Major sequelae of cirrhosis include (1) portal hypertension, (2) ascites, (3) portosystemic encephalopathy, and (4) hepatorenal syndrome.

Portal Hypertension

Portal hypertension in cirrhosis is due to intrahepatic obstruction to portal venous blood flow at the level of the sinusoid. Portal hypertension can also develop from presinusoidal (e.g., splenic vein thrombosis, schistosomiasis) and postsinusoidal (e.g., Budd-Chiari syndrome, veno-occlusive disease) obstruction. Hepatic fibrosis and regenerative nodules disrupt and obstruct normal sinusoidal vascular channels. As a consequence, pressure within the portal circuit increases (normal portal vein pressure is 7–10 mm Hg) and intrahepatic and extrahepatic shunts or

collateral vascular communications develop between high-pressure portal venous system and low-pressure systemic venous system. Splenomegaly is a result of increased portal pressure. Hypersplenism is a condition associated with portal hypertension in which formed cellular elements (red cells, white cells, and platelets) are sequestered in the spleen. Clinically important enlargement of collateral channels (varices) may occur in the distal esophagus, gastric cardia, and rectum (hemorrhoids). Bleeding from esophageal or gastric varices is a major complication of portal hypertension and is associated with a 30–60% mortality. Therapy of esophageal/gastric variceal hemorrhage may involve endoscopic occlusion or thrombosis of varices, surgical or radiographic (transjugular intrahepatic portosystemic shunt; TIPS) shunting of portal blood to the systemic venous system. Pharmacotherapy may also be used as a primary or adjunctive treatment intended to decrease pressure within the splanchnic circulation.

Ascites

Ascites or excessive fluid in the peritoneal cavity occurs in patients with portal hypertension because of alterations in rate of formation and reabsorption of hepatic lymph and because of renal retention of salt and water. There are a number of factors that are involved in the pathogenesis of ascites in the cirrhotic patient and these are listed in Table 18-6. Management of ascites requires patience and the prudent use of diuretics, and sodium restriction. Spontaneous bacterial peritonitis can develop in patients with

Table 18-6. Factors in the Pathogenesis of Cirrhotic Ascites

1. Increased hydrostatic pressure in hepatic sinusoids and splanchnic capillaries.
2. Overproduction of hepatic and splanchnic lymph secondary to (1), leading to a transudation of lymph into peritoneal space.
3. Limited or reduced reabsorption of water and protein by peritoneal lymphatics.
4. Sodium retention by the kidney secondary to hyperaldosteronism, increased sympathetic activity, alterations in metabolism of prostaglandins and kinins, and altered renal hemodynamics.
5. Impaired renal water excretion, in part caused by increased levels of ADH.

Reprinted with permission from: Boyer TD. Cirrhosis of the liver and its major sequelae. In Wyngaarden JB, Smith LH, and Bennett JC (eds.). *Cecil Textbook of Medicine* (19th ed.). Philadelphia: W.B. Saunders, 1992, p. 794.

cirrhosis and ascites. Fever, abdominal pain, decreased bowel sounds, leukocytosis, and new onset of hepatic encephalopathy may be presenting manifestations. The diagnosis is established by abdominal paracentesis and ascitic fluid white-cell count and culture. Antibiotic treatment is directed toward most frequently cultured organisms (e.g., *E. coli, S. pneumoniae,* and *S. viridous*). Prompt recognition and treatment are essential to decrease mortality.

Encephalopathy

Hepatic encephalopathy or portal-systemic encephalopathy is a reversible neuropsychiatric syndrome that can accompany advanced, decompensated liver disease. The precise etiology is unclear and may involve more than one factor. Impaired detoxifying capability of the liver, particularly for exogenous (dietary protein) and endogenous (blood) nitrogenous substances in the intestine, and portal-systemic shunting appear to be an important precondition for development of encephalopathy. Toxins such as ammonia, false neurotransmitters (biogenic amines), and gamma aminobutyric acid (GABA) have been proposed as having a pathogenic role in hepatic encephalopathy. In addition to protein in the gut, hepatic encephalopathy may be precipitated or aggravated by electrolyte or acid-base imbalance and infection (e.g., pneumonia, spontaneous bacterial peritonitis). A search for other causes of altered central nervous system function should include careful review of medications and consideration of CNS infection or sub-dural hematoma. Neurologic manifestations of encephalopathy include changes in affect, mood, orientation, and behavior. The stages of hepatic encephalopathy are outlined in Table 18-7. Treatment of hepatic encephalopathy is supportive and directed at decreasing the production and absorption of nitrogenous substrate and ammonia. Dietary protein restriction, bowel cleansing with cathartics or lactulose, and administration of neomycin may be used singly or in combination to achieve these therapeutic goals. Patients in stages III and IV (coma) are best managed in an intensive-care-unit setting where continuous monitoring can take place.

Hepatorenal Syndrome

The hepatorenal syndrome is an ominous complication of advanced liver disease and is manifest by progressive oliguria and renal failure. The pathogenesis of hepatorenal syndrome is unclear but may be related to renal cortical arterial vasoconstriction and altered blood-flow distribution. The functional and potentially reversible nature of renal failure is evidenced by the fact that renal function can be restored by liver transplantation. Despite the lack of identifiable morphologic lesion in the kidneys and the functional nature of renal failure, the majority (> 90%) of patients die with this complication. Nonetheless, the development of oliguria and declining renal function should be evaluated aggressively so that treatable conditions will not be missed. In particular, prerenal azotemia, acute tubular necrosis,

Table 18-7. Stages of Hepatic Encephalopathy

Stage	Mental Status	Motor Changes
Subclinical	No changes on routine examination; may be associated with impaired work performance or driving ability	Impaired performance on standardized psychomotor tests or bedside tests such as figure drawing or number connection
I	Mild confusion, apathy, agitation, anxiety, euphoria, restlessness, sleep disorder	Fine tremor, slowed coordination, asterixis
II	Drowsiness, lethargy, disorientation, inappropriate behavior	Asterixis, dysarthria, primitive reflexes (suck and snout), ataxic paratonia
III	Somnolent but rousable, marked confusion, incomprehensible speech	Hyperreflexia, Babinski's sign, incontinence, myoclonus, hyperventilation
IV	Coma	Decerebrate posturing; brisk oculocephalic reflexes; response to painful stimuli present early; may progress to flaccidity and absence of response to stimuli

Reprinted with permission from: Scharschmidt BF. Cirrhosis of the liver and its major sequelae. In Wyngaarden JB, Smith LH, and Bennett JC (eds.). *Cecil Textbook of Medicine* (19th ed.). Philadelphia: W.B. Saunders, 1992, p. 797.

drug nephrotoxicity, obstruction, and urinary tract infection should be excluded in evaluation of the patient with liver failure who develops renal insufficiency.

Clinical Examples

1. A 65-year-old man is admitted to the hospital with fever and right upper quadrant pain. His family notes that he has been jaundiced for 2 weeks and the patient describes the passage of tan- to clay-colored stools during this time.

Physical examination is pertinent for temperature of 38.5°C, pulse of 110 and blood pressure of 90/60. Scleral and cutaneous icterus are present. Splinting with deep inspiration and rales at the right lung base are detected. The abdomen is soft although tenderness is elicited to deep palpation in the right upper quadrant. A globular mass is felt in the right upper quadrant that is distinct from the liver edge. Bowel sounds are hypoactive.

Laboratory studies reveal WBC of 16,000 cc with 90% neutrophils. Total bilirubin is 12.3 mg/dl and AST and ALT are 120 and 160 IU/ml, respectively. Alkaline phosphatase is 4 times the upper limit of normal. Serum amylase and lipase are normal. Abdominal ultrasound reveals cholelithiasis and common bile duct diameter of 12 mm.

Discussion.   The patient presents with obstructive jaundice and ascending cholangitis secondary to choledocholithiasis. The presence of jaundice and acholic stools suggests extrahepatic biliary tract obstruction. Jaundice in the setting of right upper quadrant pain, fever, and gallstones strongly suggest common bile duct obstruction associated with bacterial cholangitis. Derangements in liver test reflect cholestasis and hepatocellular abnormalities that can be seen with biliary obstruction and infection. Furthermore, conjugated hyperbilirubinemia due to complete bile duct obstruction is associated with the presence of bilirubin but the absence of urobilinogen in the urine. Cancer of the head of the pancreas or ampulla of Vater usually presents with painless jaundice. Cholangitis would be unusual with either of these disorders. Diagnosis of choledocholithiasis can be established by endoscopic retrograde cholangiopancreatogram (ERCP) or percutaneous transhepatic cholangiogram (PTC). Stone disruption and/or extraction can be accomplished with either procedure but, in general, ERCP would be the preferred diagnostic and therapeutic procedure.

Choledocholithiasis is encountered in approximately 10% of patients undergoing cholecystectomy for gallstones. Jaundice is more common in choledocholithiasis (75%) than in cholecystitis (25%). Although a distended gallbladder associated with extrahepatic jaundice is considered to be a sign of malignant biliary obstruction, approximately 15% of patients with cholelithiasis have gallbladder distension, and as many as 40%, have the finding at surgery.

2. A 21-year-old woman presented to her family doctor with secondary amenorrhea and fatigue. Laboratory tests performed 6 months previously showed transaminases (AST and ALT) that were 2 times the upper limit of normal. She had no risk factors for hepatitis. Physical examination was remarkable for mild facial acne, spider angiomas of face and upper duct, and a palpable spleen tip.

Laboratory examination revealed hemoglobin 11.1 g/dl, WBC 7,200 cc, platelets 173×10^3/ml, and serum albumin of 3.0 g/dl. Liver tests recorded bilirubin of 2.0 mg/dl, AST 500 IU/liter, ALT 410 IU/liter, and alkaline phosphatase 580 IU/liter. Immunological studies noted positive antinuclear (1:320) and smooth-muscle (1:80) antibodies. Antimitochondrial antibody was negative. IgG antibody was elevated at 4.5 g/dl. Hepatitis (A, B, and C) serologies were negative. ERCP was normal and liver biopsy revealed chronic active hepatitis.

Discussion.   This is a case of chronic hepatitis due to an autoimmune illness. Typically, autoimmune hepatitis affects young women although men can also develop this form of hepatitis (female-male ratio is 4:1). The differential diagnosis of chronic hepatitis in someone under 35 years of age should include Wilson's disease, alpha$_1$-antitrypsin deficiency, drug-induced chronic hepatitis, and chronic viral hepatitis. Chronic hepatitis C infection has been detected in some individuals with autoimmune hepatitis. The exact relationship between HCV and autoimmune hepatitis has not been fully elucidated. Extrahepatic manifestations of autoimmune hepatitis include arthritis, rash, thyroiditis, pleuropericarditis, colitis, and glomerulonephritis. The progression of disease may be insidious and at the time of symptom development liver disease may be advanced. Primary biliary cirrhosis and primary sclerosing cholangitis may be confused clinically and biochemically with autoimmune hepatitis. Immunosuppressive therapy with corticosteroids or azathioprine is usually effective in inducing clinical, biochemical, and histological remission. In patients with severe liver disease that is complicated by variceal hemorrhage, refractory ascites, and hepatic encephalopathy, consideration should be given to liver transplantation.

Bibliography

Kelley W (ed.). *Textbook of Internal Medicine* (2nd ed). Philadelphia: Lippincott, 1989. *Excellent book with very readable and well illustrated sections on liver physiology and disease.*

Schiff L and Schiff ER (eds.). *Diseases of the Liver* (7th ed). Philadelphia: Lippincott, 1993. *Standard comprehensive reference source for liver and biliary tract diseases.*

Stein J (ed.). *Internal Medicine* (4th ed). St. Louis: Mosby-Year Book, 1994. *The portions of text devoted to the physiology and pathophysiology of gastrointestinal and hepatobiliary diseases are well done.*

19 Small Intestine

Anil Minocha

Objectives

After completing this chapter, you should be able to

Describe the normal mechanisms of intestinal absorption of water and nutrients

Describe the normal patterns of intestinal motility

Distinguish osmotic from secretory diarrhea including differences in stool composition and the effects of fasting

Discuss infectious causes of diarrhea including the usual pathogens and pathophysiologic mechanisms of the acute and chronic types

List four endocrine causes of diarrhea and explain the mechanism of each

Define the malabsorption syndrome and describe the clinical features

List and explain the major mechanisms which impair digestion and absorption of nutrients in disease states

Distinguish intestinal obstruction from pseudo-obstruction and explain the pathophysiology of each

Describe three syndromes associated with vascular insufficiency of the intestine

Discuss common tests which are used to diagnose small bowel disorders

---

The small intestine is a complex and efficient tube extending from the pylorus to the cecum. Entry of food into the small intestine is regulated by the pyloric sphincter, whereas the exit is regulated by the ileocecal valve. These anatomic modifications as well as physiologic functions like secretions and intestinal motility serve the small intestine's primary function of absorption. Abnormalities of its functions may result in a variety of syndromes, including diarrhea, malabsorption, and motility disorders.

Normal Physiology

Absorption

The small bowel mucosa is characterized by an enormous surface area (approximately two million cm^2) which assists in efficient absorption. This massive area is made possible by three structural modifications: (1) intestinal folds (plicae circulares), (2) villi, and (3) submicroscopic mi-

crovilli (Fig. 19-1). The enterocytes are joined together by tight junctions which permit selective influx of various substances. The plasma membrane of epithelial cells provides a barrier to the nonspecific movement of ions. The crypt cells are responsible for secretory activity, whereas villous cells are responsible for absorption. These two functions have different regulatory mechanisms. Therefore, the absorptive function may remain intact while the secretory function may be stimulated by toxins (e.g., cholera), etc. The nutrients are absorbed at the level of the microvilli and discharged to the bloodstream or the lymphatics. Iron and folic acid are primarily absorbed in the duodenum (Fig. 19-2). The bulk of dietary nutrients are absorbed in the jejunum. Vitamin B$_{12}$ and bile salts are absorbed primarily in the ileum.

Carbohydrates

Carbohydrates, a major component of human diet, are ingested mainly in the form of starch, glycogen, a variety of

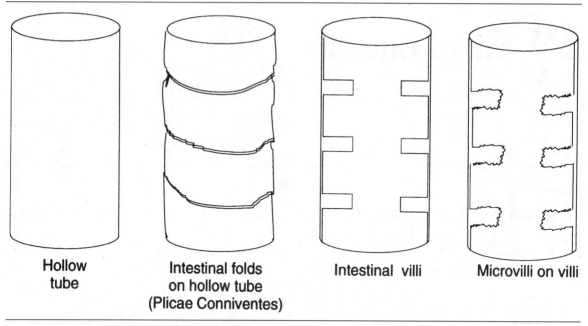

Hollow
tube

Intestinal folds
on hollow tube
(Plicae Conniventes)

Intestinal villi

Microvilli on villi

Fig. 19-1. Schematic representation of amplification of surface area of the small intestine. The combined effect of intestinal folds or plicae circulares ($\times 3$), the villi ($\times 10$), and microvilli ($\times 20$) results in increasing the surface area approximately 600-fold. The total surface area of the small intestine is approximately 200m^2, which is slightly larger than the size of a double tennis court.

disaccharides (sucrose, lactose, etc.) and monosaccharides. Starch and glycogen undergo luminal hydrolysis by pancreatic as well as salivary amylase, resulting in oligosaccharides and disaccharides. Salivary amylase (which is responsible for only a small component of carbohydrate digestion in healthy individuals) assumes a significant role in patients with deficiency of pancreatic amylase, e.g., pancreatic insufficiency. The brush border membrane of the mature enterocyte is loaded with disaccharidases which finish off the digestive process (Fig. 19-3). This hydrolysis of disaccharides results in monosaccharides such as glucose, fructose, galactose, and lactose which are then transported across into the epithelial cell. Glucose and galactose are absorbed by sodium-dependent active transport processes (Fig. 19-4). Thus the provision of glucose can drive the absorption of sodium.

Protein

Proteases secreted by the stomach and pancreas are responsible for digestion of dietary proteins as well as the proteins secreted into the intestine. Animal proteins are easier to digest than the plant proteins. Gastric pepsin plays a very minor role in protein digestion. Pancreatic proteases (trypsinogen and chymotrypsinogen) are activated in the lumen of the small intestine to trypsin and chymotrypsin. These activated enzymes convert proteins to oligopeptides, dipeptides, tripeptides, and free amino acids. Brush border enzymes (aminopeptidases and carboxypeptidase) act on the peptides with four or more amino acids to form smaller units (see Fig. 19-3). Free amino acids in the intestinal lumen are absorbed by passive as well as active transport systems. Most of the proteins are absorbed as small peptides utilizing specific transport systems. These absorbed dipeptides and tripeptides are converted into free amino acids inside the enterocyte. The free amino acids in the enterocyte diffuse into the lamina propria and then into the portal circulation.

Lipids

The major form of ingested fat is triglyceride. The lingual and gastric lipases play a minor role in the digestion of lipids, which are primarily digested in the jejunum. The enterocyte membrane into the enterocyte. Once inside the enterocyte, short-chain fatty acids diffuse directly into the portal circulation. Triglycerides, cholesterol, and lysophospholipids are resynthesized from their precursors. Within the endoplasmic reticulum, apolipoproteins, triglycerides, phospholipids, and cholesterol esters combine to form **chylomicrons.** Chylomicrons are then expelled into the intercellular space by exocytosis and are transported in the lymph.

Approximately 30% of medium-chain triglycerides can be absorbed intact by the enterocyte (presumably by passive diffusion) and exit the cell directly into the portal circulation. Most bile salts released by the gallbladder into the duodenum are reabsorbed in the terminal ileum and recirculated to the liver. This **enterohepatic recirculation** of bile salts is important for fat absorption.

Water and Electrolytes

The small intestine is presented with about nine liters of fluid each day, seven of these being endogenous secretions. Of this, 90% is absorbed in the small intestine. Since the enterocyte membrane is hydrophobic, the passive diffusion is possible only through the tight junctions. Sodium, chloride, and water are absorbed along the entire length of the small intestine. Active sodium transport occurs as a result of coupled neutral transport of sodium and chloride in exchange for hydrogen and bicarbonate. It may also be cotransported with sugars, peptides, and amino acids. Sodium and glucose share a common carrier mechanism. Thus sodium absorption may be enhanced by glucose absorption (see Fig. 19-4). Potassium is absorbed passively across the tight junctions throughout the small intestine based on the electrochemical gradient. Water diffuses passively along the osmotic gradient established by the active transport of sodium and other solutes.

Vitamins and Minerals

Absorption of fat-soluble vitamins requires the presence of bile salts and normal absorptive mechanisms for lipids. Water-soluble vitamins are absorbed by both active and passive mechanisms. **Iron** is actively absorbed in the duodenum. Iron may be absorbed as heme iron from meat and nonheme iron from vegetables. Heme iron is more efficiently absorbed than nonheme iron. Presence of acid tends to prevent the formation of insoluble iron complexes.

Folic acid is present in the diet mainly as polyglutamates. Brush border enzymes hydrolyze these polyglutamates into monoglutamates which are then absorbed. Dietary vitamin B_{12} or cobalamin is bound to enzymes in food. Once liberated from the food by gastric proteases, it

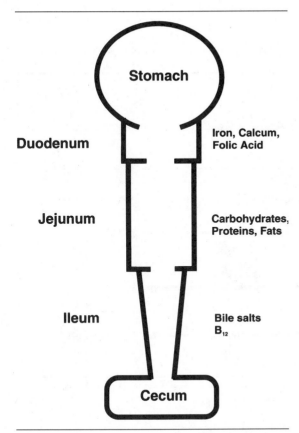

Fig. 19-2. Primary sites of absorption of major nutrients. While the entire small intestine is involved in absorption, certain nutrients may be preferentially absorbed in specific regions. Disease localized to the duodenum may produce iron deficiency anemia, while vitamin B_{12} deficiency is seen in diseases of the terminal ileum.

phospholipids and bile acids in bile emulsify large fat globules into a smaller droplet form which increases the surface area. This allows for efficient hydrolysis since enzymes can act only at the water-fat interface. Pancreatic lipase in the presence of pancreatic colipase acts upon triglycerides to form free fatty acids and glycerol. Phospholipase, secreted in an inactive form, is converted into an active form by trypsin and converts lecithin to lysolecithin and a fatty acid; cholesterol esterase digests cholesterol esters. These products of lipolysis are water insoluble and as such are incorporated into **micelles** for the purpose of transport. They passively diffuse across the

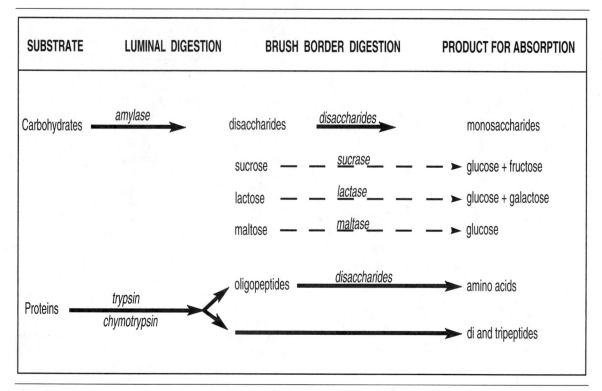

Fig. 19-3. General scheme of luminal digestion of carbohydrates and proteins.

is bound at acid pH to an intermediary protein known as the R protein. The cobalamin-R complex leaves the stomach along with free intrinsic factor. In the upper small intestine, this cobalamin R-protein complex is broken down and free cobalamin is liberated. The cobalamin now binds to the intrinsic factor. This complex is absorbed by receptor-mediated endocytosis in the ileum. When ingested in large amounts, vitamin B_{12} may also be absorbed passively by diffusion, which does not require the presence of intrinsic factor.

Intestinal Motility

The small intestinal motility assists in the function of digestion and absorption by mixing and propulsing luminal contents in a coordinated fashion. Mixing promotes digestion by enhancing the interactions between the food and the digestive enzymes. It also enhances the contact area by spreading food over a large surface area, stretching out and opening the intestinal epithelium. Movements of the villi and microvilli disturb the unstirred layer in contact with the mucosa, thus disrupting the barrier to passive diffusion.

Peristalsis propagates over short distances, usually 2–3 cm, but may go up to 10–30 cm. The peristaltic reflex is comprised of ascending contraction and descending relaxation and is the key to peristalsis. The small intestine motor patterns are organized in two fashions: (1) an interdigestive pattern occurring in a fasting state and (2) a fed pattern. The interdigestive migrating motor complex (MMC) is a cyclic motor pattern which occurs during fasting. It starts about 4–6 hours after the meal and is composed of four phases. Phase I is a quiescent period, while phase III is the most propulsive phase of the complex. Phase III has a periodicity of about once every 90 minutes. Phase II consists of random contractions and phase IV is a transition between phase III and phase I. MMC performs the housekeeper function by clearing the intestinal lumen of cellular

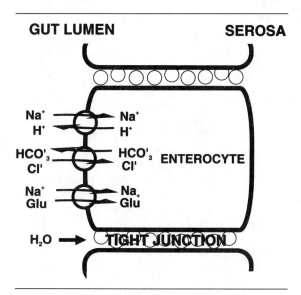

GUT LUMEN   **SEROSA**

Na^+ Na^+
H^+ H^+

HCO_3' HCO_3'
Cl' Cl' **ENTEROCYTE**

Na^+ Na_+
Glu   Glu

H_2O →   **TIGHT JUNCTION**

Fig. 19-4. The sodium/glucose cotransport mechanism. This mechanism remains intact in many diarrheal diseases. Provision of glucose enhances sodium absorption and water is dragged along by osmosis. As a result, treatment with oral rehydration formulas can effectively treat dehydration in most cases of diarrhea, thus obviating the need for intravenous fluids.

and useless bacterial debris. Feeding interrupts the MMC by a series of chaotic contractions. The motor pattern in the fed state reflects more mixing flows than propulsive flows. Subspecialized motor patterns in the small intestine include (1) giant migrating contractions which clear the ileum of the chyme by emptying it into the colon and (2) retrograde peristaltic contractions which are associated with vomiting. The small intestine, unlike the heart, does not respond to its pacemaker on a one-to-one basis. Contractile activity is determined by the relationship between (1) pacesetter potentials, (2), spikes which are the equivalent of action potentials, and (3) the contractions. The intestinal motility patterns are regulated by a wide range of integrated neural circuits within the enteric nervous system. These circuits act as a series of local control systems which are subject only to general overall control from extrinsic nerves and humoral influences. While parasympathetic activation enhances and the sympathetic stimulation inhibits the intestinal motility, neither is important in the regulation of motility in the normal state.

Pathological States

Diarrhea

Diarrhea is defined as the passage of more than 200 g per day of feces. Certain diseases may, however, produce frequent loose stools which weigh less than 150 g/day. Increased frequency of defecation without change in consistency or increase in fecal weight is known as pseudo-diarrhea. Diarrhea of small bowel origin usually consists of voluminous stools since the small intestine is the predominant site for fluid absorption in the gastrointestinal tract. In contrast, colonic pathology gives rise to small-volume diarrhea. Diarrhea may be acute or chronic. Acute diarrhea is usually a diarrhea of less than 2–3 weeks duration.

Osmotic vs. Secretory Diarrhea

Diarrhea may be classified based on alterations in intestinal secretion (secretory diarrhea) or absorption (osmotic diarrhea). Osmotic diarrhea occurs when a nonabsorbable substrate causes increased osmotic load and draws water into the intestinal lumen as well as prevents passive absorption of water. Lactose intolerance is the most common cause. Sweetening agents (e.g., sorbitol) in pharmaceuticals are the most common iatrogenic cause. Secretory diarrhea is large-volume diarrhea caused by excessive mucosal secretion of fluid and electrolytes in response to pathogens or toxins. The presence of increased levels of hormones like VIP (vasoactive intestinal polypeptide) in tumors as well as cathartics can stimulate chloride and water secretion via cyclic AMP and cyclic GMP mediated mechanisms. Since osmotic diarrhea is dependent upon the presence of osmotically active substances like unabsorbed sugars in the intestine, such diarrhea improves in a fasting state; fasting does not improve secretory diarrhea. Stool electrolytes and osmolality can distinguish between secretory diarrhea and osmotic diarrhea, although these two conditions may coexist (Table 19-1). For example, malabsorptive diseases like celiac sprue have a secretory component.

Inflammatory vs. Noninflammatory Diarrhea

Diarrhea may be categorized as inflammatory or noninflammatory based on the histologic appearance of the intestinal mucosa. Noninflammatory diarrhea is produced mainly by toxicogenic *E. coli*, viruses, cathartics, and neuroendocrine tumors. It is due to a functional impairment, whereas the inflammatory diarrhea is associated with mucosal damage. The stools in inflammatory diarrhea (e.g.,

Table 19-1. Distinguishing Features of Osmotic and Secretory Diarrhea

Property	Osmotic	Secretory
Fasting	Diarrhea improves	No effect
Stool volume	< 1 liter/d	> 1 liter/d
Stool Na	< 60mmol/liter	> 90mmol/liter
Stool osmolality	280–400 mOsm/liter	260–300 mOsm/liter
Fecal osmotic gap	> 50 mOsm	< 40 mOsm

invasive infectious diarrhea and regional enteritis) contain numerous leukocytes and may contain blood; systemic symptoms like fever may be present. Malabsorption may occur if the disorder is associated with the destruction of brush border enzymes or the villous pattern, impairment of biliary or pancreatic secretions, or lymphatic transport. Ability to secrete chloride and bicarbonate may still be maintained.

Specific Types and Etiologies

Acute Infectious Diarrhea. A variety of bacterial, viral, parasitic, and fungal agents have been implicated in the pathogenesis of acute infectious diarrhea. Infectious diarrhea may be inflammatory or noninflammatory. Noninflammatory diarrhea results from decreased intestinal fluid absorption and increased intestinal secretion. Norwalk-like virus and rotavirus are common causes of noninflammatory diarrhea. The invasive organisms like *Campylobacter* and *Shigella* often cause watery diarrhea, but this may be followed by bloody diarrhea.

Chronic Infectious Diarrhea. Infectious pathogens may result in chronic diarrhea via two mechanisms: (1) postenteric diarrhea (where the infection is resolved but its residual effects are still present) and (2) chronic persistence of infection of the small bowel. Postenteritis syndrome may be a result of persistence of injury to the mucosa or a hypersensitivity response to infection. In patients with chronic diarrhea and persistent infection, antimicrobial therapy is necessary to eradicate the infection. Small bowel tuberculosis may result in inflammatory diarrhea and malabsorption syndrome. Bowel strictures may ensue, leading to intestinal obstruction. Patients with AIDS are prone to opportunistic infections like *Cryptosporidium, Cytomegalovirus, Candida albicans, Mycobacterium avium intracellurare, Microsporidia,* and *Isosporabelli.* HIV infection may also lead to *AIDS enteropathy,* which causes diarrhea and malabsorption without any histologic changes or opportunistic infection.

Traveler's Diarrhea. Traveler's diarrhea occurs more commonly during visits to developing countries. It occurs most often in younger individuals, probably owing to adventurous eating habits or lack of prior exposure to the pathogens. Contaminated food rather than contaminated water is likely the culprit. Most cases of traveler's diarrhea are caused by bacterial infection and the most common is enterotoxicogenic *E. coli* (ETEC). ETEC produces two types of toxins: a heat-labile toxin which increases cyclic AMP and a heat-stable toxin which increases cyclic GMP. Both increase secretions from the intestine. Other bacteria implicated are enteroinvasive *E. coli, Aeromonas,* and *Vibrio* species. Viral etiologies include rotavirus and Norwalk-like virus. Protozoal infection with *Giardia lamblia* may cause only mild diarrhea or malabsorption syndrome. Traveler's diarrhea, often of an inflammatory type, may be caused by *Salmonella, Shigella, Campylobacter,* enterohemorrhagic *E. coli,* and *Clostridium difficile* as well as protozoal infections like *Entameba histolytica. Cryptosporidia* may cause a self-limited diarrhea in healthy individuals.

In approximately 20–50% of traveler's diarrhea, the etiologic agent remains unidentified. Antibiotics may be effective whether or not a definable bacterial pathogen can be identified. Traveler's diarrhea that does not resolve may progress on to "protracted" diarrhea or tropical sprue. Preventative measures against traveler's diarrhea include paying close attention to what is consumed and under what circumstances. Hot cooked foods are preferable to raw vegetables or meat; unpasteurized milk and dairy products and tap water should be avoided. Prophylaxis with antibiotics is effective but not generally recommended because the risk of adverse effects outweighs the benefits.

Cholera. Cholera caused by *Vibrio cholerae* is a waterborne diarrheal illness which ranges from mild to life-threatening in severity. The diagnosis is made by clinical presentation and stool studies. The culprit is a cholera toxin which impairs the sodium absorption and activates chloride secretion. Treatment consists of antibiotics in addition to fluid replacement. Most patients respond well to oral rehydration formulas consisting of glucose, electrolytes, and water because the glucose-coupled sodium transport system remains intact (see Fig. 19-4).

Inflammatory Diseases. These may cause mucosal damage and altered permeability leading to diarrhea. **Regional enteritis** or Crohn's disease frequently involves the small intestine. Secretagogues like histamine, leukotrienes, prostaglandins, and interleukins and neurotransmitters like substance P may also be involved in causing the diarrhea. Involvement of the terminal ileum may lead to deficiency of vitamin B_{12} and bile salts. Healing is by fibrosis and strictures may occur leading to intestinal obstruction. **Eosinophilic gastroenteritis** is characterized by infiltration of the gastrointestinal tract with eosinophils. It may be due to drugs or parasites and may also be idiopathic. Steatorrhea and protein-losing enteropathy may result. Approximately half of the patients of the idiopathic variety have other allergies, so food allergy is suspected in these patients. Treatment with corticosteroids is usually effective.

Endocrine Disorders. Hyperthyroidism may cause diarrhea by hastening the gastrointestinal transit time. Diarrhea may also result from Addison's disease. Diarrhea is seen in patients with diabetic autonomic neuropathy and may be accompanied by steatorrhea, although this is uncommon. The mechanism of diabetic diarrhea is poorly understood and may include (1) abnormal absorptive and secretory processes, (2) intestinal dysmotility, and (3) small bowel bacterial overgrowth. Endocrine tumors, like carcinoid, gastrinoma, VIPoma, and villous adenomas present with true secretory diarrhea. Metastatic carcinoid tumors produce diarrhea by excessive secretion of serotonin and other cytokines. Patients with Zollinger-Ellison syndrome (gastrinoma) may develop diarrhea because the increased hydrochloric acid secretion caused by the excess gastrin inactivates pancreatic enzymes. The watery diarrhea, hypokalemia, achlorhydria syndrome (WDHA syndrome), also known as pancreatic cholera, is associated with increased levels of vasoactive intestinal peptide (VIP) owing to a pancreatic tumor. Excessive secretion of calcitonin in medullary carcinoma of the thyroid causes diarrhea by increased intestinal secretion or hastened intestinal transit. Management of these endocrine diarrhea syndromes depends on treatment of the underlying cause. Somatostatin analogues may provide symptomatic relief in some cases.

Iatrogenic. While some drugs are more likely to cause diarrhea than others, almost any medication may result in diarrhea. Chronic ingestion of drugs like colchicine and neomycin may cause steatorrhea owing to mucosal cell damage. Cholestyramine may cause malabsorption of lipids by binding to bile acids and preventing their enterohepatic recirculation. Medications containing sorbitol as a sweetening agent are a frequent cause of diarrhea because of the nonabsorbable sorbitol. Magnesium-containing antacids and laxatives cause osmotic diarrhea. Laxatives like phenolphthalein and bisacodyl alter intestinal fluid and electrolyte transport. Nonsteroidal antiinflammatory drugs can cause inflammation and ulceration anywhere in the gastrointestinal tract. While antibiotics may result in *Clostridium difficile* enterocolitis, non-*C. difficile* antibiotic diarrhea may occur due to a direct toxic effect on the mucosa or overgrowth of some organisms. Factitious diarrhea is not infrequent, so stools should be screened for different cathartics in any patient with unexplained diarrhea.

Chemotherapy and radiation therapy may result in diarrhea by damaging intestinal epithelium. The intestinal epithelium is susceptible to damage because of its high cell turnover rate. Radiation-enteritis-induced diarrhea may occur as late as 25 years after the radiation treatment and so it is important to ask about a history of radiation therapy.

Food-specific Diarrhea. Use of raw milk may result in chronic diarrhea due to as yet unidentified organisms. Diarrhea may result from ingestion of large amounts of fruit juice or soft drinks sweetened with fructose or sorbitol. Tube feeding with enteral formulas may cause diarrhea in up to one-third of the patients. The diarrhea may be due to bacterial contamination or use of a hypertonic formula and the presence of hypoalbuminemia in malnourished patients. There may also be altered sodium absorption and chloride and water secretion in critically ill patients.

Miscellaneous. **Acute alcohol ingestion** may result in diarrhea which resolves spontaneously. Diarrhea in chronic alcoholics improves significantly with abstinence. Alcohol-induced diarrhea occurs due to damage to the intestinal epithelium, alterations in intestinal motility, as well as impaired biliary and pancreatic secretions. **Runners' diarrhea** may be seen in as many as 10–25% of people who run marathons. It is more common in women. Occult blood may be found in the stools and occasionally overt bleeding occurs. Exercise and stress decrease fluid and electrolyte absorption. Altered intestinal motility and intestinal ischemia have also been implicated. **Neoplastic lesions** of the small intestine (including carcinoma, sarcoma, and lymphoma) can infrequently cause diarrhea.

Extensive resection of the small intestine may result in **short bowel syndrome.** Pathogenesis of the diarrhea includes decreased absorptive surface, rapid transit through the intestine, and impaired bile salt enterohepatic recirculation. Undigested and unabsorbed food in the intestine may exacerbate the diarrhea by having an osmotic effect as well as producing bacterial overgrowth.

Malabsorption Syndromes (MAS)

Malabsorption may occur as a result of impaired digestive or absorptive processes (Fig. 19-5). Since the small intestine is a very efficient organ, the disease has to be extensive to cause malabsorption of most nutrients. Exceptions are iron, which is primarily absorbed in the duodenum, as well as vitamin B_{12} and bile salts, which are primarily absorbed in the ileum. In contrast to the carbohydrates and proteins, fat absorption is also dependent upon the bile

salts as well as normal gut lymphatic system. The colon plays a minor role in the absorptive process. Patients with MAS may present with a wide spectrum of clinical manifestations representing signs of malnutrition as well as those of the primary disease (including watery diarrhea or bulky, foul-smelling stools, abdominal pain, easy fatigability, and weight loss). Hyperphagia may occur. Pallor, muscle wasting and loss of subcutaneous fat, skeletal pain, and peripheral neuropathy may be noted. Hypoalbuminemia may result in edema.

Impaired Digestive Processes

Pancreatic Insufficiency. Deficiency of pancreatic tissue (e.g., chronic pancreatitis, pancreatic carcinoma, cystic fibrosis, pancreatic resection, etc.) may cause malabsorption of fats (steatorrhea) and proteins. In addition, pancreatic enzymes may be inactivated by hyperacidity

Fig. 19-5. Disorders of malabsorption classified on the basis of pathophysiology. In some disorders more than one mechanism may be involved in causing diarrhea and malabsorption.

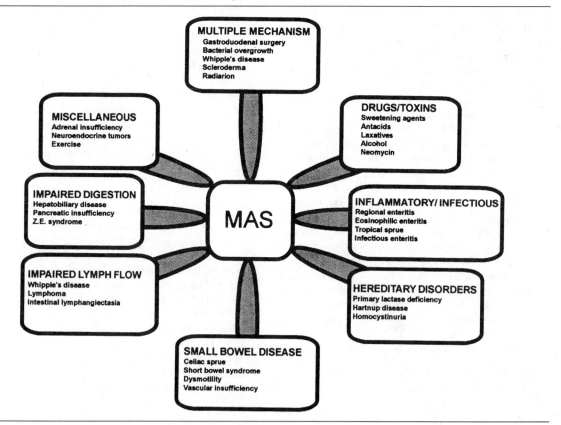

present in Zollinger-Ellison syndrome with similar results. Some degree of carbohydrate malabsorption may be seen in pancreatic insufficiency since pancreatic amylase converts starch to oligosaccharides. Treatment includes pancreatic enzyme replacements.

Bile Salt Deficiency. Deficiency of bile salts which are required for fat absorption may lead to steatorrhea. This deficiency may be caused by biliary tract obstruction, terminal ileal resection, Crohn's disease, or cholestatic liver disease.

Gastroduodenal Disorders. Intrinsic factor deficiency due to gastrectomy or pernicious anemia may lead to vitamin B_{12} malabsorption. Other gastroduodenal surgeries (including gastrojejunostomy following antrectomy and gastric bypass for obesity) may result in iron deficiency anemia.

Impaired Absorptive Processes

Deficiency of One or More Brush Border Enzymes. Such a deficiency may cause carbohydrate malabsorption. The most common of these is lactase deficiency, which may be congenital or acquired. Patients with lactose intolerance are unable to digest lactose-containing foods (dairy products). Presence of unabsorbed lactose in the gut results in abdominal cramps and diarrhea.

Gluten Enteropathy or Celiac Sprue. This is a chronic diarrheal illness characterized by damage to small intestinal mucosa and malabsorption of nutrients. The offending agent is dietary gluten, which is present in wheat, rye, barley, and oats. The major component of gluten is gliadin, which activates celiac disease. The extent and severity of the pathologic lesions can vary. Characteristically, there is villous atrophy and infiltration of plasma cells and lymphocytes in the lamina propria. Antigliadin antibodies may be seen in as many as 90% of the patients with untreated celiac disease. Removal of gluten from the diet usually results in prompt improvement of symptoms.

Tropical Sprue. It occurs due to chronic small bowel contamination with coliform bacteria that are injurious to intestinal mucosa. It is usually seen in adults. It manifests initially with acute watery diarrhea, eventually going on to malabsorption syndrome. Treatment of tropical sprue consists of pharmacologic doses of folic acid and antibiotics.

Whipple's Disease. This is a systemic bacterial illness. The as yet unidentified offending bacillus is found in a variety of organs, including the intestine. The gastrointestinal tract is almost always involved. There is obstruction of the lymphatic vessels and impaired chylomicron removal, resulting in fat malabsorption. Symptoms include weight loss, diarrhea, arthralgias, and abdominal pain. Small bowel biopsy is diagnostic. The intestine is infiltrated by characteristic periodic acid Schiff positive "foamy" macrophages. Antibiotics are the treatment of choice.

Disorders of Motility

Small intestinal dysmotility may or may not be associated with dysmotility in other parts of the gastrointestinal tract. Postvagotomy diarrhea occurs as a result of rapid small intestinal transit. Similarly, surgical procedures like gastrojejunostomy may cause diarrhea by loading the small intestine with undigested osmotically active substances (dumping syndrome).

Intestinal obstruction is a clinical syndrome occurring as a result of mechanical blockage of the normal peristaltic transport of luminal contents. Extrinsic compression owing to postoperative adhesions is the most common cause. Extrinsic compression may also result from tumors, hernias, and volvulus. Mechanical obstruction may result from luminal causes such as barium concretions, gallstones, parasites, as well as from intramural causes such as atresia, webs, or strictures related to Crohn's disease or radiation enteritis.

Bowel obstruction causes alteration of absorption/secretion homeostasis resulting in net secretion. This, coupled with vomiting, and release of cytokines causing splanchnic vasodilation results in inadequate intravascular volume and impaired tissue perfusion. There is increased intraluminal pressure and intestinal distention which may progress to bowel infarction. Bowel defense mechanisms are compromised, resulting in translocation of bacteria across the gut wall into the circulation with disastrous consequences. Patients usually complain of abdominal pain, distention, and vomiting. Stool and flatus may or may not be passed, depending on the degree of obstruction. High-pitched "metallic" bowel sounds and visible peristalsis may be noted. Abdominal x-rays show distended loops of bowel with air fluid levels (see Fig. 19-6). Management includes cessation of oral intake; correction of fluid, electrolyte, and hemodynamic disturbances; and intestinal decompression via nasogastric intubation. While stable patients with partial obstruction may respond to these conservative measures, most complete obstructions, especially those with peritoneal signs or risk of strangulation, require surgery.

Acute pseudo-obstruction or adynamic ileus occurs in postoperative patients, acute severe illnesses, intra-abdominal or systemic sepsis, and with certain drugs. This syndrome

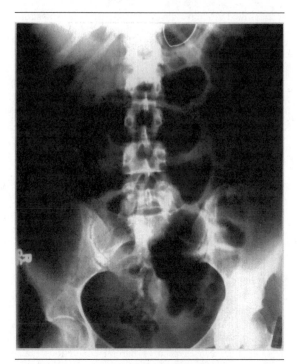

Fig. 19-6. Plain x-ray of the abdomen showing dilated loops of bowel consistent with intestinal obstruction. The small bowel obstruction in this patient occurred as a result of a stricture of the terminal ileum owing to Crohn's disease.

usually resolves with the treatment and resolution of the underlying disorder. Chronic intestinal pseudo-obstruction is a group of dysmotility syndromes mimicking intestinal obstruction in the absence of occlusion of the intestinal lumen. There may be degeneration of the intestinal smooth muscle or disruption of neural mechanisms. Any or all parts of the gastrointestinal tract may be affected. The three major types are myopathic, neuropathic, and secondary pseudo-obstruction. Absent or diminished migrating motor complexes (MMC's) are seen in the myopathic form. The neuropathic type may have increased MMC's but they are discoordinated and, as such, not effective. Secondary pseudo-obstruction may be caused by collagen vascular diseases like scleroderma and SLE, drugs (e.g., antipsychotics, antidepressants, opiates, and sedatives), endocrine disorders like hypothyroidism, and diabetes mellitus or neurological diseases like Parkinson's disease. Physical examination may reflect manifestations of malnutrition. Treatment includes correcting the cause, bowel decompression, and nutritional support. Many patients eventually require total parental nutrition (see Chap. 21).

Vascular Insufficiency Syndromes

Intestinal Angina

This occurs in patients with fixed narrowing of the splanchnic arteries due to atherosclerosis. Ingestion of food results in an increased requirement for blood flow to the intestine. When this increased demand cannot be met, transient bowel ischemia may result. Analogous to angina pectoris, this ischemia manifests as abdominal pain typically occurring after eating. This results in "fear of eating" and subsequent weight loss. Diagnosis is confirmed by angiography, and surgical repair may be helpful.

Bowel Infarction

It may occur owing to acute occlusion of a mesenteric artery due to thromboembolic phenomenon or intrinsic vascular disease. Patients typically present with abdominal pain out of proportion to other physical findings, vomiting, bloody diarrhea, and lactic acidosis. Nonocclusive ischemia may occur in the setting of reduced systemic blood flow states like shock, congestive failure, or use of drugs like vasopressors and digitalis.

Mesenteric Venous Thrombosis

It can occur in portal hypertension, hypercoagulable states, malignancies, trauma, or with bowel obstruction. Patients present with gradually worsening pain accompanied by nausea, vomiting, and diarrhea. Peritoneal signs, leukocytosis, and metabolic acidosis may develop if the condition progresses to infarction. Diagnosis is often made at laparotomy.

Methods for Diagnostic Evaluation of Small-Bowel Disorders

Patients with acute watery diarrhea and minimal systemic symptoms may undergo only symptomatic treatment without further investigation. On the other hand, patients with fever, bleeding, dehydration, or weight loss require a more detailed, individualized diagnostic workup, based on the clinical presentation. Diagnostic tests which prove useful include the following:

Stool Examination

Simple stool studies provide important clues to the diagnosis. Demonstration of the leukocytes in feces differentiates inflammatory from noninflammatory diarrhea. When an infectious etiology is suspected, the presence or absence of leukocytes in stools can distinguish toxic diarrhea from the diarrhea due to invasive organisms. Presence of blood usually suggests an inflammatory, ischemic, neoplastic or invasive infectious process. Stool cultures, as well as ova, parasite, and *C. difficile* toxin detection, should be performed when the cause of the diarrhea is not readily apparent. Sudan stain for fecal fat is a useful screening test of steatorrhea. However, elevated levels of fat in a 72-hour stool collection is the hallmark for steatorrhea. Measurement of stool electrolytes and osmolality may help in differentiating between secretory and osmotic diarrhea (Table 19-1). A cathartic screen should be part of the initial workup in cases of unexplained diarrhea.

D-xylose Absorption Test

D-xylose is a sugar that normally is absorbed unchanged into the blood and excreted in the urine. Low levels of D-xylose in blood and urine after ingestion of a standard dose suggests malabsorption due to primary small bowel disease.

Schilling Test

Vitamin B_{12} absorption is dependent upon the cleavage of vitamin B_{12}-R protein complex by the pancreatic proteolytic enzymes. Lack of these enzymes in pancreatic insufficiency typically results in a lack of rise of serum of vitamin B_{12} upon oral administration, even when intrinsic factor is provided.

Test for Bacterial Overgrowth

A culture of duodenal aspirate allows direct identification of pathogens. Alternatively, a hydrogen breath test may be performed. Luminal carbohydrates undergo fermentation by the bacteria normally present in the colon. This releases hydrogen which is absorbed into the blood and excreted in the breath. In cases of small bowel bacterial overgrowth, the ingestion of carbohydrate results in the increased levels of breath hydrogen soon after ingestion.

The lactose tolerance test determines deficiency of lactase. Patients with lactase deficiency will have little increase in plasma glucose after lactose ingestion (see Fig. 19-3). Increased breath hydrogen levels after lactose ingestion also suggest lactase deficiency.

A colonoscopy with ileoscopy may be required to diagnose inflammatory bowel disease or to exclude a neoplastic process. The diagnosis of *cryptosporidium,* Herpes simplex, and CMV infection can often be made by small bowel biopsy. Likewise, the presence of *Giardia* may be confirmed on duodenal aspirate obtained by endoscopy.

Serum hormone levels like VIP, gastrin, and calcitonin as well as urinary 5-hydroxyindoleacetic acid should be measured in case of unexplained secretory diarrhea. Serum carotene level may indicate a fat malabsorption. Malabsorption of bile acid may be assessed by ^{14}C glycolate breath test. Small bowel x-ray studies, manometry, and abdominal CT may be needed in selected patients.

Clinical Examples

1. A 28-year-old white physician presented with chronic abdominal pain and reported 6–10 stools per day. The stools were loose and without any blood or mucus. She was not taking any medications. Physical examination revealed a 5'8" female weighing 100 pounds. Laboratory studies showed anemia and hypoalbuminemia. Stool studies for WBC, ova/parasite, and cultures were negative. Sudan stain for fecal fat was positive. A 72-hour stool test for fecal fat was abnormally high. Blood and urinary D-xylose were abnormally low. An upper endoscopy and small bowel biopsy was performed. A duodenal aspirate at the time of endoscopy was negative for *Giardia* and bacterial overgrowth. The small bowel biopsy showed villous atrophy. A presumptive diagnosis of celiac sprue was made. Adherence to a gluten-free diet resulted in resolution of her symptoms.

Discussion.   This patient had diarrhea related to malabsorption syndrome. Stools negative for WBC and pathogen suggested noninfectious noninflammatory diarrhea. The presence of fat in the stool indicated malabsorption. An abnormal D-xylose test indicated that the problem is not with digestion but with the absorptive processes. Endoscopic biopsy showed villous atrophy consistent with celiac sprue. This pattern is, however, not specific for celiac sprue. Examination of the duodenal aspirate ruled out other conditions like giardiasis and small bowel bacterial overgrowth as cause for villous atrophy. Response to a gluten-free diet confirmed the diagnosis.

2. A 32-year-old white executive presented with diarrhea of 3 months' duration without any blood or mucus. She had lost 12 pounds during this period. She was not taking any medications. Abdominal exam revealed right lower quadrant fullness and tenderness without any peritoneal signs. Complete blood count was normal. Chemical profile revealed low albumin. Chest x-ray was normal. Stools were positive for leukocytes and negative for fat stain and infectious pathogens. Colonoscopy showed normal colonic mucosa. Ileoscopy with biopsies revealed severe inflammation in the terminal ileum.

Discussion.   Diarrhea and chronic inflammation resulted in the weight loss and low serum albumin in this patient. Negative fecal fat stain makes malabsorption less likely but does not rule it out completely. Stools positive for WBC and negative for pathogens suggest noninfectious but inflammatory diarrhea. Endoscopic findings suggests the diagnosis of regional enteritis or Crohn's disease. Other causes of a diseased terminal ileum (e.g., Yersinia, tuberculosis, intestinal endometriosis, and lymphoma as well as nonsteroidal anti-inflammatory drugs) are likely in view of the history, stool studies, chest x-ray, and biopsy findings.

3. A 36-year-old male with a history of Crohn's disease underwent resection of the terminal ileum for multiple intestinal strictures causing recurrent small bowel obstruction. Since his surgery, he had been having 6–8 loose stools per day without blood or mucus. Stool studies for WBC and pathogens were negative. Endoscopy revealed no evidence of active inflammation in the small or large bowel. Treatment with cholestyramine resulted in resolution of his symptoms.

Discussion.   The ileal resection in this patient caused decreased bile acid absorption. Consequently, more bile acids enter the colon and stimulate secretion of fluid and electrolytes, causing diarrhea. Cholestyramine is a bile salt binding agent. It inhibits entry of active bile salts into the colon, thus reducing their effect on colonic secretion. The bile salt pool can be maintained by increased hepatic synthesis if less than 100 cm of small bowel is resected. However, resection of greater than 100 cm causes a major decrease in reabsorption of bile salts which cannot be compensated for by increased synthesis. This results in inadequate secretion of bile salts in the bile. Fat malabsorption and steatorrhea ensue. In the latter situation, bile salt binding agents would further deplete the bile salt pool and worsen the diarrhea.

Bibliography

Avery ME and Snyder JD. Oral therapy for acute diarrhea. *N Engl J Med* 323:891, 1990. *Appropriate oral therapy for diarrhea is effective but remains underused.*

Minocha A and McClave SA. Chronic intestinal pseudo-obstruction. In Van Ness MM and Chobanian SJ (eds.). *Manual of Clinical Problems in Gastroenterology* (2nd ed.). Boston: Little, Brown, 1994. *A concise review of the intestinal pseudo-obstruction syndromes.*

Sleisenger MH and Fordtran JS (eds.). *Gastrointestinal Disease* (5th ed.). Section V. Small and Large Intestine. Philadelphia: Saunders, 1993. *The standard text on gastrointestinal diseases.*

Trier JS. Celiac sprue. *New Engl J Med* 325:1709–1719, 1991. *Review of celiac sprue.*

20 Colon

Richard F. Harty and Harry S. Ojeas

Objectives

After completing this chapter, you should be able to

Understand the absorptive and secretory mechanisms involved in ionic transport in the colon

Understand the pathophysiology mechanisms involved in the origin of diverticulosis and its complications

Explain the mechanisms in the adenoma-carcinoma transformation sequence

Explain the pathogenic mechanisms and histological features of inflammatory bowel disease

Understand the pathogenic mechanisms involved in constipation

Gain knowledge of the clinical aspects and pathogenic mechanisms of irritable bowel syndrome

Normal Function

The colon, being at the end of the gastrointestinal tract, has important but not life-sustaining functions. Unlike the small intestine, the colon does not actively transport nutrients, such as glucose and amino acids, and hence does not participate in nutrient digestion or assimilation. However, the large intestine plays an essential role in determining the volume of fecal water excretion and in transportation of residual fecal material to the rectum. Together, the small and large intestine function to maintain fluid and electrolyte homeostasis through processes of absorption and secretion across their respective epithelial surfaces.

Absorption

The daily fluid load to the gut is approximately 9 liters. The small intestine normally absorbs the majority (approximately 7 liters) of luminal fluid. Thus the jejunum and ileum have a great capacity for water and electrolyte absorption and also secretion. This latter property is exemplified in patients infected with cholera (stool volumes may reach 15 to 20 liters per day). The remaining 1500–2000 ml of liquid intestinal contents not absorbed by the small bowel are delivered through the ileocecal valve to the cecum. Remarkably, in health only 100–200 ml of water are passed in the stool each day. Figure 20-1 illustrates the importance of colonic fluid absorption in regulating fecal water excretion in health and disease states of the small and large intestine. Maximal capacity of the colon to absorb water may be as great as 5000–6000 ml/24 hours. In the presence of small intestinal disease and increased ileocecal flow, the colon can compensate, by virtue of reserve absorptive function, to preserve normal levels of stool water. When ileocecal flow exceeds the absorptive capacity of the colon, excessive amounts of stool water result in diarrhea. Likewise, colonic diseases which disrupt colonic absorptive function or promote secretion (or both) can cause diarrhea.

The preceding chapter on the small intestine has reviewed pertinent elements in enterocyte function that account for absorption at villus epithelial cells and secretion from crypt cells. Morphological and physiologic differences between the small intestinal enterocyte and large bowel colonocyte account for their functional differences. However, epithelial cells in either region of the alimentary tract utilize mechanisms of absorption and secretion that share certain similarities. Table 20-1 indicates common and distinctive transport mechanisms in the small intestine and colon.

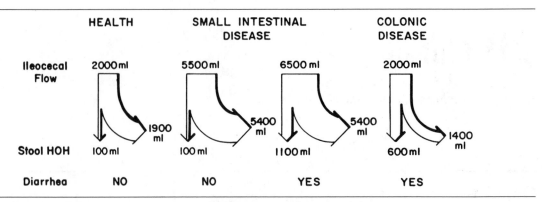

Fig. 20-1. Diagram illustrating importance of colonic fluid absorption in regulating stool water excretion in both small and large intestinal disease. An increase in stool water excretion will occur when ileocecal flow exceeds colonic absorption (panel 3) or there is an intrinsic abnormality of colonic absorptive function (panel 4). (From Binder HJ, Sandle GI, and Rajendran VM. Colonic fluid and electrolyte movement in health and disease. In Phillips SF, Pemberton JH, and Shorter RG (eds.). *The Large Intestine.* New York: Raven, 1991, pp. 141–168, copyright by Mayo Foundation. By permission of Mayo Foundation.)

Table 20-1. Electrolyte Transport Mechanisms and Their Distribution Along the Intestinal Tract

Small Intestine	Large Intestine
Electroneutral NaCl absorption	Electroneutral NaCl absorption
Cl^- secretion	Cl^- secretion
HCO_3^- secretion (mainly in proximal duodenum)	HCO_3^- secretion
Absorption of glucose and other nutrients in symport with Na^+	Electrogenic Na^+ absorption
Absorption of bile in symport with Na^+ (terminal ileum only)	Short-chain fatty acid absorption

Reprinted with permission from Dharmsathaphorn K. Regulatory controls of intestinal secretion. In Yamada T (ed.). *The Regulatory Peptide Letter,* II (1):6, 1990.

Ion Transport Mechanisms

The human colon absorbs water, sodium (Na^+), and chloride (Cl^-) and secretes potassium (K^+) and bicarbonate (HCO_3^-). As in the small intestine, electrolyte transport in the colon involves the three transcellular processes of (1) active transport, (2) secondary active transport, and (3) passive diffusion. Cellular events involved in chloride secretion and electroneutral NaCl absorption are illustrated in Fig. 20-2. In these examples, active electrolyte transport drives secretion or absorption of only one electrolyte across epithelial cells in a unidirectional manner. Ions with opposite charge and water follow the actively transported ions passively and paracellularly through tight junctions. On the apical membrane of the colonocyte, the Cl^- channel permits active secretion of Cl^- to the lumen down the anion concentration gradient. Transport pathways at the basolateral membrane

may involve transmembrane proteins such as the energy-dependent Na^+, K^+ATPase, which actively pumps Na^+ out of the cell and K^+ into the cell against their electrochemical gradients. The cotransport of Na^+, K^+, and Cl^- (Fig. 20-2a) are an example of secondary active transport.

Integration of electrolyte movement across the intestinal epithelium is coordinated, in part, by the actions of regulatory peptides, neuropeptides, and neurotransmitters at receptors located on epithelial cells. In addition, immune regulation has been shown to modulate epithelial function by locally released substances derived from effector cells in the lamina propria. The colon responds to the mineralocorticoid aldosterone and to glucocorticoids by increasing Na^+ transport. Additional neurohumoral and immunologic factors that regulate colonic electrolyte transport are noted in Table 20-2. The precise physiologic roles of a number of these agents remain to be clarified.

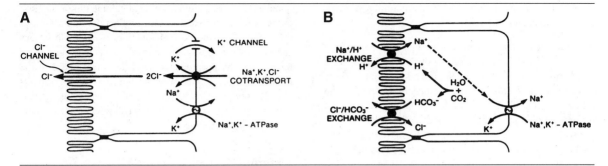

Fig. 20-2. Diagram (A) illustrates Cl⁻ secretion. The Na⁺, K⁺, Cl⁻ cotransport on the basolateral membrane serves as the Cl⁻ uptake step with the Na⁺, K⁺ATPase pump providing the driving force and recycling of Na⁺. Excess K⁺ is recycled via K⁺ channels on the basolateral membrane. Cl⁻ exits into the lumen via Cl⁻ channels. Electroneutral NaCl absorption is shown in (B). Electroneutral transport is obtained via dual exchange system comprised of an Na⁺/H⁺ exchange and a Cl⁻/HCO₃⁻ exchange working in concert. These exchange carries serve to bring Na⁺ and Cl⁻ across the apical membrane into the cell. Na⁺ is then pumped out by way of the Na⁺, K⁺ATPase. (Reprinted with permission from Barrett KE and Dharmsathaphorn K. Secretion and absorption: Small intestine and colon. In Yamada T (ed). *Textbook of Gastroenterology.* Philadelphia: Lippincott, 1991, pp. 265–293.)

Table 20-2. Neurohumoral and Immunologic Agents That Regulate Colonic Electrolyte Transport

Agent	Source	NaCl Absorption	Cl Secretion
Norepinephrine	Sympathetic and enteric nerves	↑	?↓
Epinephrine	Sympathetic nerves	↑	?↓
Acetylcholine	Parasympathetic and enteric nerves	↓	↑
VIP	Enteric nerves	↓	↑
Somatostatin	Enteric nerves	↑	↓
Histamine	Mast cells	?↓	↑
Prostaglandins	Mast cells	↓	↑
	Phagocytes		
Serotonin	Mast cells	↓	↑
Leukotrienes	Mast cells	?	↑
	Phagocytes		
Interleukin 1	Phagocytes	?	↑

↑= stimulation, ↓= inhibition, ?↓=potentially inhibitory, ?=unknown (see text for details).
Modified with permission from Binder H and Sandle GI. Electrolyte transport in the mammalian colon. In Johnson L (ed.). *Physiology of the Gastrointestinal Tract.* New York: Raven, 1994, p. 2156.

Colonic Disorders

Constipation

Definition

Constipation is a symptom rather than a specific disease. It is generally defined by the patient as defecation frequency of twice weekly or less. However, patients may differ in their perception about constipation depending on psycho-logical and social background. Other descriptive features of constipation that may be independent of bowel habits include stool consistency, sense of incomplete evacuation, and difficulty during defecation.

Mechanism

Pathophysiologic mechanisms of constipation most often involve poor colonic propulsive activity. Approach to the patient with constipation is simplified by considering colonic dysfunction in terms of either structural abnormalities or colonic motor disorders.

Structural Causes.   Any lesion or process obstructing the movement of luminal contents of the colon can cause constipation. Colon cancer is the most important of these possibilities. Left-sided colonic neoplasms that narrow the lumen are more likely to produce symptoms earlier than those located in the right colon. This is due principally to the solid consistency of the stool at the more distal sites.

Benign strictures of the colon can also cause constipation. Luminal narrowing due to fibrosis or inflammation (or both) can be related to ischemia, diverticular disease, radiation, or inflammatory bowel disease. In women, endometriosis involving the sigmoid colon can lead to fibrosis and subsequent stricture formation.

Anorectal Causes.   Anorectal diseases are frequently associated with painful defecation and constipation. This is because pain associated with inflamed hemorrhoids or anal fissure prompt avoidance of defecation. Likewise, rectal inflammation or trauma may alter bowel frequency. Tenesmus (urgency but unproductive straining at stool) is a symptom encountered in patients with rectal inflammation (e.g., proctitis). In addition to the history, the physical examination of the abdomen, perianal area, and a digital anorectal examination are essential to exclude anorectal disease in patients presenting with a complaint of constipation.

Metabolic Causes.   Impairment of colon transit can develop because of a smooth-muscle motor disorder owing to a large number of metabolic and endocrine disorders, neurogenic illnesses, collagen vascular disorders, and iatrogenic (drug-associated) conditions. The most common endocrine causes of constipation are diabetes mellitus and hypothyroidism. Autonomic neuropathy encountered in longstanding diabetes mellitus can affect smooth-muscle function of both the proximal (e.g., gastroparesis) and distal gastrointestinal tract. Diarrhea can also be a presenting symptom. The pathophysiology of diabetic diarrhea is poorly understood, but individuals with this condition need to be carefully evaluated for treatable causes (e.g., celiac disease, bacterial overgrowth) of diarrhea.

Hypothyroidism in the croaky voiced, slow-moving and apparently slow-witted individual bundled in a sweater and complaining of constipation is easy to diagnose. Subtler forms of hypothyroidism, however, may be more of a challenge and require keen diagnostic skills. Electrolyte abnormalities involving potassium, calcium, and magnesium have also been associated with reduced bowel frequency. The explanation for altered colonic motor function in states of electrolyte imbalance reflect the importance of these cations in the normal function of excitable tissues such as smooth muscle and nerves. Elevated progesterone levels seen during pregnancy and the luteal phase of the menstrual cycle have been shown to reduce smooth-muscle contractility and prolong gut transit time. Constipation experienced during these physiologic events is due, in part, to progesterone.

Irritable Bowel Syndrome

General Characteristics

Irritable bowel syndrome (IBS) is a common chronic gastrointestinal motility disorder characterized in most patients by disordered colonic motility and altered bowel habits in the absence of organic disease. Alternatively, symptoms of irritable bowel syndrome may originate from functional motility disturbances of the esophagus, stomach, or small intestine. In these instances heartburn and retrosternal fullness or nausea, early satiety, and bloating occur. IBS accounts for 30–50% of outpatient visits to gastroenterologists in the United States. It is more common in women and tends to begin in the teen years or early adulthood.

Clinical Features

Clinical presentation in patients with IBS affecting the colon fall into two broad groups: abdominal pain associated with altered bowel habits (constipation, diarrhea, or both) and painless diarrhea. The latter group constitutes the minority of the patients. Signs and symptoms associated with IBS include (a) abdominal pain relieved by defecation or associated with a change in the consistency of the stool, (b) altered frequency of bowel movements, (c) sensation of incomplete evacuation, and (d) passage of mucus upon defecation. Psychological factors such as stress have been shown to exacerbate IBS symptoms.

The most important aspect in evaluating a patient with the above complaints is to rule out organic disease. Symptoms which suggest organic disease of the gastrointestinal tract are unexplained weight loss, nocturnal diarrhea, and hematochezia. Distinction between organic or functional bowel disease may be difficult; however, the clinical features outlined in Table 20-3 are helpful in supporting or rejecting the diagnosis of irritable bowel syndrome.

Mechanisms

The pathogenesis of IBS is not well understood. Clinical and laboratory investigations have failed to detect any his-

Table 20-3. Clinical Features of Irritable Bowel Syndrome (IBS)

Supporting the Diagnosis of IBS	Against the Diagnosis of IBS
Lower abdominal pain	Onset in old age
Aggravated by meals	Steady progressive course
Relieved by defecation	Frequent awakening by symptoms
More frequent bowel movements with onset of pain	Fever
Looser stools with onset of pain	Weight loss
Does not awaken patient	Rectal bleeding from other than fissures or hemorrhoids
Visible abdominal distention	Steatorrhea
Small stools (with constipation or diarrhea)	Dehydration
Chronic symptoms consistent in pattern but variable in severity	New symptoms after a long period
Symptoms worse with periods of stress	

Reprinted with permission from Schuster M. Irritable bowel syndrome. In Fordtran J and Sleisenger M (eds.). *Gastrointestinal Disease* (5th ed.). Philadelphia: Saunders, 1993, p. 925.

tologic, microbiologic, or biochemical abnormalities in patients with IBS. Nonetheless, these patients have abnormal myoelectric and motor activities in the gastrointestinal tract. Patients with IBS also have a lower threshold for pain and induction of spastic contractions during balloon distention in the rectum. This exaggerated motor response to colonic distention may explain the symptoms that are experienced in these patients with even small volumes of colonic gas and stool.

Myoelectrical activity in the colon and elsewhere in the alimentary tract is characterized by slow waves and spike potentials. Slow waves determine the time interval during which smooth-muscle cells contract and the direction and speed of contraction. Spike potentials determine the amplitude and duration of contraction. In healthy subjects under basal (fasting) conditions, colonic slow waves occur at a frequency of 6 cycles/minute, while IBS patients have slow-wave frequency of 3 cycles/minute. This finding is present in both symptomatic and asymptomatic patients. Differences in myoelectric rhythm frequency are not uniformly recorded in IBS patients and such distinctions are felt to be arbitrary by some investigators.

The colonic motility response to a meal also differs in IBS patients. In normal subjects a postcibal gastrocolic reflex elicits increased colonic motility for 20–30 minutes followed by return to basal myoelectrical activity 1 hour after meal ingestion. In contrast, IBS patients exhibit prolonged myoelectric response to feeding that may persist for an hour or longer. The prolonged myoelectric response to feeding in IBS is capable of being modulated by anticholinergic drugs.

Diagnosis and Treatment

IBS is a diagnosis of exclusion. Symptoms associated with IBS may mimic other disease processes like cancer, inflammatory bowel disease, or infections. Physical exam is usually unrevealing but may show anxiety, abdominal tympany, and a palpable, tender sigmoid colon. All patients should have routine laboratory tests including CBC and fecal hemoccult testing. Stool examination for ova and parasites, enteric pathogens, and *Clostridium difficile* toxin should be considered when diarrhea is the presenting symptom. When indicated by history, colonoscopy or barium enema is recommended to exclude inflammatory bowel disease or right-sided colonic lesion. Upper endoscopy may also be indicated in patients with upper abdominal pain or heartburn. In some cases, abdominal ultrasound is appropriate to rule out gallbladder pathology.

Treatment consists of patient education, reassurance, and dietary counseling. High-fiber diets and supplemental fiber in the form of psyllium compounds act to provide stool bulk and hydration. This additional dietary fiber is beneficial in IBS patients with both constipation and diarrhea. Antispasmodic or antidiarrhea agents should be used intermittently and at the lowest dose needed to provide symptomatic relief.

Diverticular Disease

General Characteristics

Diverticular disease is a common acquired condition that usually is asymptomatic. Diverticular disease of the colon refers to the presence of saccular outpouchings (diverticuli) in the colonic wall caused by herniation of mucosa and submucosa through the muscularis propria at areas of weakness in the colonic wall (Fig. 20-3). Sites of diverticulum formation occur at clefts in the circular muscle layer through which blood vessels reach the submucosa.

Diverticulosis is a disease of western societies and affects one-third of persons aged 45 years and two-thirds of those 85 years or older. In rural Africa and Asia, where residents consume diets high in fiber (upwards of 100 g/day), diverticulosis is a rarity.

Diverticular disease occurs predominantly in the sigmoid colon: 65% of diverticula are confined to this area. Most of the 35% with more proximal disease also have sigmoid involvement.

Fig. 20-3. Structural dynamics of diverticular formation and vascular relationships. (A) The long branch of the vas rectum artery penetrates the colonic wall through a connective tissue gap in the circular muscle. (B) Early mucosal protrusion widens the connective tissue gap. (C) With transmural extension of the diverticulum, the vas rectum is displaced over it. As a result, the lumen of the diverticulum is separated from the vas rectum by only a thin layer of mucosa and submucosa. (From Apstein MD. Diverticular and other intestinal diseases. In Stein JH (ed). *Internal Medicine* (4th ed.). St. Louis: Mosby-Year Book, 1994, pp. 486–492. As modified from Meyers MA et al. The angioarchitecture of colonic diverticula: Significance in bleeding diverticulosis. *Radiol* 108:249–261, 1973. With permission from Mosby-Year Book and from Radiological Society of North America.)

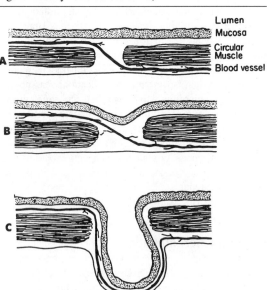

Lumen
Mucosa
Circular
Muscle
Blood vessel

Clinical Manifestations

Diverticular disease has three basic clinical manifestations: pain, diverticulitis, and bleeding.

Painful Diverticular Disease.   This is one expression of symptomatic diverticulosis: spasm without inflammation. This can mimic acute diverticulitis initially, but it requires no special treatment. Usually the patient complains of left lower quadrant pain of acute onset. It differs from acute diverticulitis due to the absence of inflammatory indicators like increased white count, fever, and rebound tenderness. It usually resolves spontaneously.

Acute Diverticulitis.   This disease usually starts as a microperforation of a diverticulum into the serosa which produces a local inflammatory reaction. Peridiverticular inflammation is accompanied by abdominal pain, fever, and an elevated white blood cell count. Localized diverticulitis may progress to abscess formation with peritonitis. Free perforation is uncommon. Fistulous connections between colonic wall and other pelvic organs, like urinary bladder, may also occur. Up to 25% of cases of diverticulitis are complicated by fistula formation.

The diagnosis of diverticulitis is usually made on clinical grounds. Noninvasive imaging of the abdomen (e.g., computerized axial tomography) may be necessary to assess the possibility of intra-abdominal abscess. Colonoscopy and barium enemas are usually contraindicated during the acute phase of illness due to the risk of colonic perforation.

Treatment consists of supportive care, antibiotics (oral or intravenous), and bowel rest. Surgery is indicated for complications like bowel obstruction, peritonitis, fistulas, and abscesses.

Lower Gastrointestinal Bleeding.   This occurs in up to 5% of cases of patients with colonic diverticula. Bleeding is usually acute and brisk, with impressive episodes of bright red blood per rectum. Bleeding occurs owing to erosion of a penetrating artery at the dome of the diverticulum. In 80% of cases, bleeding stops spontaneously but there is a 20% incidence of rebleeding in these patients. Diverticular bleeding usually occurs from the right side of the colon in contrast to diverticulitis, which usually involves the left side of the colon. Radiolabeled red cell scans and mesenteric angiography may be helpful in localizing the bleeding site.

The initial episode of diverticular bleeding is usually managed conservatively with appropriate intravenous fluid and blood replacement and careful monitoring of vital signs and clinical status. Recurrent episodes or continued bleeding may require surgery. After the initial episode of colonic bleeding the patient should undergo colonoscopy to document the presence of diverticulosis and exclude other causes of lower gastrointestinal bleeding such as arteriovenous malformations, ischemia, inflammatory bowel disease, and cancer.

Colon Polyps and Colon Cancer

Classification of Polyps

A polyp is an elevation of the colonic mucosa with tissue proliferation that protrudes from the colonic wall into the lumen. Colon polyps are classified as non-neoplastic and neoplastic. Non-neoplastic polyps include hyperplastic polyps and inflammatory polyps. These are benign and without malignant potential. Neoplastic polyps may be benign (adenoma) or malignant (carcinoma).

Adenoma-Carcinoma Sequence

Cellular dysplasia is a histologic feature common to both types of neoplastic polyps. Adenomatous polyps are benign epithelial tumors. Adenomatous epithelium is characterized by abnormal cellular differentiation resulting in hypercellularity of colonic crypts. These polyps are of special interest because of their malignant potential. A temporal sequence exists between the development of an adenoma and the appearance of colon cancer. The adenoma-carcinoma sequence is well established and typically evolves over a decade or more. Infrequently, colon cancer may develop without a previous polyp.

Knowledge of the pathogenesis of colorectal adenocarcinoma has increased dramatically in the past 10 years. This enhanced understanding has been due in large part to the application of molecular biologic techniques to defining regulation of cellular events in normal and neoplastic colonic epithelium. We now know that the polyp-cancer sequence proceeds from normal mucosa by cellular proliferation, oncogene activation, and chromosomal deletion, to adenoma formation. Increasing dysplasia in the adenomatous polyp then leads to the development of adenocarcinoma. This proposed sequence of cellular and molecular genetic events is illustrated in Fig. 20-4.

As noted previously, the time for these changes to occur is measured in years. For example, an adenomatous polyp less than 5 mm in diameter may take 10 years or longer to become malignant. On the other hand, a polyp that is 1 cm or greater in size may undergo malignant transformation in 3–5 years. Thus the larger an adenomatous polyp is the more likely it is to contain invasive cancer.

Colon Cancer

Epidemiology.   Cancer of the large bowel is the most frequent neoplasm of the gastrointestinal tract and is the second most common cause of cancer mortality in the United States. The incidence of colorectal cancer is highest in industralized nations like the United States, Western Europe, and Australia and is much lower in developing countries. The most important risk factor in the United States is age; the incidence is very low before age 40, and the relative risk increases thereafter as an exponential function of age. Increased dietary fat intake and decreased fiber in Western diets is regarded as important in the increased incidence in these nations. Genetic predisposition is also important as there is increased risk of cancer occurrence in first-degree relatives of patients with colon cancer. Hereditary polyposis syndromes, such as Gardner syndrome and familial polyposis, are associated with adenomatous polyps (100 or more) as an autosomal dominant trait. Typically, these individuals develop colon polyps in the second to third decade of life and, if untreated, colon cancer occurs 10–15 years after the onset of polyposis.

Ulcerative colitis (UC) is also a well-defined risk factor for colorectal cancer. Risk increases with severity, extent, and duration of disease. However, the adenoma-carcinoma sequence is not as clearcut as in sporadic colon cancer. Cancers in UC usually arise from flat mucosa without antecedent evidence of adenomas.

Clinical Features.   Two-thirds of colon polyps and colon cancers arise in the rectosigmoid. Colon polyps are usually asymptomatic; however, if they are large enough, may present with occult blood positive stools and/or iron-deficiency anemia. Patients with colon cancer may present with rectal bleeding, lower abdominal pain, or change in bowel habits (unexplained constipation or a change in stool caliber).

In asymptomatic patients, colon cancer may be detected by routine screening for occult blood in stool or screening flexible sigmoidoscopy. Under these circumstances, colorectal cancer may be detected at an early pathologic stage associated with improved patient survival.

Surgical excision is the optimal therapy for colon cancer. Polyps can usually be excised via endoscopy. After the colon is clear of lesions, serial endoscopy is indicated to assess recurrence.

Inflammatory Bowel Disease

Inflammatory bowel disease (IBD) consists of a heterogenous group of disorders of unknown etiology. Clinical manifestations may consist of abdominal pain, diarrhea, and rectal bleeding. Symptoms can vary depending on whether inflammation is acute or chronic, mucosal or transmural, and whether it involves the small and/or large

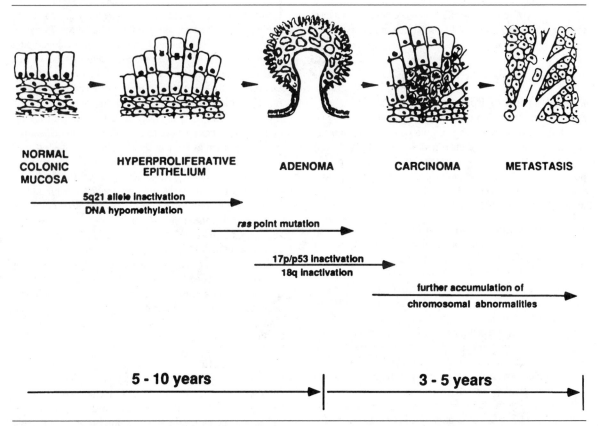

Fig. 20-4. Proposed sequence of molecular genetic events in the evolution of colon cancer. Carcinogenesis occurs from an accumulation of events. (From: Bresalier R and Toribara N. Familial colon cancer. In Eastwood GL (ed.). *Premalignant Conditions of the Gastrointestinal Tract.* Norwalk CT: Appleton & Lange, 1990, pp. 238. As modified by Bresalier R and Kim YS. Malignant neoplasm of the large intestine. In Fordtran J and Sleisenger M (eds.). *Gastrointestinal Disease* (5th ed.). Norwalk, CT: Appleton & Lange, 1993, p. 1458. With permission from R. Bresalier and Appleton & Lange.)

bowel. The two clinical entities comprising these disorders are Crohn's disease and ulcerative colitis.

Epidemiology

The incidence of IBD is approximately 3 to 20 new cases per 100,000 population in most countries. It occurs with equal ratio in males and females worldwide, but in the USA there is a 30% increased risk in women. IBD is more common in whites and especially in people of Jewish descent. It is uncommon in the extremes of age and is more common in teenagers and young adults. Family history is a definite risk factor.

Pathogenesis

Efforts to explain the etiology and pathogenesis of inflammatory bowel disease have concentrated on clinical features of these illnesses which suggest genetic predisposition, disturbed immune regulation, and certain infectious diseases. A pathogenesis model illustrating potential interactions between suspected causative factors is shown in Fig. 20-5.

Genetics.   Family and twin studies show that IBD occurs in relatives much more commonly than coincidence would predict. HLA linkage with certain extraintestinal

Potential contributors to the pathogenesis of inflammatory bowel disease

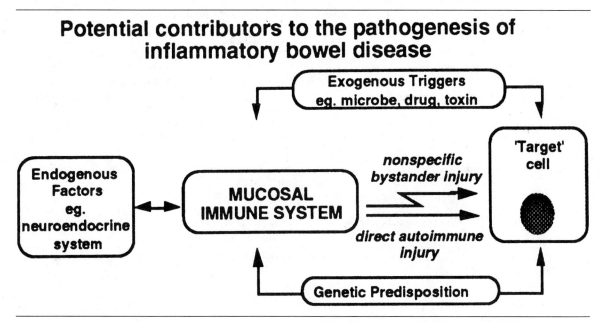

Fig. 20-5. Diagram for understanding the pathogenesis of inflammatory bowel disease. (From: Targan S. Immunopathogenesis of inflammatory bowel disease. In Mucosal Diseases of the Gastrointestinal Tract: AGA Postgraduate Course Syllabus, 1993, p. 255. With permission of the author and the American Gastroenterological Association.)

manifestations of IBD (namely, ankylosing spondylitis and uveitis) have been made with the HLA-B27 phenotype.

Immunology. It has been hypothesized that ulcerative colitis and Crohn's disease are due to disordered immunoregulation. Another theory is that increased permeability of intestinal mucosa leads to absorption of enteric antigens from the fecal stream which in turn activate local immune cells to evoke a chronic inflammatory response. Cytokines derived from intestinal lymphocytes and macrophage are felt to play a central role in the immune responses of IBD. Autoimmunity to antigens on colonic epithelium has been postulated in ulcerative colitis.

Infection. It has long been attractive to think of IBD as being due to an infectious illness. Viruses, cell wall defective bacteria, and mycobacteria have been candidate organisms. Despite rigorous investigations of each agent, Koch's postulates have not been fulfilled.

Clinical Features
Crohn's disease and ulcerative colitis differ in certain aspects (Table 20-4).

Ulcerative colitis usually manifests as bloody diarrhea and abdominal pain. It only involves the colon and almost always starts in the rectum with variable proximal extension. The colonic mucosa exhibits diffuse erythema, friability, and ulceration. Pathologically, inflammation is confined to the mucosa.

Crohn's disease may involve any part of the gastrointestinal tract from the mouth to the anus. About 40% of patients will have small bowel disease, 40% will have small and large bowel disease, and 20% will have disease limited to the colon. Regional enteritis is a term applied to Crohn's disease of the small bowel and, in particular, of the terminal ileum. The rectum is frequently spared and rectal bleeding is less common than in ulcerative colitis. Inflammation is transmural and ulceration tends to be segmental with intervening areas (skip areas) of apparently normal bowel. Pathology of involved bowel frequently demonstrates granuloma.

Complications
Ulcerative colitis may lead to severe anemia due to bleeding. In the past, a common presentation of ulcerative coli-

Table 20-4. Clinical and Pathologic Distinctions Between Ulcerative Colitis and Crohn's Disease

Ulcerative Colitis	Crohn's Disease
CLINICAL SIGNS AND SYMPTOMS	
Bloody diarrhea is typical	Blood and diarrhea may or may not be evident
Pain is crampy, lower abdominal, often temporarily relieved by defecation	Pain is steady, often in right lower abdomen, not relieved by defecation
Abdomen may or may not be tender	A tender mass in right lower abdomen is found frequently
Cigarette smoking is rare	Cigarette smoking is common
PATHOLOGY	
Disease is confined to rectum and colon	Disease may be found anywhere throughout the gastrointestinal tract
Inflammation is confined to the mucosa (except in toxic megacolon)	Inflammation is transmural
Disease is continuous for a variable extent, beginning in the rectum	Disease may be segmental with intervening areas of normal bowel

Reprinted with permission from: Kemler BJ. Inflammatory bowel disease. In Eastwood GL (ed.). *Core Textbook of Gastroenterology.* Philadelphia: Lippincott, 1984, p. 120.

tis was toxic megacolon. Presently, improved management and earlier diagnosis have combined to make this presentation less frequent. In this condition, the patient presents with fever, tachycardia, anemia, leukocytosis, abdominal pain, and abdominal distention. On abdominal x-ray, the colon, particularly the transverse colon, is dilated to greater than 6–7 cm in diameter. Failure to respond to medical therapy can be an indication for colectomy since perforation and peritonitis may occur with disastrous consequences.

The transmural nature of Crohn's disease accounts for complications such as fistulae, intra-abdominal abscess, and stricture formation. Fistulae may form between different parts of the GI tract (e.g., enterocolonic fistula), adjacent hollow viscus (e.g., enterovesical, colovaginal fistulae), and skin (e.g., enterocutaneous fistula). Perianal and perineal disease (including fissures, fistulae, and perirectal abscess) are seen more commonly in Crohn's disease.

Ulcerative colitis is associated with an increased risk of colon cancer compared with the general population. (The risk of cancer is also greater in patients with Crohn's disease but not as high as with ulcerative colitis.) In patients with ulcerative colitis, cancer risk increases with duration and extent of disease. The incidence of colon cancer begins to increase after 10 years of disease and increases by 1% per year, thereafter reaching a risk of 30% after 35 years. Patients with involvement of the entire colon, pancolitis, have a higher risk than individuals with less extensive disease. Ulcerative proctitis is not associated with increased risk of cancer. Severity of disease is not a contributing factor since cancer can develop in patients with quiescent ulcerative colitis. Cancer usually arises from flat mucosa, unlike sporadic colon cancer, which develops from adenomatous polyps. Surveillance colonoscopy is recommended in patients with ulcerative colitis greater than 8–10 years.

Extraintestinal Manifestations

Musculoskeletal. Arthritis is the most common extraintestinal manifestation of IBD. It often parallels disease activity. This is an asymmetrical and migratory arthritis affecting most often the large joint of the lower extremities. Ankylosing spondylitis also occurs. Unlike peripheral arthritis, ankylosing spondylitis does not parallel inflammatory bowel disease activity. As noted previously, ankylosing spondylitis and IBD have been associated with a high prevalence of the class I antigen HLA-B27.

Ocular. Iritis and uveitis may be manifestations of IBD. Clinical manifestations include blurred vision and headaches. Slit-lamp examination is required to establish the diagnosis.

Skin. *Erythema nodosum* is often associated with IBD. These are red, tender nodules ranging in size from one to several centimeters. They often appear in extensor surfaces of arms and legs and usually follow disease activity.

Pyoderma gangrenosum is a deep, discrete ulceration with necrotic center and surrounding violaceous-appearing skin. This distinctive ulceration typically develops on the lower extremities, but may appear elsewhere. It parallels disease activity. Oral lesions like aphthous ulcers are also seen in IBD, most commonly with Crohn's disease.

Hepatobiliary. Primary sclerosing cholangitis is a chronic cholestatic syndrome characterized by fibrosing inflammation of the biliary system, resulting in bile duct proliferation, biliary cirrhosis, and hepatic failure. It is usually associated with UC and bears no relationship to disease activity. In fact, liver disease may progress relentlessly despite colectomy. Therapy is directed at enhancing bile flow and treating episodes of cholangitis. Liver transplantation is an option in advanced liver disease. Gallstones are associated with Crohn's disease of the distal small bowel and result from bile acid malabsorption and concurrent bile cholesterol saturation.

Treatment

Medical treatment of IBD consists of salicylate derivatives like azulfidine, steroids, and immunosuppressive agents. Surgery is reserved as definitive therapy for UC and for complications of either form of IBD. Complications requiring surgery include bleeding, cancer, fistula, obstruction due to stricture, or abdominal abscess. Crohn's disease is rarely cured by surgery and tends to recur at sites of resection.

Clinical Examples

1. A 60-year-old man presents with shortness of breath, fatigue, and pallor. Laboratory tests show hemoglobin 8.5 g/dl, Hct 26%, MCV 61 Fl, and ferritin < 5 μg/ml. The patient's stool was positive for occult blood.

Discussion. The differential diagnosis of iron-deficiency anemia presenting in an adult male over 50 years of age would have to list colon cancer toward the top. Other presenting symptoms may be abdominal pain, constipation, signs of obstruction, or rectal bleeding. In this patient, colonoscopy showed a large fungating mass in the hepatic flexure. Chronic blood loss was the etiology of this patient's anemia. The outcome of surgical resection is dependent on the depth of bowel wall involvement and the presence of local or distant spread.

2. A 59-year-old woman presents with three bouts of hematochezia over a 12-hour period. Bleeding is painless and patient reports shortness of breath and mild chest pain upon arrival to the emergency room. Admission vital signs are as follows: BP 120/80 and Pulse 100 lying down; BP 90/60 and Pulse 135 sitting up. Labs: CBC Hgb 10.6 g/dl, Hct 31%, MCV 90 Fl, WBC 13.5/mm^3, Plts 191,000/mm^3, and PT 11.7.

Discussion. This middle-aged woman presents with an episode of severe lower gastrointestinal bleeding. The first priority in this patient would be to assess degree of blood loss and replace it with saline and blood transfusions as needed. The most common cause of massive lower GI bleeding is diverticular bleeding. The dome of the diverticulum erodes into a penetrating artery in the colonic wall, causing hemorrhage. This bleeding is often severe and brisk but self-limited. Continued or recurrent bleeding is an indication for surgery or radiographic therapy. Right-sided diverticuli bleed more often than left-sided ones. Other possibilities for this patient's problems are arteriovenous malformation, colon cancer (uncommon), or an upper GI source with rapid transit (like peptic ulcer disease).

3. An 18-year-old woman presents with diarrhea for the past 2 months. She also complains of diffuse joint pain, occasional fever, and abdominal pain. She has lost 10 lb. over the last month. A sigmoidoscopy was normal. An upper GI series with small bowel follow-through showed irregularity and mild stricturing of the terminal ileum. Colonoscopy showed linear ulcerations with skip areas in the right colon and terminal ileum. On biopsy, acute inflammation with granulomas was noted.

Discussion. This patient has Crohn's disease involving the right colon and terminal ileum. This is a systemic disease which may present with symptoms of fever, arthritis, and weakness. It can be differentiated from ulcerative colitis in that the rectum is spared and linear ulcers are noted beside normal mucosa (skip areas). In ulcerative colitis, the disease starts in the rectum and diffuse erythema with bleeding and friability are noted. In UC, the terminal ileum is not involved.

In this patient, infectious causes of diarrhea must be ruled out because IBD is a diagnosis of exclusion. The chronicity of her disease and the presence of granulomas point toward the diagnosis of Crohn's disease.

Bibliography

Binion D. Current concepts of IBD pathogenesis. *Res Staff Phys* Oct. 1994, pp. 11–16. *A concise overview of the possible etiologies of inflammatory bowel disease.*

Dietzen CD and Pemberton JH. Diverticulitis. In Yamada T (ed.). *Textbook of Gastroenterology.* Philadelphia: Lippincott, 1991, pp. 1734–1748. *A comprehensive text on gastroenterology with detailed sections on ion secretion and transport.*

Fordtran J and Sleisenger M (eds.). *Gastrointestinal Disease.* Philadelphia: Saunders, 1993. *A text on gastroenterology with detailed overviews on inflammatory bowel disease and colon cancer.*

Kelley W (ed.). *Textbook of Medicine.* Philadelphia: Lippincott, 1989. *A comprehensive text in internal medicine with excellent sections on irritable bowel syndrome and diverticular disease.*

Rankin GB. Extraintestinal and systemic manifestations of inflammatory bowel disease. *Med Clin N Am* 74(1): 39–50, 1990. *Excellent review of clinical features and pathogenesis of inflammatory bowel disease.*

Rogers A, et al. Diverticular disease. *Gastroint Dis Today* 3;4:8–17, 1994. *A brief, but precise, summary on the major complications of diverticular disease.*

Whelan G. Epidemiology of inflammatory bowel disease. *Med Clin N Am* 74(1): 1–12, 1990. *Excellent summary on epidemiology.*

21 Clinical Nutrition

Marie A. Bernard and Ralph T. Guild III

Objectives

After completing this chapter, you should be able to

Describe the body's response to starvation, stress, and trauma

Describe the basic nutrients required for maintenance of life

Distinguish between kwashiorkor and marasmus

Understand the components of a qualitative nutritional assessment

Describe routes of administration of nutritional support

Describe at least two eating disorders

Nutrition relates food intake to the functioning of the organism. Appropriate intake of certain nutrients is essential to maintain structure and function, especially in the presence of disease or trauma. A varied food intake has characterized man historically and complicated the definition of precise needs. Recent research has clarified nutrient requirements and identified some non-essential nutrients that become essential at some ages and stress levels. This chapter examines the metabolic response to starvation, stress, and trauma, and outlines adult nutritional requirements. Clinical nutritional disorders, nutritional assessment, support, obesity, and disordered eating are also described.

Metabolic Response to Starvation, Stress, or Trauma

Starvation

Starvation is a common occurrence among ill and hospitalized individuals and may be expected in circumstances where food or economic resources are scarce. As many as 30–40% of patients have evidence for malnutrition upon hospital admission. Hospitalized patients are at risk for worsening malnutrition, stemming from food deprivation in preparation for diagnostic testing and decreased appetite due to illness and medications. With prolonged hospitalization, patients without evidence of malnutrition on admission may develop markers of such.

During periods of inadequate caloric intake, the major sources of energy are glycogen, adipose tissue, and endogenous protein. The body requires a regular intake of energy to maintain these storage sites and to meet the energy needs of vital organs. When intake of calories is suboptimal, the metabolic needs of the body are supported initially by glycogen stores in the liver and muscle. In a nonstressed, normally nourished individual, these stores can sustain bodily functions for approximately 12 hours. However, when starvation lasts for longer than 12 hours, adipose stores are used to support metabolic needs. The body will also access adipose tissue in a shorter period of time if metabolic demands are elevated. Figure 21-1 outlines the metabolic pathways involved with starvation.

If there are prolonged periods of inadequate calorie intake, endogenous protein in muscle and visceral organs will be broken down for gluconeogenesis to meet energy needs. Individuals who are chronically ill, and therefore

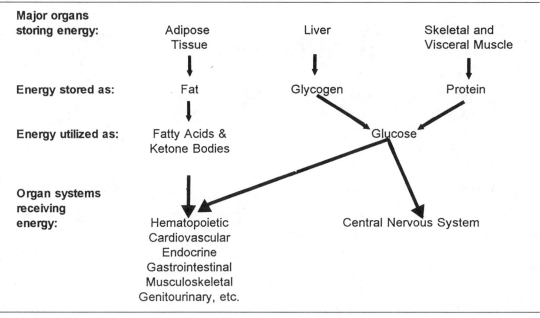

Fig. 21-1. Metabolic consequences of starvation. With starvation, the body initially utilizes glycogen stores within the liver to supply energy needs. However, with prolonged starvation, adipose tissue and endogenous protein are utilized to supply energy in the form of glucose, fatty acids, and/or ketone bodies. All organ systems can utilize either carbohydrate or fat for energy, with the exception of the central nervous system, which requires a constant supply of glucose.

consuming suboptimal quantities of calories and protein, are likely to develop protein-calorie malnutrition. These problems may be exacerbated with the development of acute illness, which increases the metabolic rate and energy needs. Table 21-1 summarizes the clinical consequences of prolonged deprivation of calories and protein.

Stress and Trauma

When the body is semistarved, nutritional deficiencies develop gradually. However, in the face of stress or trauma, such deficiencies can become evident rapidly. It has been demonstrated that metabolic demands increase 20% with simple elective surgery, 20–35% with hip-replacement surgery, 40–80% with sepsis, 50–100% with major burns.

This increase in metabolic rate associated with stress and trauma appears to be mediated by increased levels of glucagon, epinephrine, and other counterregulatory hormones. The impact of these hormonal changes may persist several days from the initiating event. In a setting of ele-

vated counterregulatory hormones, the body does not efficiently utilize adipose tissue to provide energy. Instead, endogenous protein is catabolized to meet the energy needs of the individual, unless adequate exogenous calories and protein are provided.

Table 21-1. Consequences of Malnutrition

Metabolic	Clinical
Decreased liver glycogen stores	Easy fatigability
Ketone body production	Weight loss
Adipose tissue utilization	Slowed wound healing
Endogenous protein catabolism	Increased infections (e.g., urinary tract infections, pneumonia)
	Decreased mobility
	Decreased cardiac and pulmonary function
	Pressure ulcers
	Death

Basic Nutritional Requirements

Nutritional requirements include: (1) proteins, required for structure and function of tissues, enzymes, and carrier systems and as an energy source; (2) carbohydrates, used as a primary energy substrate and as a source for dietary fiber; (3) fats, required for membrane structure and an energy source; (4) vitamins, required as components of certain molecules and as coenzymes; (5) minerals and trace elements, required for structure of certain tissues and metabolic processes; and (6) water, needed to maintain circulation and a variety of other functions. The usual adult daily requirements for protein and energy are one gram of protein and 25 kilocalories (kcal) of energy per kilogram of body weight. About 5% of the energy must be as essential fatty acids to avoid a deficiency state.

Nutritional Disorders

Kwashiorkor

Kwashiorkor is protein malnutrition. It is characteristically associated with decreased serum protein levels, edema and ascites, and increased risk for infection, pressure ulcers, and death. This syndrome may be found in third-world countries experiencing famine. Many hospitalized individuals may also suffer from a similar syndrome, such as patients who have been maintained on glucose and water during a prolonged postoperative period. The prognosis for that individual to recover is much worse than for normally nourished individuals with similar medical problems.

Marasmus

Marasmus is calorie malnutrition. It is characteristically associated with normal-body protein stores, but decreased adipose tissue. Marasmic individuals are at less risk than individuals suffering from kwashiorkor. However, should a marasmic individual be stressed with severe infection, trauma, or prolonged semistarvation, that individual would not have the adipose tissue stores to support energy needs. Thus body protein stores would be accessed to maintain vital organ function, and the individual would rapidly develop a kwashiorkorlike picture. Marasmic individuals include those who are genetically predisposed to small adipose tissue stores and long-distance runners.

Combined Protein-Calorie Malnutrition

This form of malnutrition is often found in people who have suffered from a prolonged illness. The manifestations are a combination of marasmus and kwashiorkor. The individual will present with depleted adipose tissue stores and evidence for visceral protein depletion, with decreased arm muscle circumference and decreased serum albumin concentration. The prognosis is poor without nutritional intervention to reverse the depleted state.

Other Deficiency States

There are a number of vitamins and minerals which may be deficient in chronically ill adults. These include vitamin B complex, folate, vitamin B_{12} (cyanocobalamin), vitamin C (ascorbic acid), vitamin D, and calcium. Vitamin B complex deficiency is quite common among chronically ill and hospitalized individuals. B complex vitamins are water soluble, and not stored in great excess within the body. Thus illness for several days, impairing intake of these vitamins, may lead to deficiency. Lack of B complex vitamins can lead to changes in the skin, mouth, and tongue. Vitamin C is necessary for the maintenance of skin integrity. Thus ascorbic acid deficiency may be manifested by petechiae at the base of skin follicles throughout the body. Folate and cyanocobalamin are necessary for the synthesis of thymidine in DNA. Deficiency of these vitamins will be manifest as a macrocytic anemia. Additionally, cyanocobalamin is necessary for the synthesis of serotonin, an essential neurotransmitter, perhaps explaining the neurologic deficits which occur with vitamin B_{12} deficiency. Vitamin D and calcium are necessary for the maintenance of bone health. With aging, absorption of calcium may become less efficient. This, combined with less sun exposure and a decreased conversion of vitamin D to its active form within the kidney, places older individuals at risk for a deficiency of vitamin D and calcium. This is manifest clinically as osteomalacia and osteoporosis (see Chapter 28).

Nutritional Assessment

History and Physical Findings

A good history and physical is as effective in the assessment of nutritional deficiency as any diagnostic test. Key questions include weight loss, with quantification; medications; known illness; dietary restrictions; and gastrointestinal complaints. There are several key physical findings to note. Weight and height should be measured and compared to standard tables for individuals of the same age and sex. The body mass index (BMI) weight (kg)/height^2 (in cm), is an accurate reflection of body fat, with a BMI < 18 consistent with underweight, and BMI > 30 consistent with obesity. BMI's exceeding these ranges have been associated with significant morbidity and mortality.

The appearance of the skin, hair, eyes, mouth, and extremities should be carefully noted. Very dry skin, with truncal flakiness which is evanescent with the application of skin creams, may indicate essential fatty acid deficiency. This may be found in individuals with inflammatory bowel disease or in patients who have received prolonged therapy with parenteral nutrition with inadequate fatty acid administration. Hyperpigmented skin in a band about the neck and upper chest may be consistent with vitamin B_6 deficiency (pellagra). Petechiae at the base of hair follicles suggests vitamin C deficiency. Thinning hair and alopecia are suggestive of protein-calorie malnutrition, although a number of other medical illnesses may manifest themselves similarly. Fissures at the angles of the mouth may be representative of a variety of vitamin B deficiencies. A smooth, beefy red tongue (glossitis) is also associated with a variety of vitamin B deficiencies.

In addition to the history and physical, there are a number of measurements which may help confirm an impression of the nutritional health of an individual. The most useful of these measures include skin fold thicknesses, arm muscle circumference, and serum albumin level.

Skin fold thicknesses have been measured at the triceps, biceps, subscapular, and suprailiac areas, to assess fat stores. There is significant interobserver variation in these measurements, and thus they are best obtained by a single trained individual. The usual approach is to measure the skin fold thickness three times in a single site, and take the average of the three measurements. This measure can then be compared to standard tables of skin fold thicknesses for individuals of similar age, sex, and ethnicity. This approach is quite useful in epidemiologic studies of nutrition. It is less valuable in following a single patient's nutritional progress.

Arm muscle circumference is thought to represent the protein stores of an individual. As with skin fold thicknesses, this parameter is valuable in epidemiologic studies, but less helpful for following the nutritional health of a single individual.

Biochemical markers of nutritional health include serum albumin level, transferrin, retinol binding protein, creatinine/height index, and thyroxine-binding prealbumin. The serum albumin level is a good marker of protein nutritional status, in the absence of liver disease, or nephrotic syndrome. With decrease in the serum albumin level there is an increase in morbidity and mortality. The other biochemical markers noted above are reflective of total-body protein stores, and thought to be more responsive to acute changes in those stores than serum albumin levels, since albumin has a half-life of approximately 21 days.

Plasma vitamin levels have also been measured to determine nutritional health. Plasma levels for water-soluble vitamins are often reflective of total-body stores of that vitamin. In contrast, plasma levels of the fat-soluble vitamins (A, D, E, K) may not accurately reflect total-body stores.

Nutritional Support

Rationale for Nutritional Support

Nutritional intervention utilizing the gastrointestinal tract, or the venous system, will reverse markers of malnutrition in children and adults. With severe nutritional deficiency, a number of problems develop — anemia, immobility, urinary tract infection, pneumonia, pressure ulcer, and ultimately death (see Table 21-1). The rationale for intervention is to avoid these and other consequences of progressive nutritional deficiency. In malnourished surgical patients, and selected other individuals, nutritional intervention has been shown to reduce morbidity and mortality.

Routes of Administration

The preferred means of providing nutritional supplementation is by spontaneous oral intake. Patients can reverse nutritional deficiencies simply by consuming additional calories and protein in the form of liquid supplements or by additional protein and/or carbohydrate added to the foods they ordinarily eat. If such supplementation is ineffective, a liquid formula can be provided through a feeding tube, to meet the individual's nutritional needs or to supplement spontaneous intake. Should this form of supplementation appear to be necessary for a prolonged period, a tube placed endoscopically or surgically into the stomach (gastrostomy), allows long-term feedings. If the gastrointestinal tract is nonfunctional, carbohydrates, protein, and minerals can be provided by the parenteral route — either by a standard intravenous infusion (peripheral parenteral nutrition) or by a central venous catheter placed in the superior vena cava (central parenteral nutrition). It is difficult to meet the entire calorie and protein needs of an individual by the peripheral parenteral route. Additionally, the high osmolality of the formulas leads to sclerosis and thrombosis of peripheral veins after 7–10 days. Therefore, peripheral parenteral nutrition is usually reserved for individuals requiring nutritional support for a short period. Central parenteral nutrition can be maintained for weeks to months. There are risks, both catheter related and metabolic. Thus central parenteral nutrition should only be used when the gastrointestinal tract cannot absorb adequate amounts of calories and protein.

General Guidelines for Nutrient Administration

Fluid and electrolyte balance must be carefully monitored in individuals whose sole source of nutrition and hydration is the nutritional formula. Enteral formulas tend to be a concentrated source of nutrients. Thus supplemental free water often must be administered with the enteral formula to prevent dehydration. For individuals receiving parenteral nutrition, electrolytes, trace elements, and vitamins must be provided in the parenteral formula. There are standard formulas available which provide the minimum daily requirements of electrolytes in individuals receiving at least 2 liters daily. However, the content of each formula should be evaluated and matched with the needs of the individual patient. In many instances additional supplementation is necessary. In some cases, formulas with a lower content of electrolytes or trace elements may be necessary (e.g., decreased potassium in individuals with significant renal impairment). Most enteral formulas provide the adult recommended daily requirement of vitamins in 1.5–2.0 liters of the fluid. However, vitamins must be added to parenteral formulas on a daily basis.

The following recommendations are appropriate for either parenteral or enteral feeding.

Protein

For most adult patients, 1.0–1.5 g of protein or amino acids per kilogram body weight will suffice. These should be administered with sufficient energy substrates to spare the protein for anabolism. The recommended ratio is 150–200 kcal per gram of nitrogen which would be 25–35 kcal per gram of protein. Protein is about 16% nitrogen (6.25 g of protein equals 1 g of nitrogen). For the most seriously ill, hypercatabolic patients, up to 2 g of protein per kilogram body weight may be required. The hypercatabolic state is generally characterized by a urine urea nitrogen excretion of greater than 15 g/24 hour. Special formulas containing high percentages of branched-chain amino acids may be of benefit for short periods in hypercatabolic patients. For most patients, however, a balanced formulation of amino acids is best.

Energy Substrates

The two most widely used energy substrates are glucose (3.4 kcal/g for the monohydrate form) and lipids (9 kcal/g). The brain preferentially uses glucose for energy, but most other organs utilize either glucose or fatty acids. Studies indicate that, as intake of energy rises from 25 to 35 kcal/kg body weight, both lean body mass and fat stores are repleted in about equal amounts. Above that level, fat stores are increased in excess of lean body mass. The normal maximal glucose oxidation rate is 5–7 mg/kg/minute (about 25 kcal/kg/day) for parenteral solutions. Faster administration leads to glucose intolerance. Lipids should not exceed 60% of the total daily caloric amount. However, to avoid essential fatty acid deficiency, at least 5% of daily calories should be given as lipids.

Fluid and Electrolytes

Adults with normal renal function require 25–40 ml of water per kilogram body weight per day. Increased losses, fever or other disease states may alter that amount. Sodium, potassium, calcium, magnesium, and phosphate are all required for homeostasis. Potassium and magnesium are needed to make new protein. Phosphate is essential for high-energy bonds. Calcium is needed for maintenance of the skeleton. Homeostasis and pathophysiology of these divalent minerals is described in Chapter 54.

Vitamins and Trace Elements

These nutrients should be administered in amounts approximating the usual maintenance requirements unless specific deficiencies are suspected. The fat-soluble vitamins (A,D,E,K) are toxic in excess, but excesses of the water-soluble ones (the B vitamins and C) are excreted in urine. Zinc, copper, chromium, and manganese are the trace elements administered parenterally on a daily basis. Vitamin K is not routinely included in vitamin preparations in order to avoid complicating anticoagulant therapy.

Obesity and Eating Disorders

A body mass index of greater than 30 indicates obesity and is associated with increased likelihood of hypertension, diabetes mellitus, gallbladder disease, kidney stones, certain types of cancer (e.g., endometrial cancer), and early death. Obesity is due to a number of influences: genetic predisposition, endocrine alterations, physical inactivity, and diet composition.

Treatment of obesity has been wide ranging. Surgical interventions have included jaw wiring to prevent intake, gastric stapling, and intestinal diversion. These have largely been abandoned because of the high incidence of complications. Medical interventions (including pharmacologic dosing of thyroid hormone, amphetamine administration, and the provision of other anorexiants) are either ineffective or dangerous. Behavioral interventions have included group counseling, individual counseling, hypnosis, and provision of a liquid- or a calorie-restricted defined diet. No one intervention has been found to be most effective in treating obesity. However, interventions where group support is provided, and where there is slow weight loss, coupled with efforts to change diet and exercise habits appear to have the greatest success in maintaining weight loss.

Anorexia and bulimia are also prevalent in our society. Both are most common among adolescent females. Both syndromes are associated with a distorted body image, such that the individual perceives herself as obese. The anorexic individual combats this perceived obesity by markedly limiting food intake, often associated with excessive exercise. Bulimia is associated with binge eating of excessive quantities of food, followed by purging the body by self-induced vomiting, diarrhea, or diuresis. Death is a possible consequence of both syndromes if effective psychologic intervention cannot be provided.

Clinical Example

1. A 34-year-old male required removal of a large portion of small bowel secondary to complications of an abdominal gunshot wound. Subsequently, he was unable to maintain his usual weight with oral intake and was hospitalized to start long-term parenteral feeding. His weight (154 lb.) was 90% of usual weight. His serum albumin was 3.4 g/dl and urine urea nitrogen (UUN) was 11 g/24 hours.

A permanent central venous catheter was placed surgically, and the patient was begun on parenteral feedings. The initial formulation consisted of 2.4 liters of solution daily (35 ml/kg fluid daily) containing 42.5 g/liter of amino acids and a 25% glucose concentration as well as standard amounts of electrolytes, vitamins, and trace elements. This formulation was supplemented with 500-ml infusions of a 10% lipid emulsion twice weekly. On this program, the patient maintained a weight between 155 and 160 pounds and his albumin rose to 3.7 g/dl. A repeat UUN was 11 g/24 hour. In addition to parenteral feedings, the patient was given small oral feedings of a commercially available enteral product. He was able to tolerate steadily increasing amounts of oral feedings without excessive diarrhea, after several months. He was then switched to regular food. Eventually, parenteral feedings, which had been tapered as his diet was advanced, were discontinued.

Discussion.   This formulation provided a total of 102 g (42.5 g/liter × 2.4 liters) of protein daily which is 1.5 g/kg body weight. The caloric intake calculation is slightly more complicated. The glucose contribution is 2040 kcal (250 g/liter × 2.4 liters × 3.4 kcal/g) daily. The 10% fat emulsion would provide 1100 kcal weekly (9 kcal/g for lipids plus 200 kcal/liter for the emulsifiers). Therefore average total caloric intake would be 2198 kcal daily (2040 kcal/day × 7 days plus 1100 kcal/week divided by 7 days). The kcal : N ratio would then be 129 : 1 (2198 kcal/102 g of protein which is 16% nitrogen). To calculate nitrogen balance, a factor of 4 g of nitrogen daily (to approximate nonurinary nitrogen losses) would be added to the measured UUN for a total of 15 g of nitrogen excreted. Since the intake was 17 g (16% of 102 g protein), the nitrogen balance would be a +2 g. In this example, the clinical response to feeding was a stable body weight, wound healing, and improvement of gut function.

Biochemically, the increase in serum albumin and positive nitrogen balance reflected the clinical assessment. This example presents a typical clinical situation in which parenteral feeding was appropriate initially. The subsequent recovery and transition to enteral or oral feeding would have been unlikely or impossible without the ability to support the patient through the recovery period. Some patients with short bowel syndrome will require permanent parenteral feeding, either for nutrients or fluid balance.

Bibliography

Baker JP, Detsky AS, Wesson DE, et al. Nutritional assessment: A comparison of clinical judgment and objective measurements. *N Eng J Med* 306:969–972, 1982. *This article demonstrates that critical clinical appraisal is as accurate as other methods to assess protein calorie malnutrition.*

Bernard M, Jacobs DO, and Rombeau J. *Nutritional and Metabolic Support of Hospitalized Patients.* Philadelphia: Saunders, 1986. *This is a handy spiral-bound handbook of nutrition.*

Bistrian BR, Blackburn GL, Sherman M, et al. Therapeutic index of nutritional depletion in hospitalized patients. *Surg Gynecol Obstet* 141:512–516, 1975. *A classic article delineating the prevalence of protein calorie malnutrition in hospitalized patients.*

Cahill GF Jr. Starvation in man. *N Eng J Med* 282:668–675, 1970. *A classic article on the pathophysiology of starvation in man.*

Rombeau JL and Caldwell M (eds.). *Clinical Nutrition: Enteral and Tube Feeding.* Philadelphia: Saunders, 1988. *This is one of the best textbooks on nutrition.*

Part II Questions: Digestive Diseases and Nutrition

1. Which of the following is most characteristic of an esophageal motility disorder?
   A. Progressive solid dysphagia
   B. Globus sensation
   C. Intermittent solid dysphagia
   D. Water brash
   E. Solid and liquid dysphagia

2. Which of the following have been suggested as pathogenic mechanisms in patients with duodenal ulcer?
   A. Increased basal acid output
   B. Increased sensitivity of the parietal cells to gastrin
   C. Impaired duodenal bicarbonate secretion
   D. Ingestion of anti-inflammatory drugs
   E. All of the above

3. Which phase of pancreatic secretion accounts for the majority of enzyme secretion into the duodenum?
   A. Cephalic
   B. Gastric
   C. Celiac
   D. Intestinal
   E. Humoral

4. Portal hypertension may be seen with each of the following conditions except
   A. Splenic vein thrombosis.
   B. Cirrhosis due to alcohol.
   C. Hepatic vein thrombosis.
   D. Portal vein thrombosis.
   E. Inferior vena cava thrombosis.

5. Which one of the following is *false* with respect to malabsorption syndrome (MAS)?
   A. Deficiency of bile salts leads to carbohydrate malabsorption.
   B. Steatorrhea may be seen in chronic pancreatitis.
   C. Small bowel resection may lead to decreased absorption of nutrients.
   D. Impaired vitamin B_{12} absorption may be seen in Crohn's disease.
   E. Gastroduodenal surgery may lead to iron deficiency anemia.

6. The following statements regarding diverticular disease are true except
   A. Diverticular disease occurs most commonly in sigmoid colon.
   B. Diverticulitis is most common in Western societies.
   C. Fever, increased WBC count, and left lower quadrant pain are indicators of acute diverticulitis.
   D. Diverticular bleeding is a common cause of iron-deficiency anemia.
   E. Diverticular bleeding is usually from the right colon.

7. An 80-year-old woman presents to the hospital with severe wasting apparently due to metastatic carcinoma. She is noted to have a smooth, beefy red tongue. The most likely cause is deficiency of
   A. Vitamin C.
   B. Essential fatty acids.
   C. Vitamin A.
   D. Vitamin E.
   E. Vitamin B_{12}.

III Endocrine and Metabolic Disorders

Part Editor

David C. Kem

22 Hormone Action

R. Hal Scofield

Objectives

After completing this chapter, you should be able to

Discuss the classification of hormones on the basis of structure, mechanism of action, or second messenger employed

Delineate the feedback mechanisms that regulate hormone production and describe the clinical importance of this regulation

Describe the common characteristics of hormone receptors

Outline the major classes of steroid hormones and describe their common mechanism of action

Describe the three classes of cell surface receptors

Outline the mechanisms and effectors of action for hormones that bind cell surface receptors

List the major human genetic defects in hormone receptors that lead to endocrine disease

Describe the "hormone spillover" concept and name several examples

---

Overview

This chapter outlines the different types of hormones and their receptors, the mechanism of action of the various classes of hormones and pathophysiologic processes that can affect hormonal action.

Intercellular Communication

Complex multicellular organisms must possess information systems by which cells and organs communicate. One of the primary mechanisms of communication is hormonal. At present, more than 100 different hormones have been identified in man. These substances are secreted by specific cell types and have unique target cell specificity. The target cell of a hormone may be distant from the cell secreting the hormone such that the hormone travels via the circulatory system to the target site (an endocrine effect). Alternatively, the target cells may be located adjacent to, or near, the secretory cells (a paracrine effect). Finally, the secretory cell and the target cell may be one and the same (an autocrine effect).

Hormones mediate a change in the metabolic activity of the target cell with which they interact. The ability of a cell to respond and be influenced by a given hormone is determined by the presence of a specific receptor for that hormone. Thus target cells for a particular hormone can be identified by the presence of hormone-specific receptors.

Classification of Hormones

Hormones can be classified in several ways. One convenient system is by chemical structure, such as steroid, peptide, and amine hormones. The last group includes the catecholamines that are closely akin in mechanism of action to peptide hormones as well as the thyroid hormones that are more like steroid hormones. Interaction of hormones with specific receptors usually leads to the generation of second mediators (e.g., cyclic AMP or cyclic GMP) within the target cell. Thus hormones may also be classified according to the second messengers which propagate their biologic effect. Finally, hormones can be classified into those that act at the cell surface (e.g., peptides and cat-

221

echolamines) and those that interact with receptors within the target cell (e.g., steroid and thyroid hormones).

Function of Hormones

Hormones facilitate cell-cell communication; however, at the level of complex multicellular organisms, hormones have several broadly classifiable functions. For example, reproduction is regulated by hormone production. In the adult this includes production of gametes, but the divergent development of males and females from embryonic life to young adulthood, including anatomic and functional differences, is under the control of various hormones. For example, development of male external genitalia depends on exposure of the fetus to androgens. Growth and development unrelated to reproduction are also subject to complex hormonal regulation. Intermediate metabolism, including storage of energy and conversion of food into energy, are under exquisitely tight control of the endocrine system.

Hormones may act on many processes. Thyroid hormone, for example, interacts with virtually every organ and cell type. Thus under- or overproduction of thyroid hormone can lead to protean manifestations. This is best exemplified by congenital absence of the thyroid. Left untreated, these children have profound deficits in most every aspect of growth and development. Especially severely affected is neurological development, with profound mental retardation. On the other hand, a single process (such as maintenance of serum glucose or calcium) may be affected by many hormones. Maintenance of serum glucose or calcium is a complex interplay of many hormones and organ systems.

Regulation of Hormones

Production of hormones is regulated by feedback systems. In these systems the endocrine organ receives a signal, or signals, that influence hormone production. For the pituitary and its target organs (the thyroid, adrenals, and gonads), the regulatory signal is the hormone produced by the targets (Fig. 22-1). Alternatively, the feedback regulator need not be another hormone. Glucose concentration is the major regulator of insulin and glucagon production, while tonicity of body water controls vasopressin release.

From a clinical standpoint, the feedback regulation of hormone production means that assessment of the status of a particular endocrine system usually requires simultaneous measurement of the hormone as well as an assessment of its effect. Thus serum parathyroid hormone (PTH) levels are not interpretable without knowing the serum cal-

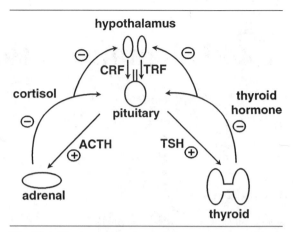

Fig. 22-1. The hypothalamic-pituitary-adrenal/thyroid axis. Adrenocorticotropic hormone (ACTH) or thyroid stimulating hormone (TSH) produced in the pituitary stimulates the target organs. Cortisol and thyroid hormone then negatively feed back on the pituitary (and also the hypothalamus) to regulate their own production. CRF = corticotropin releasing factor. TRF = thyrotropin releasing factor.

cium. For example, an elevated PTH is an appropriate response to hypocalcemia; however, the same level of PTH may be inappropriate if the calcium is elevated or in the high normal range.

Hormone Receptors

Peptide hormone receptors are on the target tissue cell surface and binding of the ligand to the receptor induces production of intracellular second messengers. Steroid, thyroid, and retinoic acid receptors lie within the cell and the hormones passively enter the target cell in most cases. With these hormones, a hormone-receptor complex mediates the biologic action by entering the nucleus and altering transcription. In either case, the receptor is intimately involved in the biologic action of the hormone.

Receptors share certain properties. (1) There is a limited amount of hormone that can be bound by a target cell. That is, receptor sites are saturable by the hormone. (2) Receptors have a high affinity for their hormone because, in general, endocrine hormones circulate at very low concentrations (paracrine and autocrine hormonal effects, however, may be dependent on hormone concentration in a very limited area). (3) A given hormone receptor must have specificity for its hormone such that the hormone exerts its effect at that receptor and not at others. Receptor specificity can extend to an entire class of hormones, however. For example, while testosterone and its metabolite dihydrotestosterone are the physiologically important androgens, other natural or synthetic androgenic hormones may bind the receptor and produce an effect. (4) Receptors have tissue specificity. Target cells either exclusively have receptors for the hormone or have the receptors in greater numbers than nontarget cells.

Abnormal Hormone Action

An event, either genetic or acquired, that alters a hormonal cascade can lead to a decrease or an increase in a regulated metabolic pathway. Thus disturbances of the hormone, the receptor, or post-receptor processes have been identified. In addition, increased concentrations of another hormone not usually bound by a particular receptor may occasionally perturb the system and lead to a pathologic state.

Steroid Hormones

Structure and Production

Steroid hormones are produced by chemical modification of cholesterol. The major classes of steroid hormones are distinguished by characteristic chemical structural changes. These classes include (1) glucocorticoids such as cortisol, (2) mineralocorticoids such as aldosterone, (3) androgens such as testosterone, (4) estrogens such as estradiol, and (5) vitamin D metabolites such as the hormonally active metabolite 1,25-dihydroxyvitamin D (Fig. 22-2). As a result of their derivation from a common precursor, these hormones all have a similar chemical structure. Synthesis of steroid hormones is the result of a series of enzymatically catalyzed steps that progressively modify the cholesterol backbone.

The activities of the various enzymes in the adrenal gland (and in other organs) that produce steroid hormones respond to specific hormonal stimuli. So, for example, the production of cortisol is under the influence of ACTH, produced in the pituitary.

Steroid Receptors

Structure

Much like the steroid hormones, the steroid receptors are structurally similar. These receptors are members of a large family of proteins which share several distinct features. Each member contains three regions of amino acid homology that are known as C1, C2, and C3. The cysteine-rich C1 domain is known to bind DNA and is highly con-

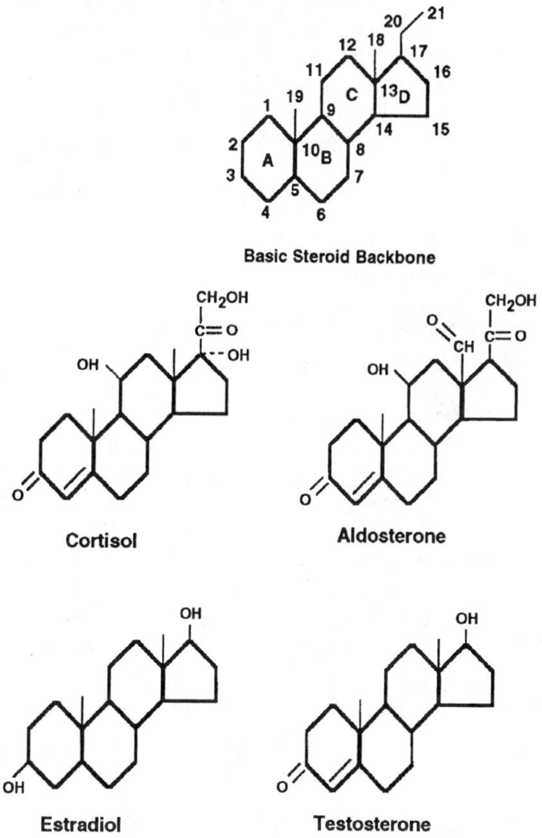

Fig. 22-2. Structure of the basic steroid backbone molecule as well as the structure of the prototypical member of the major classes of steroid hormones.

served among steroid receptors. The completely conserved cysteines within the C1 domain form two zinc-finger motifs that mediate binding to DNA. The functions of the C2 and C3 regions are not known. Several other functional domains have been identified, such as the carboxyl terminus, which serves to bind the steroid ligand.

Location of Steroid Receptors

Steroid receptors are found in low concentration in cells, ranging from 0.001% to 0.1% of the total protein. With hormone present the complex of steroid hormone and receptor is located in the nucleus. In the absence of hormone, gonadal hormone receptors seem to be primarily located in the nucleus while glucocorticoid receptors are cytosolic.

In general there are two mechanisms by which proteins

enter the nuclei of cells. One is passive diffusion through the nuclear membrane. The second is movement through a nuclear pore. The latter is facilitated by a translocation signal. Several steroid receptors have been shown to contain an amino acid sequence that functions as such a signal. The action of steroid hormones requires a nuclear location of the hormone/receptor complex.

Mechanism of Action of Steroid Hormones

Transcription in Eukaryotic Cells

Transcription of messenger RNA begins at the CAP site and upstream from this site are important regulators of transcription. Beginning only about 30 bases upstream from the CAP site are promoters. These elements include the TATA box that binds up to five transcription factors, including RNA polymerase II. Binding of these factors by the TATA box is required for transcription. Upstream of the promoters are the so-called enhancers. These sites interact with a trans element (i.e., one not part of the genomic DNA) to promote transcription. For purposes of this discussion, enhancers can be divided into steroid-responsive and steroid-independent. Thus genes whose transcription is affected by steroids have steroid response elements (SREs) in the upstream 5' region (Fig. 22-3).

Fig. 22-3. The pathway of action of steroid hormones. Hormone (labeled S) diffuses from the extracellular space into the cell and is bound by cytosolic (or nuclear) receptors. Binding of hormone induces a conformational change in the receptor such that the complex of hormone and receptor binds the steroid response elements (SREs) in the 5' region of regulated genes. This binding promotes and stabilizes binding of transcription factor (TF) to the TATA box promoter. Thus transcription of mRNA is increased.

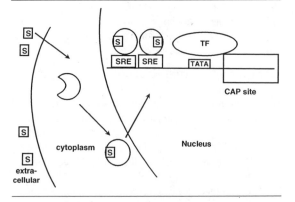

Steroid/Receptor Complex Effect on Transcription

When steroid receptor is bound to its specific hormone, the resulting conformational change enhances binding to SREs in genes regulated by the hormone. Binding affinity of a single receptor/hormone complex to its SRE is weak but is greatly enhanced by binding of a dimer to the SRE. In fact, genes may have two or more SREs such that an especially stable tetramer of the steroid hormone receptor complex can form. Binding of the upstream SREs by steroid hormone/receptor complex facilitates TATA box binding of transcription factors. With transcription factors bound more often and more stably, transcription is initiated more often and more mRNA is produced. Eventually this translates into increased protein product production and the biologic effect mediated by the hormone.

Peptide and Amine Hormones

Introduction

Unlike steroid hormones that are structurally related and arise from a single gene family, the peptide and amine hormones are a diverse group. Nonetheless, there are significant commonalities among these hormones and their receptors in mechanisms of action and structure. This section will discuss the structure and production of these hormones, their cell surface receptors, and the mechanism by which the receptor/hormone complex tranduces signal to achieve an effect.

Structure and Production

Peptide hormones range in size from several amino acids to large globular proteins with hundreds of amino acid residues. The catecholamines are amino acid analogues and are considered with the peptide hormones because of similarities in the properties of the hormones as well as their receptors. The peptide hormones are usually synthesized in the ribosomes as prohormones that are hormonally inactive. In the golgi, peptide and amine hormones are modified and packaged into secretory granules. These granules fuse with the plasma membrane (a process known as exocytosis) in response to specific stimuli to release the hormones.

Cell Surface Receptors

Structure

These receptors span the plasma membrane and have specialized extracellular, transmembrane, and intracellular domains. There are three major classes of cell surface receptor — the receptor kinases, G protein-linked receptors, and ion channel-linked receptors (Fig. 22-4). Even within the classes, however, there is wide variation. The ligand may vary from small molecules such as amino acids or catecholamines to large glycoproteins such as thyrotropin. The second messenger may differ within a class.

In the receptor kinase class, the effector mechanism is part of the intracellular portion of the receptor. The insulin receptor is the prototype of the receptor kinase class. With binding of insulin, the intracellular portion of the receptor induces phosphorylation of certain residues of the receptor itself. Thus the insulin receptor has the property of auto-phosphorylation. This auto-phosphorylation initiates additional phosphorylation of intracellular proteins that mediate insulin biologic activity.

A second class of receptors are linked to G proteins. These comprise the largest family of cell surface receptors.

Structurally, these receptors contain seven transmembrane domains of 20 to 30 amino acids. The intracellular portion of the receptor is linked to an intracellular effector such as adenylate cyclase or guanylate cyclase by virtue of a G protein complex (see Fig. 22-4).

Another class of cell membrane receptors has an ion channel specific for a cation such as sodium, calcium, or potassium as an intrinsic portion of the molecule. There are either four or six transmembrane regions and the functional unit consists of a multimer.

Some cell surface receptors have no known intrinsic function such as those described above. Included are receptors for a variety of cytokines as well as the growth hormone and prolactin receptors. The extracellular portion of several of these receptors circulate in the blood and serve as serum binding proteins for their respective hormones.

Fig. 22-4. The general structure of the three classes of cell surface receptors are shown. In the receptor kinases, binding of hormones induces intrinsic tyrosine kinase activity of the intracellular portion of the receptor. The G protein coupled receptors are linked to an effector molecule that produces a second messenger such as cAMP or IP$_3$. Conversely, the G protein complex may couple the receptor to an ion channel. On the other hand, some ion channels are part of the receptor itself and are termed ligand-gated ion channels.

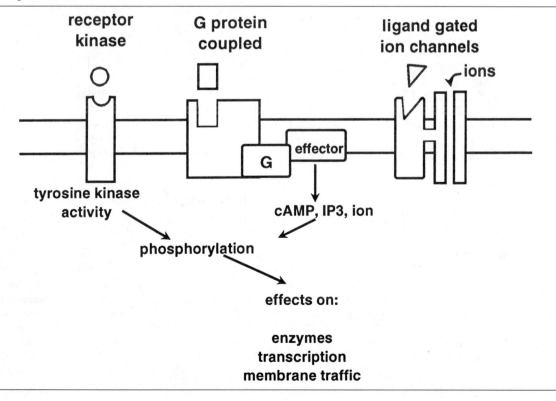

Mechanisms of Action

The hormone/receptor systems change cell metabolism by only a few processes. These include covalent modification of cellular enzymes, usually by phosphorylation/dephosphorylation of hydroxyl-containing amino acid residues. A phosphate group is transferred from adenosine triphosphate (ATP) to an amino acid residue with a hydroxyl group. In addition to serine, both threonine and tyrosine can be phosphorylated. Phosphorylation is accomplished by protein kinases while dephosphorylation is performed by protein phophatases. The catalytic activity of enzymes that are the targets of kinases and phophatases depends on the state of phosphorylation. The activity of one enzyme may be increased with phosphorylation while another enzyme may show a decrease.

Alternatively, binding of ligand to receptor may affect gene expression. The mechanisms by which gene expression is regulated by peptide hormone are poorly understood; however, it is likely that most involve activation of protein kinases that phosphorylate transcription factors that then affect transcription of mRNA. The "cAMP response element binding protein" is putatively one such factor. This protein is phosphorylated by cAMP-dependent kinases and binds specific DNA sequences of cAMP-responsive genes.

Cellular metabolism can be altered by a third mechanism, namely, regulation of membrane transport by cell surface receptor/hormone complexes. The effect is accomplished by receptors that are directly coupled to an ion channel. In addition, transport of nutrients such as amino acids and glucose is regulated by indirect mechanisms. In the case of amino acids, this regulation is influenced by insulin, glucagon, glucocorticoids, and other hormones and is dependent upon cAMP. In contrast, transport of glucose is also influenced by these same hormones, but is not mediated by cAMP.

Effector Systems for Cell Surface Receptors

Adenylate Cyclase

This is an integral membrane protein that converts ATP to cAMP, which is then used as a second messenger by receptors linked to G proteins. Production of cAMP is dependent on ligand binding to a receptor (see Fig. 22-4). This promotes dissociation of GDP from the α subunit of the G protein and allows binding of GTP by the α subunit. This results in an activated G protein that can now interact with membrane-bound adenylate cyclase and affect activity.

Activation of adenylate cyclase in this manner results in production of cAMP from ATP and subsequent activation of cAMP-dependent protein kinases such as kinase A. Kinase A activity phosphorylates other intermediate messengers leading to the biologic actions of the hormone.

The system also regulates itself as activation of the G protein results in an increase of α subunit GTPase activity. Thus GTP is metabolized and the G protein complex deactivated by reassociation with GDP.

Tyrosine Kinase

The intracellular portion of this receptor has intrinsic tyrosine kinase activity that is activated by the hormone. The receptor may catalyze phosphorylation of itself or other intracellular proteins. Phosphorylation of tyrosine residues is critical to the biologic activity of these hormone/receptor systems. The events beyond this step are poorly worked out, however, even for the extensively studied insulin receptor.

Phosphatidylinositol

These receptors are linked to and activate G proteins. The G proteins are in turn linked to phospholipase C. This enzyme produces inositol 1,4,5-trisphosphate (IP_3) and diacylglycerol (DAG), which serve as second messengers. The production of IP_3 increases intracellular calcium concentration, activates calmodulin-dependent protein kinases, and produces DAG which activates protein kinase C, even under conditions of low intracellular calcium.

Ion Channels

The ion channels may be controlled (gated) by binding of peptide hormone or neurotransmitter to the channel. These receptor/channel structures are usually large multimers that form an aqueous pore through the cell membrane. Some of these receptors require G proteins.

Hormone Receptors and Disease

Receptor Defects

There are several genetic defects in which a hormone receptor is either completely absent or is present but does not bind its ligand (Table 22-1). Severe insulin resistance in the form of several distinct syndromes may result from a mutation in the insulin receptor. Laron dwarfism results from a mutation in the growth hormone receptor. This results in no hepatic production of insulinlike growth factor I (IGF-I) which mediates many of the effects of growth hor-

Table 22-1. Selected Endocrine Syndromes Caused by a Hereditary Defect in a Receptor

Receptor	Syndrome	Clinical Features

PTH
  G protein
	Albright's hereditary
	  osteodystrophy
		Body habitus, pseudohypoparathyroid

Insulin	Type A insulin resistance	Glucose intolerance, acanthosis nigracans, hyperandrogenemia
Androgen	Testicular feminization	Male genotype Female phenotype
ADH	Nephrogenic diabetes insipidus	X-linked, polyuria, polydipsia
TSH	Thyroid hormone resistance	Hypothyroid or hyperthyroid
Vitamin D	Vitamin D resistance	Rickets
GH	Laron dwarfism	Resistant to GH

mone. Recently patients with this defect have been treated with IGF-I.

Post-Receptor Defects

The prototype post-receptor defect is Type II diabetes mellitus. This disease clearly has both genetic and environmental contributions to insulin resistance. Most commonly, the insulin molecule and the receptor are structurally and functionally normal. Thus, while the physiologic and genetic defects remain to be elucidated, they are clearly post-receptor.

Genetic defects in G proteins are known (see clinical examples). In addition, certain toxins act on G proteins. For example, the cholera toxin modifies the α subunit of a stimulatory G protein in intestinal epithelia. The final result is the massive diarrhea associated with *Vibrio cholerae* or enterotoxic *E. coli* infection.

Hormone Spillover

As discussed above, hormones and their receptors are structurally related. Overproduction of one hormone may lead to that hormone binding another hormone's receptor. This in turn leads to untoward biologic actions. There are several examples of such a scenario. Severe insulin resistance with high insulin levels may produce hyperandrogenemia in women because insulin binds IGF-I receptors in the ovary (Table 22-2).

Antibodies

Antibodies that bind hormone receptor and either block or stimulate activity of the receptor are well described (Table 22-3). Graves' disease, in which anti-TSH-receptor antibodies stimulate autonomous production of thyroid hormone is the most common (the lifetime risk of Graves'

Table 22-2. Hormone Spillover Syndromes in Which Overproduction of One Hormone Leads to that Hormone Binding a Related Hormone's Receptor

Hormone	Receptor	Clinical Features
Growth hormone	Prolactin	Galactorrhea in acromegaly*
Chorionic gonadotropin	TSH	Trophoblastic tumor-induced hyperthyroidism
IGF II	Insulin	Tumor-induced hypoglycemia
Insulin	Ovarian IGF I	Hyperandrogenemia
PTH-RP	Bone and kidney PTH	Hypercalcemia of malignancy
Cortisol	Aldosterone	Mineralocorticoid effects in Cushing's disease†

* Some patients with acromegaly have an elevated prolactin with galactorrhea on that basis, not hormonal spillover.
† In fact there is only one receptor for these two classes of steroid hormone that distinguishes them by an enzymatic function. With overproduction of glucocorticoids, the enzymatic system may be overwhelmed such that mineralocorticoid effect results from binding of the receptor by glucocorticoids.

Table 22-3. Antireceptor Antibody Syndromes

Receptor	Syndrome	Clinical Features
Insulin	Type B insulin resistance	Diabetes mellitus, acanthosis nigracans
Insulin	Antibody-mediated hypoglycemia	Fasting or post-prandial hypoglycemia
TSH	Graves' disease	Hyperthyroidism
Acetylcholine	Myasthenia gravis	Weakness

disease is 2% for women in the United States) and best known example.

Clinical Examples

1. An 18-year-old woman reported that she has never had a period. Breast development began at age 12 and proceeded normally. On physical examination she was tall (5 feet, 10 inches) but had a normal female body habitus. There was no pubic or axillary hair. A pelvic examination revealed normal female external genitalia and a blind-ending vagina without a cervix. Laboratory showed normal routine chemistries, urinalysis, and blood counts. A serum testosterone was markedly elevated for a woman, however. An analysis of the chromosomes showed 46-XY.

Discussion.   This patient provided the classic presentation of the rare disorder known as testicular feminization. These individuals have a defect in the androgen receptor. Many different mutations have been described, including some in which hormone is not bound, and others in which hormone is bound, but there is reduced binding to SRE of androgen-regulated genes. As a result, these patients have no effect of androgen despite the presence of circulating hormone. In utero, development of male external genitalia and testicular descent require androgen; thus these genetic males are born with female genitalia. On the other hand, there is no defect in the müllerian-inhibiting hormone produced by the testes, so the müllerian structures (cervix, uterus, and Fallopian tubes) regress normally.

Secondary sexual characteristics depend on the ratio of estrogen and testosterone effect. Since testosterone has no effect in these patients, secondary sexual characteristics dependent on androgen, such as body hair, are not manifest. Breast development occurs normally due to circulating estrogens which are unopposed by androgens. Patients

with this syndrome function as normal females except for infertility. However, testicles are present in the abdomen or inguinal canal. Similar to other undescended testicles, there is a high risk of malignancy and they must be surgically removed.

2. A 64-year-old white man presented with 1 week of decreasing mental status. In the 4 hours prior to admission he was incoherent. His wife reported that in the preceding 2 weeks he had mild polyuria and that for the last 2 months had occasionally coughed up blood-tinged sputum. He has smoked two packs of cigarettes a day for more than 50 years.

Laboratory showed the serum calcium to be markedly elevated at 17.3 mg/dl (normal 8.5–10.5 mg/dl). A chest radiograph demonstrated a 5-cm-diameter mass in the right upper lobe. After correction of his fluid and electrolyte status, a biopsy obtained at fiberoptic bronchoscopy showed squamous cell carcinoma of the lung.

Discussion.   Squamous cell carcinoma of the lung or upper airway is occasionally associated with hypercalcemia. While there are several mechanisms for hypercalcemia of malignancy, in the majority of patients with a squamous cell carcinoma, the tumor is producing a hormone known as parathyroid hormone-related protein (PTH-RP).

The physiologic role of PTH-RP is unknown but the protein and its mRNA are found in squamous epithelium and lactating mammary glands, where the hormone may have a paracrine or autocrine effect. The physiologic receptor for PTH-RP is unknown but may be identical to the PTH receptor. PTH-RP is structurally related to PTH in the amino terminal 13 amino acids, which mediate binding to the PTH receptor. In patients with squamous cell carcinoma producing PTH-RP, the hormone travels via the circulatory system to bone and kidney, binds the PTH receptor, and produces many biologic effects of PTH. The unregulated stimulation of the PTH receptor results in severe hypercalcemia.

Thus overproduction of PTH-RP by squamous cell carcinomas results in this hormone binding a receptor for a related hormone (PTH) that is not usually bound under normal physiology. There are several other examples of such "hormonal spillover" (see Table 22-3).

3. A 23-year-old woman presented for routine followup of mild hypertension and hypothyroidism. She was extremely short (height 4 feet, 7 inches), had a stocky body habitus with a round face and short hands, especially the fourth metacarpal (Fig. 22-5). She reported that her

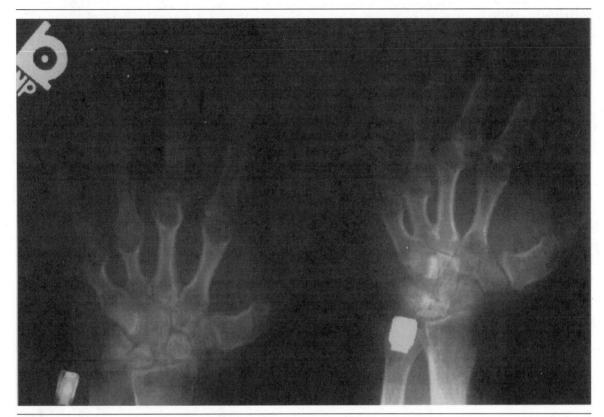

Fig. 22-5. Radiographs of the hands of a 23-year-old woman with pseudopseudohypoparathyroidism (described in case 3 of clinical examples). The characteristic features, including a short fourth metacarpal, are apparent.

brother, father, and paternal grandmother were all less than 5 feet tall. In addition, they had a body habitus similar to the patient; however, only the father had been diagnosed with hypocalcemia and hypoparathyroidism.

Discussion.   This family represents the spectrum of Albright's hereditary osteodystrophy (AHO). The father has pseudohypoparathyroidism (biochemical features of hypoparathyroidism not due to deficiency of PTH). Other family members have pseudopseudohypoparathyroidism (similar body habitus but normal calcium and phosphorus levels). All can be anticipated to have a genetic defect in the α subunit of the stimulatory G (G_s) protein associated with the parathyroid hormone receptor. Levels of both the $G_s\,\alpha$ protein and mRNA are half normal in AHO, with or without pseudohypoparathyroidism. In those with pseudohypoparathyroidism, PTH levels are elevated but the signal is not transferred to adenylate cyclase; thus the name pseudohypoparathyroidism.

This family is typical in that all affected members have the characteristic body habitus, while some have pseudohypoparathyroidism and some do not. The mechanism for this phenomenon is not completely understood, but evidence suggests that the sex of parent from whom one inherits the gene is important, i.e., imprinting. When maternally transmitted, pseudohypoparathyroidism is found. When paternally transmitted, pseudopseudohypoparathyroidism is found.

The genetically defective $G_s\,\alpha$ protein is associated with other receptors and so some patients have hypothyroidism and/or hypogonadism. The physiologic basis of the skeletal abnormalities is unknown but could be related to resistance to PTH or some other hormone whose receptor utilizes the defective $G_s\,\alpha$ subunit.

Bibliography

Baniahmad A, Tsau MJ. Mechanisms of transcriptional activation by steroid hormone receptors. *J Cell Biochem* 51:151–156, 1993. *A review of the molecular actions of steroids.*

Kahn CR, Smith RJ, Chin WW. Mechanism of action of hormones that act at the cell surface. In Wilson JD and Foster DW (eds.). *Williams Textbook of Endocrinology,* 8th ed. Philadelphia: Saunders, 1992, pp. 91–134. *A comprehensive review of peptide and amine hormones with 361 references.*

Langley JN. On nerve endings and on special excitable substances. *Proc Roy Soc* (London) 78:170–194, 1906. *This work on nicotine and curare is the origin of the idea that cells contain receptors for specific substances.*

Weinstein LS and Shenker A. G protein mutations in human disease. *Clin Biochem* 26:333–338, 1993. *A concise review of G protein-related human diseases.*

23 Adrenal-ACTH

Dale A. Freeman

Objectives

After completing this chapter, you should be able to

Understand the major regulation of glucocorticoid and mineralocorticoid synthesis

Know the causes of Cushing's syndrome

Know the signs and symptoms of Cushing's syndrome

Know the principles underlying diagnostic tests designed to differentiate Cushing's disease from other causes of Cushing's syndrome

Know the causes of Addison's disease

Know the signs and symptoms of Addison's disease

Understand how renin and aldosterone values are employed to diagnose primary hyperaldosteronism

---

Normal Adrenal Cortical Function

The adrenals are functionally two separate glands that have been anatomically merged. The medulla synthesizes catecholamines while the cortex synthesizes steroid hormones. This chapter deals with the adrenal cortex. The cortex is divided into three zones that are anatomically distinguishable from each other. The zona fasciculata and the zona reticularis are controlled by ACTH and synthesize mainly the glucocorticoid, cortisol, but also small amounts of androgens and estrogens. The outer and smallest zone, the zona glomerulosa, is specialized to synthesize aldosterone. Aldosterone, a mineralocorticoid that acts to regulate sodium balance, is mainly under the control of the renin-angiotensin system. It is important to realize that the adrenal cortex synthesizes all classes of steroid hormones, since many manifestations of adrenal disease are related to excessive production of one or more of these hormones.

Cortisol: Control of Secretion and Biologic Action

Cortisol synthesis is regulated by adrenal corticotropic hormone (ACTH) which, in turn, is controlled by the hypo-thalamic hormone corticotropin-releasing hormone (CRH), as well as other hypothalamic factors such as arginine vasopressin (AVP). Secretion of ACTH is controlled by negative feedback, has an intrinsic diurnal variation, and will increase acutely with stress.

Feedback regulation occurs when hypothalamic and anterior pituitary centers sensitive to cortisol respond to decreasing blood cortisol levels by increasing CRH and ACTH secretion respectively. Conversely, increased cortisol levels cause the hypothalamic centers to release less CRH. CRH, in turn, regulates the release of ACTH, which controls the adrenal synthesis of steroids. Additional control by cortisol occurs at the level of the pituitary and can partially offset the effect of CRH.

Circadian control of ACTH secretion occurs because the set point for hypothalamic secretion of CRH varies during the day. The physical or chemical nature of this variation is not understood. In persons who are awake during the day and sleep at night, plasma ACTH levels are greatest in the morning and lowest in the late evening. As a consequence, cortisol levels vary with a similar pattern.

Either physical or emotional stress causes CRH secretion to increase, which in turn releases ACTH and subsequently increases the plasma level of cortisol. This increase totally overrides the usual set point mechanism for controlling ACTH release. The bypassing or overriding of the set point occurs when higher CNS centers respond to the stress and induce hypothalamic CRH secretion.

Figure 23-1 depicts the regulation of CRH and ACTH secretion and of cortisol biosynthesis.

Glucocorticoids are essential for life and have a number of known metabolic effects. Like all steroid hormones, glucocorticoids bind to specific protein receptors that, when activated, bind DNA and act as transcriptional regulators. Various gene products are then induced or suppressed by the hormone-receptor transcriptional regulator. These proteins change the function of targeted cells. In the liver glucocorticoids cause glycogen levels to increase, stimulate gluconeogenesis, and increase ketogenesis, thereby increasing fuel sources for the body. In adipose tissue these steroids cause free fatty acid and glycerol levels to rise while decreasing glucose utilization and triglyceride formation. In both muscle and collagen, there is decreased protein synthesis and increased protein breakdown. Glucocorticoids also decrease the utilization of glucose by muscle.

Fig. 23-1. Control of ACTH and cortisol release. Hypothalamic corticotrophin-releasing hormone (CRF) or arginine vasopressin (AVP) cause pituitary release of adrenocorticotrophic hormone (ACTH). The adrenals respond to ACTH by releasing cortisol that in turn feeds back on both the hypothalamus and pituitary.

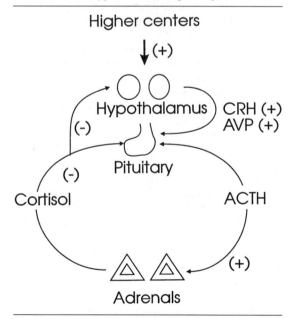

Aldosterone: Control of Secretion and Biologic Action

Aldosterone synthesis is controlled by two major regulatory systems. The major control of aldosterone synthesis is by the renin-angiotensin system. The juxtaglomerular cells of the kidney release renin in response to changes in effective blood volume or chloride flux in the distal tubule. Renin release is also stimulated by sympathetic nerve stimulation. Once released, renin — a proteolytic enzyme — cleaves angiotensin I from the α_2, globin, renin substrate. Angiotensin I is converted into the biologically active angiotensin II by a pulmonary-converting enzyme. Angiotensin II has two major actions, stimulation of aldosterone release and acting as a potent vascular smooth-muscle constrictor.

The serum potassium concentration is also a regulator of aldosterone synthesis. Increasing potassium concentration results in more aldosterone synthesis while hypokalemia markedly inhibits aldosterone synthesis. This later effect is important clinically in that hyperaldosteronism induces hypokalemia that, in turn, reduces aldosterone synthesis. Therefore, adequate evaluation of hyperaldosteronism requires measurements made after hypokalemia is corrected.

Synthesis of aldosterone is also stimulated by ACTH, but the effect is minor and transient. Aldosterone synthesis returns to normal in about 2 days despite continued ACTH stimulation. Fig. 23-2 depicts the control of aldosterone synthesis.

Fig. 23-2. Control of aldosterone release. Blood volume-sensitive cells in the juxtaglomular apparatus of the kidney release renin when they sense reduced blood volume. Renin converts a plasma protein, renin substrate, to angiotensin I. Angiotensin I is converted by angiotensin-converting enzyme (ACE) to angiotensin II. Angiotensin II acts directly as a vasoconstrictor, but also stimulates the release of aldosterone. Aldosterone causes renal sodium retention and restores blood volume, preventing further renin release.

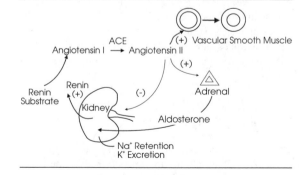

Aldosterone controls a sodium-potassium pump in the renal tubule. The effect of activating this receptor is to enhance sodium reabsorbtion and potassium secretion in the distal nephron. Like all steroid hormones, aldosterone works through a protein receptor. This receptor cannot differentiate glucocorticoid from mineralocorticoid but the kidney cell uses the enzyme 11β-hydroxysteroid dehydrogenase to alter glucocorticoids so they are not recognized by the receptor. However, if this glucocorticoid-inactivating enzyme is incapacitated by such compounds as licorice (glycyrrhizic acid) or overwhelmed by very high concentrations of cortisol, glucocorticoids will then activate the mineralocorticoid receptor.

Disease States

Cushing's Syndrome

Excessive glucocorticoid levels produce Cushing's syndrome. This can be a consequence of medical treatment; an ACTH-producing pituitary tumor; ectopic ACTH production from a tumor such as a small cell carcinoma of the lung; an adrenal tumor; or, very rarely, a CRH-producing tumor. Some symptoms and signs differ between these causes of the syndrome.

Usually iatrogenic Cushing's syndrome produces a syndrome of pure glucocorticoid excess since adrenal function is suppressed and no adrenal androgens or estrogens are produced. In such patients, a Cushingoid body habitus would be expected. The patients show central obesity since glucocorticoids cause preferential wasting of peripheral fat. This centripetal fat distribution includes the prominent supraclavicular fat pads and buffalo hump characteristic of Cushing's syndrome. The marked protein catabolism caused by glucocorticoids results in striae and fragility of the skin, muscle weakness, and poor wound healing. In-

Table 23-1. Causes of Cushing's Syndrome

Exogenous glucocorticoids — iatrogenic
Cushing's disease — pituitary microadenoma
Adrenal tumors
    Adenoma
    Carcinoma
Ectopic ACTH
    Small cell lung Ca
    Bronchial carcinoid
    Others
CRH-synthesizing tumors
    Pancreatic islet tumors
    Small cell lung Ca

hibition of glucose uptake and marked stimulation of gluconeogenesis result in diabetes mellitus. Markedly elevated glucocorticoid levels overwhelm kidney 11β-hydroxysteroid dehydrogenase and cause hypertension by acting as mineralocorticoid mimics. Catabolism of bone results in osteoporosis, exaggerated curvature of the spine, and sometimes fractures in other bones.

When Cushing's syndrome is caused by an ACTH-synthesizing pituitary adenoma (Cushing's disease), the effects of adrenal androgens are added to the list of symptoms and signs. These androgens cause both hirsutism and menstrual disturbances in women and acne in both sexes. Emotional effects of glucocorticoids are prominent in Cushing's disease and include an atypical form of depression that may lead to suicide. The psychiatric manifestations of Cushing's disease seem greater than the occasional "steroid psychosis" associated with exogenous glucocorticoid administration. A woman with many of the clinical signs of Cushing's disease is shown in Fig. 23-3.

The ectopic ACTH syndrome most commonly is associated with small cell lung cancer and differs from typical Cushing's syndrome in that manifestations of the cancer predominate. Patients typically present with generalized wasting and hypokalemia. Although typical signs of Cushing's syndrome are usually absent, urinary cortisol values may be extremely elevated. Cushing's syndrome produced by a benign carcinoid tumor is usually clinically indistinguishable from Cushing's disease of pituitary origin.

Adrenal tumors can cause typical Cushing's syndrome; however, the neoplasms produce significant quantities of other steroids and so commonly cause syndromes of feminization in men or virilization in women. Malignant adrenal tumors often produce large amounts of precursor steroids and sometimes produce no endocrine syndrome, but only the wasting and organ-replacement symptoms seen with other malignant neoplasms.

Since a CRH-producing tumor produces Cushing's syndrome by means of pituitary ACTH production, this syndrome resembles Cushing's disease. ACTH secretion from such a tumor may be partially suppressed in response to the potent glucocorticoid dexamethasone since the steroid feedback loop is still functioning at the level of the pituitary.

The various causes of Cushing's syndrome are differentiated by history, pituitary-adrenal suppression tests, and more recently by petrosal sinus testing for ACTH.

Cushing's syndrome caused by exogenous steroids should be discovered by history. Most commonly, this syndrome is associated with oral steroid treatment of rheumatic or pulmonary disease; however, topical steroids or even inhaled steroids can cause the syndrome.

The usual differential diagnostic problem is in differen-

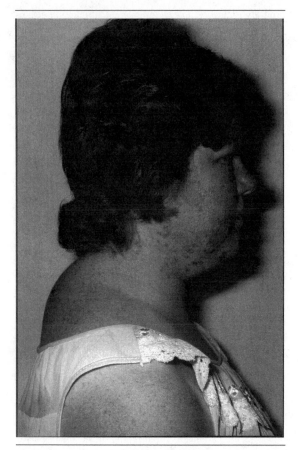

Fig. 23-3. Side view of a patient with Cushing's disease. (Note the obese "moon" face, the acne and hirsutism, and the buffalo hump.) [Picture provided with consent of the patient.]

tiating pituitary Cushing's disease from Cushing's syndrome caused by ectopic ACTH or an adrenal tumor. In either syndrome, cortisol levels will be high, the usual circadian variation in cortisol synthesis is obscured, and small doses of dexamethasone will not suppress cortisol levels. This presents a diagnostic problem in that the tumors producing Cushing's disease may be too small to be visualized on computerized tomography or magnetic resonance imaging. Also, since asymptomatic nonfunctional pituitary tumors are not rare, finding a tumor doesn't prove that it is hormonally active. The preferred diagnostic test, the dexamethasone suppression test, exploits the partial sensitivity of pituitary tumors to glucocorticoids such as dexamethasone. Hence a large dose of dexamethasone will partially suppress cortisol synthesis, owing to excess

ACTH secretion from a pituitary adenoma. In contrast, ectopic ACTH production or adrenal tumors are generally not dexamethasone-suppressible. Many medical centers have begun sampling the petrosal sinus that collects venous blood from the pituitary. Cushing's disease is associated with increased petrosal sinus ACTH concentration compared to that observed in the peripheral circulation.

Hypoadrenalism: Addison's Disease and ACTH Deficiency

Hypoadrenalism caused by Addison's disease (primary adrenal failure) is quite different from pituitary ACTH deficiency.

Addison's disease is either idiopathic (autoimmune) or associated with any number of destructive processes in the adrenal cortex. These destructive lesions can be caused by mycobacterium tuberculosis or atypical mycobacteria, histoplasmosis, or by CMV virus in AIDS patients. The adrenal can also be destroyed by hemorrhage during shock and by malignant replacement. By far, idiopathic or autoimmune Addison's disease is most common.

The clinical manifestations of Addison's disease are caused both by deficiency of glucocorticoids and mineralocorticoids and by excess pituitary synthesis of ACTH-related peptides. Gastrointestinal symptoms such as anorexia, nausea, vomiting, and weight loss are typical. Patients have impaired vigor and are lethargic and apathetic. Because glucocorticoid levels are inadequate, hepatic glucose production is decreased and hepatic glycogen is depleted. Hence patients often become hypoglycemic. The absence of mineralocorticoids causes plasma potassium to rise, sodium to be wasted, and leads to hypotension from salt loss. Pituitary production of melanocyte-stimulating hormone (MSH) leads to skin hyperpigmentation. This pigmentation is most striking on the buccal mucosa, over areas of trauma, over extensor surfaces, and in new scars. Typical buccal mucosa pigmentation is shown in Fig. 23-4.

Table 23-2. Causes of Addison's Disease

Idiopathic (autoimmune)
Infectious
    Tuberculosis
    Atypical mycobacteria
    Histoplasmosis
    Cytomegalovirus (CMV)
Shock and adrenal hemorrhage
Neoplastic destruction

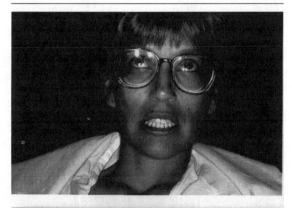

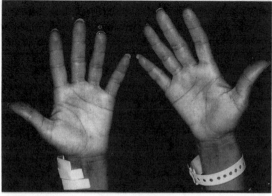

Fig. 23-4. Pigmentary changes in a patient with Addison's disease. Note the dark skin pigmentation in this normally light-complected blond woman. Note particularly the pigmentation around areas of trauma in her lips, pigmentation of her gums, the creases of her hands, and the volar aspect of her arms. [Pictures provided with consent of the patient.]

Patients with idiopathic Addison's disease often have associated vitiligo, another autoimmune disease that causes circumscribed depigmented areas of skin.

Deficiency of ACTH caused by pituitary destruction leads to a pure glucocorticoid-deficient state; however, this picture is complicated in many cases because there can also be associated deficiencies of other pituitary hormones. Pure ACTH deficiency occurs only rarely and is associated with anorexia, lethargy, and apathy. Salt balance is still maintained through the renin-angiotensin pathway, so shock from volume depletion is not a prominent feature of this syndrome. Patients on replacement hormones for panhypopituitarism can usually stop their glucocorticoid

replacement for some days without significant ill effects. In contrast, patients with Addison's disease with adrenal destruction rapidly become symptomatic.

A special form of adrenal insufficiency should be mentioned briefly. Congenital deficiencies of several enzymes required for cortisol synthesis exist. The most common is 21-hydroxylase deficiency. 21-hydroxylation is required for both mineralocorticoid and glucocorticoid synthesis, so patients with severe defects will waste salt and may die of shock. Since such infants produce large amounts of androgens, female babies with this defect are discovered early due to ambiguous genitalia, while male babies are anatomically normal and thus may not be as readily discovered. Appropriate therapy requires both glucocorticoid and mineralocorticoid replacement.

Primary Hyperaldosteronism

Overproduction of aldosterone by the adrenal glands occurs in association with discrete adenomas or with bilateral adrenal glomerulosa hyperplasia. Tumors producing hyperaldosteronism are frequently small and may be undetectable on computerized tomography. Most cases of hyperplasia are classified as idiopathic, although in one subtype (familial, dexamethasone-suppressible hyperaldosteronism) the genetic flaw has been identified.

The clinical consequences of primary hyperaldosteronism are hypertension and hypokalemia. The hypertension can be quite severe and refractory to treatment with the usual antihypertensive agents. Hypokalemia in the absence of diuretics strongly suggests hyperaldosteronism and contributes to the pathology of the disease. Hypokalemia leads to muscle weakness and may predispose to cardiac arrhythmias.

The diagnosis of primary hyperaldosteronism depends on demonstration of two characteristic features: (1) low plasma renin levels even under conditions such as upright posture and low salt intake which should stimulate renin secretion and (2) elevated plasma aldosterone levels despite saline loading which normally suppress the renin-angiotensin-aldosterone system.

Hyperaldosteronism due to an adenoma can be readily cured by surgical resection of the tumor. Medical therapy is employed in poor surgical candidates or patients with bilateral hyperplasia of the glomerulosa. The potassium-sparing diuretic spironolactone is an aldosterone (mineralocorticoid) receptor antagonist. This compound that normally would have little antihypertensive effect often effectively reduces the blood pressure of patients with hyperaldosteronism. Amiloride is also quite effective. This drug, rather than blocking the mineralocorticoid receptor, blocks the Na^+/K^+ pump that is activated/synthesized in response to aldosterone.

Isolated Hypoaldosteronism

Type IV renal tubular acidosis (RTA), is common in diabetics and is often associated with hyporeninemic hypoaldosteronism. In these patients, the juxtaglomerular apparatus does not release adequate quantities of renin. As a consequence, aldosterone levels are low and these patients typically demonstrate hyperkalemia. Since this is selective mineralocorticoid deficiency, patients generally do not develop the anorexia, fatigue, and lethargy of glucocorticoid deficiency.

Clinical Examples

1. A 43-year-old woman was referred for treatment of new onset diabetes and hypertension. In addition to these complaints she had become quite hirsute and had developed acne. On examination it was noted that she had a round face, central obesity, many bruises, and purple striae. The patient had significant proximal muscle weakness. Abnormal laboratory values included a potassium of 3.2 mg/liter, glucose of 240 mg/dl, morning cortisol of 28 µg/dl (nl = 8–24), evening cortisol of 29 µg/dl (nl = 2–15), and urinary-free cortisol of 250 µg/24 hours (nl < 105). The patient also had 17,000 WBC and no obvious source of infection. After two days on dexamethasone (0.5 mg every 6 hours) her urinary-free cortisol was 220 µg/24 hours. In contrast, when 2 mg of dexamethasone every 6 hours was given, her urinary-free cortisol fell to 80 µg/24 hours.

Cushing's disease was diagnosed and the patient was treated by transsphenoidal microsurgery to remove a microadenoma. After surgery, while still on dexamethasone, her cortisol was undetectable. She was discharged from the hospital taking hydrocortisone 20 mg orally each day. Her diabetes had resolved and her blood pressure normalized. Six months later a morning cortisol taken before her hydrocortisone dose was 12 µg/dl. One month later, while taking no hydrocortisone and after 1 mg dexamethasone given the night before, her cortisol was 2 µg/dl.

Discussion.   This patient demonstrated many of the ravages of hypercortisolism. The catabolic effects on soft tissues resulted in bruises, striae, and myopathy. Enhanced gluconeogenesis and diminished peripheral uptake of glucose resulted in diabetes. Saturation of renal 11β-hydroxysteroid dehydrogenase activated aldosterone receptors, resulting in hypertension and hypokalemia. She also demonstrated glucocorticoid-mediated leukocytosis.

Because the pituitary tumor responds to steroids but at an abnormal set point, the patient's urinary steroids did not diminish in response to a low dose of the synthetic glucocorticoid dexamethasone. However, a higher dose of dexamethasone caused partial suppression of tumor ACTH secretion. Before surgery, her cortisol values were consistently elevated and did not vary over the day as in normal persons.

Surgical removal of the tumor was curative; however, the patient did not immediately regain normal pituitary-adrenal function. Administering hydrocortisone, a short-acting glucocorticoid, once per day allowed the suppressed pituitary corticotrophs to eventually become responsive and capable of stimulating cortisol synthesis. Full recovery of the pituitary adrenal axis can take as much as one year. The tumor did not recur since the patient's cortisol levels now respond to low doses of dexamethasone.

2. A 57-year-old black man arrived by ambulance at the emergency room in shock. Blood was drawn; an electrocardiogram was taken and showed a sine wave pattern. Cardiac arrest ensued. The cardiac rhythm returned to sinus rhythm after calcium chloride administration and cardiopulmonary resuscitation. His blood pressure increased after aggressive saline infusion. Initial laboratory results included: Na^+ = 132 mEq/ml, K^+ = 8.2 mEq/liter, glucose = 37 mg/dl, bicarbonate = 12 mEq/liter. Baseline cortisol was undetectable. Despite BP of 90/50, plasma aldosterone was undetectable and plasma renin activity was > 90 ng/ml/hour (nl < 3.2).

Treatment was initiated with intravenous hydrocortisone which was subsequently given as an oral preparation. The patient also was given the mineralocorticoid fludrocortisone twice a day. After one day on this treatment his Na^+ = 142 mEq/liter, K^+ = 4.3 mEq/liter, and glucose was 122 mg/dl. His blood pressure was 140/85.

Discussion.   The patient presented with evidence of mineralocorticoid and glucocorticoid deficiency. Mineralocorticoid deficiency was evidenced by hypotension and hyperkalemia. Glucocorticoid deficiency was evidenced by hypoglycemia. Cardiac arrest was precipitated by hyperkalemia. Pigmentary changes were only noted in retrospect when it was noted that his buccal mucosa had several black spots, and he recalled noting that his skin color was darkening.

Diagnosis was confirmed when plasma cortisol was undetectable despite the presence of a potent stimulus (shock). In more subtle cases it may be necessary to demonstrate failure of the adrenal glands to respond to exogenous ACTH administration. In this patient, plasma renin was very elevated, but aldosterone was not detected, indicating complete adrenal gland failure.

Treatment consisted of a glucocorticoid and a mineralocorticoid replacement. Although hydrocortisone has some mineralocorticoid activity, fludrocortisone is a much more potent mineralocorticoid. The patient was instructed to wear a warning bracelet, double his hydrocortisone with minor stress, and keep a 3-mg syringe of dexamethasone at home, in his car, and at work. He returned to a productive life.

3. A 52-year-old white man was being evaluated for refractory hypertension. At different times he had been tried on various drugs and presently was taking clonidine 0.3 mg tid, lisinopril 40 mg qd, and extended release nifedipine 90 mg qd. Examination revealed a BP 140/102 in the left arm sitting. Further exam revealed arteriovenous crossing defects and cardiac exam revealed a S_4 gallop. Serum K^+ was 2.8 mEq/liter; urinary, K^+ was 45 mEq/24 hours; serum renin was 0.1 ng/ml/hour; and aldosterone was 65 ng/ml. After administering 500 ml saline over 30 minutes and an additional 1000 ml over 90 more minutes, aldosterone level was 61 ng/ml. Computerized tomography revealed a 1.5 cm × 2 cm left adrenal mass. Primary hyperaldosteronism owing to a left-sided adenoma was diagnosed. The patient underwent unilateral adrenalectomy. Blood pressure one day postoperatively was 160/96 when taking no antihypertensives. Two months postoperatively, his blood pressure was 140/92 on no medicines. Serum potassium was 4.7 mEq/liter.

Discussion. This is a typical presentation for hyperaldosteronism. The patient had refractory hypertension. He had low serum potassium, yet he was not conserving potassium in the urine. Plasma renin activity was quite low. Volume expansion with saline did not suppress aldosterone synthesis. Computerized tomography demonstrated an adrenal mass.

Surgical removal of the tumor significantly reduced his blood pressure. In many patients the blood pressure will not return to normal, but it will be much more easily controlled.

Bibliography

Bethune JE. The diagnosis and treatment of adrenal insufficiency. In Degroot LJ, ed. *Endocrinology* (2nd ed.). Philadelphia: Saunders, 1989, pp. 1647–1659. *A review of the clinical and laboratory features of Addison's disease.*

Freeman DA. The biochemistry of adrenal tumors. In James VHT (ed.). *The Adrenal Gland* (2nd ed.). New York: Raven, 1992, pp. 451–464. *A comprehensive review of adrenal tumor biology and biochemistry.*

Meikle AW. A diagnostic approach to Cushing's syndrome. *Endocrinologist* 3:311–320, 1993. *A coherent approach to diagnosing Cushing's disease.*

Melby, JC. Diagnosis and treatment of primary aldosteronism and isolated hypoaldosteronism. In Degroot LJ (ed.). *Endocrinology* (2nd ed.). Philadelphia: Saunders, 1989, pp. 1708–1716. *Review of mineralocorticoid excess and deficiency.*

Nelson, DH. Cushing's syndrome. In Degroot LJ (ed.). *Endocrinology* (2nd ed.). Philadelphia: Saunders, 1989, pp. 1660–1675. *A good review of diagnostic testing for Cushing's disease.*

Orth DN, Kovacs WJ, and Debold CR. The adrenal cortex. In Wilson JD and Foster DW (eds.). *Williams Textbook of Endocrinology.* Philadelphia: Saunders, 1992, pp. 489–620. *A general review of adrenal physiology and pathology.*

24 Diabetes Mellitus and Glucose Metabolism

Leann Olansky

Objectives

After completing this chapter, you should be able to

Understand the relationship between insulin and those hormones that antagonize insulin (counter-regulatory hormones) in the normal metabolic condition; this should include the physiologic responses that stimulate each hormone and the tissue effects of each hormone

Understand fuel homeostasis as related to those hormones and to feeding and fasting

Understand how this system is disturbed when diabetes or glucose intolerance develops

Discuss the etiologies of insulin-dependent and non-insulin-dependent diabetes

Understand the approach to therapy and how it is different in the different types of diabetes

Explain the chronic complications caused by diabetes and why the complications are shared by diabetic subjects of each type

Normal Physiology

Overview: Insulin vs. Counter-regulatory Hormones

Living cells require a continual source of energy to remain viable and active. Single-cell organisms achieve this end through a constant uptake of nutrients from their environment. To provide the constant delivery of energy required at the cellular level, more complex multicellular organisms like man have developed a storage and release system which permits intermittent rather than constant uptake of nutrients. In order to properly direct the flow of nutrients, a system of balancing hormones evolved. Insulin is the primary hormone involved with storage of energy and is opposed by several hormones known collectively as the counter-regulatory hormones (action opposite to that of insulin). The counter-regulatory hormones include glucagon, cortisol, epinephrine, and growth hormone. Each acts on insulin-sensitive tissues of glucose storage including liver, muscle, and adipose to release energy-rich nutrients in the form of glucose, lactate, amino acids, and free fatty acids. These hormones have overlapping activity on some of the storage tissues but function synergistically to provide both rapid and long-term delivery of nutrients to meet the needs of the organism.

The liver plays a key role in this system as a site for storage of glucose as glycogen, synthesis of triglycerides from dietary fats and glucose, and conversion of these nutrients released from storage forms into the chemical forms most easily used by cells. Glucose can be used by all tissues as an energy source. Free fatty acids and ketones may be used by many tissue but the brain has an absolute requirement for glucose and fails to function when glucose supplies fall below 1 mg/kg/minute. The brain's absolute dependency on glucose is protected by the counter-regulatory hormone system. This system prevents glucose levels from falling below a critical level that would lead to brain dysfunction, termed neuroglycopenia. Normal blood glucose levels are 70–115 mg/dl in the fasting state but some normals tolerate lower blood glucose levels without symptoms of brain dysfunction.

Insulin: Hormone of Storage

Insulin is made and released from the beta cells of the islets of Langerhans that are distributed throughout the pancreas. Insulin, like other peptide hormones, is synthesized as a longer molecule. This "pre-proinsulin" includes the signal peptide which is important for directing its proper folding and movement through the Golgi but is removed prior to storage in secretory granules. In the granules, the connecting peptide is cleaved from the proinsulin to form two separate molecules, insulin and C-peptide. The latter molecule is metabolically inert but is released in equimolar amounts with insulin and serves as a marker for insulin production by beta cells. Between feedings and when blood glucose is not elevated, insulin levels are low, usually 10 μU/ml (60 pmol/liter) or less, but never drop to zero in normal subjects. With the intake of carbohydrates, proteins, or fat, insulin is released from the beta cells into the portal circulation in transit to the liver. In response, the liver quickly switches from a glucose-producing organ to a storage depot of calories as glycogen. Excess glucose is also converted to triglycerides. Almost one half of the pancreatic insulin is extracted and the remaining insulin enters the peripheral circulation. The most important insulin-sensitive tissue is muscle as far as uptake and metabolism of glucose. Adipose tissue is much less important. The liver does take up some glucose that is stored as glycogen in the fed state but is vital for the interconversion of substrates such as glucose to fatty acids and amino acids to glucose, making the storage and mobilization of energy possible.

Insulin binds to specific receptors on the surface of target cells and triggers a series of intracellular signals. One important action is to increase the number of GLUT-4 molecules (insulin-regulable glucose transporters) on the surface of muscle and adipose tissue. The GLUT-4 transporters are stored in vesicles intracellularly and move to the surface after insulin is bound to cell surface receptors. On the surface, they facilitate glucose uptake. When insulin levels fall to basal levels, the GLUT-4 molecules return to their intracellular site and the glucose uptake falls to basal levels. Muscle glucose uptake is more responsive to insulin than is adipose tissue. Adipose tissue is the primary site for storage of triglycerides. These triglycerides are derived from dietary sources or from hepatic conversion of glucose. Lipoprotein lipase (LPL) is an important

enzyme that facilitates uptake of triglycerides by adipose tissue. The activity of LPL is greatly increased by insulin.

Glucose, amino acids, and fatty acids each lead to release of insulin from the beta cells of the pancreas. Glucose is the most potent stimulus but there appears to be a synergistic release of insulin when glucose and amino acids are coingested. Insulin is released quickly (minutes) in response to increase in portal nutrients. This "first-phase" insulin release reflects release of preformed insulin from the storage granules of the beta cells. If the nutrient flow continues, there is a sustained release of insulin. This "second phase" of insulin release can be maintained for the duration of the nutrient flux and decreases when nutrient levels fall to baseline (Fig. 24-1). Target tissues have a variable response to insulin and a characteristic uptake pattern for glucose, amino acids, or fatty acids. This peripheral uptake brings the levels of the nutrients back to baseline following a meal. Fasting glucose levels are normally 70–110 mg/dl and do not exceed 150 mg/dl under normal conditions irrespective of nutrient intake.

Insulin exerts its action by binding to receptors primarily in the liver, muscle, and adipose tissue. Insulin receptors are heterodimers of two alpha and two beta subunits held together by disulfide bonds (Fig. 24-2). The binding of insulin results in a conformational change in the het-

Fig. 24-1. Dynamics of insulin release. This is the temporal relationship of insulin release in response to infused glucose. The initial sharp peak (first phase) represents release of insulin from storage granules in the beta cells. The more slowly increasing second phase of insulin release is maintained as long as the glucose infusion continues. The second phase represents release of newly synthesized as well as stored insulin. A similar release occurs in response to oral nutrients.

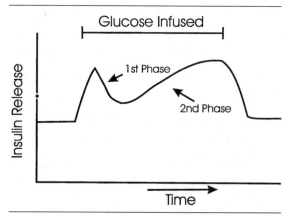

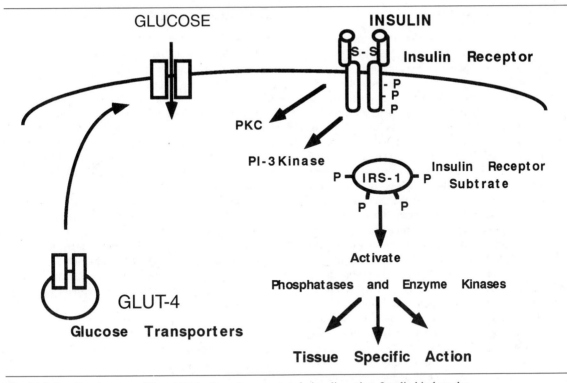

Fig. 24-2. Insulin receptor and the multiple downstream events in insulin action. Insulin binds to the portion of the insulin receptor on the outer surface of cells. This triggers a conformational change in the receptor that leads to phosphorylation of tyrosine residues (indicated as P) on the internal portions of the receptor molecules. S symbolizes the disulfide bonds that hold the subunits of the receptor together. The phosphorylated receptor, an active enzyme of the tyrosine kinase family, then phosphorylates other intracellular molecules, activating some and inactivating others. Only some of the downstream events are indicated in this figure such as mobilization of GLUT-4 (glucose transporters) from intracellular stores to the cell surface, activation of protein kinase C (PKC), and inositol tris phosphate kinase (PI3 kinase). IRS-1 is an intracellular molecule that acts as a docking protein to facilitate assemblage of many of the elements of the downstream pathway of insulin action and also appears to be activated by phosphorylation on tyrosine residues. The more distal portions of the pathway such as glycogen and fatty acid synthesis are tissue specific.

erodimer, resulting in each half phosphorylating the other. This phosphorylation occurs on tyrosine residues in the intracellular domain of each molecule. This process has come to be known as autophosphorylation. The phosphorylated insulin receptor then phosphorylates a cascade of intracellular molecules, activating some enzymes and deactivating others. These events result in the metabolic changes associated with insulin action. There is considerable tissue specificity as to which enzymes are activated in the various insulin-sensitive tissues. In muscle and adipose tissue, mobilization and transport activity of the GLUT-4

molecules is increased. The transport activity of these molecules also appears to be increased through activation of protein kinase C (PKC). In the liver, glycogen synthase is activated by a specific phosphatase that removes key phosphate residues previously added by cAMP-dependent protein kinase (PKA) in response to hormones such as glucagon and epinephrine. Some actions of insulin are mediated through a phosphoinositol kinase (PI-3 kinase) and others continue to be elucidated. These multiple downstream events in the action of insulin are referred to collectively as post-receptor insulin actions.

Counter-Regulatory Hormones

The counter-regulatory hormones defend against neuroglycopenia because of the brain's obligate need for glucose. During prolonged fasting or when energy is consumed in excess of caloric intake, nutrients may be released from stores in liver, muscle, and adipose tissue in response to counter-regulatory hormones. The earliest response to a drop in blood glucose is the release of glucagon, which, like insulin, is made and stored in the islets of Langerhans in the pancreas. The cells making glucagon, called alpha cells, are less numerous than beta cells and are located in the periphery of each islet. Glucagon has its primary effect on the liver, stimulating glycogenolysis. As glycogen is broken down glucose-6-PO_4 (G-6-P) is produced. This compound is unable to leave the cell until the PO_4 group is removed by a cell-specific phosphatase. The glucose is then released to meet the needs of the brain. If the fast persists beyond 8–12 hours, hepatic glycogen stores will be depleted and other sources must be tapped. Epinephrine leads to breakdown of muscle glycogen, which is more abundant than the stores in liver. Unlike the liver, muscle has no glucose-6-phosphatase so the derived G-6-P cannot get out of muscle cells to be used by the brain. Instead, muscle converts G-6-P to lactate, which leaves the cell, is transported to the liver, and is converted to glucose. More prolonged caloric deprivation requires breakdown of proteins to amino acids. The branched-chain amino acids are released to the blood and converted to glucose (gluconeogenesis) in the liver. The glucocorticoid cortisol is necessary for this process and increases during fasting. Also, insulin, which inhibits gluconeogenesis, is diminished, releasing its inhibition. Gluconeogenesis will support glucose production for prolonged periods of time, but at the expense of important structural proteins.

It is important that the glucose derived from the storage forms be available to the brain but that glucose uptake by other tissue be minimized. Hence another action of each of the counter-regulatory hormones is to decrease the peripheral uptake of glucose by all non-neural tissue. Energy for non-neural tissues is provided by fat. Growth hormone stimulates lipolysis (breakdown of adipose) to free fatty acids (FFA). Epinephrine and, to a lesser extent, cortisol do so as well. The liberated FFA are metabolized to ketones in the liver in a glucagon-facilitated pathway. Insulin levels are generally low under these conditions but not absent. Small amounts of insulin are required to restrain tissue breakdown beyond what is necessary for brain metabolism and to facilitate uptake of alternate energy sources such as ketones by non-neural tissues.

Diabetes Mellitus

Diabetes mellitus is the clinical syndrome that develops when insulin levels are inadequate to keep the blood sugars (and other nutrients) within the normal range. It may be due to inadequate amounts of insulin as in insulin-dependent diabetes mellitus (IDDM) or an inadequate response to normal or even elevated levels of insulin as in non-insulin-dependent diabetes mellitus (NIDDM). Normal fasting blood sugars are 70–115 mg/dl. Postprandial (fed) levels of glucose do not normally exceed 150 mg/dl. A diagnosis of diabetes has been defined by the World Health Organization as either a fasting blood glucose greater than 140 mg/dl or a 1-hour postprandial value greater than 200 mg/dl. Either criterion allows the diagnosis of diabetes mellitus to be made. Subjects with blood glucose values between normal and clearly diabetic are termed glucose intolerant. Some of these subjects will develop overt diabetes, some will become normal, but as many as half will remain in the glucose-intolerant range for many years or even decades.

Insulin-Dependent Diabetes Mellitus (IDDM)

IDDM has been called Type I or juvenile diabetes. The latter term is out of favor as this form of diabetes may develop at any age. IDDM is the result of severe insulin deficiency that ensues secondary to loss of the majority of beta cells. It is now clear that beta cells are selectively destroyed by an autoimmune process. What triggers the host immune assault on these cells is debated, but a number of factors have been elucidated. There is a genetic (inherited) susceptibility that is necessary but not sufficient for the development of IDDM. The disease is much more common in whites than in nonwhites. This susceptibility appears to reside in the human leukocyte antigen (HLA) region of chromosome 6 and is associated with HLA-DR3 and -DR4. The strongest association is with the closely linked DQ_α and DQ_β loci which code for proteins that are expressed on the surface of immune cells and the beta cells of the pancreas after exposure to a viral-induced rise in gamma interferon. Most people have an aspartic acid at position 57 of the DQ_β chain. Those that develop IDDM are more likely to have an uncharged amino acid such as serine at this position. It should be noted that many more people have these high-risk alleles than ever develop IDDM. It is likely, therefore, that other genes modify the risk associated with these alleles. Environmental triggers also influence which subjects possessing these alleles will ultimately develop IDDM. The concordance of IDDM between identical twins is only 50%, indicating important nongenetic determinants for IDDM.

The risk of developing IDDM is 6% in first-degree relatives of IDDM subjects. Rising titers of islet cell antibodies (ICA) appear to antedate and predict which relatives of IDDM subjects will develop IDDM. Armed with this ability to predict subjects who are likely to develop IDDM, trials of immune intervention are underway to manipulate the immune system of ICA+ relatives of IDDM subjects in hopes of preventing the development of overt diabetes. Immune damage appears to occur in a stepwise fashion with hyperglycemia developing only after 75% or more of the beta cells have been lost (Fig. 24-3). If the destruction is

halted when 50% of the cells remain, the subjects may never actually become hyperglycemic. It is therefore possible that IDDM will be a preventable condition in the future.

Diabetic Ketoacidosis (DKA)

DKA develops when insulin levels are quite low. DKA may be the first indication that a person has IDDM. The early symptoms are usually weight loss, frequently with increased appetite, thirst, and frequent urination. Initially blood glucose levels rise and, once a level of about 180 mg/dl is reached, glucose leaks into the urine, causing an osmotic diuresis. This stimulates thirst, which is compensated by taking in more fluid. As the condition worsens,

Fig. 24-3. Time course of beta cell injury and the developments of metabolic abnormalities. It appears that after the initial immune insult occurs to the beta cell, additional damage occurs in a stepwise fashion. The immunologic injury probably occurs as discrete but repeated episodes over a period of years to culminate as IDDM.

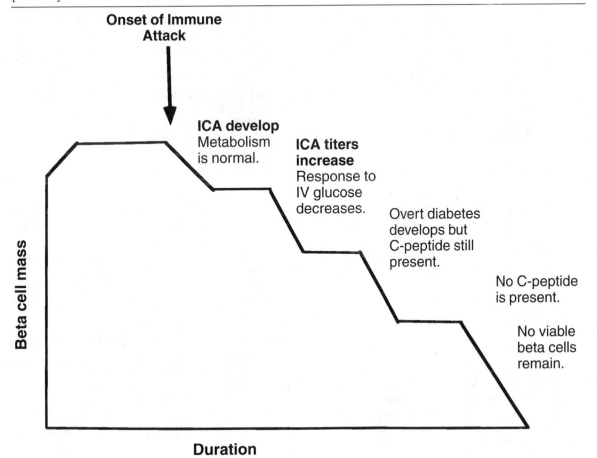

the loss of glucose and water leads to dehydration and stimulates release of catecholamines, epinephrine and nor-epinephrine, to maintain blood pressure and cardiac out-put. Epinephrine in the setting of low insulin levels leads to lipolysis and release of free fatty acids (FAA) from adi-pose tissue. The FFA are taken up by the liver and in the presence of low insulin levels are oxidized to ketones in the mitochondria. Acetoacetate (AA), β-hydroxybutyrate (BHB) and acetone are ketone bodies released into the cir-culation. Although these ketone bodies provide a critical source of energy for most tissues in the presence of intra-cellular glucopenia, their massive outpouring leads to their presence in the breath (acetone) or in the urine (AA and BHB). Acetoacetate and BHB are strong acids and deplete the body's buffering system, leading to systemic acidosis. Excretion of these anions in the urine results in a loss of balancing cations (sodium and potassium). The obligatory loss of sodium and water worsens the dehydration, causing catecholamines to rise further. Growth hormone and corti-sol also increase in response to the stress, thus accelerating tissue breakdown and further antagonizing insulin action. Glucagon is elevated due to the low insulin levels. Thus begins a vicious cycle of tissue breakdown to release stored nutrients, poor uptake of those released nutrients, production of organic acids, and loss of water and elec-trolytes. Eventually the acidosis leads to nausea and vom-iting that preclude adequate oral intake of water and the subjects become very ill. Therapy consists of replace-ment of lost water and electrolytes as intravenous saline solutions and insulin to suppress the massive gluconeo-genesis and ketogenesis and to facilitate nutrient uptake by insulin-sensitive muscle, adipose tissue, and liver. The de-velopment of DKA generally signals the requirement of long-term insulin therapy. Subjects with previously diag-nosed IDDM can also develop DKA if insulin therapy is omitted or reduced. Infection, myocardial infarction, trauma, and other stress stimulate counter-regulatory hor-mones and frequently initiate DKA in subjects taking their normal insulin doses.

Non-Insulin-Dependent Diabetes Mellitus (NIDDM)

NIDDM has been called Type II or adult-onset diabetes. Again, the latter term is out of favor as this process can be observed in teenagers and young children. Unlike IDDM, this disease results primarily from a deficient response to insulin. NIDDM is much more common than IDDM. Ninety percent of diabetes in the U.S. is NIDDM. It is fre-quently associated with obesity, more common in non-whites, and appears to increase as aboriginal peoples take on a more Western lifestyle of increased dietary fat and sedentary habits. Native Americans appear to be especially at risk, with 50% of adults developing NIDDM by age 40 in some tribes. Concordance rates for identical twins with NIDDM is 90% or more. Thus genetics and obesity are the most important factors for development of NIDDM.

Studies in the Pima tribe of Arizona have contributed to our understanding of the pathophysiology of NIDDM. Those Pima who develop diabetes can be predicted by higher insulin levels before the development of overt hy-perglycemia. Insulin levels are higher to compensate for their relatively decreased insulin responsiveness termed insulin resistance. There are some individuals with severe insulin resistance who also have a decreased number of in-sulin receptors or insulin receptors which bind insulin poorly, but the majority of subjects with insulin resistance have little or no decrease in their numbers of insulin recep-tors. Insulin resistance therefore resides in the biochemical pathways that follow insulin binding to its receptor in a majority of subjects with NIDDM. It is possible that de-fects anywhere along in the insulin cascade would appear clinically as insulin resistance. Such subjects would have elevated insulin levels prior to the development of overt di-abetes, and would develop hyperglycemia only when the beta cell can no longer keep up with the increased demand. Obesity itself contributes to development of NIDDM in susceptible subjects by increasing the insulin resistance and putting greater demand on the overworked beta cells.

Most subjects with NIDDM will not initially require in-sulin therapy. Early management should be directed toward improving insulin sensitivity and eliminating excessive demands for insulin. These goals are best met by caloric restriction with weight loss, regular exercise, and (if neces-sary) hypoglycemic pharmacologic agents. Aerobic exer-cise consumes glucose that is taken up by the exercising muscle as well as that which has been stored in the muscle as glycogen. Little if any insulin is required for that up-take. Glucose uptake by muscle that has been exercised is increased for 24–48 hours after exercise as repletion of glycogen stores occurs. Sulfonylurea agents increase the ability of glucose to release insulin from beta cells, in-crease insulin sensitivity, and facilitate GLUT-4 mobiliza-tion in response to insulin. The oral hypoglycemic agent metformin decreases hepatic production of glucose, as well as having an anorectic effect which tends to lead to weight loss. Patients with NIDDM not controlled with the above therapies or whose β-cell insulin production has been irreversibly damaged by prolonged hyperglycemia are generally treated with insulin.

Hyperglycemic Hyperosmolar Nonketotic State (HHNK)

Poorly controlled NIDDM rarely leads to DKA because insulin levels in NIDDM rarely fall to levels low enough to lead to significant ketone production. However, plasma glucose levels may rise to very high levels, resulting in a life-threatening illness. As in DKA, when the plasma glucose exceeds 180 mg/dl, water is lost in the urine via osmotic diuresis. However, because ketosis and acidosis do not develop, ketones and the obligate cations are not lost in the urine so that the loss of electrolytes is usually much less than in DKA. Patients may develop thirst but initially do not seem as "sick" as subjects with DKA. Dehydration becomes severe if thirst is inadequate or if the patient is unable to get water due to physical limitations. Epinephrine, growth hormone, cortisol, and glucagon are elevated, antagonize the action of insulin, and drive blood glucose levels higher, leading to more water loss in the urine. Intracellular water is lost as well as extracellular, resulting in hyperosmolality throughout the body fluids. In the elderly patient with moderately impaired renal function, the volume depletion can lead to diminished excretion of glucose and an additional rise in the hypertonic state. When osmolality exceeds 330 mosm/liter, brain function is compromised, patients become lethargic, and can develop frank coma. Reversal of the HHNK state primarily requires replacement of water and, to a much lesser extent, electrolytes. Large amounts of hypotonic solutions are usually required but must be administered carefully to allow equilibration to the intracellular space. Too rapid replacement of water may lead to brain edema and permanent neurologic injury. Small doses of insulin are effective in moving glucose intracellularly. This reduces plasma osmolality and shifts water into cells as well.

Chronic Diabetic Complications

The chronic complications associated with diabetes are known collectively as microvascular complications. They appear to be unique to diabetes but are indistinguishable in IDDM and NIDDM subjects. These include retinopathy, nephropathy, and neuropathy.

Retinopathy

Retinopathy is the major ophthalmic complication of diabetes and remains the primary cause of blindness in adults. Early retinopathy begins as focal areas of dilations of retinal vessels known as microaneurysms. These by themselves pose no threat to vision but with progression

increase in number. Worsening retinopathy is appreciated as small hemorrhages as well as areas of lipid exudation. The most advanced retinopathy is proliferative. Proliferative retinopathy develops in response to increasing ischemia with the release of an angiogenic substance that stimulates growth of new vessels in a process known as neovascularization. These new vessels grow in abberant locations such as into the vitreous and onto the iris. Like the neovascularization associated with tumors, these vessels lack the normal supporting connective tissue and bleed easily. When intraocular vessels bleed, vision is lost. Hemorrhages can be resorbed but tend to leave fibrous scar which is opaque. That opacity affects visual acuity. When the fibrous tissue contracts, retinal detachment is likely, which also leads to visual loss. Close ophthalmic followup of diabetic patients can prevent the progression to these later stages. Small laser burns are made across the retina to limit the production of the angiogenic hormone. This can frequently prevent neovascular changes in preproliferative retinas, avoiding the progression of proliferative retinopathy. If this strategy fails to prevent hemorrhages, other surgical therapy may help preserve vision. After resolution of a hemorrhage, fibrous tissue can be removed by a procedure known as vitrectomy. Thus vision can be improved and retinal detachment prevented.

Nephropathy

Diabetic nephropathy is the renal disease associated with diabetes. The hallmark of diabetic nephropathy is the loss of protein in the urine. Only 30–50% of people with diabetes are at risk for the development of nephropathy. The risk seems to be a genetic susceptibility because a history of nephropathy in other members of the family with diabetes greatly increases the risk of nephropathy. A family history of hypertension in nondiabetic family members also carries increased risk of nephropathy. A search for the specific genes that carry the risk of nephropathy points to the angiotensin-converting enzyme (ACE) gene but there may be others as well. In the early course of diabetes almost all subjects with IDDM and many with NIDDM have an increased glomerular filtration rate (GFR). This situation is known as hyperfiltration. After about 10 years, susceptible subjects begin to manifest trace amounts of urinary albumin (microalbuminuria) and are at risk for developing progressive diabetic nephropathy. As the process worsens the amount of protein increases to the level of grams lost in a 24-hour period. At this point, the subject usually has the nephrotic syndrome and soon the glomerular filtration rate begins to fall. This is assessed as a rise in the serum creatinine or a fall in creatinine clearance. Microscopic examination of the glomeruli reveal expansion of the mesangium and fibrous deposits called Kimmelsteil-Wilson nodules. The area for filtration is reduced, explaining the reduced GFR. Aggressive treatment of hypertension appears to slow the progression of loss of renal function once any proteinuria can be detected. In addition, the use of angiotensin-converting enzyme inhibitors have been demonstrated to have a renal protective effect beyond their antihypertensive one. Diabetes is now responsible for half the patients in the US that require renal replacement therapy for end-stage renal disease (ESRD). This consists of dialysis and transplantation.

Neuropathy

Diabetic peripheral neuropathy has a characteristic presentation as well. It is an axonal disease process with spotty demyelination and degeneration. The longest axons show the earliest changes in histology and produce the earliest symptoms and signs of nerve dysfunction. The symptoms begin in the toes usually as pain and paresthesias and progress to loss of all sensation. As the condition worsens, the dysfunction moves more centrally following a similar pattern of pain, paresthesias, and eventually anesthesia. As protective sensation is lost, subjects are at risk for foot ulcers. With the loss of proprioception, neuropathic joint destruction develops. Foot ulcers that become infected can lead to osteomyelitis, which frequently leads to amputations. Diabetes is the leading cause of nontraumatic amputations in the US and this occurs primarily in the setting of diabetic peripheral neuropathy.

All of these microvascular complications are felt to be the result of elevated levels of blood glucose. Improvement of metabolic control has been demonstrated to slow the development of each of these complications in IDDM subjects as the results of the Diabetes Control and Complication Trials (DCCT) were released in 1993. This study involved over 1400 IDDM subjects followed for 5 to 9 years on intensive (3 or more insulin injections per day or insulin pump) vs. standard insulin therapy (2 injections per day). Development of retinopathy, nephropathy, and neuropathy were reduced 50–75% by improved metabolic control as assessed by lower glycated hemoglobin in those on intensive therapy (7.1 vs. 9.0%). A similar response to tight metabolic control is expected in NIDDM subjects as well.

The mechanism of development of diabetic complications is currently argued. One of the leading theories is glycation and the development of advanced glycation end-products. Another involves the polyol pathway. See Fig.

24-4 for a schematic of each pathway. Each theory has its champions and several pharmacologic interventions have been developed based on the suspected mechanisms. These may prove important in preventing complications in those subjects where near normalization of metabolic control is not possible. The class of compounds referred to as aldose reductase inhibitors (ARIs) was developed to block the conversion of glucose to the corresponding alcohol sorbitol. This pathway forms the basis of the polyol pathway scheme to explain diabetic complications. Glucose enters non-insulin-sensitive tissues, such as the lens of the eye and peripheral nerves, in proportion to circulating blood glucose levels. These tissues contain the enzyme aldose reductase, which converts glucose to sorbitol. A second enzyme, sorbitol dehydrogenase (SDH), converts some of the sorbitol to fructose. The sorbitol and fructose cannot easily leave the cell after they are produced. It is not clear whether sorbitol and fructose have a toxic effect on the cell or produce a relative depletion of vital substrates to explain the damage to nerves. ARIs appear successful at blocking the progression of diabetic neuropathy and may even reverse it. The advanced glycation pathway is antagonized by compounds such as amino guanidine. According to this theory, damage develops from chemical attachment of glucose to free amino groups of proteins on lysine and arginine residues. Advanced glycation endproducts (AGEs) form when two glycated proteins become crosslinked (through the condensation of attached glucose moieties) to form large polymers. These large protein aggregates cannot be cleared by the usual cellular clearance mechanisms, and therefore have a longer half-life than normal. This process may be responsible for basement membrane thickening seen in the kidney and other tissues. The aggregates appear to stimulate macrophages, leading to cytokine release and increased inflammation. It is likely that both the polyol pathway and AGE formation contribute to the development of chronic complications and that each is attenuated by better control of blood glucose levels.

Macrovascular Complications

Macrovascular complications refer to the atherosclerotic process that occludes coronary and other medium-to-large-sized arteries. Unlike microvascular complications, macrovascular disease is much more common in NIDDM where lipid abnormalities are a frequent manifestation of a generalized metabolic derangement. Elevation of triglycerides and low HDL cholesterol are often associated with insulin resistance and appear to contribute to the risk of macrovascular disease in NIDDM. The risk of macrovas-

Polyol Pathway

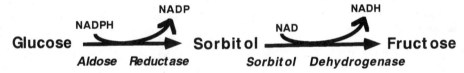

Glycation Pathway

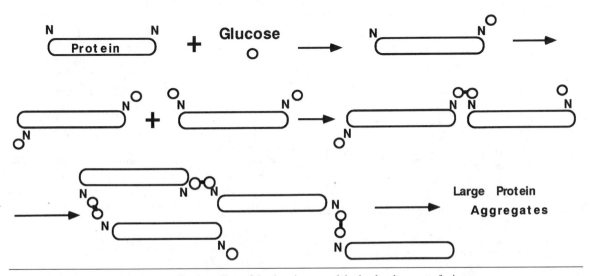

Fig. 24-4. Pathways to diabetic complications. Two of the theories to explain the development of micro-vascular complications are depicted here. N indicates free amino groups of lysine and arginine residues on protein macromolecules. Open circles represent glucose moieties attached to those amino groups.

cular complications does not have a clear association with the extent of glucose elevation. The risk of macrovascular disease appears to be no greater in IDDM without nephropathy (and the lipid abnormalities associated with nephrotic syndrome) than in nondiabetic subjects. The leading cause of death in diabetic subjects is coronary heart disease. Peripheral vascular disease along with neuropathy accounts for the increased risk of amputation in diabetics, which is estimated to be 5 to 7 times that of nondiabetics. Because of the increased risk for macrovascular disease, NIDDM subjects and all diabetics with nephropathy should try to minimize other cardiovascular risk factors such as hypertension, elevated LDL cholesterol, and smoking.

Clinical Examples

1. A 12-year-old boy stops growing and begins to lose weight, despite an increase in food intake. His schoolwork becomes poor and he frequently falls asleep in class. He has no energy and urinates on an hourly basis. He wants to go to the water fountain every 15 minutes. One morning he feels too sick to eat and complains that his stomach is upset. His parents take him to his pediatrician, who suspects IDDM. His parents are shocked because no one else in the family has had diabetes. His lab results are as follows: Glucose = 350 mg/dl, Na$^+$ is 133 mEq/liter, K$^+$ = 4.5 mEq/liter, Cl = 98 mEq/liter, HCO$_3$ = 15 mEq/liter, and ketones are positive in his serum. Blood pH = 7.20. IDDM is

confirmed and he is admitted to the hospital, where he is treated with intravenous fluids containing electrolytes and intravenous insulin. By the next day he is feeling much better and is begun on a subcutaneous regime of intermediate and short-acting insulin twice a day.

Discussion.   This is a typical presentation of IDDM. The highest incidence is in children about this age. He initially had symptoms of glucosuria that developed when insulin levels were unable to keep the plasma glucose below 180 mg/dl. This resulted in glucosuria, osmotic diuresis, and the polyuria. His thirst was stimulated and he drank frequently (polydipsia) to compensate for the loss. When the insulin levels decreased further, fat was broken down (lipolysis) to FFA and ketogenesis enhanced and DKA ensued. The nausea interfered with his ability to keep up with his water losses. This boy would be expected to have a lifetime requirement for insulin therapy.

2. A 50-year-old man had not seen a physician in 10 years because he did not think he needed to be seen. He developed burning pain in his feet and after six months went to a podiatrist. The podiatrist referred him to an internal medicine physician, who diagnosed a peripheral neuropathy which might be due to diabetes. The man admitted that there were several diabetic relatives but did not think he could have it because he felt "OK" except for the burning in his feet. On exam he was 220 lb., with a height of 5'8". His physical exam was normal except for a blood pressure of 160/100 and decreased amplitude of his deep tendon reflexes at the ankles. His laboratory data showed a plasma glucose of 250 mg/dl and normal electrolytes. A glycosylated hemoglobin was 10.5% (nl 4.0–6.5%). The internist recommended a 1500-calorie low-sodium diet and a program of walking 30 minutes a day. He was informed that if his plasma glucose and blood pressure did not respond to these measures, pharmacologic therapy would be required.

Discussion.   NIDDM may be relatively asymptomatic and, if a plasma or urinary glucose is not obtained for other reasons, can go undiagnosed for years. Not infrequently, the diagnosis is made after complications develop and the diagnosis is suspected on those grounds. The elevated glycosylated hemoglobin was indicative of an elevated plasma glucose for the preceding couple of months, but the presence of peripheral neuropathy suggested that diabetes mellitus had been present for years. He may obtain improvement in his pain with better control of plasma glucose or he may require medication for symptomatic treatment.

Bibliography

Brownlee M, Cerami A, and Vlassara H. Advanced glycosylation end products in tissue and the biochemical basis of diabetic complications. *N Engl J Med* 318:1315–1321, 1988. *This paper reviews the advanced glycation pathway for the development of diabetic complications.*

DeFronzo RA, Matsuda M, and Barrett EJ. Diabetic ketoacidosis. *Diabetes Rev* 2:209–238, 1994. *This is an excellent review of the pathophysiology of diabetic ketoacidosis and explains the rationale for treatment of DKA.*

Diabetes Control and Complications Trial Research Group: The effect of intensive treatment of diabetes on the development and progression of long-term complications in insulin-dependent diabetes mellitus. *N Engl J Med* 329:977–986, 1993. *This paper has already become a classic reference dealing with development of chronic diabetic complications. While only IDDM patients were studied, the results are expected to apply to NIDDM patients as well.*

Greene DA, Sima AAF, Stevens MJ, et al. Complications: Neuropathy, pathogenic considerations. *Diabetes Care* 15:1902–1925, 1992. *This paper explores in depth the polyol pathway and how it is thought to lead to neuropathy.*

Kahn, CR. Insulin action, diabetogenes, and the cause of Type II diabetes. *Diabetes* 43:1066–1084, 1994. *This is an extensive review of the post-receptor actions of insulin. It gives insight into pathways that could be defective in Type II diabetes. Despite the promising title, the cause of Type II diabetes remains to be elucidated.*

Lewis EJ, Hunsicker LG, Bain RP, and Rohde RD. The effect of angiotensin-converting-enzyme inhibition on diabetic nephropathy. *N Engl J Med* 329:1456–1462, 1993. *This paper is already a classic.*

Muir A, Schatz, DA, and Maclaren NK. The pathogenesis, prediction, and prevention of insulin-dependent diabetes mellitus. *Endo Metab Clin N Am* 21:199–219, 1992. *This is an excellent review of the genetics and immunology of IDDM and gives insight into prevention strategies.*

Ravid M, Savin H, Jutrin I, et al. Long-term stabilizing effect of angiotensin-converting enzyme inhibition on plasma creatinine and on proteinuria in normotensive Type II diabetic patients. *Ann Intern Med* 118:577–581, 1993. *This is one of a number of studies demonstrating a strategy for slowing progression of diabetic nephropathy and establishes the benefits of ACE-Is in NIDDMs as well as IDDMs.*

25 Reproductive System

Dale A. Freeman

Objectives

After completing this chapter, you should be able to

Understand the role of hormones and genetic inheritance in determining gonadal and phenotypic genital formation

Know the cellular targets for LH and FSH in the ovary and the testes

Know the hormonal findings and some causes of hypergonadotropic hypogonadism in women

Know the hormonal findings and some causes of hypogonadotropic hypogonadism in men or women

Know what causes elevated gonadotropin levels and infertility in men

Understand why an androgen-synthesizing tumor or adrenal androgens from congenital adrenal hyperplasia might cause infertility

What Determines Male vs. Female Phenotype?

Understanding what makes a man different from a woman is a subject of profound importance. Since a human fetus at some time in development is of indifferent phenotype, it is worth reviewing how that fetus ends up a girl or a boy.

The external genitalia of males and females derive from primordia that are the same in each sex. There are female homologues to all parts of the male genitalia and male homologues to the female genitalia. The developmental biologist Jost first made some sense of the enigma of male or female differentiation. He found that castration of a male or female embryo resulted in phenotypically female offspring. Thus the female phenotype was the default phenotype. Exposing a castrated fetus to testosterone produced a male phenotype. However, the internal genitalia were not changed by the hormonal environment of the fetus.

A number of congenital diseases indicate that Jost's basic observations were correct and provide additional understanding of this remarkable situation. In diseases where androgen synthesis is impossible, such as in 3β-hydroxysteroid dehydrogenase deficiency or 17α-hydroxylase deficiency, all fetuses are phenotypic females. Genotypic male babies

still have testes, however, and no uterus, fallopian tubes, or ovary is present. Likewise, complete dysfunction of the cellular androgen receptor leads to the syndrome of testicular feminization. These patients are XY genetic males and have intra-abdominal or labial testes, but have female external genitalia and normal female breast development at puberty (pseudohermaphrodytes). This occurs despite supraphysiologic testosterone concentrations. Genetic female babies exposed to excessive androgens during development are born with partially or almost completely virilized external genitalia (virilization of female external genitalia consists of growth of the clitoris and fusion of the labia). This occurs in 21-hydroxylase deficiency or 11β-hydroxylase deficiency, where excessive production of adrenal androgens partially virilize the fetus. These babies have normal, in this case female, internal genitalia with a uterus, fallopian tubes, and ovary.

Control of Gonadotropins and Sex Steroids

As is true for most pituitary hormones, luteinizing hormone (LH) and follicle-stimulating hormone (FSH) undergo

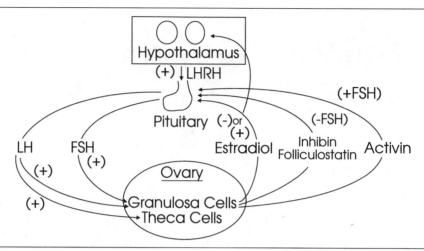

Fig. 25-1. Gonadal-hypothalamic-pituitary feedback loops in the female. Hypothalamic luteinizing hormone releasing hormone (LHRH) acts on the pituitary to release luteinizing hormone (LH) and follicle-stimulating hormone (FSH). In the ovary, theca cells respond to luteinizing hormone with increased ovarian androgen production. Granulosa cells respond to follicle-stimulating hormone by increasing conversion of androgen to estrogen and respond to luteinizing hormone by increasing progesterone production. Stimulation of the ovarian cells increases the serum concentration of the steroid hormone estradiol and the peptide hormones inhibin, folliculostatin, and activin. Inhibin and folliculostatin inhibit pituitary follicle-stimulating hormone release, activin stimulates its release, while estradiol may stimulate or inhibit both pituitary gonadotropins' release.

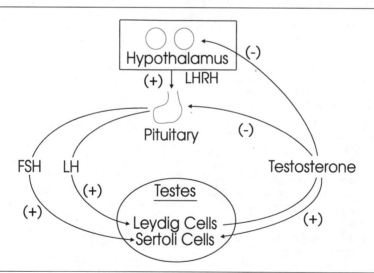

Fig. 25-2. Gonadal-hypothalamic-pituitary feedback loops in the male. Hypothalamic luteinizing hormone releasing hormone (LHRH) acts on the pituitary to release luteinizing hormone LH and follicle-stimulating hormone (FSH). In the testes, Leydig cells respond to luteinizing hormone by increasing testosterone synthesis. Sertoli cells respond to follicle-stimulating hormone and to Leydig cell testosterone. Both stimuli are necessary for initiating spermatogenesis. Testosterone inhibits subsequent gonadotropin release by feedback effects at the hypothalamus and pituitary.

feedback inhibition and primary hypothalamic positive control. Because some details of this regulation differ between males and females, each will be considered separately. Some elements of the feedback loops are common and should be mentioned here. In both sexes the hypothalamic-releasing hormone luteinizing hormone releasing hormone (LHRH) acts as a stimulus to the anterior pituitary to release both LH and FSH. Gonadal products feed back on this system, limiting further gonadotropin release. The hypothalamus of both males and females is sensitive to estradiol and to nonaromatizable androgens such as dihydrotestosterone.

To understand the hypothalamic-pituitary-ovarian axis, it is necessary to understand compartmentalization in the ovary and the various steroid and peptide products of individual ovarian cells. Steroidogenesis in the ovary is thought to require two cell types. Although any ovarian steroidogenic cell could express all enzymes required for de novo estradiol synthesis, the cells actually divide up the task. The granulosa cells convert cholesterol to progesterone, which is converted into androgens in the theca cells and then into estrogens in the granulosa cells. This peculiar division of labor probably occurs because progesterone inhibits an enzyme required for further metabolism of progesterone. It seems very likely that granulosa cells also produce the peptide hormone inhibin. Folliculostatin and activin are other ovarian peptide hormones probably of granulosa cell origin.

Feedback regulation of the ovary is exerted at the hypothalamus and the anterior pituitary. Estradiol inhibits hypothalamic LHRH and pituitary LH release. At very high and sustained concentrations, estradiol actually stimulates LH release. Inhibin and folliculostatin primarily inhibit and activin stimulates FSH release.

The female ovarian cycle is conveniently divided into a follicular and luteal phase. The follicular phase precedes ovulation. Prior to ovulation FSH induces a granulosa cell enzyme, aromatase, as well as an increase in LH receptors. Estradiol synthesized by the aromatase enzyme enhances pituitary LH and FSH release and causes the LH and FSH surge of ovulation. The high LH levels lead to luteinization of the granulosa cells. The luteinized granulosa cells produce high levels of progesterone and estradiol. In the absence of egg fertilization and production of placental gonadotropin (i.e., hCG), the corpus luteum then regresses since continued pituitary gonadotropin secretion is inhibited by ovarian estradiol and peptide synthesis.

Male hormones are not cyclic and can be thought of as two interrelated systems. Pituitary LH acts to stimulate the Leydig cells to produce testosterone which, in turn, inhibits the hypothalamus and the pituitary. Spermatogene-sis requires testosterone for maintenance, but probably requires FSH only for initiation. The FSH targets Sertoli cells which serve as nurse cells for developing sperm. The testosterone concentration required for maintenance of spermatogenesis is greater than normal peripheral testosterone concentrations. Thus maintenance of spermatogenesis requires supraphysiologic testosterone levels or enhancement of endogenous testicular testosterone concentration by LH.

Pathways for regulation of gonadotropin and gonadal steroid levels are shown in Fig. 25-1 and Fig. 25-2.

Female Hypogonadism, Infertility, and Inappropriate Ovarian Steroidogenesis

Women may come to physicians because of infertility, failure to develop secondary sexual characteristics, and/or for hirsutism or virilism either with or without infertility (hirsutism is excessive hairiness, while virilism includes this plus male pattern baldness and muscle distribution, breast atrophy, and enlargement of the clitoris). Often hypogonadism is present. It is convenient to consider gonadal insufficiency in two broad categories, hypergonadotropic and hypogonadotropic.

Hypergonadotropic Hypogonadism

This occurs when the ovary is absent, destroyed, or senescent. In all these conditions the ovarian steroid and peptide hormones that normally provide feedback inhibition to the hypothalamus and the pituitary are absent, so plasma LH and FSH are very high. If the condition resulting in ovarian failure is congenital or occurs before puberty, breast development and other secondary sexual characteristics do not develop. If this process occurs later, amenorrhea and infertility result. Turner's syndrome and the syndromes of premature ovarian failure and menopause are examples of hypergonadotropic hypogonadism.

Turner's Syndrome
This is a chromosomal disorder resulting in a phenotypic female with a 45,XO (rather than 46,XX) genotype and rudimentary nonovarian gonads. As shown in Fig. 25-3, these patients have a distinctive appearance; they are short, typically have a webbed neck, shield breasts, and have an abnormal carrying angle to their arms. In the most extreme cases, the girls are easily recognized; however, some girls with Turner's syndrome appear normal except for short

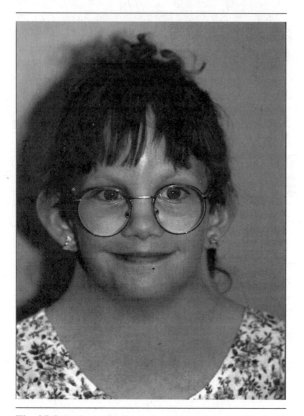

Fig. 25-3. Patient with Turner's syndrome and webbed neck. (Photo provided courtesy of Dr. Norman Levine.) [Picture provided with the consent of the patient.]

stature. Because there is no normally functioning ovarian tissue, normal puberty does not occur and most girls come to the doctor because of failure to develop secondary sexual characteristics and for primary amenorrhea. Usually the tumor-prone rudimentary gonads should be surgically removed. Secondary sexual characteristics can be induced with estrogen supplements; however, fertility cannot be achieved.

Premature Ovarian Failure

An autoimmune disease, it can occur alone or with other autoimmune diseases. These diseases include diabetes mellitus, thyroid disease, adrenal failure, pernicious anemia, and vitiligo. By definition, the failure must be before the time of normal menopause, which is between 44 and 50 years of age. If the failure occurs before puberty, secondary sexual characteristics will not develop. If ovarian failure occurs later, as it typically does, secondary amenor-

rhea is the usual complaint. Other than estrogen replacement therapy, there is nothing that can be done for this condition.

Menopause

Usually ovarian function ceases between 44 and 50 years of age. When the ovary fails, many women develop symptoms of the menopause. Hot flashes develop for some time, but eventually disappear. Menses become infrequent (oligomenorrhea), then cease. Defeminization is fairly common with involution of the estrogen-dependent vaginal mucosa and breast tissue. Other estrogen-dependent tissues, such as bone, are lost at a more rapid rate. Plasma lipoprotein patterns change from the favorable female pattern to a more unfavorable "male-type" pattern. Plasma LH and FSH concentrations are very high and serve as a marker for normal pituitary function in these women (if the LH and FSH are not elevated, something is wrong with the pituitary). Most of the undesirable side effects of menopause can be treated with estrogen supplementation. Estrogen used alone in a cyclic fashion or with progesterone in a regimen designed to prevent menstruation is now commonly prescribed for postmenopausal women.

Hypogonadism with Normal or Low Levels of Gonadotropins

This can occur as a congenital condition, in association with destructive pituitary or hypothalamic lesions or with disorders of ovarian steroid hormone synthesis. The age of onset will generally determine the patient's specific complaint. Disorders in which excessive ovarian androgens are synthesized often lead patients to seek help because of hirsutism or virilism.

Kallmann's Syndrome

This is a congenital syndrome in which patients do not synthesize the hypothalamic peptide LHRH and so do not release gonadotropins. Quite often they have defective cranial nerve I function and are unable to smell. Typically these patients come to the doctor because they fail to develop secondary sexual characteristics and/or because they have primary amenorrhea. They do not have the peculiar appearance of patients with Turner's syndrome and have a normal karyotype. Pulsatile LHRH administration can restore normal gonadal steroid synthesis and fertility. These patients must be differentiated from patients with benign (constitutional) delayed onset of puberty and from patients with destructive lesions of the pituitary or hypothalamus. Constitutional delay in puberty is often present in parents of affected individuals. This finding may aid in differentiating these patients from others presenting in this fashion. Destructive lesions are usually visible on computerized tomography or magnetic resonance images of the pituitary and hypothalamus.

Excess Steroidogenesis

Any condition in which ovarian cells produce androgenic steroid hormones independently of gonadotropin stimulation will result in hypogonadotropic hypogonadism. This can be associated with hirsutism/virilism or may occur without any symptoms except possibly dysfunctional uterine bleeding and/or infertility. A number of tumors histologically resembling normal ovarian theca cells or granulosa cells can produce these syndromes as can tumors resembling testicular Leydig cells (arrhenoblastoma and hilus cell tumors). The tumors producing predominantly androgens (arrhenoblastoma, hilus cell tumor, and many thecomas) will produce hirsutism or virilism. Tumors producing mainly estrogens tend to cause dysfunctional bleeding and, in very young girls, isosexual precocious pseudopuberty (changes of same-sex puberty occurring at an inappropriate time). Treatment is surgical removal of the ovarian tumor.

An extremely common cause of hirsutism and infertility is the polycystic ovarian disease syndrome (PCO). This syndrome is of unknown cause, but is associated with ovarian overproduction of androgens, peripheral conversion of some of these androgens into estrone, and estrone-positive feedback on pituitary LH secretion. Therefore, a cycle arises where LH secretion drives androgen production that, in turn, increases LH secretion. Since these patients are adequately estrogenized, they menstruate in response to progesterone. An extreme variant of this syndrome is ovarian hyperthecosis. Here the ovarian thecal cells take on some of the characteristics of neoplastic cells and produce large amounts of androgens, resulting in virilism. Since both polycystic ovaries or hyperthecotic ovaries are LH driven, maneuvers to suppress LH usually help the condition. Patients with polycystic ovarian syndrome are often obese and demonstrate insulin resistance. Fat tissue converts androstenedione of ovarian or adrenal origin into estrone. Weight loss often restores menstruation and fertility in these patients. Suppression of pituitary LH with oral contraceptives or LHRH antagonists prevents ovarian androgen synthesis and also can break the cycle. Surgically removing some ovarian mass may reduce the mass of androgen-producing cells and allow a normal cycle to resume.

One type of pituitary tumor, the prolactinoma, has the ability to selectively inhibit pituitary LH and FSH secretion. Patients with such tumors characteristically develop a syndrome of galactorrhea (breast milk production) and amenorrhea.

Male Hypogonadism

Male hypogonadism usually causes patient complaints of infertility, impotence (inability to have or maintain penile erection), or failure to develop or retain normal secondary sexual characteristics. Because production of sperm does not affect potency, infertile men only lacking sperm may have no complaints relating to sexual function. Disordered Leydig cell function, on the other hand, will cause both impotence and infertility. Most impotence is related to psychological factors or to vascular or neurological impairment of the penis and usually does not have an endocrine cause. Male hypogonadism, like the female variety, can be grouped into hypergonadotropic and hypogonadotropic types.

Hypergonadotropic Hypogonadism

This condition includes congenital defects such as Klinefelter's syndrome and destructive processes that affect testicular tubules, Leydig cells, or both.

Classical Klinefelter's syndrome patients are 47,XXY phenotypic males, but mosaic forms (XXY/XY) with less severe abnormalities also occur. A patient with typical Klinefelter's syndrome is shown in Fig. 25-4. These patients are almost all infertile. The testes are typically pea-sized and hard. The Leydig cells are markedly reduced in number and no germinal epithelium is present. The degree of Leydig cell failure often determines the presenting symptoms. With a near normal complement of Leydig cells, infertility may be the only presenting complaint. With less Leydig cell mass, higher LH levels result and the hyperstimulated Leydig cells produce excess estradiol. The high estradiol concentrations cause gynecomastia. If the Leydig cell failure is profound in a prepubertal boy, he may fail to develop normal secondary sexual characteristics. Klinefelter mosaics have a less severe disease, usually have larger testes, and may be phenotypically indistinguishable from normal men. They will be infertile so long as the testes is XXY genotype; however, not all of these men are azoospermic.

The testes is susceptible to damage by infections, radiation, and toxins. Usually the sperm-producing tubules are at greatest risk; however, the testosterone-producing Ley-

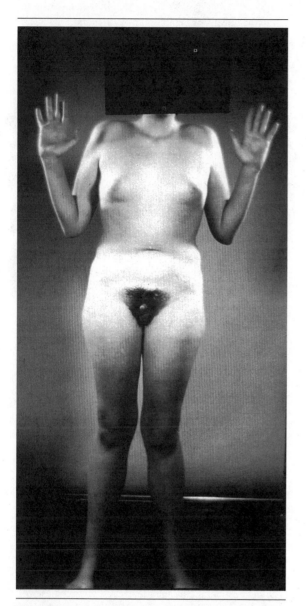

Fig. 25-4. Patient with Klinefelter's syndrome (note eunuchoid body proportions, gynecomastia, and small genitals).

dig cells may be damaged. The most common cause of secondary testicular failure is viral infection. The mumps virus is best known for causing testicular inflammation and failure, but other viruses can do this as well. The testicular tubules are very radiation sensitive while the Leydig cells are more resistant. Exposing the testes to heat disrupts spermatogenesis. Cancer chemotherapy fre-

quently damages the testicular tubules. Modern intensive chemotherapy damages Leydig cells as well. Since the tubules are affected by any of these causes, the patients are likely to have infertility as a complaint. With more severe injury, the Leydig cells become damaged and gynecomastia and/or impotence develop. The testicular damage post chemotherapy usually recovers with time if no further insults occur.

Hypogonadotropic Hypogonadism in Men

It is caused by the same processes affecting women. Kallmann's syndrome usually causes patients to present with failure to enter puberty. Pulsatile administration of LHRH can correct the defect. Destructive lesions of the pituitary or hypothalamus will, in children, result in failure to develop secondary sexual characteristics; in adult men it results in impotence and infertility. Prolactinomas in men rarely result in galactorrhea, but cause impotence, infertility, and (with sufficient time) regression of secondary sexual characteristics.

Infertility without Hypogonadism

Many causes of infertility are not directly related to the hypothalamic/pituitary/gonadal axis. The most common cause of female infertility is sexually transmitted infections of the fallopian tubes with resultant scarring. Likewise, infections, heat, radiation, and chemotherapy may affect spermatogenesis directly and spare the Leydig and Sertoli cells of the testes.

Clinical Examples

1. A 27-year-old woman was referred to the office with a 6-month history of amenorrhea and "hot flashes." The patient related that her first menstrual period was at age 13 and that she had menstrual periods every 28 days until about one year previously, when her periods became irregular and then stopped completely 6 months ago. Her only past medical history was that of hypothyroidism treated with 0.1 mg levothyroxine. On physical exam the patient was noted to have normal breasts, pubic and axillary hair. Her pelvic exam was normal. She was also noted to have vitiligo in several areas. Plasma LH and FSH determined from a pooled sample made from three separate specimens drawn 20 minutes apart revealed an LH of 63 IU/liter (nl, 5–25 IU/liter), an FSH of 80 IU/liter (nl, 5–20 IU/liter), and estradiol of 30 pmole/liter (nl, 70–220 pmole/liter).

The patient was placed on conjugated estrogens 0.625 mg daily with good relief of her vasomotor symptoms.

Discussion. This patient presented with classic symptoms of menopause at an inappropriate age. The high gonadotropin levels confirmed that ovarian function had ceased. Since LH and FSH both are intermittently released hormones, it is best to pool multiple samples spaced at least 20 minutes apart. The menopausal vasomotor symptoms were readily suppressed with estrogen. Fertility is not possible.

2. A 32-year-old woman was referred to the office for treatment of hirsutism, irregular periods, and infertility. She had always been overweight and recollected that her first menstrual period was at age 11½. Periods had averaged five times per year since about age 17. The patient noted that her facial hair had increased to the point that she shaved each day. Although married 5 years and engaged in unprotected intercourse, she had not become pregnant. Pooled plasma LH and FSH were 30 IU/liter (nl, 5–25 IU/liter) and 10 IU/liter (nl, 5–20 IU/liter) respectively. Androstenedione levels were 9 nmole/liter (nl, 3.5–7.0 nmole/liter); testosterone was 4.8 nmole/liter (nl, < 3.5 nmole/liter); and estradiol was 225 pmole/liter (nl, 70–220 pmole/liter). The patient was treated with a 1,000 kcal/day diet for 6 months. Over this time she went from 249 lbs to 207 lbs. Menstrual periods occurred at approximately monthly intervals and facial hair growth slowed.

Discussion. This patient had a fairly typical history and laboratory findings of polycystic ovarian disease. She was hirsute, had oligomenorrhea, and (as is often the case) was obese. Laboratory testing confirmed that she was adequately estrogenized, that she was hyperandrogenemic, and that she had an LH/FSH of greater than 2. Successful treatment breaks the cycle of ovarian androgen formation, conversion of estrogen to androgen, and pituitary LH hypersecretion. Since fat tissue contains much of the non-ovarian aromatase, significant body fat loss often improves the disease. If hirsutism is a problem and fertility is not desired, suppression of pituitary LH with LHRH analogues or oral contraceptives might be useful. The aldosterone antagonist spironolactone has an antiandrogen effect and may improve hirsutism as well.

3. A 23-year-old man presented with complaints of bilateral breast enlargement for about nine months. He denied impotence and recollected that he entered puberty at about age 13. He had frequent unprotected intercourse with his girlfriend, but she had not become pregnant.

The physical exam was notable for the following: The patient had a eunuchoid body habitus and somewhat feminine fat distribution. He had 4 cm (diameter) of palpable breast tissue bilaterally. The testes were hard and pea-sized. Plasma LH was 30 IU/liter (nl, 5–25 IU/liter; FSH was 53 IU/liter (nl, 5–20 IU/liter); testosterone was 7 nmole/liter (nl, 10–35 nmole/liter); and estradiol was 200 pmole/liter (nl, < 180 pmole/liter). Semen analysis detected no sperm. Karyotype analysis revealed 47,XXY.

Discussion. This patient presented with many of the symptoms, signs, and laboratory abnormalities of Klinefelter's syndrome. The patient was eunuchoid; had small, hard testes; and had significant gynecomastia. Laboratory evaluation revealed a slightly elevated LH, a markedly elevated FSH, slightly low testosterone, and slightly increased estradiol concentrations. As with most men with Klinefelter's syndrome, he was azospermic.

4. A 24-year-old man was referred because of failure to enter puberty. The patient noticed that he did not have pubic hair and had a quite small penis. He also had not needed to shave. His mother noticed that he was always a good boy, was never rebellious, and was not distracted by girls.

Physical exam revealed a 6′2″ man with sparse axillary hair, no beard or pubic hair, and much "baby" fat. His penis was 1.5 cm long and his scrotum was small, non-rugated, and contained about 1 cm soft tissue masses. He could not tell the difference in smell between coffee and peppermint. Serum LH was 2 IU/liter, (nl, 5–25 IU/liter); FSH was 3 IU/liter (nl, 5–20 IU/liter); and testosterone was 0.3 nmole/liter (nl, 10–35 nmole/liter). Karyotype analysis revealed 46,XY.

Discussion. This man had typical features for Kallmann's syndrome. Since these patients have no gonadotropins and very low levels of gonadal steroids, they tend to be less aggressive than normal adolescents and are taller than their parents since their epiphysis fail to close at a normal age. In the absence of testosterone, secondary sexual characteristics do not develop and the genital appearance remains prepubertal. These patients typically have deficient olfactory nerve function due to congenital abnormalities in the region of the inferior forebrain. Laboratory testing is used to confirm hypogonadotropic hypogonadism.

Bibliography

Carr BR. Disorders of the ovary and female reproductive tract. In Wilson JD and Foster DW (eds.). *Williams Textbook of Endocrinology*. Philadelphia: Saunders, 1992, pp. 733–798. *A good review of female reproduction physiology and pathology.*

Christensen RB, Matsumoto AM, and Bremner WJ. Idiopathic hypogonadotropic hypogonadism with anosmia — Kallmann's syndrome. *Endocrinologist* 2:332–340, 1992. *A good description of inherited hypogonadotropic hypogonadism.*

Griffin JE and Wilson JD. Disorders of the testes and male reproductive tract. In Wilson JD and Foster DW (eds.). *Williams Textbook of Endocrinology* (8th ed.). Philadelphia: Saunders, 1992, pp. 799–852. *A good review of disorders of male reproduction.*

Grumbach MM and Conte FA. Disorders of sexual differentiation. In Wilson JD and Foster DW (eds.). *Williams Textbook of Endocrinology* (8th ed.). Philadelphia: Saunders, 1992, pp. 853–952. *A comprehensive description of sexual differentiation.*

Rebar RW. Hirsutism, hyperadrenogenism and polycystic ovarian syndrome. In DeGroot LJ (ed.). *Endocrinology* (2nd ed.). Philadelphia: Saunders, 1989, pp. 1982–1993. *A review of one of the most common causes of hirsutism and infertility.*

Saenger P. The current status of diagnosis and therapeutic intervention in Turner's syndrome. *J Clin Endocrinol Metab* 77:297–301, 1993. *A good description of female gonadal dysgenesis.*

26 Anterior and Posterior Pituitary

Matthew T. Draelos

Objectives

After completing this chapter, you should be able to

Describe the clinical manifestations of oversecretion and undersecretion of the anterior pituitary hormones

Make the diagnosis of disease states characterized by over- or undersecretion of any of the anterior pituitary hormones

List the type and frequencies of anterior pituitary tumors

Describe the causes and treatment of hyperprolactinemia

Understand and describe the etiology, pathophysiology, means of diagnosis, and therapy of diabetes insipidus

Understand the etiology, pathophysiology, means of diagnosis, and therapy of SIADH

The pituitary, a small multifunctional gland located in the hypophyseal fossa of the skull, regulates crucial metabolic processes necessary to sustain life. It is composed of an anterior and posterior lobe, each with differing functions. The anterior pituitary regulates the thyroid and adrenal glands, gonads, and breast growth through the secretion of target-specific stimulatory hormones. It also controls growth and development through secretion of growth hormone (GH). The posterior pituitary regulates body fluid osmolality and water metabolism through secretion of arginine vasopressin (AVP).

Anterior Pituitary

Normal Physiology

The pituitary is surrounded bilaterally and inferiorly by the sphenoid bone. Superiorly, the pituitary is covered by the diaphragma sella, a dural sheath through which passes the hypophyseal stalk, which connects the pituitary gland to the hypothalamus. The optic chiasm lies directly above the diaphragma sella in front of the hypophyseal stalk. The anatomical location of the pituitary provides little room for tissue expansion. Expansion of the pituitary (e.g., due to a

tumor) therefore results in symptoms, the most common being headache and visual disturbances (classically bitemporal hemianopsia, due to impingement of the pituitary mass on the optic chiasm).

Hypothalamic Regulatory Hormones

Anterior pituitary hormone secretion is regulated by hypothalamic hormones which bind to cell membrane receptors on specific anterior pituitary cells (Fig. 26-1). Secretion of the hypothalamic-releasing hormones is regulated by local neurotransmitters (e.g., epinephrine, serotonin, acetylcholine), neuropeptides, and cytokines, all of which interact with the negative feedback of endocrine target organ hormones (e.g., thyroxine, cortisol, testosterone) on the hypothalamus. The endocrine target organ hormones also exert negative feedback on the anterior pituitary cells. Additionally, there is negative feedback by anterior pituitary hormones on the hypothalamic regulatory hormones. The hypothalamic regulatory hormones, all peptides, with the exception of dopamine, include:

Thyrotropin-Releasing Hormone (TRH). This hormone releases thyroid-stimulating hormone (TSH) and prolactin.

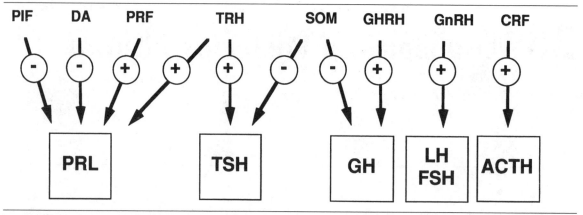

Fig. 26-1. Hypothalamic control of anterior pituitary secretion. Symbols: + indicates that substance has a stimulating (releasing) effect, while – indicates an inhibiting effect; ACTH = adrenocorticotropic hormone; CRF = corticotropin-releasing hormone, DA = dopamine; FSH = follicle-stimulating hormone; GH = growth hormone; GHRH = growth hormone-releasing hormone; GnRH = gonadotropin-releasing hormone; LH = luteinizing hormone, PIF = prolactin release-inhibiting factor; PRL = prolactin; PRF = prolactin-releasing factor; Som = somatostatin; TRH = thyrotropin-releasing hormone; TSH = thyroid-stimulating hormone.

Gonadotropin-Releasing Hormone (GnRH).   Also known as luteinizing hormone-releasing hormone or LHRH, it releases both luteinizing hormone (LH) and follicle-stimulating hormone (FSH). GnRH must be secreted in a pulsatile fashion in order to release LH and FSH.

Corticotropin-Releasing Hormone (CRH).   This stimulates the pituitary release of pro-opiomelanocortin (POMC). This prohormone is cleaved within the pituitary to yield corticotropin (ACTH) and beta lipotropin.

Growth Hormone-Releasing Hormone (GHRH). It stimulates growth hormone (GH) release.

Somatostatin   (Somatotropin-release-inhibiting Factor or SRIF).   This inhibits GH and, to some extent, TSH secretion.

Dopamine (DA).   This inhibits prolactin release. In addition to the above, poorly characterized prolactin-inhibiting and -releasing factor(s) exist.

Anterior Pituitary Peptide Hormones

The anterior pituitary secretes six well-characterized peptide hormones in a pulsatile fashion. TSH, LH, and FSH comprise the glycoprotein hormone family, each consisting of an alpha subunit and a beta subunit. The alpha subunit is common to all three hormones, whereas the beta subunit confers specificity to each. Prolactin and GH are grouped together, because each contains 199 amino acids and 16% of the amino acids are homologous for the two hormones. ACTH is classified separately. The anterior pituitary hormones include:

TSH.   Produced in the thyrotrope cells, it stimulates both the synthesis and secretion of the thyroid hormones levothyroxine (T4) and triiodothyronine (T3).

Luteinizing Hormone (LH).   Synthesized in the gonadotrope cells, LH is primarily responsible for the regulation of testosterone synthesis by Leydig cells of the testes in males and estrogen and progesterone synthesis by the ovaries in females.

Follicle-Stimulating Hormone (FSH).   Also produced by the gonadotrope cells, it stimulates spermatogenesis by Sertoli cells in males and follicular development in females.

ACTH.   This 39-amino-acid peptide is synthesized within the corticotrope cells as part of a 241-amino-acid precursor molecule, pro-opiomelanocortin (POMC). POMC is enzymatically cleaved into beta-lipotropin (beta-LPH), ACTH, an adjoining peptide, and an NH_2 terminal peptide. ACTH stimulates the adrenal cortex to secrete cortisol and sustains mineralocorticoid and androgen synthesis. The function of beta lipotropin is unclear.

GH. Produced in the somatotroph cells, GH has growth-promoting activity involving numerous tissues, including stimulation of linear growth at the epiphyseal plate of long bones. GH also has many metabolic actions involving numerous organ tissues, which can be summarized as being anabolic, lipolytic, and diabetogenic. Most, if not all, of the actions of GH are mediated through the stimulation of insulinlike growth factor-I (IGF-I, also known as somatomedin C), which is synthesized in the liver and other tissues.

Prolactin. This hormone is synthesized in the lactotrope cells of the anterior pituitary. The main site of prolactin action is the breast gland, where prolactin initiates and maintains lactation. Prolactin also binds to other tissues, but its physiologic function is unclear. Prolactin has a potent inhibitory feedback effect on GnRH release from the hypothalamus.

Feedback regulation of ACTH, TSH, LH, and FSH by peripheral hormones is covered in other chapters. IGF-I exerts negative feedback inhibit on GH secretion. Regulation of prolactin involves prolactin-releasing factors (TRH plus yet to be identified factors) from the hypothalamus as well as predominant tonic inhibition from hypothalamic dopamine. The tonic inhibition makes prolactin unique among the anterior pituitary hormones.

Pathophysiology: General Principles

Dysfunction of the anterior pituitary consists of hyposecretion or hypersecretion of the anterior pituitary hormones. The clinical manifestations therefore result from hypofunction or hyperfunction of the respective target organs. Hyposecretion of an anterior pituitary hormone is documented by low blood levels of the hormone and failure of the hormone to respond appropriately to stimulation. Conversely, hypersecretion is documented by high blood levels of the hormone and failure to respond appropriately to suppression.

Hypofunction of the pituitary, or pituitary insufficiency, may result from diseases of the pituitary, diseases affecting the hypothalamus or surrounding structures, or disturbance of the blood supply to the anterior pituitary or of the vascular flow from the hypothalamus to pituitary. General categories of causes of pituitary insufficiency include tumors of the pituitary, hypothalamus, or surrounding structures; trauma, surgery, or irradiation of the hypothalamic-pituitary region; infection involving the pituitary; vascular disease; and other less common disorders. Any of the anterior pituitary hormones may be involved individually or in combination.

Panhypopituitarism is a generalized failure of the anterior pituitary and usually presents initially as hypogonadism, followed, in order, by GH deficiency, hypothyroidism, and adrenal insufficiency. GH deficiency results in hypoglycemia, reduced growth in children, but is usually not recognized as a pathologic syndrome in adults. If, however, an adult is using glucose-lowering medication, e.g., insulin or sulfonylurea therapy in a patient with diabetes mellitus, then GH deficiency can predispose to the development of hypoglycemia.

Hypersecretion of pituitary hormones is primarily due to tumors of the pituitary, which are nearly always benign. Tumors are classified as microadenomas (diameter < 10 mm) or macroadenomas (diameter > 10 mm). Table 26-1 shows the frequency of the various pituitary adenomas. Hypersecretion of a single hormone is the rule, although secretion of two or more hormones may occur, with simultaneous hypersecretion of GH and prolactin being the most common example.

Pituitary adenomas can present with signs and symptoms of hormonal hypo- or hypersecretion, or can present with signs and symptoms due to their space-occupying characteristics.

Spontaneous hemorrhage into a pituitary tumor (pituitary apoplexy) and its resulting compression of surrounding tissue can produce severe headache, decreased vision, extraocular palsies, and other neurologic findings.

Clinical Disorders of the Anterior Pituitary

Hyperprolactinemia

Etiology. Hyperprolactinemia is the most common anterior pituitary disorder. The causes of hyperprolactinemia are numerous and are illustrated in Table 26-2. Any process that interferes with dopamine synthesis, its trans-

Table 26-1. Classification of Pituitary Tumors

Type of Tumor	Relative Frequency
Prolactin-producing	27%
Nonfunctioning	25%
Corticotrope adenoma, silent or symptomatic	15%
GH-secreting	15%
GH and prolactin-producing	8%
LH- or FSH-producing	7%
Plurihormonal	2%
TSH-producing	1%

Table 26-2. Causes of Hyperprolactinemia

PITUITARY-SECRETING ADENOMAS	ALTERED PHYSIOLOGIC STATES
Decreased delivery of dopamine to pituitary	Primary hypothyroidism
Hypothalamic destruction	Chronic renal insufficiency
Pituitary stalk section	Cirrhosis
	Stress, psychological or physical

DRUGS	NEUROGENIC STIMULATION
Dopamine receptor antagonists	Breast manipulation
Phenothiazines	Chest wall lesions
Butyrophenones	Spinal cord lesions
Metaclopramide	
Domperidone	
Sulpiride	
Other drugs	
Methyldopa	
Reserpine	
Verapamil	
Cimetidine	
Estrogens	
Opiates	

port to the pituitary, or its action at the lactotrope dopamine receptors may produce hyperprolactinemia. High levels of estrogen directly stimulate the lactotrope cells to produce prolactin and induce an acute suppression of dopamine secretion from the hypothalamus. Stress-induced hyperprolactinemia appears to be mediated via beta-endorphin, as opiates stimulate prolactin secretion. Histamine H_2 receptor antagonists and catecholamine depletors and synthesis inhibitors (reserpine and methyldopa) stimulate prolactin release. Chest wall lesions, nipple stimulation, and spinal cord lesions increase prolactin through a neuroendocrine reflex which results in the release of prolactin-releasing factors from the hypothalamus. The mechanism by which renal insufficiency produces hyperprolactinemia is not known. Hyperprolactinemia seen in cirrhosis has been attributed to the presence of false neurotransmitters.

Clinical Features. Women commonly present with amenorrhea, with or without galactorrhea. For this reason, hyperprolactinemia is usually identified earlier in women than in men. Occasionally, women with prolactinomas have spontaneous menses, but are infertile. Men usually present with decreased libido and impotence or with headache and visual disturbances secondary to the intracranial mass. Hypogonadism in both sexes appears to result from

inhibition of hypothalamic GHRH secretion by prolactin, with subsequent decreased LH and FSH secretion.

Diagnosis. Hyperprolactinemia is confirmed by demonstrating elevated blood levels of prolactin. Once drugs and other secondary causes are excluded, an anatomic evaluation of the head is performed with either a computerized tomography (CT) scan or a magnetic resonance imaging (MRI) scan.

Treatment. Removal of identifiable causes, such as drugs, is the initial step. If a prolactin-secreting adenoma is present, therapy with the semisynthetic ergot alkaloid bromocriptine is employed. Bromocriptine is a dopamine agonist which acts on lactotrope dopamine receptors to inhibit prolactin secretion and induce shrinkage of the adenoma. If necessary, surgical removal via a transsphenoidal or transfrontal approach is employed.

Acromegaly

Etiology. Acromegaly, a syndrome characterized by excessive secretion of GH, is due to a pituitary somatotroph adenoma in 99% of cases. Excessive production of GHRH, either by the hypothalamus or from a tumor elsewhere (ectopic) in the body, accounts for less than 1% of cases. Ectopic GH secretion has been described but is extremely rare.

Clinical Features. The symptoms of acromegaly result from the effects of chronically high levels of GH and IGF-I on body tissues, resulting in both growth-promoting and metabolic effects (Fig. 26-2). These symptoms begin insidiously and progress gradually. The presence of excess GH prior to the closure of long-bone epiphyses leads to increased stature, gigantism, or both. Enlargement of the facial features, hands, and feet are present in most patients. Other common symptoms include arthralgias, excessive sweating, weakness, malocclusion and the development of new skin tags. Hypogonadism (due to decreased LH and FSH secretion), hypertension, and impaired glucose tolerance may also develop.

Diagnosis. Due to the insidious nature of this disease, a delay in diagnosis of as many as 15–20 years is common. The most reliable diagnostic screening test involves the measurement of serum IGF-I, which is universally elevated in patients with active acromegaly. Confirmation consists in demonstrating elevated GH levels which fail to suppress normally in response to an oral glucose load (normal response is GH < 2 ng/ml, 60–90 minutes following the oral ingestion of 50–100 g of oral glucose solution). Following the biochemical diagnosis, the adenoma is anatomically evaluated with either a CT or MRI scan.

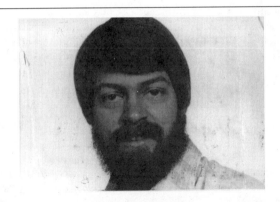

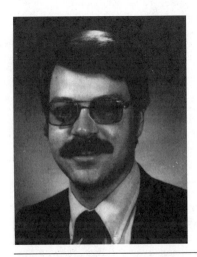

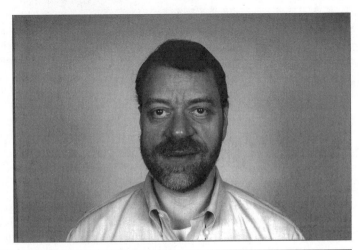

Fig. 26-2. Facial appearance of a 39-year-old man with acromegaly as seen in 1977 (top), 1981 (lower left) and 1994 (lower right). [Used with the consent of the patient.]

Treatment.   Surgery, via either a transsphenoidal or transfrontal approach, is the definitive therapy. Radiotherapy offers similar efficacy for patients with GH levels less than 50 mg/ml, but the effect is gradual, as opposed to the immediate effect seen with surgery. Bromocriptine induces symptomatic improvement in the majority of patients, but rarely reduces the serum GH level into the normal range. Recently, octreotide, a synthetic analogue of somatostatin, has been shown to reduce GH and IGF-I levels to normal in the majority of patients and to induce tumor shrinkage in greater than one-third of patients.

Cushing's Disease

It results from excess secretion of ACTH by a pituitary adenoma and is discussed in Chap. 23.

Nonsecretory Adenoma

Etiology.   Nonsecretory or "nonfunctioning" pituitary tumors are characterized by the absence of hypersecretion of a pituitary hormone. Interestingly, histologic examination of these tumors often reveals the presence of secretory granules. Although the tumors appear to synthesize and store pituitary hormones, lack of secretion results in the absence of any of the syndromes of hormone excess.

Clinical Features.   The majority of patients present with symptoms secondary to the tumor mass (headache or visual disturbance) or symptoms of pituitary hypofunction (hypogonadism, hypothyroidism, or adrenal insufficiency).

Diagnosis. The tumor is identified by CT or MRI scan (Fig. 26-3), and pituitary function is evaluated by measurement of serum prolactin, IGF-I, LH, FSH, TSH, alpha subunit, and cortisol and/or ACTH.

Treatment. Surgical excision via the transsphenoidal approach is the recommended treatment. Radiation may be employed as either primary or secondary therapy. Medical treatment of nonsecretory adenomas with bromocriptine may be used, but is unsuccessful in the majority of patients. Alpha subunit levels, if elevated, can be measured pre- and postoperatively to gauge the efficacy of surgery and provide evidence of recurrence.

Posterior Pituitary
Normal Physiology

Arginine vasopressin (AVP, also known as antidiuretic hormone, or ADH) is a peptide synthesized in the supraoptic nuclei of the hypothalamus and transported via the hypophyseal tract to the posterior pituitary. AVP is transported with a carrier protein called neurophysin.

The most important role of AVP is its antidiuretic effect on the kidney. In response to the binding of AVP to a specific receptor (the V_2 receptor) and subsequent activation of adenylate cyclase, the renal-collecting tubules increase their permeability to water, resulting in an increase in water reabsorption in the hypertonic medulla. In the absence of AVP, the permeability of the collecting tubules to water is diminished. AVP thereby conserves free water, increasing the concentration of the urine and maintaining plasma osmolality within a narrow range (285 ± 5 mOsm/kg). The absence of AVP allows excretion of free water into the tubules, a hypotonic urine, and an increase in plasma osmolality.

The primary regulator of AVP release is plasma osmolality (Fig. 26-4). Hypothalamic osmoreceptors are sensitive to small changes in plasma osmolality. Increases or decreases in plasma osmolality of as little as 1% will stimulate or diminish, respectively, release of AVP from the posterior pituitary. AVP release is also regulated through changes in plasma volume, as detected by cardiopulmonary baroreceptors. The baroreceptor system is less sensitive than the osmoreceptor system, but can override the hypothalamic osmoreceptors when activated by these receptors. A 5–10% decrease in thoracic blood volume results in neural transmission to the hypothalamus, resulting in stimulation of AVP release. This results in AVP activation of specific receptors on vascular smooth-muscle cells, V_1 receptors, which exert a significant pressor response.

Clinical Disorders of the Posterior Pituitary

Diabetes Insipidus (DI)

Definition. DI is a polyuric syndrome characterized by (1) urinary volume greater than 30 ml/kg body weight/day and (2) urine osmolality less than 300 mOsm/kg.

Fig. 26-3. Magnetic resonance images demonstrating a nonfunctioning pituitary macroadenoma (arrow) in coronal (upper) and saggital (lower) views.

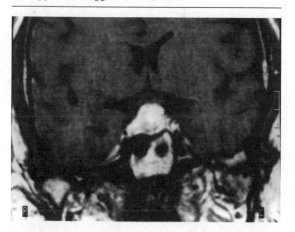
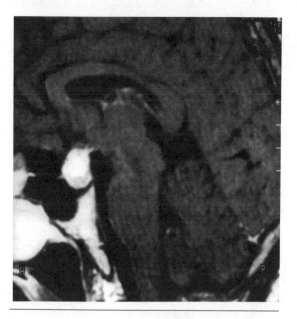

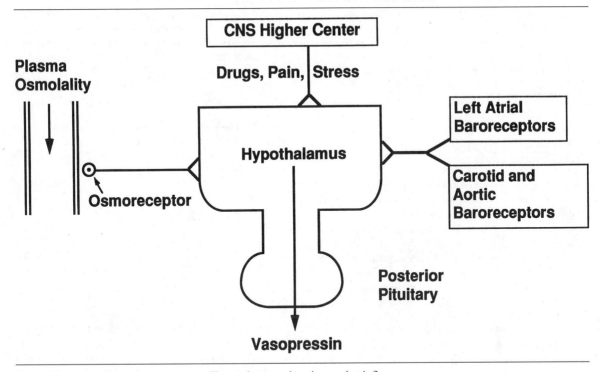

Fig. 26-4. Control of vasopressin release. Figure shows various inputs that influence vasopressin release. CNS = central nervous system.

Etiology. DI is classified as central (or neurogenic), marked by inadequate AVP release, or nephrogenic, due to impaired renal responsiveness to AVP. Central DI can result from any process (surgery, trauma, neoplasm, infection, ischemia, granulomatous disease) that damages the hypothalamus or severs the pituitary stalk. A rare hereditary autosomal dominant form also occurs. Nephrogenic DI can also be either familial (X-linked) or acquired and involves a defect in the V_2 receptor transduction system. Acquired causes include electrolyte imbalances (hypokalemia, hypercalcemia), sickle-cell disease, pyelonephritis, amyloidosis, following treatment for urinary obstruction, and drug-induced (lithium, demeclocycline, methoxyflurane).

Clinical Features. The primary symptoms of DI are polyuria, thirst, and polydipsia. The urinary volume may vary from a few liters/day, in the case of partial hormone deficiency/resistance, to as many as 18 liters/day, with complete hormone deficiency/resistance. Nocturia is invariably present. Patients with central DI characteristically show a predilection for cold or iced drinks. The onset of disease in central DI is generally abrupt, in contrast to a more prolonged onset with nephrogenic DI. The most striking clinical manifestations are seen if access to water is interrupted. Hyperosmolality rapidly develops and the central nervous system symptoms of irritability, mental dullness, ataxia, hyperthermia, and coma follow.

Diagnosis. Starting with documentation of urinary volumes exceeding 3 liters/day, the diagnosis is made by the finding of dilute urine (osmolality less than plasma) in the presence of an elevated plasma osmolality (may vary from slightly elevated to markedly elevated depending upon thirst and water intake). Central DI is characterized by inappropriately low serum AVP levels despite elevated plasma osmolality. The cardinal feature of nephrogenic DI is the failure to form concentrated urine in response to parenterally administered AVP. In contrast, the ability to concentrate the urine in response to vasopressin administration is maintained in central DI.

Treatment. The specific therapy for central DI is vasopressin replacement. The most widely used preparation is a long-acting form, desmopressin, which can be administered intranasally or parenterally on a demand basis. In nephrogenic DI, the most effective therapy includes the combination of thiazide diuretics and mild salt depletion. Thiazide diuretics induce, and salt restriction augments, a mild salt depletion that results in greater proximal tubular fluid absorption and a decrease in the volume of fluid delivered to the collecting duct. The result is a decrease in water excretion and a more concentrated urine.

Syndrome of Inappropriate ADH Secretion (SIADH)

Etiology.   This syndrome, characterized by the sustained release of AVP in the absence of osmotic or nonosmotic stimuli, is the most common cause of hyponatremia in hospitalized patients. Conditions resulting in the inappropriate secretion of AVP include central nervous system disorders (tumors, strokes, infections, trauma, metabolic encephalopathy), nonmalignant pulmonary conditions (e.g., pneumonia, tuberculosis, positive pressure ventilation), exaggerations of known stimuli to AVP release (e.g., pain, emotional stress), and neoplasms, including small-cell carcinomas of the lung, bronchial adenomas, or thymic tumors which secrete AVP or AVP-like substances. Additionally, several pharmacologic agents can stimulate AVP release or potentiate its action at the kidney, among the most common being phenothiazines, haloperidol, tricyclic antidepressants, chlorpropamide, and cancer chemotherapeutic agents.

Clinical Features.   Hyponatremia and submaximal urinary dilution are the hallmark findings. Patients are mildly volume expanded, although nonedematous. Clinical signs and symptoms depend on the degree and rate of development of the hyponatremia. Acute hyponatremia below 120 mmol/liter results in somnolence, seizures, and coma. Slowly-developing hyponatremia may be asymptomatic even with serum sodium levels below 120 mmol/liter, but symptoms may include abdominal cramps, nausea, vomiting, and headaches.

Diagnosis.   This syndrome is marked by hyponatremia in the presence of urine that is less than maximally diluted. Urinary osmolality generally exceeds 150 mosm/kg and is usually greater than the serum osmolality. In order to make the diagnosis of the syndrome of inappropriate ADH secretion, other diseases with "appropriate" or "explainable" secretion of ADH must be excluded. A careful history, physical examination, and laboratory evaluation are necessary. Measurement of serum electrolytes, urea nitrogen and osmolality, urine osmolality and sodium, and evaluation of thyroid and adrenal function are generally indicated. Normal thyroid and adrenal function must be present for this syndrome to be diagnosed, as hypothyroidism and hypoadrenalism both result in the reduced ability to dilute the urine. Additionally, congestive heart failure and hepatic cirrhosis should be ruled out, as both of these conditions may provide nonosmotic stimuli for AVP release.

Treatment.   The most important measure is to eliminate the underlying cause. Water restriction, or the use of antagonists to the action of AVP (e.g., demeclocycline) may also be employed.

Clinical Examples

1. A 63-year-old man seeks medical attention because of headaches and loss of peripheral vision. Further questioning reveals a recent loss of sex drive, decreased frequency of shaving, impotence, and decreased energy. Physical examination reveals a BP of 102/56, P 58, R 12, T 36.5. A bitemporal hemianopsia, lack of goiter, dry skin, delayed deep tendon reflexes, absent pubic hair and small testes are present. Laboratory examination reveals serum testosterone 139 ng/dl (nl, 300–1100), serum cortisol 1.7 μg/dl (nl, 5.0–25.0), free thyroxine 0.5 ng/dl (nl, 0.7–2.0 ng/dl), TSH 0.38 μU/ml (nl, 0.6–5.0 μU/ml), prolactin 8 ng/ml (nl for male, 0–10 ng/ml), somatomedin C 110 ng/ml (nl in adult, 54–389 ng/ml). An MRI scan of the head reveals a pituitary mass with suprasellar extension, measuring $22 \times 18 \times 12$ mm, compressing the optic chiasm. He was referred to a neurosurgeon for removal of the tumor.

Discussion.   The symptoms that brought this man to medical attention were those due to the mass effects of a pituitary adenoma. Further questioning revealed symptoms consistent with pituitary insufficiency. Physical examination and biochemical evidence of secondary gonadal, thyroid, and adrenal failure were identified. Corticosteroid therapy needs to be started immediately and continued after surgery. Thyroxine should also be started, but this is not as urgent as the need for corticosteroid therapy. Testosterone therapy can be started as an outpatient. These medications will be continued for his lifetime. Surgery is indicated in order to prevent further vision loss. Neither radiation nor medical therapy is generally effective to halt the growth of or shrink nonfunctioning pituitary adenomas.

2. A 28-year-old man is hospitalized for unconsciousness following a motor vehicle accident in which he sustained head trauma. The day after admission, the nurse

reports that the patient produced 3.5 liters of urine over the preceding 6 hours, despite receiving only 125 ml/hour of intravenous fluid. How should this situation be approached?

Discussion. Central diabetes insipidus must be considered in any patient who has sustained head trauma severe enough to be rendered unconscious. DI usually manifests 12–24 hours after injury, and implies damage to the supraoptic nucleus or to the hypothalamo-neurohypophyseal tract.

Three distinct patterns may follow neurosurgical or traumatic damage to the neurohypophysis, in order of decreasing frequency: (1) transient DI, (2) permanent DI, or (3) a "triphasic response," consisting of initial DI, an antidiuretic phase associated with inappropriate release of AVP from degenerating axons beginning several days after the initial insult and lasting 2–14 days, followed by permanent DI.

In the evaluation of such a patient, it is important to be certain that the polyuria represents DI and is not secondary to either fluid administration or an osmotic diuresis. Fluid intake seems unlikely in this case, since he is receiving only 125 ml/hour of intravenous fluid. The most common cause of osmotic diuresis would be glycosuria secondary to the hyperglycemia sometimes induced by high doses of corticosteroids. The diagnosis of DI requires demonstration of inappropriately dilute urine in the presence of plasma hyperosmolality (> 290 mOsm/kg).

The mainstay of therapy is administration of sufficient water to replace urinary losses. Treatment with vasopressin is indicated in all cases of post-traumatic DI, and is initiated as soon as DI is confirmed. The commercially-available, long-lasting AVP analogue desmopressin can be administered intranasally or parenterally, but in this case would be administered parenterally, as the patient is unconscious.

Serum sodium concentration, urine osmolality, and overall fluid balance must be followed carefully until stabilization or resolution of the DI.

Any patient with post-traumatic DI should be assumed to have anterior pituitary insufficiency, until proven otherwise. Such patients should be covered with appropriate doses of corticosteroids until anterior pituitary function can be thoroughly evaluated.

Bibliography

Ezzat S, Snyder PJ, Young WF, et al. Octreotide treatment of acromegaly: A randomized, multicenter study. *Ann Intern Med* 117:711–718, 1992. *Results of a multicenter study of a somatostatin analogue in the treatment of acromegaly.*

Klibanski A and Zervas NT. Diagnosis and management of hormone-secreting pituitary adenomas. *N Engl J Med* 324:822–831, 1991. *A review of the clinical diagnosis and treatment of functioning pituitary tumors.*

Melmed S. Acromegaly. *N Engl J Med* 322:966–977, 1990. *A comprehensive review of acromegaly.*

Ober KP. Diabetes insipidus. *Critical Care Clin* 7:109–126, 1993. *A review of the acute management of diabetes insipidus.*

Streeten DHP and Moses AM. The syndrome of inappropriate vasopressin secretion. *Endocrinologist* 3:353–358, 1993. *A clinical review of SIADH.*

Thapar K, Kovacs K, Laws ER, et al. Pituitary adenomas: Current concepts in classification, histopathology, and molecular biology. *Endocrinologist* 3:39–57, 1993. *A recent review of pituitary adenomas, focusing on histopathology.*

Thorner MO, Vance ML, Horvath E, et al. The anterior pituitary. In Wilson JD and Foster DW (eds.). *Williams Textbook of Endocrinology.* Philadelphia: Saunders, 1992, pp. 221–309. *Chapter from authoritative textbook of endocrinology.*

27 Thyroid

R. Hal Scofield

Objectives

After completing this chapter, you should be able to

Describe the synthetic pathway, structure, mechanism of action, and regulation of thyroid hormone including the different properties of T_3 and T_4

Contrast the pathogenesis, physical examination, and diagnosis of Graves' hyperthyroidism with subacute thyroiditis and toxic nodular goiter

List and describe the extra-thyroidal manifestations of Graves' disease

Describe the clinical manifestations of hyperthyroidism

Describe the causes of hypothyroidism

Describe the clinical manifestations of hypothyroidism

Overview

Abnormalities of thyroid gland function are among the most common of medical problems. This chapter will outline normal thyroid physiology essential for understanding thyroid pathophysiology and the major categories of thyroid disease.

Development and Anatomy

The thyroid gland arises from the pharyngeal floor at the junction of the middle and posterior third of the tongue beginning about a gestational age of one month. The primitive thyroid, at first consisting of thickened epithelium and later a diverticulum, undergoes a caudal displacement, forming the thyroglossal duct. Production of thyroxine begins during the eleventh week of gestation and pituitary production of thyroid-stimulating hormone (TSH) is detectable about this same time.

Abnormal thyroid development occasionally is clinically important. The thyroglossal duct usually disappears during the second month of fetal life, but portions may persist, resulting in thyroglossal cysts. Thyroid tissue may develop anywhere along the path of descent. Rarely, lingual or other ectopic thyroid is the only functioning thyroid tissue. The thyroid may migrate into the mediastinum

to lie retrosternal. Agenesis of the thyroid results in neonatal hypothyroidism that, if untreated, will lead to cretinism.

In the United States the average normal adult thyroid weighs about 20 g and lies just anterior and lateral to the trachea. The superiorly pointed, inferiorly blunt right and left lobes are connected by the isthmus, a thin band crossing the midline just below the cricoid cartilage.

Biochemistry

Thyroid hormone consists of iodinated, coupled tyrosines. There are several forms of this hormone which differ in the number and position of the iodine residues. The major circulating form is thyroxine (3,5,3',5'-tetraiodothyronine or T_4), while the hormonally active form is 3,5,3'-triiodothyronine (T_3). Reverse triiodothyronine (3,3',5'-triiodothyronine or rT_3) is an inactive metabolite of T_4 that is found in low concentrations in the serum. The structure of tyrosine and the thyroid hormones are given in Fig. 27-1. Relevant features of T_4 and T_3 are compared in Table 27-1.

Synthesis and Secretion

The thyroid gland extracts and concentrates iodine from the circulation. Iodine intake varies greatly throughout the

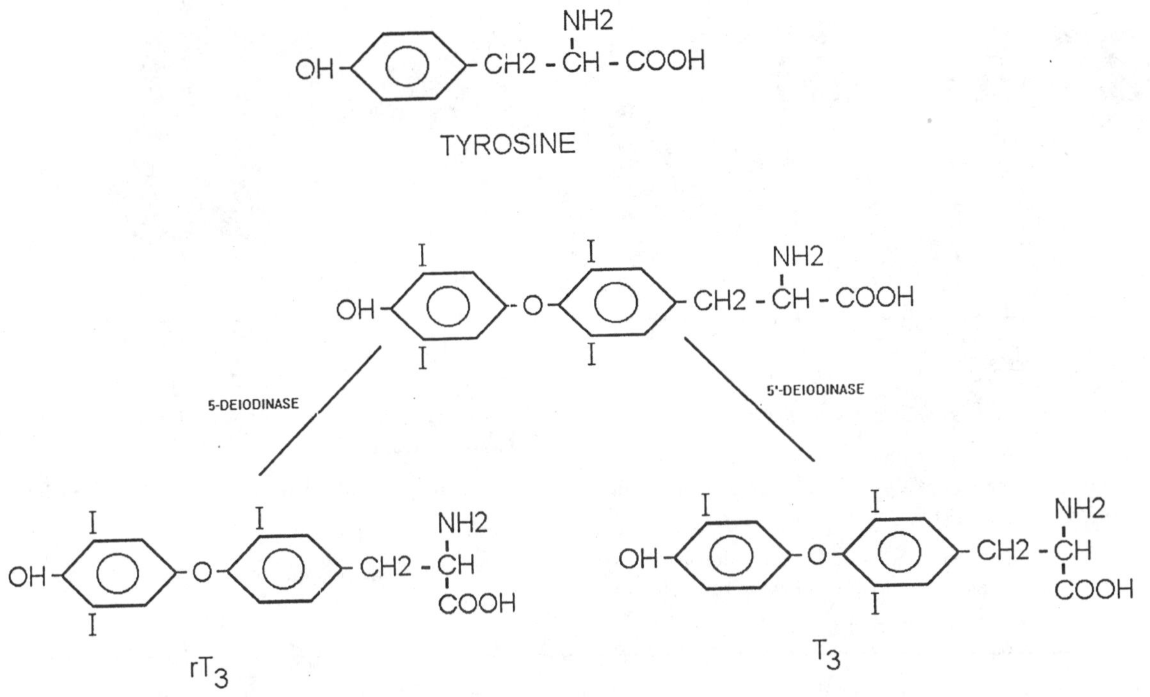

Fig. 27-1. Structure of tyrosine and thyroid hormones.

Table 27-1. Comparison of the Properties of T_4 and T_3

	T_4	T_3
Daily production (μg)	80	30
from thyroid	80	6
in periphery	0	24
Serum concentration	8 μg/dl	120 ng/dl
% free in serum	0.3	0.02
Half-life	7 days	18 hours

world, depending on the concentration of iodine in the environment, but averages approximately 500 μg/day in the United States.

After active transport into the thyroid gland, iodine is used in the synthesis of thyroid hormone, which can be divided into a two-step process. First, tyrosine residues of thyroglobulin are enzymatically iodinated by thyroid peroxidase. This is followed by intramolecular coupling of iodotyrosine to produce either T_3 or T_4 which is still part of thyroglobulin. Hormone is stored in the gland in this form, with iodothyroglobulin making up the majority of intrafol-

licular colloid. Second, proteolysis releases thyroid hormone from its linkage within thyroglobulin. Free T_3 and T_4 then enter the circulation. Thyroglobulin is also released by the thyroid gland and circulates in the serum.

Most thyroid hormone secreted from the gland is T_4, with a daily production of about 80 μg. In comparison, less than 10 μg of T_3 is secreted by the thyroid and even smaller amounts of rT_3 are secreted. During certain disease states such as hyperthyroidism or iodine deficiency the ratio of T_3 to T_4 production by the thyroid may be markedly increased. Normally, however, the majority (> 80%) of T_3, the biologically active hormone, is produced outside the thyroid by the action of 5′-deiodinase (Type I). This enzyme is found most abundantly in the liver and kidney. Its counterpart, 5-deiodinase, converts T_4 to rT_3 (see Fig. 27-1).

Mechanism of Action

The mechanism of action of thyroid hormone has been presented in Chap. 22. Briefly, thyroid hormone is transported into the cell by an active process that requires ATP. Once inside a cell, T_3 is translocated into the nucleus and binds high-affinity receptors. The complex of receptor and T_3 induces changes in mRNA production of genes regulated by thyroid hormone.

Regulation of Production

Thyroid hormone secretion is controlled by the hypothalamus and pituitary through a negative feedback loop. The critical feature is the production of thyroid-stimulating hormone (TSH) by the pituitary. This hormone can be measured in the circulation to assess thyroid hormone status. TSH is a glycoprotein with an alpha and beta subunit that increases all processes within the gland leading to synthesis and release of the hormone. TSH acts via a cell surface receptor on the thyroid linked to a G protein using cAMP as its second messenger. The pituitary secretes TSH in a pulsatile fashion with a frequency of 1–2 hours. There is a circadian rhythm with a nocturnal peak just before sleep that is unrelated to cortisol or thyrotropin-releasing hormone (TRH) secretion. TRH is a tripeptide produced in the hypothalamus and reaches the pituitary via the portal circulation in the pituitary stalk. Measurement of TRH is not clinically important.

Action of Thyroid Hormone

The cellular action of thyroid hormone is discussed in Chap. 22. Thyroid hormone has broad effects on most every cell and tissue type. Both O_2 consumption and thermogenesis are increased. Protein synthesis, including enzymatic and structural proteins, is increased. Hepatic production of glucose and lipid particles is altered as are other components of lipid and carbohydrate metabolism.

Thyroid hormone interacts with catecholamines. There is an increased sensitivity to circulating catecholamines that is mediated in part by an increased number of receptors and in part by increased post-receptor sensitivity. Several manifestations of hyperthyroidism (including tachycardia, tremor, increased sweating, and heat intolerance) are a result of this increased sensitivity to catecholamines and can be treated with beta-adrenergic receptor blockade.

Pathophysiologic Approach to Biochemical and Functional Diagnosis

A diagnosis of thyroid disease can be entertained, and often confirmed, on the basis of a careful history and physical examination. An anatomical diagnosis can usually be made by physical examination of the neck with attention to thyroid size, consistency, and contour. Both inspection and auscultation are important parts of the examination.

Once sufficient evidence has been obtained from the history and physical, biochemical assessment of thyroid status is appropriate. Circulating thyroid hormone is almost completely protein bound, so changes in binding protein concentrations affect total hormone levels independent of thyroid status. Unbound, or free hormone, is unaffected by binding protein levels and can be measured. One can assess not only the amount of thyroid hormone in the blood but also the patient's physiologic response by determination of plasma TSH levels. Consequently, measurement of TSH along with free T_4 is sufficient to ascertain thyroid status in the great majority of patients.

The thyroid's ability to concentrate iodine from the circulation can be exploited diagnostically. Very small doses of radiolabeled iodine are given orally. Then the percentage of the administered dose found in the thyroid gland is determined. In addition, the distribution of the isotope within the thyroid is important in the differential diagnosis of hyperthyroidism (Fig. 27-2).

Fig. 27-2. Examples of thyroid uptake scans from a variety of illnesses. In the upper left is a single "hot" spot of a toxic adenoma. The upper right shows the nonhomogeneous uptake by a toxic multinodular goiter. The bottom right shows homogeneous, diffuse, and increased (76%) uptake of the isotope in a patient with Graves' disease. The bottom left shows a gland with normal uptake (22%) and moderate asymmetry, which is common in the population.

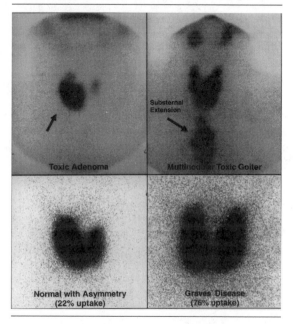

Hyperthyroidism

Excess thyroid hormone leads to characteristic biochemical, physiologic, and clinical features. Graves' disease is the usual cause of hyperthyroidism, but a number of other less common causes will be considered.

Graves' Disease

Known as Basedow's disease in some parts of the world, Graves' disease is the most common condition that produces hyperthyroidism. This disease is more common in women compared to men by about 10 to one. In the general population an incidence of 1–2 per 1000 per year has been estimated. Graves' disease usually begins in young adulthood but can have its onset at any age.

Pathogenesis

The production of autoantibodies that bind and activate the thyroid cell surface receptor for TSH are the cause of the hyperthyroidism seen in Graves' disease. These so-called thyroid-stimulating immunoglobulins (TSIs) cause production and release of thyroid hormone that is autonomous of regulation by TSH; however, the gland is not intrinsically autonomous in that it still requires external stimulation. Uptake of iodine by the thyroid is stimulated by TSIs. This abnormality can be exploited clinically in that patients with Graves' disease will have an abnormally high percent uptake of iodine.

Extrathyroidal Manifestations of Graves' Disease

While the heightened adrenergic sensitivity of hyperthyroidism from any cause can produce lid lag and widened palpebral fissure, Graves' disease has specific ocular and cutaneous manifestations that are related to the unique underlying autoimmunity.

The infiltrative ophthalmopathy of Graves' disease is found in roughly one-half of patients. The cardinal feature is exophthalmos in which the eyes protrude owing to inflammatory and cellular involvement of the retro-orbital tissues, including ocular muscles and fat. This can be progressive such that some patients are unable to close their eyes because the eyelids cannot be apposed (Fig. 27-3). There may be periorbital edema, chemosis, or injected conjunctivae.

In some patients symptoms are minor and include a foreign-body sensation, pruritus, excess tearing, or dry eyes. Most patients can be treated with more conservative measures such as lubricating eye drops or topical steroids. On

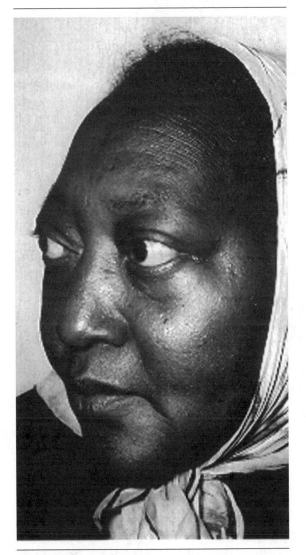

Fig. 27-3. Moderate exophthalmos due to Graves' disease. [Used with consent of the patient.]

the other hand, Graves' eye disease can be severe and even threaten vision. Corneal ulcers may develop. Extraocular muscles may become involved in the infiltrative process such that extraocular movements are compromised. An occasional patient requires systemic steroids, decompression surgery, or external beam radiation to control the disorder.

The natural history of the ophthalmopathy is independent of the hyperthyroidism. Thus treatment of hyperthyroidism does not improve eye disease. Thyroid ophthalmopathy sometimes predates or is never accompanied by hyperthyroidism. Most patients with Graves' ophthalmopathy but no hyperthyroidism have circulating TSIs, however. Occasionally ophthalmopathy is unilateral and frequently it is more pronounced in one eye.

Infiltrative dermopathy is found in only 1–5% of Graves' patients and is almost exclusively seen in the subset with eye disease. The most common form is red, raised, indurated, intensely pruritic lesions over the tibia that are known as pretibial myxedema. The lesions can coalesce to form large plaques and are rarely seen on the face or upper extremities. Thyroid dermopathy also has a course independent of hyperthyroidism. Treatment usually consists of potent topical corticosteroids.

Diagnosis of Graves' Disease

The diagnosis of Graves' disease is made on clinical grounds in patients who present with features of hyperthyroidism and Graves' ophthalmopathy. Laboratory confirmation is established by an elevated serum free T_4 and a suppressed TSH. Occasionally, serum T_3 is high but T_4 is not. This is known as T_3 toxicosis. Radioiodine uptake scanning reveals an increased percent uptake with homogeneous distribution of the isotope. TSIs can be measured but are rarely needed clinically.

Treatment of Graves' Disease

There are three options: radioiodine therapy, surgery, and antithyroid medications. Radioiodine has become the preferred treatment in the United States. The patient is given oral radioiodine. This is taken up by the thyroid and destroys thyroid tissue, resulting in decreased production of thyroid hormone. About one-quarter to one-third of patients so treated will develop hypothyroidism within the first year. Subsequently, about 2.5–5.0% per year develop this complication, which is probably not different than the natural history of Graves' disease without radioiodine treatment. After almost half a century of experience with this treatment there is no evidence of other long-term complications such as malignancy or tetragenicity. The amount of gonadal radiation delivered is not significantly greater than that of common diagnostic radiologic procedures such as barium enema. Radioiodine cannot be given to pregnant women because the isotope will cross the placenta and destroy the fetal thyroid.

Graves' disease can also be treated with antithyroid drugs such as propylthiouracil (PTU) or methimazole. These both block uptake and organification of iodine by the thyroid and PTU blocks conversion of T_4 to T_3 in the periphery. A 1- or 2-year course is given at a dose to produce euthyroidism. Then the drug is discontinued. In about 50% of patients hyperthyroidism recurs, while half will maintain a normal thyroid status, at least until the later onset of hypothyroidism. The major side effect of the antithyroid drugs is agranulocytosis, which can be life-threatening.

Surgery is largely reserved for pregnant women whose hyperthyroidism cannot be controlled with low doses of PTU or patients with cosmetically disfiguring goiters.

Subacute Thyroiditis

Also known as de Quervain thyroiditis, it is much less common than Graves' disease. Two subgroups can be based on the presence or absence of pain. Some patients present with pain in the anterior neck and constitutional features including fever. Swallowing, turning the head, or direct pressure may exacerbate the pain. Physical examination reveals a slightly enlarged, tender thyroid. Others have no pain but an otherwise similar clinical course.

The disease has several phases during which thyroid hormone production varies. During the acute phase of illness, which may last from a few days to many weeks, almost all patients have biochemical evidence of hyperthyroidism with a high T_4 and T_3 as well as a suppressed TSH. About half give a history consistent with mild hyperthyroidism. After resolution of the thyroid pain and the hyperthyroid phase, many patients are transiently hypothyroid, but most have recovery of thyroid function after several weeks or months. An occasional patient is left with permanent hypothyroidism, sometimes after recurrent episodes of subacute thyroiditis.

Pathogenesis

The hyperthyroidism results from release of preformed, stored thyroid hormone from a gland damaged by an immune assault. The pathology of this illness is distinctive. A patchy lymphocyte infiltrate is seen with formation of giant cells and granulomas. The etiology is unknown but a substantial fraction of patients give a history of an antecedent upper respiratory illness.

Diagnosis

This disease can usually be diagnosed on the basis of the history, physical examination, and biochemical hyperthyroidism with elevated T_4 and low TSH found during the acute phase. In addition to the finding of a tender thyroid in some patients and the lack of ophthalmopathy, subacute thyroiditis, especially painless, can be distinguished from

Graves' hyperthyroidism by virtue of a low uptake of iodine. A markedly elevated sedimentation rate is characteristic and helpful in distinguishing painful hemorrhage into a thyroid nodule from subacute thyroiditis.

Treatment

During the acute phase, nonsteroidal anti-inflammatory agents (NSAIDs) are indicated. These will control the pain as well as treat the constitutional symptoms. Some patients who do not respond to or cannot tolerate NSAIDs will need a short course of systemic glucocorticoids. The transient hyperthyroidism can usually be observed but some patients will need beta-adrenergic blocking agents or antithyroid drugs for control of symptoms. Also, hypothyroidism may need treatment with oral thyroxine if prolonged or severe.

Toxic Nodular Goiter

Hyperthyroidism may be produced by either a single thyroid adenoma or by a toxic multinodular goiter (MNG). Unlike Graves' disease, these conditions represent autonomous functioning of the gland. The clinical manifestations of either toxic adenoma or toxic MNG are generally less severe than in Graves' disease.

Toxic MNG is invariably preceded by nontoxic MNG. Transition is slow, usually with a gradual onset of symptoms. Older individuals and men are more likely to be affected, compared to Graves' disease. Physical examination shows a multinodular gland that has a "cobblestone" feel. At times a single larger nodule may predominate among other, smaller nodules. Goiter size can be very large (Fig. 27-4). An adenoma that produces thyroid hormone is a true neoplasm of the thyroid. Such a tumor is substantially less common than toxic MNG.

There are two patterns of iodine uptake in toxic MNG. Most commonly there is patchy nonhomogeneous uptake throughout the gland. Less common are a few areas of uptake in a gland that otherwise takes up little iodine (see Fig. 27-2). In either case, the uptake of iodine and production of thyroid hormone are independent of exogenous signals. Thus exogenous thyroxine has no effect on hormone production by toxic MNG.

Diagnosis depends on demonstration of hyperthyroidism and physical examination consistent with a single nodule or MNG. An uptake scan will confirm the presence of either entity (see Fig. 27-2).

Hyperthyroidism associated with toxic nodular goiter can be treated with radioiodine, but usually requires higher

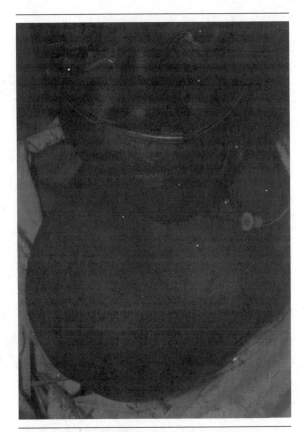

Fig. 27-4. Massively enlarged thyroid in a patient with toxic multinodular goiter. [Used with the consent of the patient.]

doses than Graves' disease. Some patients with multinodular goiter require surgery for definitive therapy.

Other Forms of Hyperthyroidism

Surreptitious or unknowing use of large doses of thyroid hormone can cause clinically apparent hyperthyroidism. There have been several "epidemics" of hyperthyroidism associated with consumption of hamburger meat made, at least in part, from bovine thyroid. Thyroglobulin production by the thyroid will be suppressed by ingestion of exogenous thyroid hormone and its measurement in the serum may help distinguish exogenous from endogenous hyperthyroidism.

Rarely there is production of TSH by a pituitary tumor.

Such individuals have hyperthyroidism with an elevated TSH. Faulty sensing of thyroid hormone by the pituitary may lead to nontumorous overproduction of TSH. This condition, known as pituitary resistance, can be differentiated from tumorous TSH production by measurement of the alpha subunit of TSH in the serum. Another rare condition is true ectopic production of TSH by the ovarian teratoma struma ovarii. Choriocarcinomas that produce large amounts of hCG can lead to hyperthyroidism by a hormonal spillover mechanism in which hCG binds to and activates the TSH receptor.

Clinical Manifestations

Table 27-2 lists some of the many signs and symptoms that can be produced by hyperthyroidism and the percent of patients affected compiled from several published series. In general, Graves' disease tends to have more severe hyperthyroidism than other forms. The prototype patient with Graves' disease is a young woman with several weeks to several months of fatigue, nervousness, palpitations, heat intolerance, increased appetite, and weight loss. She almost invariably has an enlarged thyroid. Older individuals with Graves' disease or toxic multinodular goiter may present in a less typical fashion with isolated atrial fibrillation, congestive heart failure, unexplained weight loss, or dementia. This is sometimes known as apathetic hyperthyroidism and may easily escape clinical detection.

Table 27-2. Signs and Symptoms of Hyperthyroidism and the Percentage of Patients Having Each

Symptoms	Percentage	Signs	Percentage
Nervousness	80–100	Goiter	4–100
Excess sweating	50–90	Bruit	30–80*
Heat intolerance	40–90	Lid lag	50–62
Palpitations	65–90	Tremor	40–95
Dyspnea	65–80	Damp palms	75
Fatigue	44–88	Tachycardia	60–100
Weight loss	50–85	Atrial fib	10–40
Increased appetite	10–65	Hyperkinesis	40–80
Hyperdefecation	10–33	Eye disease	50–62*

* For Graves' patients only.
Data from: Utiger RD: The thyroid: physiology, hyperthyroidism, hypothyroidism, and the painful thyroid. In Felig P, Baxter JD, Broadus AE, and Frohman LA (eds.). *Endocrinology and Metabolism.* New York: McGraw-Hill, 1986, pp. 389–510.

Hypothyroidism

Failure of the thyroid gland to produce adequate thyroid hormone is common, producing characteristic, but diverse, clinical sequelae. The most common pathogenesis is an autoimmune disorder known as Hashimoto's thyroiditis. This disease can affect any age or sex but, similar to Graves' disease, is more likely to be found in young women.

Autoimmune Thyroiditis

The thyroid shows a lymphocytic infiltrate with loss of thyroid follicles. Lymphoid follicles with germinal centers are found at times. Eventually the gland can become totally replaced by fibrosis tissue. The lymphocytic infiltrate is polyclonal and contains T cells that respond to thyroid tissue extract in vitro. These data imply that cell-mediated autoimmunity is involved in the pathogenesis of autoimmune hypothyroidism.

Evidence of a humeral immune response to the thyroid is also found. Greater than 80% of patients have circulating antibodies that bind thyroid antigens. The most abundant of these are anti-thyroid peroxidase (antiTPO) and antithyroglobulin (antiTGB). These antibodies are frequently found at low titer in healthy young women, especially those with a family history of thyroid disease, as well as in patients with Graves' disease.

The pathogenic nature of some thyroid antibodies has been demonstrated. Some patients have an antibody that binds the TSH receptor and inhibits the action of TSH. The presence of these antibodies results in hypothyroidism because TSH cannot interact with the thyroid. Other antibodies bind cell-surface proteins and prevent thyroid growth. Patients with antibodies that block TSH receptor or thyroid growth may have hypothyroidism without a goiter.

Other Causes of Hypothyroidism

Treatment of Graves' disease is the second most common cause of hypothyroidism in the United States. Sporadic cretinism is found in about 1 in 5000 births and is usually due to development defects such as thyroid agenesis or ectopic thyroid. The diagnosis can rarely be made clinically at birth but biochemical screening of neonates is now required in every state. Rarely a genetic defect in thyroid hormone synthesis is identified in congenital or adult hypothyroidism.

Hypothyroidism secondary to pituitary or hypothalamic

failure is uncommon and almost always is accompanied by failure of secretion of other pituitary hormones. Pituitary tumors or their treatment is the most common etiology, but postpartum pituitary necrosis, granulomatous disease, metastatic tumor, or pituitary infarction may be responsible.

Endemic goiter is related to dietary deficiency of iodine and is a major worldwide health problem that affects an estimated 200 million people. Once common in some areas in North America such as around the Great Lakes, the condition has almost completely disappeared in the USA with iodine supplementation of salt.

Clinical Manifestations of Hypothyroidism

The various signs and symptoms of hypothyroidism are shown in Table 27-3. Because of the protean nature of these manifestations, it is difficult to describe a typical patient with this illness. Young to middle-aged women may present with fatigue, dry skin and hair, and menstrual abnormalities. The finding of an enlarged thyroid is helpful because biochemical evaluation for hypothyroidism is of low yield in the absence of a goiter or history of treatment for thyroid disease. Similar to hyperthyroidism, the presentation of hypothyroidism may be altered in the elderly. Dementia, weight loss, or weakness can be the major complaint.

Diagnosis

Autoimmune hypothyroidism is a disease of insidious onset that can have a long subclinical course. Because of

Table 27-3. Signs and Symptoms of Hypothyroidism with the Percentage of Patients Who Have Each

Symptoms	Percentage	Signs	Percentage
Dry skin	60–100	Hair/skin changes	70–100
Cold intolerance	60–95	Puffiness	40–90
Hoarseness	50–75	Bradycardia	10–15
Weight gain	50–75	Slow tendon	
Constipation	36–65	relaxation	50
Paraesthesia	50	Prox. muscle	
Weakness	90	weakness	Common

Data from: Utiger RD. The thyroid: physiology, hyperthyroidism, hypothyroidism, and the painful thyroid. In Felig P, Baxter JD, Broadus AE, and Frohman LA (eds.). *Endocrinology and Metabolism.* New York: McGraw-Hill, 1986, pp. 389–510.

the nonspecificity and diversity of the signs and symptoms, even the patient with overt hypothyroidism can escape clinical detection. Once the diagnosis is considered, it can be easily confirmed with the simultaneous measurement of free T_4 and TSH. With overt disease T_4 is low and TSH high (greater than 10 with normal range being roughly 0.6–5.0 µU/ml). In this case, the diagnosis is unequivocal. Those with subclinical hypothyroidism may have either a high TSH and a low normal T_4 or a TSH that is only minimally elevated, i.e., between 5 and 10 µU/ml.

Treatment

Once the diagnosis is made, treatment is usually straight forward. L-thyroxine (T_4) is given by mouth once a day in a dosage sufficient to normalize the TSH. Patients can be followed most economically with periodic measurement of TSH only. L-thyroxine has a half-life of about 1 week, so 6–8 weeks should pass before measuring TSH after a change of the dose.

Clinical Examples

1. A 68-year-old healthy man was found to have a multinodular goiter. There were no symptoms or signs of hyper- or hypothyroidism. A free T_4 was 1.8 ng/dl (normal 0.8–2.0 ng/dl) and a TSH was 0.8 µU/ml (normal 0.6–5.0 µU/ml). The patient was started on 0.075 mg of L-thyroxine by mouth each day in an attempt to "suppress" the multinodular goiter.

He returned 3 months later with his daughter, who reported that he had become confused and had gotten lost in familiar surroundings. Examination showed an irregular tachycardia and an impaired mental status. Thyroid studies showed a free T_4 of 2.5 ng/dl and a TSH of < 0.01 µU/ml. An uptake scan revealed nonhomogeneous pattern with 26% of the dose in the thyroid at 24 hours while still on L-thyroxine. An EKG showed atrial fibrillation with a rapid ventricular response.

Discussion.   This patient had a multinodular goiter with autonomous production of thyroid hormone. When initially seen he was euthyroid. When thyroid hormone was given by mouth, the gland continued its autonomous production of hormone and the patient became overtly hyperthyroid.

The symptoms seen in this patient are typical of hyperthyroidism in older individuals. Many patients develop cardiac manifestations, such as worsened congestive heart failure or angina, or new onset atrial fibrillation.

2. A 31-year-old black woman first noted unintentional weight loss about 3 months prior to seeking medical attention. She lost a total of 45 lb. associated with a mildly increased appetite. She was continually tired but frequently felt agitated. In the last 2 months she was frequently hot and sweaty. Her eyes had been dry and itchy for 6 weeks, but they were not more prominent. On physical examination, she had injected conjunctivae. The thyroid was three times normal size, smooth, and nontender. There was a bruit over the thyroid gland. Her palms were damp and there was a tremor of her hands. The free T_4 was 4.3 μg/dl and the TSH was < 0.01 μU/ml. Thyroid scan showed 76%, homogeneous uptake (see Fig. 27-2).

The patient received 12.5 mCi of radioiodine and, after this treatment, began propylthiouracil and propranolol. Weight loss, fatigue, tremor, and heat intolerance all improved. At 2-month followup, the medications were discontinued and she continued to feel well until 4 months after radioiodine treatment when weight gain, fatigue, and dry skin were noted. TSH was elevated and she was started on thyroid hormone replacement.

Discussion. This patient has a typical presentation of Graves' hyperthyroidism. Her laboratory and the findings on uptake scan confirm the diagnosis. Treatment with radioiodine can take several months to be effective; and so, given her severe weight loss, propylthiouracil treatment was undertaken. The beta-blocker propranolol was used to symptomatically treat the tremor, heat intolerance, and excess sweating; beta-blockade alone, however, is not adequate treatment of hyperthyroidism.

The patient developed typical symptoms of hypothyroidism several months after radioactive iodine. These patients must be carefully monitored for the onset of hypothyroidism in the first year after treatment, and then periodically in subsequent years.

3. A 35-year-old woman was referred for an elevated cholesterol of 283 mg/dl found on routine screening by her gynecologist. She had noticed heavy periods for the last 6 months. She was a bicycle enthusiast and in the last 2 months had not been able to ride her usual 100 miles a week without considerable fatigue. Her skin was dry and the thyroid was about twice normal size without tenderness or nodules. Free T_4 was 0.8 ng/dl and a TSH of 24 μU/ml.

The patient started 0.1 mg of L-thyroxine every day and 2 months later energy level and menstruation had returned to normal. The TSH was also normal at 3.2 μU/ml. A serum cholesterol drawn 4 months after starting thyroid hormone was 202 mg/dl.

Discussion. In studies of patients referred for elevated cholesterol up to 25% are found to be hypothyroid. Symptoms referable to the thyroid may be absent or subtle. Because of its varied presentation, seriousness if left untreated, and ease of treatment, hypothyroidism must be sought in many patients.

Bibliography

Griffin JE. Review: Hypothyroidism in the elderly. *Am J Med Sci* 299:334–345, 1990. *This paper reviews the physiologic changes in thyroid economy in the elderly and the impact of these changes on clinical illness in this population.*

Levey GS and Klein I. Catecholamine-thyroid hormone interactions and the cardiovascular manifestations of hyperthyroidism. *Am J Med* 88:642–646, 1990. *An integration of the basic and clinical data in the hyperadrenergic state of hyperthyroidism.*

Wheetman AP. Thyroid-associated eye disease: pathophysiology. *Lancet* 338:25–28, 1991. *A review of the genetic, environmental, and immunologic mechanisms involved, or proposed to be involved, in ophthalmopathy. Recently evidence has been obtained that the TSH receptor is present in the retro-orbital space (Lancet 342:337–338, 1993).*

28 Metabolic Bone Disease

Mary Zoe Baker

Objectives

After completing this chapter, you should be able to

Be familiar with the various cell types and components of bone

Understand the normal physiology of bone and its remodeling

Know a clinical approach to the patient with a suspected metabolic disease

Be familiar with osteoporosis

Know about other selected metabolic bone diseases

Bone is a specialized connective tissue which has several functions. It provides structural support of the body, protection of internal organs, and sites for muscle attachments. Bone also serves as a reservoir for minerals — 99% of the body's calcium, 80% of the phosphate, and significant amounts of sodium, magnesium, and carbonate are found in bone. In concert with renal and respiratory mechanisms, bone helps maintain a normal acid-base balance via the release of phosphate and carbonate.

Anatomy and Physiology

There are two major types of bone, cortical (compact bone), which makes up 85% of the skeleton, present in the shafts of long bones, and trabecular (cancellous bone), which is found in the vertebrae, ends of long bones, and ribs. All bone is composed of cells and extracellular matrix. Unique to bone, extracellular matrix has the ability to become calcified (mineralized). While bone growth primarily occurs before the early twenties, bone formation and resorption proceeds throughout life, a process known as bone remodeling. This allows for the healing of microfractures and re-enforcement of bone along lines of increased mechanical stress.

Bone Cells

Osteoblasts

Responsible for bone formation, they arise from a pluripotent mesenchymal precursor which can differentiate into fibroblasts, adipocytes, or osteoblasts. In their mature active form osteoblasts are cuboidal with an eccentric nucleus and a prominent endoplasmic reticulum. These cells are closely connected to cells lining the bone, which are also of osteoblast lineage and are probably resting osteoblasts (Fig. 28-1). Osteoblasts are the source of bone matrix which undergoes mineralization to form bone. Mineralization is facilitated by bone-specific alkaline phosphatase which is present in high concentrations in osteoblasts.

Osteocytes

About 10–20% of osteoblasts become buried in calcified bone in spaces called lacunae at which point they become osteocytes. When they become totally encased, their metabolic activity decreases substantially. Osteocytes receive their nutrients via canaliculi which form an elaborate array of connecting tubules. This system also serves as a communication network between osteocytes and their related bone-lining cells. The exact function of osteocytes is not

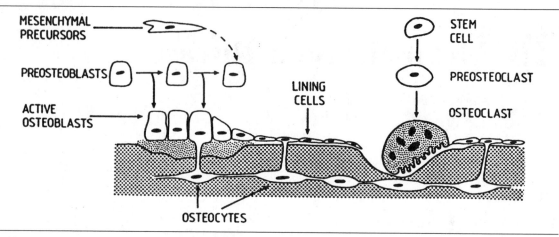

Fig. 28–1. Schematic representation of the major cells of bone. (Reprinted with permission from: Martin TJ, Ng KW, Suda T. Bone cell physiology. *Endocrinol Clin N Am* 18(4):834, 1989.)

clear. They may serve to transmit signals between osteoblasts and osteoclasts. The observation that osteocytes produce transforming growth factor beta (TGF-beta) and platelet-derived growth factor (PDGF) which stimulate osteoblastic activity raises the possibility that they may be important in bone remodeling.

Osteoclasts

They are the major bone-resorbing cell: large, multinucleated, and derived from hematopoietic mononuclear precursors. Under the influence of a variety of growth factors, vitamin D, and parathyroid hormone (PTH), these precursor cells develop into mature multinucleated osteoclasts. The mature osteoclast develops a ruffled border, which seals the cell to the bone surface, and secretes hydrogen ions and proteolytic lysosomal enzymes, facilitating resorption under the ruffled border (see Fig. 28-1). Osteopetrosis, a disease of osteoclast failure or deficiency, is characterized by defective or absent bone resorption. Radiographs of osteopetrotic bones reveal very dense bones. In its most severe form, pancytopenia occurs as bone replaces the marrow space. Some forms of osteopetrosis can be treated by bone marrow transplantation.

Bone Matrix

This is the product of osteoblasts. The major organic constituent, making up 95% of the matrix, is type I collagen.

Type I collagen is a triple helix made up of two alpha-1 and one alpha-2 peptide chains. In the alpha chains, every third amino acid is a glycine and almost every fourth is either proline or hydroxyproline. Hydroxyproline is found in only two or three proteins, the most abundant of which is collagen. In normal bone, collagen is arranged in layers giving rise to an organized lamellar pattern, which gives bone added tensile strength. When bone is formed very rapidly as in healing of fractures, in tumors, or with certain metabolic diseases, there is no organization of collagen fibers. This gives rise to bone with a disorganized "woven" pattern which is not as strong as normal bone. Other components of the extracellular bone matrix include osteocalcin (bone GLA protein) and other nonspecific macromolecules such as glycoproteins, proteoglycans, proteolipids, and phosphoproteins. Osteogenesis imperfecta is a genetic disorder of type I collagen. In its most extreme form, it is characterized by blue sclera, brittle, easily fractured bones, and early death.

Bone Mineralization

Osteoid or nonmineralized matrix is mineralized in an orderly, highly regulated way at the interface of osteoid and mineralized bone. Mineral is initially deposited as amorphous calcium phosphate which is ultimately transformed to hydroxyapatite. This process is influenced by the matrix proteins, primarily collagen and acidic phosphoproteins. Another requirement for mineralization is the availability of active vitamin D metabolites, which provide a ready supply of calcium and phosphate. Rickets in children and osteomalacia in adults results from either vitamin D deficiency or defective vitamin D metabolism. Impaired mineralization can also be caused by aluminum and fluoride intoxication, and phosphate deficiency. Excessive bone resorption, mediated by osteoclasts, results in demineralization. Once the mineral is removed from bone, degradation of the matrix occurs under the influence of collagenase and other proteolytic lysosomal enzymes.

Bone Remodeling

The term refers to the dynamic skeletal processes which occur after the epiphyseal growth plates have closed. Bone formation, mediated by osteoblasts, is closely coupled to bone resorption, an osteoclastic process. In the adult skeleton, bone formation occurs only where bone resorption has previously occurred. Bone remodeling occurs in discrete pockets referred to as bone remodeling units. Bone remodeling is regulated by hormonal factors. Table 28-1 lists the known mediators of bone metabolism, classifying them by their effects upon net bone formation. Anabolic mediators result in a net increase in bone mass, whereas catabolic mediators have the opposite effect. PTH and vitamin D have complex effects on bone, in some instances anabolic while in others catabolic. In general, however, the net effect on bone of these mediators is anabolic. One cytokine, interleukin-l, is the most potent bone-resorbing factor yet identified. At low concentrations, it appears to stimulate collagen synthesis, which would facilitate bone formation. Because it stimulates both formation and resorption, it could be a link between the two processes.

Table 28-1. Mediators of Bone Metabolism

Anabolic Mediators	Catabolic Mediators
Parathyroid hormone	Glucocorticoids
Vitamin D	Thyroxine
Estrogen	Interleukin-1
Testosterone	Lymphotoxin
Insulin	
Growth hormone	

Clinical Assessment of Metabolic Bone Diseases

Assessment of Bone Remodeling

There are a variety of biochemical markers which aid in assessing the degree of bone remodeling. These are frequently classified by their ability to reflect either bone formation or resorption. These markers can be used to diagnose bone diseases, aid in the choice of and assess the response to treatment.

Markers of Bone Formation

They reflect osteoblastic activity. Two such markers are serum alkaline phosphatase and osteocalcin, a recently discovered protein produced during bone formation. The two most common sources of alkaline phosphatase are bone and liver. Differentiating between the two can be difficult and is aided by identifying pre-existing liver disease and measuring liver-specific enzymes. It may be necessary to fractionate the alkaline phosphatase into its isoenzymes. Osteocalcin is synthesized by the osteoblast. Its blood levels are a reflection of new protein synthesis rather than release from demineralized bone matrix. This marker is therefore highly specific for bone formation. In general, both markers are elevated in bone diseases characterized by high bone turnover such as hyperparathyroidism and hyperthyroidism.

Markers of Bone Resorption

These markers are either derived from degraded bone matrix or are products of the osteoclasts. Urinary hydroxyproline (UHYP), a degradation product of collagen, is the most widely available clinical marker of bone resorption. It can be affected by diet and renal function. Another marker of osteoclastic activity is tartrate-resistant acid phosphatase, present in high concentrations in osteoclasts. Both are elevated in Paget's disease, hyperthyroidism, and multiple myeloma with bone involvement.

Bone Histomorphometry

Direct microscopic examination of sections of trabecular bone obtained from transiliac bone biopsies can establish a diagnosis and guide treatment. By studying the type and number of cells present in the bone and the marrow as well as quantifying the amount and composition of osteoid and mineral, important information about the dynamic process of bone remodeling can be obtained. In addition to traditional tissue stains, fluorochrome labeling is a valuable tool for studying bone remodeling. Tetracyclines are localized at the interface of osteoid and mineralized bone undergoing active mineralization. Different tetracyclines fluoresce at different wavelengths. This difference can be exploited to differentiate between pairs of labels given in temporal sequence. In diseases of defective mineralization such as osteomalacia, tetracycline deposition is diminished or delayed and the thickness of the osteoid seam is increased.

Assessment of Bone Density

New techniques have made it possible to determine bone density with accuracy and precision. That was not possible previously. This allows the clinician to determine the degree of osteopenia (decreased bone mass) and follow response to treatment. It also can help assess the risk of fracture in diseases with decreased bone mass, the most prevalent of which is postmenopausal osteoporosis. These methods are based upon measurement of transmission of radiation (x-rays or gamma rays) through bone and soft tissue. Dual x-ray absorptiometry has better precision and accuracy than earlier methods and a lower radiation exposure. Another method is quantitative computerized tomography or QCT. It is accurate but is more expensive and requires a higher radiation exposure. The indications for bone mass measurements are still being developed. At present unselected screening of women for osteoporosis is not recommended.

Selected Metabolic Bone Diseases

In metabolic bone diseases, the normal interactions between bone and the mediators of bone remodeling are altered. Since the hormones and minerals involved in bone homeostasis are interrelated, a deficiency or excess in one can lead to a major alteration in another. An example is osteomalacia due to malabsorption of vitamin D. This leads to a secondary elevation of PTH. Histologic examination of bone reveals osteomalacia due to the vitamin D deficiency and marrow fibrosis as a consequence of increased PTH. In addition, the clinical expression of metabolic bone diseases may vary with age. An example is intestinal malabsorption resulting in rickets in children but osteomalacia in adults.

Osteoporosis

The most prevalent bone disease in Western societies, where nutrition is adequate, is osteoporosis. It can occur in either sex and any age, but is primarily a disease of post-

menopausal women. It is a major public health problem in the United States, affecting some six million women, causing 300,000 new cases of hip fractures annually. In osteoporosis, there is a loss of bone mass with a normal ratio of osteoid to mineralized bone. Peak bone mass in women normally occurs at age 30 and in men at age 40 (Fig. 28-2). After age 30, women lose bone at a rate of 8% per decade and men at a rate of 3% per decade. Once menopause occurs, and if estrogen replacement is not given, the rate of bone loss in women accelerates rapidly. This disease does not occur as frequently in men, who reach a higher peak bone mass and maintain some testicular function throughout their life. Testosterone has anabolic effects on bone and helps preserve bone mass.

The pathogenesis of osteoporosis is not well defined but risk factors have been identified. Lifestyle and nutritional factors such as smoking, heavy alcohol and caffeine ingestion, inactivity, and poor calcium intake are associated with osteoporosis. Other risk factors include early menopause without estrogen replacement, late menarche, exercised-induced amenorrhea, a positive family history, small body habitus, and white or Asiatic ethnicity. Associated medical illnesses include hyperthyroidism, anorexia nervosa, Cushing's syndrome, and rheumatoid arthritis. The use of glucocorticoids and excessive thyroid hormone replacement can also accelerate bone loss.

Standard biochemical tests of bone and mineral metabolism are usually normal in age-related osteoporosis. Alkaline phosphatase can be elevated, after fractures. Bone turnover, as measured by bone biopsy, can be normal, high, or low.

Fig. 28-2. Bone mass changes with age and sex.

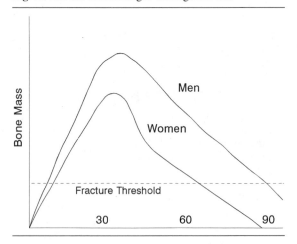

There are no good treatments which dramatically increase bone density in patients with osteoporosis. Treatment is aimed at prevention of falls and stabilization of bone mass with estrogen replacement, calcitonin treatment, and maintenance of adequate calcium intake (at least 1500 mg/day). Long-term prevention remains the most rational and successful approach in women at risk. This includes maintenance of adequate calcium intake and exercise beginning in adolescence, early initiation of estrogen replacement in the peri-menopausal period, and alteration of lifestyle risk factors.

Recently, a defect in the vitamin D receptor has been described which appears to be associated with osteoporosis, in patients homozygous for the defective gene. Heterozygotic individuals for the vitamin D receptor mutation have intermediate bone densities. This discovery may make it possible to target those women at risk to prevent the development of osteoporosis.

Osteomalacia and Rickets

Both diseases result from defective mineralization of bone. If this occurs before the epiphyseal plates have closed, rickets ensues. In rickets, defective mineralization involves the growth plate (junction between the epiphysis and metaphysis) as well as osteoid throughout the skeleton. The disease in adults following closure of the epiphyses is osteomalacia. The primary cause in both is vitamin D deficiency. Osteomalacia is the most common metabolic bone disease in the world, occurring primarily in underdeveloped regions of the world with poor dietary intake of vitamin D. Vitamin D deficiency can result from poor dietary intake, lack of sunlight exposure, malabsorption syndromes, accelerated metabolism of vitamin D (seen in people taking anticonvulsants), or defective production of $1,25\text{-}(OH)_2$-vitamin D (see below). Rickets can also be the result of inherited disorders of vitamin D metabolism. An example is the autosomal recessive disease vitamin D-dependent rickets. These patients are short, have the typical bony abnormalities of rickets, and do not respond to 25-OH vitamin D but administration of the active metabolite $1,25\text{-}(OH)_2$-vitamin D (calcitriol) promotes healing. This disease is presumed to be the result of defective renal production of 1-alpha hydroxylase and therefore $1,25\text{-}(OH)_2$-vitamin D.

Patients with these diseases demonstrate low to normal serum calcium, low serum phosphate, and elevated serum alkaline phosphatase levels. This enzyme elevation is a reflection of the high bone turnover. Bone biopsies reveal diminished deposition of tetracycline label at the mineralization front and large amounts of unmineralized osteoid.

Treatment of both dietary osteomalacia and rickets involves the administration of vitamin D with adequate dietary calcium. In "secondary" vitamin D deficiency, the underlying cause should be identified and corrected, if possible.

Renal Osteodystrophy

The kidney plays a major role in the homeostasis of calcium and phosphorous (See Chaps. 54 and 57). It is the site of production of $1,25\text{-}(OH)_2$-vitamin D (calcitriol), the active form of vitamin D via the renal enzyme 1-alpha hydroxylase. In renal failure, the activity of this enzyme is diminished, resulting in decreased production of calcitriol and decreased intestinal absorption of calcium. In addition, phosphate excretion is impaired in renal failure, leading to hyperphosphatemia which also inhibits calcitriol synthesis. The high phosphorous levels directly depress serum calcium. This hypocalcemia stimulates parathyroid hormone (PTH) secretion and leads to secondary hyperparathyroidism. In addition, accumulation of aluminum from the water used in dialysis and from aluminum-containing antacids (used as phosphate binders) occurs in chronic renal failure. Aluminum has been implicated in the development of the osteomalacia of chronic renal failure.

The skeletal abnormalities seen in chronic renal failure can be divided into two major types. A high turnover form is characterized by the pathologic lesion osteitis fibrosa cystica associated with secondary hyperparathyroidism. A low turnover form with osteomalacia is attributed to the inhibitory effects of aluminum with a contribution from the hypocalcemia and low calcitriol levels on mineralization.

Bone biopsies in patients with the high turnover form of osteodystrophy reveal increases in both osteoblastic and osteoclastic activity, bone marrow fibrosis, and a net increase in bone resorption, as a result of hyperparathyroidism. In low turnover osteodystrophy, findings typical of osteomalacia are seen with a marked decrease in osteoblastic activity. In some patients a mixed histologic picture of osteitis fibrosa and osteomalacia is seen. This may represent a transition phase from the high turnover disease to the low turnover form as aluminum accumulates in the bone.

Current management of renal osteodystrophy involves the use of low phosphate diets and calcium-containing phosphate binders to control hyperphosphatemia. Calcitriol administration and subtotal parathyroidectomy have been used to control the secondary hyperparathyroidism. Some clinicians have used desferrioxamine as a chelating agent to treat severe aluminum toxicity.

Primary Hyperparathyroidism

Caused by excess production of PTH with loss of normal feedback control of PTH secretion by calcium, it may occur as a result of a single adenoma of the parathyroid glands or from hyperplasia of the parathyroid glands (see Chap. 54). Before the advent of routine screening calcium measurements, this diagnosis was made only after the complications had occurred. Two major types of complications are observed, skeletal and renal. Renal manifestations include nephrolithiasis (renal stones) and nephrocalcinosis (diffuse deposition of calcium and phosphate in the renal parenchyma). Skeletal abnormalities range from diffuse osteopenia in the mildest forms to osteitis fibrosa cystica in advanced disease. The clinical picture of this disease is changing. Today, the initial presentation of primary hyperparathyroidism is generally asymptomatic hypercalcemia found on routine blood chemistry determination. At this stage, there may be no easily identifiable skeletal complications. The usual skeletal abnormality seen in patients with hyperparathyroidism is diffuse osteopenia, a reflection of the early effects of PTH on the bone. Currently, it is rare that to find osteitis fibrosa cystica in the patient with primary hyperparathyroidism.

Treatment of this disease has also changed with earlier diagnosis. In the past, surgery was the treatment of choice, as it is today in patients with symptoms or significant bone or renal disease. Asymptomatic hyperparathyroidism is becoming more common and with it a therapeutic dilemma. This situation is one of the indications for bone densitometry. If bone density is normal, the patient may be followed closely and treated medically with a liberal salt intake and restriction of calcium intake. If bone density is low, surgical resection might be recommended to help preserve bone mass. (It is easier to preserve bone than to attempt to rebuild it.)

Paget's Disease of Bone

A localized disorder of bone remodeling which is seen primarily in elderly white populations, this disease is initiated by an increase in osteoclastic-mediated bone resorption with subsequent compensatory activation of new bone formation by osteoblasts. The result is a disorganized mosaic of lamellar and woven bone at affected sites. This bone is less compact, more vascular, and more likely to fracture than normal bone. There are two different distribution patterns of disease, monostotic (single site) and polyostotic or multiple-site involvement. The most common skeletal sites of involvement are the tibia, femur, pelvis, spine, and skull.

There is an increased incidence of osteogenic sarcomas in Paget's disease. There is a geographic distribution of the disease, which is common in North America, Europe, New Zealand, and Australia. In general, prevalence rates decrease when moving north to south in Europe. In addition, viruslike inclusion bodies have been found in osteoclasts in affected bone, suggesting a viral etiology for this disease. Many now believe that Paget's disease is the result of a common viral infection, perhaps during early adulthood, in genetically susceptible individuals which subsequently manifests itself later in life.

These patients may have pain at involved skeletal sites. In active disease, both serum alkaline phosphatase and urinary hydroxyproline are elevated, indicating high bone turnover rate. Treatment is not indicated if symptoms are few, blood chemistries (including alkaline phosphatase) are normal, and weight-bearing bones are not involved. However, if the patient is in pain or at risk for long-bone fracture, treatment is necessary. Treatment currently involves the use of two agents, calcitonin and etidronate. Calcitonin is a small polypeptide hormone secreted by the parafollicular cells of the thyroid gland which inhibits osteoclast activity. Etidronate is a bisphosphonate which inhibits demineralization. These drugs are sometimes used in sequence. Response to treatment can be demonstrated by decreases in both serum alkaline phosphatase and urinary hydroxyproline.

Thyrotoxicosis

Hyperthyroidism is not usually thought of as a cause of metabolic bone disease, primarily because more dramatic clinical signs and symptoms dominate the clinical picture. Thyroid hormone acts on bone to stimulate osteoclastic activity in a manner similar to PTH. Hypercalcemia can be seen. Hyperthyroidism is therefore a state of high bone turnover with prolonged, untreated thyrotoxicosis leading to net bone loss. Treatment of the underlying thyroid disorder in a timely fashion will prevent significant bone loss.

Malignancy-Related Bone Disease

Bone diseases of malignancies are varied. Primary malignancies of bone such as osteosarcomas or Ewing's sarcoma can be deadly and difficult to treat. Extraskeletal malignancies often metastasize to bone. In lytic metastases, osteoclasts are activated and bone resorption is increased. Rarely, bone metastases are blastic (most often seen in prostate cancer). In these cases, cytokines produced by tumor cells stimulate osteoblasts to form new bone. Cells of the bone marrow can undergo malignant transformation. Multiple myeloma, a disease of plasma cells, can cause destructive bone lesions. Osteopenia may result from cytokine-stimulated osteoclastic activity. Other tumor products from different malignancies are capable of stimulating osteoclastic activity which can result in localized or diffuse osteopenia. Thus hypercalcemia can be seen in malignancies for a variety of reasons. One recent interesting discovery is that a PTH-related peptide secreted by certain tumors can stimulate osteoclastic activity and cause hypercalcemia. Treatment of the skeletal manifestations of malignancies are directed at the underlying disease along with specific treatment of complications such as pathologic fractures or hypercalcemia.

Clinical Example

1. A 47-year-old woman complained of diffuse musculoskeletal pain especially in her lower extremities. She had significant muscle weakness to the extent that she could no longer do her usual household duties. Her past history was remarkable for a partial gastrectomy with a Bilroth II anastomosis for peptic ulcer disease. Physical exam revealed a thin, ill-appearing woman who demonstrated difficulty arising from a chair and musculoskeletal pain with movement.

Laboratory Values

Serum calcium	7.8 mg/dl
Serum phosphorous	2.5 mg/dl
Serum albumin	3.0 gm/dl
Serum alkaline phosphatase	168 U/liter (normal: 14–103)
Serum intact PTH	256 pg/ml (normal: 10–65)
Serum 25-OH-vitamin D	6 ng/ml (normal: 10–55)
24-hour urinary calcium	15 mg/day (normal: < 250)
Chest x-ray	Old rib fractures and diffuse osteopenia

Discussion. This patient demonstrates osteomalacia as a complication of postgastrectomy malabsorption syndrome. The characteristic pain of osteomalacia includes a muscular component in addition to skeletal pain. Typically, the patient complains of pain mostly with movement and not at rest. In addition, an unexplained muscular weakness is often an accompanying finding. Spontaneous, nontraumatic fractures of the ribs or pelvis are frequently seen with osteomalacia. Osteopenia may be an additional finding. Fractures occur because of lack of repair of naturally-occurring microfractures and ineffective bone remodeling. The 25-OH-vitamin D level is markedly reduced and is the major cause of osteomalacia. Since vitamin D is a fat-soluble vitamin, fat malabsorption following partial gastrectomy leads to deficiency of 25-OH-vitamin D generally with low normal levels of $1,25\text{-}(OH)_2$-vitamin D. As a result of vitamin D deficiency, calcium absorption from the gut is decreased. In addition, there is diminished ability to liberate calcium from bone, which leads to hypocalcemia. Secondary hyperparathyroidism develops in response to hypocalcemia. This is evidenced by increased alkaline phosphatase levels indicating increased bone turnover and low 24-hour urinary excretion of calcium indicating maximal renal reabsorption of calcium.

Bibliography

Consensus development conference: diagnosis, prophylaxis, and treatment of osteoporosis. *Am J Med* 94:646–650, 1993. *The results of the most recent conference.*

Favus Murray J (ed.). *Primer on Metabolic Bone Diseases and Disorders of Mineral Metabolism* (2nd ed.). New York: Raven, 1993. *A concise overview of the biology of bone with excellent clinical descriptions of metabolic bone diseases.*

Morrison N, Qi JC, Tokita A, et al. Prediction of bone density from vitamin D receptor alleles. *Nature* 367:284–286, 1994. *The identification of a specific genetic defect which predicts bone density, a determinant of osteoporotic fractures. The first identified genetic defect in osteoporosis.*

Riggs BL and Melton LJ III. The prevention and treatment of osteoporosis. *New Engl J Med* 327:620–627, 1992. *An excellent clinical review on osteoporosis.*

Ristelli L and Ristelli J. Biochemical markers of bone metabolism. *Ann Med* 25:385–393, 1993. *An excellent review of the various bone markers with a focus on their clinical use.*

Part III Questions: Endocrine and Metabolic Disorders

1. Which of the following does not distinguish peptide and steroid hormones?
   A. Derivation from cholesterol
   B. Location of receptors in the target cell
   C. Regulation of transcription
   D. cAMP second messenger
   E. Nuclear location for effect on cellular metabolism

2. Patients with primary adrenal insufficiency typically demonstrate
   A. Diabetes mellitus
   B. Hypokalemia
   C. Sudden recent weight gain
   D. Hypotension
   E. None of the above

3. The primary metabolic difference between normal fasting and diabetic ketoacidosis (DKA) is that
   A. Insulin levels are lower in DKA.
   B. Activation of the counter regulatory hormone system occurs only in DKA.
   C. Release of FFA from adipose stores occurs only in DKA.
   D. Hepatic production of glucose is increased only in fasting.
   E. Glucose uptake by muscle is inhibited only in DKA.

4. A 43-year-old former Marine probation officer comes to your office with complaints of breast growth. Features consistent with a diagnosis of Klinefelter's syndrome include all but which of the following:
   A. Gynecomastia
   B. 0.8 cm hard testes
   C. 45,XO karyotype
   D. Twenty years of successful marriage
   E. Slightly reduced intelligence

5. If the connection between the hypothalamus and pituitary is disrupted, which of the following will occur?
   A. Decrease in the secretion of all anterior pituitary hormones
   B. Increase in prolactin and GH secretion
   C. Increase in prolactin secretion
   D. Increase in the secretion of all anterior pituitary hormones
   E. Increase in ACTH if the adrenals are intact

6. Graves' disease is produced by which of the following?
   A. Release of preformed thyroid hormone by the thyroid during autoimmune destruction of the gland
   B. Thyroid nodule that autonomously produces thyroid hormone
   C. Autoantibodies that bind T_4 receptors on the pituitary and induce production of TSH
   D. Autoantibodies that bind TSH receptors on the thyroid and induce production of thyroid hormone

7. Which of the following is *not* a factor involved in the evolution of renal osteodystrophy?
   A. Phosphate retention
   B. High PTH levels
   C. Aluminum toxicity
   D. Hypercalcemia
   E. Phosphate-binding antacids

IV Hematologic and Neoplastic Disorders

Part Editor

James N. George

29 Red Cells, Anemia, and Erythrocytosis

Sylvia S. Bottomley

Objectives

After completing this chapter, you should be able to

Describe the process of normal erythropoiesis and hemoglobin synthesis

State the factors regulating red cell production

Master the cardinal mechanisms causing hypoproliferative anemia

Explain the pathogenesis of maturation defects of erythropoiesis

Outline the major mechanisms leading to hemolytic disease and its complications

Illustrate the multifactorial basis of anemia

Distinguish primary from secondary erythrocytosis

Describe the clinical consequences of erythrocytosis

Normal Physiology of the Erythron

Lineage of Red Cells

In the special environment of the bone marrow stroma of reticular fibers and cells (fibroblasts, fat cells, endothelial cells, macrophages, and lymphocytes) the erythroid cell lineage, like all hematopoietic cell lines, derives from a pool of primitive, pluripotent stem cells which are semi-dormant with a lifelong capacity for self-renewal (Fig. 29-1). Through incompletely defined mechanisms, cellular and cytokine signals cause the pluripotent stem cell to differentiate into either a lymphoid progenitor cell to support lymphopoiesis or a multipotent progenitor cell, the CFU-GEMM, which is restricted to produce the other hematopoietic cells. In response to interleukin-3 and GM-CSF, the CFU-GEMM differentiates further, and in the case of erythropoiesis into the earliest progenitor committed to erythroid development, the BFU-E. Under the control of erythropoietin, the BFU-E matures into the CFU-E, which

is the immediate precursor of the pronormoblast, the earliest red cell precursor identifiable under the microscope.

The term "erythron" denotes the entire erythroid tissue, comprising the immature erythroid cell component in the bone marrow and the circulating erythrocytes (the red cell mass).

Red Cell Production

The erythrocyte develops in 7–8 days (Fig. 29-2). Erythropoietin induces the earliest erythroid committed progenitor cell to express genes of proteins unique to erythroid cells (i.e., certain membrane proteins including transferrin receptor, globin, enzymes of heme synthesis) and to proliferate through at least four cell divisions, yielding 16 cells that simultaneously mature as their nuclear and cell size decrease and cytoplasmic hemoglobin accumulates. Finally the nucleus is extruded, resulting in a reticulocyte. In a couple of days, the reticulocyte is released into the circulation, where during the ensuing 24 hours it produces the last 25–30% of the red cell's hemoglobin and before the residual hemoglobin-synthesizing organelles (mitochon-

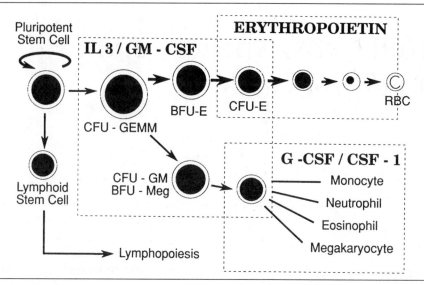

Fig. 29-1. Marrow cell generation. Illustrated are progenitor cells of increasingly restricted potentiality that ultimately give rise to the peripheral blood cells. CFU = colony-forming unit (denotes the in vitro identification of the progenitor cell); GEMM = granulocyte-erythrocyte-monocyte (macrophage)-megakaryocyte; BFU = burst-forming unit; E = erythroid; RBC = red blood cell; GM = granulocyte-monocyte (macrophage); Meg = megakaryocyte; IL3 = interleukin-3; CSF = colony-stimulating factor; G = granulocyte. (Reprinted with permission from: Hillman RS and Finch CA. *Red Cell Manual* (6th ed.). Philadelphia: Davis, 1992, p. 3.)

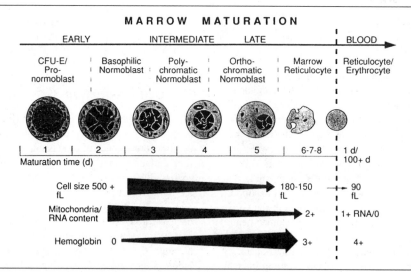

Fig. 29-2. Maturation of erythroid cells. (Reprinted with permission from: Hillman RS and Finch CA. *Red Cell Manual* (6th ed.). Philadelphia: Davis, 1992, p. 5.)

dria and ribosomes) are lost. Hence the reticulocyte content in the peripheral blood reflects the "birth rate" of new erythrocytes and is a quantitative index of erythroid marrow function.

Several nutritional factors are essential for both proliferation and maturation of the developing red cell. Folic acid and vitamin B_{12} are required in adequate amounts for methionine and thymidylate synthesis for DNA replication and sequential cell division (Fig. 29-3A). Iron is essential for ribonucleotide reductase in DNA synthesis and large amounts are needed for hemoglobin production. In the normal adult 65–75% of body iron is contained in the erythroid tissue. It is conveyed to the immature erythroid cell through the plasma by the protein transferrin and then via endocytosis of the iron-transferrin receptor complex (Fig. 29-3B). Most of intracellular iron enters the mitochondria for incorporation into heme and any excess taken up is stored within ferritin molecules as semicrystalline aggregates, recognized on the Prussian blue-stained bone marrow smear as blue dots in the cytoplasm (sideroblasts). Simultaneously with the biosynthesis of heme, polypeptide chains of alpha and beta globin, and small amounts of delta and gamma globin, are synthesized on erythroid cell ribosomes that become assembled as tetramers of heme and globin into the hemoglobin molecule. In adult erythrocytes hemoglobin A $(\alpha_2\beta_2)$ makes up 96–97% of the hemoglobin, hemoglobin $A_2(\alpha_2\delta_2)$ about 2.5%, and hemoglobin F$(\alpha_2\gamma_2)$ less than 2%.

Red Cell Survival, Breakdown, and Replenishment

The erythrocyte remains intravascular for 120 days during which there is progressive loss of membrane, critical enzymes of its glycolytic pathways, and metabolic intermediates necessary to sustain its structural and functional integrity; it is removed by the reticuloendothelial (RE) system of the spleen (and liver). At this point the erythrocyte's membrane and proteins are catabolized, the porphyrin ring of heme is degraded to bilirubin, and its iron is salvaged and transported to the marrow for reutilization in hemoglobin synthesis (see below). To maintain 25×10^{12} circulating erythrocytes (750 g of Hb) in an adult man, the marrow must produce 2×10^{11} reticulocytes (6 g Hb) per day. It can increase this production rate six- to eightfold (half a pint of blood per day) so that the red cell lifespan has to be reduced to below 15–20 days for anemia to ensue.

Regulation of Erythrocyte Production

During its 175-mile voyage through the bloodstream, the erythrocyte's principal function is as a vehicle for hemoglobin, the respiratory pigment that accepts oxygen in the lung, then transports and releases it to tissues. While reduction in tissue oxygen supply promptly engages certain general physiologic mechanisms — such as an increase in cardiac output, an increase in active tissue capillaries, or a rightward shift of the oxygen-dissociation curve (to enhance release of oxygen to tissues at lower pressures) — tissue oxygen supply is the fundamental factor or "thermostat" which regulates red cell production through the humoral mediator erythropoietin (Fig. 29-4). The principal hypoxia "sensor" tissue resides in the kidney (the proximal convoluted tubule cells or peritubular interstitial cells) and in response to oxygen requirements elaborates erythropoietin.

About 10–15% of erythropoietin is produced in the

Fig. 29-3. (A) Metabolic link of folate and vitamin B_{12} for DNA synthesis. (B) General schema of hemoglobin production. (Reprinted with permission from: Hillman RS and Finch CA. *Red Cell Manual* (6th ed.). Philadelphia: Davis, 1992, pp. 7–8.)

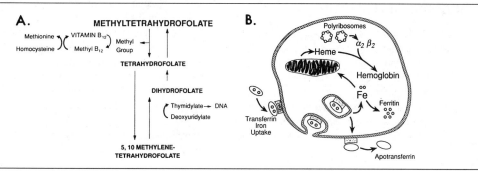

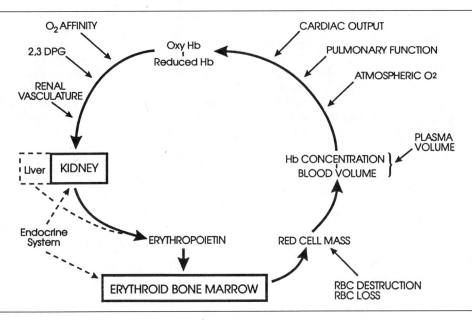

Fig. 29-4. Regulatory circuits governing red cell production. 2,3 DPG = 2,3-diphosphoglycerate; Hb = hemoglobin.

liver, accounting for the low rate of red cell production in anephric individuals. Other regulators of erythropoiesis are the hormones from the testes, the pituitary, and the thyroid and adrenal glands, since hypofunction of these tissues results in diminished rates and hyperfunction in increased rates of erythropoiesis. The precise mechanisms of action of these hormones have not been defined. Oxygen requirements play the major role in thyroidal control of erythropoiesis. Androgens enhance production of erythropoietin by increasing its release by the kidney, explaining the higher circulating red cell count in males.

Mechanisms of Anemia

The pathophysiologic approach to explain anemia (defined as the individual's hemoglobin or hematocrit falling more than two standard deviations below the established mean for age, sex, and altitude of residence) is based on the general nature of the dysfunction of the erythron. Thus either red cell production is impaired because of abnormalities of proliferation or maturation, or the loss of red cells exceeds the erythroid marrow's capacity to compensate for the anemia (Table 29-1).

Decreased Production of Red Cells

Hypoproliferative Anemia

The proliferation of erythroid cells becomes impaired with insufficient iron supply, suppression of erythropoietin production, or loss of stem cells or inhibition of their function (see Table 29-1). The morphologic evidence for these aberrations is a low reticulocyte count (index) and a hypoplasia or aplasia of the erythroid cell line in the marrow, reflecting its inability to respond to the anemia. **Iron-deficient erythropoiesis** due to body iron depletion or due to impaired iron availability in inflammatory disorders is by far the most common. The bulk of body iron is trapped within circulating hemoglobin and essentially all of the iron required (25 mg) for replacement of worn-out red cells each day is drawn from stores laid down when old cells are destroyed (Fig. 29-5). Only a small but critical fraction of iron (1 mg in man, 2 mg in the menstruating woman) is obtained from the diet to merely replenish what is lost in sloughed intestinal epithelium and exfoliated skin. Thus iron deficiency develops readily from continued blood loss (e.g., lesions in the gastrointestinal tract in men and post-menopausal women, excessive menstrual bleeding) and in Western countries less often from dietary

Table 29-1. Pathophysiologic Classification of Anemia

Type	General Mechanism	Cause (Principal Examples)
Hypoproliferative	Iron-deficient erythropoiesis	Early iron deficiency, inflammation
	Decreased erythropoietin production	Renal disease, hypometabolism
	Stem cell damage or loss	Drugs, radiation, immune, neoplastic marrow disorders, fibrosis, tumor metastasis
Maturation defect	Nuclear (megaloblastic)	Vitamin B_{12}/folate deficiency, drugs, hereditary defects, erythroleukemia
	Cytoplasmic (microcytic)	Severe iron deficiency, globin defect, porphyrin synthesis defect
Hemorrhage/Hemolysis	Acute blood loss	
	Decreased RBC deformability	Spherocytosis, microangiopathic, sickle cell anemia, Heinz bodies
	RE phagocytosis	Immune and autoimmune, hypersplenism
	Intravascular hemolysis	Immune, autoimmune, macroangiopathic, PNH*, drugs, venoms

* PNH = paroxysmal nocturnal hemoglobinuria.

Fig. 29-5. Metabolic pathways of iron (the iron cycle). RBC'S = red blood cells; Fe = iron. (Used with permission from: Duffy TP. Iron deficiency. In Spivak JL and Eichner ER (eds.). *The Fundamentals of Clinical Hematology* (3rd ed.). Baltimore: Johns Hopkins, 1993, p. 18.)

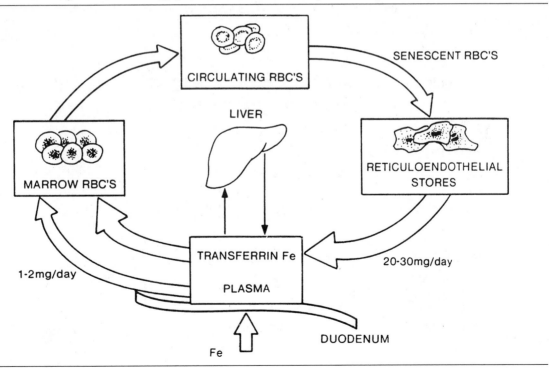

deficits and during normal growth (e.g., infancy, pregnancy). However, iron deficiency typically evolves gradually and this is readily reflected in several biochemical and morphologic indicators aiding in diagnosis (Fig. 29-6).

During chronic infections and inflammation that may also accompany certain malignancies and collagen vascular disorders, iron-deficient erythropoiesis evolves without a body iron deficit, and the associated anemia is called anemia of chronic disease. Here activated, proliferating macrophages appear to compete with erythroblasts for iron by retaining the iron they receive as they degrade the hemoglobin of expired red cells, thus impairing its reutilization (the "inflammatory block" of iron metabolism). This anemia is importantly distinguished from iron deficiency in that the serum transferrin level (IBC) is usually depressed, due to impaired protein synthesis, and iron stores are normal or increased (the iron displaced there from the missing hemoglobin) as detected by marrow hemosiderin deposits and/or the serum ferritin level. The anemia is further complicated by a blunted erythropoietin production and a moderately shortened red cell lifespan. These multiple derangements are explained by immune activation in response to foreign antigens incident to the inflammatory state, causing the production of cytokines by activated macrophages, e.g., interleukin-1, tumor necrosis factor. Such cytokines alter macrophage iron metabolism and most significantly directly inhibit the production of erythropoietin and its action in that the anemia can be overcome with the administration of large amounts of recombinant erythropoietin.

The effect of a **lack of erythropoietin** on the erythron is analogous to dysfunction of erythroid-committed progenitor cells because they represent the target tissue of the hormone. Erythropoietin production is impaired in diseases of tissues involved in its generation, namely renal and liver disease, and is blunted in response to the anemia of inflammation, as mentioned above. Rarely, antibodies to erythropoietin may arise that inhibit the biologic activity of the hormone.

Loss of stem cells or inhibition of their function reduces or may halt erythroid differentiation and proliferation. While dysfunction of erythroid-committed progenitors results in erythroid dysplasia (refractory anemia) or pure red cell aplasia, damage to or a genetic change in

Fig. 29-6. Sequential changes in the development of iron deficiency. (Reprinted with permission from: Hillman RS and Finch CA. *Red Cell Manual* (6th ed.). Philadelphia: Davis, 1992, p. 69.)

	NORMAL	IRON DEPLETION	IRON DEFICIENT ERYTHROPOIESIS	IRON DEFICIENCY ANEMIA
Iron stores →				
Erythron Iron →				
RE Marrow Fe	2 - 3 +	0 - 1 +	0	0
Transferrin IBC (μg/dL)	330 ±30	360	390	410
Plasma ferritin (μg/mL)	100 ±60	20	10	<10
Iron absorption (%)	5 - 10	10 - 15	10 - 20	10 - 20
Plasma iron (μg/dL)	115 ±50	115	<60	<40
Transferrin saturation (%)	35 ±15	30	<15	<10
Sideroblasts (%)	40 - 60	40 - 60	<10	<10
RBC Protoporphyrin (μg/dL RBC)	30	30	100	200
Erythrocytes	Normal	Normal	Normal	Micro/Hypo

more ancestral progenitor cells leads to associated leukopenia and thrombocytopenia as well (e.g., myelodysplastic syndrome, aplastic anemia). Unknown factors, known marrow toxins (e.g., drugs, chemicals, and x-rays), or viruses are implicated in these states. New proliferating clones of hematopoietic progenitors (e.g., leukemias) with a growth advantage over the normal blood cell lineages, proliferation of tumor cells invading the marrow, or a fibrosis process within the marrow space all can be said to disrupt the critical environment of normal stem cells or their immediate progeny. Stem cell function can also be inhibited by antibodies or abnormal lymphocytes (suppressor lymphocytes).

Maturation Disorders (Ineffective Erythropoiesis)

Here disruption of the orderly subcellular events during maturation of erythroid cells results in faulty erythroblasts, many of which are removed by marrow RE cells, a process called intramedullary hemolysis. Because progenitor cell function is intact and erythropoietin production in response to the anemia is appropriate, the erythroid marrow is hypercellular, but the reticulocyte count is low. This constellation of features, termed "ineffective erythropoiesis," is characteristic of all erythroid maturation defects (see Table 29-1).

Impaired nuclear maturation due to slowed cell division occurs when DNA synthesis is inhibited because of depletion of certain essential coenzymes or defects of enzymes involved in nucleic acid synthesis, or other disturbances of nucleic acid metabolism. Vitamin B_{12} (cobalamin) and folic acid represent the principal coenzymes that can be depleted in man, each in distinct settings of nutritional or metabolic aberrations as illustrated in Table 29-2. Drugs, particularly chemotherapeutic and antineoplastic agents, inhibit nucleic acid biosynthesis. Methotrexate specifically inhibits dihydrofolate reductase so that the active coenzyme tetrahydrofolate, essential for nucleic acid production, cannot be formed (see Fig. 29-3). Impairment of DNA synthesis prolongs the resting phase of the dividing precursor cells between mitosis while cytoplasmic development proceeds unimpeded. The consequence is a **megaloblastic** cell, which is larger than normal and has excessive cytoplasm and a disproportionately immature nucleus. Only a proportion of such cells mature fully into large erythrocytes and are released into the circulation (macrocytic anemia), but they have a reduced life span (see above). Maturation of leukocytes and megakaryocytes is similarly affected, so that pancytopenia commonly accompanies megaloblastic anemia. Distinct and potentially irreversible effects of vitamin B_{12} deficiency are neural deficits (particularly of peripheral sensory nerves and the dorsal and corticospinal tracts) because vitamin B_{12} is also an essential coenzyme for maintenance of membrane lipids and hence the neuronal integrity of myelin.

Impaired cytoplasmic maturation occurs when hemo-

Table 29-2. Mechanisms of Vitamin B_{12} (Cobalamin) and Folic Acid Deficiency

Disorder	Cause	Physiologic Basis
Vitamin B_{12} deficiency	Loss of intrinsic factor (e.g., pernicious anemia, infiltrative tumor of gastric fundus, gastrectomy)	Vitamin B_{12} must be complexed with intrinsic factor for absorption in the ileum
	Bacterial colonization of small intestine (e.g., blind loops, diverticulosis)	Bacteria consume the vitamin B_{12} ingested in the diet
	Diseases of the terminal ileum (e.g., ileitis, lymphoma, resection, AIDS)	Vitamin B_{12} is not absorbed because the terminal ileum is its site of absorption
	Inactivation of cobalamin (e.g., nitrous oxide anesthesia/abuse)	Nitrous oxide oxidizes the Co^+ in cobalamin
Folic acid deficiency	Dietary lack or insufficient supply for increased needs (e.g., alcoholism, pregnancy, hemolysis, hemodialysis)	Body reserves (stores) of folic acid are limited — sufficient for 5 months
	Malabsorption diseases of the small intestine (e.g., sprue)	Dietary folic acid is not absorbed
	Folic acid antagonist drugs (e.g., methotrexate, trimethoprim)	Drugs compete for enzymes that transform folate to metabolically active forms

globin synthesis is defective while cell division is relatively unaffected. The resulting erythrocytes are small and poorly hemoglobinized (microcytic-hypochromic anemia) and they also have a reduced lifespan. The commonest cause is **severe iron deficiency anemia,** when the impaired heme synthesis becomes dominant over the proliferative defect (see above) due to iron lack along with a high erythropoietin drive. Reduced or absent synthesis of structurally normal globin chains impairs hemoglobin production in **thalassemia,** the most common genetic disorder worldwide. While homozygous beta thalassemia, almost always due to point mutations in the beta globin gene(s), is manifested by severe hypochromic-microcytic anemia associated with ineffective erythropoiesis and hemolysis, in heterozygotes (synonyms are thalassemia trait, thalassemia minor), with only one of the two beta globin genes affected, the anemia is mild and resembles iron deficiency. The reduced beta globin chain production is often associated with an increase of delta and/or gamma globin chains, and therefore of Hb A_2 ($\alpha_2\delta_2$) and Hb F ($\alpha_2\gamma_2$); quantitation of these hemoglobins provides important diagnostic tests for this thalassemia. Severity of alpha thalassemia depends upon the number of functioning alpha globin genes of which there are normally four. Deletion of all four genes produces hydrops fetalis; loss of three genes causes Hb H disease — a hemolytic anemia due to damage of red cells caused by precipitates of unstable tetramers of unpaired beta globin chains that are produced at a normal rate. Deletion of two alpha globin genes produces a thalassemia minor that is clinically indistinguishable from beta thalassemia trait while deletion of a single alpha globin gene produces only a slight microcytosis without anemia, hence called "silent carrier" and is common in American blacks. Incompletely defined defects of heme biosynthesis impair hemoglobin production in the **sideroblastic anemias** and enormous amounts of iron characteristically accumulate in mitochondria of erythroblasts (called ring sideroblasts), impeding their development. Within the spectrum of these disorders, inherited defects produce a uniformly hypochromic-microcytic anemia and in the X-linked form are due to mutations in erythroid-5-aminolevulinate synthase, the first and rate-limiting enzyme of heme synthesis. Acquired sideroblastic anemia is usually a clonal disorder and typically manifests only a small population of hypochromic-microcytic red cells in the peripheral blood; the mean corpuscular volume (MCV) is commonly increased. The ineffective erythropoiesis in both, homozygous thalassemia and most sideroblastic anemias, promotes an indolent but relentless increased intestinal iron absorption, and milder hereditary sideroblastic anemia in particular may present as an iron overload state mimicking hemochromatosis.

Increased Destruction of Red Cells (Hemolysis)

The rate of red cell loss (hemorrhage) or destruction (hemolysis) must exceed the production capacity of the normal marrow, which is 6- to 8-fold basal, for anemia to develop; thus a mild hemolysis or hemorrhage will not produce readily detectable anemia. Signs of increased red cell generation (e.g., reticulocytosis, marrow erythroid hyperplasia) are therefore the major clues for compensated hemolytic disease. Among the numerous causes of hemolysis, red cells succumb to premature destruction through one of three general pathophysiologic mechanisms (see Table 29-1).

Decreased Erythrocyte Deformability/Fragmentation

The normal red cell does not survive beyond 120 days in individuals who have had splenectomy. However, the red cell's survival for 120 days in the presence of the spleen is largely dependent upon its ability to deform, or change from its round, biconcave, 7-micron disc shape into an elongated shape that can traverse from the red pulp of the splenic cords through the 0.5- to 2.5-micron spaces between endothelial cells lining the venous sinuses of the spleen. A prolonged sojourn of a less deformable red cell in splenic cords (where viscosity is high and pH, glucose concentration, and partial pressure of oxygen are low) reduces its limited metabolic resources and favors premature phagocytosis. Increased cell size (e.g., macrocytes of megaloblastic anemia), a decreased membrane-to-volume ratio (e.g., spherocytes of hereditary spherocytosis and of antibody-mediated partial red cell phagocytosis), an increased membrane-to-volume ratio (e.g., target cells of hypochromic anemias and spur cells of liver disease), increased cytoplasmic viscosity (e.g., hemoglobin aggregation due to hypoxia in sickle cell anemia), and damage of the bilayered membrane of the red cell (e.g., fragmented cells of angiopathic hemolysis and the presence of Heinz bodies from oxidant drugs) all reduce its deformability.

Enhanced Erythrocyte Phagocytosis
Antibodies of the IgG class may develop to certain drugs or as autoantibodies (e.g., in association with collagen vascular diseases, or lymphoid malignancies, or without other disease = idiopathic), and bind to autologous red cells with or without complement so that the red cells are aggluti-

nated by anti-IgG and/or anti-C3 in the Coombs test. IgM autoantibodies are most often encountered with EBV or mycoplasma infections and in association with B-cell neoplasms. They are usually cold-reactive, i.e., they cause overt red cell agglutination when refrigerated (hence called cold agglutinins) and mediate hemolysis by binding complement on the red cell. Antibody- or complement-coated red cells are removed in part or entirely by splenic and/or hepatic macrophages after binding of the Fc fragment of the antibody and/or complement on the red cells to the Fc fragment receptor and/or complement receptor on macrophages. Partial phagocytosis is common and removes more membrane than cytoplasm, resulting in spherocytes. These functions of the RE system lead to a "work" hypertrophy of the organs of red cell destruction (splenomegaly and hepatomegaly). On the other hand, an enlarged spleen from other causes (e.g., congestive or infiltrative splenomegaly) can sequester normal red cells excessively (**hypersplenism**).

Intravascular Hemolysis

The red cell may be prematurely destroyed by outright lysis within the circulation in only a few instances: (a) mechanical disruption in angiopathic states mentioned above; (b) antibody-mediated hemolysis when complement is bound to the red cell and becomes fully activated; (c) complement-mediated hemolysis without antibody, unique for the paroxysmal nocturnal hemoglobinuria defect; (d) an oxidant stress sufficiently severe (usually from oxidant drugs) to disrupt the integrity of the membrane; and (e)

lysins generated by certain bacteria (e.g., *C. welchii*) or venoms reaching the circulation. Hemoglobin is released into the plasma (hemoglobinemia) and the mechanisms of its subsequent disposal are depicted in Fig. 29-7. Low serum haptoglobin and hemopexin (these become depleted initially), methemalbuminemia, and hemoglobinuria and/or hemosiderinuria are the specific laboratory parameters measured to detect intravascular hemolysis. Prolonged hemosiderinuria also leads to iron deficiency.

Complications of Hemolytic Anemia

In hemolytic states of chronic or life-long duration several distinct complications can develop: (a) formation of bilirubin stones due to the increased production of bilirubin; (b) gout because of the overproduction of uric acid incident to increased nucleic acid catabolism from the high erythroid cell turnover in the bone marrow; and (c) in hereditary hemolytic anemias, an abrupt increase in anemia accompanying a viral illness, e.g., B19 parvovirus infection (aplastic crisis), due to depletion of folic acid when the dietary supply becomes insufficient for the increased cell turnover (megaloblastic crisis), or due to enhanced hemolysis from intercurrent infection or certain drugs (hemolytic crisis).

Multifactorial Basis of Anemia

In settings of complex illness in particular, more than one mechanism for anemia is very common, each adding to the severity of anemia and occasionally one mechanism in part

Fig. 29-7. (A) Fate of hemoglobin released into plasma. (B) Sequential indicators of acute intravascular hemolysis. (Reprinted with permission from: Hillman RS and Finch CA. *Red Cell Manual* (5th and 6th eds.). Philadelphia: Davis, 1985, p. 20 and 1992, p. 103.)

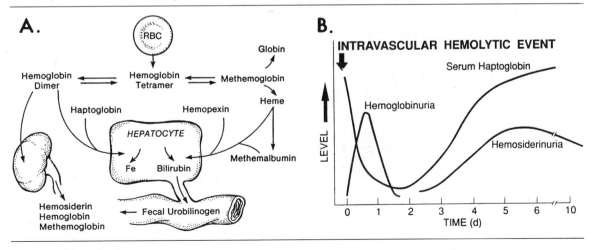

masking the cardinal features of another. For example, in chronic renal disease the major defect of erythropoietin lack may be complicated by the unavailability of iron due to a chronic infection, by the lack of iron due to chronic blood loss, by the lack of folate which is removed by hemodialysis, or by a hemolytic process due to an oxidant drug. Another common example is encountered in patients with liver disease, in whom any or all of the following causes of anemia may coexist: acute or chronic blood loss, folate deficiency, chronic infection, ethanol toxicity, ring sideroblast defect, spur cell hemolysis, hemolysis due to hypophosphatemia, hypersplenism, as well as the liver disease itself. A third instance is infiltration of the bone marrow by tumor cells impairing erythropoiesis and a concomitant increased peripheral destruction of red cells (e.g., due to an antibody) but the latter seeming masked by the lack of a reticulocytosis because the erythroid marrow cannot respond to the accelerated loss of red cells.

Physiologic Effects of Anemia

The severity of anemia and the rate at which it has developed determine the hypoxia effects on other systems and hence on symptoms. Rapid blood loss (hemorrhagic anemia) may proportionately produce the symptoms of tachycardia, hypotension, and shock. With slow evolution of anemia, remarkable adaptation occurs that includes increased levels of 2,3-DPG allowing oxygen unloading at a lower saturation of hemoglobin, and few if any symptoms appear in the absence of physical exertion. Once anemia is sufficiently severe, the status of the cardiovascular system (the principal physiologic compensatory mechanism for anemic hypoxia) determines clinical manifestations, e.g., shortness of breath, increased heart rate, palpitations, angina, and in older individuals heart failure; other symptoms are referable to the muscular and central nervous system, e.g., fatigue, irritability, dizziness, and headache. Cardiac output remains relatively constant until the hemoglobin falls below 10 g/dl when less than the normal 4 ml of O_2/dl of circulating blood can be made available to tissues (each gram of Hb carrying 1.34 ml of O_2 when completely saturated). Then cardiac output increases in proportion to the hemoglobin deficit, blood flow is redistributed to the most vital centers, renal blood flow may be reduced by 50%, and cutaneous flow is markedly decreased. Unless severe cardiac or pulmonary disease is present or the hemoglobin level is below 6 to 7 g/dl, blood transfusion is usually not justified. In many chronic anemias a very low hemoglobin can be tolerated, especially by younger individuals, until a specific therapeutic response can be obtained.

Mechanisms of Erythrocytosis
Relative Erythrocytosis

If the hemoglobin and hematocrit alone are relied upon, an apparent or relative erythrocytosis caused by a reduction in plasma volume may be misinterpreted as a raised red cell volume. Thus isotopic measurements of the circulating red cell and plasma volumes are necessary to establish the presence of true or absolute erythrocytosis. Sometimes only a high-normal red cell volume and low-normal plasma volume explain a modest increase in hematocrit. Common but transient settings for a contracted plasma volume include depletion of extracellular fluid volume of any cause. Sustained relative erythrocytosis typically occurs in a middle-aged man with a hard-driving personality, often with a history of smoking and cardiovascular disease, especially essential hypertension. In this circumstance the pathophysiologic mechanism for the reduced plasma volume is not defined but is commonly accentuated by diuretic agents.

Absolute Erythrocytosis
Appropriate Increase of Red Cell Production

An absolute increase in circulating red cells (or red cell mass) is most often encountered as a physiologic response to tissue oxygen deficits (Table 29-3). In this case, oxygen delivery is compensated by an erythropoietin-mediated increase in red cell production, and one finds a direct relationship between the red cell mass and arterial oxygen saturation. The classic example of a physiologic erythrocytosis is that which develops in individuals after sojourns at high altitudes. The common clinical conditions are many pulmonary disorders, cardiac abnormalities accompanied by a right-to-left shunt, and the reduced oxygen saturation of hemoglobin due to excess carboxyhemoglobin in heavy smokers. Uncommonly mutations of globin structure may impart to the hemoglobin molecule an increased affinity for oxygen, impairing its release to tissues. In this situation the hemoglobin P_{50} is shifted to the left (P_{50} refers to the partial pressure of oxygen at which hemoglobin is 50% saturated with oxygen.)

Inappropriate Increase of Red Cell Production

Here one finds no direct relationship between the red cell mass and arterial oxygen saturation, and the latter is normal. **Large amounts of erythropoietin** may be produced and released by several types of neoplasms or through local renal ischemia caused by certain benign lesions of

Table 29-3. Causes of High Hemoglobin/Hematocrit

RELATIVE ERYTHROCYTOSIS (SPURIOUS ERYTHROCYTOSIS)

ABSOLUTE ERYTHROCYTOSIS

Physiologically appropriate erythropoietin overproduction
  Hypoxemic states (decreased PaO_2)
    High altitude
    Pulmonary disorders
    Intermittent hypoxia (supine hypoventilation, sleep
     apnea)
    Right-to-left cardiac shunt
  Abnormal hemoglobin function (normal PaO_2)
    High oxygen-affinity hemoglobin
    Carboxyhemoglobinemia (smokers)
    Congenital methemoglobinemia
    Diphosphoglycerate (DPG) mutase deficiency
Physiologically inappropriate erythropoietin over-
  production
  Neoplasms (kidney, cerebellum, liver, uterus,
    adrenal)
  Renal lesions (renal artery stenosis, cysts, hy-
    dronephrosis, transplant-associated)
  Hereditary defects
Autonomous erythropoiesis
  Polycythemia vera
  Hereditary defects of erythroid progenitors

the kidney (see Table 29-3). Removal of such lesions or repair of a renal artery stenosis corrects the erythrocytosis. Excessive production of erythropoietin also occurs as a rare recessively inherited defect. In **polycythemia vera,** a genetic change is acquired in a multipotent progenitor cell and gives rise to a clone of progeny committed to the erythroid as well as granulocytic and megakaryocytic cell lines which proliferate excessively and independently of the normal humoral controls, the erythroid cell line proliferating most markedly. This panmyelosis is usually evidenced by some hepatosplenomegaly due to extramedullary hematopoiesis in these organs, as well as by leukocytosis and thrombocytosis. Serum erythropoietin levels are characteristically normal or low. The very massive red cell overproduction possible in this disorder may double the circulating red cell mass, iron supply becomes a rate-limiting factor, and the erythrocytes are often microcytic-hypochromic. It is the continued iron depletion achieved by phlebotomy therapy that serves best as a brake on the excessive erythroid proliferation. After 5–20 years this process slows down, may be followed by bone marrow fibrosis, and/or may terminate in acute leukemia. Recent reports indicate that genetic defects of the erythropoietin receptor or post-receptor events in the erythroid progenitor

cell may underlie apparent autonomous familial erythrocytosis, without leukocytosis and thrombocytosis.

Consequences of Erythrocytosis and Polycythemia Vera

The harmful effects of excess red cells are due mainly to increased blood viscosity that rises sharply with a hematocrit over 50% (Fig. 29-8), impairing cardiac hemodynamics and reducing oxygen transport, which in turn can

Fig. 29-8. Effect of the hematocrit on blood viscosity and oxygen transport. (Reprinted with permission from: Babior BM and Stossel TP. *Hematology: A Pathophysiological Approach* (3rd ed.). New York: Churchill Livingstone, 1994, p. 21, as modified from: Erslev AJ and Gabuzda TG, *Pathophysiology of Blood.* Philadelphia: Saunders, 1975, p. 31.)

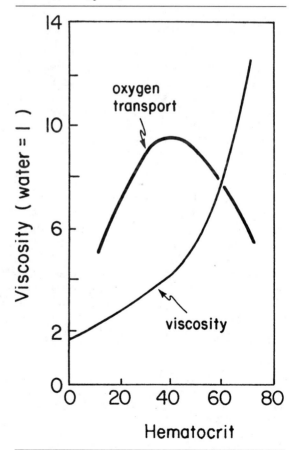

further increase the erythrocytosis. The symptoms are similar to those of anemia. The cardiovascular stress from hypervolemia may manifest as chest pain or fullness, increased heart rate, shortness of breath, or claudication; effects on the central nervous system may result in irritability, lightheadedness, or fatigue. In polycythemia vera, the high blood viscosity, particularly when coupled with the thrombocytosis and coexisting atherosclerotic vascular disease, notably promotes arterial and venous thrombosis and infarctions. The paradox of simultaneous hemorrhagic manifestations may also accompany the disease because of impaired platelet function as part and parcel of this myeloproliferative disorder (see Chap. 34). Complications of operative procedures from hemorrhage and/or thrombosis are very significant, and elective surgery should be planned several months after hematologic control. The excessive cellular proliferation also leads to increased production of uric acid and gouty arthritis in 5–10% of patients.

Clinical Examples

1. A 51-year-old biochemist was referred for evaluation of anemia noted on a blood count which he had requested for reasons of not feeling well. He reported fatigue, a 20-lb. weight loss, achiness of muscles and joints and intermittent fever (to 101°F) for some 6 weeks. Nine months earlier a heart murmur was found on annual employee examination but he had not yet obtained the advised cardiologic evaluation. Examination was remarkable for: temperature 38.2°C, pulse 100, BP 120/70; a petechial hemorrhage on the left lower palpebral conjunctiva; a grade iv systolic murmur along the left sternal border radiating to the axilla as well as a small apical thrill; and palpable liver and spleen, both 3 cm below the costal margins. Laboratory data: Hb 11.2 g/dl, Hct 35.8%, MCV 86 fl, reticulocytes 1.0%, WBC $8.3 \times 10^3/mm^3$ with 73% neutrophils, 2% bands, 21% lymphocytes, 3% monocytes and 1% basophils; platelets $287 \times 10^3/mm^3$; sedimentation rate (Wintrobe) 30 mm; serum iron 30 g/dl (normal 70–150), TIBC 188 g/dl (normal 280–350), transferrin saturation 16% (normal 25–45), serum ferritin 450 ng/ml (normal 20–200).

Previous records nine months ago showed Hb 16 g/dl, Hct 48.2%, MCV 99 fl. Chest x-ray revealed mild cardiomegaly and echocardiogram a large vegetation on the posterior mitral valve with mitral valve prolapse. Several blood cultures grew *peptostreptococcus* after a few days, and the patient received four weeks of intravenous penicillin with resolution of the fever and his symptoms. The anemia, however, resolved only after another three to four weeks.

Discussion.   The patient's primary illness was a subacute bacterial endocarditis and mild to modest anemia is common with this disorder as it is with most chronic infections. The lower MCV than his usual (as documented earlier) is consistent with impaired iron reutilization and hence production of smaller red cells. In this setting, the serum iron is typically low, the iron being retained in macrophages. The low TIBC (which denotes serum transferrin) is typical of chronic inflammatory disorders, and in contrast to iron deficiency where the TIBC is normal or increased. The raised serum ferritin reflects an increased amount of storage (RE) iron and is also typical of anemia of chronic inflammatory disease. The delayed recovery of such anemia following treatment is characteristic.

2. A 62-year-old and previously healthy housewife had undue fatigue for three weeks. For three days she also experienced shortness of breath and palpitations during her normal activities. Her husband had noted her to be unusually pale. Physical examination revealed pallor of the skin, nail beds, and conjunctivae; scleral icterus; a grade ii systolic ejection murmur over the precordium; and the spleen palpable 3 cm below the costal margin. There was no lymphadenopathy. Laboratory data: Hb 9 g/dl, Hct 27%, MCV 116 fl; WBC $13 \times 10^3/mm^3$, WBC differential – 65% neutrophils, 5% bands, 25% lymphocytes, 5% monocytes; platelets $450 \times 10^3/mm^3$, reticulocytes 30%; the peripheral blood smear showed numerous spherocytes and prominent basophilia. Blood chemistries were remarkable for the total bilirubin of 6 mg/dl (conjugated fraction 0.4 mg/dl, unconjugated fraction 5.6 mg/dl) and the LDH 300 U. The direct Coombs test was positive with IgG antiserum but not with an anticomplement antiserum.

Discussion.   The patient's symptoms in the face of only a moderate degree of anemia indicate a relatively abrupt onset. The reticulocyte count reflects an effective erythropoietic response to the anemia, with a marrow production rate of approximately 6 times normal. The raised unconjugated bilirubin denotes increased hemoglobin breakdown, hence hemolysis rather than blood loss from hemorrhage causing the anemia. The spherocytes are typical of warm antibody-mediated hemolysis, and is established in this case by the IgG antibodies detected in the Coombs test. Such antibody-coated red cells are largely removed by the spleen, which explains the splenomegaly (a "work-hypertrophy" of splenic tissue). In the absence of other associated or underlying disease, the diagnosis would be idiopathic autoimmune hemolytic anemia.

3. A 46-year-old man had a routine medical examination before employment. He had smoked cigars and cigarettes for the past 25 years and had a nonproductive cough and mild fatigue. He appeared plethoric, but otherwise the physical examination was normal. The hemogram showed: Hb 19 g/dl, Hct 58%, MCV 98 fl; WBC $7.5 \times 10^3/mm^3$; platelets $280 \times 10^3/mm^3$. Other laboratory data were: red cell volume, 44 ml/kg (increased); plasma volume, 38 ml/kg (normal); PaO_2, 75 mm Hg; $PaCO_2$, 35 mm Hg; arterial oxygen saturation 85%; carboxyhemoglobin, 15% (increased); hemoglobin P_{50}, 23 mm Hg (decreased). Spirometry studies were normal. He stopped smoking, and 3 months later the hemoglobin was 16 g/dl and hematocrit 48%.

Discussion. The erythrocytosis could be attributed in part to the reduced arterial oxygen saturation caused by the presence of carboxyhemoglobin. In addition, the carboxyhemoglobinemia caused an increased affinity of hemoglobin for oxygen (low P_{50}), impairing oxygen release to tissues and thus also mediating a compensatory increase in red cell production. The diagnosis of smoker's erythrocytosis was confirmed, since it reversed when smoking was stopped.

Bibliography

Hillman RS and Finch CA. *Red Cell Manual* (6th ed.). Philadelphia: Davis, 1992. *This manual provides an introduction to the area of red cell disorders and a concise guide to their diagnosis and management, stressing the pathophysiologic approach.*

Krantz S. Erythropoietin. *Blood* 77:419–434, 1991. *A review article concerned with the chemistry and structure of erythropoietin, its production, and mechanism of action.*

Krantz S. Pathogenesis and treatment of the anemia of chronic disease. *Am J Med Sci* 307:353–359, 1994. *The recent advances toward understanding the pathogenesis of the anemia of chronic disease and its treatment are reviewed.*

Lee GR, Bithell TC, Foerster J, et al. *Wintrobe's Clinical Hematology* (9th ed.). Philadelphia: Lea & Febiger, 1993, Vol. 1. *A current large hematology text covering all aspects of diseases of the red blood cell in detail.*

Papayannopoulou T and Abkowitz J. Biology of Erythropoiesis, Erythroid Differentiation and Maturation. In *Hematology: Basic Principles and Practice* (2nd ed.). Hoffman R, Benz EJ Jr, Shattil SJ et al. (eds.). New York: Churchill Livingstone, 1995, pp. 242–254. *Best single and comprehensive review of erythropoiesis.*

Smith JR and Landaw SA. Smoker's polycythemia. *N Engl J Med* 298:6–10, 1978. *The landmark study of 22 patients with smoker's erythrocytosis, defining the criteria for diagnosis.*

Spivak JL and Eichner ER. *The Fundamentals of Clinical Hematology* (3rd ed.). Baltimore: Johns Hopkins, 1993. *A clinically oriented text of the major blood disease categories from a physiologic perspective.*

Stamatoyannopoulos G, Nienhuis AW, Majerus P, et al. *Molecular Basis of Blood Disease* (2nd ed.). Philadelphia: Saunders, 1994, Chaps. 3–10. *This text details the molecular aspects of hematopoiesis and the molecular pathology of the abnormal hemoglobins, the thalassemias, red cell membrane disorders, red cell enzyme defects and diseases of iron metabolism.*

Wasserman LR, Berk PD, and Berlin NI. *Polycythemia Vera and the Myeloproliferative Disorders.* Philadelphia: Saunders, 1995. *The most current text detailing the pathogenesis, manifestations, and treatment of polycythemia vera and spurious erythrocytosis as well as of the other myeloproliferative diseases.*

Young NS and Alter BP. *Aplastic Anemia Acquired and Inherited.* Philadelphia: Saunders, 1994. *The most comprehensive presentation of aplastic anemia and related bone marrow failure states in adults and children.*

30 Disorders of Myelopoiesis

Dennis L. Confer

Objectives

After completing this chapter, you should be able to

Identify two essential characteristics of hematopoietic stem cells

Describe how colony forming unit (CFU) assays define the stages of committed myeloid precursors

Discuss the differences between neutrophil phagocytes and monocyte/macrophage phagocytes

Describe the oxygen-dependent and oxygen-independent microbicidal systems of the human neutrophil

Identify at least three functions of the red blood cell (RBC)

State the three broad categories of clonal myeloid diseases

Discuss the distinguishing features of at least three of the seven subtypes of acute myelogenous leukemia

Define the term "myelodysplastic syndrome"

Recall the four disorders classified under the heading of myeloproliferative diseases

All blood cells are descendants of hematopoietic stem cells. In order for stem cells to succeed with the perpetual task of blood production, they must (1) proliferate, that is, self-renew and (2) differentiate, which means they give rise to progeny that are committed to develop into recognizable blood cell types. Although differentiated blood — white cells, red cells, and platelets — are readily recognized, stem cells themselves are difficult to identify. Morphologically they are effectively invisible because they strongly resemble mature lymphocytes. Phenotypically they are known to reside among a group of marrow cells that expresses the surface molecule CD34 and, while many CD34-positive cells also coexpress HLA-DR, hematopoietic stem cells do not.

The first branch point for the differentiating stem cell is "lymphoid or myeloid?" The former commits it to the lymphoid system from which arise the T and B cell systems of cellular and humoral immunity, respectively. The latter branch routes the stem cell into the myeloid compartment, which is the subject of this chapter.

Committed Precursors of the Myeloid Compartment

Myelopoiesis is strikingly complex. Most of what is known has been gleaned through laboratory experiments in which isolated bone marrow cells were placed into culture under various conditions and analyzed for outcome. Through such experiments, it has been possible to identify the various stages of committed myeloid precursor cells. For example, one primitive myeloid precursor, termed CFU-GEMM (Colony Forming Unit-Granulocyte, Erythrocyte, Monocyte, Megakaryocyte) is capable of producing colonies that contain all myeloid elements. Other well known myeloid precursors include those committed to development of granulocytes and monocytes (CFU-GM), to development of erythrocytes (CFU-E), and to development of megakaryocytes (CFU-Meg). The relationships between the various myeloid precursors and their mature progeny are depicted in Fig. 30-1.

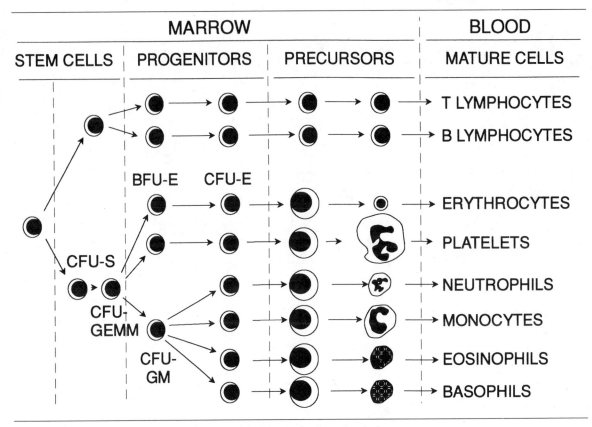

Fig. 30-1. Hematopoiesis. All formed elements of the blood arise from the pluripotent stem cell.

Granulocyte/Monocyte Compartment

All granulocytes and monocytes arise from a common committed precursor cell, the CFU-GM. Macrophages are also included in this compartment because they represent differentiated monocytes, often with characteristics specific for the tissue of their residence (for example, peritoneal macrophages have characteristics that distinguish them from pulmonary macrophages). All of the cells in this compartment are phagocytes, which means they have the capacity to engulf and in some way process particulate material. (The eosinophil is a bit of an exception because it may attempt to engulf things, i.e., parasites, that are several hundred times its size. This process, referred to as "frustrated phagocytosis," ends up with the eosinophil releasing its granule contents onto the surface of the parasite, which causes irreparable damage to the parasite membrane.)

Except for the designation "phagocyte" and the origin from a common precursor, there is little similarity between granulocytes and monocyte/macrophages. The granulocytes are essentially cytocidal cells whose primary duty is to engulf and destroy microbes. In contrast, monocyte/macrophages play a much more complex role that involves regulation of and interaction with numerous other cells involved in human defenses. The intricate interplay between monocyte/macrophages and mature lymphocytes can be thought of as bridging the gap between the mature components of the myeloid and lymphoid compartments.

Granulocytes

The granulocytes consist of basophils, eosinophils, and neutrophils. Of these, the neutrophils constitute the vast majority and have been studied in the greatest detail. The primary function of neutrophils is the phagocytosis and destruction of bacteria and yeast. For this purpose, the neutrophils are well armed. Their armaments fall into two classes: the oxygen-dependent systems, which utilize various forms of reactive oxygen to damage microbial structures, and the oxygen-independent systems, which consist of digestive enzymes and various toxic proteins.

The ability of neutrophils to produce toxic oxygen species is extremely important (Fig. 30-2). The first step in this process involves the generation of superoxide anion by the enzymatic reduction of molecular oxygen. The en- zyme complex responsible for this step is deficient in the various forms of chronic granulomatous disease (CGD), a congenital defect leading to recurrent bacterial infections and oftentimes death before adulthood. Superoxide molecules can be enzymatically or spontaneously converted into hydrogen peroxide, which is a well known disinfectant. The combination of superoxide and hydrogen peroxide, in the presence of iron, causes formation of the highly reactive hydroxyl radical, which is probably the most po-

Fig. 30-2. The reduction pathway of molecular oxygen. The hydroxyl radical is the most potent granulocyte oxidant.

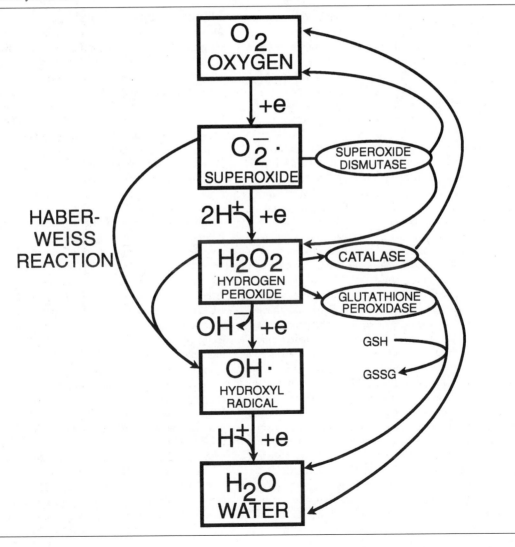

tent antimicrobial oxidant in neutrophils. Additionally, however, to protect the host from the effects of excessive production of toxic oxygen species, neutrophils also maintain systems for removal of oxidants. Superoxide in the presence of water will spontaneously dismute into hydrogen peroxide and oxygen. This reaction is dramatically accelerated by the enzyme superoxide dismutase. Of the systems for removing hydrogen peroxide, the best known is the enzyme catalase, which converts hydrogen peroxide to oxygen and water. However, more active metabolically in the functioning neutrophil is the enzyme glutathione peroxidase that reduces hydrogen peroxide directly to water (see Fig. 30-2).

In addition to the toxic oxygen capabilities of the neutrophil, the intracellular granules contain a variety of enzymes and microbial toxins. Once a microbe is phagocytized, granules fuse with the primary phagosome, dumping their contents onto the microbe and damaging the membrane and cellular components. An important concept in the microbicidal capacity of neutrophils is redundancy. The normal neutrophil maintains several systems that have apparently evolved to provide a potent and multipronged attack against invaders.

Neutrophils are short-lived cells that enter the bloodstream from the bone marrow and circulate for only a few hours before entering peripheral tissues. The exact duration of their persistence in these peripheral tissues is unknown, but is probably on the order of a few hours. The normal adult produces between 50 and 75 billion neutrophils per day, which amounts to more than a half a million per second. The measured neutrophil count quantitates only the "circulating pool." An almost equal number of cells reside in the "marginating pool," which constitutes cells loosely associated with the vascular endothelium that, by videomicroscopy, appear to roll along the surface of the endothelium. The marginated neutrophil pool can be quickly demarginated by administration of adrenergic agents, by emotional stress, or by exercise. In this way, the simple act of running up a flight of stairs may effectively double a person's measured white blood cell count. Another reserve pool of neutrophils exists in the bone marrow as mature neutrophils that have not yet been discharged from the marrow space, but can enter the bloodstream promptly in the presence of an appropriate challenge, such as an acute infection. The marrow reserve pool can also be mobilized with the administration of corticosteroids.

The minor granulocytes in human blood, the eosinophils and basophils, are less well studied. Eosinophils are involved in many allergic reactions and also have a role in the defense against parasitic infections. Like neutrophils,

eosinophils can generate reactive oxygen products, but their major armaments are highly cationic proteins contained in their eosinophilic granules. When the eosinophil attaches to a parasite, in the act of frustrated phagocytosis the granular proteins are discharged into the intercellular space, where they attach preferentially to the parasite and provoke membrane damage.

Basophils are the rarest of granulocytes and their exact function is unknown. They are known to participate in immediate hypersensitivity reactions probably through their interactions with IgE antibodies. It is also postulated that basophils have a role in protection against parasitic infections.

Monocytes and Macrophages

In contrast to the granulocytes, monocytes and macrophages have a far more important role in the regulation of hematopoiesis and the immune response. Among the important cytokines and growth factors released by monocytes and macrophages are interleukin-1, interleukin-6, tumor necrosis factor (TNF), transforming growth factor-beta (TGF-beta), fibroblast growth factor (FGF), platelet-derived growth factor (PDGF), interferons, and several hematopoietic growth factors. The rich array of active products prepares monocyte/macrophages for important roles in the regulation of hematopoiesis, the control of immune responsiveness, and the oversight of local wound repair.

Although monocyte/macrophages can phagocytose and kill microbes (similar to the granulocytes), they carry the process further through their important role as antigen-presenting cells (APCs). In this capacity, monocyte/macrophages digest foreign microbes down to the peptide level, at which point the foreign peptides are bound by HLA molecules and presented to specific T cells to provoke an immune response. In order for a T cell receptor to recognize antigen, it must also recognize the specific HLA molecule on the surface of the monocyte/macrophage. If the T cell recognizes the HLA molecule but not the foreign peptide, then no immune response is evoked. Similarly, recognition of the foreign peptide, but not the specific HLA molecule, also fails to induce an immune reaction. It is further important to recognize that CD8-positive lymphocytes (cytotoxic/suppressor subset) interact preferentially with HLA Class I molecules (HLA-A, -B, and -C), while CD4-positive lymphocytes (helper/inducer subset) interact with HLA Class II molecules (DR, DP, and DQ) on the antigen-presenting cell. Finally, several additional molecules on both the APC and the T lymphocyte are necessary to "glue" the cells together and control the cellular responses. (See Chaps. 31 and 35 for further discussion of APC-lymphocyte interactions.)

Erythroid Compartment

Erythropoiesis can be considered as a component of myelopoiesis, as red cells, white cells, and platelets have a common ancestor progenitor cell. However, because erythropoiesis and its disorders, including the spectrum of anemias, are so important to clinical hematology, these are described separately (see Chap. 29).

Megakaryocyte/Platelet Compartment

Platelets are the smallest formed elements in blood. They are actually not cells; rather, they are cytoplasmic fragments that bud from parent megakaryocytes within the marrow space. The critical role of the platelet in hemostasis is covered in Chap. 34.

Megakaryocytes and platelets contain, among numerous other constituents, potent tissue growth factors. Platelet-derived growth factor (PDGF), as the name implies, was originally isolated from peripheral blood platelets. This growth factor stimulates fibroblasts to proliferate and to synthesize extracellular matrix proteins. In certain marrow disorders, as will be discussed subsequently, the inappropriate release of PDGF and other tissue growth factors can lead to marrow fibrosis.

Clonal Disorders of Myeloid Compartment

The common clonal disorders of the myeloid marrow are grouped into three categories. These are the acute leukemias, the myelodysplastic syndromes, and the myeloproliferative diseases (Table 30-1). These three categories are well worth committing to memory, because they are very descriptive of their inclusive disorders. The first category includes frank leukemias involving myeloid marrow elements. The second category (the myelodysplastic syndromes) includes disorders characterized by abnormal, that is, dysplastic, development of myeloid cells. In contrast, the myeloproliferative diseases are conditions in which essentially normal marrow elements proliferate to an abnormal degree.

All of the diseases in these three categories are clonal, which means that each appears to arise initially from a single abnormal cell in the marrow space. It is hypothesized that a genetic event occurs (or more likely a series of

events accumulate) that results in the transformation of a single cell. The transformed cell becomes autonomous, meaning that it proliferates without being subject to all of the normal regulatory controls. Conceptually, if the abnormal cell proliferates without differentiating, it gives rise to an acute leukemia syndrome. If the cell proliferates, but differentiates abnormally, it may give rise to a myelodysplastic syndrome. If the abnormal cell retains the capacity to differentiate normally, then myeloproliferative disease is the end result (see Table 30-1).

Demonstrating clonality in a marrow disorder requires some type of marker, and is not always straightforward. Chromosomal evidence of clonality is present when (1) an abnormal karyotype is identified, (2) the abnormal karyotype is present (sometimes with or without additional abnormalities) in all metaphases of cells representing the marrow disorder, and (3) normal cells do not demonstrate the abnormal karyotype. Thus the Philadelphia chromosome (which is a translocation between chromosomes 9 and 22) will be present in the leukemic cells of an individual with chronic myelogenous leukemia, but is absent from all normal tissues of that individual, and serves to demonstrate the clonality of chronic myelogenous leukemia. Conversely, the leukemic cells of a person with Down syndrome may all show trisomy 21, but that is not proof of clonality because all cells in that person will show this same abnormal karyotype.

Table 30-1. Classification of Clonal Myeloid Disorders

ACUTE MYELOGENOUS LEUKEMIA	
M1	AML without differentiation
M2	AML with differentiation
M3	Acute promyelocytic leukemia
M4	Acute myelomonocytic leukemia
M5	Acute monocytic leukemia
M6	Erythroleukemia
M7	Acute megakaryoblastic leukemia
MYELODYSPLASTIC SYNDROMES	
RA	Refractory anemia
AISA	Acquired idiopathic sideroblastic anemia
CMML	Chronic myelomonocytic leukemia
RAEB	Refractory anemia with excess blasts
RAEB-t	Refractory anemia with excess blasts in transformation
MYELOPROLIFERATIVE DISEASES	
P. vera	Polycythemia vera
CML	Chronic myelogenous leukemia
ET	Essential thrombocythemia
AMM	Agnogenic myeloid metaplasia

In many clonal disorders of the bone marrow, the chromosomal karyotype is grossly normal. In many of these instances, clonality has been demonstrated by examining women with the disorder for evidence of "nonrandom X chromosome inactivation." In order for this to be possible, it is necessary that the two X chromosomes of the affected woman differ in some way. Classically, this difference has been demonstrated by isoenzymes of glucose-6-phosphate dehydrogenase (G-6-PD). When one X chromosome carries a different isoenzyme than the other, it is possible to examine the bone marrow or peripheral blood for evidence of clonality. Thus the condition is nonclonal, then random inactivation of the X chromosome dictates that approximately 50% of the sample will demonstrate one isoenzyme, and 50% will demonstrate the other. If, however, the condition is clonal and arises from a single cell, with one active X chromosome, then all of the sample will show a single G-6-PD isoenzyme. In recent years, newer molecular biology-based techniques have become available to also demonstrate clonality in acute leukemias, myelodysplastic syndromes, and myeloproliferative diseases.

Acute Myelogenous Leukemias

Classification

There are seven primary categories of acute myelogenous leukemia, according to the FAB (French-American-British) classification. These are labeled AML-M1 through AML-M7 (see Table 30-1). In order for a disease to be labeled acute myelogenous leukemia, there must be greater than or equal to 30% blast cells in the bone marrow and these must be demonstrated to be myeloid in origin. When these criteria are met, then the leukemia is subclassified to one of the seven subtypes according to morphological criteria, often supplemented by chromosome data.

Overall, the clinical similarities among the different categories of AML outweigh their distinctions, but there are some important differences. For example, with AML-M3, acute promyelocytic leukemia (also called acute progranulocytic leukemia and APL), a characteristic feature is disseminated intravascular coagulation (DIC) caused by the release of procoagulant substance from the APL granules. Frequently, DIC is present at the time of diagnosis and is almost always made worse by (induction) chemotherapy. In fact, death due to hemorrhage is a serious problem with APL.

Essentially all patients with APL have a characteristic chromosome abnormality involving a translocation between chromosomes 15 and 17. The translocation involves a region of the chromosome that includes a receptor for retinoic acid. This is particularly interesting because treatment of APL patients with a retinoic acid analogue causes the leukemic cells to differentiate into mature granulocytes. While patients are receiving retinoic acid, as the leukemic cells differentiate, evidence of DIC disappears and chemotherapy can then be given without the risk of disseminated intravascular coagulation and hemorrhage.

Acute monocytic leukemias also behave somewhat distinctly. In general, when there is a monocytic component to the acute leukemia, the prognosis is worse. This may be because monocytic leukemias are more frequently tissue invasive. Leukemic infiltration of the skin, the mucosal tissues, and the central nervous system is more common with monocytic leukemia. Infiltration and bleeding of the gingiva is a typical finding in monocytic leukemia.

Etiology

The cause of acute myelogenous leukemia is unknown. It occurs in about three persons per 100,000 population per year. Factors that are known to increase the risk include exposure to alkylating agents (such as chlorambucil), exposure to ionizing radiation, certain congenital defects (such as Down syndrome), and environmental exposure to benzene. Of all the chemicals present in the modern workplace, benzene is the only one that has been clearly shown to increase the risk of acute leukemia. This increase is approximately fourfold for individuals repeatedly exposed to benzene for a period of several years. Thus the rate of acute leukemia among benzene workers is approximately 12 per 100,000 per year. This means that acute leukemia is still rare among benzene workers, but when it occurs it is most likely a result of the benzene exposure.

Symptoms and Signs

The symptoms of acute myelogenous leukemia are nonspecific. They are primarily those that reflect bone marrow failure, namely, symptoms of anemia, thrombocytopenia, and neutropenia. These symptoms are sufficiently vague that a person with acute leukemia may visit a physician more than once before the diagnosis is established. The correct screening test for acute myelogenous leukemia is the complete blood count (CBC). This will essentially always reveal some abnormality of the white blood cell count, the hemoglobin level, or the platelet count. Obviously, an abnormal CBC does not usually mean a disease as serious as acute leukemia, but it is the clue that points the doctor in the correct direction. In order to definitively diagnose acute leukemia, one must perform a bone marrow aspiration and biopsy. The marrow specimen is submitted for morphology, including special cytochemical stains, for chromosome analysis, and for evaluation of cell surface markers using flow cytometry.

Treatment

Acute myelogenous leukemia is treated with aggressive chemotherapy, which is divided into an induction phase and a consolidation phase. The induction treatment is designed to place the leukemia into a complete remission. However, individuals in remission frequently (> 75% of the time) harbor residual leukemic cells, so that aggressive chemotherapy is continued and is referred to as the consolidation treatment. The most aggressive form of consolidation is marrow transplantation.

Myelodysplastic Syndromes

The myelodysplastic syndromes are a heterogenous group of disorders. The common features within this group are (1) a hypercellular bone marrow, (2) evidence of myelodysplasia, and (3) varying degrees of marrow failure. These disorders were once termed "preleukemias." This term has been largely abandoned, however, because it implies that these disorders always evolve into acute leukemia, and this is not so.

Patients with myelodysplastic syndromes typically present with some evidence of marrow failure, i.e., anemia, leukopenia, or thrombocytopenia. In the peripheral blood smear, there is frequently evidence of dysplasia, with hyposegmentation of neutrophils, diminished or absent granulation of both granulocytes and platelets, and abnormally shaped red cells, particularly oval macrocytes. The diagnosis of a myelodysplastic syndrome is made by bone marrow aspiration and biopsy. Treatment of these disorders is difficult. Chemotherapy as used for acute leukemia worsens the marrow failure and only occasionally restores normal hematopoiesis. For the most part, these disorders are treated supportively, unless marrow transplantation is a viable option.

Refractory Anemias

There are three myelodysplastic syndromes that are termed refractory anemias. These are refractory anemia (RA), refractory anemia with excess blasts (RAEB), and refractory anemia with excess blasts in transformation (RAEB-t). Of these, RAEB-t most closely resembles frank acute leukemia. The percentage of blasts in the marrow exceeds 20% in RAEB-t, but fails to reach the level of 30% required for a diagnosis of leukemia. In RAEB and RA, the percentage of marrow blast cells is less than 20% and less than 5%, respectively.

Acquired Idiopathic Sideroblastic Anemia

This disorder is characterized mainly by failure to produce adequate red blood cells and is often stable and long-lived. The peripheral blood smear typically shows red cell "dimorphism," i.e., the simultaneous presence of normal red cells intermixed with a population of severely hypochromic red cells. The diagnosis is confirmed by the presence of "ring sideroblasts" in the Prussian blue-stained marrow aspirate. Ring sideroblasts are erythroblasts in which numerous iron-positive granules are arrayed in a halo around the nucleus.

Chronic Myelomonocytic Leukemia

Chronic myelomonocytic leukemia (CMML) is the rarest of the myelodysplastic syndromes. It is characterized by leukocytosis and an absolute increase in the circulating monocytes to greater than 10^9/liter. The Philadelphia chromosome, which characterizes chronic myelogenous leukemia, is absent in this disorder. CMML carries a poor prognosis, with survival ranging from many months to a few years.

Myeloproliferative Diseases

In contrast to the myelodysplastic syndromes, myeloproliferative diseases tend to feature excessive production of blood cells that are morphologically normal. Patients are often discovered "by accident" at the time of a routine examination or when volunteering to donate blood. Symptoms, when they occur, are usually the result of excessive marrow expansion, e.g., bone pain, splenomegaly, etc., or because of marked elevations of peripheral blood counts, e.g., hyperviscosity symptoms, thrombosis, hemorrhage, etc. Therapy for myeloproliferative diseases is aimed at controlling the excessive production of blood cells. This is usually accomplished with some minor form of oral chemotherapy. Except when marrow transplantation is performed, these disorders are incurable. Conceptually, the reason for this is that the abnormal stem cells in myeloproliferative diseases differ only marginally from the normal counterparts. Therefore, any treatment sufficient to eradicate the abnormal stem cells will almost certainly eradicate normal stem cells, rendering the recipient devoid of any normal marrow function.

Chronic Myelogenous Leukemia

Chronic myelogenous leukemia (CML) is characterized by a moderate to a marked increase of peripheral blood neutrophils along with a striking "left shift." It is not uncommon for asymptomatic patients to be discovered with a white cell count in excess of 100,000/microliter (100 ×

10^9/liter). The hemoglobin is usually normal, while the platelet count may be elevated, normal, or depressed. An absolute increase in peripheral blood basophils is characteristic.

Chronic myelogenous leukemia was the first malignant disorder in which a chromosome abnormality (the Philadelphia chromosome) was identified. It is now known that the Philadelphia chromosome is an abnormal chromosome 22 with a small translocation from chromosome 9. The missing portion of chromosome 22 is found on the chromosome 9 which donated its material. The 9;22 translocation moves the Abelson proto-oncogene (c-ABL) from chromosome 9 into a region of chromosome 22 known as the "breakpoint cluster region" (BCR). The resulting gene, BCR-ABL, is transcribed, messenger RNA is produced and translated into a fusion protein which exhibits tyrosine kinase activity.

CML is a disease that changes over time. It is characterized by an initial chronic phase that lasts on the average two to three years. As the chronic phase wears on, CML begins to show signs of "acceleration": poor responsiveness to therapy, persisting splenomegaly, increasing peripheral blood basophilia, and increasing "left shift." These changes eventually evolve into "blast crisis," the terminal phase of CML similar to an aggressive, de novo acute leukemia. Remissions are difficult to achieve, however, and when they occur they tend to be of short duration.

Bone marrow transplantation is the only treatment which has eradicated chronic myelogenous leukemia. Marrow transplantation is most successful when undertaken in the chronic phase of CML, and disease-free survival is best when transplantation is undertaken during the first year following diagnosis.

Polycythemia Vera

Polycythemia vera (P. vera) is the typical myeloproliferative disease. It is characterized by orderly but excessive proliferation of red blood cells along with granulocytes and platelets. It usually presents in older individuals, with symptoms and signs of excess circulating red cells and attendant increased blood viscosity. Splenomegaly, due to extramedullary hematopoiesis, is characteristic. The diagnosis is confirmed by demonstrating an inappropriate increase of the red cell mass, in the absence of decreased arterial oxygen saturation or an alteration in hemoglobin-oxygen affinity. Supporting laboratory evidence includes raised white cell and platelet counts, an increase in the leukocyte alkaline phosphatase (LAP), and the vitamin B_{12}-binding capacity. The treatment of polycythemia vera must prevent the consequences of the hyperviscosity and is accomplished with phlebotomy and occasionally with mild chemotherapy.

Essential Thrombocythemia

Among the myeloproliferative diseases, CML is primarily a proliferation of granulocytes, polycythemia vera is mainly a proliferation of red blood cells, and essential thrombocythemia (ET) is a proliferation of megakaryocytes with accumulation of platelets. Patients may present without symptoms or because of bleeding or thrombosis. Paradoxically, bleeding is common despite markedly elevated platelet counts. Conceptually, this is because too many platelets make for inefficient hemostasis.

Platelet counts are well in excess of 10^{12}/liter (1,000,000/microliter), and mild leukocytosis is not uncommon. Iron deficiency anemia may occur due to occult bleeding in the gastrointestinal tract.

Agnogenic Myeloid Metaplasia (AMM)

This disorder, also called myelofibrosis, is characterized by slow evolution of peripheral blood cytopenias as a result of an extensive marrow fibrosis. These cytopenias are frequently made worse by marked splenomegaly due to extramedullary hematopoiesis. The latter is marginally beneficial in the face of the marrow fibrosis as the massively enlarged spleen sequesters blood cells, further aggravating the cytopenias.

AMM was once thought to represent an abnormal proliferation of marrow fibroblasts. It has now become clear that it is more correctly a cousin of essential thrombocythemia. Oftentimes the marrow shows only megakaryocytes surrounded by intense fibrosis. However, analysis of the fibroblasts shows absence of clonality. It is presumed that the megakaryocytes, which are clonally derived, release large amounts of platelet-derived growth factor (PDGF) and other fibroblast growth factors. Thus abnormal marrow cells, and not abnormal fibroblasts, drive fibrosis of the marrow cavity.

Agnogenic myeloid metaplasia can be difficult to treat. Chemotherapy only worsens the cytopenias. Transfusions may fail because cells are sequestered promptly in the spleen. Sometimes splenectomy is beneficial, but the procedure carries a significant risk when the spleen is very large; if it is a major site of hematopoiesis, its removal may be a "therapeutic wash."

Clinical Examples

1. A 22-year-old college student was evaluated because for several weeks he had felt increasing fatigue, sensations of fever but without chills, and sweats at night. His appetite had been poor and he had lost several pounds in the last several weeks. During the past week he had noted a

tendency to bruise easily and the occurrence of spontaneous petechiae around the feet and ankles. On physical
examination, temperature was 101.5°F, and pulse was 92.
Several bruises were noted over the legs and thighs; there
were many petechiae over the feet and ankles. The spleen
was palpable 3 cm below the left costal margin. Rectal examination showed fluctuance and tenderness at one point;
the stool guaiac was negative. Neurological examination
was normal. Initial laboratory data revealed the hemoglobin 8.2 g/dl, hematocrit 25%, WBC 41,850/mm^3 with a
differential of 2% neutrophils, 9% lymphocytes, 3%
monocytes, and 86% large atypical cells. The platelet
count was 12,000/mm^3. The blood chemistry profile was
normal with the exception of the serum LDH of 2,250
U/ml (normal < 200), and the serum uric acid of 11 mg/dl
(normal < 7.0). A bone marrow aspirate was not successful, yielding only a few drops of blood without identifiable
spicules. Touch preparations of the marrow biopsy revealed sheets of large mononuclear cells. Marrow biopsy
sections revealed a markedly hypercellular marrow with
rare granulocytic, erythroid, and megakaryocytic elements
and most of the cells were immature mononuclear forms.
The atypical cells in the peripheral blood were characterized as myeloblasts by special stains and flow cytometry.

Initial management included treatment of the perirectal
abscess, red cell and platelet transfusion, measures to prevent urate nephropathy, and then induction chemotherapy.
A complete remission was achieved by the chemotherapy
and was followed by an allogeneic marrow transplant from
a matched sibling donor. Five years later the patient remains well and without recurrence of the leukemia.

Discussion. The young man demonstrated the typical
presenting features of AML. His symptoms were related
principally to infection due to severe neutropenia, and
bleeding because of severe thrombocytopenia. In addition,
the disease was characterized by a high white cell count,
consisting mainly of myeloblasts. The increased turnover
of these cells led to the high serum value of LDH (which
does not cause any problem) and of uric acid (which can
cause renal failure from acute urate nephropathy). The
management was first supportive, followed by intensive
induction combination chemotherapy. Since the leukemia
was the M2 type of AML, it was not anticipated that central nervous system complications would occur; so routine
CNS prophylaxis was not required. Most such patients will
achieve a complete remission with induction chemotherapy,
yet most who achieve a remission suffer a subsequent relapse and die from their leukemia. The best opportunity for
cure is to perform a marrow transplant while the patient is
in the initial complete remission from the acute leukemia.

2. A 43-year-old business man saw his physician for a
routine physical examination. Although he had no "chief
complaint," he had tired more easily in recent months and
this had prompted him to see his physician; however, he
continued to work very hard in his profession. There were
no other symptoms and he reported no weight loss. Physical
examination was normal except that the spleen was palpable 3 cm below the left costal margin. Laboratory data revealed that the white blood cell count was 22,000/mm^3
with a differential of 41% neutrophils, 15% bands, 4%
metamyelocytes, 8% myelocytes, 2% promyelocytes, 1%
myeloblasts, 20% lymphocytes, 4% monocytes, 1% eosinophils, and 4% basophils. The remainder of the hemogram
was normal: hemoglobin 14.7 gm/dl, hematocrit 48%,
platelet count 342,000/ml. The red cell morphology was
normal and no nucleated red cells were seen; several
large platelets were noted. The initial impression was
chronic myelogenous leukemia (CML), diagnosed almost
incidentally. The diagnosis was confirmed by bone marrow examination, demonstrating the Philadelphia chromosome t(9; 22). Initially no treatment was given, but when
the white count increased and symptoms of tiredness also
increased, treatment was begun with hydroxyurea. Because the patient had no siblings with his tissue type, a
matched unrelated volunteer donor was identified for allogeneic marrow transplantation, which was successfully
performed eight months after diagnosis.

Discussion. CML is a specific disease characterized by
a specific chromosomal translocation leading to the abnormally regulated production of the BCR-ABL gene product;
other myeloproliferative syndromes are less sharply defined and may be less distinct, one from another. The high
white count is characteristic of CML, with the differential
approximating the differential of marrow granulocytes.
The increase of circulating basophils is also characteristic.
Despite the benign appearance of this illness at diagnosis,
the disease is inevitably fatal without bone marrow transplantation. Over a period of 1–10 years, marrow failure
occurs or other signs of accelerated disease appear, which
may resemble acute leukemia of either the AML or ALL
type.

Bibliography

Boulad F and Kernan NA. Treatment of childhood
    acute nonlymphoblastic leukemia: A review. *Cancer
    Invest* 11:534–553, 1993. *Although a review of child-
    hood AML, much of the information is applicable at all
    ages.*

Goasguen JE and Bennett JM. Classifications of acute myeloid leukemia. *Clin Lab Med* 10:661–681, 1990. *A nice review of the FAB classification and its nuances.*

Goasguen JE and Bennett JM. Classification and morphologic features of the myelodysplastic syndromes. *Semin Oncol* 19:4–13, 1992. *The same two authors above tackled the myelodysplastic syndromes and provide an understandable explanation.*

Rigenberg HS and Doll DC. Acute nonlymphocytic leukemia: The first 48 hours. *S Med J* 83:931–940, 1990. *A review of the early steps in management of AML and the AML-associated emergencies.*

Sachs L and Lotem J. The network of hematopoietic cytokines. *Proc Soc Exp Biol Med* 206:170–175, 1994. *An understandable review of cytokine involvement in hematopoiesis.*

31 Lymphocytes and Lymphoproliferative Disorders

Regina Resta and Michael A. Kolodziej

Objectives

After completing this chapter, you should be able to

Understand normal B cell function and immunoglobulin synthesis

Understand normal T cell function and the basis of cellular immunity

Recognize the importance of each normal lymphoid organ in immunity

Identify the clinical characteristics of acute lymphoblastic leukemia, its differentiation from acute myeloblastic leukemia, and the general principles of treatment

Identify the clinical characteristics of chronic lymphocytic leukemia, its characteristic morphology, and the general principles of management

Differentiate Hodgkin's disease from non-Hodgkin's lymphoma, particularly with respect to the importance of staging and histology, and how these impact on the treatment of these conditions

Appreciate the diverse clinical presentations of multiple myeloma and the pathophysiology responsible for each

Normal Lymphocyte Biology

General Considerations

Lymphocytes are the cells that specifically recognize antigen, proliferate, and generate an immune response. Before addressing the uncontrolled proliferation of lymphocytes that results in **lymphomas** and **leukemias,** it will be helpful to review normal lymphocyte biology. Morphologically identical lymphocytes are divided into the distinct subsets of **B cells, T cells,** and **NK cells** on the basis of their function and cell surface proteins.

B Cells

The cell surface immunoglobulin molecule, the B cell antigen receptor, consists of a **heavy chain** and a **light chain,** both chains having a **constant (C)** and a **variable (V)** re-gion. Each B cell bears an immunoglobulin molecule of a single antigen specificity. This molecule is generated through a well regulated series of **rearrangements** (DNA splicing, excision, and rejoining) of the immunoglobulin variable region genes during the development of the B cell in the bone marrow. It is this series of multiple possible rearrangements of the immunoglobulin gene that generates some of the diversity of the antibody repertoire. Also contributing to this diversity is the imprecision of the rearrangements, the association of different heavy and light chains in each B cell to form the antigen binding site, and the ability of B cells to mutate their variable region genes when they are stimulated by antigen (**somatic hypermutation**).

The initial stages of B cell maturation, from stem cell to pro-B cell to pre-B cell to surface IgM$^+$ immature B cell, occur in the bone marrow. B cells that recognize self-antigen are eliminated in the bone marrow to ensure self-

313

tolerance. Immature B cells emerge from the marrow and can encounter antigen in peripheral lymphoid organs. Antigen recognition induces B cell proliferation, and these clonally expanded B cell populations differentiate into either antibody-secreting plasma cells or long-lived memory cells. B cell response to most antigen requires interaction between the B cell and antigen-specific T cells. The T cell secretes **cytokines** that signal the B cell to proliferate. In the absence of T cell-B cell interaction, the B cell may become **anergic.**

T Cells

T cells recognize antigen only as peptide fragments presented by antigen-presenting cells (APCs), not as soluble proteins recognized by B cell immunoglobulin. The T cell antigen receptor consists of a heterodimer (α:β or α:δ), and the receptor genes rearrange in the thymus according to a defined program which is similar to what occurs in B cells in the marrow. Once naive T cells leave the thymus and enter peripheral lymphoid organs, they encounter antigen presented by APCs. APCs (macrophages, B cells, and dendritic cells) take up antigen, degrade it, and present it on the cell surface as a peptide fragment bound tightly by an **MHC** (major histocompatability complex) molecule. MHC class I molecules are expressed on the surface of most nucleated cells; MHC class II molecules are present only on APCs and thymic stromal cells.

Cytotoxic T cells (CTLs) kill endogenous cells infected with virus or bacteria when the foreign peptide is presented on the infected cell surface by MHC class I molecules. CTLs express the cell surface molecule **CD8,** which associates with the T cell receptor (TCR) and binds the MHC class I molecule. Thus CD8, MHC, and the TCR form a trimolecular complex surrounding the antigen and linking the CTL to the infected cell.

Helper T cells and **inflammatory T cells** express **CD4** instead of CD8 and recognize antigen only when it is presented by MHC class II molecules. Inflammatory T cells are activated to secrete cytokines that stimulate macrophages to kill intracellular pathogens, while helper T cells are activated to stimulate B cells to make antibody.

NK Cells

NK Cells (Natural Killer Cells)

These are large granular lymphocytes that kill their targets by granule exocytosis and secretion of toxins, similar to CTLs. NK cells are neither T nor B cells. They recognize antibody-coated cells via NK cell Fc receptors; they also recognize some virally infected cells and tumor cells through a mechanism that is not yet worked out, but may involve specific recognition of a ubiquitous cell surface molecule with subsequent activation that can then be inhibited by recognition of a self-MHC class I molecule. NK cells do not require MHC molecules on their targets, and in fact selectively kill cells with low MHC class I levels.

Normal Lymphoid Organ Architecture

Lymphocytes, macrophages, and other accessory and antigen-presenting cells are normally localized in specific organs. The architecture of these organs is not fixed because many lymphocytes recirculate and exchange between these organs and the circulation. Lymphoid organs can either be generative (where lymphocytes arise or mature) or peripheral (where mature lymphocytes encounter and respond to antigens). The bone marrow and thymus are generative organs, while the lymph nodes and spleen are peripheral organs in the immune system.

Primary Lymphoid Organs

Bone Marrow.   In adults, **hematopoiesis,** or the generation of all blood cells, occurs in the **bone marrow.** All blood cell lineages originate from the proliferation and differentiation of **stem cells.** The red marrow of the flat bones (i.e., sternum, vertebrae, ribs, and ilium) consists of a spongelike framework between boney trabeculae. The spaces in this framework are filled with fat cells, stromal cells, and hematopoietic stem cells that give rise to all the cellular elements of blood: **leukocytes** (white blood cells, including lymphocytes, monocytes, and polymorphonuclear leukocytes), **erythrocytes** (red blood cells), and **platelets.** We will be concerned primarily with the generation and differentiation of lymphocytes and monocytes in this chapter. The early stages in B cell development occur in the bone marrow.

Thymus.   Hematopoietic stem cells from the bone marrow seed the **thymus,** a bilobed lymphoid organ with multiple lobules in the anterior mediastinum where T lymphocytes mature. The thymus consists of T lymphocytes in a network of dendritic cells, macrophages, and epithelial cells. Precursor cells that are destined to become T cells enter the thymic cortex, or rim, via blood vessels. It is unknown whether the cells that enter the thymus are already committed to becoming T cells and somehow home to the thymus or whether B cells also enter and simply do not stay or survive there. The immature thymocytes mature and are selected as they migrate from the cortex to the inner **medulla. Negative selection** is the process of eliminating T cells that recognize self-antigens; in **positive selection** T cells that recognize foreign antigen are stimulated to mature. Ninety-eight percent of the cells that enter the thymus die there in a process known as **apoptosis,** a programmed cell death in which the nucleus condenses and the DNA fragments in a characteristic way. Mature T cells leave the thymus via lymphatics and venules.

Peripheral Lymphoid Organs

Lymph Nodes.   Located along lymphatic ducts, lymph nodes serve as sites for the sampling of antigens that enter lymph via the lymphatic channels that drain most organs. **Peyer's patches** are lymphoid aggregates located along the mucosa that are organized similar to lymph nodes. Lymph enters the nodes via afferent lymphatics that enter the subcapsular sinus and then percolates through the cortex and the medulla, finally leaving the node via an efferent lymphatic at the hilum. Antigen from the lymph is trapped throughout the node by antigen-presenting cells (macrophages and follicular dendritic cells). Naive T and B cells enter the node from the bloodstream via specialized **high endothelial venules (HEVs);** T cells migrate to the **paracortical** T cell area, and B cells to the cortical **follicles.** Most entering lymphocytes do not encounter antigen which they specifically recognize and leave via the efferent lymphatic. T cells that do encounter their specific antigen in the node become **activated** and proliferate and eventually leave the efferent lymphatics as **effector** T cells. B cells that encounter their specific antigen are similarly activated and form areas of intense cell proliferation in the follicles called **germinal centers;** some of these activated B cells migrate to the medullary cords and become antibody-secreting **plasma cells,** and eventually leave via the efferent lymphatic to return to the bone marrow.

Spleen.   This is the other major peripheral lymphoid organ and, although different in appearance from the nodes, it shares the same architectural principles. In the spleen, blood-borne antigen is trapped and presented to lymphocytes; in lymph nodes, antigen enters via lymph. The spleen contains **red pulp,** where blood cells are filtered and destroyed, and the lymphoid **white pulp.** Blood enters the white pulp via arterioles that feed into the **marginal sinus.** The marginal sinus is surrounded by a T cell area, the **periarteriolar lymphoid sheath (PALS),** and a B cell area with germinal centers where B cells mature.

Malignant Diseases of Lymphocytes

General Considerations

The common malignant disorders of lymphocytes are leukemias, lymphomas, and multiple myeloma. Leukemia is defined as a malignant disease of hematopoietic cells dominated by peripheral blood/bone marrow involvement; lymphoma is defined as a malignant disease of hematopoietic cells dominated by lymph node involvement. It is important to remember, however, that leukemia and lymphoma are not mutually exclusive clinical entities, and the clinical presentations of lymphocytic leukemias and non-Hodgkin's lymphoma overlap considerably. This is best explained by the fact that lymphocytes are often migratory cells, taking up residence in bone marrow, lymph nodes, spleen, or extralymphatic lymphoid sites like Peyer's patches. Accordingly, patients with leukemia, in which the clinical disorder is dominated by the blood and bone marrow picture, often have lymphadenopathy and splenomegaly, while patients with lymphoma may have a "leukemic phase," or peripheral blood involvement. The factors which dictate the predominant tissue location for any given malignancy are poorly understood, but probably include the specific mechanisms of malignant transformation, or expression of cellular factors such as adhesion receptors. In the sections that follow, the malignant disorders of lymphocytes will be discussed in terms of the dominant clinical features for each disorder.

Disorders Diagnosed by Peripheral Blood Abnormalities

Acute Lymphocytic Leukemia
Acute lymphocytic leukemia (ALL) is characterized by the presence of primitive lymphoid cells (lymphoblasts) in excess number in the bone marrow and blood (Plate 1). In addition to an excess number of lymphoblasts, there is often a deficiency in normal myeloid cells, erythroid cells, and megakaryocytes in the marrow with corresponding neutropenia, anemia, and thrombocytopenia. The distinction of primitive lymphoblasts from myeloblasts (the malignant cell in acute myeloid leukemia) on examination of peripheral blood smear is often difficult, as primitive blast cells share many morphologic features. Although expert pathologists might make the distinction by morphology alone, other techniques used to accurately identify the

hematopoietic lineage of leukemic blast cells include cytochemistry, flow cytometry, and cytogenetics. **Cytochemistry** has been the traditional technique to identify blast lineage; it involves histochemical staining reactions which are specific for myeloid cells like myeloperoxidase, and periodic acid Schiff (PAS) and terminal deoxynucleotidyl transferase (TDT) which are positive in lymphoid leukemia. **Flow cytometry** takes advantage of the fact that lymphoid and myeloid cells have specific cell surface markers, which can be detected with monoclonal antibodies linked to fluorescent dyes. **Cytogenetics** can identify the typical chromosomal changes present in either myeloid or lymphoid leukemia; for example, the most common chromosomal abnormality in myeloid leukemia is the (8;21) translocation, whereas the (4;11) translocation is a common translocation in adult lymphoid leukemia.

Based on the morphologic appearance of the lymphoblasts on peripheral blood and bone marrow smears, there are three morphologic subtypes of ALL: **L1,** the most common type in children; **L2,** the most common type in adults; and **L3,** an uncommon B cell leukemia, often overlapping Burkitt's lymphoma. Acute lymphocytic leukemia can also be classified by the immunologic origin of the malignant lymphocyte: **B cell, T cell, common ("calla" or CD10 positive), and null cell.** It has recently been shown that common and null cell are primitive B cell tumors. The immunologic subtype correlates with clinical behavior and response to therapy.

Acute lymphocytic leukemia is an explosive illness. Untreated, survival is less than 2 months. Most patients have minor symptoms, with fatigue being the most common symptom, followed by infection and bleeding These are related to the anemia, leukopenia, and thrombocytopenia seen in acute leukemia. Physical signs are nonspecific, but many patients have lymphadenopathy or splenomegaly, or physical findings consistent with pancytopenia. The different immunophenotypes of ALL have distinctive clinical presentations. T cell ALL is typically a disease of adolescent males who present with a large mediastinal mass. Common ALL is a disease of children. B cell ALL often presents with bulky abdominal masses or central nervous system disease. Overwhelmingly, though, the clinical picture is most dominated by the laboratory findings, which include anemia, thrombocytopenia, and leukocytosis. In some patients, leukopenia is actually observed, but examination of the bone marrow shows replacement by leukemic lymphoblasts.

Successful treatment of acute leukemia necessitates eradication of all acute leukemia cells using high-dose chemotherapy. This allows repopulation of the bone marrow with normal progenitors. This initial phase of therapy is called **induction.** After intensive therapy and before marrow recovery, the patient experiences marrow aplasia and pancytopenia. During this time, there is tremendous risk of hemorrhage and disseminated infection. Appropriate support includes transfusion and broad-spectrum antibiotics. A single course of induction therapy is inadequate for most adults. Post-induction therapy might include low-dose oral chemotherapy (**maintenance therapy**), intermediate-dose intravenous chemotherapy (**consolidation therapy**), or high-dose chemotherapy, of the same intensity or greater intensity as induction (**intensification therapy,** such as bone marrow transplantation). The precise therapeutic plan is determined by considering the previous prognostic factors. Adverse prognostic factors include age > 7 years, male sex white blood cell count > 30,000/ml, immunophenotype other than common ALL, central nervous system involvement, and presence of chromosomal abnormalities. The prognosis for adult ALL is not as favorable as that for ALL in children, which is commonly cured. About 60% of children and 20% of adults are cured by standard chemotherapy, and perhaps as many as 50% by bone marrow transplantation.

Chronic Lymphocytic Leukemia

In contrast to acute lymphocytic leukemia, chronic lymphocytic leukemia (CLL) is typically an indolent illness occurring in older persons. The malignant cells of CLL look like mature lymphocytes, but many of them are smudged (Plate 2). Though they look mature, they are immunologically immature and functionally impotent. In addition, although they are B lymphocytes, they commonly express inappropriate surface antigens and may possess specific chromosomal abnormalities, the most common being trisomy 12. The sine qua non for a diagnosis of CLL is persistent lymphocytosis greater than 5000/ml.

CLL is the most common of the leukemias, and is a disease of adults over 55 years of age. A typical presentation (seen in about one-third of CLL patients) is an asymptomatic patient with isolated lymphocytosis. The extent of lymphocytosis correlates imprecisely with symptoms, and "sludging" of CLL cells in the microcirculation almost never occurs. Patients with CLL may complain of fatigue or weight loss. They also may have symptoms from bulky adenopathy or splenomegaly, which is confirmed by physical examination. Fever is rarely, if ever, a symptom of CLL. When fever is present, bacterial infection should actively be sought. Bacterial infections are common in CLL due to acquired hypogammaglobulinemia. Anemia and thrombocytopenia may be seen. Both of these abnormalities have at least two mechanisms in CLL. Both may be autoimmune in etiology, thought due to immune dysregulation with production of autoantibodies. These immune cytopenias respond well to therapy of CLL. A much more ominous finding in CLL are cytopenias due to bone marrow replacement. This carries a very adverse prognosis.

Because of the clinical diversity of CLL, extending from a clinically benign laboratory abnormality to a rapidly progressive disease fatal in less than two years, a clinical staging system is important. The most common staging system employed in CLL is the **Rai system** (Table 31-1). There is very good correlation between stage and survival. Other prognostic factors include chromosomal abnormalities and rate of rise in the white count (not absolute white count). About 20% of patients develop an aggressive lymphoma in the terminal stages of their disease (**Richter's syndrome**). This is generally refractory to therapy.

Table 31-1. Staging of Chronic Lymphocytic Leukemia

Rai System Stage	Clinical Features
0	Lymphocytosis
I	Lymphocytosis
	Lymphadenopathy
II	Lymphocytosis
	Splenomegaly*
III	Lymphocytosis
	Anemia*,†
IV	Lymphocytosis
	Thrombocytopenia*,†

* Lymphadenopathy may be present or absent.
† Anemia and thrombocytopenia must be on the basis of decreased marrow production rather than immune destruction.

CLL is very often an indolent disease. Many patients require no treatment for many years. Treatment is generally initiated to control signs and symptoms; it is not curative. Standard therapy involves the administration of **oral chemotherapy** (like the alkylating agent, chlorambucil, and prednisone). Most patients respond over the course of months. Combination intravenous chemotherapy can result in more rapid response but is only occasionally justified. If symptoms are confined to a single bulky lymph node, local radiation therapy can be very helpful. Newer forms of chemotherapy include the nucleotide analogue fludarabine, which inhibits a purine salvage pathway. It may be more effective than standard oral chemotherapy. Supportive care in CLL includes transfusion and antibiotic therapy as appropriate. Intravenous immunoglobulin replacement therapy is sometimes used to prophylax against recurrent bacterial infections in patients with profound hypogammaglobulinemia.

Disorders Dominated by Lymph Node Abnormalities

Non-Hodgkin's Lymphoma

Lymphoma is, first and foremost, a disease of lymph nodes; lymph node biopsy is accordingly the diagnostic test of choice. Based on lymph node appearance, lymphomas are divided into two general categories, Hodgkin's disease and **non-Hodgkin's lymphoma**. In non-Hodgkin's lymphoma, the appearance is further described on the basis of two features: **presence of nodules or follicles and size of cells.** These two descriptive factors are then entered into a standard classification system, like the **Rappaport system** or the **Working Formulation** (Table 31-2). Within these classifications, there are three general groups of non-

Table 31-2. Histological Classification of Non-Hodgkin's Lymphoma

	Rappaport Classification	Working Formulation Classification
Low grade	Diffuse lymphocytic, well differentiated	Small lymphocytic
	Nodular lymphocytic, poorly differentiated	Follicular, small cleaved cell
	Nodular, mixed lymphocytic and histiocytic	Follicular, mixed small and large cells
Intermediate grade	Nodular histiocytic	Follicular large cell
	Diffuse lymphocytic, poorly differentiated	Diffuse, small cleaved cell
	Diffuse, mixed lymphocytic and histiocytic	Diffuse, mixed small and large cells
	Diffuse histiocytic	Diffuse, large cell
High grade	Diffuse histiocytic	Immunoblastic
	Lymphoblastic	Lymphoblastic
	Diffuse undifferentiated (Burkitt or non-Burkitt)	Small noncleaved cell (Burkitt or non-Burkitt)

Hodgkin's lymphomas. **Low-grade lymphomas** are slow growing, often widespread at diagnosis, and incurable by conventional chemotherapy. Nodular lymphomas fit into this group. **Intermediate-grade lymphomas** are somewhat faster growing, but potentially curable by conventional chemotherapy. Diffuse lymphomas and lymphomas composed of large cells fall into this category. **High-grade lymphomas** behave very aggressively, much like acute lymphocytic leukemia. The "blastic" lymphomas (immunoblastic and lymphoblastic) and Burkitt's lymphoma are high grade. Histology is the single most important prognostic factor in non-Hodgkin's lymphoma.

As with leukemia, the signs and symptoms of lymphoma are fairly nonspecific. The presence of fever, weight loss, or night sweats (termed **B symptoms**) carries an adverse prognosis. Some patients complain of pruritus, which is not necessarily due to lymphoma in the skin. Lymphadenopathy and splenomegaly are very commonly found on physical examination. Non-Hodgkin's lymphoma may involve extra-nodal sites, such as the stomach, the central nervous system, and the testis; this happens rarely in Hodgkin's disease, and appears to be particularly common in non-Hodgkin's lymphomas in patients with the acquired immunodeficiency syndrome. Just as immunophenotype can predict clinical behavior in acute lymphocytic leukemia, so can histology predict clinical behavior in non-Hodgkin's lymphoma. Nodular lymphomas tend to be extensively disseminated at diagnosis, involving multiple lymph nodes and often the bone marrow. Intermediate lymphomas may involve extranodal sites such as the stomach. High-grade lymphomas present with bulky adenopathy and central nervous system involvement. Anemia and thrombocytopenia are common in lymphoma patients, either due to bone marrow involvement by tumor or immunologic destruction. Lymphoma cells may be seen in the blood, most commonly in the low-grade lymphomas, but also in high-grade lymphomas.

Staging is a description of the extent of lymphoma, and the common staging system employed in both Hodgkin's disease and non-Hodgkin's lymphoma is the **Ann Arbor system** (Table 31-3). Higher stage is afforded by involvement of more lymph node groups and the spleen is considered an infradiaphragmatic node group. Involvement of the bone marrow or liver is stage IV and carries an adverse prognosis. In addition to advanced stage, other adverse prognostic factors in lymphoma patients include older age, bulky disease, and elevated lactate dehydrogenase (LDH). Histology and stage dictate the appropriate therapy for non-Hodgkin's lymphoma. Low-grade lymphomas are not curable with chemotherapy. Accordingly, treatment is used

Table 31-3. Ann Arbor Staging System for Lymphoma

Stage	Clinical Features
I	Involvement of a single lymph node group or single extralymphatic site (IE)
II	Involvement of two or more lymph node groups on the same side of the diaphragm, or a single extralymphatic site and a lymph node group on the same side of the diaphragm (IIe)
III	Involvement of lymph node groups on both sides of the diaphragm
IV	Involvement of the liver or bone marrow, or other extralymphatic sites

The notation of "B" is added if the patient has any of the following symptoms: (1) unexplained fever > 38°C, (2) night sweats, (3) loss of > 10% body weight in prior 6 months. In the absence of these symptoms, the stage is noted as "A."

to control symptoms or prevent catastrophes. Oral chemotherapy, similar to that used for chronic lymphocytic leukemia, is typically employed first. Radiation therapy is used if the lymphoma is localized or if symptoms are due to a particular site of disease (like ureteral obstruction). Intermediate-grade lymphomas are treated with aggressive combination intravenous chemotherapy, like the combination CHOP (cyclophosphamide, doxorubicin, vincristine, and prednisone). Approximately 30–50% of patients with this lymphoma are cured with this therapy. High-grade lymphomas carry a much worse prognosis and are generally treated in a fashion akin to acute leukemia. In both Burkitt's lymphoma and lymphoblastic lymphoma, central nervous system prophylaxis is an important component of therapy.

Hodgkin's Disease

Although **Hodgkin's disease** shares with non-Hodgkin's lymphoma the Ann Arbor staging system and the clinical propensity to involve mostly lymph nodes, it is an entirely distinct entity. The diagnosis of Hodgkin's disease requires the identification of **Reed-Sternberg cells** in the diagnostic biopsy. Reed Sternberg cells are binucleate "owl's eye" cells, often seen in the background of lymphocytes and eosinophils. There are four classical histological patterns, termed the Rye classification, in Hodgkin's disease: lymphocyte depleted, mixed cellularity, nodular sclerosing, and lymphocyte predominant. These have some prognostic importance, but are not nearly as important as histology in non-Hodgkin's lymphoma.

The symptoms of Hodgkin's disease are very similar to those of non-Hodgkin's lymphoma, including B symptoms and pruritus. Lymphadenopathy is the predominant clinical sign. However, in Hodgkin's disease the involvement of lymph nodes is very orderly and contiguous. For example, it is common to involve lymph nodes in the neck and axilla on the same side, but rare to involve lymph nodes in the neck and pelvis without involvement of the lymph nodes in between. Hodgkin's disease is also almost exclusively a lymph node-based disease. Involvement of extranodal organs is unusual unless adjacent to a very large mass of nodal Hodgkin's disease. Hodgkin's disease is virtually never present in the blood. However, anemia and thrombocytopenia can be seen, as can eosinophilia.

Staging, using the Ann Arbor system (see Table 31-3), is the same as for non-Hodgkin's lymphoma. The stage is the single most important prognostic factor in Hodgkin's disease. Because stage is so important, a thorough evaluation of the patient for sites of lymphoma is undertaken in every patient with Hodgkin's disease. This evaluation includes radiographic studies (CT scans of chest, abdomen, and pelvis) and bone marrow examination initially, and staging laparotomy with biopsies of all lymph node groups, the liver, and splenectomy in selected cases.

Treatment of Hodgkin's disease is based mostly on stage. Localized disease, stages I and II, is treated with radiotherapy encompassing affected lymph node groups plus the next contiguous node groups (**extended field**). Disseminated disease, stages III and IV, is treated with combination intravenous chemotherapy like MOPP (nitrogen mustard, vincristine, procarbazine, and prednisone) or ABVD (doxorubicin, bleomycin, vinblastine, and dacarbazine). Greater than 80% of patients with localized and 60% of patients with disseminated Hodgkin's disease are cured.

Disorders Diagnosed by Marrow Abnormalities

Multiple Myeloma

Multiple myeloma is a disease of malignant plasma cells. These plasma cells often have secretory activity, releasing their product, a **monoclonal immunoglobulin,** into the plasma. Serum protein electrophoresis (SPEP) often yields the first clue to a plasma cell neoplasm (Fig. 31-1) The SPEP separates proteins electrophoretically; overproduction of an immunoglobulin is visualized as a protein spike. Immunofixation identifies the spike as monoclonal and defines the immunologic isotype (IgG kappa, for example). About 20% of cases of myeloma do not have a serum monoclonal protein, but do have a urine protein which may be free immunoglobulin light chains. Urine protein electrophoresis is a mandatory component of the workup of myeloma. The presence of a monoclonal protein alone is insufficient to make the diagnosis of multiple myeloma, since a sizable percentage of normal people (especially the elderly) have a monoclonal protein of unclear significance. The critical diagnostic test in myeloma is bone marrow examination, which typically documents greater than 20% plasma cells, many of which are immature or in sheets or clusters (Plate 3). There are numerous clinical manifestations of multiple myeloma which can generally be divided into mass effects of the malignant plasma cells and secretory effects of the paraprotein or other myeloma cell produced cytokines (Fig. 31-2). Replacement of the marrow by myeloma cells leads to bone marrow failure, with resultant anemia and thrombocytopenia. Like the malignant cells in chronic lymphocytic leukemia, the malignant plasma cells in myeloma are incompetent, resulting in decreased production of normal antibodies, which in turn leads to infection. Bone disease is common and may manifest as lytic, "punched out" lesions, diffuse osteopenia or, more rarely, osteoblastic lesions. The lesions are thought to occur owing to the lymphokine **OAF (osteoclast activating factor)** elaborated by the malignant plasma cell. X-rays are the best test to evaluate bone disease; bone scans are often negative in the face of extensive bone disease. Hypercalcemia can be severe. Plasma cell destruction of vertebral bodies can lead to spinal cord compression.

Secretory effects of the paraprotein can be devastating due to their toxicity to normal tissues as well as "bystander effects." Renal disease, including renal failure, is often the overwhelming clinical feature of myeloma. The causes include tubulo-interstitial disease, hypercalcemia, and amyloidosis. Occult renal dysfunction can be unmasked by nephrotoxic insults such as intravenous contrast. Immunoglobulin or light chains can be deposited in tissue leading to organ dysfunction (heart, kidneys, GI tract). These aggregates, **amyloid,** can be visualized by biopsy of affected organs. Antibodies can be directed to supporting structures of peripheral nerves leading to peripheral neuropathy. Coating of the red cells leads to **Rouleaux** formation. Coating of platelets may lead to abnormal bleeding. Extreme overproduction of the paraprotein can lead to hyperviscosity with neurological dysfunction.

Multiple myeloma is, like chronic lymphocytic leukemia, generally a slow-growing disease affecting older patients that cannot be cured by conventional chemotherapy. Also like chronic lymphocytic leukemia, asymptomatic patients may be appropriately observed without

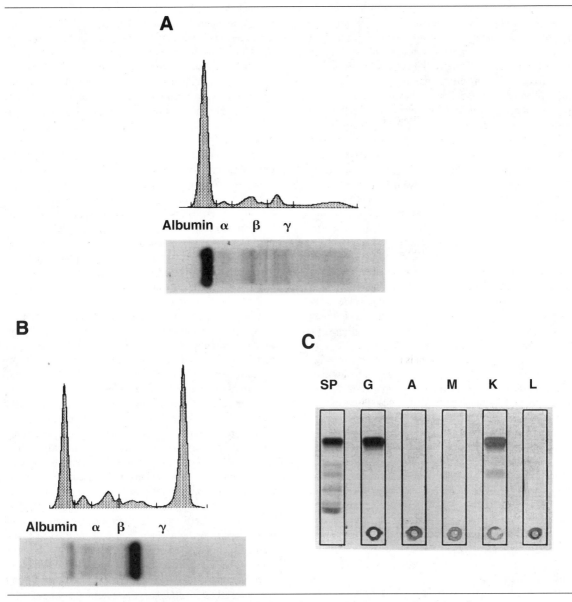

Fig. 31-1. Serum protein electrophoresis and immunofixation. The normal electrophoretic pattern of serum and the corresponding densitometric tracing is shown in (A). Notice that the albumin band is darkest on the electrophoresis and so has the highest peak on the densitometric tracing. The gamma band, representing immunoglobulin, is broad and comparatively small. An electrophoresis and tracing from a patient with multiple myeloma are shown in (B). Notice that the intensity of the gamma band is dramatically greater and corresponds to a peak on the densitometric tracing. In (C), immunofixation, performed by reacting the immunoglobulin paraprotein with antiserum directed against the specific immunoglobulin isotypes (G for the gamma heavy chains of IgG, A for the alpha heavy chains of IgA, M for the mu heavy chains of IgM, K for the kappa light chains, and L for the lambda light chains) identifies this particular paraprotein as IgG kappa.

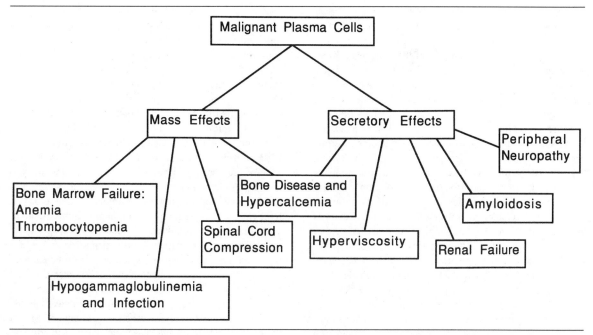

Fig. 31-2. Pathophysiology of multiple myeloma. The clinical consequences of multiple myeloma can best be characterized by "mass effects" related to the large number of malignant plasma cells or "secretory effects" related to the overproduced immunoglobulin.

therapy for a period of time. The mainstay of therapy is oral chemotherapy (melphalan, an oral alkylating agent, plus prednisone). More aggressive intravenous chemotherapy can be used if a more prompt response is desired, but this affords no survival benefit. Radiation therapy is used for painful bone lesions or if fracture threatens. Use of bone marrow transplantation is experimental, but may offer the only chance for long-term survival. The majority of patients with myeloma die of their disease.

Clinical Examples

1. A 22-year-old male university student comes to your office because he has noticed a progressive fullness in his left supraclavicular region. He has not felt completely well for about 2 months, feeling more tired than usual, having the sensation of fever intermittently accompanied by heavy sweats at night, and having lost weight from 180 to 160 lb. He has delayed seeking medical advice because he attributed his symptoms to the stress of a full summer term course load plus a full-time construction job. He had inter-

preted the left supraclavicular mass as a result of a job-related minor shoulder injury. Your examination is normal with the exception of a very firm, nontender 4 × 3 cm left supraclavicular mass. Blood counts, urinalysis, and routine serum chemistry data are normal. However, a chest x-ray demonstrates a mass of 10-cm diameter in the anterior mediastinum.

Discussion. This young man presents the characteristic clinical features of malignant lymphoma, although these features are not specific. The progressive symptoms of fever, sweats, and weight loss could also be the result of a chronic infectious illness. Similarly, the mass, presumably representing a supraclavicular lymph node enlargement, may also be the result of chronic granulomatous infection. The normal blood counts make chronic lymphocytic leukemia unlikely; the large mediastinal mass makes malignant lymphoma most likely. The appropriate diagnostic procedure is a lymph node biopsy. This demonstrates Hodgkin's disease, nodular sclerosing type. Further clinical evaluation is required to diagnose the extent of the Hodgkin's disease. Routine procedures include CT scans to more accurately define the size of the mediastinal mass and to detect additional mediastinal lymphadenopathy as well as abdominal lymphadenopathy. Bone marrow biopsies may also be done. The results of these studies demonstrate the presence of retroperitoneal lymph nodes but a normal bone marrow. The clinical stage is then designated as IIIB. This clinical stage is considered too extensive for treatment by radiation therapy, and chemotherapy provides a better opportunity for cure. The treatment is intensive, using a combination of chemotherapeutic agents administered in maximal doses, accepting a risk of neutropenia and secondary infection. After four months of chemotherapy there is no evidence for residual Hodgkin's disease when all diagnostic studies are repeated. Two further months of chemotherapy are administered. The patient is now considered to have a complete remission. Whether this remission is in fact a cure can only be determined after several years of followup without evidence of recurrence. The long-term sequelae of the treatment even in cured patients represents a slight increased risk for the development of a second, treatment-induced malignancy. The risk of this is very low in patients treated only with chemotherapy, but it is greater in patients treated with a combination of radiation therapy and chemotherapy.

2. A 78-year-old woman is admitted to the hospital after a fall at home resulting in a fractured left hip. X-rays in the emergency room demonstrated not only the hip fracture but also the presence of several osteolytic lesions in the left femur. When the fracture was stabilized and pain was controlled, a more detailed history revealed that this woman had experienced progressive fatigue over several months with difficulty in maintaining her usual routine of household chores. Particularly she had difficulty with washing floors because of low back pain. An additional symptom was progressive constipation. Initial laboratory data demonstrated a hemoglobin of 9.2 mg/dl, hematocrit 28%, MCV 88 fl, WBC 4200/ml with a normal differential count, platelet count 92,000/μl, normal urinalysis, and abnormal serum chemistry values including serum calcium 11.2 mg/dl, serum creatinine 1.8 mg/dl, and BUN 35 mg/dl, total protein 8.2 g/dl, and albumin 2.4 g/dl. Additional x-ray examinations revealed osteolytic lesions in the skull and diffuse osteoporosis involving the thoracic and lumbar vertebrae.

Discussion.   These presenting features are all characteristic of multiple myeloma, but not diagnostic. Pancytopenia with normocytic anemia could be due to marrow failure of several etiologies. Hypercalcemia and renal failure are also not specific for multiple myeloma. Osteolytic

lesions are characteristic of myeloma but may be due to another malignant disease, such as breast cancer. A defining feature of multiple myeloma is to examine the serum and urine for the presence of monoclonal immunoglobulins. In this woman the abnormal serum proteins on the routine chemical analysis provide the most important clue. On serum protein electrophoresis, a monoclonal protein was identified in the gamma globulin region, and quantified at 4.8 gm/dl. Immunofixation identified this as being restricted to IgG heavy chains and kappa light chains. A 24-hour urine demonstrated 3.2 g of protein in 1000 ml (in spite of the "negative proteinuria" in the routine urinalysis). Upon electrophoresis this was found to represent a monoclonal band identified by immunofixation as kappa light chains. A bone marrow aspirate and biopsy demonstrated an increased number of mature-appearing plasma cells. Therefore this patient fulfills diagnostic criteria for myeloma, and the extent and symptomatic problems with the disease demand treatment. Her age, however, does not allow her to be considered as a candidate for the most intensive chemotherapy supported by bone marrow transplantation. In most patients, oral chemotherapy will control the multiple myeloma and cause regression of the disease as manifested by decreased amounts of immunoglobulin light chains in the urine and decreased serum immunoglobulin paraprotein. However any therapeutic result will only be temporary, followed by relapse and chemotherapy-resistant disease. Additional important therapy is local radiation to the osteolytic lesions in weight-bearing bones to prevent further pathologic fractures. Also careful attention to hydration is an important component for management of the hypercalcemia.

Bibliography

Dighiero G, Travade P, Chevret S, et al. B cell chronic lymphocytic leukemia: Present status and future directions. *Blood* 78:1901–1914, 1991. *A current review of the biology and treatment of CLL.*

Janeway C and Traven P. *Immunobiology: The Immune System in Health and Disease.* New York: Current Biology, Ltd., Garland Publishing, 1994. *An excellent current text summarizing the advances in basic immunology.*

Kyle RA. Multiple myeloma: review of 869 cases. *Mayo Clin Proc* 50:29, 1975. *The classic reference in myeloma, probably the best reference for clinical manifestations of the disease. Treatment is better summarized in more recent references in myeloma.*

The Non-Hodgkin's Lymphoma Pathologic Classification Project: National Cancer Institute sponsored study of classifications in non-Hodgkin's lymphomas: Summary and description of a working formulation for clinical usage. *Cancer* 49:2112–2135, 1982. *The basis for the current pathologic classification system in lymphoma. A very rich resource for pathologists and clinicians interested in staging and natural history, treatment is better covered in more recent references.*

Preti A and Kantarjian H. Management of adult acute lymphoblastic leukemia: present issues and key challenges. *J Clin Oncol* 12:1312–1322, 1994. *An up-to-the-minute summary of treatment and controversies in acute lymphocytic leukemia in adults.*

Urba W and Longo D. Medical progress: Hodgkin's disease. *N Engl J Med* 326:678–687, 1992. *A thorough review of Hodgkin's disease, including controversies surrounding pathogenesis.*

32 Oncogenesis and the Genetic Basis of Cancer

Thomas H. Carter

Objectives

After completing this chapter, you should be able to

Understand the conceptual difference between oncogenes and tumor suppressors

State the major examples of oncogenes and their relationship to pathways of signal transduction for growth factors

List the three classes of mutation that activate oncogenes in human tumors and know major examples

Describe the classes of mutation that affect tumor suppressor genes

Have an appreciation for the role of clonal evolution in tumor progression

Know general mechanisms that produce damage in the DNA of cancer cells

Understand hereditary cancers in terms of germline and somatic mutations

Have sufficient knowledge to deduce whether particular methods are suitable for testing various oncogenic mutations. (For example, to detect common mutations in a *ras* gene, how applicable is analysis by cytogenetics? . . . immunoblot? . . . PCR?)

Control of Cellular Growth

Elaborate mechanisms regulate the growth and elimination of cells. Normal cells exhibit one of three growth behaviors: They rest in a mitotically quiet state, they grow and divide, or they undergo apoptosis (programmed cell death). Cancerous cells accumulate abnormally and invade surrounding tissues. Despite the apparent diversity of tumors, which arise from nearly every cell type in the body, cancer cells share a common set of biochemical derangements. These derangements include the regulation of the cell cycle, differentiation, and apoptosis. Biologists increasingly view oncogenesis as one process — the accumulation of genetic lesions affecting normal mechanisms of development, tissue renewal, and response to injury. This discussion summarizes how this basic understanding will relate to the care of patients with cancer and to cancer prevention.

Most cancer cells contain multiple mutations. Basic research in the genetic basis of cancer addresses the following questions: (1) Which genes undergo mutation and how do the mutations convert a normal cell into a neoplastic one? (2) What produces oncogenic damage of the DNA in the first place? The answers to these questions enable us to attack a vitally important medical problem — how to prevent the lethal consequences of this genetic damage. This information has growing importance in the diagnosis and treatment of cancer. The next few years may provide clinical tests to assess who has a high risk of breast or colon cancer. This knowledge may have a major impact on the effectiveness and cost of cancer prevention practices.

This chapter will define oncogenes and tumor suppressor genes, review the kinds of mutations that are characteristic for important cancer genes, and consider the causes of these mutations. Examples are provided that illustrate the cellular pathophysiology of cancer and genetic-based tests that have clinical applications. Terms in the text marked with an asterisk are defined in the glossary (Table 32-1). Table 32-2

Table 32-1. Definitions of Commonly Used Terms in Oncogenesis

ALLELES	Different forms of a gene at the same genetic locus on homologous chromosomes.
AMPLIFICATION	Formation of multiple copies of a gene or a chromosomal region. Tumor cells may amplify an oncogene to hundreds of copies. The increased "gene dosage" may cause overproduction of the gene product.
AUTOCRINE	Refers to the production of a growth factor or hormone that influences the growth or metabolism of the same cell that produces it.
CARCINOGEN	A substance that causes cancer. Some chemical carcinogens act directly, but others require metabolism in vivo before becoming effective. Many carcinogens act by causing mutations*.
CLONE	A family of cells derived from one parent cell. An abnormal chromosome or mutation may serve as a clonal marker, identifying cells within a clone. Most human tumors appear to arise from a single cell and hence are mono-clonal.
CODING REGION	The coding region is that part of a nucleic acid sequence that contains codons determining a protein sequence. Exons are DNA sequences retained in the mRNA after splicing; they include the coding region and represent the expressed portion of the gene.
DELETION	Mutation consisting of a loss of DNA. Small deletions, such as the loss of a few bases, represent one form of point mutation that may cause either modest sequence changes in the encoded protein or large changes by shifting the translational frame and causing premature termination of protein synthesis. Moderate-sized deletions may affect only some domains of an encoded protein — this occasionally activates an oncogene. Large deletions, on the other hand, may involve hundreds of genes on a chromosome — they may totally eliminate a tumor suppressor gene in the deleted segment. Methods to detect large deletions include analysis for LOH* or cytogenetic examination.
DNA REPAIR	The process whereby damaged DNA is a substrate for enzymes that attempt to restore the original sequence. Repair may lead to complete restoration of the DNA (error-free repair) or may result in alteration or deletion of bases (error-prone repair).
ENHANCER	A DNA sequence that increases the activity of promoters (sites where RNA synthesis begins). The location of enhancer sequences may be within or on either side of the coding region of genes.
GTP-BINDING PROTEINS	A family of proteins that includes the products of the *RAS* oncogenes and the heteromeric G proteins. Many serve as cytoplasmic components of signal transduction pathways.
GROWTH FACTOR	A polypeptide hormone that acts to regulate growth or differentiated properties of cells. Growth factors interact with cells through specific receptors on the cell surface. Their binding to receptors activates a variety of intracellular enzymes that mediate signal transduction* and elicit specific cellular responses.
HETEROZYGOSITY	When different alleles* of a gene are present on homologous chromosomes. This contrasts with homozygosity, when only one allele is present (in one or multiple copies). See LOH*.
IMMORTALIZATION	The process that allows cells to proliferate indefinitely in culture. Immortalization appears to be a characteristic step of transformation* in vitro.
LOH	Loss of heterozygosity, a somatically acquired mutation found by comparing tumor cells with normal cells from one individual. It generally occurs as a consequence of mutations affecting large chromosomal regions that contain tumor suppressor genes. For example, deletions may cause the loss of a wild-type allele for tumor suppressor gene. If sufficiently large, this deletion may also cause the loss of neighboring genetic markers — tumor cells lose one copy of any marker that is heterozygous in the germline. A highly polymorphic marker is most informative because many individuals are heterozygous. Typical markers are RFLPs* and microsatellites*.
MICROSATELLITES	DNA sequences scattered throughout the genome that consist of nucleotide repeats. One may readily assess microsatellites by PCR. The length of a repeat at a given locus may vary among individuals (i.e., it is polymorphic) but microsatellite lengths display stable Mendelian inheritance. These features make microsatellites powerful genetic markers for linkage analysis in family studies and for mapping regions that undergo selective loss during tumor development (loss of heterozygosity*). In addition, tumors defective in mismatch repair may display a high mutation rate in which microsatellites throughout the genome change length (microsatellite instability).

Table 32-1. Definitions of Commonly Used Terms in Oncogenesis (continued)

MUTATION	A change in one or more of the DNA bases in a gene. Mutations in coding exons may lead to altered protein products; mutations in noncoding regions may lead to altered amounts of protein. Activation of human proto-oncogenes usually involves point mutation*, translocation*, or amplification*.
ONCOGENE	A gene whose protein product actively drives neoplastic transformation of a cell. The normal form of the gene (c-*onc* or proto-oncogene) is altered in cancer cells by mutations that cause a gain in function.
POINT MUTATION	A small-scale mutation, such as a base change or an insertion or deletion of a few bases. Consequences can range from a change in one amino acid to a complete loss of the protein product.
PCR	Polymerase chain reaction, a technique for amplifying a short stretch of DNA in the test tube. The method depends on the use of two flanking oligonucleotide DNA primers and repeated cycles of primer extension using a DNA polymerase.
PROTEIN KINASE	An enzyme that catalyzes the transfer of phosphate groups to proteins. Phosphorylation and dephosphorylation are major mechanisms for reversibly controlling the function of proteins. Many oncogenes encode protein kinases. Most protein kinases are specific for the addition of phosphate to either tyrosine residues (tyrosine kinases) or serine and threonine residues. Many tyrosine kinases are components of cell surface receptors (receptor tyrosine kinases), while many serine/threonine-specific kinases are intracellular components of signal transduction.
PROTO-ONCOGENE	One of a set of normal cellular genes, many identified by sequence homology to transforming genes in RNA tumor viruses. Proto-oncogenes typically encode proteins that control cellular proliferation, survival, and differentiation. Activation of oncogenic potential in human tumors occurs by point mutation*, amplification*, or rearrangement*.
REARRANGEMENT	Changes in the order of genes or gene segments. Genetic rearrangement occurs in the normal process that generates antibody molecules. Abnormal rearrangements can induce mutations such as translocations or deletions that affect cancer genes.
RECESSIVE	At the cellular level, a condition manifest only in cells homozygous for the mutant gene (i.e., carrying a double dose of the abnormal gene). Recessive is the opposite of dominant, where the effect occurs in cells that are heterozygous (i.e., carrying one mutant and one normal allele).
RETROVIRUS	A class of virus in which the genome consists of RNA and replication involves reverse transcription into DNA. A subset of retroviruses were termed RNA tumor viruses because of the ability to induce malignancies in animals. These viruses serve as carcinogens through their ability to insert into the host cell genome, to incorporate cellular sequences into virus particles, and to introduce mutations in pirated cellular sequences.
RFLP	Restriction fragment length polymorphism, a genetic marker determined by naturally occurring variations in the DNA sequence at a recognition site for a restriction endonuclease. Analysis for a RFLP typically involves cutting the DNA with the restriction enzyme and performing a Southern blot.
SIGNAL TRANSDUCTION	Biochemical reactions inside a cell that transmit information between the surface of the cell and its interior. Cellular responses relevant to oncogenesis include changes in the expression of specific genes, regulation of the cell cycle, and apoptosis.
STEM CELL	A hypothetical cell that has the capacity to produce a tumor. The stem cell passes genetic lesions on to all cells in the neoplastic clone.
TRANSCRIPTION FACTORS	Proteins that bind specific sequences of DNA and influence the expression of genes. Examples include the products of both oncogenes (*MYC*) and tumor suppressor genes (*p53*).
TRANSFORMATION	Commonly used to describe the multiple changes that occur on conversion of normal cells to cancer cells. This complex phenotype includes abnormalities in appearance (morphologic transformation) and growth regulation in tissue culture (loss of contact inhibition, loss of anchorage-dependent growth, loss of requirements for added growth factors, etc.). Fully transformed cells can produce a tumor when injected in an appropriate animal.

Table 32-1. Definitions of Commonly Used Terms in Oncogenesis (continued)

TRANSLOCATION	The displacement of one part of a chromosome to a different chromosome or to a different part of the same chromosome. When a translocation joins the coding regions of two genes, the breakpoint may encode a fusion protein (or chimera) with abnormal activity. If the coding region remains intact, it may come under the influence of a foreign control region that causes inappropriate expression.
TUMOR SUPPRESSOR GENE	A gene whose inactivation contributes to the development of cancer (also referred to as an antioncogene). In cancer cells, these genes are the targets of mutations that cause a loss of function. Recurrent losses of a gene provide evidence for its classification as a tumor suppressor.
TUMOR VIRUS	Although viruses do not cause most human tumors, virally induced transformation has provided important model systems for understanding cancer. The term "tumor virus" traditionally applied to viruses with direct transforming activity in experimental settings. In contrast, some viruses assist in oncogenesis by indirect mechanisms — as appear to be true for several viruses strongly associated with human tumors. The two classes of tumor viruses induce transformation by genes of different origins. RNA tumor viruses are retroviruses* that induce cancer via mutant forms of host genes. DNA tumor viruses interact with cellular proteins through proteins of viral origin.

An asterisk marks words that are defined in this glossary.

Table 32-2. Cancer Genes with Clinical Utility

Gene	Disease	Utility	Mutational Mechanism	Biochemical Features
ONCOGENES				
N-*MYC*	neuroblastoma	prognosis and therapy	amplification	transcription factor
BCR/ABL	chronic myelogenous leukemia	diagnosis	translocation	intracellular tyrosine kinase
RET	medullary thyroid carcinoma (MEN2)	cancer prevention (prophylactic surgery)	point mutations	receptor tyrosine kinase
NEU (*ERBB-2*) (*HER-2*)	breast carcinoma	prognosis	amplification	receptor tyrosine kinase
ERBB-1	breast carcinoma	prognosis	overexpression	receptor tyrosine kinase
TUMOR SUPPRESSOR GENES				
RB-1	retinoblastoma	screening and prevention	multiple	cell cycle regulator
p53	Li-Fraumeni syndrome	prognosis (point mutations)	multiple	transcription factor
MAJOR NEW CANCER GENES				
MLL	acute leukemias	prognosis	translocations	?
MSH2	hereditary nonpolyposis colon cancer	prediction of risk		DNA mismatch repair
BRCA1	inherited breast/ ovarian syndrome	prediction of risk		?

provides a summary of clinically important examples of cancer genes.

Which Genes Are Targeted by Oncogenic Mutations?

We classify a gene as an oncogene* or tumor suppressor gene* depending on whether mutations* increase or decrease the function of the gene product in cancer cells. Deletion* of an entire gene is typical of tumor suppressors, not oncogenes.

Oncogenes — Mutations Causing a Gain of Function

The first cancer genes characterized in detail were termed oncogenes. Mutations of these genes activate cancer-promoting activity by increasing the level of gene expression or by increasing the biochemical activity of the encoded protein molecules. Thus either quantitative or qualitative changes of the gene products contribute a positive effect in cancer cells — a **gain of function.**

RNA Tumor Viruses

Animal models involving RNA tumor viruses* led to the idea that an individual gene can be capable of producing the complex cellular changes that are characteristic of cancer. In 1911, Peyton Rous showed that a virus could transmit sarcomas between chickens. Virologists subsequently found numerous examples of transmissible tumors. The amount of genetic information carried by the causative retroviruses* is tiny compared to the large host cell genome (10^4 versus 10^9 nucleotides). This consideration led to the formulation of the oncogene hypothesis, which stated that malignant transformation* results from single genes (generically designated v-*onc*) carried by retroviruses. Considerable experimental evidence now supports this idea.

The transforming genes of RNA tumor viruses originate from DNA sequences of host cells. This insight came in the late 1970s when researchers showed that viral oncogenes are homologous to cellular genes (proto-oncogenes*, designated c-*onc*). Sequence comparison showed that retroviruses had pirated and mutated host genes. The ability of retroviruses to mutate cellular genes derives from the fact that they insert into the host genome during their replication cycle. Although retroviruses activate oncogenes in animals, investigators have not found this mechanism to

occur in humans. Nevertheless, the study of RNA tumor viruses serves to identify genes that are targets for other forms of mutation in humans.

Growth Factor Signaling Pathways

Potent biochemical pathways communicate signals from the environment of a cell to regulate mitosis and differentiation. Derangement of these pathways provides a major theme in oncogenesis. Figure 32-1 shows how gain-of-

Fig. 32-1. Mutations affecting growth factor pathways can result in uncontrolled growth. The upper panel shows schematically how a normal growth factor pathway operates. Extracellular information, such as the presence of a soluble peptide hormone, interacts with the cell through a surface receptor. Signal transduction relays information through the cytoplasm to the nucleus and ultimately induces an appropriate cell response, such as mitosis. The lower panel illustrates four sites known to serve as targets of gain-of-function mutations in cancer cells. (A) When a cell produces both a growth factor and its cognate receptor, the cell may divide independently of its environment — a form of cellular activation termed autocrine stimulation. (B) Mutations in cell-surface receptors may mimic the effect of adding growth factor to a cell. Structural alterations of receptor tyrosine kinases may cause high kinase activity even in the absence of growth factor. (C) Mutations that alter intracellular molecules may also cause constitutive signal transduction. (D) Mutations that alter the expression or structure of nuclear proteins, like transcription factors, may mimic part of the mitogenic signal of growth factors.

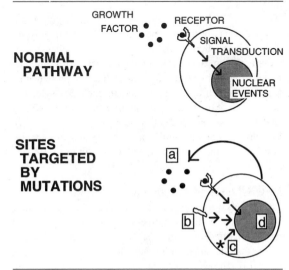

function mutations may result in unregulated signal trans-duction* in a growth-stimulatory pathway.

Growth Factors.   Extracellular ligands transmit regulatory information to the cell. Tumor cells can drive their own growth by producing excess growth factor* together with a receptor for that factor — creating a feedback loop termed **autocrine*** stimulation (see Fig. 32-1a). Transformation* can result from this uncontrolled self-stimulation.

Receptors.   Cells express receptors for peptide growth factors at their surface. Many are trans-membrane proteins with tyrosine-specific protein kinase* activity that normally depends strictly on the presence of growth factors. In autocrine stimulation, the receptors are structurally normal but may be overexpressed. In the ligand-*in*dependent situation, on the other hand, mutant receptors have structural abnormalities that mimic the effect of growth factors (see Fig. 32-1B).

Signal Transduction Molecules.   Like receptors, intracellular signaling molecules may undergo mutations that lock them into conformations with elevated activity. For example, GTP-binding proteins* involved in growth factor signaling are mutated to become v-*ras* oncogenes (found in viruses passed through *ra*ts which induce *sarco*mas). Alterations of the human *RAS* products are among the most common mutations clinically. Likewise, intracellular protein kinases may become oncogenic when mutated to constitutively active forms, as in the cases of *BCR-ABL* and v-*raf.*

Nuclear Responses.   Mitogenic stimuli regulate numerous events in the nucleus. Growth factors rapidly induce transcription factors* that control other genes required for normal cells to divide. Later responses include fluctuations in the levels of cyclins, which are proteins that regulate the cell cycle at checkpoints for DNA synthesis and mitosis. Mutant components of a transcription factor (AP-1) can serve as potent oncogenes (v-*fos* and v-*jun*). Likewise, overexpression of a cyclin results from mutations found in parathyroid and other tumors (*PRAD1* gene).

New Classes of Oncogenes

Researchers are uncovering genes that contribute to tumor formation by mechanisms other than by driving mitosis. In tissues that undergo significant turnover, homeostasis requires that the rate of cell production be exactly balanced by cell death. Mutations that prevent programmed death may contribute to the accumulation of malignant cells; this

effect may result from the inappropriate expression of *BCL-2* in nodular non-Hodgkin's lymphomas. Normal cellular behavior also requires appropriate differentiation. A mutant receptor for retinoic acid appears to block cellular differentiation in acute promyelocytic leukemias; this mutation may underlie the dramatic response to treatment with all *trans*-retinoic acid. Other oncogenes probably determine invasiveness and the ability of tumors to recruit new blood vessels, but knowledge in this area has lagged.

Mutations That Activate Oncogenes

The mutations that activate proto-oncogenes in most human cancers consist of point mutation*, gene amplification*, or translocation* (Fig. 32-2) — human cancers do not involve retroviral mechanisms for mutating proto-oncogenes like animal models. Proto-oncogenes generally undergo activation by qualitative or quantitative changes in the protein product. The mechanism of activation is specific for each gene.

Altered Protein Structure.   Mutations affecting the coding regions* of a gene can result in a structurally altered protein. The *RAS* genes are activated by point mutations* located at specific codons. Amino acid changes that eliminate a GTPase activity critical for negative regulation fix the protein in an active conformation. The GTP-bound form provides a constitutive growth signal. Methods useful for detection of point mutations include PCR* and hybridization to allele-specific oligonucleotides.

The synthesis of fusion protein may result from a chromosomal rearrangement* that joins coding regions of two genes. The *BCR-ABL* oncogene arises by a translocation that joins coding regions from chromosomes 9 and 22 (t(9;22)). The chimeric protein has constitutive protein kinase activity that promotes growth of the malignant clone* in chronic myelogenous leukemia. Numerous gene fusions involve transcription factors. For example, in t(l;19) of certain lymphocytic leukemias the DNA-binding region of a transcription factor important in immunoglobulin expression (E2A) is replaced by a homeobox domain; this swap of DNA-binding domains apparently targets gene promoters for an abnormal pattern of transcription. Researchers discover new fusion genes by identifying recurrent translocations in tumors and cloning the breakpoints. After characterizing a gene fusion, one may develop specific tests to screen clinical samples for the mutation at the RNA level (e.g., PCR-based methods) or protein level (Western blot).

Excessive Levels of Expression.   Inappropriate transcription may occur if mutations affect gene control elements. Burkitt's lymphoma expresses the c-*MYC* gene (on

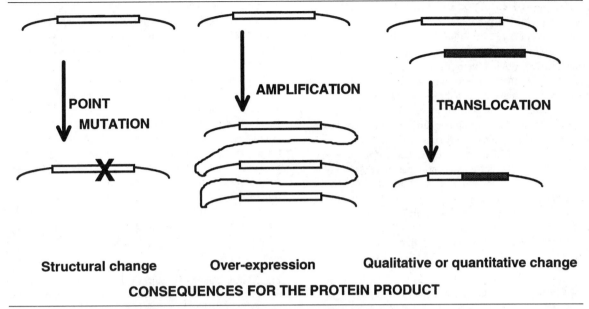

POINT MUTATION

AMPLIFICATION

TRANSLOCATION

Structural change **Over-expression** **Qualitative or quantitative change**

CONSEQUENCES FOR THE PROTEIN PRODUCT

Fig. 32-2. Three types of mutation convert proto-oncogenes to oncogenes in human cancers. Point mutations that occur in the coding region of a proto-oncogene may produce a structurally abnormal protein that is functionally overactive. Amplifications result in overexpression of a protein by gene dosage. A translocation may result in a structurally abnormal protein if the breakpoint joins the coding regions for different genes — resulting in a fusion or chimeric protein. Alternatively, translocations can bring an intact coding region into proximity of a new control element, causing inappropriate expression of a structurally normal protein. Mutational mechanisms that activate oncogenes cause a gain of function by altering either the quality or quantity of the gene product.

chromosome 8) as a result of translocations that join it to control elements for one of the immunoglobulin genes (on chromosomes 2, 14, and 22); the immunoglobulin enhancer* elements derange transcription of c-*MYC*. Cytogenetic analysis is a practical way to detect large chromosomal rearrangements such as t(8;14). On the other hand, neuroblastoma overexpresses N-*MYC* as a result of amplification. A method to measure an increase in gene copy number is Southern blotting.

Clinical Utility of Oncogene Testing

Analysis of oncogene activation has prognostic and therapeutic importance in a small but growing number of situations. The Philadelphia chromosome*, which bears *BCR-ABL,* is a hallmark of chronic myelogenous leukemia; cytogenetic testing for its presence helps to establish the diagnosis. Amplification of N-*MYC* establishes a poor prognosis in neuroblastoma and influences the deci-

sions for treatment. Immuno-histochemistry can detect overexpression of *ERBB-2* (or synonymously, *HER-2* or *neu*), which predicts a high risk of relapse after resection of localized breast carcinoma. Point mutations in a receptor tyrosine kinase, *RET,* underlie susceptibility to multiple endocrine neoplasia, type 2A; PCR-based tests now guide the use of prophylactic surgery to prevent thyroid carcinoma.

Tumor Suppressors — Mutations Causing Loss of Function

Some tumor samples contain mutations that delete certain genes entirely, so we infer that the gene products normally inhibit cancerous growth. The **loss of function** of these genes, termed tumor suppressor genes (or anti-oncogenes), represents a step toward cancer.

RB-1 — A Prototype for Tumor Suppressor Genes

Retinoblastoma is a rare tumor that provides a paradigm for an approach now applied to the study of many common cancers. This ocular tumor of childhood occurs in familial and sporadic forms. These forms differ in the risk for a second tumor; patients with the sporadic form have tumors that are solitary (unilateral disease), while those with the familial form often get multiple tumors of the same tissue (bilateral disease) and other tissues (osteosarcoma).

Epidemiologic data provided the basis of a hypothesis published in 1971 to explain retinoblastoma. One might explain the hereditary and sporadic forms of disease if the responsible gene were autosomal and if it affected individual cells in a recessive* manner. This model proposed the mutation of both alleles* in cancer cells (Fig. 32-3).

The identification of a gene for retinoblastoma provided dramatic confirmation of this two-hit hypothesis. A collection of very rare patients with retinoblastomas and birth defects provided a clue to the gene's location. Cytogenetic studies showed constitutional deletions involving large portions of chromosome 13. While the endpoints varied from patient to patient, all deletions shared a common region, as seen by aligning individual deletions to define the smallest region of overlap (SRO, Fig. 32-4). This region apparently contained a gene for retinoblastoma. Studies of retinoblastoma families allowed more precise mapping of the disease locus; linkage analysis identified polymorphic markers close to the disease gene. The study of tumor tissue provided additional evidence for the cancer-inducing role of this region. Tumors in both familial and sporadic forms often showed loss of genetic material from this region, termed **loss of heterozygosity*** (LOH*). This refers

Fig. 32-3. Model for the role of a tumor suppressor gene in retinoblastoma. The upper panel depicts hereditary disease. One allele of the gene is mutant in the germline; all cells of an affected individual acquire this mutation. During development of the retina, some cells undergo mutation of the normal allele and acquire a growth advantage, eventually forming tumors. Mutation of the normal allele is frequent enough to result in multiple tumors in many individuals. The lower panel represents sporadic disease. The germline of the individual contains two normal alleles. Mutations affecting each allele of the retinoblastoma gene would have to occur to produce a neoplastic retinoblast. The occurrence of two mutations in the same cell would be rare, so individuals with sporadic retinoblastoma would be unlikely to develop a second tumor.

Fig. 32-4. Location of a cancer gene indicated by large deletions associated with retinoblastoma. Very rare children with birth defects and retinoblastoma had constitutional deletions of chromosome 13. The suspected retinoblastoma gene lay in a region shared by all deletions, termed the smallest region of overlap (SRO). Additional evidence implicating this location came from more typical forms of retinoblastoma (see text).

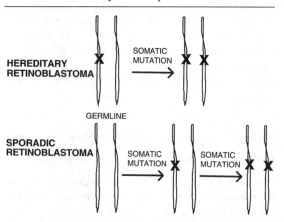

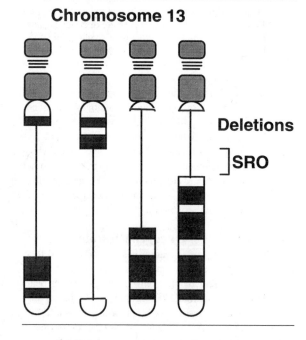

Chromosome 13

Deletions

]SRO

to somatically acquired mutations in cancerous clones causing the loss of markers on one copy of a chromosome. The identification of closely linked markers led to the cloning of the *RB-1* gene by a positional strategy. Molecular studies confirmed the presence of mutations as predicted.

Molecular techniques now permit the accurate prediction of which children are at high risk in families with retinoblastoma. This prognostic information guides screening and therapy, as illustrated in the second clinical example at the end of this chapter.

Loss of Tumor Suppressors in Human Cancer

Investigators seek the locations of new tumor suppressor genes by genetic, cytogenetic, and molecular techniques. They closely examine childhood and familial malignancies by cytogenetic and linkage studies to find markers in the germline DNA that segregate with the disease. They also study common sporadic cancers for consistent loss of chromosomal material in tumor tissue. New methods that are important in these studies include fluorescent in situ hybridization (FISH) and PCR of microsatellite markers. Analysis of many kinds of cancer has implicated numerous chromosomal loci as containing tumor suppressors. Recently cloned tumor suppressor genes include those involved in Wilm's tumor and neurofibromatosis type 1.

The *p53* Gene. A 53 kDa protein encoded by the *p53* gene is defective in the majority of human tumors and is the most frequently mutated cancer gene. Some tumors contain deletions of both alleles of *p53,* which indicates that loss-of-function mutations are oncogenic. By this and other experimental criteria, we may consider *p53* a tumor suppressor. Paradoxically, some oncogenic mutations result in accumulation of p53 protein; these particular mutant proteins form complexes with the product of the normal allele in heterozygous cells and ablate p53 function (a phenotype termed "dominant negative"). Rare germline mutations of *p53* result in an inherited susceptibility to a variety of tumors, including breast cancer and sarcomas that appear in middle age (Li-Fraumeni Syndrome).

Rb and p53 Regulation of Cell Division and Cell Death. Rb (the protein produced from the *RB-1* gene) and p53 play important roles in terminal differentiation,

and their loss appears to remove an important barrier to neoplastic growth. Recent experiments have shown that cells exit proliferation during normal differentiation through the ability of Rb to sequester growth-promoting transcription factors (e.g., E2F). Consequently, the loss of Rb function can result in a failure to exit the cell cycle. The p53 protein normally provides a safeguard against this inappropriate proliferation. One of the functions of normal p53 is to link the systems that detect untimely DNA synthesis and the genes that induce either cell death or cell cycle inhibition. Thus Rb and p53 cooperate to regulate differentiation, the cell cycle, and apoptosis.

Cancer cells can lose the function of Rb and p53 in several ways. Human tumors often contain mutations of both Rb and p53. Inactivation of p53 may also result from overexpression of an inhibitor termed mdm2; amplification of the *MDM2* gene occurs in sarcomas, glial tumors, and bladder cancer. Interestingly, DNA tumor viruses target both p53 and Rb for inactivation (Fig. 32-5). During a viral infection, viral proteins apparently control the cell cycle of the host by inactivating p53 and Rb. If expressed out of the context of viral replication, these proteins can transform cells. Proteins encoded by human papilloma viruses appear to play a role in cervical carcinoma by inactivating Rb and p53 (Table 32-3).

Fig. 32-5. DNA tumor viruses inactivate tumor suppressor proteins of the host cell. Human papilloma viruses (HPV) encode proteins of viral origin (E6 and E7) that bind to and inactivate p53 and Rb proteins. In the setting of a productive viral infection, this mechanism allows the virus to control the cell cycle. In certain tumors, these viral "oncoproteins" appear to contribute to neoplastic transformation. By knocking out the "brakes" for cell division, these viral oncoproteins promote runaway growth.

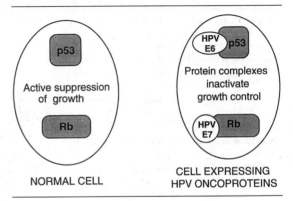

Table 32-3. Viruses Associated with Human Neoplasms

Virus	Disease
Human papilloma virus	Cervical carcinoma
	Benign genital warts
HTLV-1	Adult T cell leukemia
Hepatitis B virus	Hepatocellular carcinoma
Epstein-Barr virus	Burkitt's lymphoma
	Nasopharyngeal carcinoma
	Lymphoma in the immuno-compromised host

Cancer Arises by Multiple Steps

Germline Mutations

In familial cancer syndromes, germline cells carry the mutation. Individuals generally acquire one mutant allele at the time of conception, so all cells in these individuals have one copy of mutant gene. Only a few cells of an affected individual become neoplastic, so additional events evidently occur in the diseased subset of somatic cells.

Somatic Events

Genetic alterations that occur in somatic cells presumably promote cancer by conferring a selective advantage for growth or survival. The progeny cells undergo multiple rounds of mutation and selection, eventually acquiring fully transformed properties (Fig. 32-6). By analogy to

Fig. 32–6. The multi-step origin of cancer. Multiple genetic events convert a cell to a neoplastic phenotype. A dozen steps may be necessary for some types of cancer. For hereditary cancer syndromes (top), a germline mutation shifts the status of the cells to the right.

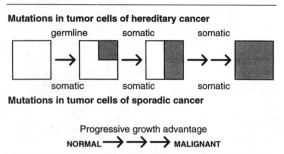

Mutations in tumor cells of hereditary cancer

Mutations in tumor cells of sporadic cancer

Progressive growth advantage

NORMAL → → → MALIGNANT

normal tissues, we may consider a tumor to contain a stem cell* that is capable of renewing itself and expanding to a population of progeny cells. Cells arising from a single precursor are termed **monoclonal.** As mutations accumulate, multiple subclones appear with different characteristics. This model predicts that subclones share some markers in common to the parent stem cell, and it explains why tumor cell populations are heterogeneous and why they tend to become increasingly malignant (Fig. 32-7).

In clinical experience, multi-step oncogenesis may explain why tumors progress from indolent to aggressive behavior. The phases of chronic myelogenous leukemia provide a good illustration, as discussed in a clinical example at the end of this chapter. Patients with chronic lymphocytic leukemia occasionally deteriorate with sudden conversion to an aggressive large cell lymphoma (Richter's syndrome) or leukemias. Patients with certain tumors that initially respond to chemotherapy (such as lymphomas, myeloma, and small cell carcinoma of the lung) often re-

Fig. 32-7. Clonal evolution during oncogenesis. The stages of tumor development, depicted as a series of mutations and biologic selections, lead to increasingly malignant features.

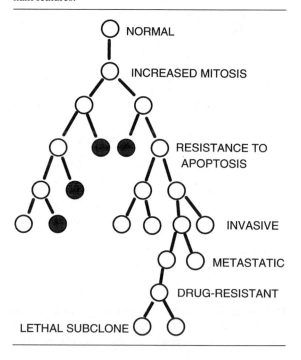

NORMAL

INCREASED MITOSIS

RESISTANCE TO APOPTOSIS

INVASIVE

METASTATIC

DRUG-RESISTANT

LETHAL SUBCLONE

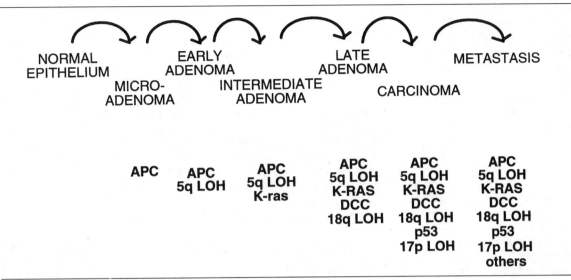

Fig. 32-8. Accumulation of mutations during the development of colorectal carcinoma. Clinicians may sample tumor cells throughout early and late stages of this neoplasm. Some mutations, identified by loss of heterozygosity (LOH*) suggest the inactivation of tumor suppressor genes. Other mutations cause a gain of function, such as alterations of the *RAS* oncogenes resulting in specific amino acid changes that lock the encoded protein into a constitutively active form.

lapse with an acquired drug resistance. The natural history of colonic neoplasms provides an excellent example of multi-step oncogenesis (Fig. 32-8).

What Produces Oncogenic Damage in DNA?

Insights Provided by Epidemiology

In 1775, an English physician made one of the first scientific observations of this problem. Sir Percival Pott suggested that the cause of scrotal cancer in chimney sweeps might be exposure to chimney soot. Subsequent epidemiologic studies have linked a variety of malignancies to occupational exposures. Epidemiologic studies indicate that the most common preventable cause of cancer in industrialized countries is cigarette smoking. International variation in the incidence of cancers can provide additional clues about the environmental and behavior factors in cancer causation. Esophageal cancer is frequent in a geographic belt across Asia. Melanoma rates vary with latitude, implicating a role for solar exposure of the skin.

Breast and colon cancer have elevated incidences in industrialized countries.

A combination of epidemiologic and molecular approaches can provide new insight into causes of mutation. Studies of *p53* mutations in large populations, for example, provide clues about the role of different carcinogens.* Hepatocellular carcinoma is the most common cancer in portions of Africa and Asia. One factor appears to be hepatitis B virus, which shares a similar geographic distribution (see Table 32-3). In certain regions, hepatocellular carcinoma is also associated with contamination of food with a fungal byproduct, aflatoxin. Analysis of *p53* mutations in aflatoxin-associated cases shows predominantly a specific base change. Other tumors, such as lung and colon cancers, show different *p53* mutations. This variability suggests that different carcinogens may leave characteristic signatures in the damaged DNA of tumors.

Contribution of Host Factors

Tumor surveillance by the immune system has an important role in the development of cancer. A general decline in immune responsiveness accompanies aging, which may contribute to the increased incidence of cancers in the elderly. Recipients of immunosuppressive therapy for organ transplantation are at risk for non-Hodgkin's lymphoma; moreover, these tumors can regress upon reduction of immunosuppressive therapy. AIDS patients also have elevated risk for non-Hodgkin's lymphoma.

Excessive tissue turnover may contribute to mutation — the risk of genetic accidents seems to increase with the number of cell divisions. Squamous cell carcinoma of the bladder occurs in association with Schistosomiasis or prolonged use of indwelling catheters; chronic turnover of the bladder epithelium and inflammation may favor tumor development. Patients with cirrhosis are at increased risk for liver cancer, with chronic hepatocyte turnover being a possible factor. Adult T cell leukemia is strongly associated with a retrovirus (T cell lymphadenotropic virus-I; HTLV-I; see Table 32-3), although fewer than 1% of infected individuals develop the disease. HTLV-I appears to induce tumors indirectly, perhaps by altering the control of lymphocyte growth, inducing lymphoid hypertrophy, and increasing the population of cells susceptible to mutations.

Chronic stimulation of the immune system drives lymphocytes through the risky process of gene-segment rearrangement. Normal genetic rearrangement occurs between segments of antigen receptor genes. Errors by this recombinase can cause aberrant rearrangements such as translocations. In Burkitt's lymphoma this mechanism occasionally joins the control elements of immunoglobulin genes and the c-*MYC* gene. Burkitt's lymphoma in Africa is also notable for its association with Epstein-Barr virus (EBV) and its geographic overlap with endemic malaria. Although the precise pathogenesis of African Burkitt's lymphoma is unclear, perhaps chronic immune stimulation by malaria cooperates in some way with EBV to induce this lymphoma (see Table 32-3).

Mechanisms that maintain DNA integrity are important in cancer risk. Inherited deficiencies in DNA repair* can predispose to tumor formation. For example, a predisposition for chromosomal breakage appears to underlie lymphoid malignancies in Bloom's syndrome, ataxia telangiectasia, and Fanconi's anemia. The biochemical defect in Bloom's syndrome involves DNA ligase. A cellular system appears to monitor the genome for damage prior to mitosis. In the absence of *p53* function, cells proceed through the cell cycle in the face of unrepaired DNA damage, which may place cells at increased risk for new mutations. Another defect underlies a common form of inherited cancer, hereditary nonpolyposis colon cancer (HNPCC). A deficiency in DNA mismatch repair influences the stability of microsatellites*, causing changes in the length of these nucleotide repeats. Inherited and somatic mutations occur in several genes involved in mismatch repair in a subset of colon carcinomas.

The inherent capability of the host to metabolize chemicals can influence their carcinogenic potential in complex ways. Enzymatic activation and clearance play important roles in the biologic effects of chemical carcinogens. Experiments have shown that carcinogen metabolism can vary with animal species, age, sex, hormonal status, nutrition, and other environmental factors.

Agents of DNA Damage

One typically defines chemicals as carcinogens by an ability to induce tumors in animal testing. Active forms of many carcinogens are reactive electrophilic species that attack nucleophilic sites, such as nitrogen, oxygen, or sulfur atoms in cellular macromolecules. Metabolic conversions play important roles in both activation and elimination of carcinogens. These conversions involve cytochrome P450-dependent mono-oxygenases, peroxidases, and conjugation enzymes. Cellular responses to injury induced by carcinogens can either repair or compound DNA damage. We may identify chemicals that induce mutations by the Ames' test, named after its developer; this procedure classifies mutagens by detecting the reversion of defined mutations in bacteria. The mutagenic activity of some compounds is proportional to their cancer-inducing activity, which supports the idea that the critical target of many carcinogens is DNA.

Radiation of different energies causes DNA damage by one of two general mechanisms (Fig. 32-9). (a) Ionizing radiation consists of energetic particles or photons (> 10 eV) that affect biologic targets in a stepwise fashion. Interaction with water molecules forms a series of water radicals. Subsequently, these reactive species attack macro-molecules in the cell. (b) Ultraviolet radiation (UV, photons in the 2–10 eV range) is not energetic enough to be ionizing, but it is absorbed by certain molecules to produce an excited state. Pyrimidine bases in DNA absorb UV and become chemically reactive. They can react with water to produce an altered base, with neighboring pyrimidines to form dimers or with proteins to form covalent cross-links. A sensitivity to UV and skin tumors results from an inherited defect in the excision of pyrimidine dimers (xeroderma pigmentosum).

a.) Ionizing radiation

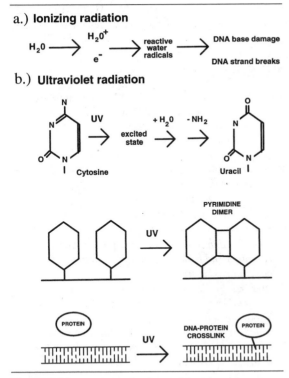

b.) Ultraviolet radiation

Fig. 32-9. Mutagenic mechanisms of the two major classes of radiation. (a) Ionizing radiation affects biologic targets largely by producing water radicals. (b) Ultraviolet radiation produces an excited state by direct interaction with target molecules, such as pyrimidine bases in DNA. Subsequent reaction with water can result in DNA base changes (top). Other reactions can produce covalent cross-linkages with adjacent bases on the DNA (middle) or with proteins (bottom).

Clinical Examples

1. A 55-year-old woman is diagnosed with chronic myelogenous leukemia (CML) in chronic phase. Cytogenetic analysis of a bone marrow aspirate shows t(9;22). She enrolls in a research protocol and receives alpha-interferon. The disease goes into apparent complete remission. Cytogenetic analysis of her marrow is normal, but a PCR-based method detects persistence of *BCR-ABL* fusion transcripts. After two years, she presents acutely ill with a high white count consisting of blasts with lymphoid markers. Cytogenetic analysis again shows t(9;22) and new chromosomal abnormalities.

Discussion. The Philadelphia chromosome (one product of the translocation) is a clonal marker for neoplastic cells in CML. It bears a gene fusion that joins *BCR* (named for the *b*reakpoint *c*luster *r*egion) and *ABL*, which encodes a tyrosine kinase. This cytogenetic abnormality occurs in hematopoietic cells but not other cell types, such as fibroblasts; its presence in only a subset of tissues indicates that t(9;22) arises as a somatic mutation. It is a marker of the malignant clone during various stages of the disease: during the chronic phase it is seen within differentiated myeloid cells, during the acute phase it is seen in undifferentiated cells (blast cells with either myeloid or lymphoid phenotypes), and during remission it can sometimes be detected in otherwise normal-appearing marrow. The translocation appears in cells of myeloid or lymphoid lineages in CML — this finding suggests that this mutation originates in a pluripotent stem cell as an early step during oncogenesis. The PCR method for detecting *BCR-ABL* is much more sensitive than cytogenetics; however, its prognostic value during clinical remission needs to be established in prospective studies.

The presence of the Philadelphia chromosome in this patient's blast cells is consistent with progressive CML (i.e., blast crisis). Extra copies of the Philadelphia chromosome are common in blast crisis, suggesting a gene dosage effect for the *BCR-ABL* oncogene. Increasing aneuploidy and chromosomal rearrangements provide evidence that subclones have acquired additional mutations.

2. A 4-year-old girl presents with visual difficulties and is diagnosed with retinoblastoma involving both eyes. Her father had retinoblastoma as a child and was diagnosed with osteosarcoma recently. The patient is treated by enucleation of the more severely affected eye, and radiation to the other eye. Genetic analysis of the family is performed, and a younger brother is determined to carry markers linked to the *RB-1* allele shared by his father and sister. He is followed very closely with ophthalmologic examinations over the next several years. Small tumors arise in both eyes, and these are treated by laser.

Discussion. Hereditary cancer syndromes typically predispose an individual to multiple tumors. Different syndromes vary in the predilection for few or many tissues. When multiple tissues are at risk in a given syndrome, the spectrum of tumor types is termed a cancer cluster. Hereditary retinoblastoma shows a narrow tissue tropism, with tumors restricted mainly to the retina; osteosarcomas do occur, but they are much less frequent and arise later in life. Hereditary syndromes that involve bilateral organs typically place both sides at risk, as is true for retinoblastoma.

The available therapy can cure retinoblastoma. Susceptible individuals require followup for only a few years, until the child outgrows the period of risk for the ocular tumor. Frequent eye exams detect second tumors early enough to allow treatment that preserves vision and avoids iatrogenic complications (e.g., radiation-induced malignancies). Genetic counseling should be an integral part of therapy. In the hereditary form of retinoblastoma, one should evaluate all siblings of a patient. A genetic study of the family may predict individuals at risk for the disease. Management of this syndrome owes its success to the availability of highly effective screening and therapy.

There is currently no explanation for the predilection of retinal cells (and, to a lesser extent, bone cells) to this form of cancer. Many tissues normally express the Rb protein, and acquired mutations affect it in sporadic tumors of other organs, such as small cell carcinoma of the lung. Numerous other cancer genes display unexplained tissue tropisms.

Note an apparent paradox in the use of the terms "recessive" and "dominant." The person inherits a predisposition for retinoblastoma in an autosomal pattern that is dominant. At the level of the cell, however, the mutant gene behaves in a manner that is recessive — only when genetic lesions inactivate both *RB-1* alleles does the cell become cancerous.

Bibliography

Brock DJH. Molecular Genetics of Cancer. In *Molecular Genetics for the Clinician.* Cambridge, England: Cambridge University Press, 1993, pp. 136–167. *This 22-page chapter provides a clear overview of inherited cancers, oncogenes, and tumor suppressors.*

Cell 64 (2):235–350, 1991. *A large portion of the January 25 issue of this journal was devoted to reviews on basic aspects of the molecular biology of oncogenesis.*

Tannock IF and Hill RP (eds.). *The Basic Science of Oncology* (2nd ed.). New York: McGraw-Hill, 1992. *A 420-page text that provides an extensive introduction to the causation and biology of cancer, including the biologic basis for cancer treatments.*

Varmus HE and Weinberg RA. *Genes and the Biology of Cancer.* New York: Scientific American Library, 1993. *Two prominent researchers wrote this beautifully illustrated monograph for a nontechnical audience. The 215-page book covers the molecular biology of cancer from its conceptual and historical roots.*

33 Cancer: Biology and Clinical Course

Vikki A. Canfield

Objectives

After completing this chapter, you should be able to

Identify genetic and environmental risk factors for the development of several common cancers

Define and describe the importance of staging of cancer

Describe the pattern of spread and appropriate staging tests for common cancers

Describe the roles of the following treatment modalities in the treatment of cancer: surgery, irradiation, and chemotherapy

Describe factors influencing the ability to cure disseminated cancers with chemotherapy

Pathobiology

Cancer develops because genetic changes of normal cells allow them to escape from normal growth and differentiation patterns. As discussed in Chap. 32, these changes are often multiple and sequential. They can be inherited or acquired because of environmental factors which induce genetic changes. Since cancer arises as a malignant transformation in any tissue, cancer refers to a spectrum of diseases with great variability in presentation and natural history. The common feature among all cancers is the abnormal growth pattern which allows invasion into adjacent normal tissues and spread to distant organs. Progressive uncontrolled growth of the cancer will lead to death in most patients.

Genetic changes involved in the etiology of cancer affect DNA structure and repair mechanisms. Therefore, actively dividing cells are more susceptible to environmental carcinogens than are nondividing cells. Some cancers may arise in tissues where there is chronic irritation or inflammation because these provide a stimulus to growth and cell division. Other cancers arise in tissues where there is continuous environmental exposure to potential carcinogens, such as the lung and gastrointestinal tract.

Understanding how tumors grow is of practical benefit for understanding the clinical approach to cancer treatment. A model of tumor growth is demonstrated in Fig. 33-1. In this model, tumor growth is initially exponential but, as tumor size increases, the time increases between each tumor volume doubling, even without change in the time between mitoses of individual cells. This diminished tumor growth, defined by the increased interval between volume doubling, is related to a variety of factors. Tumors may outgrow their blood supply and tumor cells may compete for limited nutrients, leading to an increase in cell death. In addition, restricted nutrient supply may limit the percent of the total tumor cell population which is participating in tumor growth. This model allows a hypothesis that small tumors may be more susceptible to chemotherapy or irradiation because a larger percentage of cells may be dividing. Also, a derivative of this hypothesis is that when a larger, slower growing tumor is treated, the remaining surviving tumor cells may resume a more rapid growth phase. These phenomena have been clinically observed

339

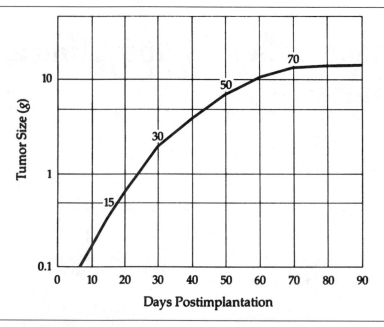

Fig. 33-1. Gompertzian model of tumor growth. Tumor growth is initially exponential but then levels off with time. (Reprinted with permission from: Frei E. Pathobiology of cancer. *Scientific American Medicine,* Dale DC, Federman DD, eds. Section 12, Subsection III. © 1995. Scientific American, Inc. All rights reserved.)

and have been effectively incorporated into cancer management strategies.

Although a cancer is typically considered monoclonal, arising from a series of transformation events within a single cell, there is typically heterogeneity of cells within a tumor. Some of this heterogeneity is caused by further genetic changes within the malignant cells. Tumor cells are thought to be genetically unstable with an increased mutation rate. Subclones of the original tumor may have a faster growth rate or increased ability to metastasize or invade. Clinically, cancers often appear to evolve to a more aggressive phenotype, which may be the basis for the evolution of drug resistance and the failure of most tumors to be eradicated by chemotherapy.

As tumor cells lose the normal control mechanisms which restrict their growth and development within a normal tissue, they can become locally invasive and can also spread to distant organs. Some of the biologic features of tumor cells which allow this uncontrolled growth are the presence of receptors on the tumor cell surface for basement membrane and stromal cell glycoproteins allowing their attachment and invasion. Some tumor cells also pro-

duce a collagenase enzyme which can hydrolyze connective tissue and facilitate invasion. Tumors can also produce angiogenic factors which stimulate new capillary growth to provide additional required blood supply. Once tumor cells have entered regional lymph nodes, the interconnection of lymphatic and capillary systems implies that distant tumor dissemination has occurred. However, only a small fraction of tumor cells released into the blood will produce a distant metastatic lesion; most tumor cells are recognized as foreign cells by immune surveillance mechanisms and are destroyed or their growth inhibited.

The organ distribution of metastatic disease is not random or determined simply by anatomic features such as blood supply. There are specific relationships between tumor cells and target organ susceptible to the development of metastatic lesions. These susceptibilities are referred to as "metastatic tropisms." Examples are that breast cancer commonly metastasizes to bone, lung cancers commonly metastasize to the adrenal glands and brain, mesenchymal tumors such as sarcomas commonly metastasize to the lung, and colon cancer commonly metastasizes to the liver.

Clinical Features, Prevention, and Screening

Because cancer describes a very heterogeneous group of disorders, the clinical features are as widely diverse as the tissues and organs involved. However, some symptoms are common to any tumor exhibiting rapid growth, and result simply from the accelerated tumor metabolism. These include the systemic symptoms of fatigue, weight loss, loss of appetite, and fever. Local symptoms are simply related to local anatomic functions, such as altered bowel habits in colorectal cancer and cough or dyspnea in lung cancer. Beyond these systemic and local symptoms, there are syndromes described as "paraneoplastic" because they do not appear to be directly related to local factors or hypermetabolism (Table 33-1). Many of these are related to ectopic hormone production by the tumor; some are related to immune phenomena such as tumor antigen complexes with antitumor antibodies.

Because cancers are often difficult to treat and more difficult to cure, there is emphasis on understanding risk factors which predispose to the development of cancer to allow preventive measures and further to allow screening tests which can provide early detection. Examples of some risk factors are presented in Table 33-2. Some, such as tobacco use, can be avoided. Some, such as hepatitis B, can be prevented with proper immunization. Others (such as those resulting from therapy involving alkylating agents, radiation, and immunosuppression) may be unavoidable.

There are many so-called preneoplastic lesions which put patients at increased risk for the development of cancer. For some cancers, primarily epithelial ones, preneoplastic pathologic changes can occur. These preneoplastic events are usually induced by environmental risk factors and identified pathologically. Examples include breast cancer: atypical hyperplasia; cervical cancer: dysplasia; oral cavity: leukoplakia and erythroplasia; colon: polyps; and skin: actinic keratoses.

Major public health efforts have been mounted for screening tests for early detection of treatable cancers. Some of these are listed in Table 33-3. To be effective, a screening test must be sensitive and specific, must be safe and well tolerated by the patient, and must be relatively inexpensive. Some of these screening procedures have been very effective, such as the pelvic examination and Papani-

Table 33-1. Examples of Paraneoplastic Syndromes

Clinical Syndrome	Mechanism	Tumor Types
ENDOCRINE		
Cushing's syndrome	ACTH secretion by tumor	Lung cancer (all histologic types)
Inappropriate ADH	AVP secretion by tumor	Lung cancer (especially small cell type)
Nonmetastatic hypercalcemia	Parathyroid hormone-related peptide secretion by tumor	Lung cancer (especially squamous cell tumors)
NEUROLOGICAL		
Subacute cerebellar degeneration	Antipurkinje antibodies	Lung, prostate, colon, ovary, cervix, Hodgkin's
Dermatomyositis/polymyositis	Unknown	Lung, stomach, ovary
Myasthenic syndrome (Lambert-Eaton)	Autoimmune	Small cell lung cancer, stomach, ovary
RENAL		
Nephrotic syndrome Membranous glomerulonephritis	Tumor specific antigen/antibody complexes	Many different carcinomas
SKIN		
Acanthosis nigricans	Unknown	Gastric or other abdominal carcinomas
OTHER		
Fever	Unknown	Hodgkin disease, renal carcinoma, osteogenic sarcoma
Hypertrophic pulmonary osteoarthropathy	Unknown	Lung cancer, lung metastases from other cancers

Table 33-2. Common Risk Factors for Cancer

Risk Factor	Cancer Incidence Increased
Increased age	Most carcinomas and hematologic malignancies
Sex	Female: breast, ovary, uterus
	Male: testis, prostate
Tobacco use	Lung, head & neck, esophagus, bladder, pancreas, kidney, uterine cervix
Obesity	Endometrium, breast
Alcohol use	Oral cavity, pharynx, esophagus, larynx, liver
Heredity	A variety of syndromes associated with high incidence of cancer, but only identified as cause in small percentage — i.e., familial polyposis — colon cancer, retinoblastoma, MEN, etc.
Pesticides	Lymphoma, lung
Benzene	Leukemia
Asbestos	Lung, mesothelium
Hepatitis B	Liver
Ionizing radiation	Most sites

Table 33-3. Summary of American Cancer Society's Recommendations for the Early Detection of Cancer in Asymptomatic People

Test or Procedure	Sex	Age	Frequency
Sigmoidoscopy, preferably flexible	M&F	50 and over	Every 3–5 years
Fecal occult blood test	M&F	50 and over	Every year
Digital rectal examination	M&F	40 and over	Every year
Prostate exam*	M	50 and over	Every year
Pap test	F	All women who are or who have been sexually active, or have reached age 18, should have an annual Pap test and pelvic examination. After a woman has had three or more consecutive satisfactory normal annual examinations, the Pap test may be performed less frequently at the discretion of her physician.	
Pelvic examination	F	Over 18	Every 1–3 years with Pap test
		Over 40	Every year
Endometrial tissue sample	F	At menopause if at high risk†	At menopause and thereafter at the discretion of the physician
Breast self-examination	F	20 and over	Every month
Breast clinical examination	F	20–40	Every 3 years
		Over 40	Every year
Mammography‡	F	40–49	Every 1–2 years
		50 and over	Every year
Health counseling and cancer checkup§	M&F	Over 20	Every 3 years
		Over 40	Every year

*Annual digital rectal examination and prostate-specific antigen should be performed on men age 50 and older. If either is abnormal, further evaluation should be considered.

† History of infertility, obesity, failure to ovulate, abnormal uterine bleeding, or unopposed estrogen or tamoxifen therapy.

‡ Screening mammography should begin by age 40.

§ To include examination for cancers of the thyroid, testicles, ovaries, lymph nodes, oral region, and skin.

Reprinted with permission from: Fink DJ. Cancer detection: The cancer-related checkup guidelines. In Holleb AI, Fink DJ, and Murphy GP (eds.). *American Cancer Society Textbook of Clinical Oncology* (1st ed.). Atlanta, Ga.: American Cancer Society, 1991, p. 155.

Table 33-4. Staging of Breast Cancer: An Example of TNM Staging

STAGE GROUPING FOR BREAST CANCER

0	Tis	N0	M0
I	T1	N0	M0
IIA	T0	N1	M0
	T1	N1	M0
	T2	N0	M0
IIB	T3	N0	M0
	T3	N0	M0
IIIA	T0	N2	M0
	T1	N2	M0
	T2	N1	M0
	T3	N1	M0
	T3	N2	M0
IIIB	T4	Any N	M0
	Any T	N3	M0
IV	Any T	Any N	M1

TNM STAGING

Primary Tumor (T)

Tx	Primary tumor cannot be assessed
T0	No evidence of primary tumor
Tis	Carcinoma in situ. Intraductal carcinoma, lobular carcinoma in situ, or Paget's disease of the nipple with no tumor
T1	Tumor 2 cm or less in greatest dimension
T1a	0.5 cm or less in greatest dimension
T1b	More than 0.5 cm but not more than 1 cm in greatest dimension
T1c	More than 1 cm but not more than 2 cm in greatest dimension
T2	Tumor more than 2 cm but not more than 5 cm in greatest dimension
T3	Tumor more than 5 cm in greatest dimension
T4	Tumor of any size with direct extension to chest wall or skin
T4a	Extension to chest wall
T4b	Edema (including peau d'orange) or ulceration of the skin of breast or satellite nodules confined to same breast.
T4c	Both T4a and T4b
T4d	Inflammatory carcinoma

Lymph node (N)

Nx	Regional lymph nodes cannot be assessed
N0	No regional lymph node metastasis
N1	Metastasis to movable ipsilateral axillary lymph node(s)
N2	Metastasis to ipsilateral axillary lymph node(s) fixed to one another or to other structures
N3	Metastases to ipsilateral internal mammary lymph node(s)

Distant metastasis (M)

Mx	Presence of distant metastasis cannot be assessed
M0	No distant metastasis
M1	Distant metastasis (includes metastasis to ipsilateral (supraclavicular lymph nodes)

Reprinted with permission from: Scanlon EF. Breast Cancer. In Holleb AI, Fink DJ, and Murphy GP (eds.). *American Cancer Society Textbook of Clinical Oncology* (1st ed.). Atlanta, Ga.: American Cancer Society, 1991, pp. 183–84.

colaou staining of cervical epithelial cells to detect cancer of the cervix. In women having regular examinations, cervical cancer is essentially eradicated. Mammography for the early detection of breast cancer is also extremely effective but the indications are less well defined.

Diagnosis and Staging

A cancer is typically suspected because of the presence of a mass lesion. The most important principle of diagnosis is that a tissue biopsy is required for pathologic interpretation. This is essential not only because the diagnosis of a cancer is uncertain without pathologic confirmation, but also because the histology of the tumor provides information for therapy and prognosis.

After a pathologic diagnosis has been made, further diagnostic studies are required to define the extent of disease. This is typically referred to as establishing the "stage" of the cancer and provides further important information for therapy and prognosis. An initial key question is often the distinction between localized and metastatic cancer, providing the information on whether surgical resection is appropriate or not. There are many systems developed to describe the extent of cancers originating in different organs. One common system takes into account the size of the primary tumor, the extent of lymph node invasion, and the presence of metastatic disease. This system is applicable for many solid tumors and is commonly referred to as the TNM staging system, which describes initial tumor size (T), regional lymph node involvement (N), and the presence or absence of distant metastases (M). The TNM stages are usually grouped into numbered stages where patients have similar prognosis. An example for breast cancer is included in Table 33-4. Another common staging system is the Ann Arbor Staging System for lymphomas (see Chap. 31).

Tests done for staging are dependent on our knowledge of the natural history and pattern of spread of a particular type of tumor. For example, for breast cancer, staging consists of a physical exam, chest x-ray, routine blood chemistry measurements which may reflect bone involvement (by alkaline phosphatase activity) and abnormal liver function, and an axillary lymph node dissection at the time of breast surgery. Other tests such as bone scans are reserved for those patients who have symptoms or suspicious findings on routine evaluation or those who have locally advanced tumors. Patients with lymphomas are staged with CT scans of the chest, abdomen, and pelvis as well as with bone marrow biopsies. Patients with sarcomas are often staged with CT scans of the chest because of the propensity of these tumors to spread to the lung even when they appear to be locally limited, and because therapy for apparently localized sarcomas can be quite morbid and would not be helpful if metastases are already present.

Principles of Cancer Therapy

A generation ago, surgery was the only potentially curative measure for malignant disease. Localized tumors could be completely resected and thereby cured; incomplete resection because of undetected spread was inevitably followed by recurrent cancer and often death. While surgery remains the major modality for cure among the common cancers (such as breast cancer, lung cancer, and colon cancer), there are notable exceptions and some cancers can be cured by radiation and/or chemotherapy. Examples are testicular tumors in men, which are curable by intensive chemotherapy even after extensive metastasis has occurred, and squamous cell tumors of the head and neck and anus. The sensitivity of cancer to chemotherapeutic agents may be greater at an earlier stage, which may be related to the growth characteristics of tumor cells as described above. Since many cancers have clinically undetectable dissemination at the time of diagnosis, chemotherapy has been used following potentially curative surgery as an additional therapeutic effort to produce a cure. This approach to chemotherapy, following surgery in a patient with no demonstrable residual cancer, is termed "adjuvant therapy." Adjuvant therapy has been shown to increase the cure rate following conventional surgery in both breast and colon cancer, as well as in bone sarcomas.

Typically, however, chemotherapeutic agents are used to treat disseminated cancers. Principles of chemotherapy include the use of drugs which interfere with DNA synthesis or repair, or interfere with the provision of precursors for DNA or RNA synthesis. This implies that chemotherapy is most effective against cells in replicating cycles, but some agents are able to also kill noncycling cells. Because damage to normal tissue is an inevitable toxicity of chemotherapeutic agents, treatment is often given with combinations of drugs which have different mechanisms of action and toxicities. Chemotherapy drugs may also have synergistic anti-tumor effects. Because normal tissues which have the greatest growth faction are the ones most adversely effected, clinical side effects include neutropenia and thrombocytopenia from bone marrow suppression, stomatitis and intestinal toxicity from intestinal epithelial toxicity, sterility, and alopecia.

A variety of clinical and biologic factors influence our ability to cure cancers with chemotherapy. These factors are outlined in Table 33-5.

Table 33-5. Factors Affecting Curability of Human Cancers with Conventional Chemotherapy

Type of Cancer	Morphology	Growth Rate	Growth Function	Influence of Tumor Size	Significance of Resistant Cells
CURABLE Choricarcinoma Wilms' tumor Pre-T cell acute lymphocytic leukemia Burkitt's lymphoma Hodgkin's disease Acute promyelocytic leukemia Diffuse histiocytic lymphoma Testicular cancers	Undifferentiated	Relatively rapid	Relatively	Moderate	Unimportant
RARELY CURABLE T cell acute lymphocytic leukemia Acute myelocytic leukemia Small cell carcinoma of lung Squamous cell carcinoma of upper aerodigestive tract Adenocarcinoma of ovary Osteosarcoma Ewing's sarcoma Embryonal rhabdomyocarsoma	Partially differentiated	Less rapid	Relatively low	Critical	Important
NOT CURABLE Breast cancer Lung carcinomas other than small cell Carcinomas of esophagus, stomach, pancreas, liver, biliary tract, and colon Carcinomas of endometrium and cervix Carcinomas of kidney, bladder, and prostate Carcinoma of thyroid Gliomas Melanoma Carcinoids Chronic myelogenous leukemia Chronic lymphocytic leukemia Multiple myeloma	Partially differentiated	Less rapid	Low	Critical	Very important

Adapted from: Stockdale FE. Cancer Growth and Chemotherapy. In Rubenstein E and Federman DD (eds.). *Scientific American Medicine.* New York: Scientific American, 1993, p. 5.

An important concept of management of the patient with cancer is the supportive care of patients who have incurable disease. Although intensive treatment with chemotherapy, surgery, or radiation may be inappropriate, important supportive care is required and provides immeasurable benefits for patients and their families. In these patients, the physician must weigh the balance between therapeutic effect on the tumor, relief of the patient's symptoms, and the side effects and cost of therapy. These are decisions which often cannot be made by the physician alone, but are made in consultation with the patient and family.

Clinical Examples

1. A 28-year-old African-American female has had multiple sexual partners. She presents for an annual physical examination. A PAP smear is done and is abnormal with severe dysplasia present. Colposcopy is done and biopsies are made of a suspicious area. A diagnosis of microinvasive cervical cancer (4-mm invasion) is made. The patient has normal liver chemistries, CBC, chest x-ray, CT scan of the pelvis, and exam under anesthesia is normal. She undergoes total abdominal hysterectomy with pelvic lymph node dissection. No other tumor is found.

Discussion. The PAP smear is an example of a screening test which relies on our ability to detect pre-neoplastic and neoplastic cytological changes. Patients who have abnormal PAP smears should be further evaluated with colposcopy and biopsies. Patients who have cancer diagnosed at an early stage, like this patient, have a very good chance of being cured with surgery or radiation therapy. Patients with dysplasia can be treated with cervical conization (removal of a cone-shaped portion of tissue from the cervix including the transformation zone) and followed closely so if they do develop carcinoma it will be caught at an early stage.

2. A 52-year-old postmenopausal Native American female notes a lump in her left breast while taking a shower and seeks medical attention. On physical exam she has a 3 × 2 cm mass in the upper outer quadrant of the left breast. A mammogram did not show any suspicious areas, but you refer her to a breast surgeon for evaluation. An excisional biopsy shows invasive intraductal carcinoma. After discussion of therapeutic options, the patient elects to undergo a lumpectomy and axillary dissection followed by radiation therapy. On final pathology the tumor measures 2.3 × 2.6 cm. Margins are negative for tumor, indicating complete resection. A specimen is sent for evaluation for the presence or absence of receptors for estrogen and progesterone. These are both present. Three of 18 axillary nodes contain microscopic foci of tumor. The patient is started on adjuvant therapy with tamoxifen, 20 mg po/day.

Discussion. Patients are often the first ones to find an abnormality like a breast lump. Typically lumps found incidentally by patients are over 1–2 cm, whereas screening mammography may detect tumors as small as 0.5 cm. This patient however, had a nondiagnostic mammogram. Not all cancers produce mammographic changes and patients who have a palpable lump should have a biopsy even if the mammogram is normal.

Patients with small tumors (less than 4–5 cm) can often be treated with a breast conserving approach with limited surgery (lumpectomy) and local radiation therapy. Randomized trials have shown that survival is similar with the two approaches — mastectomy or lumpectomy plus irradiation.

Patients who have axillary lymph nodes involved with breast cancer are at risk for recurrent cancer. The presence of tumor in the nodes suggests that tumor cells have spread via blood and lymphatics even when they cannot be detected. Clinical trials have shown that giving chemotherapy or tamoxifen (an anti-estrogen) to post-menopausal, node-positive, hormone receptor-positive patients can prolong their survival and decrease their chance of recurrence. Current research studies are evaluating whether combinations of chemotherapy and hormonal therapy are better than hormonal therapy by itself.

Bibliography

Bertino JR. Ode to methotrexate, the Karnofsky Memorial Lecture. *J Clin Oncol* 11:5–14, 1993. *A historical perspective on the development of methotrexate and the use of chemotherapy to treat cancer.*

Bishop JM. Molecular themes in oncogenesis. *Cell,* 64: 235–248, 1991. *A review of molecular events involved in carcinogenesis.*

DeVita V, Hellman S, and Rosenberg SA. *Principles and Practice of Oncology.* Philadelphia: Lippincott, 1993. *The most comprehensive textbook for medical oncology.*

Early Breast Cancer Trialists Collaborative Group. Systemic treatment of early breast cancer by hormonal cytotoxic or immune therapy. *Lancet* 339:1–15, 71–85, 1992. *A review and meta-analysis of all adjuvant therapy trials for breast cancer.*

Holleb AI, Fink DJ, and Murphy GP. *American Cancer Society Textbook of Clinical Oncology.* Atlanta: American Cancer Society, 1991. *Concise overviews. Good reviews of epidemiology and staging at all sites.*

Rubenstein E and Federman DD. *Scientific American Medicine.* New York: Scientific American, 1992. *Good discussions of pathobiology of cancer and molecular carcinogenesis.*

Toribara NW and Sleisenger MH. Current Concepts: Screening for colorectal cancer. *N Engl J Med* 332: 861–867, 1995. *An overview of the scientific basis for cancer screening.*

34 Hemostasis and Thrombosis

James N. George

Objectives

After completing this chapter, you should be able to

Distinguish initial primary hemostatic mechanisms and secondary coagulation mechanisms

Understand the steps in platelet production and the unique features of platelet circulation

Understand the structure, tissue distribution, and function of von Willebrand factor

Distinguish von Willebrand factor and coagulation factor VIII

Understand the structure and function of tissue factor and its role in the initiation of coagulation

Understand the normal control mechanisms of blood coagulation, and how abnormalities of regulatory proteins can cause an increased risk for thrombosis

Understand the mechanism and frequency of pseudo-thrombocytopenia

Understand the clinically important mechanisms of an abnormally prolonged partial thromboplastin time that are not associated with an increased bleeding risk

---

This chapter will summarize normal hemostatic mechanisms and their control systems as a basis for understanding the pathophysiology of abnormal bleeding and thrombosis. The pathophysiology of bleeding and thrombotic disease provides an outline for the clinical approach to diagnosis and management of these disorders.

Normal Hemostatic Mechanisms

The hemostatic response to injury can be divided into two reactions: (1) Primary hemostasis involves the immediate responses of platelet adhesion and aggregation and vessel contraction. These reactions can effectively seal a small lesion. (2) Secondary hemostasis involves the activation of plasma coagulation factors resulting in the formation of fibrin. Fibrin reinforcement of the initial platelet aggregate is essential to prevent bleeding from larger lesions.

Primary Hemostasis

The vessel wall and circulating blood platelets are the two components of the initial, primary hemostatic response.

The endothelial cells lining the vessel wall have specific properties that inhibit hemostatic reactions and maintain the fluid state of blood. When the endothelial lining is broken, subendothelial fibers and cells trigger the initiation of hemostatic reactions.

Platelets are produced by bone marrow megakaryocytes. Megakaryocytes arise from a stem cell which can also differentiate into cells of erythroid, granulocyte, or monocyte/macrophage lineages. Differentiation of megakaryocytes results in giant polyploid cells with up to 32 sets of chromosomes and vast cytoplasm which demarcates into zones of nascent platelets. The mechanism of actual platelet production is obscure, but platelets likely fragment from megakaryocytes within the marrow sinusoids. Humoral regulation of megakaryocyte development involves multiple cytokines. The principal factor is thrombopoietin, which is synthesized by liver, endothelium, and other tissues. Platelets circulate as discs of 2–3 microns diameter in a normal concentration of 150,000–350,000 per microliter; their survival is approximately 10 days. About one-third of platelets in normal subjects are pooled within the spleen where they are slowly but continuously exchangeable with the circulating plasma. The splenic pool is exaggerated in most instances of splenomegaly, and therefore this is a common cause of mild thrombocytopenia.

Platelets are continuously involved in microscopic hemostatic reactions, sealing the gaps that normally occur in capillary epithelium. Evidence for their role in maintaining endothelial integrity is the sudden asymptomatic appearance of innumerable petechiae on the feet, ankles, and lower legs when severe thrombocytopenia suddenly develops. This distribution of petechiae in dependent regions parallels intravascular hydrostatic pressure, because the greater pressure makes the small vessels more vulnerable to endothelial breaks. The initial reaction of hemostasis is the adhesion of platelets to subendothelial fibers of collagen and von Willebrand factor. Von Willebrand factor in the subendothelial matrix readily binds to its platelet constitutive receptor, GP Ib, while soluble plasma von Willebrand factor does not. Following adhesion to subendothelium and subsequent aggregation, platelets secrete more adhesive proteins, such as fibrinogen and von Willebrand factor, that reinforce the stability of the platelet aggregate. Aggregation is principally mediated by fibrinogen linkages to the platelet receptor, GP IIb-IIIa. Platelets are also actively involved in accelerating the secondary hemostatic reactions of plasma coagulation.

Secondary Hemostasis

The coagulation sequence resulting in the formation of the fibrin clot is a cascade of sequential enzymatic reactions that are progressively amplified to generate the final key enzyme, thrombin (Fig. 34-1). Coagulation factors are traditionally designated by Roman numerals, and their active enzyme form is designated by the addition of a small letter "a." For example, factor X is the normal zymogen, or proenzyme, form present in plasma, while the active enzyme form, produced by a proteolytic cleavage of factor X, is known as factor Xa. Coagulation has been described as a cascade or waterfall of sequential enzymatic, proteolytic reactions, culminating in the generation of thrombin from prothrombin. However, many crossover and feedback reactions amplify this system, as suggested by Fig. 34-1. Traditionally, coagulation reactions have been divided into two pathways: one termed *intrinsic* because the major reactants are contained within the plasma; the other termed *extrinsic* because its initiation requires tissue factor, a membrane surface protein of perivascular fibroblasts which bind factor VII. This distinction helps to define the laboratory assessment of hemostasis because the two basic clinical assays, the **partial thromboplastin time** (PTT) and the **prothrombin time** (PT), measure the components

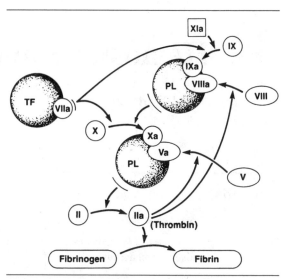

Fig. 34-1. Plasma coagulation reactions in normal hemostasis. Three distinct reactions occur on lipoprotein surfaces that are shown as large spheres: (1) the association of factor VII with tissue factor (TF) on subendothelial fibroblasts; (2) the activation of prothrombin (factor II), and (3) the activation of factor X on the platelet (PL) surface. The vitamin K-dependent factors are all similar in structure and are indicated by the small circles. Factors V and VIII, large molecules that are similar to each other in structure and function, are indicated by the ellipses. In this figure, factor XII, prekallikrein, and high-molecular-weight kininogen are omitted because they are not required for normal in vivo hemostasis. (Used with permission from: George JN and Kolodziej MA. Hemostasis and Fibrinolysis. In Stein JH et al. (eds.). *Internal Medicine* (4th ed.). St. Louis: Mosby-Year Book, 1994, p. 694.)

of the intrinsic and extrinsic systems respectively. A normal partial thromboplastin time also requires the presence of three proteins that are not necessary for in vivo coagulation: factor XII, prekallikrein, and high-molecular-weight kininogen. For this reason, the coagulation scheme shown in Fig. 34-1, the sequence of in vivo coagulation, differs from the in vitro coagulation reactions shown in Fig. 34-4.

The sequence of events initiating coagulation in vivo begins with the exposure of blood to tissue factor and its immediate saturation by factor VII. Tissue factor is constitutively present on the surface of subendothelial fibroblasts, forming a hemostatic "envelope" surrounding blood vessels. Factor VII bound to tissue factor is exquisitely sensitive to activation by the trace amounts of activated coagulation factors (which are proteolytic enzymes) present in normal plasma, factors Xa and VIIa. Once factor VII bound to tissue factor is activated to factor VIIa, it can further activate factors X and IX, and thus the coagulation cascade explodes suddenly and swiftly. Another important amplification feedback loop is the ability of thrombin to convert factors V and VIII to much more active cofactors by limited proteolysis. Both the intrinsic and extrinsic pathways of factor X activation are required for normal hemostasis, as demonstrated by severe bleeding abnormalities with deficiencies of either factors VIII or IX or factor VII.

Control Mechanisms of Blood Coagulation

An enzymatic system that is as potentially explosive as blood coagulation obviously must be regulated by multiple tight controls. These control mechanisms are outlined in Table 34-1 and Fig. 34-2. Deficiencies in these control mechanisms are associated with an increased risk for thrombosis.

Blood Flow

Swiftly flowing blood is the most effective means of dispersing activated coagulation factors not incorporated in

Table 34-1. Control Mechanisms of Blood Coagulation

Dispersal of activated coagulation factors by flowing blood
Inactivation of activated coagulation factors
    Antithrombin III: in combination with endothelial cell surface proteoglycan (heparan sulfate), inhibits thrombin and factors Sz, IXa, VIIa, and XIa
    Protein C and its cofactor, Protein S: proteolytic cleavage of factors VIIIa and Va
Digestion of the fibrin clot by plasmin

Fig. 34-2. Natural coagulation inhibitors: antithrombin III and protein C. The solid arrows represent the procoagulant reactions; the broken arrows represent the inhibitory reactions. Antithrombin III inhibits the active serine protease enzymes, factors XIa, IXa, Xa, VIIa, and IIa (thrombin). The inhibitory activity of antithrombin III is greatly enhanced by heparinlike molecules on the endothelial cell surface. Protein C is activated to a proteolytic enzyme, protein Ca, by thrombin with an endothelial cell membrane protein, thrombomodulin (TM), serving as a cofactor. Protein Ca then specifically inactivates factors Va and VIIIa with protein S as a required cofactor. (Used with permission from: George JN and Kolodziej MA. Hemostasis and Fibrinolysis. In Stein JH et al. (eds.). *Internal Medicine* (4th ed.). St. Louis: Mosby-Year Book, 1994, p. 695.)

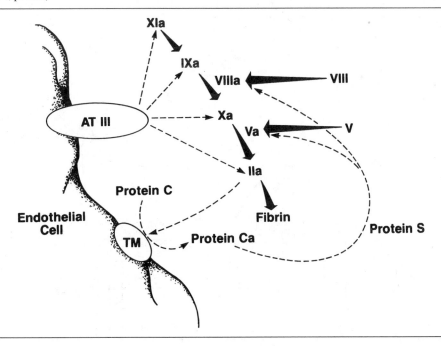

the platelet aggregate and evolving clot. The protective effect of normal blood flow is clearly demonstrated by the importance of stasis as the greatest risk factor for thrombosis.

Antithrombin III

Antithrombin III binds irreversibly to the serine protease coagulation enzymes: factors XIa, IXa, Xa, VIIa, and thrombin. Antithrombin III alone is relatively ineffective, but its activity is dramatically accelerated by heparan-sulfate proteoglycans on the surface of vascular endothelium. This acceleration is the basis for the therapeutic effect of heparin.

Protein C

Protein C is a vitamin K-dependent plasma protein (like factors II, VII, IX, and that is cleaved by thrombin to form

a serine catalytic-site protease, designated protein Ca (or APC, for activated protein C). When thrombin is bound to the constitutive endothelial cell surface protein thrombomodulin, its substrate specificity changes from fibrinogen to protein C. Therefore this key coagulation control mechanism is initiated by the switch of thrombin from its central role as the ultimate procoagulant enzyme to an anticoagulant enzyme. Activated protein C proteolytically degrades factors Va and VIIIa, inhibiting their function. This activity of protein Ca requires the cofactor function of another vitamin K-dependent plasma protein, protein S.

Fibrinolysis

Fibrinolysis describes the process of digestion of the fibrin clot by the enzyme plasmin (Fig. 34-3). This process helps

Fig. 34-3. Mechanism and control of fibrinolysis. Once the fibrin clot is formed, it becomes the active cofactor for its own dissolution by providing the specific surface on which fibrinolytic reactions occur. Tissue plasminogen activator (tPA) is secreted from endothelial cells and circulates in an inactive complex with another endothelial cell-secreted protein, plasminogen activator inhibitor-1 (PAI-1). tPA binds to fibrin where it becomes a binding site for plasminogen (Pg) from plasma. Thus plasminogen is converted to the active fibrinolytic enzyme plasmin (P) directly on the fibrin surface. Plasmin digests fibrin into multiple soluble fragments, termed fibrin degradation products. Any plasmin escaping into the plasma is immediately neutralized by alpha$_2$-plasmin inhibitor (PI). Alpha$_2$-plasmin inhibitor itself is covalently linked to fibrin by factor XIIIa. Thus the complete sequence of plasmin production and control is organized within the developing fibrin clot. The solid arrows indicate the profibrinolytic reactions. The broken arrows indicate the reactions inhibiting fibrinolysis. (Used with permission from: George JN and Kolodziej MA. Hemostasis and Fibrinolysis. In Stein JH et al. (eds.). *Internal Medicine* (4th ed.). St. Louis: Mosby-Year Book, 1994, p. 698.)

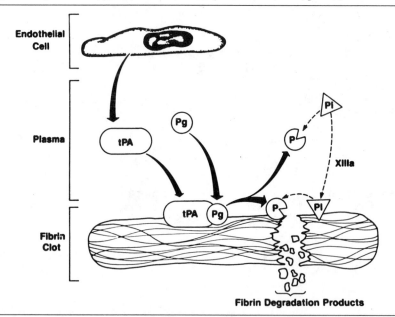

to restrict the clot to the site of hemostasis and to clear away the fibrin as the process of vessel restructuring and wound healing begins. Plasmin is formed from a circulating plasma protein, plasminogen, by an enzyme released from endothelial cells, tissue plasminogen activator (tPA). There are other enzymes capable of activating plasminogen: urokinase, which is present in most tissues, and streptokinase, a therapeutic material derived from streptococcal bacteria. tPA appears to be the physiologic intravascular activator of plasminogen. As in coagulation, surface binding of the reactants serves to localize fibrinolysis to the specific site where plasmin is required. In this case, fibrin itself serves to bind and accelerate the activity of tPA, restricting plasmin formation to the fibrin clot.

Also similar to coagulation, there are significant control mechanisms for the fibrinolytic reactions. These include the restriction of tPA activity to the fibrin surface and the presence of plasma inhibitors of tPA and plasmin. Plasminogen activator inhibitor-1 (PAI-1) is synthesized and secreted by endothelial cells and its concentration in plasma is greater than the concentration of tPA. Therefore all tPA normally circulates in an inactive complex with PAI-1. Any plasmin that escapes the fibrin clot into plasma is immediately neutralized by $alpha_2$-plasmin inhibitor. Plasmin bound to fibrin is 100-fold less sensitive to $alpha_2$-plasmin inhibitor than when it is free in plasma.

Clinical Approach to Patients with Bleeding Disorders

The history and physical examination should allow a distinction to be made between disorders of platelets and small blood vessels (primary hemostasis) characterized by mucocutaneous bleeding, petechiae, and superficial purpura from disorders of coagulation (secondary hemostasis) characterized by delayed recurrent oozing and hematoma formation. From the history and physical examination, a preliminary diagnosis can be made based on the type of bleeding, the duration of the abnormality and the family history (indicating a congenital or acquired disorder), and the expected frequency of certain diseases. Laboratory studies should only be initiated after a thorough clinical evaluation has been performed and a preliminary diagnosis established.

Defective Primary Hemostasis

Clinical Evaluation

Petechiae, tiny dot hemorrhages, represent the leakage of red blood cells from small vessel lesions and are the characteristic lesions of defective primary hemostasis. "Purpura" may refer to the appearance of many petechiae, and also refers to larger superficial hemorrhages. "Purpura" is distinct from the term "hematoma," which implies a substantial mass of extravasated blood and is characteristic of defective coagulation (secondary hemostasis). The bleeding symptoms in disorders of primary hemostasis are typically purpura (often described as easy bruising), epistaxis, gingival bleeding, and menorrhagia.

The most common cause of purpura is the vascular fragility caused by atrophy of subcutaneous supporting tissue, termed senile purpura. This is not a disease associated with other bleeding problems, but an inevitable accompaniment of old age and chronic illness. The appearance of large, superficial, nonpalpable purple blotches on the back of the hands and forearms is predictable with thin, shiny, inelastic skin and the vulnerability of these areas to minor trauma.

Thrombocytopenia is a common cause of bleeding, and mild thrombocytopenia that is not associated with increased bleeding is even more common. Bleeding can occur even without trauma in the more vascular organs. Hemarthroses and large slowly-forming hematomas in less vascular regions such as the retroperitoneum, which are so characteristic of coagulation disorders, do not occur. Inflammatory vasculitis can also cause petechiae, but in contrast to thrombocytopenic petechiae these are often palpable, may occur in clusters that are not distributed in dependent regions, and may be associated with prodromal (burning or stinging) symptoms.

Laboratory Evaluation

The most important test is the platelet count. It is typically performed with an automatic cell counter, and the routine use of these counters has greatly increased the recognition of asymptomatic and unexpected thrombocytopenia. Automated cell counters have a risk for reporting falsely low platelet counts when platelets clump in the blood sample, and this can be caused by IgG platelet agglutinins in normal subjects or in patients with any disease. Also cell counters may not detect very large platelets in patients with hereditary giant platelet syndromes. Therefore it is absolutely essential to confirm an abnormal platelet count by examination of the peripheral blood smear.

A diagnostic test of platelet function is the bleeding time. With a reproducible skin incision on the forearm, 1 mm deep and several mm long, the primary hemostatic mechanisms involving platelets and small vessels can stop bleeding independent of coagulant reactions. Patients with a coagulation defect, such as hemophilia or following anticoagulation with heparin or warfarin, typically have normal bleeding times. A platelet count of over 75,000/ul is sufficient to allow a normal bleeding time. However, the bleeding time only has value as a diagnostic aid and cannot predict the risk of hemorrhage. The inability of the bleeding time to predict the risk for excessive bleeding is often not appreciated in clinical practice, leading to overuse and misinterpretation — such as in presurgical evaluations. The measurement of platelet aggregation in response to agents such as ADP, epinephrine, collagen, and thrombin is of limited clinical value. Like the bleeding time, these tests cannot predict the risk of bleeding. The ubiquitous use of aspirin, which causes an irreversible inhibition of platelet aggregation in response to low concentrations of these agonists, frequently makes interpretation impossible.

Common Disorders

Congenital Disorders. The most common congenital disorder of primary hemostasis is von Willebrand disease. The incidence of von Willebrand disease is difficult to define because of the inconsistency of the laboratory diagnostic tests in these patients, but it may be as frequent as 1 in 100–1000 normal subjects. In typical heterozygous (type I) von Willebrand disease, the platelet count is normal but the bleeding time is long due to a deficiency of normal von Willebrand factor required for platelet adhesion to the damaged vessel wall. Plasma von Willebrand factor can be measured by both immunologic and functional assays. Soluble plasma von Willebrand factor, in contrast to von Willebrand factor in the subendothelial matrix, does not interact with platelets unless its structure is altered by a cationic reagent. The reagent used in routine evaluation of von Willebrand factor function is the antibiotic ristocetin: ristocetin causes platelets to agglutinate in the presence of von Willebrand factor. All factor VIII in plasma is bound to von Willebrand factor and therefore factor VIII activity may also be decreased in von Willebrand disease.

Acquired Disorders. The initial evaluation is essentially limited to an estimate of platelet number. A platelet count of less than 150,000/ul is abnormal, but bleeding does not occur from thrombocytopenia alone unless the platelet count is less than 50,000–75,000/ul. Spontaneous bleeding with many petechiae does not occur unless the platelet count is less than 10,000/ul. If thrombocytopenia is confirmed by examination of the peripheral blood smear, the next diagnostic study is a bone marrow aspiration to determine the presence or absence of megakaryocytes. A deficiency of megakaryocytes indicates that marrow failure is the cause of the thrombocytopenia. Thrombocytopenia due to marrow failure is often associated with other evidence of marrow disease affecting granulocytes and red cells. Common causes are chemotherapy for malignant or immune disease, or involvement of the marrow with a neoplastic disease, such as leukemia. Viral infections, particularly with HIV, can cause thrombocytopenia due to marrow suppression. Marrow megakaryocytes are typically present in normal numbers in patients with HIV infection, in spite of evidence for poor platelet production.

The presence of megakaryocytes is usually interpreted as evidence that platelet production is adequate and that the thrombocytopenia is caused by excessive peripheral platelet destruction, or by pooling of platelets in a large spleen. The most frequent cause of thrombocytopenia due to increased platelet destruction is immune thrombocytopenic purpura (ITP), which is an acute and self-limited disease of young children and a less common chronic disease of adults. A very common cause of mild thrombocytopenia is hepatic cirrhosis with portal hypertension and congestive splenomegaly. In these patients mild thrombocytopenia (platelet counts of 50,000–150,000/ul) is the rule. Platelet production and survival, and even the total-body number of platelets, are typically normal; the abnormality is simply the increased fraction of the platelets pooled within the spleen.

Defective Secondary Hemostasis

Clinical Evaluation

The nature of excessive bleeding in patients with coagulation disorders is distinct from the bleeding that occurs with platelet-blood vessel abnormalities. A few large, deep tissue hematomas occur rather than innumerable tiny petechial hemorrhages. Small vessel breaks that may cause petechiae are easily sealed by platelets alone, as demonstrated by the normal diagnostic bleeding time in most patients with coagulation defects. When a larger vessel lesion occurs, platelets can only temporarily arrest bleeding. In the absence of a firm fibrin network, the initial platelet plug eventually breaks down and more blood oozes out. For example, in hemophilia it is characteristic for no excessive hemorrhage to occur initially after trauma, and many patients consider the second or third day to be the time of greatest risk. The bleeding may then recur intermittently for many days. Certain bleeding problems are common to both disorders of primary and secondary hemostasis (nosebleeds, menorrhagia, gastrointestinal bleeding, hematuria) but it is important to recognize the distinct and characteristic features of each defect: petechiae and superficial purpura in platelet-small blood vessel abnormalities, and the delayed formation of large, deep hematomas and hemarthroses in coagulation disorders.

Laboratory Evaluation

The laboratory evaluation is based on assays that activate the coagulation sequence at different sites (Fig. 34-4). The reagents used for the partial thromboplastin time initiate the reactions by activation of factor XII. A normal partial thromboplastin time requires three factors that are unnecessary for hemostasis in vivo: factor XII, prekallikrein, and high-molecular-weight kininogen (note the difference between Figs. 34-4 and 34-1). Moreover, platelets are not required in these coagulation assays because exogenous phospholipid is supplied. Coagulation is initiated in the prothrombin time by a reagent termed thromboplastin which contains both tissue factor and phospholipid.

It is important to understand that the partial thromboplastin time and the prothrombin time may have different inherent sensitivities to the same defects in their common pathways. For example, the partial thromboplastin time is more sensitive to heparin, even though heparin's greatest

Fig. 34-4. Plasma coagulation reactions in in vitro laboratory assays. This diagram outlines the coagulation factors required for each of four basic laboratory tests. Note the difference between this diagram and Fig. 34-1. Factor XII, prekallikrein, and high-molecular-weight kininogen are required for a normal partial thromboplastin time but not for normal in vivo hemostasis. Platelets and tissue factor are required for normal in vivo hemostasis but are supplied by exogenous reagents in the laboratory assays. (Used with permission from: George JN and Kolodziej MA. Evaluation of Hemostasis and Thrombosis. In Stein JH et al. (eds.). *Internal Medicine* (4th ed.). St. Louis: Mosby-Year Book, 1994, p. 746.)

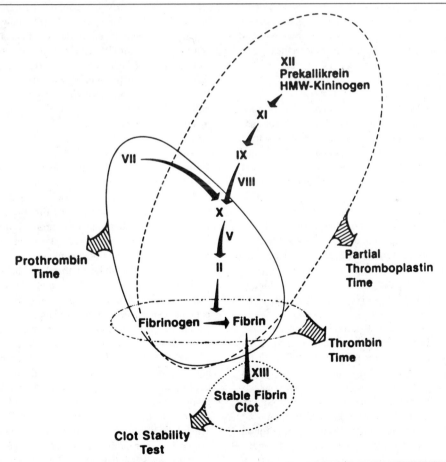

inhibitory effects are on thrombin and factor Xa, and the acquired coagulation inhibitor known as the lupus anticoagulant, which inhibits the reaction of factors X, V, and prothrombin. In contrast, the prothrombin time is often more sensitive to the coagulation abnormalities in patients with liver disease, even though all procoagulant proteins are synthesized in the liver. Both the partial thromboplastin time and the prothrombin time have been valuable contributors to the evaluation of hemostasis for many years because their degree of sensitivity is clinically relevant: In most patients they become abnormal at levels of coagulation factor deficiencies that are associated with an increased risk for clinically important bleeding (about 20–30% of normal).

The partial thromboplastin time and the prothrombin time measure the time required to form a fibrin clot. The subsequent conversion of this fibrin polymer into a permanent covalently bonded structure is essential to form a firm clot in vivo but is not measured in the routine coagulation assays. This final coagulation reaction is assessed by clot stability, which evaluates the function of factor XIII, a transglutamase enzyme that catalyzes the formation of covalent bonds between the fibrin monomer molecules.

Common Disorders

Congenital Disorders. It is most common for congenital disorders to involve only a single coagulation factor, while acquired disorders involve multiple factors. Congenital disorders, such as hemophilia, should be apparent from a lifelong history of bleeding problems and similar problems in other family members, but sometimes these diseases can be very mild and the history can be misleading. The absence of apparent spontaneous bleeding, or of excessive bleeding with minor trauma, does not rule out mild hemophilia and does not mean that serious bleeding may not occur with a surgical procedure. Of all possible congenital coagulation disorders, hemophilia A (factor VIII deficiency) is by far the most common; hemophilia B (factor IX deficiency) is one-tenth as common. Other disorders are much more rare.

The basic assays, the partial thromboplastin time and the prothrombin time, are sufficient to initiate the evaluation, though specific assays for factor VIII and factor IX activity are commonly performed simultaneously when the history is suggestive of hemophilia. Because coagulation inhibitors (antibodies formed against transfused factors VIII or IX in patients with hemophilia A or B) seriously affect transfusion therapy, a screening test for an inhibitor should be performed in each patient with the diagnosis of a coagulation factor deficiency.

The management of the hemophilias, both factor VIII and IX deficiencies, has been revolutionized in the past 20 years by the availability of therapeutic concentrates of the specific coagulation factors that are stable in home freezers. This has allowed patients to infuse themselves intravenously at the first symptom of bleeding and has virtually emancipated patients with severe hemophilia from the hospital and clinic. Often the initial symptoms of bleeding are subtle and subjective, distinguishable from the chronic painful symptoms of hemophilic arthritis caused by repeated hemarthroses only by long experience, and the patient can judge the indication for factor VIII or IX infusion with much better accuracy than can a physician. Early treatment has prevented many hospitalizations and much of the time lost from school and work. The availability of the coagulation factor concentrates has also made possible the consideration of surgery based solely on its medical indications, because hemostasis can be controlled with complete confidence. The infectious risks of the concentrates are great, since they are commercially produced from pools of plasma from up to 25,000 individual donors. Therefore essentially all frequently treated hemophilias were infected with HIV and hepatitis C before screening and sterilization techniques were available. Coagulation factor production by monoclonal antibody affinity isolation and recombinant DNA technology is now feasible and will likely remove all infectious risks in the future treatment of hemophilia.

Acquired Disorders

Evaluation of these disorders is more difficult because the possible abnormalities are much more diverse. Liver disease is the most common cause of acquired coagulation disorders. In chronic severe liver disease, all coagulation factors may be abnormal and thrombocytopenia occurs due to pooling in the enlarged spleen. Unrecognized vitamin K deficiency may be a common cause of significant bleeding in severely ill hospitalized patients. Lupus anticoagulant is a term used for an antibody to prothrombin bound to phospholipid. It was originally described in patients with systemic lupus erythematosus, but it also occurs in many other diseases and in otherwise normal subjects. Many of these patients also have anti-phospholipid antibodies measured by immunologic techniques. Lupus anticoagulants are usually first noticed when a routine partial thromboplastin time is prolonged, and it is confirmed by the demonstration of a coagulation inhibitor by mixing patient plasma with an equal volume of normal plasma. The lupus inhibitor is not associated with an increased risk of bleeding, but may be associated with an increased risk for thrombosis (see below).

Evaluation of Patients with Thrombosis

Thrombotic disease can usually be related to acquired abnormalities related to impaired blood circulation. Old age and immobility are by far the most common factors that predispose to venous thromboembolic disease. The recognition of the frequency of venous thrombosis in hospitalized patients has led to more aggressive attention to early mobility and this simple adjustment has been a major therapeutic advance. Specific congenital hematologic abnormalities that are associated with an increased risk for thrombosis may be identified in some patients. Deficiencies or abnormalities of three plasma proteins involved in the control of coagulation reactions (antithrombin III, protein C, and protein S) appear to allow increased thrombosis because of failure to inhibit activated coagulation factors. Congenital abnormalities of factor V that make it resistant to proteolysis by protein C have recently been described as the most common cause of hereditary thrombosis. As in the assessment of bleeding disorders, clinical evaluation must be the primary basis for diagnosis. For example, an initial occurrence of deep venous thrombosis in the lower leg does not warrant an investigation for a hemostatic defect. However a recent onset of recurrent severe thromboembolic complications suggests the possibility of an underlying malignancy, and a thorough evaluation is essential. Patients with congenital hemostatic disorders that predispose to thrombosis often do not have a history of lifelong symptoms; many patients have their first thrombotic episode only after a triggering event such as trauma or enforced bed rest. Affected relatives may then be identified who have no clinically apparent problem. A recent survey of a normal population suggested a prevalence of protein C deficiency of 1 in 250, though none of the identified subjects had a history of thrombotic disease. Whether these asymptomatic, affected relatives may benefit from anticoagulant therapy is unknown.

Evaluation of Patients with Laboratory Abnormalities of Hemostasis Not Associated with Clinical Bleeding Problems

Since laboratory studies of hemostasis are often ordered as part of a routine evaluation, unexpected abnormalities are occasionally discovered in patients who have had no problems with excessive bleeding (Table 34-2). Pseudothrom-

Table 34-2. Laboratory Abnormalities of Hemostasis Not Associated with Clinical Bleeding Problems

Pseudothrombocytopenia due to EDTA-active platelet agglutinin
Coagulation abnormalities
  Prolonged partial thromboplastin time due to deficiencies of factor XII, prekallikrein, or high-molecular-weight kininogen
  Prolonged partial thromboplastin time (and possibly also prothrombin time) due to a lupus anticoagulant, an antibody to phospholipid and prothrombin
  Prolonged partial thromboplastin time and prothrombin time due to extreme erythrocytosis causing an increased ratio of citrate anticoagulant to plasma in the blood collection tube

bocytopenia can be caused by an antibody that agglutinates platelets in vitro in the presence of the anticoagulant EDTA. Since EDTA is the conventional anticoagulant for clinical laboratory blood counts, the platelets agglutinate in the tube of blood and the number of individual platelets recognized by the automated cell counter is falsely low. Platelets are actually normal in number and morphology on the peripheral blood smear made from a finger stick, and platelet counts are also normal in unanticoagulated blood sampled directly into the ammonium oxalate diluting fluid. This is an example of the critical importance of examining the peripheral blood smear to confirm the presence of thrombocytopenia reported by a routine automated count. EDTA-active agglutinins occur in about one in 1000 subjects, both normal persons and patients with a wide variety of diseases. They have no clinical importance.

The initial coagulation reactions required for a normal partial thromboplastin time involve three proteins that are unnecessary for normal hemostasis in vivo: factor XII, prekallikrein, and high-molecular-weight kininogen. The association of each of these plasma proteins with in vitro coagulation was originally recognized by the observation of a prolonged partial thromboplastin time in subjects with entirely normal hemostasis. The lupus anticoagulant also causes a prolongation of the partial thromboplastin time with no clinical bleeding.

A simpler in vitro artifact is the abnormality of coagulation tests that predictably occurs in patients with extreme erythrocytosis. In these samples the ratio of liquid sodium citrate anticoagulant to plasma is too great, and the standard amount of calcium added for the coagulation assay is inadequate to neutralize the citrate and allow the calcium-dependent coagulation reactions to proceed. The problem can be easily corrected by removing an appropriate volume of the citrate anticoagulant from the commercially prepared tube. For example, if the hematocrit is 65%, the amount of plasma in a blood sample is only two-thirds of the amount of plasma in a normal blood sample with a hematocrit of 45%. Therefore one-third of the citrate anticoagulant should be removed from the tube before blood collection.

Clinical Examples

1. A 22-year-old man is evaluated for continued oozing for 3 weeks after having two wisdom teeth extracted. His past history is normal. He has been healthy without any symptoms of excessive bleeding, but he is not circumcised, he has not had teeth extracted previously, and he has not had major trauma requiring sutures. His parents are healthy, but one older brother had prolonged bleeding that may have been the cause of his death after an automobile accident. Physical examination is normal except for the large, purple, boggy hematomas over each tooth extraction site. Laboratory data reveal normal blood counts and normal blood chemistry values including normal liver function tests. Tests of hemostasis demonstrate a normal platelet count, a normal prothrombin time (12 seconds), and a slightly prolonged partial thromboplastic time (41 seconds; normal, 21–37 seconds). Specific assays for coagulation factors demonstrate a factor VIII activity level of 108% and a factor IX level of 9%. A mixture of 50% patient plasma with normal plasma demonstrated a factor IX level of 63%. Bleeding was controlled with local measures, oral administration of an antifibrinolytic agent, and infusion of single donor units of fresh frozen plasma to achieve plasma factor IX levels of 20%.

Discussion.   The low factor IX level is diagnostic of hemophilia B. The 9% value indicates sufficient factor IX for normal hemostasis except following significant trauma, accounting for the patient's normal history. However once trauma occurs, bleeding may be very difficult to stop.

The family history is consistent with the X-linked male-expressed inheritance of hemophilia B, and also illustrates that the risk of bleeding from hemophilia is consistent within a family.

Factor IX (and VIII) levels of 9% may be at the margin of causing an abnormal partial thromboplastin time. With substantial clinical suspicion of a congenital bleeding disorder, specific coagulation factor assays must be performed.

The factor IX assay on the mixture of patient and normal plasma demonstrates that no inhibitor of (acquired antibody to) factor IX is present. This is an important observation because it predicts that plasma infusion therapy will be beneficial.

Treatment with commercially available concentrates of factor IX have significant risks of infection since they are produced from pools of plasma from up to 20,000 donors. Sterilization procedures inactivate the HIV and hepatitis C viruses, but in this patient (who will require few transfusions in his lifetime) any risk at all is inappropriate. Also the factor IX concentrates may have a risk of causing thrombosis. The minimum therapy is most appropriate.

2. A 33-year-old man is evaluated for definitive antithrombotic therapy following a serious episode of pulmonary embolism. He had been well until age 18 when he underwent surgical repair of a chronic left-knee injury caused by repeated athletic injuries. During that postoperative period he had deep venous thrombosis involving the left thigh, treated with intravenous heparin followed by 3 months of oral warfarin. Two years later he had a recurrent episode of left-thigh venous thrombosis, and following this episode warfarin was given for one year. The current hospitalization was for acute chest pain and dyspnea 3 days following his return to Oklahoma City from Tokyo. Pulmonary embolism was diagnosed by a high probability ventilation-perfusion lung scan and the demonstration of extensive venous thrombosis in his right thigh. Laboratory studies to investigate a possible congenital abnormality of hemostatic control system were normal.

Discussion.   Venous thromboembolism is a common disease. Common predisposing factors are immobilization (such as enforced bedrest or long automobile or airplane travel), venous stasis, inflammation, and previous thrombosis. The first three factors were present with the knee surgery. Currently prophylaxis with low doses of heparin would be used for this type of surgery, but this was not always given 15 years ago and may not always be effective. Immobilization in the small airline seats for transoceanic flights is another significant risk factor.

The diagnosis of pulmonary embolism can be difficult, as there are no absolutely diagnostic studies other than invasive pulmonary angiography. In this man the previous history and the concurrent diagnosis of thigh venous thrombosis makes the diagnosis of pulmonary embolism nearly absolute.

Recurrent thromboembolic disease in an otherwise healthy young man raises the possibility of a congenital abnormality of the mechanisms of coagulation control. However even in the most suspicious cases, these are documented in less than 50% of patients.

At this time, lifetime anticoagulation with warfarin is indicated. This patient has suffered a life-threatening episode with this pulmonary embolism, and potentially life-threatening disease with each previous proximal leg venous thrombosis. Current data demonstrating the efficacy of low-dose warfarin make this a safe, feasible lifetime therapy.

Bibliography

Dahlback B. Physiological anticoagulation: Resistance to activated protein C and venous thromboembolism. *J Clin Invest* 94:923–927, 1994. *A concise review of the proteins involved in the regulation of coagulation, with description of congenital abnormalities which increase the risk for thrombosis. Emphasis is on the recently described mutations of factor V which cause resistance to activated protein C.*

Furie B and Furie BC. Molecular and cellular biology of blood coagulation. *New Engl J Med* 326:800–806, 1992. *This review provides the recent knowledge on the structure and function of proteins involved in blood coagulation. Clinical implications of structural abnormalities are described.*

Furie B, Limentani SA, and Rosenfield CG. A practical guide to the evaluation and treatment of hemophilia. *Blood* 84:3–9, 1994. *This article is particularly helpful as a fundamental clinical approach to this classic disorder.*

George JN, El-Harake MA, and Raskob GE. Chronic idiopathic thrombocytopenic purpura. *New Engl J Med* 331:1207–1211, 1994. *This concise review describes the pathogenesis of ITP in adults and the approach to management of this common, chronic disorder.*

George JN and Shattil SJ. The clinical importance of acquired abnormalities of platelet function. *New Engl J Med* 324:27–39, 1991. *This review describes platelet function and tests used to evaluate platelet function. The specific focus is on the extremely common occurrence of abnormal platelet function and its infrequent clinical importance.*

Hirsh J. Heparin. *New Engl J Med* 324:1565–1574, 1991. *A comprehensive discussion of one of the most widely used therapeutic agents in America.*

Hirsh J. Oral anticoagulant drugs. *New Engl J Med* 324: 1865–1975, 1991. *A very thorough review of the structure, function, and appropriate clinical use of warfarin.*

Hoyer LW. Hemophilia A. *New Engl J Med* 330:38–47, 1994. *This review of hemophilia describes the molecular abnormalities of factor VIII, recent advances in clinical management, and the future for potential gene therapy.*

Part IV Questions: Hematologic and Neoplastic Disorders

1. Ineffective erythropoiesis refers to abnormal red cell production characterized by
   A. Marrow erythroid hyperplasia and an increased reticulocyte count.
   B. Marrow erythroid hyperplasia and a normal or decreased reticulocyte count.
   C. Marrow erythroid hypoplasia and an increased reticulocyte count.
   D. Marrow erythroid hypoplasia and a normal or decreased reticulocyte count.
   E. Marrow erythroid aplasia and absent reticulocytes.

2. Each of the following is typical of myelodysplastic syndromes, except
   A. The marrow is usually hypercellular.
   B. The peripheral blood shows evidence of marrow failure.
   C. The marrow aspirate shows greater than 30% blasts.
   D. The clinical course is variable.
   E. They are clonal disorders.

3. A 65-year-old white male presents to his general practitioner's office for his annual physical examination. His only complaint is of mild fatigue. Physical examination shows generalized lymphadenopathy and splenomegaly. Laboratory analysis shows a normal hemoglobin and platelet count, but marked leukocytosis with a WBC of 65,000/ml. Examination of the blood smear shows that the vast majority of the blood cells are mature lymphocytes, with occasional smudged cells. What is the likely diagnosis?

   A. Acute lymphocytic leukemia
   B. Chronic lymphocytic leukemia
   C. Multiple myeloma
   D. Hodgkin's lymphoma
   E. Infectious mononucleosis

4. Which type of mutation would be *least* likely to affect an oncogene in either human or animal tumors?
   A. Gene loss by deletion
   B. Amplification
   C. Translocation
   D. Point mutation
   E. Retroviral transduction

5. Characteristics of tumors which are curable with chemotherapy include all of the following except
   A. Presence of resistant cells is not important.
   B. Morphology is undifferentiated.
   C. Growth rate is rapid.
   D. Tumor size is small.
   E. Growth fraction is high.

6. A patient with liver cirrhosis, portal hypertension, and congestive splenomegaly has a platelet count of 70,000/μl. Which of the following statements about this patient is *false?*
   A. Bone marrow megakaryocytes appear normal.
   B. An abnormally increased fraction of platelets is sequestered in the spleen.
   C. Platelet survival is shortened to less than half normal.
   D. Radioisotope study demonstrates that the total body number of platelets is normal.
   E. Platelet morphology on the peripheral blood smear is normal.

V Rheumatologic and Immunologic Disorders

Part Editor
Morris Reichlin

35 Organization of the Immune System: Mechanisms of Immune Injury

John B. Harley

Objectives

After completing this chapter, you should be able to

Appreciate the capacity of defects in the immune system to lead to clinical illness

Know the structure of immunoglobulin molecules in broad outline

Understand how such incredible antibody diversity is generated

Appreciate parallels between diversity in T cell receptors and antibody molecules

Appreciate the roles of the histocompatibility molecule and T cell receptor in governing the immune response

Appreciate the critical role complement plays in health and disease

Appreciate the complicated interrelationships between complement molecules

Understand how intricate the molecular interplay is between infectious agents and the immune system

---

A human being is home to trillions of microorganisms. Our gastrointestinal tract, airways, eyes, ears, and skin are particularly obvious sites of carriage. Others are not so obvious, such as the ganglia, for example, where *Herpes zoster* is latent after primary infection. Our survival is clearly related to our ability to defend ourselves against viruses, bacteria, fungi, and parasites. The diverse strategies for pathology presented by these organisms is staggering. All told there must be tens of thousands of distinguishable pathogens now known. Whether this is the major portion only a minor fraction of the universe of organisms potentially pathogenic to man cannot be known. Clearly, people who cannot resist and defeat pathogenic organisms have serious, often life-threatening problems. When the underlying cause of recurring infections cannot be definitively addressed, an early death from infection is a constant possibility.

Given the organisms that we face and their incredible sophistication, it is astonishing that we survive at all. How is it then that we manage to thrive in such a dangerous world? Virtually everyone is the beneficiary of a very sophisticated **immune system.** A variety of barriers, mechanisms, cellular processes, protein cascades all act in concert to defend the host against the armamentarium arrayed against it. The immune system has two very different fundamental components, the **innate immune system** and the **adaptive immune system.**

Innate Immunity

The defenses against pathogenic microorganisms that are present in a host who has not been previously exposed to the pathogen (or any of its close relatives) are innate.

These include the barriers to infection, such as the skin and mucosa. Also, the **complement system, natural killer** cells, and **phagocytic cells** with their respiratory burst leading to pathogen destruction all contribute to innate immunity.

The failure of skin and mucosa to serve as a barrier leads to chronic sustained infection, as occurs with many dermatoses and much mucositis. Failure of phagocytosis to destroy microorganisms is found in chronic granulomatous disease and other defects in phagocytic cells as discussed in Chap. 39.

Complement

A complicated cascade of proteins, complement subsumes a variety of functions. The initiation of the complement system is through the **classic** or **alternate** pathway. The **alternate pathway of complement activation** nonspecifi-

cally initiates the complement cascade (Fig. 35-1). There is a low level of spontaneous conversion of complement component C3 to C3b. The protein called B, with help from D, binds to C3b and forms a complex of C3b,Bb on cell surfaces. C3b,Bb is stabilized by P and converts more C3 to C3b. On cell membranes of the host, other proteins act to control this alternate pathway, including H, MCP, and DAF. These proteins are not found on the membranes of infectious agents and hence on them the alternate pathway proceeds unimpeded. C3b,Bb also activates C5 and sequentially proceeds until C9 polymerizes on the surface of cells and forms pores. The osmotic gradient across the cell membrane is destroyed, which causes swelling and lysis.

There are a few interesting features of this cascade that influence inflammatory responses in other ways. Some of the fragments generated by cleaving the intact complement molecules, particularly C4a, C3a, and C5a act as me-

Fig. 35-1. The complement cascade is part of the innate immune system and activated by the alternate or classical pathway.

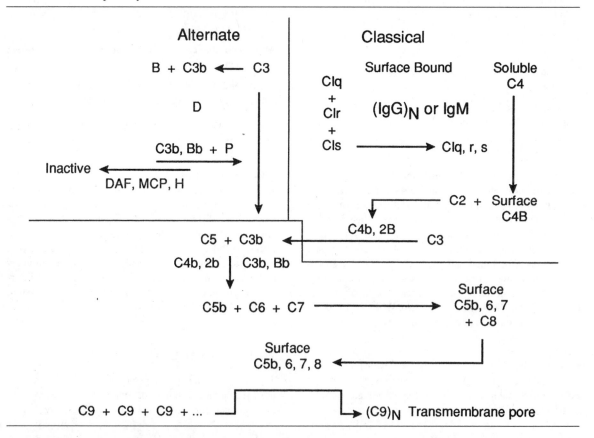

diators of inflammation. Many cells have receptors for C3b and some have receptors for C4b. Complement deposition on cells or as part of immune complexes facilitates phagocytosis of complexes or cells. Also, C3b deposition tends to solubilize complexes that would otherwise be insoluble.

The **classic pathway of complement activation** is triggered by immunoglobulin. Immunoglobulin is part of the adaptive immune system and in this way the complement cascade amplifies the specific identification of antigen. Here C1q binds to IgM or two (or more) IgGs and then activates C1r and C1s to generate the convertase for C4. C4b then binds to a surface and converts C2 to C2b. The molecule created by the noncovalent association of C2b and C4b or C2b,C4b is a convertase for C3.

At this point the classical and alternate pathways converge. Starting with C3 the same components are used, whether the pathway was activated nonspecifically or by immunoglobulin. C4b,2b and C3b,Bb are referred to as C3/C5 convertases. They generate more C3b from C3, which acts to amplify complement activation. They also generate C5b from C5, which carries complement activation toward cell lysis. C6 and C7 bind to C5b with C7 anchoring the complex to a membrane. The anchor is made more secure by C8. Then the complex is capable of polymerizing C9 to construct a membrane pore, thereby destroying the osmotic gradient across the cell membrane.

Deficiencies of complement components increase the risk of certain diseases, sometimes in ways that are not understood. Deficiency of the early components of the classical pathway C1q, C2, or C4 predispose affected individuals to systemic lupus erythematosus. C4 deficiency, though rare, appears to confer the highest risk of lupus and most of the known C4 deficient individuals are affected. C2 deficiency is the most common clinically relevant deficiency, with an allele frequency estimated at one in a hundred. Since complete deficiency of C2 requires that both genes be dysfunctional, C2 deficiency is expected and is observed at one in ten thousand individuals. C3 deficiency causes increased susceptibility to serious infection and is very rare. C6, C7, and C8 deficiency dispose to serious intravascular sepsis, especially by *Nisseria* species.

The infection of some organisms is mediated by the complement system. There are receptors for C3b and C4b, as mentioned above. Complement receptor CR1 is found on erythrocytes, monocytes, macrophages, and B cells and binds to C3b and C4b. CR2 is only found on B cells. Epstein-Barr virus, which causes infectious mononucleosis, and Burkitt's lymphoma, among other B cell lym-

phomas, binds to CR2 on the B cell surface and thereby gains entry into the cell. The tissue trophism of viruses is mediated by specific interactions with cell surface molecules.

The complement system has such incredible potential for amplification that a variety of molecular systems is arrayed against it to keep it in check. One imagines that without these the spontaneous generation of C3b would lead to the consumption of all available complement and much needless destruction. Decay accelerating factor (DAF) is one of these and operates with other cofactors to accelerate the destruction of active C3b. Paroxysmal nocturnal hemaglobulinuria is associated with a deficiency of decay accelerating factor. The molecular mechanism of this disorder is now known and has a number of interesting features.

In paroxysmal nocturnal hemaglobulinuria there is a population of red blood cells that appear to be especially sensitive to complement lysis as well as lysis induced by osmotic change. This has been shown to be a clonal disorder, meaning that hematopoietic cells which express the defect appear (from a few different experimental arguments) to have been derived from a single precursor cell. Other cell surface molecules, in addition to decay accelerating factor, appear to be deficient, also. All of these cell surface molecules are anchored to the cell surface by a covalent bond with phosphoinositol glycolipid. The cells involved have a genetic defect in the synthesis of this bond which is inherited from one generation of cells to the next and hence none of the cell surface molecules requiring this linkage are formed. The cell surface molecules attached by a phosphoinositol glycolipid linkage are not present on the cell surface of the progeny of the stem cell which first expressed the defect.

Natural Killer Cells

These are a cell type that have the capacity to destroy other cells. In experimental systems they provide resistance to some infections and some transformed cell types. Natural killer cells are thought to be part of the innate resistance to infection and to some cancers.

Adaptive Immunity

The other major division of the immune system has the important flexibility and the plasticity to respond specifically to substances and organisms never previously encountered by the host. Though there are many aspects of immune function that remain to be discovered, experimental evidence from the last few decades has established how the immune system achieves its incredible diversity.

In outline, the system works as follows. In early development, which means before birth for most mammals, the host becomes **tolerant** or **anergic** to the intercellular environment. This means that the host will not subsequently mount an immune response to substances with the appropriate antenatal exposure. However, later in life the introduction of a foreign substance or organism into the host will lead to a vigorous specific immune response. The two central elements of this system are **immunoglobulin** and the antigen-specific **T cell receptor.**

Immunoglobulins

Trillions of different immunoglobulins are possible. All of the immunoglobulins actually observed are referred to as the **repertoire.** Normal adults have an impressive repertoire of immunoglobulins. On the other hand, neonates appear to have a more limited capacity to generate diverse immunoglobulins. Perhaps this is why immunoglobulin G is transported by the placenta from the mother into the circulation of the third-trimester fetus. This gives the neonate the benefit of the immune experience of his or her mother. This is also why many hereditary immune deficiency syndromes do not present with clinical illness until between 3 and 6 months of age, when this maternal immunoglobulin has been catabolized by the liver from the neonatal circulation.

There are five types or **classes** of immunoglobulin found in the circulation: immunoglobulins M, D, G, A, and E (or IgM, IgD, IgG, IgA, and IgE). All of these immunoglobulins are composed of "heavy" and "light" chain polypeptides. The heavy chains are different between classes. There are two types of light chains, called kappa and lambda, and they are found in association with every type of heavy chain.

IgG is the most abundant immunoglobulin in the circulation. A schematic of its structure (Fig. 35-2) shows how the structural features are related to each other. Within classes, immunoglobulin is constructed with a portion that tends to be the same (or very similar) from one molecule to the next which is called the **constant region.** In IgG the constant region is composed of three immunoglobulin constant-region domains. These are globular structures in which many of the features, such as the positions of cysteine residues in intermolecular disulfide linkage, are relatively preserved. The constant regions are not exactly the same, one to the next, but they are clearly related and constitute the carboxyl termini of the polypeptide chain. It is

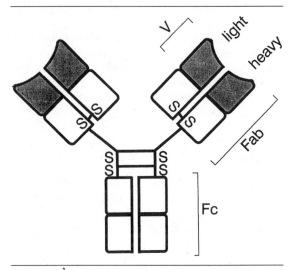

Fig. 35-2. A schematic of immunoglobulin G or IgG. The variable region (V) which binds antigen is shaded and composed of contributions from the heavy and light polypeptide chains of IgG. Sulfhydryl bonds between heavy and light chains and the two between heavy chains are indicated (S-S). The two major proteolytic fragments are indicated as Fab (or fragment with antigen binding activity) and as Fc (or crystallizable fragment). The Fc may be bound by specific receptors on phagocytes, natural killer cells, and other cells.

widely suspected that gene duplications relatively distant in evolution account for the structure we now observe.

The **variable** region of the molecule (V in Fig. 35-2) is found at the amino terminal ends of the polypeptides. The variable regions from the heavy and light chains come together to form the **antigen-combining site.** After immunization with tetanus toxoid, for example, IgG is synthesized that binds to tetanus toxoid by virtue of constructing a unique antigen-combining site. The variable region is a truly extraordinary property of immunoglobulins.

How we have so many immunoglobulins has been recently explained and is one of the major scientific achievements of the last two decades. Some thought that this **generation of diversity** occurs because all of the variable regions are encoded by the genome, but others retorted that the human genome was too small to accommodate all of the immunoglobulins which appeared to be possible. Some thought that encoded sequences were somehow mutated, but others retorted that undirected mutation would be without precedent.

The astonishing explanation involves both mutation and

multiple encoded sequences. The variable region for the gamma heavy chain, for example, is composed of different component parts called **V, D,** and **J** (Fig. 35-3). Each one of these is selected from a collection of encoded **germline** genes. It appears that any of the few thousand V regions can combine with any of the few dozen D regions and any of the few J regions. Already, by mixing and matching the heavy chains more than a hundred thousand choices are possible. A similar process occurs to both the heavy and light chains. The light chains, however, do not have a D region. In addition, there are variations in the sites of joining segments together, extra or deleted codons, and errors made between the V, D and J segments, again multiplying the possibilities further. It is also clear that **somatic mutation** occurs which changes the immunoglobulin produced by mutating the DNA encoding for the immunoglobulin. How this is restricted to such a very small part of the genome is the subject of much current research.

All immunoglobulin is made in B lymphocytes. The precursors to these cells appear to originate in the fetal liver in man, after which they populate the spleen, lymph nodes, and bone marrow. This whole business of assembling the particular V, D, and J regions occurs in B cells and their precursors. B cells differentiate into plasma cells and become cellular factories for the production of immunoglobulin.

Each of the major classes of immunoglobulin subsume a somewhat different role. **IgM** is usually the first immunoglobulin to be specifically produced and detectable in the blood after antigen exposure in the **primary immune response** (Fig. 35-4). It is usually of lower affinity than the antigen-specific classes of immunoglobulin which follow. IgM is a pentameric molecule containing 10 heavy polypeptide mu chains and 10 light chains. Each pair of heavy chains binds a pair of light chains to constitute a unit of the pentamer. Except that mu chains have four constant

Fig. 35-3. Generation of immunoglobulin heavy-chain variable-domain diversity by randomly constructing a coding region composed of different V, D, and J choices. In this example V964, D3, and J4 have been recombined and coded for as heavy-chain variable domain. Multiplication of the number of choices in each category gives the total number of different possibilities.

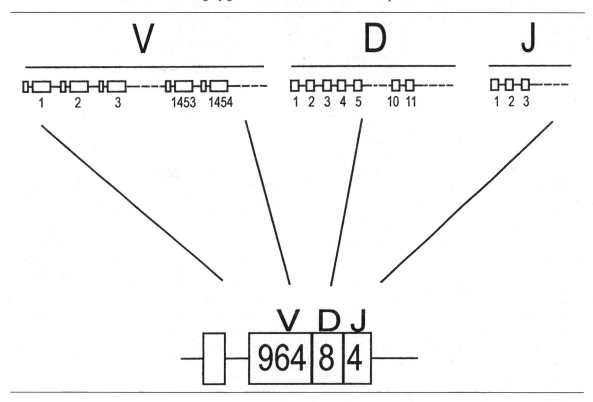

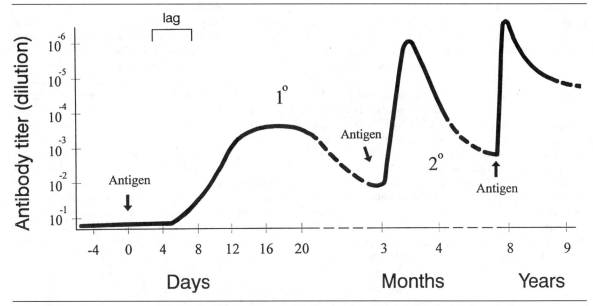

Fig. 35-4. The humoral immune response after immunization or infection. A few days after exposure (lag) to a foreign antigen (non-self) which has not been previously encountered by the host, adaptive immune response immunoglobulin specifically directed against the antigen is first detectable. This primary immune response (1°) is predominantly IgM and composed of low-affinity antibody. In the absence of antigen the antibody titer gradually falls. With subsequent exposure a secondary immune response (2°) is induced composed of high-affinity IgG. Without antigen this response is gradually reduced over time, but is rapidly reinduced with subsequent exposure, even many years later.

domains, while the gamma chains of IgG have only three domains, each unit of the pentamer is similar to the structure given in Fig. 35-2. The five units are then covalently bound to one another by disulfide bonds. The low affinity of the binding of the antigen-combining region has been somewhat compensated by having 10 binding sites.

If the impetus for differentiation is present, then the DNA that codes for the variable region on the mu heavy chain is transferred to the gamma heavy chain. What was IgM becomes IgG. This may happen as part of the primary immune response or may occur when the host is exposed to an antigen for the second time. This is called the **secondary immune response** or the **anamnestic response** (to emphasize that this is not the first encounter with this antigen) (see Fig. 35-4). Now larger quantities of specific immunoglobulin are synthesized. Since they have the advantage of already having an expanded pool of specific B cells, further differentiation and somatic mutation leads to much higher affinity antibody.

Even long after the antigen has been cleared, memory B cells persist and are available to be stimulated by antigen. In this way our immune system maintains a life history of previous exposures. The presence of specific IgM or IgG antibodies is used clinically to help determine whether a process underway (and usually undiagnosed) could be due to a particular organism. Most laboratories will ask for blood specimens collected at least 3 weeks apart, often referred to as **acute** and **convalescent titers.** For example, imagine that you are evaluating a flulike illness in a young woman who is in the first trimester of pregnancy. IgM antibody to rubella might be seen in the first specimen. This, with a rising IgG antibody titer to rubella in the second trimester, would help confirm the diagnosis. If she had no history of German measles and had not been immunized, then you would be very concerned that she had a rubella infection at the time when it is known to cause very serious fetal malformations.

IgA is the immunoglobulin of mucosal surfaces and secretions. The alpha heavy chain-producing B cells are concentrated in the respiratory tract, the gastrointestinal tract, and in the saliva, tears, colostrum, and milk. There is a secreted form of IgA that is different from that found in the circulation.

IgE is responsible for much allergy, mostly because there are receptors on mast cells for IgE. When IgE is bound by antigen, these receptors induce the release of histamine and other mediators that are associated with the well-known symptoms of allergy and atopy. The epsilon heavy chain is the distinctive structural feature which makes an immunoglobulin molecule IgE. The molecular mechanism which is responsible for generating the DNA coding sequence for epsilon is particularly interesting. The variable region, which was previously part of a mu or gamma heavy chain, for example, is far removed from the epsilon constant-region sequence. All of the intervening DNA which codes for other heavy-chain constant regions is removed, thereby bring the variable region next to the epsilon constant region. This mechanism is referred to as immunoglobulin class switch and also occurs for the switch from IgM to IgG or IgA.

Cell Surface Immunoglobulin Receptor

During maturation to become a plasma cell, the B cell interacts with antigen by a cell surface receptor. This cell surface receptor is the immunoglobulin molecule with a domain that traverses and thereby anchors the immunoglobulin in the membrane. After the receptor binds antigen, a signal is transmitted which activates and triggers the B cell to divide. In this way the cell population that binds to antigen selectively expands. Control of this process is extremely important. Factors which appear to play a role are the concentration of antigen and the presence of co-stimulatory signals, particularly those from T lymphocytes.

Adaptive Humoral Immune Mechanisms of Defense

When first confronted with antigen, the adaptive humoral immune system must respond before the host is overwhelmed by infection. The infection must be sufficiently slow or innate immunity must delay the progress of the infection until the mechanisms of the adaptive immune system can identify, expand, and (hopefully) destroy the intruder. Immunoglobulin facilitates the destruction of organisms and toxins by a number of mechanisms. The binding of antibody may **neutralize** a toxin by preventing it from binding to cells. Immunoglobulin may agglutinate organisms

and slow infection. Some immunoglobulin may coat organisms for **opsonization.** Receptors on phagocytes bind the constant regions of some IgG-facilitating phagocytosis. Natural killer cells may also bind to constant regions of immunoglobulin and destroy organisms by **antibody-dependent cellular cytotoxicity.** Mast cells may be activated after cross-linking of their surface IgE. Finally, the complement system may be activated by immunoglobulin and impede infection as discussed above.

Role of T Lymphocytes

There are only a few basic ways that the adaptive immune system specifically recognizes antigen. First, receptors on B cells which are composed of surface immunoglobulin may specifically bind antigen and expand their number, as discussed above. Second, immunoglobulin free in solution may bind antigen, form complexes of antigen and antibody, and thereby facilitate the binding of complexes to cells with appropriate receptors. Third, there is another system of antigen recognition for which **T lymphocytes** assume the central and major role. T cells have both a regulatory role and an effector role. To begin to understand how they work, we must begin with antigen processing.

HLA System

When B cells bind and internalize antigen, the antigen is also partially digested and transported to the surface as peptides in association with **histocompatibility** molecules (Fig. 35-5) or (as usually referred to) **human leukocyte antigens** or **HLA.** These molecules and the peptides found noncovalently bound to them are part of the central control mechanisms of the adaptive immune system. Nearly all cells have **Class I histocompatibility molecules** on their surfaces, while only B cells, macrophage, dendritic cells, and a few other "activated," injured, or growing cell types also express **Class II histocompatibility surface molecules.**

There are three major types of Class I histocompatibility antigens expressed on cell surfaces in man, usually referred to as HLA-A, HLA-B, and HLA-C. These are single-chain transmembrane molecules that noncovalently associate with beta-2 microglobulin. The endogenous peptide is bound in a groove formed by two alpha helices on a platform of beta-pleated sheets. Each variant of the class I molecules binds a different set of peptides. The extent of polymorphism in the human population is staggering. For HLA-B, for example, over 70 variants are known.

The Class II histocompatibility molecules present exogenous peptides, which are peptides that are derived from

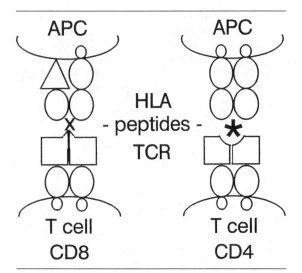

Fig. 35-5. Trimolecular complexes. Antigen presenting cells (APC) have Class I and/or Class II HLA molecules. Class I molecules contain beta-2-microglobulin (triangle). The HLA bind peptides (X and *). The T cell receptor (TCR) recognizes peptide bound by Class I HLA for CD8 cytotoxic T cells or by Class II HLA for helper-inducer T cells. Other accessory molecules also mediate important signals between cells. Some of these interactions control the consequence of the TCR binding to peptide and HLA.

outside the cell. Immune complexes, for example, which are internalized into macrophage and other cell types, are partially digested. The derived peptides are bound by Class II molecules and presented in this way.

The Class II molecules are complicated. There are three types: HLA-DR, HLA-DQ, and HLA-DP. Each molecule is composed of two transmembrane polypeptide chains, alpha and beta, which come together to generate a structure similar in its major features to the antigen-binding groove of the Class I molecule (see Fig. 35-5). Class II molecules are also very highly **polymorphic,** which means that there are many different choices or **alleles** commonly found in the population. The polymorphisms in Class II have important differences compared to Class I molecules. First, for HLA-DR beta there are four different coding regions; an individual chromosome has only a subset of these. HLA-DR alpha is virtually monomorphic, meaning that the same alpha chain is used for all of the human HLA-DR molecules.

Second, for HLA-DQ and HLA-DP the alpha and the beta chains are usually different on the two chromosomes

of an individual. Both HLA-DQ and HLA-DP are theoretically able to form four molecules from all the possible combinations of their respective alpha and beta chains. Two of these would be from the same chromosome and two would be cross products. The latter molecules would ordinarily not be found in either parent and have the potential to confer unique immune capabilities to each individual. This is another feature which makes each of our immune systems relatively unique. Indeed, your HLA molecules are very unlikely to be identical to the HLA molecules of someone who is not a close relative.

A whole host of human diseases is associated with particular HLA alleles. These include, for example, most of the idiopathic inflammatory disorders, several suspected autoimmune diseases, as well as other disorders (Table 35-1). HLA molecules are also responsible for the immune reactions of and against transplanted organs.

T Cell Receptors

T lymphocytes have cell surface molecules called T cell receptors that bear many similarities to immunoglobulin. The T cell receptor is composed of variable alpha and beta chains. Diversity is generated by a mechanism of coding sequence rearrangement parallel to what we have discussed above for immunoglobulin (see Fig. 35-3). Each T cell receptor beta chain, for example, is composed of one from a group of V regions, one from the D regions and one from the J regions. Somatic mutation does not appear to be an important contributor to the diversity found in T cell receptors, an aspect for which they differ from immunoglobulin. The T cell receptor binds peptides bound to (or presented by) HLA molecules. The trimolecular complex

Table 35-1. Disease Associated with HLA

Disease	HLA Association	Relative Risk
Insulin-dependent	DR3 & DR4	3.0
diabetes mellitus	DR2	0.3
Pemphigus vulgaris	DR4	14.0
Graves' disease	DR3	4.0
Hashimoto's thyroiditis	DR5	3.0
Systemic lupus	DR3	3.0
erythematosus	DR2	2.0
Ankylosing spondylitis	B27	90.0
Goodpasture's syndrome	DR2	15.0
Multiple sclerosis	DR2	4.0
Rheumatoid arthritis	DR4	4.0

of the HLA molecule, the antigen peptide, and the T cell receptor is at the center of immune control and decision making (see Fig. 35-5). This complex is important for every antigen-dependent T cell response.

Superantigens

The trimolecular complex provides another, somewhat surprising, opportunity for a pathophysiologic mechanism. Some microorganisms elaborate substances, now called **superantigens,** that bind to particular trimolecular complexes, those which satisfy certain structural requirements. When this happens, aspects of the control of the immune system are lost and the results can be catastrophic. For example, in the late 1970s a mysterious illness appeared that has been called toxic shock syndrome. During menses young women would develop hypotension and circulatory collapse. Some died. After many years of brilliant research we now know that this illness was caused by staphylococcal organisms growing in tampons and producing a toxin, the toxic shock syndrome toxin. This toxin binds to some beta chains of the T cell receptor and to some HLA molecules. This bridging of the T cell receptor to the HLA in this nonphysiologic way liberates cytokines from large numbers of lymphocytes, leading to the clinical presentation observed. Public health measures have been taken to prevent recurrence of this illness. Other substances produced by bacteria, mycoplasma, and viruses cause pathology by mechanisms that share features with toxic shock syndrome.

Peripheral Blood T Cells

In the peripheral blood there are two major types of mature T cells, those that express a molecule called CD4 and others that express CD8. The CD4 positive T cells bind peptides presented by Class II HLA and CD8 T cells bind peptides presented by Class I HLA (Fig. 35-5).

The CD4 positive T cells are referred to as helper-inducer T cells. They may encourage B cells to mature and develop specific immunoglobulin. They may proliferate after interaction with antigen presented with HLA. A subpopulation of these cells appears to be involved in the decision whether an immune response will become a **humoral immune response** (meaning the development of immunoglobulin predominates) or a **cellular immune response** (meaning that the specific immune response is restricted to T cells). The CD4 molecule is also known to be the receptor for the gp120 molecule of human immunodeficiency virus.

The CD8 positive T cells are cytotoxic and immunosuppressive cells. When they bind to a cell expressing a peptide,

a signal is produced which destroys cells by disrupting the membrane barrier or by triggering the cell to undergo an automatic process of self-destruction, called **apoptosis.**

The control of the adaptive immune system is mediated by the specific interactions with antigen which occur with surface and soluble immunoglobulin and with the HLA-bound peptides that are recognized by T cell receptors. Many other components influence, attenuate, or accentuate the participation of certain cells in the immune response, but they are fairly useless in the absence of specific recognition.

Cytokines

These are soluble mediators that influence the actions and responses of cells. **Interferons** influence cellular metabolism in ways that increase resistance to some viral infections. They may also change the state of cell activation and influence the type of immune response that predominates. **Interleukins** help govern the immune response as well as the growth and differentiation of many cell types. Many different interferons and interleukins are now known. Cytokines, interferons, and interleukins exert important influence upon the control of the immune system.

Allergic Reactions, Hypersensitivity, and Tissue Injury

The classic types of immune reactions which initiate tissue damage have been divided into four categories by Gell and Coombs. Although this classification scheme has been in use for more than three decades, it remains a useful framework upon which to consider clinical phenomena. (See Chaps. 36–38 and 41.)

Anaphylactic (Type I) Reactions

Here local or systemic reactions are induced by a particular antibody, often IgE. These disorders include the troublesome problems of hay fever, allergic asthma, angioedema, and allergic urticaria. Anaphylaxis is a systemic response to antigen, often occurring within seconds or minutes after exposure. Patients experience bronchospasms, urticaria, and hypotension which may progress to circulatory collapse.

Cytotoxic (Type II) Reactions

These occur when antibodies interact with antigens found on cell surfaces. The antigen may be an intrinsic part of the cell or may be bound to the cell. Antibodies to red blood cell surface molecules may induce transfusion reactions by this mechanism. Maternal antibody may cross the placenta, destroying red blood cells of the fetus or neonate which carry antigens found in the father but not the mother. Some drugs may attach to cell surfaces and lead to hemolytic anemia, leukopenia, or thrombocytopenia by this mechanism.

Immune Complex-Mediated (Type III) Reactions

In serum sickness, antibodies bind to the heterologous serum components (from another animal). The antibody and antigen form complexes which deposit in various organs and tissues whereupon they induce an inflammatory response. This mechanism may be important in some types of vasculitis and almost certainly is important in some patients with systemic lupus erythematosus or polyarteritis nodosa.

Delayed-Type Hypersensitivity (Type IV) Reaction

T lymphocytes may also recognize antigen. When they do, a mononuclear cell infiltrate may accumulate at the site of antigen concentration and lead to the elaboration of toxic products and tissue injury. Contact dermatitis, such as poison ivy, is an example of this type of immune response. Some forms of transplant rejection and the tuberculin skin reaction after infection by *Mycobacteria tuberculosis* are also mediated by this mechanism.

Autoimmunity

The adaptive immune system is confronted by the overwhelming central problem of distinguishing **self** and **non-self.** Infectious organisms are generally non-self and the apparent purpose for having an adaptive immune system. The awesome plasticity of adaptive immunity enables any individual to generate a specific immune response against a virtually infinite variety of infectious agents.

The immune system must be prevented from attacking the constituents of the host or self and sophisticated systems are available to ensure this function. During development, mechanisms prevent the generation of self-reactive T and B cells. B cells do most of their maturation in the bone marrow and in experimental systems; those that bind a self-antigen in the bone marrow are destroyed. T cells that bind peptides found on HLA in the thymus during T cell development are also destroyed. Both B and T cells require the cell surface expression of costimulatory molecules and their binding by ligand produced by the T or B cell. In the absence of this interaction, the specific T or B cell undergoes self-destruction and does not proliferate.

A system so complicated, even though it is fundamental for survival, cannot operate free of error all of the time. Immune responses occur which appear to be directed against constituents of self. Both the humoral immune system and cellular immune system have been implicated. **Autoimmune diseases** result when the mechanisms in place fail to prevent adaptive immunity directed against self. There must now be nearly a hundred disease processes in which an autoimmune process is proven or at least implicated in pathogenesis. These include autoimmune thyroid disease (both Graves' disease and Hashimoto's thyroiditis), type 1 diabetes (which is also called juvenile onset or insulin-dependent diabetes), myasthenia gravis, systemic lupus erythematosus, subacute sclerosing panencephalitis, and multiple sclerosis. HLA genetic associations have been described for many. For some disorders the evidence is convincing that autoimmunity is fundamental to their pathophysiology. For others, such evidence has not been collected or is much less convincing. Nevertheless, this is an area of active research which will hopefully produce better diagnostics and therapy in the years to come. Collectively, these disorders affect tens, perhaps hundreds, of millions causing untold worldwide suffering.

Clinical Examples

1. Your nephew is 8 years old and having a great time in second grade. In late January a third of his class, including your nephew, develop fevers, chills, myalgias, and cough so severe they stay home from school. The onset of illness is within 72 hours for all affected. Children are home from one to six days. A few have a persistent cough. The public health officials comment on the epidemic in the news. Very few people over the age of 20 and no one in your medical school class are affected. What is the primary mode of host defense? Will your nephew be susceptible to this illness again? Why are most over the age of 20 unaffected?

Discussion.   This acute febrile illness is probably of viral etiology, most likely influenza. A specific immunoglobulin directed against a specific influenza virus strain is the primary mode of host defense. It is not likely that your nephew will be susceptible to another infection by this antigen strain although he may become infected with another strain of influenza virus. The observation that most people over 20 years of age are unaffected suggests prior exposure to an antigenically similar virus many years ago.

2. Your best friend has fevers, big lymph nodes, and profound fatigue. The student health service tells him that his spleen is also big, that he has unusual cells called atypical

lymphocytes in his blood, that a blood test called the "heterophile" is positive, and that he needs to rest in bed for a few weeks or even months. He goes home and takes some ampicillin that is in his medicine cabinet. Three days later, just as the fevers start to wane, he develops a rash on his chest, arms, and legs. It is red, raised in splotches and scares him. What is his diagnosis? What caused his illness? What are the immune mechanisms operating here? What is a heterophile test? Why did he get the rash?

Discussion. Mononucleosis is the most likely diagnosis. Epstein-Barr virus, which is a herpes virus, causes mononucleosis. Epstein-Barr virus infects B cells via the CR2 receptor. The B cells proliferate and secrete immunoglobulin escaping the normal control mechanisms of the immune system. The T cells then proliferate to limit and control the infection. The atypical lymphocytes in your friend's peripheral blood are likely to be T cells. When B cells are "polyclonally" activated they produce antibodies with specificities not ordinarily found in the circulation. An antibody which agglutinates sheep red blood cells is one of these and is called the heterophile antibody. About 90% of patients with mononucleosis develop a rash if they are treated with ampicillin. The mechanism is not fully understood, but may involve the antibodies against ampicillin that are found in these patients with polyclonal activation of B cells.

3. You and your identical twin went on a hike in the woods yesterday with a group of friends. You have an erythematous pruritic rash in streaks on your legs above your socks and below the hem of your shorts. What is this? Your twin is not affected. Why not?

Discussion. This is probably poison ivy. You probably have had a previous exposure which sensitized you and now have a delayed-type hypersensitivity response to oleoresin, the inducing antigen in poison ivy. Your identical twin should be capable of developing a response to poison ivy. Perhaps your twin wore long pants and was not exposed. Perhaps your twin washed with soap and water before the oleoresin could initiate delayed-type hypersensitivity. Perhaps your twin has not previously had a sensitizing exposure. If he or she is now sensitized, then when the two of you do this again, your responses are more likely to be similar.

Bibliography

Austen KF, Claman HN, and Frank MM. (eds.). *Immunological Diseases* (5th ed.). Boston: Little, Brown, 1994. *These authors have assembled a cadre of world-recognized experts who present the role of the immune system in clinical illness. This is a useful and comprehensive text for physicians and students with particular interest in immune disorders.*

Bjorkman PJ and Parham P. Structure, function and diversity of class I major histocompatibility molecules. *Ann Rev Biochem* 59:253–288, 1990. *Includes recent advances toward creation of a physical and detailed structural understanding of the histocompatibility molecules which promise to provide a fundamental understanding of the immune system.*

Janeway Jr CA, and Travers P. *Immunobiology: The Immune System in Health and Disease* (1st ed.). New York: Garland Publishing, 1994. *This is a comprehensive basic text which describes the fundamental features of the immune system as they are now understood.*

Silverstein AM. *History of Immunology* (1st ed.). London: Academic, 1989. *This text provides a fascinating look at immunology's complicated history.*

36 Immediate Hypersensitivity Diseases

James H. Wells

Objectives

After completing this chapter, you should be able to

Know the role of mast cells in immediate hypersensitivity disease

Explain the action of mast cells and other cells during the early and late phases of immediate hypersensitivity

State the role of TH1 and TH2 subpopulations of thymic-derived lymphocytes in determining whether immediate hypersensitivity develops

Understand the variable role of IgE in immediate hypersensitivity

Identify the various known mediators and their effects in producing immediate hypersensitivity disease

Have some understanding of the term "atopy" and its basis

Overview

Variability is a hallmark of this group of diseases but they share several common features.

Early "Mast Cell" Phase

As the name implies, immediate hypersensitivity reactions typically occur rapidly and even explosively. Examples include anaphylactic reactions or attacks of allergic rhinitis or asthma in highly sensitive subjects following a challenging exposure. The common denominator of the acute phase of these and other immediate hypersensitivity reactions is the role of inflammatory mediators released by mast cells. Even though the events leading to mediator release and the resulting clinical signs and symptoms may vary, tissue mast cells are the important source of the mediators which produce acute inflammation during the first few hours, minutes, or sometimes even seconds. Initially, edema is the main inflammatory tissue event.

Late Phase

There is often much more to immediate hypersensitivity phenomena than the early acute phase, especially when the early phase is brisk and strong. Some of the mast cell mediators attract, recruit, and activate other cells to produce the late phase of the acute reaction which usually begins between 3 and 8 hours after challenge. At this stage, the inflammatory cell population generally includes granulocytes with many basophils and a prominent eosinophilia. Occasionally the early phase is mild when compared with the late phase of the acute reaction.

Chronic Patterns

Immediate hypersensitivity diseases may follow a chronic course rather than being acute and episodic. Or they may be chronic with repeated acute exacerbations, as is often seen with rhinitis, asthma, urticaria, and atopic dermatitis. During chronic immediate hypersensitivity inflammation, the tissue infiltrate is pleomorphic, containing many lymphocytes, monocytes, and still with an eosinophilia. Even after prolonged inflammation, surprisingly little tendency toward fibrosis is seen.

Variability

Several immediate hypersensitivity phenomena may occur due to immunologic reactions involving several different types of antibodies. Alternatively they may be due to totally nonimmunologic mechanisms.

Immediate hypersensitivity processes with both variable and common features will be discussed in this chapter, along with some common diseases they produce or are associated with, e.g., anaphylactic reactions, urticaria/angioedema, and atopic dermatitis. Rhinitis and asthma will be dealt with in the following chapter on allergic respiratory diseases.

Normal Physiology

Immune Response

Protective Functions

The normal immune system protects against antigenically foreign materials and micro-organisms which are potentially harmful. Examples include viruses, bacteria, fungi, parasites, and some autogenous neoplasms.

Components of Response

Some components of the immune system such as macrophages and complement are more primitive and less specific than others. The development of B lymphocyte-derived specific antibodies and specifically sensitized T lymphocytes with helper, suppressor, cytotoxic, and memory functions is phylogenetically more sophisticated. It depends on an initial sensitizing exposure to antigen that begins with recognition and processing of the antigen by various phagocytic cells. This begins a selective process of sequential involvement of various other cells which results in a heterogeneous immune response. Often antigen-specific antibodies in several antibody classes as well as cell-mediated immunity occur, but generally one type of response predominates.

Heterogeneity of Response

The nature of this immune response varies with the nature of the stimulus and with the immune capabilities (both inherited and acquired) of the individual. Various aspects of the immune response (e.g., cellular vs. antibody) are not mutually exclusive, but the dominant response often partially down-regulates other responses.

After antigen processing by the initial phagocytic cell, the antigen is presented to T lymphocytes in a form which selects predominantly either a helper-inducer population (with CD4+ cell surface antigen phenotype) or a cytotoxic-suppressor population (CD8+ phenotype).

Viruses and cellular antigens on tumor cells generally invoke a CD8+ T cell-driven protective response which is cytotoxic for those tissue invaders.

Processed bacterial and other soluble antigens are more selective for CD4+ T cells which become helper-inducer cells as well as memory cells for either antibody formation or delayed-type hypersensitivity (DTH). IgG and IgM are most protective against high-grade pathogenic bacteria. IgA protects mucus membranes, and DTH responses are more effective in destroying intracellular organisms, fungi, and viruses.

CD4+ helper T cells contain two subpopulations, TH1 and TH2, which tend to be mutually inhibitory. This classification is based on the distinct patterns of cytokines which they secrete and by which they act. (Cytokines are soluble short-range messengers which many immune cells use to communicate and influence each other.)

TH1 cells are involved in DTH reactions and may be recognized by production of interleukin-2 (IL-2) and gamma interferon. TH2 cells carry out a helper function in antibody production by B cells. TH2 cells produce cytokines IL-4 and IL-5 among many others. TH2 cytokines are essential for heavy-chain switching by B cells, thus determining whether G, A, or E immunoglobulin classes will replace IgM production. The switch to IgE is regulated by IL-4 from TH2 cells and depends on the genetic capacity of the host as well as immunization procedures. When immunization procedures are changed to favor IgG production, IgE is usually down-regulated. IL-5, in addition to stimulating activated B cells, also stimulates growth and activation of eosinophils.

IgE

Network of Inflammation

TH2 cells which induce IgE production also enhance growth and differentiation of mast cells and eosinophils. In turn, mast cells and basophils stimulate TH2-dependent functions including IgE production. Thus there is a network of interacting T cells, mast cells, basophils, and eosinophils present in ongoing IgE-mediated reactions which initiates, orchestrates, amplifies, and prolongs the reaction.

In non-IgE-mediated mast cell-driven reactions many of

these interactions between networking cells apparently operate also, although the nature of initiating events is often less clear than when IgE is involved.

Associated Conditions

While IgE antibodies may seem of little positive value compared to other immune responses, they are produced in large amounts in response to parasitic diseases, such as intestinal worms and trichinosis, and help to limit or control these infections. High serum levels of IgE are often found in patients with these infections. Elevated levels may also occur in allergic patients, in patients with immune defects which impair suppressor cells, and in a variety of other less easily classifiable conditions.

Characteristics

IgE is synthesized primarily in those lymphoid tissues near the respiratory and gastrointestinal tracts. It has a molecular weight of 190,000 and is inactivated by heating at 56°C for 2–4 hours. Its production is under control of both suppressor and helper regulator T cell populations. After appearance in the circulation, IgE remains there briefly, having a serum half-life of 2.3 days. Thereafter, IgE attaches through the Fc portion of the molecule to specific binding sites on various cells.

Binding of IgE

IgE is a homocytotropic antibody, meaning that it will fix to the tissues of man and other primates, but not those of other species. This sensitizes the tissue for antigen-induced mediator release. The Prausnitz-Küstner (PK) procedure is performed by injecting serum that contains specific IgE antibodies into a skin site of a nonsensitive recipient, allowing time for fixation of antibodies, then injecting specific allergen into the site to demonstrate local skin test reactivity. During the first few days after serum injection, 95% or more of the IgE content leaves the injection site by diffusion. The optimum time for fixation of the remainder is 1 to 2 days. After fixation, IgE displays a high affinity for its binding sites on mast cells and basophils, with a tissue half-life of about 14 days. Skin sites passively sensitized with high-titered sera may remain so for months.

While IgE receptors on mast cells and basophils are of high affinity, there are low-affinity IgE receptors on B lymphocytes, monocytes, eosinophils, and platelets. These low-affinity receptors play an important role in the extended inflammation that may prolong acute reactions begun by mast cells. As mast cell products attract and recruit other cells into an inflammatory network, IgE production is enhanced and the activities of cell surface IgE receptors of both high and low affinity are also stimulated.

Other effector mechanisms of the cells that bear the receptors are activated when IgE binding to the receptors increases, thus promoting inflammation.

Mast Cells and Basophils

Triggering

IgE-mediated reactions are initiated by interaction of an antigen molecule with two cell-bound IgE molecules (bridging). (Alternatively in the laboratory anti-IgE may be used in place of the antigen.) This triggers degranulation of mast cells and basophils and production of inflammatory biochemical mediators. Additionally, mechanisms other than those involving IgE and IgE receptors can also initiate degranulation.

Cellular Characteristics

Mast cells and basophils both are derived from the same bone marrow precursors, but mast cells mature in connective tissues and are longer lived (weeks to months) than basophils, which mature in the bone marrow and live for days. Mast cells are normally found in all connective tissues, while basophils are recruited into tissues by immunologic inflammatory reactions.

Mast cells are especially numerous beneath the skin, in the respiratory, gastrointestinal, and genitourinary tracts, and in and around nerves and vessels. They are therefore situated near potential portals of entry for environmental invaders such as parasites, other pathogens, inhaled and ingested substances, stings, and bites. Mast cells in different anatomic locations may belong to different subpopulations. While all mast cells contain tryptase, those in the skin contain much chymase, while lung mast cells have little. Other physiologic differences have been described as well. Mast cells have been implicated in a variety of functions such as angiogenesis and wound healing, bone remodeling, tumor resistance, and an array of pathologic conditions, including peptic ulcer disease, atherosclerosis, inflammatory bowel disease, rheumatic disorders, and allergy.

Mediators

Mast cells and basophils release a similar but not identical profile of inflammatory mediators, and possess other similarities and differences in structure and responses. Both contain preformed histamine and other mediators in cytoplasmic granules which are released nonlytically from the granules during cell activation. Other mediators are newly generated by these cells at the same time.

Some of the known initial mediators from mast cells and

basophils include histamine, various products of arachi-donic acid metabolism (e.g., leukotrienes, prostaglandins, and other inflammatory and chemotactic factors), eosino-phil chemotactic factor of anaphylaxis (ECF-A), neutrophil chemotactic factor of anaphylaxis (NCF-A), kallikrein and other enzymes, adenosine, and platelet-activating factor (PAF). Various cytokines are also produced.

In addition to causing various kinds of inflammation, many mediators also participate in other important processes. Some appear to be part of normal regulatory mechanisms for glandular, vascular, and smooth-muscle function. For example, histamine is a controlling regulator of acid secretions by the stomach. It acts through cell membrane receptor sites (H2) that are functionally distinct from those involved in immediate hypersensitivity (H1) and thus are blocked by different antihistamine drugs.

Pathophysiology of Immediate Hypersensitivity Diseases

Terms

"Hypersensitivity" indicates an immunologic reaction that is harmfully overintense and often directed against an agent from which protection seems unnecessary. "Al-lergy," another term for hypersensitivity, was coined by Von Pirquet in 1906 from the Greek words for altered state of reactivity and refers to the hypersensitive state brought about by a sensitizing exposure. The antigens involved in allergic sensitization and reactivity are referred to as aller-gens. Many allergens are protein in nature, although simple chemicals and drugs may sensitize haptenically. Allergic or hypersensitivity reactions may occur through any of the four Gell and Coombs classification mechanisms.

Triggering Mechanisms

Immediate hypersensitivity reactions are initiated by phar-macologically active chemical mediators produced by mast cells and basophils. Several mechanisms can produce an immediate hypersensitivity reaction. The classic mech-anism (Gell and Coombs type I) involves the interaction of an allergen molecule with two specific IgE antibodies which have been fixed to the cell surface, thus sensitizing the cell. However, reactions that are clinically similar may be produced by other mechanisms, both immunologic and nonimmunologic, that do not involve IgE. Immunologically, subclass IgG4 has been reported to contain antibodies that can sensitize cells in a way similar, but not identical, to IgE

and to participate in allergic reactions in some cases. This mechanism of cytophilic IgG-dependent immediate hyper-sensitivity is probably of minor importance in humans. Additionally, when IgG and IgM antibodies activate the complement system (IgE does not), the fragments C3a and C5a which are produced are capable of releasing media-tors. These fragments, called anaphylatoxins, may also be produced nonimmunologically through alternate-pathway complement activation. An additional nonimmunologic mechanism, not involving antibody or complement, is via direct membrane activation. Some drugs act directly on the cell membranes of mast cells and basophils to release me-diators; examples include opiate drugs, polymyxin, thi-amine, and curare. When injected into the skin, these drugs will cause wheal and flare reactions similar in appearance to those produced by allergens in subjects with IgE hyper-sensitivity. These various mechanisms of mast cell media-tor release are depicted in Fig. 36-1.

Semantically, there is disagreement on whether all reac-tions caused by the mediators of type I hypersensitivity should be classified as immediate hypersensitivity, regard-less of whether or not IgE was involved in mediator re-lease. For the purpose of this discussion, they will be so classified.

Variable IgE Involvement

The immediate hypersensitivity diseases include allergic rhinitis, bronchial asthma, urticaria/angioedema, systemic anaphylaxis, and atopic dermatitis. Except for allergic rhinitis (by definition), IgE has variable involvement in these diseases; it is part of the mechanism in some cases and not in others. Allergic rhinitis has a nonallergic counter-part, nonallergic eosinophilic rhinitis, in which mediators are released nonimmunologically. When IgE is involved, skin testing is useful in identifying causative allergens as long as they are immunologically recognizable as whole allergens.

Atopy

Description

A familial tendency to develop immediate hypersensitivity diseases is often apparent. For example, respiratory allergy occurs in approximately 12–14% of offspring when nei-ther parent is allergic. When one parent is allergic, about 30% of the children will be affected, and when both parents have respiratory allergy, so will 50–60% of the children.

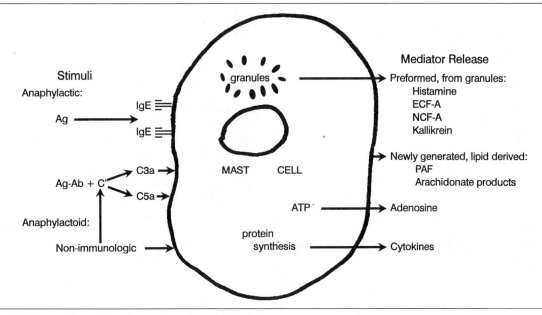

Fig. 36-1. Mechanisms of mediator release from mast cells.

This hereditary tendency to develop asthma, rhinitis, and other immediate hypersensitivity diseases was named "atopy" by Coca in 1923. Hereditary predisposition is most often seen in rhinitis, asthma, and atopic dermatitis, less frequently in urticaria and angioedema. The effect of heredity is poorly defined in anaphylaxis. It is unclear whether severe anaphylaxis, caused, for example, by penicillin or *Hymenoptera* stings, is more common in persons with other indications of an atopic tendency or not. However, it is clear that anaphylactic reactions are not confined to such individuals.

Basis

Atopic allergy affects 15–20% of the U.S. population. Some aspects of atopy are due to a propensity of affected families and individuals for producing IgE to common environmental allergens (pollen, molds, dusts, danders, etc.). The mode of inheritance for IgE-mediated disease is not yet clear. IgE production is influenced both by genes which control the general IgE response and by those which determine responsiveness to individual allergens.

When genetic influences are strongly at work, they tend to be most apparent in allergy beginning in early life. A study at the University of Iowa of 1125 consecutive patients with respiratory allergies illustrates this point (Fig. 36-2). IgE-mediated respiratory allergies began most com-

monly during childhood, and this was especially pronounced in patients with positive family allergy histories. Early onset also tended to favor greater numbers of allergic sensitivities. However, in this study as in others, it is clear that allergy can begin at any age.

High total levels of IgE have been shown to correlate with allergic immediate hypersensitivity disease. Numerous exceptions occur, however. Almost all normal persons have detectable, though low, serum IgE levels. As a group, atopic allergic patients have higher serum IgE levels than normals, but with considerable overlap (Fig. 36-3). For this reason, IgE levels cannot be used as a definitive test for either the presence or absence of atopic allergic disease.

Even when a hereditary tendency for IgE sensitization exists, its expression is dependent on other factors. Heavy natural exposure to potential allergens appears to favor sensitization. Also host factors such as diseases which impair the normal ability of suppressor T cells to downregulate IgE production may likewise favor sensitization. Clinical examples may be found in transplant and other immunosuppressed patients who develop drug allergy to unlikely agents.

There are additional hereditary influences to those governing IgE that operate in disease production. An example is asthma, which shows familial tendencies even when in-

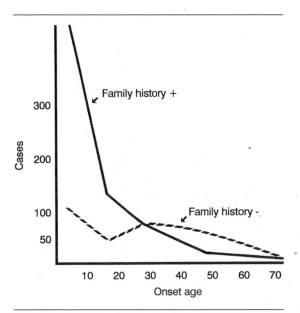

Fig. 36-2. Relationship of age of onset of respiratory allergies to family history. (Reprinted with permission from: Smith JM. Epidemiology and natural history of asthma, allergic rhinitis, and atopic dermatitis (eczema). In Middleton E, Reed CE, Ellis EF, et al. (eds.). *Allergy: Principles and Practice* (3rd ed.). St. Louis: Mosby-Year Book, 1988, p. 911.)

heritance of allergy is discounted. Currently atopic immediate hypersensitivity diseases are considered to result from both genetic and environmental influences.

Whatever the role of heredity, individuals who tend to strongly express immediate hypersensitivity reactivity differ importantly from those who do not. Factors favoring strong immediate hypersensitivity reactivity may include production of large amounts of allergen-specific IgE, along with the TH2 helper cell-associated cytokine inflammatory responses which stimulate mast cell, basophil, and eosinophil activity as already described. Other possible explanations include easier release of mediators and a greater responsivity to such mediators in subjects prone to immediate hypersensitivity reactions. Cytokines called "histamine-releasing factors" are among the regulators that govern immediate hypersensitivity phenomena. Additionally, the intensity of the reaction will be influenced by various circulating hormones and autonomic reflexes, which will be discussed in the next chapter. Studies of the factors that control immediate hypersensitivity inflammatory re-

sponses will be a rich area of scientific investigation for many years.

Mediators of Immediate Hypersensitivity Diseases

Early Phase

When an immediate hypersensitivity reaction occurs, the acute or early phase is caused by the chemical actions of mast cell mediators. Two main groups of mediators are produced within seconds to minutes from separate sources. One group is present as preformed mediators stored in cytoplasmic granules, while the other group is newly generated mainly from the phospholipid layer of the cell membrane. The major mast cell (and basophil) mediators are listed in Table 36-1.

Most of these mediators either cause inflammation directly or attract and influence other inflammatory cells to prolong and amplify the reaction. Some do both. The most active primary inflammatory mediators of the early, mast cell phase of immediate hypersensitivity which have been identified are histamine, various prostaglandins (PGs) and leukotrienes (LTs), platelet-aggregating factor (PAF), adenosine, and cytokines. The most active of the chemotactic principles are eosinophil chemotactic factor of anaphylaxis (ECF-A), neutrophil chemotactic factor of anaphylaxis (NCF-A), LTB4, PAF, histamine, and PGD2. Tryptase and PGD2 production occur during activation of mast cells but not basophils and hence may be used to differentiate between reactions driven by these two cell types.

As a mediator of immediate hypersensitivity, histamine was one of the early mediators to be associated with mast cells. It is preformed by decarboxylation of histidine and stored in the metachromatic granules of mast cells and basophils. Once elaborated it exerts brief, intense actions and is then rapidly degraded by tissue enzymes. Histamine is important in many immediate hypersensitivity reactions as reflected by the frequent usefulness of antihistamines in treating many of their manifestations.

Arachidonic acid is released from membrane phospholipids during mast cell and basophil activation and is converted into at least 20 products with a spectrum of actions, both inflammatory and chemotactic. Some are thought to be of primary importance in asthma. The precursors of PAF and arachidonic acid are attached to each other in equimolar proportions during membrane storage. PAF is generated from its precursor at the same time that arachidonate is made available for oxidation.

There is obviously much redundancy in the pro-

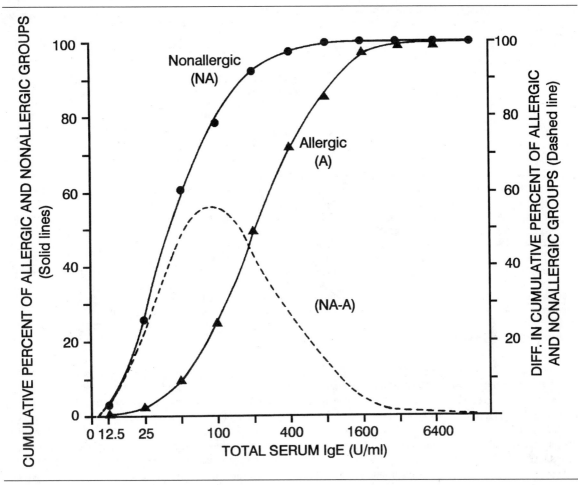

Fig. 36-3. Total serum IgE levels in allergic and nonallergic populations (solid lines) and differences in cumulative frequency between the two populations (dashed line). From: Marsh DG, Bias WB, and Ishizaka K. Genetic control of basal serum immunoglobulin E level and its effect on specific reaginic sensitivity. *Proc Nat Acad Sci USA* 71:3588, 1974. (Reprinted with permission of the authors.)

inflammatory effects of the various mediators, and it has not been possible to assign a pivotal role to any single mediator in production of immediate hypersensitivity. Rather, immediate hypersensitivity diseases seem to result from the combined effects of many mediators, which may be to some degree variably produced in different individuals, thus contributing to clinical variability.

Late Phase

Following a brisk, acute immediate hypersensitivity reaction, signs and symptoms often subside completely within several hours. In about 50%, however, the reaction may be prolonged or wane and then worsen again. This "late phase" of inflammation may be observed with skin testing, or following nasal or bronchial allergen inhalational challenge, or sometimes even with systemic allergic reactions. Its beginning is usually apparent between 3 and 8 hours after challenge.

The cause of late-phase inflammation is inflammatory cells which have been attracted by chemotactic materials elaborated during the early phase. A second wave of mediator release occurs during the late phase which does not in-

Table 36-1. Major Mast Cell and Basophil Mediators

Mediators	Actions
PREFORMED (GRANULAR)	
Histamine	Spasmogenic (for smooth muscle), vascular, glandular, chemotaxis, pruritus
ECF-A	Chemotaxis of eosinophils
NCF-A	Chemotaxis of neutrophils
Kallikrein	Kinin activation for vascular effects & edema
Neutral proteases (including tryptase*)	Degradative enzymes
NEWLY GENERATED	
Cyclooxygenase products of arachidonic acid	
PGD2*	Spasmogenic, vascular, chemotaxis of eosinophils and neutrophils
PGF2 alpha	Spasmogenic
Thromboxane A2	Spasmogenic, platelet aggregation
Lipoxygenase products of arachidonic acid	
LTC4, LTD4	Spasmogenic, vascular, glandular
LTB4	Chemotaxis of neutrophils
PAF	Platelet aggregation, spasmogenic, vascular, chemotaxis of eosinophils and neutrophils
Adenosine	Inflammatory, enhances mediator release
Cytokines: IL-4, IL-5, TNF	Promote IgE production & allergic inflammation

* Produced by mast cells and not basophils.

clude tryptase or PGD2; hence mast cells are thought to be no longer importantly involved. The cells initiating the late phase are mainly eosinophils, basophils, and often neutrophils at first with round cells adding later to prolonged or chronic episodes. The chemo-attractants most responsible for the eosinophilia in the late phase are ECF-A, PGD-2, and PAF.

During the late phase, basophils contribute many of the same mediators to the reaction as did mast cells during the early phase, excepting tryptase and PGD2. Neutrophils and eosinophils are rich sources of inflammatory substances such as lysosomal enzymes and, in the case of eosinophils, major basic protein (MBP) and other positively charged proteins. Granulocytes and eosinophils both generate additional arachidonate products.

In IgE-mediated reactions, low-affinity IgE receptors on eosinophils, macrophages, and platelets are thought to assist in inflammatory cell recruitment.

Significance of Prolonged Immediate Hypersensitivity Reactions

Late-phase reactions are more likely to occur after intense early-phase reactions than after weak ones. There is mounting evidence that these late cellular events contribute im-portantly to disordered physiology, particularly in the bronchial hyper-reactivity of asthma (see next chapter). During late phase (or chronic immediate hypersensitivity reactions) the inflamed tissues become hypersensitive to a variety of nonspecific minor irritants, making control of symptoms more difficult. Examples include magnification of symptoms caused by air pollution in allergic rhinitis or by exertion in asthmatics. Occasionally patients experiencing anaphylaxis who are successfully treated then relapse several hours later, probably due to late-phase mechanisms in some cases.

Most of the drugs used to control immediate hypersensitivity reactions do so either by affecting mediator release or by modifying the effect of mediators on target tissues, or by doing both. However, often drugs such as antihistamines and bronchodilators that are very effective in the early phase become less effective after late-phase cellular inflammation and edema have become established, while anti-inflammatory drugs such as corticosteroids become more effective.

Clinical Syndromes

Allergic rhinitis and asthma will be discussed further in Chap. 37.

Urticaria and Angioedema

Urticaria (hives) typically appear as pruritic, reddened cutaneous elevations that blanch with pressure. Individual lesions come and go, usually lasting less than 24 hours, and disappear without residuals. Histologically, small venules and capillaries in the superficial dermis are dilated, and localized edema due to vascular permeability is present. A low-grade inflammatory infiltrate may be present and tends to correlate in cellularity and composition with the phase and severity of the skin lesion. Such infiltrates tend to be sparse in comparison with more intense vasculitides. Urticaria and angioedema may occur separately or in conjunction with each other. Angioedema results from a similar process deeper in the dermis and subcutaneous tissues, swelling is more extensive, and erythema and itching are less prominent or absent. Sometimes resolution requires as long as several days.

When allergy is the cause, a food or drug is most frequently incriminated and is often obvious. However, in some patients hives become a chronic problem, and in this setting allergy is seldom found. Chronic urticaria can occasionally be linked to one of a wide array of conditions; these may include infections, other inflammatory processes including collagen vascular diseases, neoplasia, emotional stress, or exposure to physical agents such as heat, cold, water, pressure, or sunlight. However, more than 80% of the time no cause is ever found for chronic urticaria.

Anaphylaxis

A severe, often life-threatening, systemic allergic reaction, anaphylaxis may variably involve the skin (hives, flushing, itching), the gastrointestinal tract (nausea, vomiting, cramps, diarrhea), the respiratory tract (wheezing, upper airway angioedema), and the cardiovascular system (hypotension, arrhythmia). When anaphylaxis proves fatal, death is usually due to shock, severe asthma, or upper-airway closure. Allergies to a wide variety of substances through every conceivable route of exposure have been reported as causes. Drug treatment, especially with penicillin, is the most frequent.

In some cases, allergic mechanisms are not involved. Such reactions are termed anaphylactoid. An example is nonimmunologic mediator release that occasionally occurs following injections of contrast medium during radiographic dye studies.

Severe reactions caused by injectable medications usually begin within 30 minutes of injection, but occasionally ensue later. Food allergy reactions may or may not begin abruptly, but some more protracted reactions, which ultimately proved fatal after hours, have been reported.

Atopic Dermatitis or Atopic Eczema

A chronic inflammatory skin disorder that often has an association with other signs of atopy, it usually begins during the first 2 years of life and frequently remits by age 6, although it may either appear or remit later in childhood or adolescence. Occasionally it persists into adulthood and then tends to be lifelong.

Clinically, atopic dermatitis often affects mainly the antecubital and popliteal fossae, although the face and neck are not uncommonly involved, as well as other sites. Its usual appearance is that of a dry, scaly, chronic inflammation of the skin, which can become wet and oozing, crusted, and more inflamed when it is flared by scratching or secondary infection.

Atopic dermatitis is a problem in only a small minority of atopically allergic persons; however, the majority who have this skin condition will at some time develop asthma or allergic rhinitis and tend to be highly allergic. Controversy has existed for decades regarding the importance of IgE mediation in the development of this process. In many patients IgE cannot be incriminated. However, patients are occasionally encountered who appear to flare with exposure to food or inhalant allergens and recently renewed interest has been expressed in the possible role of food allergy in some children. Rigidly controlled clinical studies, including double-blinded food challenges, have confirmed that in some highly allergic eczema patients one or several foods cause an acute inflammatory dermatitis and a flare of eczema.

Regardless of the role of IgE, these patients tend to have dry, itchy skin, which itches even more after mechanical abrasion and ultimately thickens (lichenifies) from the inflammation caused by chronic excoriation. The self-inflicted trauma that actually produces most of the skin damage in these patients is termed the scratch-itch cycle. Therapeutically, measures to reduce dryness and itching, prevent scratching, and control inflammation are generally indicated and valuable. When food allergy as a cause of the dermatitis is identified, prolonged strict avoidance of the food is required, at the same time ensuring that proper nutrition is maintained.

Clinical Examples

1. A patient with known valvular rheumatic heart disease was admitted for treatment of subacute bacterial en-

docarditis caused by an organism that antibiotic sensitivity testing indicated would require penicillin for effective treatment. History disclosed an urticarial reaction to penicillin 10 years previously. Skin testing was carried out with dilute solutions of penicillin G and penicilloyl-polylysine (PPL) and was negative. Using the skin tests as the first dose, gradually increasing doses of penicillin G were given every 15 minutes until the patient was receiving 20 million units/day. On the third day, he developed urticaria which responded to antihistamines without cessation of penicillin treatment.

Discussion.   After a Type I allergic reaction to penicillin such as the hives which occurred 10 years previously, the levels of the IgE antibodies which caused it often decline over a period of years. The present reaction was caused by an anamnestic response of IgE antibodies directed toward penicillin or one or more of its metabolites. Such anamnestic reactions begin more than 48 hours after penicillin is started and are not rapidly life-threatening. Negative skin tests with penicillin G and PPL (which contains the major penicillin metabolite) predict over 95% probability against potentially fatal anaphylaxis within 48 hours of beginning penicillin treatment, while a positive skin test would indicate high risk for such a reaction. Penicillin G and PPL are unique among small-molecular-weight drugs (haptens) in being available as clinically useful reagents for Type I skin tests.

Anaphylactic drug reactions are common in persons without other evidence of atopy. Penicillin can also cause non-anaphylactic reactions; penicillin allergy by each of the four Gell and Coombs mechanisms can occur.

2. During an evaluation for hematuria, a patient underwent intravenous pyelography. After injection of the radio-iodinated contrast medium (RCM) for kidney visualization, the patient complained at once of itchy palms, then generalized pruritus. Hypotension, flushing, hives, and wheezing rapidly ensued. Injections of 0.3 cc of epinephrine (1:1000) subcutaneously and of diphenhydramine 50 mg intravenously caused rapid clearing of signs and symptoms.

Discussion.   This was an anaphylactoid reaction, not involving IgE or other antibodies. No skin test or blood test will predict RCM reactions, and test dosing has been tried without success. Standard RCM dyes release mediators in susceptible individuals. Significant anaphylactoid reactions occur in about 2% of RCM dye studies. If additional RCM studies were needed in this patient, the risk of re-reaction might be as high as 30%; risk can be reduced to acceptable levels by premedication according to a protocol containing corticosteroids, diphenhydramine, and ephedrine. There are also newer dyes, nonionic or lower in osmolality, which are safer for high-risk patients.

The acute anaphylactoid reaction was treated appropriately; epinephrine is the first drug to give when an allergic reaction causes hypotension or respiratory embarrassment. Mild reactions consisting of only hives may be treated with antihistamines alone. Corticosteroids, which were not given, do not benefit acute symptoms.

A reaction to RCM dye does not indicate allergy to iodine or seafood, which are "old wives' tales" often heard.

Note.   Because characteristic reactions to certain drugs are common clinical problems, protocols have been developed and tested for dealing with these problems with least possible risk. Published protocols deal specifically with penicillin desensitization and evaluation of reactions to aspirin, local anesthetics, ingested metabisulfites, and RCM dyes. Also more generic protocols for various drug challenges and desensitization procedures have evolved. The reference by Patterson is particularly useful for such problems.

Bibliography

Galli SJ. New concepts about the mast cell. *N Eng J Med* 328:257–265, 1993. *Role of mast cells in inflammation.*

Middleton E, Reed CD, Ellis EF, et al. (eds.). *Allergy. Principles and Practice* (4th ed.). St. Louis: Mosby, 1993, Vols. I and II. *Broad scope. In-depth, basic-science approach to allergic disorders.*

Patterson R, Grammer LC, Greenberger PA, and Zeiss CR (eds.). *Allergic Diseases: Diagnosis and Management* (4th ed.). Philadelphia: Lippincott, 1993. *Authoritative clinical allergy text useful for practicing physicians.*

Reisman RE and Lieberman P (guest eds.). Anaphylaxis and anaphylactoid reactions. *Immunol. Allergy Clin N Am* 12:501–689, 1992. *Common clinical problems including specific drug reactions.*

37 Allergic Respiratory Diseases

James H. Wells

Objectives

After completing this chapter, you should be able to

Apply the principles of Chap. 36 to immediate hypersensitivity diseases of the respiratory tract

Understand the application of the concept of mediator release to the development of allergic rhinitis and bronchial asthma

Understand the concept of bronchial hyper-reactivity in bronchial asthma

Apply the concept of early- and late-phase immediate hypersensitivity inflammation to asthma and rhinitis

Describe the heterogeneity that these diseases and their underlying pathophysiologic mechanisms display, as discussed in these chapters

Overview

This chapter deals mainly with airway disease in which eosinophilic inflammation is present and IgE-mediated mechanisms must be considered: allergic rhinitis and nonallergic eosinophilic rhinitis (NER), bronchial asthma, and allergic bronchopulmonary aspergillosis. In contrast, different findings and mechanisms occur in hypersensitivity pneumonitis, which is discussed because it, like bronchial asthma, is a respiratory disease in which extrinsic environmental antigens play an important role.

There are, however, numerous other diseases in which immunologic mechanisms produce injury to the respiratory tract, such as Wegener's granulomatosis, Goodpasture's Syndrome, various infectious processes, and many of the autoaggressive diseases. These will be dealt with elsewhere.

The Normal Airway

Structure and Function

The nose and the tracheobronchial tree may be viewed as a central duct system which during inspiration delivers air to the alveoli, where the pulmonary blood is oxygenated and carbon dioxide removed for elimination by exhalation. During inhalation, a vital function of this duct system is to serve not merely as a conduit, but also as an air conditioner. Inspired air must be properly warmed, humidified, and cleansed as it passes through these ducts to protect the more sensitive distal portions of the pulmonary apparatus.

The Nose

The internal nares are separated from each other by the nasal septum. Along the lateral walls, the turbinates are formed by bony ridges, which run from front to back. Except for an area of squamous epithelium near the external nares, the nasal mucosa is a pseudostratified, ciliated, columnar epithelium. The mucosa and submucosa contain both simple and compound mucinous and serous glands. These glands normally secrete as much as 1,500–2,000 ml/day, to form the mucus blanket that overlies the ciliated epithelium. The two-layered mucus blanket consists of a thin layer of mucin lying on top of a weak electrolyte solution through which the cilia project. Over the inferior and middle turbinates, the submucosa is vascular. The arteries and veins run parallel to the mucosa in the direction of the long axis of the turbinate. Between the arteries and veins beneath the respiratory surface lie a valveless network of capillaries and distensible cavernous sinusoids. The amount of blood in this plexus is controlled by arteriovenous anastomoses and by the tone of draining veins, which in turn are controlled by autonomic nerves and circulating hormones.

There is sensory afferent innervation of the nasal epithelium as well as autonomic innervation of vessels and glands, which have receptors for alpha and beta adrenergic and cholinergic agonists as well as histamine, other inflammatory mediators, and various hormones. It is also known that the nasal nerves contain neuropeptides along with the classical adrenergic and cholinergic transmitters; these neuropeptides also contribute to nasal airway control. Sympathetic stimulation constricts blood vessels, while parasympathetics induce watery secretion and vasodilatation of the microvascular plexus.

As air passes through the nose, particles are removed by becoming trapped in the mucus blanket. During normal nasal breathing, particles larger than 20 microns are virtually all removed from the air by the nose. The beat of the mucosal cilia carries the blanket posteriorly to the nasopharynx where it is swallowed, thus disposing of any entrapped materials. Heat exchange is regulated mainly by capillary blood flow, while the caliber of the turbinates is controlled by the amount of blood pooling in the venous sinusoids. When the turbinates are engorged, air turbulence is increased, thus facilitating heat exchange, humidification of the air, and removal of pollutants.

A "nasal cycle" occurs normally in most individuals, whereby the caliber of each internal nasal airway changes phasically in reciprocal fashion by means of shifts in vascular engorgement over the turbinates. This is under autonomic control and may be exaggerated in some cases of nasal disease.

A variety of other nasal reflexes has been identified. Some reflexes begin with sensory stimulation of the nose, then discharge through efferent pathways which produce sneezing, sniffing, salivation, laryngeal constriction, and even change in cardiac and pulmonary physiology, as occurs in the "diving reflex" with cold-water immersion. Others produce changes in nasal function due to recumbent posture, exercise, or various ambient climate conditions.

The Tracheobronchial Tree

The tracheobronchial tree is also lined with a ciliated epithelium, contains both serous and mucus glandular elements, and has an overlying mucus blanket. This mucus blanket also is carried by ciliary action toward the pharynx to be discarded. Because of reabsorption of water, only about 10 ml of mucus per day normally reaches the larynx. Many small particles which have escaped removal during passage through the nose will impact in the bifurcating bronchial tree during inspiration. The airway branches as many as 24 times between the trachea and the alveolar ducts. It is therefore unlikely for particles larger than 5 microns in diameter to reach the alveoli.

The walls of the trachea and large bronchi are supported by horseshoe-shaped cartilaginous rings. More distally, they give way to cartilage plates, which decrease progressively in size and disappear in airways with diameters of 1 mm and smaller. The airways also contain loose connective tissue and smooth muscle. The smooth muscle extends downward to alveolar ducts, and because of the concentric muscle fiber arrangement can cause airway narrowing and obstruction when it contracts. The bronchial tree is normally in a chronic state of very slight cholinergically-mediated bronchoconstriction which is considered to be the normal resting tone of the smooth muscle.

As in the upper airway, neurohumoral regulation of bronchial function occurs via autonomic and sensory nerves and circulating hormones. This is shown in Fig. 37-1. The parasympathetic cholinergic efferent nerves and sensory afferent nerves go to and from the lung via the vagus nerve along with nonadrenergic, noncholinergic (NANC) efferent nerves. The fibers of all these nerves innervate both large and small airway structures, including smooth muscle, vessels, and epithelium. Sympathetic efferent nerves mainly innervate parasympathetic ganglia in the lung and release norepinephrine to modulate their function. Sympathetic stimulation to the lung itself is via circulating catecholamines acting on adrenergic receptors which are found with increasing density out into peripheral airways. The beta receptors outnumber the alpha, and are of greater functional importance in control of airway smooth-muscle function. Beta adrenergic agonists exert a bronchodilator effect.

Neuropeptides are found along with the classical neurotransmitters in sensory, parasympathetic, and sympathetic nerves, as well as in NANC nerves. Some examples are shown in Fig. 37-1. VIP (vasoactive intestinal peptide) and PHM (peptide histidine methionine) are potential bronchodilators. Sensory fibers contain substance P, neurokinin A, and CGRP (calcitonin gene-related peptide) all with bronchoconstrictive, vascular, and other inflammatory actions. Populations of neuron systems contain specific combinations of neuropeptide transmitters, and the effects of nerve and reflex activation reflect the profile of classical neurotransmitters and neuropeptides released during depolarization. This net effect of corelease is termed cotransmission.

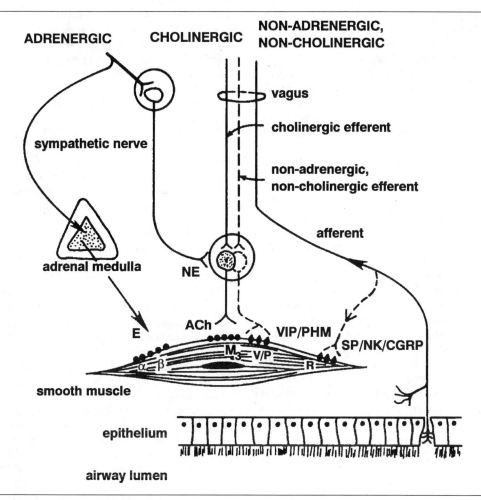

Fig. 37-1. Innervation of human airway smooth muscle. Neurotransmitters shown include epinephrine (E), norepinephrine (NE), acetylcholine (ACh), and neuropeptides (see text). (Reprinted with permission from: Casale TB. Neurogenic control of inflammation and airway function. In Middleton E, Reed CE, Ellis EF, et al. (eds.). *Allergy: Principles and Practice* (4th ed.). St. Louis: Mosby, 1993, p. 651.)

Irritative stimuli, such as noxious air pollutants or inhaled or endogenously released histamine and other inflammatory mediators, stimulate bronchial sensory nerves to initiate reflex responses. One example is the classical cholinergic "cough reflex" with efferent pathways via vagal parasympathetic nerves. This results in liberation of acetylcholine and various neuropeptides, which have also been identified in these nerves. These neurotransmitters act on receptors on glands, vessels, and smooth muscle in the airway. This produces glandular hypersecretion, hyperemia of the respiratory membranes, bronchoconstriction,

and cough, all of which are potentially protective against airway irritants.

A second type of irritant reflex is an axon reflex involving only the sensory nerve. When the bronchial irritant stimulus causes firing of an afferent sensory fiber, depolarization proceeds to a nerve fiber branch and then not only continues centrally, but also passes antidromically back along the other nerve fiber branch. When the sensory neuron depolarizes, its combination of several neurotransmitters will be released not only at central synapses and nerve terminals, but also at points (nodes) along the peripheral dendrites as well. This enables localized inflammation to spread to adjacent respiratory membranes up and down the airway. Since multiple mediators may be variably released, the result is an effect of cotransmission.

Neuropeptides have also been identified in eosinophils, mast cells, and other inflammatory cells. Once elaborated, they may serve as neurotransmitters, hormones, or paracrine mediators. Normally in the airway they contribute to regulation of airway function. However, when inflammation is present, neuropeptides along with classical neurotransmitters are capable of affecting inflammatory cell function and vice versa.

Associated Structures

The paranasal sinus ostia open into the nose. The middle ears communicate with the superior oropharynx by means of the eustachian tubes. Normally the passageways into the middle ears and sinuses remain open enough of the time that pressure inside these membrane-lined cavities can equalize with the outside atmosphere. During inflammatory conditions when the eustachian tube is persistently blocked by tissue swelling, oxygen reabsorption by the membranes which line the middle ear leads to a partial vacuum within the cavity, then to replacement of the vacuum with a serous effusion. Common examples of processes which lead to serous otitis media include viral infections and allergy. The ocular conjunctivae are also commonly affected by inflammatory processes which affect nasal membranes and may be considered to be part of the upper respiratory tract in this regard.

Mediator-Producing Cells

Mast cells are found in connective tissue throughout the body including the nasal and bronchial submucosa, and in association with blood vessels and nerves in both the nose and lung. Basophils and other inflammatory cells are readily attracted by mast cell products following mast cell activation. Mediators produced by mast cells and basophils were discussed in the previous chapter.

Allergic Rhinitis, Nonallergic Eosinophilic Rhinitis, and Asthma

Mechanisms of Inflammation

Eosinophilic Inflammation

These are all diseases in which eosinophilia is a hallmark of disease activity. In each condition increased numbers of

eosinophils may be identified in respiratory tissues and in secretions by their distinctive granules which take up acid dyes such as eosin. Eosinophilic rhinitis, both allergic and nonallergic, is generally associated with little or no increase in blood eosinophilia. Asthma is frequently associated with increased eosinophil levels in blood, and the magnitude of the blood eosinophilia tends to reflect disease activity.

As described in the previous chapter, the respiratory eosinophilia of these diseases is the result of stimulation by several mediators, especially ECF-A from mast cell granules, PAF from a precursor linked to arachidonic acid and coliberated with it from mast cell membrane phospholipid, and the arachidonate product PGD-2.

Variable Involvement of IgE

IgE-mediated allergies are present to some degree in about two-thirds of asthmatics. About 90% of patients with eosinophilic rhinitis (without asthma) are allergic, while the remaining 10% have nonallergic eosinophilic rhinitis, often referred to as NER. The diagnosis of NER is one of exclusion; it is made when a patient presents with rhinitis and nasal eosinophilia, undergoes allergy evaluation, and is found to be nonallergic.

Even in subjects with proven IgE-mediated allergies which are important in their disease, the degree of importance varies. In patients with strictly seasonal allergy, or allergy only to a pet, their disease causation may be virtually 100% allergy-related. In most affected individuals, however, non-IgE-mediated events, stimuli, and exposures can also provoke disease. An example is the effect of viral respiratory infections, which can provoke asthma in an allergic person. But in some nonallergic individuals, and even in allergic patients, the basis for some symptom production may be obscure. Thus to varying degrees there is an idiopathic basis for these inflammatory processes.

Regardless of whether IgE is involved in disease production, many aspects of allergic and nonallergic asthma and eosinophilic rhinitis appear the same. Similarities in histology, cytology, mediator production, reflex control, and functional changes indicate considerable overlap in the inciting mechanisms of these disorders.

Histology and Cytology

The sequence of cellular events during the progression of a disease episode has been studied with antigen challenge in IgE-sensitive subjects. An acute antigen challenge generally consists of inhalation of an aerosol of ragweed, grass, animal danders, or some other allergen solution, given to a subject who is not currently symptomatic. If the subject is allergic to the challenge material, over 90% will develop symptoms and functional changes referable to rhinitis, asthma, or both within seconds to minutes. Known as the "early phase," this initial acute response includes an increase in respiratory secretions and tissue edema in which no unusual cellularity is obvious at first. Tissue mast cells degranulate at this time, so they may not be seen but their products are present. During the next several hours an inflammatory tissue infiltrate appears which is reflected in about 50% of patients by the "late phase" of symptoms 3–8 hours after initial challenge. Tissue biopsies at this time contain many eosinophils, neutrophils, and basophils. All of these cells may also be seen in appropriate stains of nasal secretions. They are also present, along with the predominant alveolar macrophage, in bronchoalveolar lavage fluid. With repeated daily challenges, or during an allergy season, a pleomorphic inflammatory infiltrate will remain in respiratory tissues and secretions. It is characterized by an obvious increase in eosinophil content. Increases in basophils, mast cells, lymphocytes (including activated T cells), and monocytes are typically observed. Neutrophilia is often absent except after an acute allergen challenge.

In chronic asthma the subepithelial basement membrane is thickened due to deposition of collagen by myofibroblasts; chronic inflammation with eosinophilia persists, but granulation tissue and fibrosis or other severe destructive changes are not seen.

In patients dying in status asthmaticus after severe chronic asthma, there is edema and inflammatory infiltrate of bronchial walls, thickened subepithelial basement membranes, goblet cell hyperplasia, and hypertrophy and hyperplasia of smooth muscle and capillaries in the airways. Mucus plugs containing inflammatory cells occlude airways. Sputum may also contain Charcot-Leyden crystals from eosinophil cytoplasm, and casts of small airways called Curschmann spirals. The epithelium is damaged and has sloughed in many areas, leaving subepithelial tissues and nerve fibers unprotected. Denuded areas have been shown by special staining to contain concentrations of eosinophil-derived MBP, indicating a likely role for eosinophils in inflicting the damage responsible for the slough.

Mediator Release

Histamine is thought to be of prime importance in allergic rhinitis through its actions on blood vessels, glands, and afferent sensory nerves. The basis for this postulate is that many patients benefit from drugs that are competitive antagonists of histamine. However, as discussed in the previous chapter, other mediators are released and also contribute to tissue changes.

In bronchial asthma, histamine is only one of the important mediators, as evidenced by only occasional therapeutic response to antihistamines in asthmatic bronchospasm. Other important mediators of bronchoconstriction, mucus secretion, and bronchial edema include products of arachidonic acid. Many mediators have direct actions on target tissues, while the chemotactic mediators act through the cells they attract. Specific mediator actions were summarized in Table 36-1.

Neural Aspects

The fascinating interplay between mediator release and autonomic neural activity has been extensively studied in asthma.

With allergen challenge, mast cell mediator release initiates the asthmatic response. However, in addition to their direct inflammatory effects, many mediators (including histamine) initiate depolarization of sensory nerves. This triggers the various irritant reflexes previously described. The products of cholinergic efferent and NANC excitatory nerves have two important effects: one is to directly participate in asthmatic inflammation; the other is to enhance the release of inflammatory mediators from the cells that produce them. The actual extent to which the mechanisms of mediator release and irritant reflexes trigger and recruit one another appears variable in asthma and allergic rhinitis (Fig. 37-2).

Allergy-induced asthma, flares of asthma due to viral infection, and occupational asthma due to certain chemicals are examples in which inflammation is often intense, resulting in prolonged increase in asthmatic activity. However, asthmatics are also sensitive to inhaled substances which initiate responses via irritant sensory neural reflexes. Examples include inhalation of certain air pollutants, pungent odors, cholinergic drugs and histamine aerosols. These neurally-initiated bronchoconstrictive reflexes are generally acute, but engender little or no tissue inflammation and therefore do not induce prolonged asthmatic activity. However, increased inflammation from allergy, viral infections, etc. leads to heightened sensitivity and responsiveness of these reflexes.

Functional Changes

In allergic rhinitis the mucosa is swollen and congested. Its color is typically pale due to edema, and a bluish discoloration from stasis of blood in venous sinusoids is often seen. Excessive glandular activity results in hypersecretion of watery mucus. Additionally, many patients complain of mucus membrane pruritus and paroxysms of sneezing.

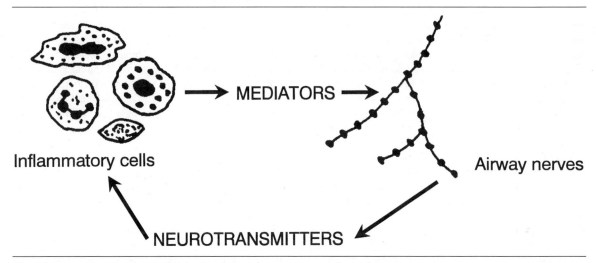

Fig. 37-2. Interaction between inflammatory cells and airway nerves. (Reprinted with permission from: Barnes PJ. New concepts in the pathogenesis of bronchial hyperresponsiveness and asthma. *J Allergy Clin Immunol* 83:1020, 1989.)

In bronchial asthma there is increased resistance to airflow due to smooth-muscle constriction, edema, and inflammation in both large and small airways. Hypersecretion of mucus occurs. During an attack, areas of the mucosa may be shed and the submucosa denuded especially in areas of high eosinophil concentration. Because of impaired mucociliary clearance, ineffective coughing due to bronchospasm, and mucosal dehydration, mucus plugs may form and occlude the airways. These events are reflected in wheezing dyspnea, which can be chronic and unremitting or (more likely) episodic and fluctuating widely in degree.

In mild to moderate asthma, pulmonary function testing shows airway obstruction which improves or normalizes within a few minutes of inhaling a beta adrenergic aerosolized drug. More severe asthma, especially if chronic, is often less responsive to bronchodilators alone.

As described previously in this chapter and the last, with deliberate allergen challenge (nasal, bronchial, or skin test) most allergic individuals react with "early-phase" inflammation, while about 50% also manifest a "late phase." Figure 37-3 shows typical biphasic airway responses of a patient with allergic asthma after inhalation of a pollen extract. An inhaled corticosteroid prevented the late-phase response but not the early.

Nasal Priming

If pollen-sensitive patients are experimentally treated out of season by repeated daily applications of a solution of the pollen to the membranes of the same nostril, the strength of the solution required to provoke definite allergic changes in that nostril becomes progressively less. A single control challenge to the other nostril (after repeated treatments of the first nostril) shows no corresponding elevation in sensitivity. This indicates that increasing allergic sensitivity brought about by repeated allergen exposures is to some extent a local phenomenon. The mechanism is thought to involve inflammation due to an extended late-phase allergic response.

Bronchial Hyperreactivity

An identifying feature of asthma is bronchial hyperreactivity. Even when their disease is quiescent, asthmatics will respond more quickly and vigorously to graded bronchoconstrictive stimuli than will normal individuals. Commonly used stimuli include exercise or inhalation of histamine, acetylcholine analogues, respiratory irritants, or allergens. Such studies may even identify pre-asthmatics. It appears that some degree of bronchial hyperreactivity is lifelong and probably genetic in many asthmatics. Figure 37-4 shows typical histamine inhalation challenge results in asthmatics with varying degrees of asthma severity.

There are also acquired aspects. Nonspecific airway reactivity tends to increase with repeated or continuing exposures to inflammatory stimuli, due to increasing tissue responses as already described. The duration of heightened asthmatic airway sensitivity after viral infections is often weeks to months. After heavy allergy exposure it may persist for days to weeks. After exposure to oxidative air pollu-

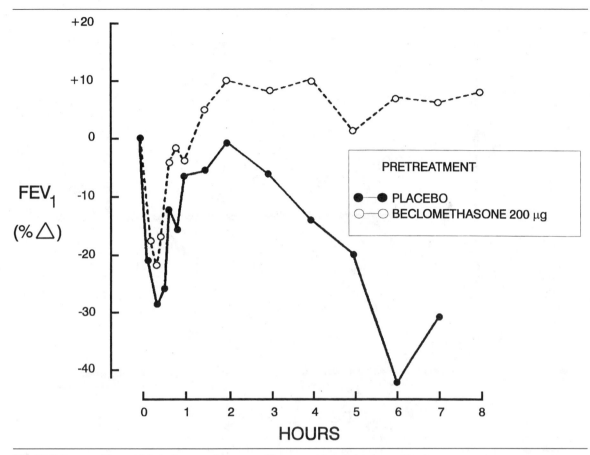

Fig. 37-3. Repeated bronchial challenges with grass pollen extract inhalation in an allergic asthmatic. Initially both an early and a late response occur (solid line). After pretreatment with beclomethasone, an inhaled corticosteroid, a late response is abolished but not the early response (dashed line). (Reprinted with permission from: Crockroft DW. The bronchial late response in the pathogenesis of asthma and its modulation by therapy. *Ann Allergy* 55:857, 1985.)

tants such as ozone and nitrogen dioxide, airway reactivity may return to normal in a few days. In contrast, exposure to sulfur dioxide, histamine, methacholine, or an exercise challenge will all cause an acute response but no subsequent increase in airway reactivity.

Changes in Pulmonary Function

During an asthma attack, deterioration in pulmonary function occurs that reflects increasing airway resistance, and this results in air trapping and hyperinflation. Thus, although vital capacity and air flow rates worsen, total lung capacity tends to increase due to elevation of residual volume.

Gas exchange is also impaired in asthma. Mucus plugging and bronchospasm occlude airways, impairing or preventing ventilation of alveoli. Since blood flow to these areas is reduced by reflex vasoconstriction, but does not stop completely, areas of low ventilation/perfusion ratios and shunting occur. Systemic arterial hypoxemia results and is a common feature of asthma. If shunting is widespread, the reflex pulmonary vasoconstriction it produces can lead to acute pulmonary hypertension. This occurs only in very severe asthma, which is also true of carbon dioxide retention. Typically, carbon dioxide elimination is not impaired, even though moderate to severe hypoxemia may be present.

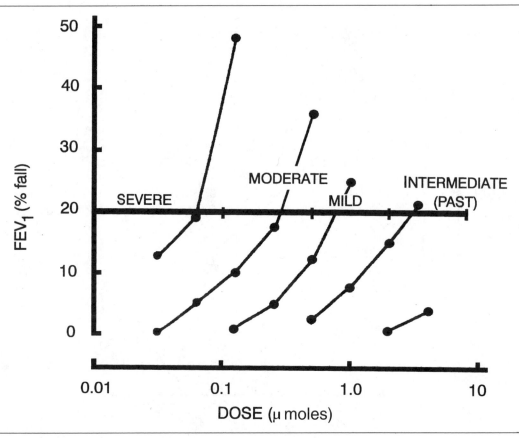

Fig. 37-4. Dose-response curves to histamine in subjects with severe, moderate, and mild asthma, in a subject with past asthma, and in a subject without asthma. (Reproduced with permission from: Woolcock AJ. Expression of results of airway hyperresponsiveness in airway responsiveness. In Hargreave FE and Woolcock AJ (eds.). *Airway Responsiveness: Measurement and Interpretation.* Mississauga, Ontario: Astra Pharmaceuticals, 1985, p. 80.)

Clinical Aspects

Epidemiology

Allergic rhinitis affects about 15% of the population. The incidence of asthma is about 4–5% and increasing. Approximately 30% of patients with allergic rhinitis give a history of asthma or at least episodic wheezing. Allergic rhinitis or asthma can begin at any age, but most patients have onset of symptoms before the age of 20.

Triggers

The most frequent causes of nasal allergy are seasonal pollens, airborne fungal spores, house dust, and animal dan-

ders. Only rarely does food allergy contribute to airway symptoms.

The majority of asthmatic patients are sensitive to these same allergens. This is especially true in children and young adults. However, production of asthma by seemingly nonallergic causes is also common. Viral infections, air pollution, and heavy exertion will frequently produce exacerbations. With increasing age, there is a general tendency for allergy to be less prominent and for nonallergic triggers such as respiratory irritants and adverse atmospheric conditions to be more important. A minority of asthmatics can have severe flares after ingesting aspirin and other nonsteroidal anti-inflammatory agents. Finally, in many patients, despite having frequent flares, the factor(s) responsible for exacerbations cannot be identified.

Occupational Disease

In highly industrialized societies, occupational respiratory diseases are recognized as an increasing problem. Many types can occur, including allergic rhinitis and asthma. Multiple potential occupational sensitizers have been recognized. They include such diverse agents as molds among handlers of organic materials, drugs and biologicals in the pharmaceutical industry, flour inhaled by bakers, and simple haptenic chemicals such as toluene diisocyanate where polyurethane is produced and trimellitic anhydride in plastic manufacturing. Respiratory disease with such agents is complex, and appears to result from immediate hypersensitivity, other immune mechanisms, primary irritant properties of the agent, or some combination. Variable individual susceptibility of workers is also common in industrial sensitization.

Diagnosis

The presence of allergic rhinitis may be strongly suspected from symptoms of watery, itchy nose and eyes, nasal congestion, and sneezing episodes. Asthma may likewise be strongly suspected in patients with episodes of wheezing, dyspnea, or cough.

In differentiating allergic rhinitis and asthma from other respiratory conditions, the finding that more than 15–20% of the cells in respiratory secretions are eosinophils during symptomatic periods is helpful. This does not prove an allergic etiology, but is rather a marker for mediator release.

With asthma, the history of fluctuating symptoms is also diagnostically useful, as is the bronchial hyperresponsiveness that is a part of this disease. Asthmatics will not only develop bronchoconstriction more readily than patients with other bronchopulmonary diseases, they will also show greater improvement in pulmonary function with bronchodilator treatment, unless severe asthma is present. Significant reversal of obstruction (15–20% improvement) by an inhaled beta adrenergic drug is consistent with a presumptive diagnosis of asthma. Provocative tests are occasionally used. Thus a patient with suspected probable asthma but with normal airway function can be diagnosed with probable asthma by a positive histamine, methacholine, or exercise-challenge test.

Treatment

Therapy of allergic respiratory disease begins with identification of environmental triggers and then counseling about how to avoid them, either partially or completely. Diagnostic tests for allergen-specific IgE may be useful in identifying agents to be avoided. Skin tests are more sensitive than currently available blood tests. Medications include antihistamines and decongestants for allergic rhinitis and bronchodilators for mild asthma. Aerosolized anti-inflammatory drugs are then added for resistant or more serious symptoms. Brief courses of systemic corticosteroids are indicated for occasional severe flares and are usually well tolerated acutely. Some patients with severe chronic asthma require chronic systemic corticosteroid therapy for control. In such cases, serious long-term side effects of steroid therapy may eventually appear.

With a sufficiently aggressive medical regimen, asthma that is not complicated by some other process is a potentially completely reversible form of obstructive bronchopulmonary disease. In severe asthma, however, a poor initial response to bronchodilator drug treatment reflects the importance of bronchial edema, inflammation, and mucus plugging in addition to smooth-muscle spasm. When bronchodilators alone are insufficient, corticosteroids are employed to combat inflammation.

Severe asthma that is unresponsive to bronchodilators is termed status asthmaticus and is a medical emergency. Respiratory acidosis with carbon dioxide retention is either present or will ensue unless vigorous treatment is successful. The onset of hypercapnia is a sign that overall pulmonary ventilation has been profoundly impaired. Carbon dioxide retention and respiratory acidosis herald impending death. Treatment by assisted ventilation must be considered as a life-saving measure at this point.

Allergic rhinitis or allergic asthma which remains troublesome despite reasonable avoidance measures and medications may be considered for immunotherapy. The latter is aimed at reducing specific inhalant IgE-mediated sensitivities and consists of frequent, regular injections of allergenic extracts. The allergen dose is gradually increased to a "maintenance dose" which is then continued at regular intervals. Treatment courses are typically given for several years and the majority of well-selected subjects report clinical improvement. The immunologic basis for improvement is not entirely understood, but it may relate to eventual reduction in allergen-specific IgE levels, an increase in allergen-specific IgG "blocking" antibodies, reduction in allergen-induced mediator release, and change in the allergen-induced pattern of cytokine release by TH2 cells away from an "atopic" pattern (see Chap. 36).

Allergic Bronchopulmonary Aspergillosis

This condition can occur as a complication of asthma. It is caused by colonization of an asthmatic patient's bronchial tree by the fungus *Aspergillus* and the subsequent development of hypersensitivity responses. This characteristically results in a marked increase in persistent asthmatic symptoms as well as transient infiltrates on chest x-ray, marked peripheral blood eosinophilia, fever, and weight loss. These patients have much higher total levels of serum IgE antibodies than are usually seen in uncomplicated allergic asthma. They not only have specific antibody for *Aspergillus* of the IgE class but also have precipitating antibodies that are usually IgG. In addition, cell-mediated immune mechanisms are suspected to play a part in the inflammatory response that often leads to bronchiectasis and pulmonary fibrosis. The main treatment is long-term corticosteroid therapy, which seems to eradicate the fungus by reducing production of the bronchial secretions that act as the growth medium.

Hypersensitivity Pneumonitis (Allergic Alveolitis)

Like bronchial asthma, hypersensitivity pneumonitis can be caused by hypersensitivity to various inhaled fungi and other organisms, organic dusts, and chemicals. However, more peripheral lung tissues and different mechanisms are involved. The prototype is farmer's lung caused by thermophilic actinomycetes in moldy hay. Many other agents have been implicated, and examples are given in Table 37-1.

Immediate hypersensitivity is usually not present, but precipitating antibodies are often demonstrable. Immune complex deposition and cell-mediated immunity are thought to be involved.

The reaction occurs 4–6 hours after acute exposure and consists of cough, dyspnea, fever, leukocytosis, and pulmonary function changes that reflect reduction in lung volumes and increased stiffness of lung tissue. With continued or repeated exposure, pulmonary fibrosis develops. When hypersensitivity is not intense, a chronic low-level exposure can result in the insidious development of pulmonary disability without other symptoms.

Clinical Examples

1. A 14-year-old boy came to the emergency room for treatment of an acute exacerbation of asthma. His mother reported a history of his wheezing in infancy with respiratory infection. Since the age of 4, he has had allergic rhinitis, which is worse in the fall of the year. At the age of 5, he began having wheezing episodes that were controlled by

Table 37-1. Examples of Hypersensitivity Pneumonitis

Exposure Source	Disease
Moldy sugar cane*	Bagassosis
Moldy hay*	Farmer's lung
Mushroom compost*	Mushroom worker's lung
Contaminated air systems*,†	Ventilation pneumonitis
Contaminated humidifiers*,†	Humidifier lung
Moldy cheese†	Cheese worker's lung
Moldy grain†	Malt worker's lung
Mold on redwood†	Sequoiosis
Moldy cork dust†	Suberosis
Moldy sawdust†	Woodworker's lung
Rats (urine protein)	Animal handler's lung
Parakeets (droppings)	Budgerigar disease
Oyster dust	Oyster shell lung
Pigeons (droppings)	Pigeon breeder's disease
Pituitary snuff	Pituitary snuff user's lung
Wheat weevils in grain	Miller's lung
Misc. chemicals	Various industrial and occupational diseases

* Thermophilic actinomycetes.
† Other fungi.

an inhaled bronchodilator used regularly in the fall and occasionally the rest of the year. The present episode began with fever and coughing 3 days previously. He was using a metered-dose inhaler containing a bronchodilator at excessively frequent intervals. He was constantly wheezing and very dyspneic.

Arterial blood gases on room air: PaO_2 = 52 mm Hg; $PaCO_2$ = 40 mm Hg; pH = 7.40. A chest x-ray was normal.

He did not respond to nebulized bronchodilators in the emergency room and was admitted for treatment with oxygen, fluids, antibiotics, bronchodilators, and corticosteroids. Gradual improvement began about 12 hours after admission.

Discussion.   Atopic allergy or asthma can develop at any age but usually this occurs by the age of 10. Although some children outgrow their diseases, many do not. This patient had asthma caused by allergic (at least during ragweed season in the fall) and nonallergic mechanisms (as with his current, probably viral, respiratory infection). This is common.

The patient had become unresponsive to bronchodilators and, by definition, was in status asthmaticus, a medical emergency. Overuse of inhaled bronchodilators commonly accompanies flares of asthma, as the bronchodilators become less effective. It has also been proposed that this overuse may contribute to the increased death rate from asthma which has been recently observed.

The patient's normal $PaCO_2$ was ominous. Earlier in the attack he would have demonstrated a low $PaCO_2$ due to hyperventilation. When seen, he was ventilating more poorly and was at high risk for rapid deterioration. Had that occurred, he might have required mechanical ventilation.

His asthma control will be improved in the future if he also regularly uses inhaled anti-inflammatory drugs as asthma preventives. Examples include aerosols of synthetic corticosteroids or blockers of mediator release, such as cromolyn or nedocromil.

2. A 50-year-old man with frequent bouts of asthma presented for evaluation of an unexpected severe asthma attack. His history included several decades of asthma and sinus disease, requiring regular daily medications and frequent antibiotics and systemic corticosteroids for flares. On the day of the visit, he had taken a proprietary nonsteroidal anti-inflammatory drug (NSAID). Within 30 minutes he noted acute rhinorrhea and nasal congestion, red watery eyes, and abrupt onset of severe dyspnea. He was treated with an epinephrine injection in a nearby emergency room and responded quickly. His examination revealed bilateral mucus polyps occluding both internal nares and diffuse mild musical wheezing in both lungs.

Discussion. Aspirin triad consists of (1) asthma, (2) nasal polyps or severe chronic sinus disease, and (3) severe flares of the asthma after ingesting aspirin or other NSAIDs. Patients at high risk for this disorder are middle-aged with chronic troublesome asthma. About half of such patients will react to an aspirin challenge with bronchospasm, which sometimes is life-threatening. Reactions occur within 2 hours, often sooner, and cross-reactions between aspirin and other NSAIDs with prostaglandin synthetase-inhibiting effects commonly occur. Cross-reactions due to other salicylates or acetaminophen are not likely. These reactions are biochemical, not immunologic in nature. Diagnosis is by history (as in this case) or by cautious, graded challenge with aspirin during repeated spirometric measures. Approximately 10% of all asthmatics react, children less commonly than adults.

Bibliography

Busse WW and Holgate ST. *Asthma and Rhinitis.* Boston: Blackwell, 1995. *Very comprehensive, particularly about basic-science aspects.*

McFadden ER. Evolving concepts in the pathogenesis and management of asthma. *Advan Int Med* 39:357–394, 1994. *Informative and insightful.*

Middleton E, Reed CD, Ellis EF, et al. *Allergy. Principles and Practice* (4th ed.). St. Louis: Mosby, 1993, Vols. I and II. *Broad scope. In-depth basic-science approach to allergic disorders.*

Naclerio RM. Allergic rhinitis. *N Engl J Med* 325: 860–869, 1991. *Up-to-date summary.*

Patterson R, Grammer LC, Greenberger PA, and Zeiss CR (eds.). *Allergic Diseases. Diagnosis and Management* (4th ed.). Philadelphia: Lippincott, 1993. *Authoritative clinical allergy text useful for practicing physicians.*

38 Systemic Rheumatic Diseases

Morris Reichlin

Objectives

After completing this chapter, you should be able to

Understand that systemic rheumatic diseases are mediated by autoimmunological mechanisms

Realize that there are autoantibodies that mediate tissue damage and others that do not

Know that some autoantibodies are specific for a single disease

Recognize that in ankylosing spondylitis, the central point is to try to understand how this Class 1 allele (HLA B27) is involved in disease pathogenesis

Realize that autoantibodies to RNA proteins in SLE partition patients into subsets with varying course and prognosis

Know that antibodies to aminoacyl tRNA synthetases are associated with both polymyositis and interstitial lung disease

Appreciate that limited and diffuse scleroderma have different autoantibody profiles

Understand that antineutrophil cytoplasmic antibodies (ANCA) are a feature of diseases with necrotizing vasculitis

This chapter examines a group of rheumatic diseases in which the primary tissue lesion is inflammatory but whose etiology and pathogenesis are for the most part unknown or only incompletely understood. Included in this discussion will be systemic lupus erythematosus, the seronegative spondyloarthropathies, scleroderma, poly- and dermatomyositis, Sjögren's syndrome, rheumatic fever, and systemic vasculitis. A separate chapter has been devoted to rheumatoid arthritis.

Invasion of joint spaces by micro-organisms and deposition of crystals in joint structures are well-known mechanisms of joint inflammation. Infection of joints is referred to as infectious arthritis; gonococci, pneumococci, staphylococci, myobacteria, and fungi are some of the better-known offenders. Gout is the most common condition in which arthritis is caused by crystal deposition in joints.

Neither of these mechanisms has been demonstrated to play a role in the inflammation occurring in the diseases under consideration. Attempts to recover micro-organisms from the inflammatory lesions in these diseases have given mostly negative results. Isolated reports of success have

not been confirmed even when attempted again by the same investigators. It is still possible that the inflammatory reaction in these diseases is due to direct tissue invasion by micro-organisms that cannot be cultivated by currently available techniques or to the dissemination of nonviable fragments of micro-organisms into tissues. Histopathologic examination of the inflammatory lesions in these diseases shows them to be comprised predominantly of varying mixtures of immunologically competent cells including T and B lymphocytes, plasma cells, and macrophages. It is generally believed that the tissue inflammation occurring in them is mediated by immunologic mechanisms.

There are several ways in which immunologic reactions can cause tissue inflammation, injury, or dysfunction. These include organ or tissue-specific antibodies, immune complex deposition with complement activation, and delayed hypersensitivity or cell-mediated immunity due to thymus derived (T) cells which become activated at the tissue site.

The chronic and aggressive nature of the inflammatory

reaction occurring in these diseases and the failure to identify any etiologic factor have led many to consider autoimmunity as a possible cause. Autoimmunity in the form of autoantibody formation is frequently observed in some of these diseases, especially systemic lupus erythematosus (SLE). Disease-specific families of autoantibodies are found not only in SLE but also in scleroderma, dermato- and polymyositis, and in Sjögren's syndrome. These autoantibodies will be described in this chapter.

A major question is whether these autoantibodies are only epiphenomena (a result of the disease or the generalized immunologic hyperactivity that is associated with most of these diseases) or whether they, or cell-mediated immunity with corresponding specificities, are the essential feature(s) of the disease mechanism.

Another problem is that most of these autoantibodies are not absolutely specific for the disease or manifestations of a disease in which they may have a role, nor do they occur in every patient with the disease. Many of them are present to some extent in a wide range of other diseases and even in presumably healthy individuals. However, it seems likely that either anti-native DNA antibodies directly or as DNA/anti-DNA complexes mediate the renal injury in SLE, and that IgG rheumatoid factors which undergo self-aggregation into complexes may mediate some of the extra-articular manifestations of rheumatoid arthritis and also contribute to the intensity of joint inflammation.

A frequently proposed concept of autoimmunity in the rheumatic diseases, which also takes into account that many of these diseases show a varying genetic predisposition, is as follows. As a result of some environmental insult, perhaps a viral infection, the genetically predisposed individual fails to eliminate the offending agent in a normal manner. A generalized immunologic hyperactivity results, perhaps enhanced by amino acid sequence similarity between the inciting agent(s) and self-molecule(s) (molecular mimicry), and possibly related to defective suppressor T lymphocyte function or polyclonal B cell activation (or both). The loss of normal suppressor function permits autoantibody formation to occur. Whether or not disease results depends on the antigenic specificities of the autoantibodies formed, the amount and type of antibody formed, and the avidity of the antibodies for their antigen. The antibodies present in a given disease may then have a variable relation to the disease. Some may be only a result of the disease or the immunologic hyperactivity; some may have a close relation to some etiologic factor or particular pathogenic mechanism, and then be more or less disease-specific, their detection being useful as a diagnostic test; others may be an essential part of the disease mechanism.

These concepts are applicable to all the systemic rheumatic diseases.

Seronegative Spondyloarthropathies

This designation includes ankylosing spondylitis, Reiter's syndrome, some forms of juvenile chronic arthritis, and certain other diseases. Some of these were referred to in the older literature as rheumatoid variants; ankylosing spondylitis was previously called rheumatoid arthritis of the spine. This view was considerably changed when it was found that most of the patients with these diseases were seronegative for rheumatoid factor. This has been reinforced by the finding that these diseases are strongly associated with the human histocompatibility antigen HLA-B27, suggesting a major role for genetic factors in etiology and pathogenesis. For example, 95% of whites with ankylosing spondylitis are HLA-B27 positive in contrast with a 7% incidence of this antigen in the normal population. These conditions are now considered distinct diseases, entirely separate from rheumatoid arthritis.

Ankylosing spondylitis is a chronic inflammatory disease affecting sacroiliac joints, spinal structures, and (less frequently) other joints. It is clinically recognized most often in young men; in its most severe forms, it can lead to complete spinal immobility and severe postural deformity. Reiter's syndrome is a symptom complex consisting of arthritis, urethritis, conjunctivitis, and mucocutaneous lesions. The disease often seems to be a consequence of certain infections such as chlamydial infections of the genitourinary tract, *Shigella* dysentery, and others (much as rheumatic fever is a result of streptococcal infections).

The synovitis in Reiter's syndrome is generally less cellular than in rheumatoid arthritis, but the synovitis in ankylosing spondylitis, when it affects peripheral joints, is similar to rheumatoid arthritis but with more tendency to extend to the capsule and periarticular structures. This was one of the reasons for its originally being considered rheumatoid arthritis of the spine.

The remarkable association of these diseases with the HLA-B27 antigens is the strongest disease association found for any of the histocompatibility antigens. A definitive explanation for this relation has been elusive. Some proposed explanations include: HLA-B27 itself or a closely linked gene product binds a bacterial or viral product and causes the disease; the B27 gene or a closely linked gene determines an inappropriate or inadequate immune response to some agent, and this initiates the disease process; and finally, the explanation for which there are now supporting data. There is, uniquely among the HLA-B alleles, sequence similarity between the characteristic B27 amino acid sequence and proteins of gram-negative bacteria. This "molecular mimicry" may give rise to a sustained immune response which is perpetuated by the presence of the B27 molecule in all tissues.

Collagen-Vascular Diseases

This designation usually includes systemic lupus erythematosus (SLE), polyarteritis nodosa (PN), dermato- and polymyositis (DM, PM), and progressive systemic sclerosis (PSS), also called scleroderma. SLE is a chronic disease usually affecting young women and characterized by multisystem involvement (arthritis, dermatitis, pleuritis, pericarditis, nephritis, cerebritis, etc.) and recurrent, often severe, febrile episodes. PN is also a disease affecting multiple body systems, with necrotizing vasculitis being the underlying pathologic lesion. PM and DM are characterized by muscle inflammation and degeneration, as well as dermatitis in the case of DM. PSS is characterized by thickening and hardening of the skin, plus fibrosis and degeneration of synovium, digital arteries, esophagus, intestinal tract, heart, lung, and kidneys. In the latter condition, fibrosis rather than inflammation is the dominant lesion.

These diseases are usually classified together as collagen-vascular or connective-tissue diseases. However, the original reason for grouping them together was that early pathologic observations suggested they were characterized by a common pathologic lesion widely distributed in blood vessels of the body which was fibrinoid necrosis or degeneration of collagen fibers. An underlying abnormality in the collagen fibers or connective tissues of the body that causes these diseases was suspected. However, despite extensive efforts, this has never been demonstrated. The connective tissues and blood vessels of the body serve as sites for the inflammatory and fibrotic lesions of these diseases, but otherwise appear normal. There are some other conditions, such as the Ehlers-Danlos syndrome or osteogenesis imperfecta, that are a result of molecular abnormalities of structural components of connective tissue. These latter diseases are more appropriately referred to as connective-tissue diseases.

Systemic Lupus Erythematosus

Antibodies to nuclear antigens are common in these diseases and are true autoantibodies; the nuclear antigens in-volved are of multiple specificities. The pattern of autoantibody formation in terms of the recognized nuclear antigens varies from one disease to the other. Accounting for this variation has an important bearing on attempts to explain these diseases as being autoimmune. For example, antibodies to single-stranded or denatured DNA occur in many chronic diseases and are likely to be a reaction to the disease. High-titered, high-avidity antibodies to native DNA are confined to SLE and often accompany and are believed to cause nephritis. Antibodies specific for nucleoprotein (DNA + protein) are common in SLE, are characteristic of drug-induced SLE, and occur with some frequency in rheumatoid arthritis. Their recognition is a useful diagnostic procedure, but their role in disease activity is doubtful.

As listed in Table 38-1, a variety of autoantibodies occurs in patients with SLE in addition to antibodies to DNA. Those with the highest specificity for the disease are anti-native DNA, anti-Sm, and anti-ribosomal "P" proteins.

Table 38-2 lists antibodies which are characteristic of SLE. As seen, none of them occurs in all the patients, although in some series antibodies to native DNA occur in as many as 90% of the patients. Most of these antibodies do not occur in other systemic rheumatic diseases, in normals, or even in first-degree relatives of SLE patients. In addi-

Table 38-1. Autoantibodies in Systemic Lupus Erythematosus

ANTIBODIES AGAINST CELLS AND PARTICLES

Red blood cells, lymphocytes, platelets, neural membranes, ribosomes, and lysosomes

ANTIBODIES AGAINST SOLUBLE SUBSTANCES

DNA (both native and single-stranded forms), gamma globulin, a family of RNA protein antigens (Sm, nuclear RNP, Ro/SSA, and La/SSB), DNA histone, RNA (both single- and double-stranded), cardiolipin, clotting factors, histones, and the ribosomal "P" proteins

Table 38-2. Characteristic Autoantibodies of SLE

Specificity	Occurrence (%)
Native DNA	70–90
Sm	20–25
U_1RNP	40
Ro/SSA	40
La/SSB	15
Cardiolipin	30
Ribosomal P	15

tion to the high-disease specificity of the autoantibodies in this table, they are also associated with disease subsets and are helpful not only in diagnosis but in identifying patients at risk for specific complications. These disease subsets are listed in Table 38-3.

As seen, anti-nDNA antibodies occur in acute, severe disease and are present in more than 80% of active untreated nephritis patients. Anti-nDNA varies with disease activity and failure of therapy to cause diminution or disappearance of these antibodies is a poor prognostic sign. These antibodies are concentrated in renal glomerular lesions of SLE patients and some mouse monoclonal anti-nDNA antibodies are capable of inducing the disease in normal mice. Much research is focused on determining the molecular features of those anti-nDNA subpopulations which are capable of inducing nephritis in mice and these, not surprisingly, are described as pathogenic anti-nDNA. These antibodies are diagnostically specific and closely associated with disease activity, especially nephritis, probably because they can directly cause tissue damage either by direct binding to cells or as immune complexes.

Antibodies to the ribosomal P proteins have received much attention not only because of their high-disease specificity but because of their association with neuropsychiatric disease. While they occur in only 15% of SLE patients, they are frequently, but not always, found in SLE patients who suffer from psychosis and/or depression. Recent work also suggests that in SLE patients with hepatitis where viral infection, drugs, or alcohol are not present, the majority of such patients have antibodies to the ribosomal P proteins. Recent work suggests a pathophysiologic mechanism for this hepatitis since the ribosomal P protein also exists in a membrane-bound form accessible for reaction with the anti-P antibodies.

While antibodies to the Ro/SSA and La/SSB antigen occur more frequently in primary Sjögren's syndrome than in SLE, they do occur in 40% and 15%, respectively, of SLE patients. Their presence is associated with a diverse array of clinical subsets, as seen in Table 38-3. Notable is a very strong association with inflammatory skin disease. This skin disease which characterizes subacute cutaneous lupus erythematosus, is also found in neonatal lupus, homozygous C_2 and C_4 deficiency, all of which exhibit a similar widespread subacute dermatitis in which characteristic annular and psoriasiform lesions are present in a photosensitive distribution. The morphology of the annular skin lesions is seen in Fig. 38-1. The fact that this dermatitis occurs in neonatal lupus, which is associated with the transfer of anti-Ro/SSA across the placenta, strongly suggests that the anti-Ro/SSA is the proximate cause of the skin disease. Virtually all patients with SCLE have high levels of antibodies to Ro/SSA.

A common feature of the systemic rheumatic disease is frequent overlap between and among the various individual diseases. Antibodies to URNP or U_1RNP are frequently present when SLE patients are found to have features of either scleroderma or polymyositis. Some scholars of these diseases designate these overlap syndromes mixed connective-tissue disease or MCTD, the major defining feature of which is the presence of antibodies to U_1RNP.

Finally, much attention has focused in recent years on patients with antibodies to cardiolipin (ACL) or other phospholipids. While 30% of SLE patients have these anti-

Table 38-3. SLE Autoantibodies and Associated Clinical Findings

AAb to	Association
nDNA	SLE and nephritis
	Acute, severe disease
Ribosomal P	SLE psychosis/depression, hepatitis
Ro/SSA and La/SSB	Sjögren's syndrome
	Subacute cutaneous lupus erythematosus (SCLE)
	Photosensitivity
	Neonatal lupus erythematosus (mothers of children with NLE)
	Homozygous C_2 and C_4 deficiency
	Interstitial pneumonitis
nRNP (U_1RNP)	Overlap with myositis and scleroderma
	Raynaud's phenomenon
Cardiolipin	Thrombocytopenia, recurrent fetal loss, and thrombosis (arterial and venous)

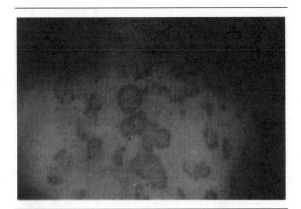

Fig. 38-1. Annular subacute cutaneous LE. The red rings of annular SCLE on this middle-aged man's back are merging to produce a polycyclic array. (Reprinted with permission from: McAuliffe DP and Sontheimer RD. In Wallace DJ and Hahn BH (eds.). *Dubois' Lupus Erythematosus* (4th ed.). Baltimore: Lea & Febiger, 1993, p. 303.)

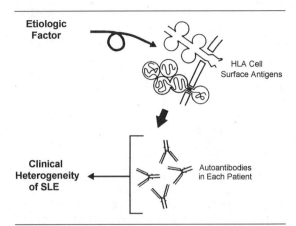

Fig. 38-2. Model for disease heterogeneity in systemic lupus erythematosus (SLE). The etiologic factor(s) of SLE potentiates a susceptible individual to express the SLE phenotype. Then the HLA composition or alleles at linked loci are related to the particular set of autoantibodies produced. The particular autoantibodies and their concentration interact in sometimes complicated ways to influence, at least partially, the different clinical manifestations found in individual SLE patients. (Reproduced with permission from: Harley JB et al. A model for disease heterogeneity in systemic lupus erythematosus. *Arthrit Rheumat* 32:826, 1989.)

bodies, the associated recurrent fetal loss, thrombosis, and thrombocytopenia are greatly enriched in SLE patients with antibodies to cardiolipin. When these antibodies and this triad of associated clinical features are present, in the absence of defining signs or symptoms of SLE, the patients are said to have the "primary anti-phospholipid syndrome." Many of these patients with ACL also have a lupus anticoagulant (LAC) defined by an inhibitor of in vitro coagulation tests not corrected by mixing with normal plasma. Thus we have the paradox of a lupus anticoagulant associated with a greatly increased prevalence of thrombosis. Biochemical studies have attempted to define the procoagulant activity of LAC but the mechanism is still obscure.

A model for the interplay of genetic factors, autoantibodies, and disease expression in SLE is depicted in Fig. 38-2. The essence of this model is that certain Class II MHC antigens promote autoantibody production by facilitating antigen presentation. These autoantibodies interacting with other factors, perhaps environmental, then mediate disease expression.

Poly- and Dermatomyositis

The inflammatory myopathies, PM and DM, are important and serious causes of muscle weakness although these diseases are uncommon and together have a prevalence of about 1:10,000. The characteristic features are proximal muscle weakness, release of muscle enzymes into the circulation, characteristic electromyographic changes, and a biopsy which features fiber degeneration, regeneration, and widespread infiltration of mononuclear cells. Although the clinical, pathologic, and biochemical distinction between PM and DM is beyond the scope of this chapter, the presence of a characteristic inflammatory dermatitis on extensor surfaces of the knuckles (Gottron's papules) and a violaceous discoloration of the eyelids (heliotrope) causes clinicians to diagnose DM when such features accompany the inflammatory myopathy. In recent years, a family of myositis-specific antibodies has been defined. These antibodies are highly disease-specific and define subsets within the polymyositis spectrum of diseases. The most common of these is antibody to the enzyme histidyl tRNA synthetase or the Jo_1 antigen. More than half of these patients also have interstitial lung disease and other features such as Raynaud's phenomenon and an erosive arthropathy occur commonly. This constellation of symptoms has been called the Jo_1 syndrome. In addition, autoantibodies characteristic of this syndrome have been recognized which are directed at components of the cellular translation system; the enzymes and particles which effect protein synthesis. How these disease-specific antibodies are related to the pathogenesis of the inflammatory myopathies remains unknown. That these antibodies are highly disease-specific and useful in diagnosis and disease classification is established.

Scleroderma

Scleroderma is a chronic fibrosing syndrome affecting the skin, lungs, gastrointestinal tract, heart, and kidney. There are two major clinical forms: diffuse and limited. Almost all patients (> 90%) have Raynaud's phenomenon usually early in the course, and affliction of the internal organs is much more common in the diffuse form of the disease than in the limited form of the disease. In the limited form of the disease, some patients develop a constellation of symptoms which is designated CREST syndrome for calcinosis, Raynaud's phenomenon, esophageal motility disturbance, sclerodactyly, and telangiectasia. Most scleroderma patients, whether diffuse or limited, have capillary dropout and dilatation which can be visualized by wide-angle microscopy of the nail bed. While the pathogenesis of this disease is obscure, it is widely believed that microvascular damage (exemplified by the changes seen in the nail bed) is an early and widespread event in the development of this disease. Also recognized in the past decade is a family of disease-specific autoantibodies listed in Table 38-4.

Two types of autoantibodies are characteristic of diffuse disease. These are antibodies to an enzyme topoisomerase I, which mediates unwinding of DNA. This antigen was formerly called scleroderma 70 related to its molecular weight used in Western blots for detection of this antibody. Sera containing this antibody produce a speckled pattern of nuclear fluorescence. There is also a series of nucleolar antigens which are targets of autoantibodies found in scleroderma sera. Although sophisticated biochemical tests are required to define the precise antigenic specificity of such sera, a high-titered nucleolar antibody titer in association with the features of scleroderma strongly supports the clinical diagnosis of this condition.

Antibodies to the centromere antigen(s) visualized on the chromosomes of dividing cells are highly characteristic of limited scleroderma and occur in more than 80% of such patients.

It is now known that these antibodies, especially those directed against the centromere, occur years before the onset of clinical symptoms and are therefore not the result of the disease per se. What role, if any, these antibodies play in the pathogenesis of the microvascular injury or the tendency to deposit collagen in affected tissues is unknown. It is conceivable that even if they play no role in pathogenesis, these autoantibodies may be a marker for etiological or disease-specific pathogenetic events in scleroderma.

Sjögren's Syndrome

Sjögren's syndrome is a clinical triad consisting of dry eyes (keratoconjunctivitis sica), dry mouth (xerostomia), and a connective-tissue disease, usually rheumatoid arthritis. The pathology of the disease is characterized by dense infiltration of affected organs by mononuclear cells composed primarily of lymphocytes, with some plasma cells and histiocytes. Two forms of the disease exist: primary, in which no connective tissue disease is present, and secondary, in which the dry eyes and mouth are accompanied by either rheumatoid arthritis, PSS, SLE, or PM.

It has been recognized in recent years that many organs in addition to the lacrimal and salivary glands are infiltrated by mononuclear cells. Thus there may be lymphadenopathy, splenomegaly, pulmonary infiltrates, and various renal lesions, but principally renal tubular acidosis, interstitial nephritis, and (less frequently) glomerulonephritis. There is also a remarkable frequency of nonthrombocytopenic purpura, vascular ulcers, peripheral neuropathy of the mononeuritis multiplex type, and even central nervous system involvement. This central nervous system disease is much more frequent and serious than previously recognized and may take numerous clinical forms. Among these are dementia, stroke, cerebellar degeneration, a multiple sclerosis-type picture, psychosis, depression, and gross disturbances in cognitive function.

Aside from the obvious association with connective-tissue diseases, all of which are thought to have autoimmune features, there is an impressive array of autoantibodies in

Table 38-4. Scleroderma-Specific Antibodies

Specificity	% Positive	Clinical Subset
Scleroderma 70 or topoisomerase I	20	Diffuse scleroderma
Various nucleolar antigens (RNA polymerase I, fibrillarin, Nor 90)	25	Diffuse scleroderma
Centromere	80–90	Limited scleroderma

this disease. Rheumatoid factors occur in 90–95% of both primary and secondary Sjögren's syndrome. Hyperglobulinemia is the rule; antinuclear factors occur in 50–60% of these patients, and precipitating antibodies to Ro/SSA and La/SSB occur in 60 and 30%, respectively, in Sjögren's syndrome. With sensitive ELISA methods, even more patients with Sjögren's syndrome have elevated levels of anti-Ro/SSA and anti-La/SSB antibodies.

As previously stated, these antibodies also occur in a proportion of SLE patients and, not surprisingly, almost all patients with both SLE and Sjögren's have these antibodies in high titer. While the etiology of Sjögren's syndrome remains obscure, genetic factors play a role, perhaps in controlling the production of autoantibodies. The DR3 antigen is greatly enriched in these patients and DQ1/DQ2 heterozygosity is strongly associated with high levels of both anti-Ro/SSA and anti-La/SSB antibodies.

Rheumatic Fever

Rheumatic fever is clearly caused by group A streptococcal infections. Bacteriologic or serologic evidence of preceding streptococcal infection is invariably present in cases of rheumatic fever; prevention of streptococcal infections by prophylactic use of penicillin prevents rheumatic fever. The pathogenesis of the disease, however, remains unsettled. The streptococci possess antigens that cross-react with human heart muscle. Infection with these organisms does cause formation of antibodies reactive with human heart muscle, and this could explain the myocarditis of rheumatic fever but not the valvulitis. Deposition of immune complexes containing streptococcal antigens or tissue antigens has been suggested as a possible mechanism for the valvulitis. Rheumatic fever is a rarely made diagnosis at the present time, in sharp contrast with its wide prevalence in years up to and including World War II. Apparently, widespread use of antibiotics has altered its incidence. Recently, sporadic outbreaks of this disease have appeared once more.

Vasculitis and ANCA

There are a series of clinical syndromes in which necrotizing vasculitis is the underlying pathologic lesion. The vessels involved may be as large as muscular arteries or as small as capillaries, but the unifying feature is an inflammatory destruction of the vessel wall with occlusion. When the vasculitis affects the skin, hemorrhage into the skin is a common and diagnostic feature, especially when the platelet count is normal and no bleeding diathesis is present. The inflammatory infiltrate may be neutrophilic, mononuclear, or granulomatous. It has long been known that "vasculitis" can be caused by immune complex deposition with complement activation; and when these are demonstrated by direct immunofluorescence of the tissue lesion, the pathogenesis of those lesions is understood. Such a mechanism underlies the vasculitis of patients with systemic lupus erythematosus, rheumatoid vasculitis, mixed cryoglobulinemia, many cases of hypersensitivity angiitis, and some cases of polyarteritis nodosa. This is almost always the case in cases of polyarteritis nodosa which are associated with hepatitis B and C infection.

There is a group of patients with vasculitis who do not have immune complexes deposited in the lesions but who do have antineutrophil cytoplasm autoantibodies or ANCA. There are two types of ANCA specificities based on their immunofluorescent pattern on alcohol-fixed human neutrophils as seen in Fig. 38-3. In one pattern, the cytoplasm is stained; this is called cANCA and the antigenic target has been identified as Proteinase 3. In a second pattern, there is a perinuclear redistribution of the cytoplasmic enzymes myeloperoxidase and elastase and is called pANCA.

Autoantibodies of these two types have different clinical associations, and their description follows. Wegener's granulomatosis is a vasculitis leading to sinus, pulmonary, and renal disease. Immunoglobulins are not found in the vascular lesions found in the lung and kidney, but 90% or more of such patients, when active and untreated, have a

Fig. 38-3. Indirect immunofluorescence microscopy detection of cANCA (A) and pANCA (B) using alcohol-fixed neutrophils. (Reproduced with permission from: Jennette JC and Falk RJ. Antineutrophil cytoplasmic autoantibodies and associated diseases. *Am J Kidney Dis* 15:517, 1990.)

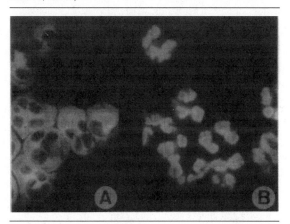

positive cANCA. In some patients with Wegener's, the cANCA titer varies with disease activity; in others, it does not. About 20% of Wegener's patients are also positive for pANCA. Other diseases in which cANCA is frequently positive are polyarteritis nodosa and the Churg Strauss syndrome. In Churg Strauss syndrome, there is granulomatosis involvement of vessels in skin and nerves in more than half the cases but almost uniform involvement of the lungs with asthma and eosinophilia. The major pANCA positive disease is cresentic glomerulo-nephritis in which rapidly progressive renal disease is the major finding and pANCA is more frequent than cANCA. A positive pANCA is found in low frequency in all the vasculitides and lacks the high specificity that cANCA has for Wegener's granulomatosis.

The pathogenesis of ANCA-associated diseases is visualized as follows. It has been shown that p or cANCA reacts with neutrophils activated by various cytokines such as tumor necrosis factor (TNF) or interleukin-1 (IL-1). Such bound ANCA causes neutrophils to undergo a respiratory burst and release toxic oxygen species which cause tissue damage. These activated neutrophils with bound ANCA also degranulate, releasing their lysosomal enzymes which can also mediate tissue damage. While this mechanism has been shown to be operative in vitro, more work is needed to establish whether this represents the in vivo pathway of pathogenesis.

Notwithstanding, recognition of these autoantibodies has provided new tools for the diagnosis and care of patients with the vasculitis syndromes described which heretofore could be diagnosed only on clinical findings supplemented by tissue biopsy.

Clinical Example

1. A 19-year-old white female presented with a 3-month history of pain in her hands, wrists, elbows, and shoulders. She also had noted some swelling in her wrists and the large knuckles of her hands and was stiff for 1 hour upon arising. She also had sharp pain on deep inspiration in her left lateral chest which has been intermittently present the past 3 days. Finally, she has had some redness over her nose and upper cheeks which began after spending a day at the beach one week ago. Her physical exam showed her to be well developed, well nourished, and in no distress. The positive findings on her physical exam were swollen, tender metacarpophalangeal and interphalangeal joints in both hands; both wrists were boggy, tender, and restricted to 45 degrees of flexion and extension. Her scalp and hair were normal. She had an erythematosus rash over the bridge of her nose and upper cheeks (malar) in the shape of a butter-

fly. There was no atrophy or scaling. Her chest and heart exam were completely normal and no rubs were heard. Her lab work showed a normal CBC and urinalysis except that her total white blood count was 3500/cumm and her absolute lymphocyte count was 900/cumm. Further studies showed a Westergren erythrocyte sedimentation rate of 90/mm/hr, a positive ANA of 1:3240 with a nuclear homogenous pattern, a positive anti-nDNA by Crithidia of 1:30, normal complement levels, and her rheumatoid factor was negative. A chest x-ray was normal.

She was treated with hydroxychloroquine and Naproxen and had a satisfactory resolution of her symptoms.

Discussion. The combination of a photosensitive dermatitis, symmetrical polyarthritis, leukopenia, a positive ANA, and a positive anti-nDNA establish a diagnosis of systemic lupus erythematosus. There was also a suggestion of pleuritis, but the absence of a rub and a normal chest x-ray leave the nature of her chest pain still unknown. The presence of both granulocytopenia and lymphopenia is also suggestive of SLE. The absence of rheumatoid factor and the presence of a rash make the diagnosis of rheumatoid arthritis unlikely. Also, anti-nDNA is not found in patients with rheumatoid arthritis.

Bibliography

Kelley WN, Harris ED, Ruddy S, and Sledge CB (eds.). *Textbook of Rheumatology* (4th ed.). Philadelphia: Saunders, 1990. *Major American textbook with excellent coverage (see relevant chapters) of polymyositis, dermatomyositis, scleroderma, vasculitis, Sjögren's syndrome, and antiphospholipid syndrome.*

Koopman WJ and McCarty DJ (eds.). *Arthritis and Allied Conditions* (12th ed.). Philadelphia: Lea & Febiger, 1993. *Chapters 68, 70, 73, 74, 75, and 78 provide excellent information on polymyositis, dermatomyositis, scleroderma, vasculitis, Sjögren's syndrome, and antiphospholipid syndrome.*

Reichlin M. Disease specific autoantibodies in the systemic rheumatic diseases. In Rose N and Mackay I (eds.). *The Autoimmune Diseases.* London: Academic, 1992. Vol. II, pp. 195–209. *Reviews the disease-specific antibodies of systemic lupus erythematosus, systemic scleroderma, polymyositis, dermatomyositis, and Sjögren's syndrome.*

Wallace DJ and Hahn BH (eds.). *Dubois' Lupus Erythematosus.* Philadelphia: Lea & Febiger, 1993. *Covers every aspect of systemic lupus erythematosus. Chapters 6–13 (on immunologic abnormalities) provide especially good reviews of pathophysiology of autoimmune diseases.*

39 Immunodeficiency

Samuel R. Oleinick

Objectives

After completing this chapter, you should be able to

Identify lymphocyte cell surface markers and cell membrane receptors

Understand mechanisms for leukocyte adhesiveness and communication

Enumerate the different cytokines and their action in regulating the immune response

Relate deficiencies of complement components and regulatory proteins to specific immune deficiency disorders

Identify the common congenital immunodeficiencies and describe the genetic defects

Become familiar with aspects of common variable immunodeficiency

Appreciate the spectrum of secondary immunodeficiency diseases, including AIDS

Develop an approach to the clinical investigation and diagnosis of patients with immunodeficiency disorders

Understand laboratory studies to document immunodeficiency

Appreciate the expanding array of therapeutic interventions for specific immunodeficiency diseases

Overview

Organization of the immune system (innate and adaptive) is explicated in Chap. 35. The morphology and function of the cellular components of immunity are also discussed in Chap. 31. Proper functioning of these mechanisms provides protection against the onslaught of infective microorganisms and endogenously arising malignant cells. This present chapter will concern itself with congenital and acquired deficiencies of the immune mechanism, identify wherever known the molecular basis for the dysfunction, and describe the consequences to the afflicted patient.

Lymphocyte Markers

An understanding of lymphocyte markers is necessary to comprehend many of the immune deficiency states and to become familiar with the laboratory tests currently available or under development which are utilized for clinical diagnosis of immunodeficiency.

Cell Surface Markers

A number of markers identify the various lymphocyte subclasses. Immunoglobulins on the lymphocyte surface identify B lymphocytes. These immunoglobulins are antigen receptors. B lymphocytes give rise to the antibody-generating plasma cell lineage. Class II transplantation antigens (HLA-D/DR/DQ/DP or Ia antigens) are present on mature B cells, but they also can be found on some monocytes and on activated T cells. B lymphocytes can also be identified by certain CD (CD = cluster of differentiation or cluster designation) markers on their plasma membranes such as CD19 and CD20.

The various T lymphocyte subclasses can be recognized by using monoclonal antibodies to various surface markers appearing on the specific T cells. Monoclonal antibodies can recognize CD3+ cells (all T cells). Other such antibodies identify CD4+ cells (helper cells) and CD8+ cells (cytotoxic/suppressor cells). There are also monoclonal antibodies identifying monocyte surface antigens, and others which can discriminate NK cell surface antigens. Table

39-1 lists significant CD molecules which can be identified on leukocyte surfaces.

Lymphocyte Membrane Receptors

Most mature B cells have complement receptors. A proportion of B cells have receptors for the Fc portion of IgG, for mouse red blood cells, or for Epstein-Barr virus on their surface. Most T cells have a receptor (CD2) for sheep red cells on their surface. Distinct subpopulations of T cells have a receptor for the Fc portion of bovine IgG (T gamma cells) or a receptor for the Fc portion of bovine IgM (T mu cells), respectively. T lymphocytes also demonstrate antigen-specific receptors on their surfaces. The T cell receptor for antigen is a double-chain (alpha/beta or gamma/delta) structure whose variable regions are complementary to peptide antigens. These alpha/beta or gamma/delta chains are linked to the invariant CD3 molecule forming a trimolecular complex. T cells also have a receptor for the T cell-secreted growth factor, interleukin-2 (IL-2). Null (K) cells have a receptor for the Fc portion of IgG.

Intercellular Adhesiveness and Communication

Certain bimolecular heterodimer complexes, **integrins,** occur on leukocytes. They bind to counter-receptors on other leukocytes and on vascular endothelial cells. These complexes facilitate cell-cell adhesiveness. If lymphocyte-monocyte or lymphocyte-lymphocyte binding occurs through this pairing, signal transduction and cell differentiation or activation can ensue. In the interaction between T lymphocytes and antigen-presenting cells, these interactions provide costimulating signals which supplement the cell stimulation signals generated by the interaction of the T cell receptor and CD4 or CD8 molecules with the antigen-MHC complex. Thus these interactions can be seen to be of great importance in the generation of immune responses. If integrins bind to adhesion molecules or to selectins on vascular endothelial cells, homing of lymphocytes to areas of inflammation or to lymphoid organs is facilitated.

Counter-receptors for these integrins are intercellular **adhesion molecules** which are members of the immunoglobulin gene superfamily and share domains with immunoglobulins. These adhesion molecules occur on vascular endothelial cells and on mononuclear cells (antigen-presenting cells). The major adhesion molecules of the immunoglobulin supergene family are ICAM-1 (intercellular adhesion molecule 1 = CD54), ICAM-2, ICAM-3, and VCAM-1 (vascular cell adhesion molecule 1). The integrin LFA-1 binds to ICAM-1 and the integrin VLA-4 binds to VCAM-1. CD2 on T lymphocytes and LFA-3 (CD58) on monocytes and lymphocytes are also members of the immunoglobulin supergene family and are another set of receptors and counter-receptors. Table 39-2 enumer-

Table 39-1. Significant CD Molecules on Leukocyte Surfaces

CD2	All T cells; acts as sheep cell rosette receptor; acts as ligand for LFA-3 on antigen presenting cells
CD3	Component of TCR for antigen recognition
CD4	Marker for helper/inducer T cells; interacts with TCR-antigen-MHC II complex; receptor for HIV
CD8	Marker for suppressor/cytotoxic T cells, interacts with TCR-antigen-MHC I complex of molecules
CD10	Pre-B cells marker; common acute lymphoblastic leukemia antigen (CALLA); also present on granulocytes
CD11	Three forms:
	CD11a Alpha chain of the integrin LFA-1 on leukocytes
	CD11b Alpha chain of CR3 on many different leukocytes
	CD11c Alpha chain of CR4 on many different leukocytes
CD18	Beta chain of all three different CD11 adhesion molecules
CD19	Mature B cells
CD21	CR2 on B cells; EBV receptor
CD25	IL-2 receptor on activated T and B cells and on macrophages
CD34	Hematopoietic stem cells
CD35	CR1 on phagocytic cells
CD44	Ligand on T cells for surface-bound invariant chain (Ii) which appears on antigen-presenting cells
CD45RA	Marker of "naive" CD4 and CD8 T cells
CD45RO	Marker of "memory" CD4 and CD8 T cells

CD=cluster of differentiation; LFA=lymphocyte function associated antigen; TCR=T cell receptor; CR1, CR2, CR3, CR4=complement receptors; MHC=major histocompatibility antigen; HIV=human immunodeficiency virus; EBV=Epstein-Barr virus; IL-2=interleukin-2.

Table 39-2. Costimulatory Signals Between Antigen-Presenting Cells (APC) and T Cells

On T Cell	On APC Cell
TCR Complex Plus CD4 or CD8	Antigen Complexed to Class I or Class II MHC Molecule
CD28 or CTLA-4	B7-1 (CD80); B7-2 (CD86)
LFA-1	ICAM-1, ICAM-2, or ICAM-3
CD2	LFA-3
VLA-4	VCAM-1
Receptor?	HSA

MHC=major histocompatibility complex molecule; CTLA=cytolytic T-lymphocyte associated antigen; TCR=T cell receptor; LFA=lymphocyte function associated antigen; ICAM=intercellular adhesion molecule; VLA=very late activation antigen; VCAM=vascular cell adhesion molecule; HSA=heat stable antigen. Modified from: Rosen FS, Wedgwood RJ, Eibl M, et al. Primary immunodeficiency diseases. Report of a WHO scientific group. *Immunodeficiency Rev* 3:204, 1992.

ates the molecular interactions which provide cell-cell adherence, stimulating signals, and costimulating signals between antigen-presenting cells and T lymphocytes.

Selectins are cell surface glycoproteins with an amino terminal lectin domain. Their ligands are oligosaccharide molecules on glycoproteins and glycolipids which are present on neutrophils, monocytes, some lymphocytes, and on vascular endothelial cells. These selectins facilitate the binding of leukocytes to vascular endothelium at sites of inflammation and also direct the homing of lymphocytes to lymphoid tissues. Three selectins have been described and characterized: E-selectin expressed by stimulated endothelial cells, P-selectin identified on stimulated platelets and endothelial cells, and L-selectin on lymphocytes, monocytes, and neutrophils.

Cytokines

Cytokines are molecules produced in lymphocytes (**lymphokines**) or monocytes (**monokines**) which regulate the development and function of cells of the immune and hemopoeitic systems. Other cytokines are produced by fibroblasts, stromal cells, platelets, or osteocytes. Thirteen **interleukins** (IL-1 through IL-13), three **interferons** (IFNα, IFNβ, and IFNγ), four stimulating factors for proliferation of leukocyte subsets or red blood cells (G-CSF, M-CSF, GM-CSF, and erythropoeitin), and tumor necrosis factor alpha (TNFα), TNFβ (lymphotoxin), and transforming growth factor beta (TGFβ) have been described and characterized as to molecular structure and function.

Interleukin-4 (IL-4) differentiates precursor T helper cells (Th0 cells) into Th2 cells which cooperate with B cells in the humoral immune response. Interleukin-12 (IL-12) influences Th0 cells to differentiate into the Th1 cells which are important in the generation of delayed hypersensitivity responses to antigens and which also produce IL-2 and gamma interferon. IL-12 also activates NK cell cytolytic functions. Receptor molecules for certain of these cytokines have also been identified on the surface of lymphocytes and other cells.

In Vitro Functional Activities of Lymphocytes

Examination of the function of lymphocytes in laboratory assays such as those listed below can assist in diagnosing and dissecting immunodeficiency disorders.

Proliferation with mitogen stimulation (concanavalin A, phytohemagglutinin, pokeweed mitogen)
Proliferation in mixed lymphocyte cultures
Helper function for antibody-synthesizing cells
Suppressor function for antibody-synthesizing cells
Cytotoxic function of sensitized T cells
K cell cytolytic activity in antibody-dependent cell-mediated cytotoxicity
Release of lymphokines (interleukins; macrophage migration inhibitory factor; macrophage activating factor; chemotactic factors for mononuclear cells, neutrophils, and eosinophils; skin reactive factor; lymphotoxin (TNFβ); blastogenic factor; cloning inhibitory factor; lymph node permeability factor; interferons; and transfer factor)
Natural killer cell activity against tumor cell lines

Complement

Chapter 35 describes the complement system and its role in immune reactions. Genetically acquired deficiencies of complement may lead to characteristic syndromes. C1 esterase inhibitor deficiency leads to hereditary angioneurotic edema. Homozygous C1, C2, C4, C5, and C7 deficiencies are commonly associated with connective-tissue diseases such as SLE, polymyositis, or sclerodermalike syndromes. The most common of these is C2 deficiency, in which roughly one-third of the patients develop an SLE-like syndrome. Homozygous C3 deficiency is extremely rare but is associated with recurrent bacterial infections. Deficiencies of the late complement components C6, C7, and C8 are associated with disseminated *Neisseria gonorrhoeae* and systemic *Neisseria meningitides* infections.

Classification of Immunodeficiency

Immunodeficiency states may be primary (of unknown cause) or secondary to another disease. The primary deficiency may be congenital or acquired in later life.

Congenital Immunodeficiencies

They occur predominately as antibody deficiency diseases (50%). Another 20% are various combined cellular and antibody disorders, 18% are phagocytic cell defects, 10% are pure T lymphocyte abnormalities, and 2% are complement deficiencies. Table 39-3 lists the most prominent of these

Table 39-3. Classification of Primary Immunodeficiency Disorders

ANTIBODY DEFICIENCIES

Bruton's agammaglobulinemia
Hypogammaglobulinemia with hyper IgM
X-linked hypogammaglobulinemia with increased IgM
Selective deficiency of IgG subclasses
IgA deficiency
Immunoglobulin heavy-chain deletions
Kappa-chain deficiency
Common variable immunodeficiency

T CELL OR COMBINED IMMUNODEFICIENCIES

Severe combined immunodeficiency
Adenosine deaminase deficiency
Purine nucleoside phosphorylase deficiency
Bare lymphocyte syndrome
Reticular dysgenesis
CD3 gamma-chain deficiency
X-linked lymphoproliferative disease

DEFECTS OF ACCESSORY CELLS

Chronic granulomatous disease
Leukocyte adhesion deficiency types 1 and 2
Myeloperoxidase deficiency
Glucose-6-phosphate dehydrogenase deficiency
Natural killer cell deficiency

COMPLEMENT DEFECTS

Isolated deficiencies of C2, C1, C4, C3, C5, C6, C7, C8
Properdin deficiency

OTHER SYNDROMES

Ataxia telangiectasia
Di George syndrome
Wiskott-Aldrich syndrome

Modified from: Nelson DL and Kurman CC. Molecular genetic analysis of the primary immunodeficiency disorders. *Ped Clin N Am* 41:657, 1994.

primary immunodeficiencies. Some of the mechanisms include

1. Bruton's agammaglobulinemia (X-linked agammaglobulinemia) patients lack B lymphocytes, except for pre-B cells in the bone marrow, and have profound deficiencies in immunoglobulins. The genetic defect leads to a failure to produce Bruton's thymine kinase (BTK) which is required for the signaling for B cell maturation.

2. Selective deficiency of one or more IgG subclasses: IgG1 or IgG3 deficiency is associated with inability to make antibodies to microbial protein antigens; IgG2 deficient patients have impairment of synthesis of antibodies to bacterial polysaccharides.

3. Di George syndrome: aplasia or dysplasia of the thymus with failure of maturation of T lymphocytes; CD4 cells are numerically reduced and PHA-induced proliferation is impaired.

4. Chronic mucocutaneous candidiasis: T cell defect.

5. Severe combined immunodeficiency: in the X-linked disease, T and B cells are dysfunctional because they lack the gamma chain for the IL-2 (and other interleukin) receptors. This leads to gross impairment of both cellular and humoral immunity. In the adenosine deaminase deficiency subtype there is accumulation of toxic levels of an inhibitor of methylation reactions in lymphocytes leading to profound lymphopenia and impaired cellular and humoral immunity.

6. Bare lymphocyte syndrome: lymphocytes fail to synthesize class II MHC molecules on their surfaces, leading to defective lymphocyte differentiation, defective antigen recognition, and impaired cell-mediated and antibody immunity.

7. Chronic granulomatous disease patients have dysfunctional granulocytes which are unable to kill phagocytized microorganisms; patients with myeloperoxidase deficiency, G6PD deficiency, Chediak-Higashi syndrome, and leukocyte adhesion deficiency (failure to synthesize the CD18 chain of intercellular adhesion molecules) also show defects in intracellular killing.

8. Leukocyte adhesion deficiency: because lymphocytes, neutrophils, monocytes, eosinophils, and NK cells in this disorder lack intercellular adhesion molecules, the function of these cells is greatly impaired and patients succumb to bacterial and viral infections.

9. Wiskott-Aldrich syndrome: these boys have an inability to make antibodies to polysaccharide antigens; they also manifest thrombocytopenia and eczema.

10. Ataxia telangiectasia: when lymphocytes produce T cell receptor (TCR) alpha and beta chains and when B

lymphocytes switch from IgM to IgG, IgA, or IgE immunoglobulin heavy-chain synthesis, breaks in DNA occur which allow for gene rearrangement; patients with ataxia telangiectasia have a defect in the repair mechanism for these DNA breaks; thus both T cells and immunoglobulins are defective and cell-mediated immunity is impaired; these patients present also with childhood onset of cerebellar ataxia, muscle atrophy, conjunctival and cutaneous telangiectases, and frequent malignancies.

11. Persons with absence of late complement components (C6, C7, or C8) are susceptible to recurrent *Neisseria* infections or their systemic dissemination.

Table 39-4 and Fig. 39-1 describe the known genetic abnormalities in primary immunodeficiency diseases.

There remain many disorders of immunodeficiency in which the reason for the absence of cellular elements of the immune system or dysfunction of these elements is incompletely understood. A partial listing of proposed explanations is as follows: (1) absence or failure of stem cells, (2) defective signaling for maturation, or (3) defects of enzymes of the purine metabolic pathway. In addition, immune suppression of precursor cells or of the maturation of these precursor cells into functional immunocompetent cells may occur. Both nonimmune and immune mechanisms may operate in the same patient. For example, perhaps 1 out of every 600 persons has selective deficiency of IgA in plasma and secretions. Some of these persons are unable to synthesize or secrete IgA because of defective B lymphocytes. Other such persons have T cells that suppress IgA-synthesizing B cells as well as having defective B lymphocytes. Certain of these patients also have deficiencies of IgG subclasses IgG2 and IgG4.

Common Variable Immunodeficiency

These patients present with humoral immunodeficiencies of one or several immunoglobulin isotypes (IgG, IgA, or IgM) and may also have defects in cell-mediated immu-

Table 39-4. Genetic Abnormalities in Primary Immunodeficiency Diseases

Disease	Chromosome	Defective Gene Product	Impaired Function
X-linked agammaglobulinemia (XLA)	Xq	Bruton's tyrosine kinase (BTK)	Signaling for B cell maturation
Immunoglobulin deficiency with hyper IgM	Xq	CD40 ligand (membrane structure on activated T cells which binds to CD40 on B cells)	Signaling for B cell isotype switching
Adenosine deaminase deficiency (subclass of SCID)	20	Adenosine deaminase	Allows buildup of S-adenosylhomocysteine which is active in blocking cell methylation reactions, especially in lymphocytes
Purine nucleotide phosphorylase deficiency	14	Purine nucleotide phosphorylase	
X-linked severe combined immunodeficiency (XSCID)	Xq	IL-2 receptor gamma chain (which also is a component of IL-4 & IL-7 receptors)	Activated T & B cells will lack these functional receptors and cannot respond to IL-2, IL-4, or IL-7
CD3 gamma chain deficiency	11	Defective CD3 gamma chain	The T cell receptor complex (TCR) will fail to respond to antigens or mitogens
Chronic granulomatous disease (CGD)	Xp	Heavy chain of cytochrome b245 (phagocyte oxidase)	Inadequate respiratory burst in phagocytic cells
Leukocyte adhesion deficiency (LAD)	21	CD18	Defect in adhesion molecules or complement receptors on leukocytes (LFA-1, CR3, and p150,95)

Modified from: Buckley RH. Breakthroughs in the understanding and therapy of primary immunodeficiency. *Ped Clin N Am* 41:665, 1994.

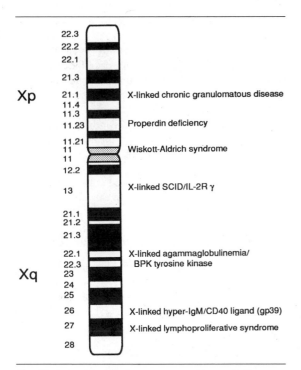

Fig. 39-1. Model of X chromosome and locus assignments of X-linked immunodeficiency diseases. (Reprinted with permission of W.B. Saunders Co. from: Voss SD, Hong R, and Sondel PM. Severe combined immunodeficiency, interleukin-2 (IL-2), and the IL-2 receptor: Experiments of nature continue to point the way. *Blood* 83:626, 1994.)

nity. B lymphocytes are present but do not differentiate into plasma cells. The onset of infections is later than in Bruton's agammaglobulinemia but is similar: encapsulated pyogenic bacteria, staphylococcus, giardia, pneumocystis, and enteroviruses. Relatives may have autoimmune diseases and malignancies. The genetic basis is not identified, but an abnormality in the MHC region of chromosome 6 is suspected. Suppressor cells for the immunoglobulin-synthesizing B cells or for the effector T cells of cell-mediated immunity can be found. These suppressor cells may be T lymphocytes or monocytes/macrophages.

Secondary Immunodeficiencies

Table 39-5 presents a classification of these disorders. Acquired immunodeficiency syndrome (AIDS) due to infection by the human immunodeficiency virus (HIV) is the prototype of acquired immunodeficiency diseases. The virus infects and destroys helper T cells (CD4 cells). The CD4 molecule on the lymphocyte surface is the receptor for the gp120 protein of the virus. Early in the course of infection there is selective inability of the patient's immune system to mount a response to the virus. Subsequently, all functions of the immune system which rely upon helper T lymphocytes are impaired, along with a dysregulation of immunoglobulin synthesis leading to hyper-immunoglobulinemia often without appropriate antibody formation.

The patient may be seen at any stage of a spectrum of clinical findings. Early, there may be an acute mononucleosislike syndrome. Conversely, the patient may only have serologic or virologic evidence of infection without symptoms. The infection may be further advanced, producing lymphopenia and/or deficiency of helper T cells, and perhaps thrombocytopenia. There next may be persistent generalized lymphadenopathy. Further progression of the infection is associated with other evidence of disease. There may be severe constitutional symptoms of fever, weight loss, and chronic diarrhea. There may be neurologic disease presenting as dementia, spinal cord disease, or peripheral nerve involvement. There may be secondary infectious diseases: *Pneumocystis carinii* pneumonia, *Mycobacterium* tuberculosis or atypical mycobacterial infections, salmonella bacteremia, nocardiosis. There may be fungal infections such as candidiasis, cryptococcosis, or histoplasmosis, or protozoan infections such as toxoplasmosis, cryptosporidiosis, isosporiasis, or intestinal amebiasis. There may be disseminated parasites such as extra-intestinal strongyloides, or viral infections such as extensive herpes simplex or herpes zoster, cytomegalovirus, or progressive multifocal leukoencephalopathy. Secondary malignancies are also part of this state: Kaposi's sarcoma, primary lymphoma of the brain, or non-Hodgkin's lymphoma.

Therapy is directed at treating the specific infection or malignancy, but four antiretroviral drugs which block virus replication are available: zidovudine (AZT), didanosine (ddI), zalcitabine (ddC), and stavudine (d4T). A viral protease inhibitor, saquinavir, and other anti-HIV drugs as well as drugs to reconstitute the immune system are under investigation.

Other Secondary Immunodeficiencies

Autoreactive cells which destroy precursors of differentiated lymphocytes may be generated by malignancies and infections, or by drugs, by aging, and during systemic lupus erythematosus. In other instances where autoreactive cells are found, the proximate cause is not known. Certain secondary immunodeficiencies such as anergy associated with Hodgkin's disease, polyclonal immunoglobulin deficiency seen in multiple myeloma, and anergy associated with disseminated fungal infections manifest suppressor cells for the immunoglobulin-synthesizing B cells or for the effector T cells of cell-mediated immunity. These suppressor cells may be T lymphocytes or monocytes/macrophages.

Clinical Consideration

Immunodeficient patients come to the physician with infections. Rarely, the immunodeficiency is an asymptomatic finding. A careful history often directs the physician toward a broad categorization of the defect, since certain groups of infections are associated with deficiencies of particular components of the immune response (Table 39-6).

Table 39-5. Classification of Secondary Immunodeficiency Diseases

NUTRITIONAL DEFECTS

Protein-calorie malnutrition
Vitamin deficiencies
Trace metal deficiencies (especially zinc)

MALIGNANCIES

Multiple myeloma: suppressor monocytes/macrophages
Hodgkin's disease: suppressor T cells or suppressor monocytes/macrophages

INFECTIONS

Acquired immunodeficiency syndrome (AIDS): see text
Disseminated fungal infections: increased suppressor T cells
Tuberculosis with pleural effusions: sequestration of reactive T lymphocytes in the effusion fluids
Infectious mononucleosis: increased suppressor T cells during active disease
Influenza, measles, paramyxoviruses: acute self-limited depression of T cell-mediated immunity

COLLAGEN-VASCULAR DISEASES

In the prototype disease, systemic lupus erythematosus, there are autoantibodies for suppressor T lymphocytes, a decreased autologous mixed lymphocyte reaction, a decreased B-lymphocyte primary immune response, impaired clearance of antibody-coated particles, and perhaps a decrease in helper T lymphocytes

BURNS

Loss of plasma immunoglobulins

PROTEIN-LOSING ENTEROPATHY

Gastrointestinal loss of plasma immunoglobulins and circulating lymphocytes

NEPHROTIC SYNDROME

Loss of plasma immunoglobulins

TREATMENT WITH CORTICOSTEROIDS OR CYTOTOXIC DRUGS

IDIOSYNCRATIC REACTIONS TO MEDICATIONS

(immunoglobulin deficiency with diphenylhydantoin, etc.)

MISCELLANEOUS

Sarcoidosis: sequestration of reactive T lymphocytes in granulomas in the lung; heightened resting autologous mixed lymphocyte reaction
Splenectomy: suboptimal antibody responses to particulate antigens such as the pneumococcus; absence of the major reticuloendothelial (phagocytic) organ of early life; defects of the alternative pathway of complement activation
Sickle-cell disease with splenic infarction: defects of the alternative pathway of complement activation
Myotonic dystrophy: hypercatabolism of IgG

Table 39-6. Infections Associated with Various Immunodeficiency States

INFECTIONS ASSOCIATED WITH DEFICIENCIES OF HUMORAL IMMUNITY

Encapsulated pyogenic bacteria
Streptococcus (including *S. pneumoniae*)
Meningococcus
Haemophilus
Pseudomonas
Staphylococcus
Giardia lamblia (enteritis)
Pneumocystis carinii (pneumonia)
Viruses having a viremic phase (hepatitis, polio, and echoviruses)

INFECTIONS ASSOCIATED WITH GRANULOCYTE DEFECTS

Catalase-positive organisms such as *Staphylococcus aureus, Serratia marcescens,* as well as other bacteria, *Candida albicans,* and *Aspergillus* are problems in chronic granulomatous disease
Pyogenic bacteria are risks in neutropenia and in Chediak-Higashi syndrome

INFECTIONS ASSOCIATED WITH A DEFICIENCY OF T CELL-MEDIATED IMMUNITY

Bacteria
Mycobacterium
Salmonella
Listeria monocytogenes
Francisella tularensis
Brucella
Treponema pallidum
Pseudomonas mallei
P. pseudomallei
Fungi
Aspergillus
Candida
Cryptococcus neoformans
Phycomycetes
Histoplasma capsulatum
Coccidioides immitis
Viruses
Herpes simplex
H. zoster
Cytomegalovirus
Rubeola (measles)
Vaccinia
Helminths
Schistosoma
Strongyloides
Protozoa
Toxoplasma gondii
Plasmodia
Unclassified
Pneumocystis carinii

Reprinted with permission from: Kaufman CE and Papper S (eds.). *Review of Pathophysiology.* Boston: Little, Brown, 1983, p. 225.

Table 39-7. Useful Tests for the Evaluation of Immunodeficient States

ROUTINE LABORATORY TESTS

Complete blood count (with differential count and platelet count and morphology)
Serum protein electrophoresis
Cultures (identify the infecting microorganism)

ROENTGENOGRAPHY

Chest
    Acute and chronic lung changes
    Thymus shadow
Nasopharynx, for tonsillar tissue
Sinuses, for inflammation

TEST FOR T CELL FUNCTION

Screening: Delayed hypersensitivity skin testing
    Recall antigens (streptokinase, mumps, *Candida* especially valuable)
    Phytohemagglutinin (PHA) — investigational
Specialized
    T cell count (monoclonal antibody cell-sorter techniques for T cell subclasses: CD3 marker for post-thymic T cells; CD4
        marker for helper/inducer T cells; CD8 marker for suppressor/cytotoxic T cells)
    Lymphocyte transformation (PHA, concanavalin A, specific antigens)
    Migration inhibition factor (MIF) production
    Specific immunization (DNCB, KLH)*
    Mixed lymphocyte cultures

TEST FOR B-CELL FUNCTION

Screening
    Quantitative immunoglobulin levels (IgG, IgA, IgM, IgE, and IgG subclasses: IgG1, IgG2, IgG3, IgG4)
    Diphtheria, tetanus, polio, measles, mumps antibody titers
    Isohemagglutinin titers (IgM antibodies)
Specialized
    B-cell count (using flow cytometry techniques with monoclonal antibodies directed against CD19 or CD20 markers,
        kappa or lambda light chains, for surface immunoglobulins)
    Immunization studies (KLH*, pneumococcal, or *Haemophilus influenzae* polysaccharides)
    Lymphocyte transformation (pokeweed mitogen will require T cell help for B cell stimulation; *Staphylococcus aureus,*
        lipopolysaccharide, or Epstein-Barr virus do not require T cell help for B cell transformation)

EFFECTORS OF IMMUNITY

Complement (total hemolytic complement, components, inhibitors, inactivators, stabilizers, etc.)
Neutrophils (count, morphology, appearance of granules, chemotaxis, phagocytosis, NBT test*, chemiluminescence, perox-
    idase stain, bactericidal assay). Surface CD markers for intact adherence molecules (CD11–CD18 complexes)
Macrophages (morphology, phagocytosis, chemotaxis)
In vitro leukotactic or chemotactic assays

TISSUE EXAMINATION

Bone marrow aspiration
Lymph node biopsy
Tonsils, appendix, small bowel biopsy
Rectal biopsy

Adapted from: Kaufman CE and Papper S (eds.). *Review of Pathophysiology.* Boston: Little, Brown, 1983, p. 226.
* DNCB = dinitrochlorobenzene; KLH = keyhole limpet hemocyanin; NBT = nitroblue tetrazolium.

Clinical Evaluation of the Patient with Immunodeficiency

Careful history and family history should be taken, especially stressing age of onset of infections, frequency and type of infection, offending microorganism, and clues to diseases associated with immunodeficiencies. Among these associated diseases and abnormalities are allergies; autoimmune/collagen-vascular diseases; ectodermal dysplasias of skin, hair, and nails; endocrinopathies; hematologic abnormalities; malabsorption; malignancies; skeletal abnormalities (e.g. short-limbed dwarfism); eczema; telangiectasia; and ataxia. For example, in addition to infections, patients with common variable immunodeficiency may have involvement with a seronegative rheumatoid arthritis-like disorder, or with systemic lupus erythematosus, Sjögren's syndrome, scleroderma, dermatomyositis, hemolytic anemia, thrombocytopenia, chronic active hepatitis, or sialadenitis. Physical examination should especially direct attention to enumerating the sites of infection, character of associated inflammation, status of lymphoid tissues (lymph nodes, tonsils, spleen, and liver), and stigmata of cutaneous, mucosal, and skeletal abnormalities. On the basis of these results, hypotheses can be tested further by selectively performing some of the tests listed in Table 39-7.

Therapy

Replacement of deficient immunoglobulins can be achieved by periodic treatment with intramuscular or intravenous human gamma globulins. Occasionally, plasma infusions from individual donors may be required. Bone marrow transplants from HLA identical relatives or from HLA matched bone marrow registry donors have been successful in such varied primary immunodeficiency disorders as severe combined immunodeficiency (SCID), Wiskott-Aldrich syndrome, bare lymphocyte syndrome, purine nucleoside phosphorylase deficiency, incomplete Di George syndrome, chronic granulomatous disease, Chediak-Higashi disease, and leukocyte adhesion deficiency. Worldwide, approximately 800 bone marrow transplants have been done for immunodeficiency diseases with a 60% success rate. A recent study describes the improvement of patients with common variable immunodeficiency by intravenous or subcutaneous administration of recombinant IL-2 conjugated to polyethylene glycol. In the adenosine deaminase variant of severe combined immunodeficiency, the missing enzyme can be passively provided by red blood cell infusions (normal red cells contain adenosine deaminase) or by infusions of bovine ADA modified by polyethylene glycol. Somatic cell gene therapy with cloned human genes is a recent and exciting innovation. Children have been successfully treated with the ADA gene transduced ex vivo by a retrovirus into their peripheral blood leukocytes. The leukocytes were then reinfused and survived and multiplied in the patients. Additional children have had this procedure performed on umbilical cord stem cells. In the complete Di George syndrome, transplantation of fetal thymus gland is necessary for reconstitution.

Clinical Example

1. An 8-year-old boy was seen because of recurrent sinus infections, bronchitis, and pneumonia since infancy. In infancy he was treated briefly with gamma globulin. He had required high-dose intravenous antibiotics for a recent pneumonia and sinusitis.

Physical examination was unremarkable except for some growth retardation and coarse rales in his lungs. No arthritis or skin rashes were noted. Previous workup for cystic fibrosis was negative. Chest x-ray showed a pneumonitis and pleural reaction. Paranasal sinus x-rays showed an air-fluid level in the right maxillary sinus (acute sinusitis). Sputum culture grew out *Haemophilus influenzae*. White blood count varied from 7.8 to 10.8×10^3 per cubic millimeter with 50–62% poly-morphonuclear leukocytes and 3–11% bands (stabs).

Serum protein electrophoresis showed almost complete absence of gamma globulin. Quantitative immunoglobulin levels were: IgG, 86 mg/100 ml (normal, 700–1,400); IgA, less than 1.1 mg/100 ml (normal, 100–350); and IgM, 11 mg/100 ml (normal, 60–220). There was no secretory IgA detected in saliva.

The patient was blood type O positive but he had no anti-A or anti-B isohemagglutinins. Agglutinins for typhoid, paratyphoid, and proteus were negative. A battery of skin tests for delayed hypersensitivity (cell-mediated immunity) was positive for functional T lymphocytes (positive PHA skin test) and for recall (anamnestic) cellular immunity (positive mumps skin test).

Discussion. Chronic respiratory infections in childhood (especially recurrent pneumonias and unexplained bronchiectasis) should prompt an investigation for cystic fibrosis and immunoglobulin-deficiency disorders. The early onset of infections, persistence of infections to present age 8, male sex, almost total absence of immunoglobulins of all classes, and intact cell-mediated immunity establish the diagnosis of Bruton's agammaglobulinemia. Although this is a genetic X-linked disorder, fewer than half of the patients will have a positive family history. Recent molecular biology techniques have been employed to identify maternal carriers of the genetic defect. Treatment is lifelong replacement with gamma globulin and antibiotics as needed. Despite this, upper-airway infections recur. Recurrent pulmonary infections lead to pulmonary insufficiency. Gastrointestinal infections, collagen-vascular diseases, viral hepatitis, and encephalitis may be troublesome.

Bibliography

Buckley RH. Breakthroughs in the understanding and therapy of primary immunodeficiency. *Pediatr Clin N Am* 41:665–690, 1994. *Thorough review of known genetic abnormalities and current status of therapy.*

Chapel HM for the Concensus Panel for the diagnosis and management of primary antibody deficiencies: Concensus on diagnosis and management of primary antibody deficiencies. *Brit Med J* 308:581–585, 1994. *A practical article on evaluation and therapy.*

Cournoyer D. Gene therapy of the immune system. *Ann Rev Immunol* 11:297–329, 1993. *Review of the state of the art in somatic cell gene therapy.*

European Group: Bone marrow transplantation (BMT) in Europe for primary immunodeficiencies other than SCID: a report from the European group for BMT and the European group for immunodeficiency. *Blood* 83:1149–1154, 1994. *The current status of bone marrow transplantation for immunodeficiency disorders.*

Hong R. Update on the immunodeficiency diseases. *Am J Dis Child* 144:983–992, 1990. *Good description of basics of the immune system, specific diseases of immunodeficiency, and available therapies.*

Pacheco SE and Shearer WT. Laboratory aspects of immunology. *Pediatr Clin N Am* 41:623–655, 1994. *An orderly, comprehensive, and practical approach to laboratory tests evaluating the immune system.*

Rosen FS, Cooper MD, and Wedgwood RJP. The primary immunodeficiencies. *N Engl J Med* 333:431–440, 1995. *Exhaustive review of up-to-date information.*

Weissman IL. Developmental switches in the immune system. *Cell* 76:207–218, 1994. *Excellent article on the thymus and lymphocyte development.*

40 Osteoarthritis

Haraldine A. Stafford

Objectives

After completing this chapter, you should be able to

State the different types of normal joints

Illustrate the structure of normal joints

Describe the components of articular cartilage and how they are maintained

Understand the anatomy, histology, and chemistry of the articular tissues that are responsible for normal diarthrodial joint functioning and biomechanics

Understand how the pathologic processes that occur in osteoarthritis lead to clinical disease

Understand how the proposed pathogenetic mechanisms result in osteoarthritis

---

The musculoskeletal system is uniquely endowed for movement. In a very regulated fashion, each part has a major role. The neuromuscular units generate the force to make purposeful movements. The skeleton provides the scaffolding for the neuromuscular units. The joints allow contiguous bones to move freely and align properly. The goals of this chapter are to review normal joint structure and function and explore how osteoarthritis interferes with functioning of the musculoskeletal system.

Normal Joint Structure and Function

Classification

There are three classes of joints, their classification depending on the histologic features of the joint and the range of motion permitted. The synarthrodial joints are the suture lines of the skull. These joints are composed of thin fibrous tissue which separate adjoining cranial plates. Synarthroses allow for minimal motion between cranial plates and provide sufficient space for orderly growth of the plates. The amphiarthrodial joints are composed of fi-

brocartilage. The intervertebral disc, pubic symphysis, and sacroiliac joints are examples of amphiarthrodial joints. These joints have increased mobility as compared to the synarthroses. The diarthrodial joints are the most abundant type of joint, and allow for the greatest mobility between bones. It is this type of joint that will be the focus of the rest of the chapter.

Diarthrodial joints possess a synovial membrane and contain synovial fluid; thus they are referred to as synovial joints. These joints are further subclassified according to shape. There are ball-and-socket joints, e.g., the hips; hinge joints, e.g., the interphalangeal (IP) joints; saddle joints, e.g., the first carpometacarpal (CMC) joint; and plane joints, e.g., patellofemoral joints. The type of joint motion is determined by the shape and size of the opposing bone surfaces. These motions include flexion (bending) and extension (straightening), abduction and adduction (away and towards the midline), and rotation.

Organization of the Diarthrodial Joint

The anatomy, histology, and chemistry of the articular tissues are responsible for normal diarthrodial joint functioning. These functions include effortless movement over the joint's complete arc of motion, distribution of load appropriately, and maintenance of stability during use. The shape of the joint is crucial to normal joint functioning. The highly regulated chondrocyte is responsible for creating the extracellular matrix (ECM) which is important for the biomechanical properties of the articular cartilage. Ligamentous conjoining of the articulating surfaces as well as neuromuscular control of joint motion are responsible for joint stability.

Anatomy of the Diarthrodial Joint

The supporting structures of the joint (i.e., its capsule and the muscles, tendons, and ligaments) are responsible for joint stability (Fig. 40-1). The mass of stabilizing muscle surrounding a joint is determined by the joint's mobility; joints with excessive mobility (e.g., the shoulder) have a bulky musculature. Joints with limited mobility (e.g., the IP joints) are stabilized predominantly with ligaments (fibrous tissue that connects bone to bone). Tendons (the fibrous tissue at the ends of muscle) insert in the joint capsule, and provide the link between muscle and bone.

Fig. 40-1. Diagram of a normal diarthrodial joint. A fibrous capsule envelops the joint. It merges externally with the periosteum, ligaments, tendons, and fascia, and is covered internally with synovium which also lines the joint cavity. The articulating surfaces have incongruent shapes and are covered by hyaline cartilage. The properties of these tissues are responsible for the functional attributes of the diarthrodial joint. (Reprinted from: the Clinical Slide Collection on the Rheumatic Diseases, copyright 1991. Used by permission of the American College of Rheumatology and the American Physical Therapy Association.)

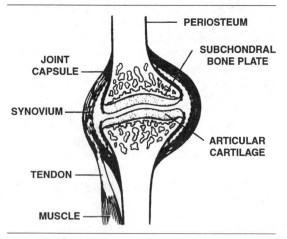

They transmit the force of the muscle to the bones. Both ligaments and tendons are made of collagen and elastin.

The synovium is a thin tissue that covers all intra-articular structures except articular cartilage, menisci, and localized bare areas of bone. It contains the type A or "macrophagelike" cell, which has predominantly phagocytic function, and the Type B or "fibroblastlike" cell, which has primarily synthetic function. Synoviocytes produce many macromolecules which are important to the integrity and function of the normal joint.

Articular or hyaline cartilage is the highly specialized tissue of diarthrodial joints that allows for their effortless motion and load absorption. Its smooth surface permits gliding of one bone over another. Its unique structure allows for extreme compressive stress, impact absorption, and tolerance of shear forces. These unique properties are related to the composition and structure of its ECM, a dense collagen network containing a high concentration of proteoglycans and a large amount of water.

Chemistry of Cartilage

Twenty percent of the tissue weight of cartilage is derived from proteinaceous macromolecules including collagens, proteoglycans, and glycoproteins. Water and inorganic salts constitute the remaining tissue weight. Collagens belong to a family of proteins that have a similar primary sequence and associate in a triple helix. These collagens differ from each other by differences in their primary sequence, which results in varying degrees of nonhelical portions. Collagen, especially type II, is the major macromolecule of cartilage, and it constitutes the fibrillar portion of cartilage. Type II collagen molecules become cross-linked and aggregate in a regular staggered fashion to form the collagen fibril (Fig. 40-2). This quaternary structure is responsible for cartilage's tensile strength and is essential for the maintenance of its volume and shape. Other minor collagens are also present in cartilage. The proteoglycans constitute the nonfibrillar component of cartilage. The aggregating type of proteoglycan, aggrecan, is the major form of proteoglycan in cartilage. It is composed of a protein backbone with numerous glycosaminoglycan side chains (Fig. 40-3). The glycosaminoglycans are long chains of repeating polydimeric saccharides, chondroitin-4-sulfate and chondroitin-6-sulfate (sulfated dimers of N-acetylgalactosamine and glucuronic acid), and keratin sulfate (a sulfated dimer of N-acetylglucosamine and galactose). Aggrecan noncovalently interacts with hyaluronic acid, a high-molecular-weight glycosaminoglycan consisting of many repeating disaccharide units (N-acetyl-glucosamine and glucuronic acid). Their interaction is stabilized by link proteins, low-

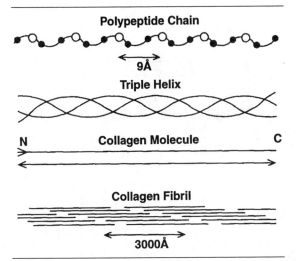

Fig. 40-2. Organization of the collagen fibril. The primary sequence of the collagen polypeptide chains have a unique repeating amino acid triplet, Gly-X-Y. Three polypeptide chains of a specific collagen type associate to form a triple helical collagen molecule. Cross-links form between the collagen molecules. The cross-linked collagen molecules aggregate in a staggered fashion to form the collagen fibril. (From: *Biochemistry* by Lubert Stryer. Copyright © 1975 by Lubert Stryer. Used with permission of W. H. Freeman and Company.)

molecular-weight proteins resembling the most N-terminal globular domain of aggrecan. Up to 200 aggrecan molecules can bind to one hyaluronic acid molecule. The composition and size of these proteoglycan aggregates vary within cartilage. The composition and absolute amount of aggrecan in the ECM changes with age. Low-molecular-weight proteoglycans have also been identified in cartilage, although their exact function is not known.

Cartilage Homeostasis

Cartilage homeostasis is maintained by the chondrocyte. Under physiologic conditions, chondrocytes maintain a dynamic steady state where cartilage synthesis is balanced by cartilage degradation. However, changes in the loading of the joint may lead to alterations of the cartilage matrix. Subphysiologic levels of mechanical stress are associated with enhanced catabolic activity of the chondrocytes, whereas physiologic levels of mechanical stress promote anabolic activity. Supraphysiologic mechanical stress leads to dysfunction of the chondrocytes, with resultant cell injury and necrosis. Chondrocytes also respond to growth factors and cytokines. Growth factors stimulate chondrocytes to synthesize more ECM components. Cytokines, e.g., IL-1 and TNF-α, stimulate chondrocytes to synthesize proteolytic enzymes which degrade the components of the ECM. With aging, the proteoglycan content of cartilage decreases, causing reduced water-binding capacity and resultant decreased tensile strength.

Biomechanics

The major load on cartilage results from the contraction of muscles that stabilize or move the joint. For example, normal walking produces loads of 3–4 times body weight across the knee joint. Without adaptive mechanisms to protect the knee joint, cartilage would be destroyed and joint failure would occur. Articular cartilage is an excellent shock absorber; nonetheless, it is too thin to be the sole absorber of the joints. The subchondral bone and the surrounding muscles help to absorb the transmitted load by absorbing energy. Any process which causes muscle weakness or trabecular bone stiffening or loss will decrease the efficiency of energy absorption.

Once the load is transmitted to the joint, articular features come into play. The shape of the opposing joint surfaces is important for load absorption. In the normal joint in the unloaded state, the surfaces of the opposing cartilages are incongruent, i.e., they lack precise fit (see Fig. 40-1). With loading, the opposing surfaces change their shape (the process of deformation) so that the contact area between opposing surfaces is maximized. This deformation reduces the stress (force per unit area) on any given section of cartilage.

The articular cartilage has excellent biomechanical properties by virtue of its collagen network and ECM. The proteoglycan aggregates are highly negatively charged macromolecules which attract water and electrolytes. The amount of water absorbed is determined by the restraints placed by the collagen network. Water accounts for some 70–80% of the cartilage weight and is responsible for the load-bearing properties of cartilage. When a load is applied to articular cartilage, deformation occurs, and water bound to the proteoglycan can be displaced towards the synovial cavity. As the underhydrated proteoglycans are forced together, negative repulsive forces take over and resist further loss of water and further deformation. As the load is removed, water returns from the surrounding tissue to hydrate the proteoglycans and restores the original form of tissue. Consequently, the biomechanical properties of cartilage to withstand an applied load are based on the collagen-proteoglycan composition and the hydration status of the tissue.

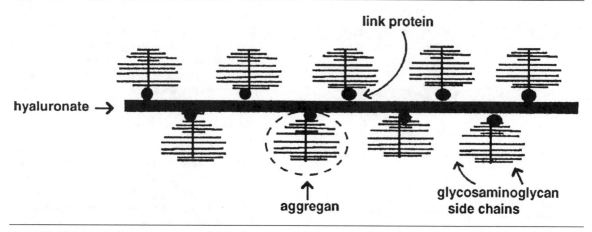

Fig. 40-3. Major noncollagenous macromolecules in the extracellular matrix (ECM) of articular cartilage. The major proteoglycan aggrecan noncovalently interacts with hyaluronic acid and the link proteins. These macromolecules along with the collagens are responsible for the biomechanical properties of articular cartilage.

Osteoarthritis

Definitions

Osteoarthritis (OA) is a chronic disease that is confined to the joints; it has no systemic component comparable to that seen with rheumatoid arthritis (RA). Historically, it was termed "degenerative joint disease" (or wear-and-tear arthritis); postmortem studies emphasized age-related degeneration of cartilage as the central feature of the disorder. In the 1960s, further pathologic and anatomic studies pointed out that degeneration is not the cardinal pathologic feature. In fact, attempted repair is more likely to be the focus of pathology. Moreover, the OA process is considered to be a dynamic, age-related reaction pattern of a joint responding to insult or injury.

OA is the most common disorder of the joint, affecting many animals in the animal kingdom, including humans. The economic impact of OA on humans and animals is substantial — 30-fold greater than that observed for RA. OA accounts for significant work disability; the number of persons retiring annually because of OA is greater than 5%, and is only surpassed by heart disease.

OA is not a single disease entity; it comprises a group of conditions that share common pathologic and radiologic features. OA was originally defined by pathologists who differentiated between two forms of arthritis, the hypertrophic and the atrophic forms. Atrophic disorders were characterized by synovial inflammation with erosion of bone and cartilage, and were later classified as RA and septic arthritis. Hypertrophic arthritis was characterized by focal loss of cartilage, with hypertrophy of the underlying bone and cartilage, and ectopic bone at the joint margins. This form of arthritis was never subdivided, and became synonymous with what we now call OA.

Classification

There are two major classification schemes describing OA based on disease etiology or articular distribution of disease. The traditional scheme divides OA into two categories, primary and secondary. Primary (idiopathic) OA arises de novo without underlying joint pathology. Secondary OA arises as a consequence of underlying joint pathology, e.g., after RA or associated with pseudogout. Classically, secondary OA usually affects younger individuals, occurs in approximately 20% of all OA cases, and often presents in an atypical fashion, i.e., at an unusual joint site or with uncharacteristically severe pain. OA described in this fashion is further characterized by the number of joints involved; there is single-joint (monoarticular) or generalized (polyarticular) arthritis.

This traditional scheme is now considered oversimplified, and is being replaced by a scheme which takes into account the individual's characteristics and the specific joint involvement. This schema includes knee/hand disease, isolated hip disease, and polyarticular disease. Knee OA is seen predominantly in two groups: young individuals, often male, who have a history of knee injury or meniscectomy and middle-aged and older individuals who have OA at other sites, and may or may not be obese. Hip OA develops in all age groups, and is frequently the only joint involved. Hand OA affects the distal and proximal interphalangeal joints (DIP and PIP joints, respectively) and the joint at the base of the thumb (first CMC) almost exclusively. The other joints of the hand and wrist are much less frequently involved in OA, but are the predominant joints involved in RA. Hand OA is often associated with other joint involvement, especially the knee. A destructive form of OA may develop in elderly females, and often involves multiple sites.

Epidemiology

Prevalence

The prevalence of OA increases with age. Radiographic prevalence of knee OA based on population surveys showed that less than 0.1% of individuals 25–34 years old, 10–30% of individuals 64–75 years old, and greater than 30% of individuals 75 years or older have OA changes. Additionally, the number of joints with OA increases with age. Pathologic data reveal that the prevalence of pathologic OA is greater than that appreciated by radiologic evaluation. Autopsy-proven cartilage damage is present in almost everyone over 65 years old. Pathologically defined OA with cartilage erosions, subchondral reaction, and osteophytosis is identified in the knees of 60% of men and 70% of women who died in their 60s and 70s. Discordance between the radiologic and pathologic prevalence estimates is due to the inability of plain radiographs to detect mild pathologic changes and to examine the entire joint.

The prevalence of arthritis varies with the joint(s) involved. In women 60–70 years old, radiographic evidence of OA is present in 75% of their DIP joints as contrasted to the 10–30% prevalence cited for knee arthritis. Hip OA is not as common as hand or knee OA.

Gender differences exist for OA. For knee and hand OA, females are affected more often than males. In contrast, for hip OA, males are affected as frequently as females. Differences in hip and knee/hand disease suggest that there may be differences in etiology between these forms of OA.

Racial differences exist for both the prevalence of OA and the pattern of joint involvement. In the aforementioned radiographic surveys, black females were twice as likely as white females to have knee OA. Hip OA is seen less frequently in Hong Kong Chinese, South African blacks, East

Indians, and native Americans than in whites. Certain Native American tribes have increased prevalence of hand OA as compared to whites. The cause of these difference is unknown, but could possibly reflect genetic differences or differences related to joint usage.

Risk Factors

Introduction. The individual risk factors can be classified by their proposed pathogenetic mechanisms. There are factors leading to an increased susceptibility to OA (susceptibility factors) and factors resulting in abnormal biomechanics (mechanical factors) at specific joint sites. In addition, some factors may affect both susceptibility and biomechanics.

Susceptibility Factors. As described above, age is the most powerful risk factor for OA. The proposed mechanism for this association is not totally understood, but probably reflects changes in the chemistry of articular cartilage with age.

Obesity is frequently associated with OA of the knee, less strongly with hip, and probably not associated with hand OA. The reason for the association is not known. It is surmised that metabolic factors rather than excessive mechanical loading lead to OA. If excessive loading were the cause of OA, then the hips and ankles (which are also weight-bearing joints) would be affected with OA as frequently as the knee. However, hip OA is observed less frequently and ankle OA rarely observed in obesity-associated OA.

Hereditary factors are important, particularly in polyarticular OA, as shown in twin and family studies and in a mouse model of OA. These factors are apparently polygenic and are transmitted as an autosomal dominant trait for females and a recessive autosomal trait for males. Recent studies have identified different mutations in the type II collagen gene in families with generalized OA and with precocious OA.

The female predominance of OA, especially in polyarticular OA, and the increased prevalence in postmenopausal females, has led investigators to suggest that female hormones may play a role in this disease. However, hormone replacement in postmenopausal females has so far failed to retard OA. Consequently, the role of female hormones in the generation of OA is unclear.

Mechanical Factors. Trauma, especially related to sports injuries, is a common cause of monoarticular OA. The knee is a frequent site of trauma-related OA, predominantly secondary to cruciate ligament damage and meniscal tears. Major injury at one joint can also lead to OA at other joints, presumably by altering biomechanics at the other sites.

Altered joint shape can lead to the development of OA. This has been well documented with childhood hip disorders, e.g., Perthes disease, slipped capital epiphysis, and congenital dislocation of the hip. Presumably, altered joint biomechanics are responsible for the development of OA.

Repetitive use of specific joint groups has been associated with OA. Examples include cotton pickers and weavers. This is most frequently a cause of hand and knee arthritis, and is probably due to injury of joints through occupational or avocational activities.

Pathogenesis

OA was previously thought to be a consequence of aging; however, many joints remain normal even into extreme old age. Consequently, its pathogenesis is more complex and reflects an interplay of joint anatomy, physiology, biochemistry, and mechanics. Although the most obvious changes in OA occur in the articular cartilage, OA should not be thought of solely as a disease of the cartilage. OA represents disease of the entire joint. Consequently, the primary abnormality may reside in the articular cartilage, synovium, subchondral bone, ligaments, or neuromuscular unit.

OA may develop when there is a problem with the mechanical load on the joint or a problem with the underlying constituents of the joint. In the first case, the articular cartilage and underlying subchondral bone are normal, but excessive loading forces are placed on the tissues which causes them to fail. Repetitive-impact loading and eccentric load distribution are examples. In the second case, the loading forces are normal, but the articular cartilage or subchondral bone are abnormal so that they cannot withstand normal stresses. There are a variety of conditions, inheritable and acquired, that lead to abnormal cartilage or subchondral bone (Table 40-1). Many of these can be complicated by the development of OA. Mutations in the type II collagen gene have been identified in some of these conditions, e.g., familial chondrodysplasia. Abnormal collagen is produced which is unable to sustain normal joint loading. If the adjacent subchondral bone is destroyed or metabolically altered, it will be unable to respond to a load appropriately. The cartilage subsequently becomes overstressed, which leads to injury of its collagen network and resulting OA. Once initiated regardless of the precipitant, OA progresses because of the pathologic alterations that develop in all the articular tissues.

Pathology

The pathology of OA is characterized by both joint damage and repair. The most striking pathologic changes occur at the load-bearing areas of the joint but all articular tissues are affected. Disruption of the collagen network is a sen-

Table 40-1. Causes of Abnormal Articular Tissues That May Result in OA

Diseases That Cause Abnormal Cartilage	Diseases That Cause Abnormal Bone
METABOLIC DISEASES	**INFLAMMATORY DISEASES**
Calcium crystal deposition diseases	Rheumatoid arthritis
Hemachromatosis	Seronegative spondyloarthropathy
Ochronosis	Septic arthritis
Wilson's disease	Gout
Hemophilia	**INFARCTIONAL DISEASES**
Gout	Sickle cell disease
HERITABLE DISEASES	Systemic lupus erythematosus
Stickler syndrome	Gauchers disease
Chondrodysplasias	Osteonecrosis
Epiphyseal dysplasias	**MISCELLANEOUS DISEASES**
Familial calcium crystal deposition diseases	Acromegaly
MISCELLANEOUS DISEASES	Osteopetrosis
Septic arthritis	Paget's disease
	Bone fracture

tinel event in OA. As a rule, anabolic changes predominate early in OA, whereas catabolic activity predominates later in the course of the disease.

Cartilage

Gross evidence of early cartilage injury is reflected by roughened or eroded articular cartilage (Fig. 40-4). Later in the course of OA the cartilage becomes cracked, with frank ulcerations and clefts. In the end-stage OA joint, the subchondral bone may be totally devoid of cartilage. The radiologic features correlate with the pathology and include joint-space narrowing, osteophytosis (presence of osteophytes), subchondral sclerosis (increased bone density), cyst formation, and abnormalities of bony contour (Fig. 40-5).

The corresponding histologic findings reflect the chemical and cellular events that occur after cartilage has been injured. Early in the disease there is a net increase in the thickness of the cartilage as a result of increased amounts of water and ECM components, especially proteoglycans. Water content is increased as a consequence of damage to the collagen network of the tissue. Chondrocytes replicate, forming cell clusters, and synthesize more ECM components. These findings reflect an attempt at hypertrophic cartilage repair.

With disease progression, there is thinning of the hyaline cartilage and decreasing proteoglycan concentration, presumably secondary to increased catabolism by lysosomal proteases and neutral metalloproteinases. Certain cytokines may produce the heightened catabolic activity. Cartilage subsequently softens and becomes hypocellular, its surface integrity is lost, and vertical clefts develop (fibrillation). The fibrillated cartilage is lost with joint movement, and underlying subchondral bone becomes exposed. The cartilage produces fibrocartilage in an attempt to repair itself. The fibrocartilage eventually fails secondary to inferior mechanical stability, and full-scale loss of cartilage occurs.

Fig. 40-4. Characteristic pathologic features of an osteoarthritis joint. Diagrammatic evidence of injury and repair is shown. The joint capsule is thickened and the synovium is edematous secondary to inflammation. The articular cartilage is thinned, leading to altered shape of the opposing surfaces. The subchondral bone is sclerotic and contains cysts. Osteophytic lipping is seen at the joint margins. Diagram of a normal joint is given for comparison. (From: *Atlas of Clinical Rheumatology,* by PA Dieppe, PA Bacon, AN Bamji, I Watt. Gower Medical Publishing Ltd., London, UK, 1986.)

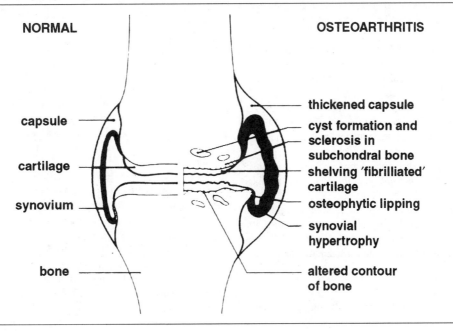

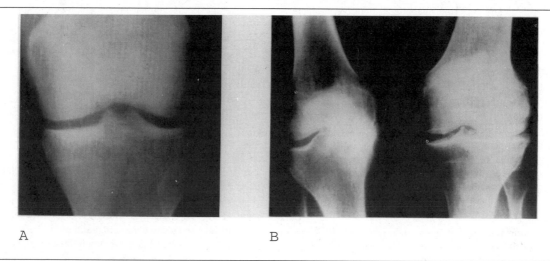

A   B

Fig. 40-5. Characteristic radiologic features of an osteoarthritic joint. Frontal views of a normal knee (A) and bilateral knees involved with OA (B). There is marked narrowing and sclerosis of the medial and lateral joint spaces of the left and right osteoarthritic knees, respectively. (Reprinted from: the Clinical Slide Collection on the Rheumatic Diseases, copyright 1991. Used by permission of the American College of Rheumatology.)

Bone

Remodeling and hypertrophy of bone are cardinal pathologic features of OA; however, bone destruction can also occur. Early in the OA process, new bone is synthesized beneath the articular cartilage in the subchondral area by proliferating osteoblasts. This appositional bone growth results in the radiographic sclerosis. The appositional bone can interfere with intraosseous blood flow. This leads to venous engorgement and increased medullary pressures, which in turn increases the stiffness of the bone and can lead to bone necrosis. Bone cysts representing focal areas of bone necrosis form beneath the articular cartilage and weaken the integrity of the remaining bone. Microfractures of the trabeculae can occur and further weaken the subchondral bone. This bone pathology results in an increased load being transmitted to the remaining cartilage, which can accelerate joint failure.

Growth of cartilage and bone at the joint margins leads to the formation of osteophytes. These osteophytes alter the shape of the joint and interfere with motion. The presence of osteophytes alone is not sufficient to diagnose OA; they can be a normal consequence of aging.

Soft Tissues

The synovium often shows mild, chronic inflammatory changes (synovitis) secondary to Type A synoviocytes

phagocytizing cartilage and bone debris. The joint capsule thickens as a result of injury and subsequent scarring. Surrounding muscle may become atrophic from disuse.

Clinical Features

Symptoms

Joint Pain (Cardinal Symptom). Pain can vary with respect to joint site; the hip is usually the most painful, whereas the hand joints are the least painful. The onset of pain is usually slow and insidious. The severity of pain tends to coincide with the severity of radiographic changes, although some radiographically abnormal joints appear to be symptom-free.

The typical OA pain is usually described as diffuse, often intermittent, related to use, and worse later in the day. Pain can be described as sharp or dull, and exacerbated with activity. Although use-related pain is the most frequently described symptom, rest and night pain have also been described. As the severity of OA increases, the character of the pain can change. In severe OA, pain can be constant and unrelenting. Pain is reported more frequently by women and by individuals who are depressed or anxious.

The pathogenesis of pain in OA as in other disorders is probably multifactorial and evokes a combination of local, systemic, and central neurologic factors. The anatomic changes in the joint that occur as a function of OA can lead to abnormal mechanical stresses being applied to the periarticular structures. This can cause localized tenderness. As this condition persists, a secondary periarticular disorder, e.g., bursitis or tenosynovitis, may arise. Appositional bone formation can obstruct venous outflow and lead to increased intraosseous pressure. These changes can cause severe and prolonged rest and night pain. Periosteal elevation resulting from osteophyte formation may also cause pain. Mild synovitis is seen in some patients with OA, and the elaboration of inflammatory mediators may account for pain from this source. Muscle weakness arising from disuse of a contiguous joint may result in pain as the muscle is used. Referred pain (pain perceived at a distant site resulting from shared innervation of nearby structures) is frequently associated with OA. The perception of pain is individual-specific, and reflects the presence of central factors involved in the pathogenesis of pain.

Stiffness after Prolonged Inactivity.   This symptom is experienced by most patients with OA. It is a vague complaint used to describe difficulty in initiating movement, difficulties in moving a joint through its expected range of motion, or an ache or pain on movement. This is usually mild in OA, i.e., $< 30°$. The pathogenesis of joint stiffness in OA is not known and probably is not explained by synovitis. It is more likely that stiffness in OA has a mechanical explanation.

Progressive Loss of Function Secondary to Limited Mobility.   This is often seen in OA, and it leads to significant disability. The pathogenesis of limited mobility is probably complex. The altered shape of the OA joint and the associated capsule thickening may limit free movement. Additionally, pain often causes the individual to stop moving the joint. This leads to muscle weakness and flexion contractures from unopposing flexor muscles.

Cracking of Joint on Movement (Crepitus).   This symptom is often noted by patients, especially those with severe OA of the hip or knee. The pathogenesis of crepitus is probably due to the roughening of the joint surface secondary to cartilage loss, and osteophytosis, both of which interfere with the normal frictionless motion of the joint.

Signs
Findings on physical exam include tenderness to palpation at the joint margins and sometimes at the periarticular structures. There is often enlargement of the joint secondary to capsular thickening and osteophytes. Signs of mild inflammation (warmth, redness, and effusions) may be seen in OA, especially with DIP and PIP joint disease. More frequently, noninflammatory, cool effusions are detectable. The pathogenesis of these effusions remains obscure. Restricted, painful movements associated with coarse crepitus can be seen.

As the disease progresses, certain joint deformities can be seen. Varus angulation (bow-legged deformity) of the knee arises secondary to medial joint-space damage, and ligamentous laxity and instability. Leg-length discrepancy occurs secondary to destruction of the hip joint, with subsequent migration of the femoral head into the pelvic acetabulum.

Natural History of OA
In the majority of cases, OA progresses very slowly. Symptoms are often intermittent and exacerbated by change in activity level or new trauma. Some patients may have flares of their arthritis without any apparent antecedent event. Disease evolution appears to be fastest in the hand, slowest in the knee, and intermediate in the hip: This again suggests that there are differences in pathogenesis of OA at different joints. OA in any hand joint usually becomes clinically silent after a few years; once the swelling becomes firm and fixed and the joint movement becomes reduced, then the pain remits. However, joints can flare sequentially, producing symptoms for longer periods of time. In a minority of patients, rapid progressive disease occurs with marked bone destruction occurring over months rather than years. In another subset of patients, joint disease can improve both radiographically and symptomatically. The reason for the discrepancy between patients is unknown but again reflects the heterogeneity of this group of disorders.

Complications
Since OA is a disease confined to the joint, complications are related entirely to local processes and to the pain and disability resulting from damaged joints. Local complications result from the expanded joint margins and distorted anatomy. These include nerve entrapment syndromes and secondary periarthritis. Severe disease can result in secondary fractures, osteonecrosis (collapse of bone secondary to bone necrosis), and secondary arthritis in other joints. Traumatic fractures occur secondary to muscular weakness. Fibromyalgia (a syndrome characterized by poor sleep habits, depression, and chronic pain) and depression can result as a consequence of chronic pain and/or disability.

Clinical Examples

1. A 35-year-old white male who was previously in excellent health came in complaining of bilateral knee pain. He described the pain as an intermittent, dull ache that became worse on stair climbing and squatting, but that had been present for several months. On prompting, the professional baseball player recalled that he had experienced sharp knee pains for at least one year that were aggravated by knee movement. No other family members were affected with arthritis. His exam showed tenderness to palpation at the patellofemoral joints, and with compression of each patella. Radiographs of the knees showed minimal patellofemoral joint-space narrowing and sclerosis.

Discussion.   The clinical and x-ray findings are consistent with patellofemoral OA. This case is an example of abnormal stresses being placed across a normal joint secondary to repetitive-impact loading. In the absence of a family history of OA, it is unlikely that he has a heritable form of OA leading to precocious disease. A professional baseball catcher loads 10 times his body weight on his patellofemoral joints each time he squats. For a 150-1b. individual, this translates to 1500 lb. loaded on his articular cartilage 100–200 times a day for many years! Even with normal cartilage, this will eventually result in OA.

2. A 70-year-old female with longstanding rheumatoid arthritis came to the office complaining of right shoulder pain. The patient reported that she had chronic shoulder pain for 30 years. She noted that the character of the pain has changed gradually over the last 6 months, the pain becoming more severe with use and worse late rather than early in the day. Her exam was notable for typical deformities of rheumatoid arthritis; mild weakness of the right shoulder musculature as compared to the left; and right shoulder joint tenderness with palpation and movement, associated with restricted motion. X-rays showed destruction of the shoulder joint and marked osteophytosis.

Discussion.   This patient presented with osteoarthritis superimposed on rheumatoid arthritis. Clinical features of OA consist of use-related pain and change in the character of her chronic pain. This case is an example of normal stresses being placed on an abnormal joint. The subchondral bone is destroyed by the rheumatoid process and muscle atrophy is present secondary to disuse. Consequently, the subchondral bone and the surrounding muscle cannot help absorb the transmitted load and an increased load is transmitted to the articular cartilage. The cartilage becomes overstressed, and this eventually leads to OA.

Bibliography

Felson DT. The course of osteoarthritis and factors that affect it. *Rheum Dis Clin N Am* 19:3:607–616, 1993. *A nice review describing the natural history of OA and the factors that influence it.*

Howell DS, Treadwell BV, and Trippel SB. Etiopathogenesis of osteoarthritis. In Moskowitz RW, Howell DS, Goldberg VM, et al. (eds.). *Osteoarthritis Diagnosis and Management.* Philadelphia: Saunders, 1992, pp. 233–252. *A discussion of the etiologies and pathogenesis of OA.*

Mankin HS and Brandt KD. Biochemistry and Metabolism of Cartilage in Osteoarthritis. In Moskowitz RW, Howell DS, Goldberg VM, et al. (eds.). *Osteoarthritis Diagnosis and Management.* Philadelphia: Saunders, 1992, pp. 109–154. *A comprehensive review of cartilage metabolism in OA.*

Williams CJ and Jimenez SA. Heredity, genes and osteoarthritis. *Rheum Dis Clin N Am* 19:3:523–544, 1993. *A current review that addresses the latest research on heritable diseases that lead to OA.*

41 Rheumatoid Arthritis

Leslie S. Staudt

Objectives

After completing this chapter, you should be able to

Explain the clinical nature of rheumatoid arthritis

Understand the composition and significance of a rheumatoid factor

Understand the current theories of disease initiation, including genetic predisposition

Characterize the synovial pathology in rheumatoid arthritis

Understand the mechanical forces which cause joint deformity

Discuss the inflammatory process mediating extra-articular disease

Definition and Clinical Features

Rheumatoid arthritis (RA) is a systemic disease generally estimated to affect 1% of the adult population. Its incidence increases with increasing age but onset can occur at all ages, including childhood. It is at least twice as common in women as in men. A not uncommon scenario is a woman of child-bearing age presenting with a several month history of new-onset arthritis. It is a chronic, typically life-long, illness with a highly variable course. It may be, at one extreme, insidious in onset and smolder for years, having little effect on the patient's daily activities or have an explosive onset with rapidly progressive joint destruction resulting in marked functional impairment. With active disease or significant deformity, many patients encounter difficulty with performing job activities and the majority are unable to maintain gainful employment after 10–20 years of disease. The basic activities of daily living such as buttoning clothes, putting on shoes, opening jars, cooking, arising from a chair, climbing stairs and walking become problematic. Life expectancy is shortened. RA is an expensive disease both to the individual and to the community in terms of emotional costs, the expense of therapy, and loss of manpower.

Common to all patients and inherent in the basic definition of the disease is an ongoing inflammatory, destructive arthritis involving both small and large joints in a symmetric fashion. The most commonly affected joints and the most characteristic of the disease are the metacarpophalangeal (MCP), proximal interphalangeal (PIP), and wrist joints of the hands while the distal interphalangeal (DIP) joints are frequently spared. The pattern of joint involvement helps to clinically distinguish RA from other arthritides such as osteoarthritis which most commonly involves the DIP and PIP joints and spares the MCP and wrist joints. If one considers that the synovial lining layer of the joint is the center for the pathologic process, then it makes sense that the joints affected would be diarthrodial (synovial) joints. Other frequently affected joints include the elbows, shoulders, hips, knees, ankles, feet, and cervical spine.

Joint inflammation produces pain, morning stiffness, stiffness after rest (gelling), and loss of function. On examination, there is warmth and swelling (effusion) of the involved joints (Fig. 41-1). Analysis of joint fluid obtained by needle aspiration characteristically reveals an inflammatory (> 2000/mm³) white cell count with a predominance of polymorphonuclear cells. Radiographic evaluation, normal in the initial stages of the disease, will show erosive bony changes and joint-space loss as the disease progresses and the joint sustains ongoing damage (Fig. 41-2). Tendon laxity results in joint instability. All of these

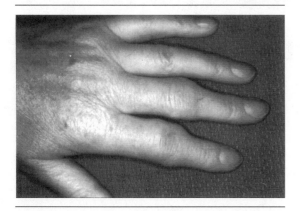

Fig. 41-1. Swelling can be seen in the proximal interphalangeal (PIP) joints of the second and third fingers, a typical location in RA. On examination, there would be an associated tenderness and pain with movement in these joints. (Reprinted from: the Clinical Slide Collection on the Rheumatic Diseases, copyright 1991. Used by permission of the American College of Rheumatology.)

changes taken in toto lead to irreversible deformity with contracture and subluxation. The associated muscle groups atrophy, leading to weakness, further compounding the individual's functional deficits. Complications of joint involvement may even be life-threatening such as brainstem or spinal cord damage from instability of the atlantoaxial articulation.

It should not be forgotten that RA is a systemic disorder which may, in addition to its effects upon the joints, involve other organ systems. These nonarticular manifestations vary widely in type and severity between individual patients. Generalized symptoms, resulting from the inflammatory nature of the disease, can include fever and malaise. The classic rheumatoid nodule, composed of a necrotic core surrounded by pallisading fibroblasts and a capsule, is typically located subcutaneously over extensor surfaces (Fig. 41-3) but may occur internally, such as in the lung parenchyma. Eye manifestations range from dryness to episcleritis to the more serious scleritis with its potential for loss of vision. A mild anemia is common; more serious hematologic abnormalities are rare but may in-

Fig. 41-2. Bilateral hand films demonstrate the extensive, symmetric joint destruction which can occur over time. The right first metacarpophalangeal (MCP) joint has been surgically pinned. There is joint space loss and extensive alteration of the normal joint architecture in the wrists. Erosive bony changes can be seen in the MCP and PIP joints. Juxta-articular osteopenia is evident.

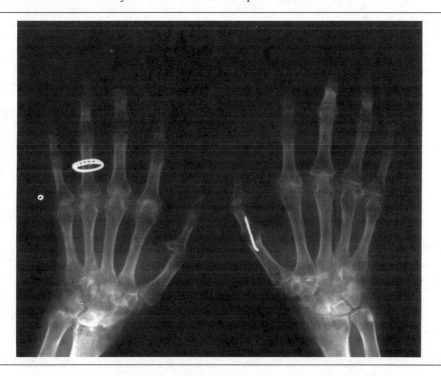

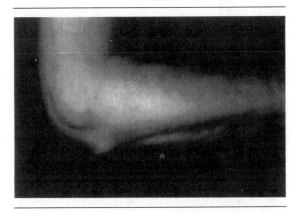

Fig. 41-3. A typical rheumatoid nodule is located subcutaneously over the extensor surface of the forearm. Not present in all RA patients, they are associated with high titers of rheumatoid factor and a more aggressively destructive disease course. These nodules must be distinguished from the tophi of gout, xanthomatosis of hyperlipidemia, and other rarer causes of nodule formation which may have a similar appearance. (Reprinted from: the Clinical Slide Collection on the Rheumatic Diseases, copyright 1991. Used by permission of the American College of Rheumatology.)

clude potentially life-threatening neutropenia. Various pulmonary and cardiac complications can occur, with pleuritis and interstitial pulmonary fibrosis leading the list. Vasculitis, a rare but life-threatening complication, is typically seen in patients with longstanding, severely-deforming disease.

Rheumatoid Factor

Hallmark of the disease, present in approximately three-fourths of patients, is a positive rheumatoid factor (RF). It is an autoantibody to an antibody, specifically to the Fc portion of the immunoglobulin G (IgG) antibody. It is typically an immunoglobulin M (IgM) molecule although immunoglobulin A (IgA) and IgG have been identified. It was originally identified when patient sera were found to agglutinate red blood cells. Erythrocytes, coated with IgG, will agglutinate when RF-positive sera is added as the multivalent IgM antibodies cross-link the IgG molecules. Clinically, a positive RF portends a more rapid and destructive disease course and carries a higher incidence of extra-articular disease manifestations compared to those patients who are RF-negative. It should be noted that, while commonly present, rheumatoid factors are not spe-

cific for rheumatoid arthritis and may be found in other chronic inflammatory diseases, particularly in chronic infections such as endocarditis or tuberculosis. Rheumatoid factors can also be identified in a small number of normal individuals with the percentage of positive RF and the titer both increasing with advancing age.

Diagnosis

The American Rheumatism Association criteria for the diagnosis of rheumatoid arthritis have a specificity of 87% and a sensitivity of greater than 90% in correctly identifying RA patients. As with most disease criteria, these were primarily developed to provide a common basis for enrolling patients in clinical trials and not for clinical practice. The seven criteria are morning stiffness of the joints for greater than one hour, arthritis of at least three joint areas at one time, arthritis in the joints of the hand, symmetric involvement, rheumatoid nodules, a positive serum rheumatoid factor, and bony erosions or juxtaarticular osteopenia present on hand radiographs. An individual must have had arthritic symptoms of over 6 weeks duration and meet four of these seven criteria to be classified as having RA. With the right clinical picture and with no features suggesting an alternative diagnosis, a clinician may well make the diagnosis in a patient who fails to meet these criteria, particularly early in the disease course.

Joint Structure

The articular joint structure is composed of opposing bony end-plates each covered by articular cartilage with the whole structure surrounded by the joint capsule. The synovium, a layer normally of only one to three cells in thickness, lines all the internal surfaces of the joint space except those directly overlying cartilage. It is a highly vascular structure, allowing for diffusion between the plasma, the interstitium, and the synovial fluid of nutrients and small proteins, and disposal of waste products by the sera and lymphatics. The cells composing the synovium have been designated Type A with a potential for phagocytic, macrophagelike activity and Type B with a protein-synthesizing capacity. The synovium, precisely because of this vascularity and cellularity, serves as the stage for the immunologic process in RA.

The cartilage, in contrast, is an avascular structure dependent upon the diffusion of nutrients from the synovial fluid. It is relatively protected against the early destructive forces of the disease. Composed primarily of proteoglycans, collagens, and water, it serves to absorb impact, to distribute load across the articulating joint surfaces, and as a smooth surface for joint range of motion. The bone provides structural support. The capsule maintains joint integrity and, with the ligaments, acts to stabilize the joint with movement. A more complete description of normal joint structure and function can be found in Chap. 40.

Pathogenesis

Disease Initiation

The initial step in the immunologic process leading to RA simplistically requires three things: a susceptible host, the appropriate antigen (one which has the potential to trigger disease in that patient), and intact T cell function. Initially macrophages (antigen-presenting cells) take up and process (partially degrade) the antigen. A portion of the processed antigen is then extruded onto the surface of the macrophage attached to the class II major histocompatibility (MHC) molecules. It is in this form that the antigen is presented to the T lymphocyte initiating the immune response.

The specific triggering antigen for RA is not known. There may be more than one potential antigen with the ability of each to initiate the disease being dependent on the individual's susceptibility to that particular antigen. Currently an infectious (particularly a viral) agent is considered the most likely candidate. Since RA is seen in all races, countries, and socioeconomic standings, something ubiquitous, such as an infection, seems more likely than environmental exposures or toxins. Additionally, there are already several well-documented associations between known infections and specific inflammatory arthritic syndromes such as Lyme disease following infection with the spirochete *Borrelia burgdorferi,* Reiter's syndrome following bacterial dysentery or genitourinary infection with *Chlamydia trachomatis,* and the short-lived arthritis associated with parvovirus B19. Agents under current consideration include the Epstein-Barr virus, members of the parvovirus family, and various mycobacteria. Antibodies to specific Epstein-Barr virus antigens can be documented in the majority of RA patients although these antibodies may simply reflect polyclonal B cell activation rather than specific antigen exposure. A similar question arises regarding the detection of antibodies to heat-shock proteins from mycobacteria in patients with RA. The detection of parvoviruslike particles in rheumatoid synovium is enticing but does not prove causality, particularly as symptom onset rarely follows infection.

The search for an etiology of RA has not been limited to infections. Endogenous protein molecules as the antigenic stimuli have been considered. Collagen, while attractive theoretically and previously the center of much speculation, has fallen out of favor from lack of supporting data. An abnormal IgG molecule is an appealing possibility, particularly in light of the high prevalence of rheumatoid factor positivity in RA patients, but definitive evidence is lacking.

Host susceptibility is principally determined by a person's immunogenetic makeup, particularly the expression of MHC Class II molecules which comprise receptors on the antigen-presenting cells. A striking number of patients with RA are HLA-DR4 and/or HLA-DR1 positive. These specific MHC Class II alleles are additionally associated with a more destructive disease course and a higher incidence of nonarticular disease manifestations.

Host susceptibility determination can be narrowed down still further to specific segments of the HLA-DR4 and DR1 alleles. There are five subtypes of HLA-DR4, but the association with RA is only seen in two of these, specifically Dw4 and Dw14. Comparisons of amino acid sequences have revealed a shared epitope located at amino acids 70–74 in the third hypervariable domain of the beta chain. It is this specific sequence, composed of a glutamine-leucine-arginine-alanine-alanine (in DR1 and Dw14) or a glutamine-arginine-arginine-alanine-alanine (in Dw4), which is held responsible for conferring RA susceptibility. Variations of this sequence by as little as two amino acids are not associated with disease.

T cell activation is key to the inflammatory process in RA. Its importance is clinically striking in those RA patients who contract the acquired immunodeficiency syndrome (AIDS) — a disease characterized by dysfunction of the T cell system — and experience remission of their RA. In contrast, B cells, while contributing to ongoing inflammation through antibody production, do not appear necessary to the initiation of the process. Abnormalities in their function fail to prevent RA as exemplified by RA development in patients with agammaglobulinemia. Ways to produce controlled modifications of T cell activation or function with monoclonal antibodies or selective chemotherapeutic agents are being investigated as therapeutic modalities.

Inflammatory Mediators and Destructive Forces

Activation of T cells sets into motion a cascade of inflammatory mediators. Many of the components of this intense reaction have been identified, but the relative importance of each and their complex interactions are less than perfectly understood.

Early in the disease angiogenesis begins. This production of new blood vessels is driven by macrophage production of endothelial-growth factors. Fibroblast-growth factor, for example, induces the endothelial cells to invade and form capillaries. This proliferating endothelium in turn produces plasminogen activator and metaloproteinases such as collagenase, which further fosters invasion, and likewise joint destruction, by matrix degradation. Alteration in the microvasculature permeability results in protein and fluid extravasation into the synovium, with the resulting tissue edema.

These new vessels are additionally acted upon by specific cytokines, including interferon gamma, interleukin-1, and tumor necrosis factor. In response, the synovial endothelium expresses surface addressins, glycoprotein molecules which act to bind lymphocytes to the vessel wall via receptors on the lymphocytes. These addressin molecules may provide for selective recognition of specific lymphocyte subsets. Once adhered, the lymphocytes migrate into the synovial stroma.

Activated T cells predominate in the synovium. There is a striking increase in the number of CD4 (helper) cells and a concomitant decrease in CD8 (suppressor) cell number. Only a restricted number of T cell receptor subtypes are represented within this group, suggesting selective clonal expansion in addition to selective migration.

B cells, following activation by T cells, proliferate, undergo differentiation and secrete rheumatoid factor (RF), the autoantibody to the Fc portion of IgG molecule. The RF then perpetuates the inflammatory cascade through the formation of immune complexes. These complexes primarily contain IgM rheumatoid factors which have the ability to bind and activate complements, thereby releasing mast cell mediators, attracting polymorphonuclear leukocytes, and triggering platelet aggregation leading to microthrombi and ischemia. Immune complexes have been found enriching the surrounding cartilage and are believed to serve as the attractant for synovial invasion into this adjacent tissue.

In contrast to the predominance of lymphocytes within the synovium, polymorphonuclear leukocytes (PMNs) are the principal cells in the synovial fluid. Similar to the method of ingress into the synovium of T cells, the endothelium is induced by the cytokines interleukin-1 and tumor necrosis factor to produce specific leukocyte-binding molecules on their cell surface and allow migration. The PMNs are drawn into the joint space by chemoattractants including C5a — a product of the activation of complement, leukotriene B4 — a product of the cyclo-oxygenase pathway, and platelet-activating factor, all enriched in the synovial fluid. The large number of PMNs within the joint space have great destructive potential. Activated through the ingestion of cellular debris and immune complexes, they degranulate, releasing proteinases, collagenase, and elastase, thereby promoting the degradation of collagen. Oxygen free radicals are produced. Prostaglandins and leukotrienes are produced by the metabolism of arachidonic acid released by the mobilization of membrane phospholipids. The sum of these effects of PMN activation is the perpetuation and enhancement of the inflammatory response.

Cytokines, soluble proteins acting in the microenvironment, function as the intercellular messengers for the immune response. Produced by a variety of activated cells, they interact with specific cell surface receptors. Each individual cytokine may exert different and sometimes opposing effects on different cells simultaneously. Within the synovium, the cytokines, which predominate, originate not from the lymphocytes, but from the macrophages and fibroblasts. The products of these cells may actually suppress expression of the lymphocyte cytokines in patients with RA but additionally may act to stimulate the selective proliferation of the T helper (CD4-positive) subset. As a gross oversimplification, while the T cell can be viewed as the cell of RA initiation, the macrophage is the cell which modulates propagation of the disease.

Macrophages and fibroblasts, like the T cells and PMNs, migrate into the synovium following endothelial adhesion. Once there, they become activated through the ingestion of debris, and the effects of cytokines and immune complexes. They produce such cytokines as interleukin-1 (IL-1), interleukin-6 (IL-6), tumor necrosis factor (TNF), platelet-derived growth factor (PDGF), fibroblast growth factor (FGF), and transforming growth factor (TGF). IL-1 and TNF act primarily to stimulate production of degradative enzymes such as collagenase, prostaglandin, and stromelysin and the acute-phase proteins such as C-reactive protein. IL-1 additionally induces fibroblasts to produce the cytokine IL-6, another inducer for the production of acute-phase proteins. PDGF and FGF, in high concentration in synovial fluid, are potent stimulators of fibroblast chemotaxis and proliferation, inducing collagenase production and thereby promoting cellular invasion. TGF is actually a family of related proteins, each with differing functions. TGF-alpha stimulates bone reabsorption and inhibits new bone formation. It too stimulates fibroblast proliferation. The role of TGF-beta, typically associated with wound repair, is more difficult to ascertain; while it aids in cellular proliferation and angiogenesis, by promoting biosynthesis and suppressing the production of collagenase it also appears to counteract many of the degradative effects induced by the other cytokines.

Cytokines produced by the T cells, down-regulated by the macrophages partially through the effects of TGF-beta, include IL-2, IL-3, and interferon-gamma (INF-gamma), and typically deal with promoting T and B cell function. INF-gamma, the most abundant of the three, induces HLA-DR on endothelial cells and suppresses collagen synthesis. IL-2 promotes T cell proliferation and the production of hydrogen peroxide. IL-3 appears only in extremely low concentrations.

There are numerous other mediators of the inflammatory articular process. The coagulation cascade and its final product, fibrin, contribute to joint destruction. What initiates the cascade is unclear but probably involves immune complexes. Fibrin, deposited throughout the joint surface, fosters ischemic changes and potentially serves as an inflammatory trigger. Bradykinin is released, increasing vascular permeability. Histamine, from mast cell degranulation, and serotonin, produced by platelets, contribute to this vascular leakage. Complement consumption within the joint leads to the release of C5a and C3a. C5a mediates both chemotaxis and PMN lysosomal-enzyme release. Neuropeptides, specifically substance P, stimulate the production of prostaglandins and metaloproteinases, thereby promoting inflammation.

Joint Destruction and Deformity

The net result of the inflammatory process is a tremendously hypertrophied synovial tissue, called pannus, with the ability to invade surrounding tissue, irreversibly destroying tissue. Cartilage is eroded, with subsequent radiographic joint space loss. Bony erosions occur initially at the site of direct contact between bone and pannus, that is, at the joint margin where the bone lies unprotected by overlying cartilage (Fig. 41-4). Demineralization of periarticular bone and generalized osteoporosis occur. Over time, normal joint structure is lost with complete joint collapse (see Fig. 41-2) and, in some cases, total loss of normal motion.

Joint contracture may develop relatively early in the disease course, before radiographic evidence of destruction. Pain frequently produces a prolonged immobilization of the joint, often unconsciously on the patient's part. Lack of use results in muscle weakness and eventual atrophy, further decreasing joint functional capacity. Joint stability is lost as the surrounding ligaments and tissue are stretched from chronic swelling and weakened by enzymatic degra-

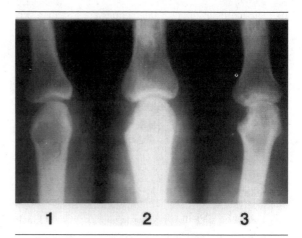

Fig. 41-4. Progressive destructive changes in this MCP joint can be seen over time from panels 1 to 3. Initially, there is soft tissue swelling (1) progressing to joint-space loss and cortex thinning (2) to a marginal erosion over the radial aspect of the metacarpal head (3). (Reprinted from: the Clinical Slide Collection on the Rheumatic Diseases, copyright 1991. Used by permission of the American College of Rheumatology.)

dation. This, along with the abnormal mechanical stresses, leads to many of the classic deformities of RA such as ulnar deviation of the fingers as the result of synovitis at the MCP joints (Fig. 41-5). Instability of the knee and involvement of the feet causes gait instability and an increased risk for falls. Tenosynovitis, inflammation of the synovial sheath lining the tendons, may result in eventual rupture of the involved tendon with resulting loss of the ability to extend the joint.

Extraarticular Involvement

The inflammatory process, while most marked and best understood in the joint, is not limited to articular spaces. The pathogenesis of the extraarticular disease manifestations, with some variability depending on the organ involved, is similar to that in the joints. Rheumatoid vasculitis illustrates this phenomenon with immune complexes and inflammatory cells detected in the involved vessel walls. A panarteritis develops with resulting intimal proliferation, microthrombi formation, and local tissue ischemia. Inflammatory mediators and degradative enzymes are released. The clinical result of this process is dependent upon the size of vessel involved along with the tissue it supplies. Ar-

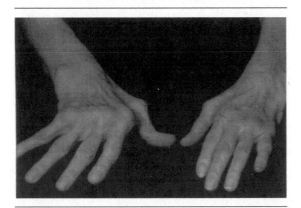

Fig. 41-5. Destructive forces in the right hand have led to ulnar deviation of the fingers and significant muscle atrophy of the dorsal musculature. Chronic swelling can be seen in the MCP joints. This picture is atypical for RA in the asymmetry although subtle changes can be seen in the left hand. (Reprinted from: the Clinical Slide Collection on the Rheumatic Diseases, copyright 1991. Used by permission of the American College of Rheumatology.)

terial involvement in the extremities produces digital ischemia. Compromise of the vascular supply to a nerve produces neuropathy. Visceral organ disease might result in liver dysfunction, renal failure, or bowel ischemia. Skin manifestations of vascular insufficiency may cause ulceration or palpable purpura. The rheumatoid nodule itself is the result of a venulitis.

A similar scenario can be evoked to explain nearly all nonarticular manifestations. Localized inflammatory reactions in the eye may lead to episcleritis, scleritis, or corneal ulceration. Inflammation may develop of the pleura or pericardium. Interstitial lung disease and myocarditis, although uncommon, can occur. Felty's syndrome, a rare complication, is a triad of RA, splenomegaly, and neutropenia, often complicated by recurrent infections. The pathogenesis is antigranulocyte autoantibody production, with immune complex formation resulting in sequestration, splenic degradation, and impaired granulocyte function.

Clinical Examples

1. A 30-year-old mother of two complained of pain and swelling of her hands for several months. The pain made caring for her infant difficult, particularly in the previous few weeks. It was worse in the mornings or if she got up

during the night. She additionally noted stiffness and discomfort in her knees with stair climbing, after prolonged sitting, and with extended walking. Her right knee was particularly troublesome the prior few days. She noted occasional pain in her feet and ankles. She had tried taking acetaminophen and over-the-counter ibuprofen without appreciable benefit.

She had no past medical history and took no medications regularly. She related having a maternal great-aunt with a "crippling arthritis." She felt tired but denied other problems. Her physical examination was normal except for her joints. She demonstrated warmth over her hands and wrists with swelling and tenderness to palpation over the metacarpophalangeal (MCP) joints and several proximal interphalangeal (PIP) joints bilaterally, worse on the right than the left. There was pain with range of motion of her wrists. Grip strength was diminished secondary to pain. Her right knee had a moderate effusion but good range of motion. Both knees were warm. She was tender over her metatarsophalangeal (MTP) joints. She had no palpable nodules.

Her laboratory studies demonstrated an elevated erythrocyte sedimentation rate, a lab result which was nonspecific but suggested ongoing inflammation. She had a slight normocytic, normochromic anemia. Her rheumatoid factor was positive at a titer of 1:80. Antinuclear antibody (ANA) testing was negative. Aspiration of her right knee yielded 10 cc of yellow, cloudy fluid with an inflammatory-range white cell count of 12,000/mm^3 with 90% polymorphonuclear leukocytes on differential. Examination for crystals and gram stain and culture of the joint fluid were negative. Radiographs of her hands were normal.

Discussion.   This woman's presentation was typical for new-onset RA. She clearly had a symmetric, polyarticular inflammatory arthritis involving both large and small joints. Systemic lupus erythematosus was in the differential but was unlikely with a negative ANA and the lack of other manifestations. Crystal-induced arthritis and osteoarthritis would be highly unusual in a woman of this age. Infectious etiologies were possible but the course and clinical picture was atypical for disseminated gonococcal infection, Lyme disease, or parvovirus. This presentation might be seen early in the course of a spondyloarthropathy but the positive rheumatoid factor made this unlikely as a diagnosis.

2. A 55-year-old female with a 15-year history of rheumatoid factor-positive, nodular RA, currently being treated with a nonsteroidal anti-inflammatory, low-dose prednisone and hydroxychloroquine, complained of a persis-

tent, nonproductive cough on routine followup. She denied fever, chills, chest pain, peripheral edema or shortness of breath. She did note some allergic rhinitis symptoms. She had a 50 pack-years smoking history.

Pulmonary and cardiac examination were normal. She had long-standing deformities of multiple joints with ulnar deviation, MCP subluxation and swan-neck changes in her hands, poor grip strength, subluxation and fusion of the wrists, bilateral contractures of the elbows, decreased range of motion of her shoulders, crepitance and bony enlargement of the knees, decreased range of motion in her ankles, and MTP joint subluxation. Rheumatoid nodules were present over the olecranon processes and hand joints. Her joints were cool with palpable boggy synovium.

Chest radiograph demonstrated a quarter-sized, noncalcified discrete mass in the right lung parenchyma. CT-guided needle biopsy of the mass yielded normal lung tissue with necrotic debris, fibroblasts and inflammatory cells, primarily lymphocytes; there was no evidence of malignancy. She was advised to quit smoking; she did and her cough gradually improved.

Discussion. Rheumatoid nodules, while typically located subcutaneously over extensor surfaces, may develop anywhere with the lung parenchyma being one of the most frequent noncutaneous sites. They sometimes affect organ function but often, as in this case, create a diagnostic dilemma. Noncalcified lung masses must always be evaluated to rule out malignancy.

3. A 65-year-old male with a 25-year history of rheumatoid factor-positive, nodular RA presented to the local emergency room with new-onset of painful digital tip lesions, difficulty walking, abdominal pain, frequent stools, and generalized malaise. His current medications included indomethacin and low-dose prednisone. He had previously undergone bilateral knee replacements, an ankle fusion, metatarsal head resection, and surgery on his MCPs.

Physical examination demonstrated an ill-appearing elderly male with painful digital infarctions and impending gangrene. Shotty cervical adenopathy was noted. Abdominal exam showed a palpable liver edge, a palpable spleen tip, and nonlocalized, diffuse tenderness. Neurologic exam demonstrated a right foot drop. His had long-standing multiple joint deformities but little active synovitis. RA nodules were present. A stool sample was positive for occult blood.

Laboratory studies revealed anemia (hematocrit of 30%), a reduced white count of 1500/mm³ with only 40% granulocytes, and a platelet count below normal at 110,000/mm³.

His erythrocyte sedimentation rate was elevated at 90 mm/hour (normal < 20 mm/hour). Rheumatoid factor was positive with a titer of 1:1280. Abdominal ultrasound verified splenomegaly and mild hepatomegaly. Colonoscopy revealed areas of friable mucosa consistent with ischemia. Upper gastrointestinal studies revealed only esophageal irritation.

He was treated with high doses of intravenous steroids and cyclophosphamide but, over the following week, his condition dramatically deteriorated with worsening abdominal pain, bloody diarrhea requiring transfusion, and renal insufficiency. On the seventh hospital day, he was found to be febrile, confused, and hypotensive. He died within 24 hours from gastrointestinal sepsis despite broad-spectrum antibiotics.

Discussion.   This patient had two concomitant complications of rheumatoid factor-positive RA, Felty's syndrome and rheumatoid vasculitis. Felty's syndrome, occurring in only 1% of the RA population, is typified by granulocytopenia and splenomegaly. Most often, it is diagnosed on routine blood work, and may or may not be complicated by bacterial infection. Primarily a late complication, it is not unusual for the synovitis to be relatively inactive at the time of onset. Lymphadenopathy, anemia, and thrombocytopenia can occur in patients with Felty's.

Rheumatoid vasculitis, another manifestation of immune complex formation, was the cause of the digital infarctions, bowel ischemia, and neurologic deficit. Extensive organ involvement such as this is a rare but life-threatening complication requiring aggressive immunosuppression. It is one of the few complications more common in men.

Bibliography

Albani S, Carson DA, and Roudier J. Genetic and environmental factors in the immune pathogenesis of rheumatoid arthritis. *Rheum Dis Clin N Am* 18:729–740, 1992. *A review of the immunogenetics and initiation of RA.*

Harris ED Jr. Etiology and pathogenesis of rheumatoid arthritis. In Kelley W, Harris E, Ruddy S, et al. (eds.). Textbook of Rheumatology (4th ed.). Philadelphia: Saunders, 1993, pp. 833–873. *An extensive review of known RA pathogenesis.*

Harris ED Jr. Rheumatoid arthritis: Pathophysiology and implications for therapy. *New Engl J Med* 322:1277–1289, 1990. *An overview of the immunologic stages of disease initiation and perpetuation, and the potential for therapeutic intervention at each stage.*

Ollier W and Thomson W. Population genetics of rheumatoid arthritis. *Rheum Dis Clin N Am* 18:741–759, 1992. *A summary of HLA influences in RA.*

Wilder RL. Rheumatoid arthritis: A. Epidemiology, Pathology, and Pathogenesis. In Schumacher H, Klippel J, and Koopman W (eds.). *Primer on the Rheumatic Dis-*

eases (10th ed.). Richmond, VA: William Byrd Press, 1993, pp. 86–89. *An overview of RA pathogenesis.*

Yocum DE. Immunopathogenesis of RA: What happens in the rheumatoid joint. *J Musculoskel Med* 11:47–55, 1994. *A simple review of the inflammatory mediators of joint inflammation.*

42 Gout and Crystal Disease

Ira N. Targoff

Objectives

After completing this chapter, you should be able to

Understand the normal metabolism of uric acid, including the mechanisms of production and routes of excretion

Understand the different mechanisms leading to elevated levels and accumulation of uric acid (primary vs. secondary problems and overproduction vs. underexcretion)

Know the conditions that can develop as a consequence of hyperuricemia, and understand the mechanisms involved

Know the joint conditions associated with calcium pyrophosphate dihydrate deposition, and factors that may contribute to this

Know about other crystals that have been associated with joint diseases, and the nature of the conditions

The typical clinical picture of gout was described in ancient times, and many famous figures throughout history are believed to have suffered from it. The association with uric acid has been known for 200 years. We now know more about gout than almost any other rheumatic disease, although certain questions remain.

Deposition of certain types of crystals in joints can lead to an inflammatory arthritis, of which **gout,** caused by **monosodium urate monohydrate** (MSU) crystals, is most common. MSU crystal deposition can result not only in acute gouty attacks, but also nodular urate deposits (**tophi**), chronic arthritis, and **kidney stones,** or other renal injury. It is important to be familiar with gout not only because of its frequency, but also because it can usually be effectively controlled, with prevention of future attacks and tissue damage, by available medications. The ability to properly treat it depends on a knowledge of its pathophysiology.

Calcium pyrophosphate dihydrate (CPPD) deposition in joints can result in an acute attack similar to that of gout, and other crystals have also been associated with joint disease. It is important to recognize these, although we cannot yet control formation of these crystals.

Hyperuricemia

One must keep in mind the difference between **hyperuricemia,** the elevated blood urate itself, and gout, the resulting arthritis. Many patients with hyperuricemia do not develop gout. This is of importance in treatment, since suppression of joint inflammation and control of hyperuricemia must be considered separately.

Normal Urate Physiology

Total body uric acid, about 1200 mg in normal men, is determined by a balance between production and excretion, with an average turnover of about 700 mg/day. At the pH of plasma and most tissue fluids, it exists as its ionized form, urate, but uric acid predominates in the urine. The average serum urate concentration before puberty is about 3.5 mg/dl, rising to 5 mg/dl in males after puberty, but not in females until after menopause. The limit of solubility in plasma is 6.5–6.8 mg/dl at 37°C. A higher concentration represents supersaturation, and is considered abnormal (hyperuricemia) independent of its frequency in the population, although this level is also close to the mean plus two standard deviations for normal men (usually approximately 7.0 mg/dl of urate).

Production

Uric acid is derived from **purine** (mainly adenine and guanine) breakdown, and is the irreversible final product that must be excreted, since humans cannot further metabolize it. The body's purines come from three sources: (a) the **diet;** (b) breakdown of existing **cellular purines** from nucleic acids, coenzymes such as NAD, etc.; and (c) **de novo** metabolic synthesis of purines.

Diet (excluding alcohol) usually contributes only enough purines to affect the serum urate level by about 1–2 mg/dl,

and thus by itself does not usually lead to gout, nor can dietary restriction alone effectively control hyperuricemia in most patients with gout. Examples of foods rich in purines include organ meats, some fish, beans, and peas.

Guanine and the intermediate purine hypoxanthine can be irreversibly metabolized to xanthine and then to uric acid, or "salvaged" for reuse by a reaction with phosphoribosyl-pyrophosphate (**PRPP**) that is catalyzed by hypoxanthine-guanine phosphoribosyl transferase (**HGPRT**), thus saving the energy requirement of de novo synthesis (Fig. 42-1). Adenine may also be salvaged by a reaction with PRPP catalyzed by a separate enzyme.

De novo synthesis involves the conversion of PRPP to

Fig. 42-1. Purine metabolism and uric acid synthesis. The interactions of de novo synthesis and the salvage pathways as well as the point of action of enzymes of importance in uric acid metabolism are shown. Enzymes: (1) amidophosphoribosyl transferase, (2) hypoxanthine-guanine phosphoribosyl transferase (HGPRT), (3) PRPP synthetases, (4) adenine phosphoribosyl transferase, (5) adenosine deaminase, (6) purine nucleoside phosphorylase, (7) 5′ nucleotidase, and (8) xanthine oxidase. HGPRT deficiency or PRPP synthetase overactivity lead to increased PRPP, which increases de novo synthesis. HGPRT deficiency also leads to increased formation of uric acid from hypoxanthine and guanine, and less feedback inhibition by nucleotides. (From: the *Primer on the Rheumatic Diseases,* tenth edition, copyright 1993. Used by permission of the Arthritis Foundation. Adapted with permission from: Seegmiller SE, Rosenbloom FM, and Kelley WN: Enzyme defect associated with a sex-linked human neurological disorder and excessive purine synthesis. *Science* 155:1682–1684, 1967. Copyright 1967 American Association for the Advancement of Science.)

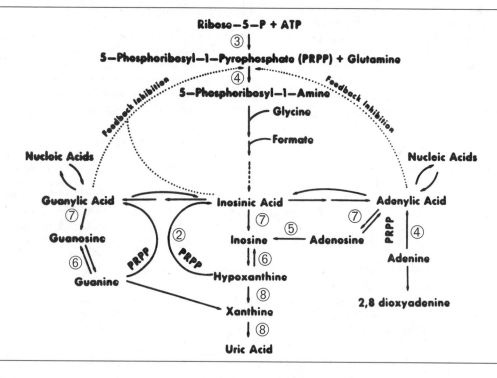

inosinic acid through a series of steps. The **rate-limiting reactions** controlling this pathway are the formation of PRPP (catalyzed by **PRPP synthetase**), and the initial step using PRPP (catalyzed by **amido-phosphoribosyl-transferase**). Purine nucleotides (the end-products of the pathway) can inhibit these enzymes, and therefore slow de novo synthesis. However, such inhibition of the transferase can be countered by the substrate PRPP, thus increasing synthesis.

Excretion

Uric acid is excreted by two major routes: 2/3 is excreted by the kidneys in the urine and about 1/3 is excreted into the gut and destroyed by intestinal bacteria.

The renal handling of urate involves four sites. All except the small amount that is protein bound is **filtered** at the glomerulus. Most of this is **reabsorbed** in the first portion of the proximal tubule. In a more distal portion of the proximal tubule there is a **urate secretory site,** where other weak organic acids such as salicylate are also secreted. Distal to this is a **post-secretory reabsorptive site.** About 7.5% of the filtered uric acid is excreted.

Mechanisms Leading to Hyperuricemia

Hyperuricemia results from either increased synthesis (**overproduction**) or decreased renal clearance (**underexcretion**) of uric acid, or a combination. In either case the plasma urate concentration will rise until enough is excreted to reach a steady state and extracellular fluid may become supersaturated with urate, which can be deposited in tissues. **Primary** hyperuricemia results from innate defects in uric acid metabolism, while in **secondary** hyperuricemia there is another recognized condition that has led to it.

Overproduction

Primary. 10–25% of those with primary gout are clearly overproducers, and can be identified by high uric acid excretion in a 24-hour urine collection (> 800–1000 mg/day on a normal diet). Some of the remaining patients with primary gout may overproduce uric acid, but are not detected due to increased gut excretion.

A small proportion of overproducers have known **inherited enzymatic defects** leading to increased synthesis of uric acid, with extreme hyperuricemia, kidney stones, and severe, early-onset gout. The best studied of these are two **X-linked** disorders of purine metabolism: (a) **deficiency of HGPRT,** and (b) various altered forms of PRPP synthetase that cause **overactivity.** By different mechanisms,

both increase the level of PRPP, which, as noted above, can increase urate synthesis. Other metabolic defects causing overproduction have been identified, such as **glucose-6-phosphatase deficiency,** but others remain to be elucidated.

HGPRT deficiency prevents salvage of hypoxanthine and guanine, thus leaving more PRPP available for de novo synthesis and more hypoxanthine and guanine for uric acid formation. Although the nucleotides that provide negative feedback are not decreased, lack of nucleotide formation by salvage results in less nucleotide than expected for the amount of hypoxanthine and guanine. **Complete HGPRT deficiency** leads to a severe neurologic condition marked by mental retardation and self-mutilation known as **Lesch-Nyhan syndrome,** which overshadows the uric acid abnormalities. Those with **partial deficiency** mainly show severe, early-onset hyperuricemia and its consequences without neurologic problems, even if only a small percent of activity remains. Multiple specific defects in HGPRT molecular structure have been identified in different families, with varying residual activity.

PRPP synthetase overactivity can result from any of a variety of gene defects that can cause increased catalytic activity or decreased responsiveness to inhibitors. These may result in varying degrees of hyperuricemia and severity of complications, with decreased inhibition usually being worse. Neurologic problems may occur, and females can be affected in some forms. All result in increased PRPP and increased de novo urate synthesis.

Glucose-6-phosphatase deficiency, which leads to glycogen storage disease, also is associated with hyperuricemia and gout, in part through overproduction. Increased PRPP may play a role, as well as decreased feedback inhibition due to depletion of nucleotides. It can also lead to increased lactic acid and ketones that impair uric acid secretion (see below). Other glycogen storage diseases can also decrease ATP and increase uric acid production.

Secondary.   Conditions associated with marked **cellular proliferation** and **increased turnover** of nucleic acid purine can lead to secondary hyperuricemia and eventually gout. These conditions may include hematologic malignancies (such as chronic leukemia and multiple myeloma), polycythemia vera, chronic hemolytic anemias, pernicious anemia, and psoriasis. Marked hyperuricemia may be seen in response to treatment of malignancies with chemotherapy, due to cell death and nucleic acid release.

Alcohol consumption increases plasma urate and is often associated with gout. Several mechanisms may be involved, among them an increase in de novo synthesis due to decreased nucleotide feedback by ATP, resulting from increased adenine nucleotide usage.

Underexcretion

Primary. About 75–85% of patients with gout have a defect in uric acid excretion, leading to decreased renal uric acid clearance, with less excretion than expected for a given serum level. Nonrenal excretion, in contrast, tends to be increased. The exact abnormalities leading to underexcretion in primary gout are unknown. Mechanisms at different sites have been proposed (secretion, reabsorption, or filtration), and may vary in different patients. Usually, impaired uric acid clearance is the only renal functional abnormality recognized.

In at least some patients with primary underexcretion, an inherited defect appears to be responsible. A **familial predilection** to gout has long been recognized, with varying frequency of affected relatives between populations studied. Certain populations have an overall high frequency of gout, such as the Maori of New Zealand with 10% of males affected. It cannot be excluded that apparent primary gout in some patients is due to an environmental factor.

Secondary.   Interference with urate excretion by **decreased renal function** of any cause commonly leads to secondary hyperuricemia, and may cause gout. The kidney injury caused by **chronic lead poisoning** is particularly noteworthy, since the hyperuricemia appears to be greater than expected for the degree of overall renal impairment, and gout is common [**saturnine gout** (i.e., lead-related)]. This may be due to increased tubular reabsorption of uric acid. However, other risk factors for gout are often found in these patients, especially alcohol consumption, since saturnine gout has been associated with consumption of "moonshine whiskey" made with equipment containing lead.

Certain weak organic acids, such as **lactic acid,** can compete with uric acid for renal tubular secretion, and impair its clearance. **Alcoholic binges** can decrease uric acid excretion acutely by increasing lactic acid formation, thus precipitating acute gouty attacks. **Salicylate** in low doses (less than 2 g/day) competes for secretion of urate, although high levels interfere with tubular reabsorption, thus increasing excretion and lowering the serum level. **Ketones,** generated by fasting or diabetes, can also compete for secretion.

Several medications other than salicylate may cause hyperuricemia and gout through effects on excretion. Examples include thiazide diuretics, which enhance tubular reabsorption and suppress tubular secretion; pyrazinamide (used in tuberculosis treatment), which strongly inhibits secretion; and cyclosporine (an immunosuppressant).

Associated Conditions

Certain chronic medical conditions have long been associated with hyperuricemia and gout (and with each other), including obesity, diabetes, hypertension, hyperlipidemia, and atherosclerosis. In some cases the reason is clear (e.g., treatment of hypertension with thiazides, diabetic or hypertensive renal disease), but in others it is not completely explained. Some associations may depend on common predisposing factors.

Consequences of Hyperuricemia

Asymptomatic Hyperuricemia

Although chronic hyperuricemia may result in gout, kidney stones, or tophi, greater than 80% of patients with hyperuricemia will never develop these problems. The risk depends on the **serum urate level** and the **duration** of elevation, with a risk of less than 1%/year at less than 9 mg/dl. If such problems arise, they can usually be treated successfully at that point, preventing permanent joint or kidney injury. Therefore, hyperuricemia without other problems (**asymptomatic hyperuricemia**) is usually not treated, unless elevations are so extreme (> 13 mg/dl, enzyme defects) that the risk of problems is very high or there is risk of acute uric acid nephropathy (for example, during the initiation of cancer chemotherapy).

A previous concern with this approach was that continued deposition of urate in kidney tissue (**chronic urate nephropathy**) due to uncontrolled hyperuricemia might lead to the gradual loss of renal function, but studies have failed to demonstrate significant functional deterioration independent of associated hypertension or diabetes. Another concern was the increased coronary disease and atherosclerosis in patients with hyperuricemia, but this appears to be due to the associated risk factors discussed above, so that lowering uric acid would not prevent it.

Acute Gouty Attacks

Hyperuricemia is usually present for years (commonly greater than 20–30) before gouty attacks occur. Most hyperuricemia does not develop until after puberty in males, with first gouty attacks most common in the fifth or sixth decade. In women, hyperuricemia usually does not develop until menopause, and gouty attacks are less common and appear later. With higher urate levels, gout is more likely, and tends to develop earlier, explaining the appearance of gout in the teens and twenties in patients with enzyme defects.

Clinical Presentation

The usual first manifestation of gout is as acute, inflammatory **monoarthritis** (arthritis involving a single joint). The first metatarsophalangeal (MTP) joint is most commonly affected, involved in up to 50% of first attacks. Other common first sites are also in the lower extremity (ankle, heel, instep, knee). If hyperuricemia persists, involvement of more proximal sites and the upper extremities may occur, and **polyarticular** (multiple-joint) attacks become more common. Acute inflammation may also occur in the synovially lined bursae (such as the olecranon bursa) and tendon sheaths.

Typical acute gouty attacks have a distinctive course, showing (a) sudden onset, reaching a peak within hours; (b) marked inflammation and pain; and (c) spontaneous resolution after days to weeks, even in the absence of treatment. During the attack, the cardinal signs of inflammation are seen in the joint: (a) extreme pain and tenderness, typically with sensitivity even to the pressure of bed sheets; (b) swelling, with development of an effusion (accumulation of fluid) in the joint and edema of the surrounding soft tissues; (c) increased heat of overlying skin; (d) erythema of the overlying skin; and (e) loss of function, with restriction of the range of joint motion. Signs of a systemic response, such as fever or leukocytosis, may be seen. After the attack, the joint becomes normal clinically (no symptoms and no abnormalities on examination), and remains so (the **intercritical period**) until the next attack. The episodic course often alerts the clinician to consider the diagnosis of gout or crystal disease.

Clinical features alone cannot establish the diagnosis, even when hyperuricemia is present. The urate level may even be normal during an acute attack. The diagnosis is confirmed by aspiration of synovial fluid from the affected joint, and demonstration of MSU crystals in the fluid. During an acute attack, most crystals will be found engulfed in whole or part by neutrophils. MSU crystals can be identified by their **needle** shape, and by their optical property under **compensated polarized light microscopy** of **strong negative birefringence** (see Plate 4). Birefringence results in the crystal appearing bright against the dark background when polarizer and analyzer are perpendicular. A negatively birefringent crystal appears yellow when its long axis is parallel to the axis of slow vibration of the red compensator, and becomes blue when turned perpendicular.

Initiating Events

MSU crystals may form when blood or tissues are supersaturated, and may be deposited in synovium, cartilage, bone, or surrounding tissue. The factors responsible for initiating crystallization and determining where urate is deposited are not entirely understood, and multiple factors may be involved. Factors that are believed important include the cooler temperature of the extremities (lowering urate solubility); resorption of fluid without dissolved urate during recumbency (increasing local urate concentration), which may explain the clinical observation that attacks often wake the patient from sleep; interaction of crystals with proteoglycans or unidentified factors in synovial fluid; and gravitational effects and physical stress such as weight bearing, which may contribute to the early deposition in the lower extremities and the predilection for the MTP.

MSU crystals in the synovial fluid or membrane involved in the acute attack may derive from preformed local deposits either by rupture of the deposits or by release of crystals from their surface, or the crystals may be newly formed at the time of the attack. Factors that raise or lower serum (and tissue) urate concentration can initiate an acute attack, presumably by affecting MSU crystal formation or release. Factors that raise urate level (such as alcohol, dietary indiscretion, starvation, or medications) can precipitate attacks.

Acute attacks are a risk of undertaking urate lowering therapy, and initiating such therapy during an acute attack can prolong it and make it more difficult to treat. Lower urate levels may shrink crystals, allowing them to escape from the matrix of the deposit ("crystal shedding"). Such therapy is started only when an acute attack has completely subsided, and during the first 6–12 months is usually accompanied by colchicine administration to prevent new attacks.

Inflammatory Response

MSU crystals can be found in synovial fluids from symptom-free joints between attacks in greater than 50% of patients with gout, and even a small percentage of those with asymptomatic hyperuricemia. Generally, these crystals are not found within neutrophils. If crystals are present in the joint, why is there no gout attack?

For an acute attack to occur, an inflammatory response to the crystals must be generated. **Neutrophils** are key cells in the response to crystals, and they predominate in the synovial fluid during an attack. However, mononuclear cells may also play a role in initiation of the attack. **Phagocytosis** of crystals by neutrophils or other immune cells can lead to release of inflammatory mediators that can amplify and perpetuate the response, including chemotactic factors, prostaglandins, and the proinflammatory interleukins (IL-1, IL-6). This can induce further infiltration with inflammatory cells, and synovial proliferation. One factor that can affect whether phagocytosis occurs is the type of proteins that coat the crystal in the joint. Coating with complement products or immunoglobulins promotes phagocytosis, and coating with apolipoproteins B or E can protect against it. An acute attack is suppressed with medications such as colchicine or nonsteroidal anti-inflammatory drugs that affect neutrophils and inflammatory mediators, rather than by addressing the urate itself.

Chronic Arthritis and Tophi

Although there are patients who have only a single attack, especially if predisposing factors can be removed (medica-tions, alcohol), most patients will have recurrent attacks if untreated. The length of time to the second attack varies, but the intercritical period becomes shorter over time. The attacks become longer, and eventually may not subside completely. In advanced stages, acute attacks are less prominent, and chronic lower-grade inflammation with progressive joint damage is seen.

Tophi, solid nodular deposits of urate, usually appear in joints and soft tissue after attacks have occurred for years without urate lowering therapy. Tophi may be found around joints such as the MTP or the finger joints, and may deform and enlarge the shape of the joint (Fig. 42-2). X-rays may show **erosions,** punched-out holes in the bones at or near the joint, due to tophi. The bone edges may grow around the deposit giving the appearance of **overhanging edges,** not seen in the erosions of rheumatoid arthritis (Fig. 42-3). Tophi may occur at the olecranon bursae, the pinna

Fig. 42-2. Tophi at the joints. Large tophaceous deposits can appear as masses, often in the area of the joints. This patient's left hand shows two large nodules around the index metacar-pophalangeal joint (compare to the right hand).

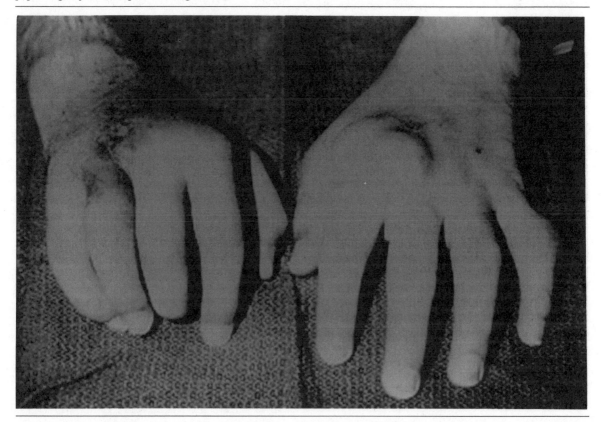

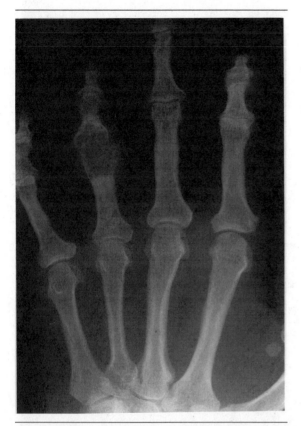

Fig. 42-3. X-ray of tophi at hand joints. The fourth proximal interphalangeal joint has been destroyed by a large tophaceous deposit. The bone is not simply eroded, but the remaining edges of bone are "overhanging," pushed out farther than their original position, especially evident in the proximal radial edge of the joint. The surrounding mass of the tophus is evident when compared to other proximal interphalangeal joints.

of the ear (frequently mentioned, but uncommon in practice), or in atypical locations, such as the spine, where their mass can cause problems. The skin over tophi can ulcerate, with drainage of the tophaceous material. This appears chalky and, with compensated polarized light microscopy, shows innumerable MSU crystals without neutrophils, each yellow or blue depending on its orientation on the slide.

An atypical clinical picture of gout is common among elderly women, especially those taking thiazide diuretics. This is marked by early polyarticular involvement and tophi, especially involving finger joints with osteoarthritis (OA), despite having milder and fewer or no acute attacks.

Many of these patients take nonsteroidal anti-inflammatory drugs such as ibuprofen that can modify gouty inflammation. The lack of characteristic features of gout often leads to incorrect or delayed diagnosis.

Kidney Effects

Uric acid stones are much more frequent in patients with gout (about 20%) than in the general population or those with asymptomatic hyperuricemia. The frequency of calcium oxalate stones is also increased, apparently forming around a uric acid center. It is not unusual for the stones to precede arthritis. Overproducers or others with increased urinary uric acid, including those taking medicines that increase uric acid excretion or those who do not drink adequate fluids, are at increased risk for stones. Urine pH is an important factor affecting uric acid solubility (**low pH = low solubility**). Maintaining high fluid intake and alkalinizing the urine can help prevent stones in those at risk.

When the urate level is very high, or there is very high uric acid formation, uric acid may precipitate in the renal-collecting tubules (where pH is lower), leading to renal failure (**acute uric acid nephropathy**). The risk is highest in patients undergoing chemotherapy, and can usually be prevented with allopurinol, which inhibits uric acid formation. This should be distinguished from chronic deposition of urate in the kidney interstitium (chronic urate nephropathy), noted above, which usually has little or no effect on renal function.

Lowering of Urate Levels

In patients with recurrent attacks, stones, or tophi, reduction of serum urate levels to below the saturation point can prevent formation of urate crystals, eventually leading to dissolution of urate deposits already present, avoiding subsequent tissue damage. Elimination of alcohol or medications may be sufficient in some cases, but urate-lowering drugs are usually required. These work either by increasing uric acid excretion (**uricosuric** agents) or decreasing its production. The most widely used uricosuric, probenecid, inhibits reabsorption of urate in the proximal tubule. **Allopurinol** is used to decrease uric acid production by inhibiting the enzyme **xanthine oxidase,** which converts hypoxanthine to xanthine and xanthine to uric acid.

Other Crystal-Induced Arthritis

Other crystals can occur in joints, and some, such as calcium pyrophosphate dihydrate (CPPD) and basic calcium phosphates (BCP, hydroxyapatite), are associated with disease. Crystals differ in their ability to induce inflammation. Those with high surface negative charge and an irregular surface may have more inflammatory potential, possibly related to membrane interactions. Other factors are probably also involved.

Calcium Pyrophosphate Dihydrate
Crystal Deposition and Chondrocalcinosis

The primary site of CPPD deposition is cartilage, in contrast to synovium for MSU, but it may later be found in other structures, including synovium, tendons, ligaments, and joint capsules. CPPD deposits may be visible by x-ray, commonly as lines of calcification within the nonvisible cartilage, referred to as **chondrocalcinosis** (CC). CPPD is the usual reason for CC, although it can less often be due to other crystals. CC in a joint that has no symptoms is common, whether or not symptoms are present in other joints, and CPPD-associated arthritis may occur without visible CC.

CC is common in fibrocartilage and may also occur in hyaline articular cartilage. The knee is the most common site, often bilateral, and affecting both medial and lateral menisci (Fig. 42-4). CC is also frequently seen in the wrist (including the triangular cartilage) (Fig. 42-5), symphysis pubis, hip, shoulder, and spine and intervertebral discs.

Fig. 42-4. X-ray of the knee in a patient with CPPD crystal deposition. A linear calcification (open arrow) is evident in the lateral compartment space of the right knee, representing chondrocalcinosis due to CPPD deposition. Additional spots of calcification may also be seen above it. There has been loss of the cartilage of the medial compartment (solid arrow); a space equal to that of the lateral compartment should have been present. Loss of cartilage space is typical of osteoarthritis, a common problem in patients with CPPD deposition.

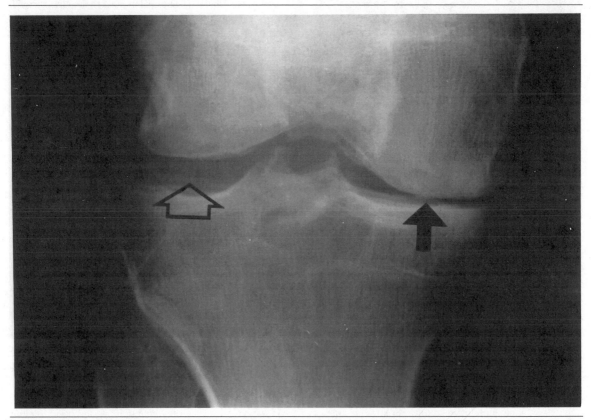

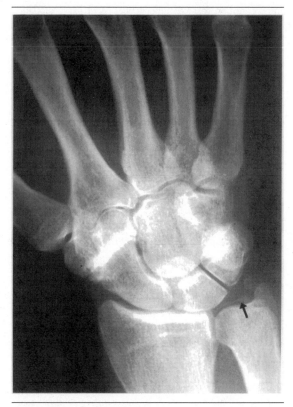

Fig. 42-5. X-ray of the wrist in a patient with CPPD crystal deposition. A linear calcification is seen just distal to the ulna, representing chondrocalcinosis (arrow).

Clinical Manifestations

Several types of clinical presentations have been associated with CPPD crystal deposition, resembling those of other rheumatic diseases, both inflammatory and degenerative. A role for CPPD in inflammatory arthritis is clear; attacks may be reproduced by intra-articular injection of crystals. The relationship of CPPD deposition to degenerative disease is more complicated. It is not clearly established whether the CPPD is a direct cause of cartilage degeneration, is a contributor to it, and/or is a consequence of it. However, its distinctive features suggest that it differs from simple OA.

Pseudogout. Patients with CPPD crystal deposition may have acute attacks of inflammatory arthritis similar to those of acute gout, termed "pseudogout." It typically involves a single joint, most commonly the knee. It can also occur in the wrist, shoulder, or other joints, but only rarely the first MTP. As in gout, the attacks come on within hours, are inflammatory in nature, and subside spontaneously after days to weeks.

Synovial fluid aspirated from an affected joint confirms the inflammation, showing a high white blood cell count similar to that of gout, with a high percentage of neutrophils (80–90%). CPPD crystals are seen in the fluid, usually engulfed by neutrophils. Unlike MSU, CPPD crystals are smaller, **rhomboid** in shape, and demonstrate **weak positive birefringence.** These synovial fluid crystals can be released from preformed CPPD deposits by crystal shedding, physical disruption of deposits, or by changes in the surrounding connective tissue. The latter may result from inflammation due to other causes, such as joint infection or gout, which may coexist with CPPD.

Acute arthritis results from the inflammatory response to the crystals. Neutrophils are important in this response, as in gout, and a similar chemotactic factor is released. The acute attack is suppressed by addressing this inflammatory response, by medicines similar to those used for acute gouty attacks (colchicine, anti-inflammatories). Sometimes the attack can be controlled by draining the synovial fluid, thus removing crystals.

Other Associated Clinical Syndromes. CPPD deposition has also been associated with a "pseudo-rheumatoid arthritis" picture, and OA with or without associated acute attacks ("pseudo-osteoarthritis").

The rheumatoid arthritis-like syndrome is characterized by chronic inflammation involving multiple joints, with synovial hyperplasia, symmetrical involvement, and other features suggestive of RA. Further confusion may occur if rheumatoid factor is present, which occurs in a small percent of normal elderly people (usually in low titer), and misdiagnosis is common. CC or CPPD crystals in joint fluid suggest crystal-induced disease, while high-titer rheumatoid factor or typical bony erosions would suggest true rheumatoid arthritis.

The most common symptomatic arthritis associated with CPPD, and the one which causes the most long-term disability, resembles OA. Significantly, the joint distribution of CPPD-associated OA differs from that of typical OA. Although the knee is commonly affected in both, the wrist, shoulder, and metacarpophalangeal joints are commonly involved in CPPD-deposition, but not in typical OA. Other distinctive clinical features of CPPD-associated OA have been observed, such as a tendency for patello-femoral involvement and subchondral bony cyst formation. Some patients with this form of arthritis may develop acute attacks or may have had earlier acute attacks. In a small number, the joint disease may be severe and deforming enough to resemble that seen in neuropathic arthritis.

Mechanisms for Deposition

The mechanisms involved in CPPD deposition are not completely understood, and they may be different in different patients. Local increases in calcium or pyrophosphate (PPi) concentration or generation, or changes in the regional connective tissues that promote deposition, have been suggested. Unlike hyperuricemia in gout, there is no metabolic indicator of a tendency to CPPD deposition, but there are clinical associations with CPPD deposition that may provide clues to the mechanisms involved, including associated metabolic diseases, increasing age, previous trauma, and the occurrence of a familial form.

Associated Diseases. CPPD deposition has been associated with a variety of metabolic diseases, including hyperparathyroidism, hemochromatosis, hypomagnesemia, hypothyroidism, and others. The associated arthritis is generally similar to that of other CPPD patients. Acute attacks may follow surgical treatment for hyperparathyroidism, possibly due to crystal shedding as the serum calcium falls. The arthritis of hemochromatosis is marked by degeneration of the middle metacarpophalangeal joints and distinctive "hook osteophytes," but these may be seen in some patients with idiopathic CPPD deposition as well. Hypophosphatasia, in which deficiency of alkaline phosphatase leads to an elevation of PPi, has also been associated with CPPD deposition.

The mechanisms for these associations are not clear. They suggest that calcium, iron, or magnesium abnormalities may directly or indirectly promote CPPD deposition. However, treatment of the associated condition and normalization of these levels does not generally affect the course of the arthritis or result in dissolution of the CPPD deposits.

Other Contributing Factors. CPPD deposition is relatively common, and increases in frequency with age. CC is seen in about 4% of adults, but in 15% over 65 years and greater than 40% over 85. OA and previous surgery to the joint are commonly associated with CPPD deposition, supporting a role for changes in the local connective tissues.

Other patients with CPPD deposition have an inherited form of the disease. Several different patterns of familial CPPD deposition disease have been described, suggesting different defects involved. Autosomal dominant is the most common form of inheritance. Most cases of CPPD deposition, however, especially in the United States, are idiopathic and sporadic.

Possible Metabolic Abnormalities. Although joint fluids may have elevated PPi concentrations in pseudogout, they are also elevated in uncomplicated OA and other conditions. Most PPi is generated during metabolic reactions that use ATP or other nucleoside triphosphates, and convert them to the monophosphate plus PPi. Studies suggest local production of PPi comes from the chondrocyte, either within the cell and then transported to the matrix or through cell surface enzymes ("ectoenzymes"). Increased activity of the ectoenzyme nucleoside triphosphate pyrophosphohydrolase, which can produce PPi, has been found in cartilage from patients with CPPD deposition. This is an area of current research interest.

Basic Calcium Phosphates (BCP)

Although often referred to as apatite, BCPs include hydroxyapatite ($Ca_5(PO_4)_3OH \cdot 2H_2O$, partially carbonate-substituted), octacalcium phosphate ($Ca_8H_2(PO_4)_6 \cdot 5H_2O$), and tricalcium phosphate ($Ca_3(PO_4)_2$), often occurring as mixtures. They have been associated with several forms of joint disease. As with CPPD, there are no biochemical markers, and the reasons and mechanisms for deposition are unclear, but may involve changes in connective tissues that promote crystal deposition, changes in calcium and/or phosphate balance, or other factors.

Calcific Periarthritis

Calcification due to BCP visible by x-ray in structures surrounding the shoulder (tendons, bursae, etc.) is common, and often without symptoms. In some patients, release of crystals, often associated with radiographic changes in the deposits, leads to acute bursitis or tendinitis, with severe pain, inflammation, and restricted motion referred to as calcific periarthritis. It may resemble other crystal-induced disease, with spontaneous resolution over days to weeks, and later recurrence. A similar tendinitis or bursitis may occur in the hip, foot, or other joints. The reason for the predilection for the shoulder may relate to characteristics of the blood supply, connective tissue, or other factors.

Acute Arthritis

An acute self-limited arthritis picture has been associated in some instances with BCP in the joint. The mechanism of acute attacks is believed similar to that of MSU and CPPD, with phagocytosis, release of mediators, and amplification of the response. The presence of crystals does not by itself confirm that the crystals are inducing this arthritis, since they may be released with acute inflammation of other causes, but it can be suggestive in certain clinical situations. BCP crystals cannot be identified by polarized light microscopy as can MSU or CPPD, because the individual BCP crystals are much smaller. They have a tendency to form aggregates, which can be visible as discs using light microscopy with Alizarin red staining, but this is less specific than for MSU or CPPD, and confirmation with electron microscopy or other more sophisticated techniques is needed.

Osteoarthritis

BCP crystals are commonly found in OA joints, and BCP may be deposited in the cartilage or synovium. Joints with crystals tend to be more severely affected than crystal-negative joints, although there are no specific differences in the clinical picture. The role of the crystals in the progression of the OA in such cases is unknown. CPPD may coexist with BCP in OA.

"Milwaukee Shoulder"

BCP has been associated with a destructive arthritis, usually of the shoulder, most commonly in elderly women, that differs from usual OA. A series of cases was described from Milwaukee, and a similar syndrome has been found by others. The knee or other joints may also be affected. Extensive destruction with complete tears of rotator cuff tendons occur, and degeneration of the glenohumeral joint. Cuff tears are not common in typical OA, and OA usually shows more prominent osteophytes and sclerosis. Although pain and loss of shoulder function occur, little evidence of inflammation is seen, with low white blood cell counts in the synovial fluid, despite large effusions. The fluid does show abundant BCP crystals in most cases. Collagenase and other proteases have been found in synovial fluids in some cases, possibly released after phagocytosis of crystals by synovial cells. Such enzymes may mediate the connective tissue loss.

Other Crystals

Arthritis has been associated with calcium oxalate crystals in patients with renal failure. Crystals can be deposited in bones, joints, and surrounding tissue, especially in the hands, and can cause acute arthritis, usually noninflammatory. Other crystals are found in joints, such as cholesterol crystals, dicalcium phosphate, calcium carbonate, protein crystals, and others, but rarely cause clinical problems.

Clinical Example

1. A 55-year-old man had intermittent attacks of pain and swelling in multiple joints for five years. For the last year, joint pains were more persistent and he developed nodular enlargements on two of his fingers and on his elbows. He was admitted to the hospital because of a more severe attack affecting his ankles, knees, and left wrist. He drank alcohol moderately and was treated for hypertension for 10 years. Aspiration of the fluid from his left knee showed a white blood count of 15,000 cells/mm^3, and many needle-shaped crystals with strong negative birefringence, most within PMNs. Aspirate from the nodule on his left elbow contained densely packed aggregates of the same crystals. X-rays of his feet showed multiple punched-out lesions in the bones around the MTP joints, some with overhanging cortical margins. Laboratory results included: urinalysis 1+ protein; 2–3 WBC/HPF; creatinine 1.6 mg/dl; uric acid 10.2 mg/dl; and rheumatoid factor test = negative.

Discussion.   Signs of advanced disease included more persistent attacks, polyarticular and upper extremity involvement, tophi, and gouty MTP erosions. Alcohol was a probable contributing factor, and hypertension a common associated condition. The history was typical, the uric acid elevated, but the demonstration of MSU crystals in joint fluid or tissue was necessary to establish the diagnosis, and was accomplished here from both fluid and tophus. Their presence in neutrophils is typical of an acute attack. The white blood cell count in the fluid indicated inflammation, typical of acute gout. Recurrent attacks and tophi indicate that long-term antihyperuricemic therapy is necessary. The mild renal disease (elevated creatinine and proteinuria) may relate to the associated hypertension. Chronic urate nephropathy (urate deposits in the renal medulla) may occur, but renal functional impairment in gout is usually related to age, hypertension, vascular disease, nephrolithiasis, infection, or other factors.

Bibliography

Crystalline deposition diseases. *Rheum Dis Clin N Am* 14:253–477, 1988. *This single-theme issue includes 14 individual articles, written by recognized authorities and active investigators, providing in-depth information about aspects of crystal diseases. Some articles provide good background for looking into research topics.*

Klippel JH and Dieppe PA (eds.). *Rheumatology.* London: Mosby-Year Book Europe, 1994, pp. 7.12.1–7.16.8.

This new rheumatology textbook uses numerous color pictures and innovative techniques to enhance the presentation. It provides detailed information, yet is clear and understandable for students, a good next step for further study of clinical aspects.

McCarty DJ and Koopman WJ (eds.). *Arthritis and Allied Conditions* (12th ed.). Philadelphia: Lea & Febiger, 1993, pp. 1773–1894. *McCarty introduced the use of compensated polarized light microscopy for synovial fluid (1961), and first described pseudogout and CPPD (1962). This major rheumatology textbook has several excellent, authoritative chapters on crystal diseases.*

Schumacher HR, Klippel JH, and Koopman WJ (eds.). *Primer on the Rheumatic Diseases* (10th ed.). Atlanta: Arthritis Foundation, 1993, pp. 209–225. *This book provides an overview of rheumatology, and the section on crystal diseases contains several basic, brief chapters that individually review gout, CPPD deposition, and apatite conditions, including their clinical features, pathogenesis, and treatment.*

Part V Questions: Rheumatologic and Immunologic Disorders

1. Deficiencies of individual complement components are associated with all the following except
   A. systemic lupus erythematosus.
   B. infections by *Neisseria species.*
   C. both A and B.
   D. classical pathway of complement activation.
   E. development of malignant lymphoma.
2. The late phase of immediate hypersensitivity
   A. is visible within 3 hours of allergen exposure.
   B. occurs in 75% of those who have an early-phase response.
   C. occurs in asthma but not allergic rhinitis.
   D. leads to fibrosis when long-standing.
   E. depends on chemotaxis.
3. The pathophysiology of asthma does not necessarily include
   A. mediator release.
   B. IgE.
   C. respiratory eosinophilia.
   D. potential reversibility.
   E. bronchial hyperreactivity.
4. The nephritis of systemic lupus erythematosus is most closely associated with which autoantibody?
   A. Anti-Sm
   B. Anti-U_1RNP
   C. Anti-native DNA
   D. Anti-Ro/SSA
   E. Anti-La/SSB
5. Match the following infections in Column I with the immune defect in Column II.

Column I	Column II
i. Disseminated *Neisseria* infections	A. Defective humoral immunity
ii. Fatal pneumococcal bacteremia	B. Defective cellular immunity
iii. Recurrent pneumococcal pneumonia	C. Splenectomy
iv. Recurrent staphylococcal pneumonia	D. Absence of C6
v. Chronic *Candida* infections	E. Defective granulocyte function

6. Which of the following statements is true regarding OA?
   A. Is a dynamic process reflecting injury and repair
   B. Only affects the elderly
   C. Is correctly described as a wear-and-tear arthritis
   D. Is always asymptomatic
   E. Symptoms correlate closely with radiographic changes
7. All of the following contribute to joint instability and deformity in RA, except
   A. joint capsule distention.
   B. ligamentous damage.
   C. muscle disuse and atrophy.
   D. tendon rupture.
   E. joint denervation.
8. Hyperuricemia in patients with gout may be related to any of the following except
   A. an enzymatic defect leading to overproduction of purines.
   B. increased turnover of nucleic acid purines.
   C. administration of a thiazide diuretic.
   D. chronic lead poisoning.
   E. increased absorption of purines from a normal diet.

VI Pulmonary Diseases

Part Editor
Paul V. Carlile

43 Pulmonary Gas Exchange

D. Robert McCaffree

Objectives

After completing this chapter, you should be able to

Understand the process of movement of atmospheric gas into the alveoli

Comprehend the exchange of oxygen and carbon dioxide between the alveoli and blood, including an understanding of gas exchange in an "ideal alveolus" expressed via the alveolar gas equation and some of the factors involved in diffusion of gas in the alveolar-capillary unit

Explain the concept of the alveolar-arterial oxygen gradient

Understand oxygen content and the oxyhemoglobin dissociation curve

State the four abnormal states associated with hypoxemia and some of the key differentiating characteristics

Basic Physiology

The entire cardiac output flows through the lung's capillaries and is exposed to atmospheric air over an enormous surface area. As a result, the lung is ideally suited for gas exchange.

Air moves through the larger airways by **bulk flow** and through very small airways and alveoli by **diffusion.** Oxygen movement from alveoli into capillary blood and carbon dioxide movement from capillaries to alveoli also occur by diffusion. The PO_2 in capillary blood leaving the alveolus ($Pc'O_2$) is normally equal to the PO_2 in the alveolus (PAO_2), around 100 mm Hg at sea level. The PaO_2 drops to about 90 mm Hg in arterial blood, and it is considerably lower inside cells and mitochondria. (Fig. 43-1).

Ideal Alveolar Gas Equation

Anatomically there are millions of gas exchange units (alveoli and their associated capillaries), each with its own alveolar and capillary gas tensions and its own ventilation and perfusion rates. However, the physiologic effects reflect weighted averages of all these gas exchange units.

Therefore, for convenience, we commonly simplify the lung into models of one or more gas exchange compartments (the most complex model has 50 compartments). The simplest model treats the lung as one alveolus ("ideal" alveolus) and pools all the capillaries into one systemic artery. By assessing the relationship between the alveolar gas and arterial gas pressures, we can then describe overall gas exchange.

We routinely measure arterial PO_2 (PaO_2), but directly measuring alveolar PO_2 (PAO_2) is more difficult. However, the PAO_2 can easily be *calculated* in an average or "ideal" alveolus. The general equation is

$$PAO_2 = PIO_2 - PACO_2 \times \left(FIO_2 + \left(\frac{(1 - FIO_2)}{R} \right) \right) \quad (43\text{-}1)$$

where **PIO_2** is the PO_2 of inspired gas, **$PACO_2$** is the alveolar PCO_2 (which is essentially the same as the *arterial* PCO_2, or $PaCO_2$), **FIO_2** is the fraction of inspired oxygen (0.21 in room air), and **R** is the gas exchange ratio (which, in the steady state, is the same as the metabolic respiratory quotient).

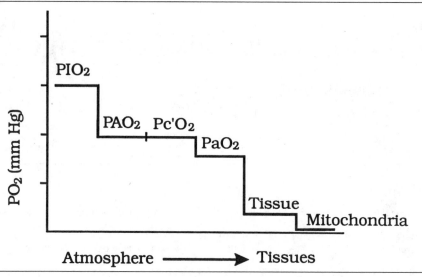

Fig. 43-1. Representation of the decrease in partial pressure of oxygen from inspired air (PIO$_2$) to the alveolus PAO$_2$, and pulmonary capillary (Pc′O$_2$) to the arterial blood (PaO$_2$) and finally to the tissues and mitochondria. (Reprinted with permission from: Kaufman CE and Papper S (eds.). (*Review of Pathophysiology*. Boston: Little, Brown, 1983, p. 396.)

The PIO$_2$ is the product of the FIO$_2$ and the dry gas pressure (barometric pressure minus water vapor pressure) or, at sea level, PIO$_2$ = 0.21 × (760 mm Hg − 47 mm Hg) = 150 mm Hg. The metabolic respiratory quotient (which is the ratio of CO$_2$ production to O$_2$ consumption) ranges between 0.7 and 1.0, with a typical value of about 0.8.

A simplified approximation of the alveolar gas equation which is useful clinically is

$$PAO_2 = PIO_2 - PaCO_2 \times 1.25 \qquad (43\text{-}2)$$

(Notice that PaCO$_2$ has been substituted for PACO$_2$.) This equation is less accurate when the FIO$_2$ approaches 1.0.

Alveolar-Arterial Oxygen Difference $(P[A - a]O_2 = PAO_2 - PaO_2)$

Calculating the difference between the partial pressure of oxygen in the alveolus (the alveolar PO$_2$, or PAO$_2$) and the partial pressure of oxygen in arterial blood (the arterial PO$_2$, or PaO$_2$) provides a relatively simple measure of the effectiveness of oxygen exchange in the lung. This mea-

sure is called the **alveolar arterial oxygen difference,** written as P(A − a)O$_2$, and is commonly referred to as the A − a gradient. In the ideal situation, the entire cardiac output comes in contact with ventilated alveoli, and blood leaving the alveolus has the same PaO$_2$ as alveolar gas, so the P(A − a)O$_2$ is zero. In the actual normal lung, 2–4% of the cardiac output bypasses the alveoli in a right-to-left shunt and there is some mismatching of ventilation and perfusion. (Shunting and ventilation-perfusion mismatching are discussed below.) Consequently, the normal P(A − a)O$_2$ is about 10 mm Hg; this value increases with age and with FIO$_2$. (Because of the latter, the measurement is of little use in a person not breathing room air.) The age-adjusted P(A − a)O$_2$ can be estimated using the following equation:

$$P(A-a)O_2 = 2.5 + 0.21 \times (\text{age in years}) \qquad (43\text{-}3)$$

A good rule of thumb is that a P(A − a)O$_2$ of greater than 20 mm Hg on room air is abnormal.

An abnormal P(A − a)O$_2$ indicates that there is significant impairment of gas exchange, usually due to a parenchymal abnormality of the lung.

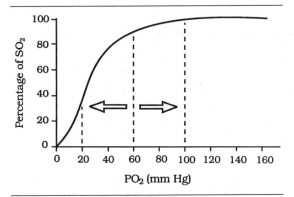

Fig. 43-2. The oxyhemoglobin dissociation curve. Consideration of the shape of the curve is important in clinical decisions. If the partial pressure of oxygen (PO_2) is 60 mm Hg or greater, increasing the PO_2 will not greatly affect hemoglobin saturation (SO_2). On the other hand, any decrement of the PO_2 below 60 mm Hg will cause marked decrease in hemoglobin saturation. (Reprinted with permission from: Kaufman CE and Papper S (eds.). *Review of Pathophysiology.* Boston: Little, Brown, 1983, p. 397.)

Oxygen Content and the Oxyhemoglobin Dissociation Curve

The total oxygen content of blood includes oxygen that is bound to hemoglobin (forming oxyhemoglobin) and a comparatively small amount which is dissolved in plasma. **Oxygen content** in arterial blood (CaO_2) is expressed as ml O_2/100 ml blood, and is calculated as follows:

$$CaO_2 = O_2 \text{ bound to hemoglobin} + O_2 \text{ dissolved in plasma} \quad (43\text{-}4)$$

$$= Hb \times 1.39 \times \frac{SaO_2}{100} + 0.0031 \times PaO_2 \quad (43\text{-}5)$$

where **Hb** is hemoglobin concentration in gm/100 ml, **1.39** is the oxygen-carrying capacity of hemoglobin in ml O_2/g Hb, **SaO2** is the percentage of hemoglobin that is bound to O_2 (= O_2 saturation), **0.0031** is the solubility coefficient for O_2 in plasma in ml O_2/100 ml/mm Hg, and **PaO2** is the partial pressure of oxygen in arterial blood in mm Hg.

The **oxyhemoglobin dissociation curve** shows how the oxygen content of blood (or oxygen saturation) is related to the PaO_2. The *sigmoid shape* of this curve (Fig. 43-2) is important physiologically. The curve is steep below a PaO_2 of 60 mm Hg but flattens out above a PaO_2 of 60 mm Hg.

For example, if the PaO_2 increases from 20 to 60 mm Hg, the oxygen saturation increases from 30 to about 90%. However, a further 40 mm Hg increase in PaO_2 to 100 mm Hg results in only a 5% increase in saturation, to about 95%.

The steep part of the curve is important physiologically. When venous blood arrives at the alveolus with a low PaO_2, a large amount of oxygen can be loaded onto the hemoglobin with a small increase in PaO_2. When the blood gets to the tissues, a great deal of oxygen is released from the hemoglobin with each small drop in PaO_2.

The flat portion of the curve is important clinically. As lung disease progresses and the arterial PaO_2 falls, there is not a significant change in the saturation of hemoglobin until the PaO_2 falls below 55 or 60 mm Hg.

Thus the shape of the oxyhemoglobin dissociation curve means that oxygen is readily bound to hemoglobin in the alveolus and easily released to be used by peripheral tissues, and it reflects a buffer against the effects of decreased PaO_2 associated with lung disease.

Increases in temperature and in hydrogen ion concentration (lower pH) shift the dissociation curve to the right, while colder temperatures and higher pH shift the curve to the left. These shifts serve useful adaptive purposes, by enhancing O_2 delivery to the tissues and by promoting O_2 uptake by the pulmonary capillary blood in the presence of fever or acidosis.

Another major influence on the dissociation curve is the level of 2,3-diphosphoglycerate (2,3-DPG), with higher levels resulting in a rightward shift. Some disorders associated with impaired tissue oxygen delivery, such as heart failure and anemia, are associated with increased levels of 2,3-DPG.

The concept of oxygen content is important in understanding abnormalities of gas exchange. If a flask with 100 ml of blood having a PaO_2 of 30 mm Hg is emptied into a flask with 100 ml of blood having the same hemoglobin concentration of 15 g/100 ml and a PaO_2 of 96 mm Hg, what is the PaO_2 of the resulting 200 ml of blood? Although it may seem natural to merely average the individual PaO_2s, the answer obtained by this method (63 mm Hg) is incorrect (Fig. 43-3). Instead, we must deal with oxygen content. The oxygen content of the blood in the first flask is 12.4 ml O_2/100 ml blood, obtained by using the oxyhemoglobin dissociation curve (or a table) to find the oxygen content which corresponds to a PaO_2 of 30 mm Hg. Similarly, the oxygen content of the blood in the second flask is 19.8 ml O_2/100 ml. The oxygen content of the mixture is therefore (12.4 + 19.8) ml O_2/200 ml blood or

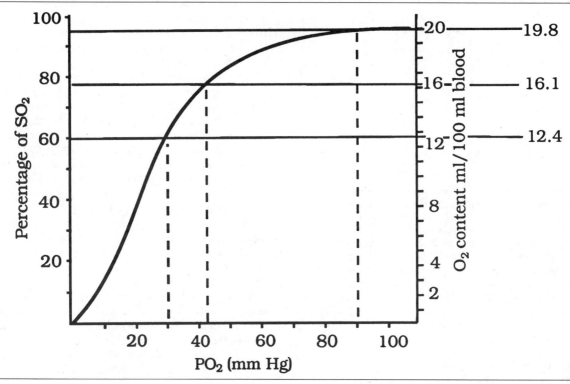

Fig. 43-3. Relation between the partial pressure of oxygen (PO_2), the hemoglobin saturation in the blood (SO_2%), and the content of oxygen in blood with a hemoglobin concentration of 15 g/100 ml. (Reprinted with permission from: Kaufman CE and Papper S (eds.). *Review of Pathophysiology.* Boston: Little, Brown, 1983, p. 397.)

16.1 ml O_2/100 ml blood. A content of 16.1 ml O_2/100 ml corresponds to a PaO_2 of 42 mm Hg. The PaO_2 of blood that results from mixing blood with different PaO_2s is determined by the average of the oxygen contents of the blood, not the average of the PaO_2s (see Fig. 43-3).

Pathophysiology: Causes of Hypoxemia

Hypoxemia is defined as an arterial blood PO_2 below the normal range of 80–90 mm Hg. As the PaO_2 falls, the hemoglobin O_2 saturation also falls, especially with PaO_2 values at or below 60 mm Hg (see Fig. 43-3). There are four main causes of hypoxemia: hypoventilation, low

ventilation-to-perfusion ($\dot{V}_A/\dot{Q}$) ratios, shunt, and diffusion impairment. There is a fifth cause of hypoxemia which is not necessarily associated with abnormalities of gas exchange: breathing a low PIO_2, i.e., due to low barometric pressure (such as at high altitude) or low FIO_2. Since this cause of hypoxemia does not involve any disease of the respiratory system, it will not be discussed.

Hypoventilation and Hypoxemia

Carbon Dioxide Elimination by the Lungs — Basic Principles

Carbon dioxide is eliminated by the process of **alveolar ventilation.** Carbon dioxide is present in the pulmonary alveoli, and its concentration in alveolar gas may be expressed either as partial pressure, $PACO_2$, or as fractional concentration, $FACO_2$. Alveolar ventilation, $\dot{V}_A$, is the quantity of air that is expired from the alveoli each minute and is equal to the difference between the total quantity of expired air ($\dot{V}_E$) and the quantity of air that is expired from dead space ($\dot{V}_D$).

$$\dot{V}_A = \dot{V}_E - \dot{V}_D \qquad (43\text{-}6)$$

$\dot{V}_D$ includes the ventilation of the conducting airways, trachea and bronchi, as well as alveoli which are ventilated but not perfused.

The quantity of carbon dioxide eliminated by the lung each minute (CO_2) is equal to the volume of gas expired from the alveoli ($\dot{V}_A$) multiplied by the fractional concentration of carbon dioxide in the alveolar gas ($FACO_2$). Thus

$$CO_2 = \dot{V}_A \times FACO_2 \qquad (43\text{-}7)$$

where $FACO_2 = PACO_2$ divided by the total pressure of all gases (excluding water vapor).

Since CO_2 is equalized between alveolar gas and capillary blood, even in the presence of conditions that impair diffusion (unlike the case with O_2), the partial pressure of carbon dioxide is equal in alveolar gas and arterial blood. This equation can be rearranged to relate $PaCO_2$ to alveolar ventilation and CO_2 production, or metabolic rate:

$$Pa\,CO_2 = PACO_2 = 0.863 \times \frac{CO_2}{\dot{V}_A} \qquad (43\text{-}8)$$

where 0.863 is simply a constant that includes barometric pressure, water pressure, and a temperature correction factor.

Hypoventilation and Hypoxemia

As seen from the above discussion, alveolar (or arterial) PCO_2 is inversely related to alveolar ventilation (and directly related to CO_2 production). If alveolar ventilation ($\dot{V}_A$) decreases, then less oxygen is delivered to the alveoli and less carbon dioxide is removed. The tissues will continue to consume O_2 and produce CO_2 at the same rate despite the change in ventilation. Ultimately, a new steady state will result with a higher $PACO_2$ and a lower PAO_2. If the alveolar ventilation falls sufficiently to cause an increase in $PACO_2$ to 80 mm Hg, PAO_2 would fall to 53 mm Hg (calculated from the alveolar gas equation). Even if the $P(A-a)O_2$ is normal (e.g., 10 mm Hg), this would cause severe arterial hypoxemia (Fig. 43-4).

$$\begin{aligned} PaO_2 &= PAO_2 - P(A-a)O_2 \\ &= 53\text{ mm Hg} - 10\text{ mm Hg} \\ &= 43\text{ mm Hg} \end{aligned} \qquad (43\text{-}9)$$

Thus if alveolar ventilation doubles (assuming CO_2 is constant), $PACO_2$ is halved, and if alveolar ventilation decreases by one half, $PACO_2$ doubles. Clinically, hypoventilation is said to be present when the $PaCO_2$ is higher than normal (i.e., more than 46 mm Hg). Conversely, a diagnosis of hypoventilation cannot be made in the presence of a normal $PaCO_2$.

Hypoventilation can occur with or without lung disease. When hypoventilation occurs without lung disease, it is

Fig. 43-4. The effect of hypoventilation on PaO_2, assuming $P(A-a)O_2$ of 10 mm Hg. (Reprinted with permission from: Kaufman CE and Papper S (eds). *Review of Pathophysiology.* Boston: Little, Brown, 1983, p. 398.)

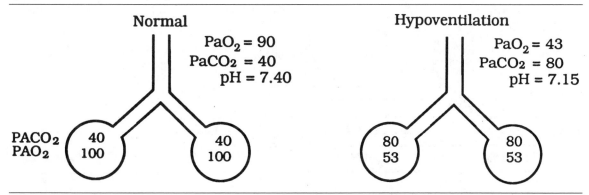

usually associated with either drug intoxications, central nervous system disorders, neuromuscular disorders, or chest wall injuries. In these cases, the P(A – a)O$_2$ is usually normal. Hypoventilation is more commonly seen with chronic obstructive lung disease and is then associated with an elevated P(A – a)O$_2$. **An increased FIO$_2$ will correct the hypoxemia of hypoventilation.** The hypoxemia that occurs in hypoventilation is caused by the increased PACO$_2$ which results in a decreased PAO$_2$. By reviewing the alveolar gas equation, one can see that simply increasing the PIO$_2$ sufficiently can increase the PAO$_2$ and cause a subsequent rise in PaO$_2$ (see note below). In summary, hypoventilation (1) causes an increased PACO$_2$ and PaCO$_2$; (2) causes a decreased PAO$_2$ and PaO$_2$; (3) is associated with a normal P(A – a) O$_2$ when it occurs in the absence of parenchymal lung disease; and (4) PAO$_2$ and PaO$_2$ (but not the hypoventilation) can be corrected by raising FIO$_2$. Note that while an increase in FIO$_2$ will correct the hypoxemia of hypoventilation, patients with acute hypoventilation may progress to apnea. Therefore, the treatment for acute hypoventilation is endotracheal intubation and mechanical ventilation.

Shunt

Shunting occurs when blood passes from the right side of the heart to the left side of the heart without contacting a ventilated alveolus. Normally 2–4% of the cardiac output bypasses the alveoli, primarily through the bronchial circulation and thebesian veins. Pathologic shunting occurs with (1) anatomical shunts, such as arterio-venous malformations of the lung and some congenital heart diseases (atrial and ventricular septal defects with right-to-left shunting of blood) and (2) with pulmonary diseases, such as pneumonia and pulmonary edema (in which alveoli are flooded with inflammatory exudate or edema fluid) or atelectasis (in which alveoli are totally collapsed). Hypoxemia occurs because the shunted blood, which has the low oxygen content of mixed venous blood, mixes with oxygenated blood leaving ventilated alveoli, resulting in an abnormally low arterial oxygen content.

Figure 43-5 is a model of shunting. $\dot{Q}_T$ is the total cardiac output and $\dot{Q}_S$ is the portion of the cardiac output that bypasses the ventilated alveolus as shunt. The blood leaving the shunt has the oxygen content of mixed venous

Fig. 43-5. A model of shunting. In this model, there is a 50% shunt (see text for explanation). (Reprinted with permission from: Kaufman CE and Papper S (eds.). *Review of Pathophysiology.* Boston: Little, Brown, 1983, p. 400.)

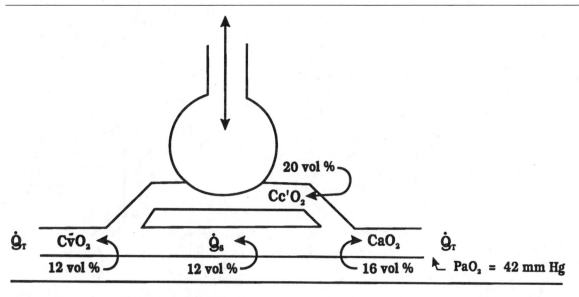

blood (CO_2), which mixes with the blood leaving the capillaries with a high oxygen content ($Cc'O_2$). The mean oxygen content that results from the blend (CaO_2) will determine the PaO_2. For example, if half of the cardiac output goes to normally ventilated alveoli and half goes to alveoli that are unventilated (due to atelectasis or pulmonary edema, for example), given a CO_2 of 12 ml O_2/100 ml blood and a $Cc'O_2$ of 20 ml O_2/100 ml blood, then the CaO_2 is the average of the two contents: $(12 + 20)/2$ or 16 ml O_2/100 ml blood. This oxygen content corresponds to a PaO_2 of 42 mm Hg. One should be aware that the **P(A − a)O$_2$ is increased in shunt.** In addition, the $PaCO_2$ is usually normal or low, since ventilation can be increased to normally functioning alveoli, making up for the alveoli not participating in gas exchange. **Large shunts respond poorly to an increase in FIO$_2$.** This is because of the sigmoid shape of the oxyhemoglobin dissociation curve. Blood leaving the ventilated alveolus in Fig. 43-5 has a saturation of about 98%, with an FIO_2 of 0.21. Increasing the FIO_2 can increase the saturation by only about 2%. Since mixed venous blood does not contact ventilated alveoli, it varies little with changes in FIO_2. Thus increases in FIO_2 have only a small effect on PaO_2 in patients with shunt and cause only a fraction of the increase in PaO_2 that would be expected with the other causes of hypoxemia (Fig. 43-6).

Ventilation-Perfusion ($\dot{V}_A/\dot{Q}$) Inequality

In an average sized individual alveolar ventilation is typically about 4 liters/minute, and cardiac output averages about 5 liters/minute, for an overall $\dot{V}_A/\dot{Q}$ ratio of 0.8. Although ventilation and perfusion are reasonably well matched in the normal lung, with the $\dot{V}_A/\dot{Q}$ ratios of most lung regions clustered around 0.8, some mismatch does

Fig. 43-6. The effects of various inhaled oxygen percentages on the PaO_2 with different levels of shunt. As can be seen, with a 50% shunt there is little increase in the PaO_2 even with 100% O_2, whereas with a 10% shunt (close to normal) 100% O_2 leads to a PaO_2 of almost 500 mm Hg.

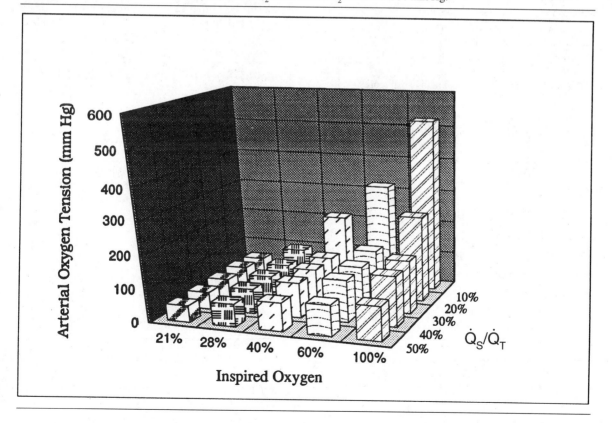

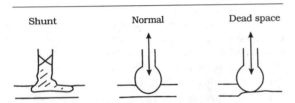

Fig. 43-7. The continuum of ventilation-to-perfusion matching from (shunt) to (dead space). (Reprinted with permission from: Kaufman CE and Papper S (eds.). *Review of Pathophysiology.* Boston: Little, Brown, 1983, p. 401.)

occur. $\dot{V}_A/\dot{Q}$ ratios as high as 3.0 are found in the lung apices, and ratios of about 0.6 occur in the bases of normal upright subjects.

When the lungs are diseased, a much wider range of values for $\dot{V}_A/\dot{Q}$ is found, from an infinitely high $\dot{V}_A/\dot{Q}$, alveoli that are ventilated but not perfused (dead space) to a $\dot{V}_A/\dot{Q}$ ratio of zero, which is shunt (Fig. 43-7).

Effect of $\dot{V}_A/\dot{Q}$ Inequality on Arterial PO_2

A low ventilation-perfusion ($\dot{V}_A/\dot{Q}$) ratio is the most common cause of hypoxemia encountered clinically. High $\dot{V}_A/\dot{Q}$ ratios are associated with an elevated PAO_2 and do not contribute directly to hypoxemia. The hypoxemia caused by $\dot{V}_A/\dot{Q}$ mismatch is due entirely to low $\dot{V}_A/\dot{Q}$ alveoli.

Fig. 43-8 depicts a lung model with two alveoli. One has

Fig. 43-8. A two-compartment model of the effect of low $\dot{V}_A/\dot{Q}$ areas on oxygen content and PaO_2. Vol% = ml O_2 per 100 ml blood. (Adapted from: Kaufman CE and Papper S (eds.). *Review of Pathophysiology.* Boston: Little, Brown, 1983, p. 401.)

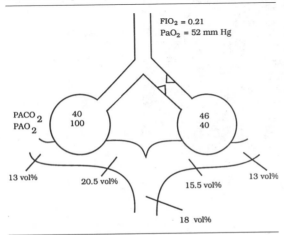

a normal $\dot{V}_A/\dot{Q}$ ratio and the other has a low $\dot{V}_A/\dot{Q}$ ratio. The low $\dot{V}_A/\dot{Q}$ alveolus is essentially a hypoventilated alveolus; the difference is that the PCO_2 in a low $\dot{V}_A/\dot{Q}$ alveolus cannot increase above the level of the mixed venous PCO_2. However, oxygen consumption continues, and the PAO_2 in the low $\dot{V}_A/\dot{Q}$ alveolus is markedly decreased. The low PAO_2 in the low $\dot{V}_A/\dot{Q}$ alveolus causes a correspondingly low content in the blood as it leaves the alveolus; thus CaO_2 and PaO_2 are abnormally low.

In contrast to the low $\dot{V}_A/\dot{Q}$ unit, a high $\dot{V}_A/\dot{Q}$ unit, one with ventilation in excess of perfusion, may have a PAO_2 of 110–130 mm Hg and a $PaCO_2$ of 20–30 mm Hg. High $\dot{V}_A/\dot{Q}$ regions do not contribute to hypoxemia, nor can a high $\dot{V}_A/\dot{Q}$ unit compensate for the effects of a low $\dot{V}_A/\dot{Q}$ unit. Although the PAO_2 of a high $\dot{V}_A/\dot{Q}$ unit may exceed 100 mm Hg, little additional oxygen can be added to blood perfusing these regions because of the shape of the oxyhemoglobin dissociation curve.

The hypoxemia caused by low $\dot{V}_A/\dot{Q}$ alveoli responds very well to even small increases in FIO_2. The left panel of Fig. 43-9 depicts the effect of an FIO_2 of 0.24 on PaO_2 in the patient in Fig. 43-8. The small increase in FIO_2 increases the PaO_2 from 52 to 89 mm Hg. On 100% oxygen (Fig. 43-9), right panel) the PAO_2 in low $\dot{V}_A/\dot{Q}$ alveoli is normal. Thus the effect of low $\dot{V}_A/\dot{Q}$ alveoli on PaO_2 is completely eliminated by 100% oxygen.

Effect of ($\dot{V}_A/\dot{Q}$) Inequality on Arterial PCO_2

The effect of $\dot{V}_A/\dot{Q}$ maldistribution on $PaCO_2$ can be understood by recalling Eq. (43-6):

$$\dot{V}_A = \dot{V}_E - \dot{V}_D = (f \times V_T) - (f \times V_D) \qquad (43\text{-}10)$$

where f is respiratory frequency, V_T is tidal volume, and V_D is the dead-space volume. Further rearrangement yields the relationship

$$\dot{V}_A = f(V_T - V_D) = \dot{V}_E \left(1 - \left[\frac{V_D}{V_T}\right]\right) \qquad (43\text{-}11)$$

where V_D/V_T is the dead space-to-tidal volume ratio, or the fraction of each breath that is wasted ventilation. Substituting into Eq. (8), we have

$$Pa\,CO_2 = 0.863 \times \frac{CO_2}{\dot{V}_E} \left(1 - \left[\frac{V_D}{V_T}\right]\right) \qquad (43\text{-}12)$$

The volume of dead space includes the conducting airways, alveoli with infinite $\dot{V}_A/\dot{Q}$ ratios, and alveoli with

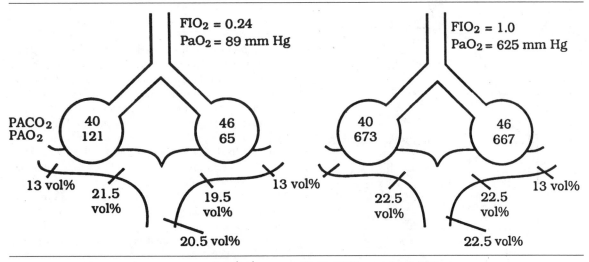

Fig. 43-9. The effect of enriched oxygen on low $\dot{V}_A/\dot{Q}$ areas and PaO_2. Vol% = ml O_2 per 100 ml blood. (Reprinted with permission from: Kaufman CE and Papper S (eds.). *Review of Pathophysiology*. Boston: Little, Brown, 1983, p. 402.)

very high $\dot{V}_A/\dot{Q}$ ratios that exert a dead-space-like effect. Thus an increase in V_D/V_T resulting from mismatching of ventilation and perfusion may lead to an increase in arterial PCO_2 (Eq. (12)). In reality, many patients with lung disease and $\dot{V}_A/\dot{Q}$ inequality do not have an elevated $PaCO_2$. This is because the effects of $\dot{V}_A/\dot{Q}$ mismatch can be overcome relatively easily by increasing $\dot{V}_E$ (Eq. (12)). Thus arterial PCO_2 may be normal, increased, or decreased — depending on whether the level of ventilation has compensated, undercompensated, or overcompensated for the wasted ventilation that results from $\dot{V}_A/\dot{Q}$ inequality.

Summary

Ventilation-perfusion ($\dot{V}_A/\dot{Q}$) mismatch (1) causes a decreased PaO_2 due to low $\dot{V}_A/\dot{Q}$ alveoli; (2) is associated with an increased $P(A - a)O_2$; (3) characteristically responds well to even small increases of FIO_2; and (4) is completely corrected by 100% oxygen.

Diffusion Impairment

The flow of a gas through a membrane by diffusion (V_{gas}) is inversely proportional to the thickness of the membrane (T) and directly proportional to the surface area of the membrane (A), the diffusion constant (D), and the pressure gradient of that gas across the membrane ($P_1 - P_2$):

$$V_{gas} \approx A \times D \times \frac{(P_1 - P_2)}{T} \qquad (43\text{-}13)$$

The diffusion constant (D) is proportional to the solubility divided by the square root of the molecular weight. Carbon dioxide diffuses through tissue 20 times more rapidly than oxygen because of its high solubility; thus its diffusion is not affected by diseases that impair diffusion. These diseases are thought to impair diffusion by thickening the alveolar membrane or by decreasing the surface area available for diffusion, or both. When diffusion impairment is present, the PAO_2 is normal, but it takes longer for capillary blood to come into equilibrium with the alveolar gas.

As seen in Fig. 43-10, the capillary PO_2 is normally equal to the PAO_2 after 0.25 second of exposure to alveolar gas, one-third of the time available. In the presence of moderately abnormal diffusion, equilibration may not occur until just before the blood leaves the alveolus, but the PaO_2 is still normal. However, on exercise, cardiac output increases and transit time decreases, leaving inadequate time for equilibration and causing a fall in PaO_2. **A precipitous fall in PaO_2 during exercise is felt to be characteristic of diffusion impairment.** A patient with grossly abnormal diffusion has a low PaO_2 even at rest and suffers a further fall in PaO_2 with exercise. The hypoxemia of diffusion impairment can be corrected by increasing

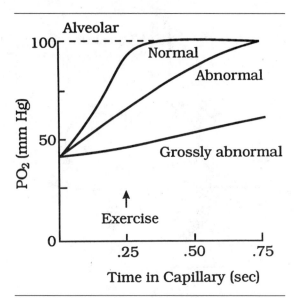

Fig. 43-10. How exercise might accentuate hypoxemia in the presence of a diffusion abnormality. (Reprinted with permission from: Kaufman CE and Papper S (eds.). *Review of Pathophysiology.* Boston: Little, Brown, 1983, p. 403.)

FIO_2. As PAO_2 increases, the pressure gradient from alveolus to capillary increases, increasing diffusion. It is said that any decrease in PaO_2 due to impaired diffusion will largely be corrected by an FIO_2 greater than 0.40. In some instances, however, as in alveolar filling with edema or exudate or severe thickening of the alveolar-capillary membrane, it is difficult to distinguish between impaired diffusion and shunt.

It should be noted that the role of diffusion impairment in hypoxemia is controversial. Certainly, most experts would agree that diffusion impairment is rarely the sole cause of hypoxemia. Indeed, the hypoxemia of many disease states, which was once thought to be due to diffusion impairment, is now known to be due to $\dot{V}_A/\dot{Q}$ mismatch. However, there is evidence to suggest that diffusion impairment may contribute to the hypoxemia seen in some of these diseases.

In summary, diffusion impairment (1) causes a decreased PaO_2 and a normal PAO_2; (2) causes an increased $P(A-a)O_2$; (3) is associated with a normal or low $PaCO_2$; (4) responds well to an increased FIO_2; and (5) is rarely the sole cause of hypoxemia.

No discussion of diffusion would be complete without mention of the **diffusing capacity of the lung for carbon monoxide** (DL_{CO}). Originally advanced as a clinical test for the detection of diffusion impairment, the DL_{CO} is not useful in distinguishing among the causes of hypoxemia since diffusion impairment has such a small role in producing clinical abnormalities of gas exchange. Rather, the DL_{CO} should be used as a measure of the amount of functioning vascular bed in the lung and is usually reduced in certain types of pulmonary vascular and parenchymal lung diseases. The DL_{CO} is the rate of transfer of CO from alveolus to blood (CO) divided by the partial pressure difference between alveolar gas (PACO) and pulmonary capillary blood (PcCO): DL_{CO} (ml/minute/mm Hg) = CO/(PACO–PcCO). CO is normally not present in blood, and since it is rapidly bound to hemoglobin, it accumulates in plasma very slowly when breathed in low concentrations. Therefore, the partial pressure of CO in capillary blood can be taken as zero, which simplifies the test for clinical application. The DL_{CO} is typically decreased in emphysema due to destruction of the vascular bed, and may be one of the earliest abnormalities in various types of interstitial lung disease and pulmonary vascular disease. Anemia decreases DL_{CO} by altering the number of binding sites for CO, and high levels of CO in the blood of heavy smokers may decrease DL_{CO} by creating a back pressure to CO diffusion. DL_{CO} is normal or near-normal in asthma unless the maldistribution of ventilation relative to perfusion is severe.

Key Points

The four abnormal states associated with hypoxemia are hypoventilation, shunt, low $\dot{V}_A/\dot{Q}$ ratios, and diffusion.
Only pure hypoventilation is associated with a normal $P(A-a)O_2$.
Only shunt is *not* corrected by 100% oxygen.
Hypoxemia due to low $\dot{V}_A/\dot{Q}$ ratios responds best to small increases in FIO_2.

Clinical Examples

(All patients live in Oklahoma City where PIO_2 = 143 mm Hg.)

1. A 21-year-old female plumber was found unconscious next to an empty bottle of barbiturates. In the emergency room, she was comatose and cyanotic. Her arterial blood gases revealed a PaO_2 of 40 mm Hg and a $PaCO_2$ of 80 mm Hg on room air.

Discussion. The first question that should be asked in evaluating this patient is, "Why is she hypoxemic?" We know from her $PaCO_2$ that she is hypoventilating, but is all of her hypoxemia due to her hypoventilation? A quick calculation of her $P(A - a)O_2$ will give that answer. $PAO_2 = 143$ mm Hg $- (80 \times 1.2) = 47$ mm Hg. Measured PaO_2 is 40 mm Hg. Therefore, $P(A - a)O_2$ is 7 mm Hg. Thus the $P(A - a)O_2$ is normal, suggesting that there is no significant abnormality of the pulmonary parenchyma. Therefore her hypoxemia is due completely to her hypoventilation, which in turn is probably due to an overdose of barbiturates. However, no matter what the cause of her hypoxemia, the most important thing to do first is to place her on supplemental oxygen. This will raise the PaO_2 even in hypoventilation. The patient will, however, if she continues to hypoventilate, develop other problems; therefore the attending physician should move quickly to endotracheal intubation and mechanical ventilation.

2. A 42-year-old male truck driver gagged and became short of breath while eating olives. In the emergency room, no breath sounds were heard over the right lung and the chest x-ray revealed atelectasis of the right lung. Arterial blood gases revealed a PaO_2 of 41 mm Hg, a $PaCO_2$ of 32 mm Hg, and pH of 7.47.

Discussion. A quick calculation of his $P(A - a)O_2$ reveals that his $PAO_2 = 143$ mm Hg $(32 \times 1.2) = 105$ mm Hg. His measured PaO_2 is 41 mm Hg. Therefore his A – a gradient is 105 mm Hg minus 41 mm Hg, or 64 mm Hg. Thus his $P(A - a)O_2$ is markedly increased, and his chest radiograph reveals that he does have pulmonary parenchymal problems. His hypoxemia is probably due primarily to shunt secondary to the atelectasis.

The patient was placed on a 28% Venturi mask. Unfortunately, the physicians did not realize that the cause of his hypoxemia was primarily shunt. (His PaO_2 came up only to 45 mm Hg.) Had they realized that hypoxemia secondary to shunt does not respond readily to oxygen, they would have placed the patient on a nonrebreathing mask to obtain the highest possible FIO_2 and then moved to correct the cause of the shunt.

3. A 63-year-old man who had smoked two packs of cigarettes a day for the past 45 years complained of chronic shortness of breath. Arterial blood gases revealed a PaO_2 of 50 mm Hg and a $PaCO_2$ of 39 mm Hg.

Discussion. This man's $P(A - a)O_2$ is $96 - 50 = 46$ mm Hg [$PAO_2 = 143 - (39 \times 1.2) = 96$ mm Hg, and the measured $PaO_2 = 50$ mm Hg]; thus he does have a parenchymal pulmonary problem. However, the only thing that can be determined from the blood gases is the fact that he is not hypoventilating. The history suggests that this man has chronic lung disease and that the most likely cause of his hypoxemia is ventilation-to-perfusion maldistribution. In contrast with the previous patient, this patient was placed on 28% oxygen and responded well, his PaO_2 going up to 78 mm Hg. This illustrates that hypoxemia due to low V_A/Q responds nicely to enriched oxygen administration, and small amounts of oxygen can be beneficial.

Bibliography

Farhi LE. Ventilation-perfusion relationships. In Farhi LE and Tenney SM (eds.). *Handbook of Physiology, Section 3: The Respiratory System.* Bethesda, MD: American Physiological Society, 1987. Vol IV: Gas Exchange. *Thorough review with theoretical considerations and practical applications.*

Hughes JMB, Glazier JB, Maloney JE, et al. Effect of lung volume on the distribution of pulmonary blood flow in man. *Respir Physiol* 4:58–72, 1968. *Early description of the distribution of blood flow and the effects of gravity and lung volume.*

Riley RL, Cournand A, and Donald KW. Analysis of factors affecting partial pressures of oxygen and carbon dioxide in gas and blood of lungs. *Methods J Appl Physiol* 4:102–120, 1951. *Classic three-compartment analysis of gas exchange.*

Wagner PD. Diffusion and chemical reaction in pulmonary gas exchange. *Physiol Rev* 57:257–312, 1977. *Comprehensive review of this aspect of gas exchange.*

West JB (ed.). *Ventilation, Blood Flow, and Diffusion. Pulmonary Gas Exchange.* New York: Academic, 1980. Vol. I. *Thorough treatment of most aspects of gas exchange.*

44 Respiratory System Mechanics

Paul V. Carlile

Objectives

After completing this chapter, you should be able to

Explain the determinants of normal lung volumes

Explain the determinants of forced expiratory flow

State the pathophysiologic mechanisms producing a restrictive ventilatory defect

State the pathophysiologic mechanisms producing an obstructive ventilatory defect

Distinguish the flow-volume loops of obstructive and restrictive ventilatory defects

Use the algorithm for interpretation of spirometry

Respiratory system mechanics is the study of factors governing the movement of air in and out of the lungs. Among other things, it encompasses (1) the elastic properties of the lung parenchyma and chest wall under static conditions; (2) the flow-resistive properties of the airways; and (3) the forces generated to overcome these mechanical elements. The physiologic classification of lung disease is based on alterations in respiratory system mechanics. Clinical assessment of respiratory system mechanics may aid in the early diagnosis of respiratory disease and provides an objective assessment of the severity and progression of disease and response to treatment.

Overview of Lung Mechanics

The lungs are elastic structures. When a distending pressure is applied, they undergo a change in volume but return to their previous **unstressed** or **relaxed** volume when the distending pressure is removed. In addition they are connected to the atmosphere by a flow-resistive element, the airways. Therefore, the mechanical properties of the lungs may be represented by a resistive element and an elastic element in series — simply stated, a balloon attached to one end of a tube. To inflate the lungs, the distending pressure must be raised by increasing the pressure at the airway

opening (P_{ao}) or decreasing the pressure **around** the lungs (pleural pressure, P_{pl}):

$$\text{Distending pressure} = P_{ao} - P_{pl} \qquad (44\text{-}1)$$

The increase in distending pressure necessary to inflate the lungs can be partitioned into two component elements: $P_{ao} - P_{pl} = (P_{ao} - P_{alv}) + (P_{alv} - P_{pl})$, where P_{alv} is alveolar pressure. The portion necessary to produce flow ($\dot{V}$) through the resistive element is ($P_{ao} - P_{alv}$) and equals flow multiplied by airway resistance (R_{aw}). The mechanical properties of the elastic element are described by its **compliance,** the change in volume per unit change in distending pressure. The component of distending pressure necessary to overcome lung elastic recoil is ($P_{alv} - P_{pl}$) and equals the tidal volume (V_T) divided by lung compliance (C_L). Therefore, at any point in the respiratory cycle:

$$\text{Distending pressure} = \left(\dot{V} \times R_{aw}\right) + \left(V_T \div C_L\right) \qquad (44\text{-}2)$$

These concepts are illustrated in the left panel of Fig. 44-1, which shows the changes in lung volume, airway opening pressure, pleural pressure, and distending pressure for a single respiratory cycle during spontaneous breathing. Since it is often necessary in clinical medicine to inflate the lungs using a positive-pressure ventilator,

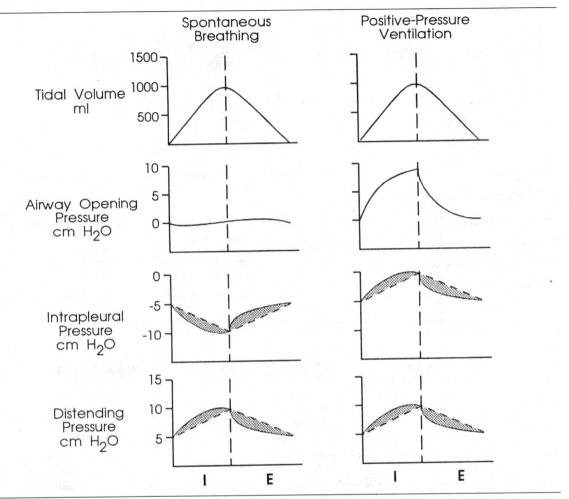

Fig. 44-1. The tidal volume, airway opening pressure, pleural pressure, and distending pressure are shown for a single respiratory cycle during spontaneous breathing (left panel) and positive-pressure ventilation (right panel). In the bottom panels the component of distending pressure necessary to overcome lung elastic recoil is represented by the straight dashed line. Since the solid line represents the distending pressure necessary to produce flow and overcome elastic recoil, the difference between the two lines at any point in the respiratory cycle equals $\dot{V} \times R_{aw}$ (shaded area). When flow is absent at end-inspiration and end-expiration, the entire distending pressure is accounted for by lung elastic recoil. I = inspiration, E = expiration.

changes in these parameters during positive-pressure ventilation are illustrated in the right panel. The changes in distending pressure and tidal volume are identical in the two situations. During spontaneous breathing distending pressure is increased by the contraction of the inspiratory muscles, which lowers pleural pressure. In contrast, the increase in distending pressure is generated by an increase in airway opening pressure during positive-pressure ventilation. When the inspiratory muscles relax or the ventilator cycle terminates, expiration occurs passively due to the potential energy stored in the elastic tissues. When airway resistance is increased by disease, an increase in distending pressure is necessary to maintain the same tidal volume and flow. Similarly, when lung compliance is reduced by disease, an increase in distending pressure is necessary if tidal volume is to remain constant. The increased distending pressure represents an increase in work of breathing for the inspiratory muscles during spontaneous breathing.

Static Elastic Properties of Lung and Chest Wall

Lung Volumes

A spirometer is a simple volume-displacement device that measures the volume of air moving in and out of the lungs. A spirometric tracing of inspired and expired air is shown in Fig. 44-2. The subject's breathing is recorded from left to right. The initial sinusoidal excursions (tidal volume) represent quiet breathing. Functional residual capacity (FRC) is the volume of gas contained in the lungs at the end of a quiet expiration when the respiratory muscles are relaxed. FRC can be divided into expiratory reserve volume (ERV) and residual volume (RV). The tidal breaths are followed by a maximal inspiration, a maximal expiration, and a return to quiet breathing. The volume of gas contained in the lungs at the end of a maximal inspiration is total lung capacity (TLC), whereas the gas contained in the lungs at the end of a maximal expiration is residual volume. The difference between TLC and RV is vital ca-

Fig. 44-2. A spirometric tracing showing the subdivisions of lung volume. TV = tidal volume, RV = residual volume, ERV = expiratory reserve volume, FRC = functional residual capacity, VC = vital capacity, TLC = total lung capacity. (Modified from: Kaufman CE and Papper S. (eds.) *Review of Pathophysiology.* Boston: Little, Brown, 1983, p. 406.)

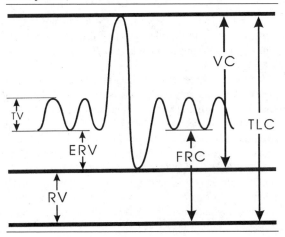

pacity (VC). Since a subject can exhale completely from TLC to RV, vital capacity and its subdivisions can be readily measured with a spirometer. However, RV cannot be exhaled from the lungs and must be measured using other techniques.

Pressure-Volume Relationships

The **pressure-volume curves** of the lung, chest wall, and respiratory system (lung and chest wall combined) are shown in Fig. 44-3. These curves are obtained by plotting the distending pressures of these structures at different volumes under static conditions. Under **static** conditions the distending pressure of the lung is alveolar pressure minus pleural pressure, and the distending pressure for the chest wall is pleural pressure minus body surface (atmospheric) pressure. The subject is instructed to inspire maximally, exhale a preset volume into a spirometer, and then relax against a closed airway with glottis open. Under these conditions P_{alv} and P_{pl} can be estimated by the pressures in the mouth and esophagus respectively. This is repeated at different lung volumes. The static distending pressure for the respiratory system is mouth minus body surface pressure.

Certain features of these curves should be noted. The respiratory system curve becomes flat near TLC and RV, indicating increased elastic recoil. The increase in elastic recoil near TLC is due mainly to increased lung elastic recoil, whereas the increase in elastic recoil near RV is due mainly to the chest wall. The relaxed volume of the chest wall is about 70% of TLC, whereas the relaxed or unstressed volume of the lung is below RV. The relaxed volume of the respiratory system is FRC, the point at which the outward recoil of the chest wall is equal (but opposite in sign) to the inward recoil of the lung.

Determinants of Lung Volumes

Total lung capacity is reached when the outward force generated by the inspiratory muscles can no longer overcome the inward recoil of the respiratory system. It follows that weakness of the inspiratory muscles or increased lung or chest wall elastic recoil would decrease TLC. Processes that result in the removal, destruction, or filling of alveolar air-spaces obviously decrease TLC.

Residual volume is reached in young, normal subjects when the inward force generated by the expiratory muscles is equal to the outward recoil of the chest wall. It follows that decreased expiratory muscle strength may increase RV. Similarly, processes that result in the removal, destruction, or filling of alveolar air-spaces decrease RV.

Functional residual capacity is determined by the passive mechanical properties of the lung and chest wall, and

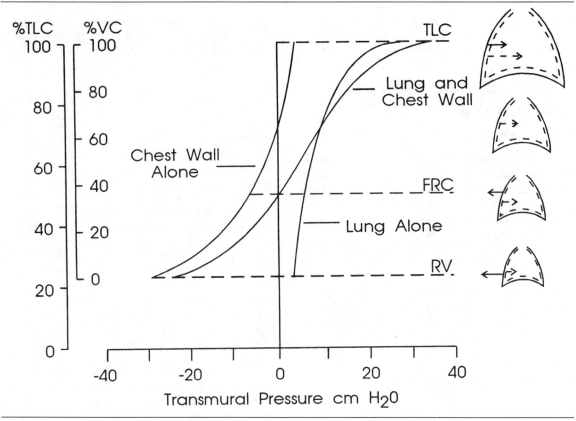

Fig. 44-3. Pressure-volume relationships of the lung, chest wall, and respiratory system (lung and chest wall combined). The direction and magnitude of elastic recoil of the chest wall (solid lines) and lungs (dashed lines) are shown on the right. FRC = functional residual capacity, TLC = total lung capacity, RV = residual volume. (Modified from: Kaufman CE and Papper S (eds.). *Review of Pathophysiology.* Boston: Little, Brown, 1983, p. 406.)

alterations in the elastic properties of either structure will shift FRC. For example, decreased lung elastic recoil may increase FRC, whereas increased lung or chest wall elastic recoil will decrease it.

Compliance

The relative steepness or flatness of pressure-volume curves is commonly represented by the **compliance.** Compliance is defined as the change in volume per unit change in distending pressure, and graphically it is the slope of the pressure-volume curve at any point. Thus chest wall compliance (C_W) is low near residual volume, and lung compliance is low near TLC. By convention C_L is usually measured as the slope of the curve between FRC and FRC

+ 500 ml. C_L and C_W each average ≈ 200 ml/cm H_2O in normal adults, and the compliance of the respiratory system (C_{RS}) — the lungs and chest wall combined — is ≈ 100 ml/cm H_2O.

It should be noted that the measured value for compliance depends not only on the inherent elasticity of the lung and chest wall but also on their initial volume. Consider for example a patient with a normal C_{RS} of 100 ml/cm H_2O over the tidal volume range (FRC + 500 ml). If distending pressure increases by 5 cm H_2O, the volume of **each** lung increases by 250 ml and the total increase in volume is 500 ml. Therefore, each hemithorax has a compliance of 50 ml/cm H_2O. However, if one lung is removed, an increase in distending pressure of 5 cm H_2O will produce a volume change of only 250 ml in the remaining lung, and an increase in distending pressure of 10 cm H_2O would be required to increase volume by 500 ml. Although the elasticity of the remaining lung is normal, the measured C_{RS} has fallen by half (500 ml ÷ 10 cm H_2O), and the amount of elastic work performed by the respiratory muscles to generate the same tidal volume has doubled. This illustrates how alveolar filling, collapse, or removal affects compliance and elastic work even if remaining lung units are normal.

Nature of Lung Elastic Recoil

The elastic recoil of the lung consists of two kinds of forces — tissue forces and surface tension forces. The elasticity of lung tissue is due principally to elastin fibers in alveolar walls and surrounding small airways. Collagen, which has limited distensibility, contributes much less to lung elasticity but probably serves to limit lung expansion at high volumes.

Surface tension plays a major role in lung elastic recoil. It arises from the attractive forces present between molecules at the air-fluid interface of alveolar lining fluid. Surface tension behaves like an elastic sheet that is continually stretched and trying to contract. The surface tension of alveolar lining fluid is much less than that of water or plasma due to the presence of **surfactant,** a mixture of phospholipids (principally dipalmitoylphosphatidylcholine or DPPC), neutral lipids, and proteins present in alveolar lining fluid. Surfactant is synthesized, stored, and secreted into alveolar lining fluid by **type II** pneumocytes. When the alveolar air-fluid interface expands during lung inflation, surfactant is adsorbed onto the surface, where it spreads rapidly. On deflation the surfactant molecules are compressed as the area of the air-fluid interface is reduced, resulting in very low values for surface tension at low lung volumes. According to the LaPlace relationship the pressure required to keep a spherical structure such as an alveolus open is inversely related to its radius of curvature: $P = 2T/r$, where P is pressure, T is surface tension, and r is radius. The ability of surfactant to lower surface tension at low lung volumes stabilizes alveoli and diminishes the tendency of small alveoli to empty into larger ones with which they communicate.

Abnormalities of Elastic Recoil

Abnormalities of Lung Elastic Recoil
Lung elastic recoil is increased by reduced surfactant activity resulting from decreased synthesis or inactivation.

The best-known clinical disorder associated with decreased surfactant synthesis is the respiratory distress syndrome of the newborn. Surfactant production may also be impaired following the interruption of pulmonary perfusion, as in pulmonary thromboembolism. Hydrostatic pulmonary edema and adult respiratory distress syndrome are associated with surfactant inactivation due to alveolar flooding. The consequences of decreased surfactant activity include decreased lung compliance due to increased surface tension and alveolar collapse (atelectasis), decreased lung volumes (TLC, RV, and FRC), and increased elastic work of breathing.

The decreased lung compliance of interstitial or infiltrative lung diseases (Fig. 44-4) results from two mechanisms — decreased distensibility and "lung shrinkage." Pathologically these diseases are characterized by alveolar filling with inflammatory exudate and/or replacement of alveoli by fibrosis, and this loss of alveolar units or lung shrinkage decreases compliance (see above) and increases elastic work. In addition, these disorders may alter the connective tissue elements of the lung, resulting in increased lung elastic recoil. As a result, TLC, RV, and functional residual capacity are decreased, and the elastic work of breathing is increased in these disorders.

Emphysema destroys alveolar walls, resulting in decreased lung elastic recoil (see Fig. 44-4) and increased total lung capacity and FRC. The decrease in lung elastic

Fig. 44-4. Static deflation pressure-volume curves of the lung in emphysema and interstitial pulmonary fibrosis. (Modified from: Bates DV. *Respiratory Function in Disease.* Philadelphia: Saunders, 1989.)

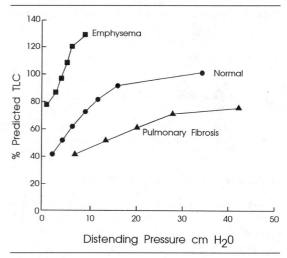

recoil also has important consequences for expiratory airflow, which are discussed below.

Abnormalities of Chest Wall Elastic Recoil

Chest wall compliance is decreased by obesity and by chest deformities such as ankylosing spondylitis and scoliosis. The main physiologic consequences of a stiffened chest wall are reductions in TLC and FRC and increased elastic work of breathing.

Air Flow

Airway Resistance

For air to flow from the airway opening into alveoli during inspiration, the respiratory muscles must not only overcome lung elastic recoil but also generate a driving pressure necessary to pull air through airways. This driving pressure is the difference between airway opening pressure and alveolar pressure, and the ratio of driving pressure to $\dot{V}$ is airway resistance. Airway resistance is related to airway geometry and the type of gas flow. R_{aw} increases with increasing length (l) and varies inversely with the airway radius (r) raised to the fourth power. This means that small changes in radius have a marked effect on flow:

$$R_{aw} \approx \frac{l}{r^4} \qquad (44\text{-}3)$$

Airway resistance results from friction between the molecules of flowing gas and between gas molecules and airway walls. If each gas molecule moves with a constant velocity and relationship to other molecules, laminar or **Poiseuille** flow is present, and airflow and pressure drop are linearly related.

$$P_{ao} - P_{alv} = R_{aw} \times \dot{V} \qquad (44\text{-}4)$$

If flow is disorganized or **turbulent,** a greater drop pressure is required for a given $\dot{V}$. Airflow is turbulent in the large airways even during quiet breathing, whereas Poiseuille flow is found only in small distal airways.

Determinants of Airway Caliber

Airway caliber is affected by factors intrinsic to the airways and by lung volume. Airways are narrowed by contraction of the smooth muscle within their walls, by mucosal edema and inflammation, and by intra-luminal mucus. Like lung parenchyma, the airways are elastic and can be compressed or distended by forces across their walls. Since the airways are tethered to surrounding lung parenchyma, an increase in lung volume exerts an outward traction on the airway walls, resulting in increased cross-sectional area and decreased R_{aw}. If lung elastic recoil is decreased, as in emphysema, the tethering effect of the lung parenchyma is less, and the airways are narrower at any given lung volume.

Maximal Expiratory Flow

Considerable information regarding airway function can be obtained by measuring maximal or forced inspiratory and expiratory flow over the range of vital capacity. To perform a forced vital capacity (FVC) maneuver, the subject inhales to total lung capacity, exhales as forcefully and rapidly as possible to residual volume, and then returns to TLC by a rapid forceful inhalation. During forced inspiration, flow increases rapidly above residual volume because the inspiratory muscles function most advantageously at low lung volumes. As inspiration progresses, flow remains high because airway resistance falls as lung volume increases. Near TLC flow decreases as the inspiratory muscles shorten, and inspiratory force decreases.

During **forced expiration** the driving pressure for flow is alveolar pressure minus airway opening pressure. P_{alv} is the sum of pleural pressure and lung elastic recoil pressure (P_{el}):

$$P_{alv} = P_{pl} + P_{el} \qquad (44\text{-}5)$$

Whereas P_{pl} is a function of muscular effort, P_{el} is a function of lung volume and the lung's inherent elasticity. The relative importance of lung volume versus muscular effort in the generation of maximal expiratory flow is shown in Fig. 44-5. If a subject performs the vital capacity maneuver repeatedly with different levels of effort, a family of flow-volume loops is produced. Near total lung capacity expiratory flow increases with each increase in effort, whereas at lower lung volumes increasing effort increases expiratory flow up to a limiting value. Since this limit cannot be exceeded by increased effort, expiratory flow is said to be **effort-independent** over the lower three-fourths of vital capacity.

Since expiratory flow is independent of muscular effort over the lower three-fourths of the vital capacity (once a finite level of muscular effort is exceeded), lung elastic re-

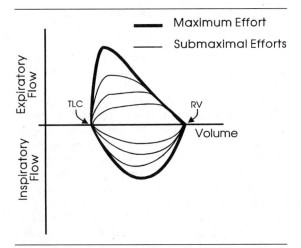

Fig. 44-5. Flow, plotted on the ordinate, as a function of lung volume, on the abscissa, with varying degrees of effort. The flow-volume loops cross the volume axis at total lung capacity (TLC) and residual volume (RV), and the horizontal distance along the volume axis is vital capacity. The heavy line represents a maximal effort, and the lighter ones represent submaximal efforts. (Modified from: Kaufman CE and Papper S (eds.). *Review of Pathophysiology.* Boston: Little, Brown, 1983, p. 410.)

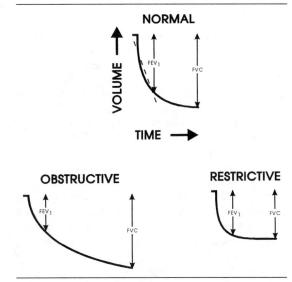

Fig. 44-6. The volume-time curves from a normal subject and patients with obstructive and restrictive defects. The slope of the dashed line on the normal curve equals the average flow rate between the 75% and 25% points of the forced vital capacity (FEF_{25-75}). FVC = forced vital capacity, FEV_1 = forced expiratory volume in one second. (Modified from: Kaufman CE and Papper S (eds.). *Review of Pathophysiology.* Boston: Little, Brown, 1983, p. 408.)

coil becomes the major determinant of driving pressure. If lung elastic recoil is decreased, as in emphysema, expiratory flow will be reduced by the decrease in driving pressure. This is the second mechanism by which emphysema and decreased lung elastic recoil impair maximal expiratory flow.

Volume-Time Curve

The expiratory portion of the FVC maneuver is frequently displayed as a plot of volume versus time (Fig. 44-6). The volume-time curve proceeds from left to right beginning at TLC and following the course of a forced expiration to RV. Thus the vertical distance between the beginning and end of the curve is proportional to FVC. Expiratory flow is assessed by the forced expiratory volume in one second (FEV_1), which represents the average flow rate over the first second of the maneuver, and the average flow rate over the middle half of the forced vital capacity (FEF_{25-75}). FEF_{25-75} is calculated as the slope of a line drawn between

points on the curve corresponding to 75% and 25% of the vital capacity and has the dimensions of volume divided by time, or flow.

Respiratory Muscle Function

Functional Anatomy

During quiet breathing the diaphragm is the primary generator of inspiratory force. Muscle fibers arising from the lower ribs and vertebral column course upward to insert into a central tendon. Contraction of the diaphragm results in a caudal descent of the central tendon and a vertical increase in thoracic volume. Descent of the diaphragm increases intra-abdominal pressure, resulting in outward movement of the abdominal wall, a useful bedside sign of diaphragm activity. Since the abdominal contents provide an impediment to diaphragm descent, contraction of the diaphragm produces an upward force on the lower ribs, displacing them upwardly and laterally and increasing the transverse diameter of the lower rib cage.

The intercostal muscles are thin, flat muscles located between the ribs. Electromyographic data indicate that the external intercostal muscles are active during inspiration, whereas the internal intercostal muscles are active during expiration. The degree to which these muscles contribute to quiet breathing is debated. The observation that paralysis of the intercostal muscles results in decreased or paradoxical movement of the rib cage suggests that they are active during normal inspiration.

The scalene muscles originate from the cervical vertebrae and insert into the upper surfaces of the first two ribs. Contraction of the scalenes elevates the upper rib cage, producing an inspiratory action. These muscles are active during normal quiet breathing. The sternocleidomastoids attach to the mastoid processes on one end and the clavicle and manubrium on the other. By elevating the sternum, the sternocleidomastoids produce an inspiratory action on the upper ribs. The sternocleidomastoids are inactive during quiet breathing but are frequently recruited in patients with respiratory distress.

Activation of the anterior abdominal muscles moves the abdominal wall inward, increases intra-abdominal pressure, and forces the diaphragm cephalad in an expiratory direction. Expiration is passive during quiet breathing because of lung elastic recoil, but the abdominal muscles become active at high levels of ventilation or in the presence of obstruction to airflow.

Respiratory Muscle Mechanics

Length-Tension Relationship

Like all muscles, respiratory muscles obey the length-tension relationship. The tension developed by a contracting muscle is greatest when its resting length is maximal. Resting length of the inspiratory muscles varies inversely with lung volume, and inspiratory pressure is greatest at RV. Conversely, resting length of expiratory muscles and expiratory pressure are greatest at TLC.

Hyperinflation

Hyperinflation signifies an increase in FRC and is commonly present in diseases of airflow obstruction. Hyperinflation serves a useful purpose in these disorders by increasing airway size and lung elastic recoil, both of which facilitate expiratory flow. However, hyperinflation makes the inspiratory muscles less efficient by decreasing their resting length. As a result, inspiratory muscle excitation and energy consumption must increase to produce the same external work.

Oxygen Supply/Demand Balance and Inspiratory Muscle Failure

As is true for the brain and heart, meeting the substrate requirements (oxygen and fuel) of the inspiratory muscles is essential to sustain life. If respiratory muscle work is increased by high ventilatory requirements or abnormal lung mechanics, oxygen supply must be increased to meet the increased metabolic demand. Alternatively, oxygen supply may be inadequate if O_2 delivery is reduced by low cardiac output, anemia, or low PaO_2. If such an energy imbalance occurs, the respiratory muscles may not be able to sustain force generation indefinitely and could fail. Clinical and experimental observations suggest that this is most likely to occur when increased work of breathing occurs in conjunction with impaired oxygen delivery or respiratory muscle inefficiency due to hyperinflation. Inspiratory muscles are thought to be more susceptible to fatigue than expiratory muscles since they are not aided by lung and chest wall elastic recoil and frequently operate at a mechanical disadvantage because of hyperinflation. If the inspiratory muscles fail as force generators, fresh gas is no longer delivered to alveoli at an adequate rate, resulting in hypercapnia and hypoxemia.

Clinical Evaluation of Respiratory Mechanics

Spirometry

The forced vital capacity and its timed subdivisions such as FEV_1 and FEF_{25-75} are readily measured by having a patient perform a forced vital capacity maneuver (see above) into a spirometer, which measures the volume of inspired and expired air over time, or into a pneumotachograph, which measures instantaneous flow during inspiration and expiration and calculates volume by integration of the flow signal. Both tabular data and graphical tracings in the form of the flow-volume loop and expiratory volume-time curve are generated. Although an assortment of measurements and calculations can be made, those that have proven the most valuable in clinical practice are the FVC, FEV_1, ratio of FEV_1 to FVC (FEV_1/FVC), and FEF_{25-75}. Diseases which affect lung mechanics typically produce a decrease in airflow (**obstructive ventilatory defect**) or a reduction in the amount of air-containing lung (**restrictive ventilatory defect**). A few diseases, or a combination of two or more processes, will produce features of both defects. Diseases of the lungs, pleura, chest wall, or respiratory muscles which cause restrictive defects produce **propor-

tionate reductions in lung volume and expiratory flow (FEV_1 and FEF_{25-75}), whereas obstructive disorders such as asthma and emphysema reduce FEV_1 and FEF_{25-75} out of proportion to lung volume. Calculation of the FEV_1/FVC ratio, which normalizes the FEV_1 for any reduction in lung volume, has proven very useful in differentiating obstructive and restrictive ventilatory defects.

Maximal Voluntary Ventilation

Routine spirometric testing frequently includes a measurement of the maximal voluntary ventilation (MVV). As its name implies, the MVV is the amount of air that an individual can ventilate with maximal effort over a brief period. It is measured by having the individual breathe as deeply and rapidly as possible for 12–15 seconds. The test is quite dependent on patient motivation and can be fatiguing in debilitated patients. However, it is a useful way to evaluate respiratory impairment and helpful in assessing the respiratory response to exercise. The MVV is usually reduced in both obstructive and restrictive disorders and is generally equal to 30–40 times the FEV_1. Although the MVV tends to be better preserved in restrictive disorders, an exception to this is neuromuscular disease, where the MVV may be less than 30 times the FEV_1.

Bronchodilator Response

It is common clinical practice to perform spirometry before and after administration of a bronchodilator aerosol, which relaxes bronchial smooth muscle, to determine the amount of improvement or **reversibility** in the FVC and FEV_1. Most obstructive disorders have some component of bronchial smooth muscle constriction and may show improvement in the FVC and/or FEV_1 after bronchodilator. A 12% increase from baseline in the FVC or FEV_1 accompanied by an absolute increase of at least 200 ml is considered significant, although much larger changes in the FVC and/or FEV_1 are frequently encountered in asthma. The presence of acute reversibility in FVC and/or FEV_1 following inhaled bronchodilator may provide useful diagnostic information, but the absence of such improvement does not preclude a therapeutic response to chronic bronchodilator therapy.

Determination of Lung Volumes

Since RV is the volume of gas remaining in the chest after a complete exhalation, it cannot be measured by spirometry. However, it can be measured by **body plethysmography** or **inert gas dilution.** In practice, the measurement of FRC is more reproducible using these techniques, and if ERV has been determined by spirometry, RV is calculated from the difference of FRC and ERV (see Fig. 44-2). Total lung capacity can then be calculated as the sum of RV and vital capacity. Chest radiographs are usually done after a full inspiration to TLC and provide a useful qualitative estimate of TLC to the clinician.

Assessment of Respiratory Muscle Strength

Respiratory muscle strength can be assessed by measurement of maximal inspiratory and expiratory pressures. Using a mouthpiece attached to a pressure manometer, the patient exerts a maximal inspiratory or expiratory effort against a closed airway. Maximal inspiratory pressure (MIP) is normally measured at RV, and maximal expiratory pressure (MEP) is measured at TLC. These measurements are indicated in patients with known neuromuscular disease to assess the presence of respiratory muscle involvement and in patients with unexplained restrictive defects on spirometry. In patients with neuromuscular disease MIP and MEP may be abnormal before the vital capacity is reduced. They are also useful to evaluate patients prior to weaning from positive-pressure ventilation. Although simple to perform, these tests are highly dependent on patient motivation and effort.

Derivation and Use of Prediction Equations

Normal or predicted values for pulmonary function parameters are fundamental to the meaningful interpretation of spirometry and lung volume measurements in an individual patient. Normal values for lung function vary with height, gender, racial or ethnic origin, and age. FVC, FEV_1, FEF_{25-75}, TLC, RV, and FRC vary directly with height and are smaller in women than men. Normal values are calculated by using prediction equations, which are derived by statistical analysis of pulmonary function tests performed on a large number of healthy subjects.

Prediction equations provide a context for comparing measurements from an individual patient to the mean value of measurements obtained from normal individuals of same age, height, and gender. However, considerable variability about the mean value exists in the normal reference group, and normal individuals have measurements that fall above and below the mean. Thus it becomes necessary to define a "lower limit of normal" (LLN) for the reference group. A common practice is to use the fifth percentile as the LLN so that 95% of the values from subjects in the normal reference group are above the LLN. The fifth percentile can be calculated directly using the data from the reference group or estimated by statistical methods. Another common practice, though lacking a statistical basis, is to use 80% of the predicted value as the LLN for FVC and FEV_1. Although this method is a reasonably good approximation of the fifth percentile for FVC and FEV_1, the LLN for the FEF_{25-75} and measures of instantaneous flow is closer to 60% of predicted. The FEV_1/FVC ratio varies inversely with age but is relatively independent of height and gender. The lower limit of normal ranges between ≈ 0.75 for a 20-year old to ≈ 0.68 for a 60-year old.

Interpretation of Pulmonary Function Tests

Obstructive Disorders

Disorders causing an obstructive pattern produce characteristic alterations in the shape of the volume-time curve (see Fig. 44-6) and flow-volume loop (Fig. 44-7). An obstructive defect is characterized by a reduction in expira-

Fig. 44-7. Flow-volume loops. Expiratory flow is upward in direction, and inspiratory flow is downward. The dashed line represents expiratory flow following the administration of an inhaled bronchodilator. (Modified from: Kaufman CE and Papper S (eds.). *Review of Pathophysiology.* Boston: Little, Brown, 1983, p. 410.)

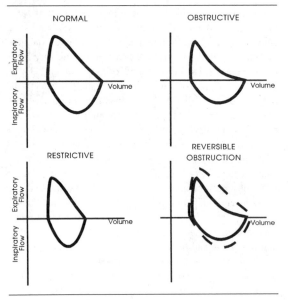

tory flow rates not attributable to decreased lung volume. Measurements of flow such as FEV_1 and FEF_{25-75} are reduced, and the FEV_1/FVC is low. Total lung capacity may be normal but is increased if lung elastic recoil is decreased, as in emphysema. FRC and RV may be normal but are typically increased. FVC is often normal but may be reduced in obstructive disorders by a large increase in RV. In this circumstance the FVC is reduced not by a decrease in the amount of air-containing lung but by **trapping** of gas in the residual volume. Just as the FEV_1 and FEF_{25-75} may improve after administration of an inhaled bronchodilator in a patient with bronchoconstriction, FVC may increase if the improvement in airway narrowing relieves or reverses gas trapping.

Restrictive Disorders

The volume of air within the lung may be reduced by several mechanisms: (1) space-occupying abnormalities within the thorax (e.g., pleural effusion, tumor); (2) parenchymal infiltration (e.g., alveolar filling with fluid or inflammatory exudate, interstitial fibrosis); (3) parenchymal destruction or removal; (4) alveolar collapse; (5) respiratory muscle weakness; and (6) abnormal recoil or deformity of the chest wall. FVC and TLC are decreased in restrictive disorders, but the changes in FRC and RV are variable. RV may be high when there is expiratory muscle weakness, but it is reduced by parenchymal infiltration, destruction, or removal. FRC is reduced by parenchymal infiltration, destruction, or removal or by any disease causing decreased chest wall or lung compliance but is normal in respiratory muscle weakness if the elastic properties of the lung and chest wall are undisturbed. Because the volume of air within the lungs is reduced, the FEV_1 is also reduced, but the FEV_1/FVC ratio will be normal. If the restrictive defect is caused by a process that increases lung elastic recoil and the driving pressure for expiratory flow, the FEV_1/FVC ratio may even be slightly increased.

Algorithm for Interpretation of Spirometry

Interpretation of spirometry begins by looking at the FEV_1/FVC ratio (Fig. 44-8). If the ratio is reduced, an obstructive defect is present. A normal FVC is indicative of a pure obstructive defect, whereas a low FVC could indicate an obstructive defect with gas trapping or a combination of obstructive and restrictive processes. These alternatives could be distinguished by measurement of TLC. A com-

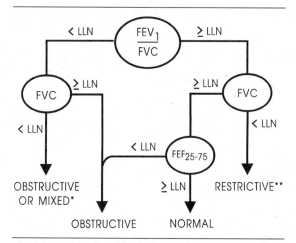

Fig. 44-8. Algorithm for the interpretation of spirometry. FEV_1 = forced expiratory volume in 1 second, FVC = forced vital capacity, LLN = lower limit of normal range, FEF_{25-75} = forced expiratory flow between the 75% and 25% points in the FVC. *Measurement of total lung capacity (TLC) would be needed to distinguish a mixed ventilatory defect from an obstructive defect with air trapping. **Restrictive defects should normally be confirmed by measurement of TLC. (Modified from: Kaufman CE and Papper S (eds.). *Review of Pathophysiology*. Boston: Little, Brown, 1983, p. 409.)

bined obstructive and restrictive defect would be associated with a reduction in TLC, whereas TLC is normal or increased in the presence of an obstructive defect with gas trapping. A normal FEV_1/FVC ratio and decreased FVC is indicative of a restrictive defect. Ideally, the presence of a restrictive defect should be corroborated by measurement of TLC.

Clinical Example

1. A 56-year-old male gives a history of gradually worsening dyspnea on exertion over the past 4 years. The patient reports that he is able to walk on level ground at a slow pace but becomes dyspneic climbing stairs or ambulating at a faster pace. He has smoked two packs per day since age 18 but decided to quit 6 weeks ago. There is no history of asthma, chest pain, hemoptysis, heart disease, hypertension, paroxysmal nocturnal dyspnea, or orthopnea.

Physical examination results are: BP 116/88, HR 88, respirations 20/minute, afebrile. Lung auscultation reveals decreased breath sounds with prolonged expiratory phase and scattered wheezes and rhonchi. Heart examination reveals that the cardiac pulsations are most easily palpated in the subxiphoid region and S_1 and S_2 are faint with no murmur or gallop. There is no cyanosis or clubbing of the extremities, but trace edema is present. Chest x-ray reveals overexpanded lungs and flattened diaphragm.

Pulmonary Function Tests

Test	Measured	Predicted	% Predicted
FVC, L	3.82	5.16	74
FEV_1, L	1.51	3.66	41
FEV_1/FVC	0.40	0.71	
FEF_{25-75} L/min	0.52	3.94	13
FRC, L	5.80	2.97	195
TLC, L	8.94	7.15	125
RV, L	5.12	1.98	259
RV/TLC	0.57	0.31	

Following Inhaled Metaproterenol (a Bronchodilator)

Test	Measured	% Predicted	% Change
FVC, L	4.39	85	+15
FEV_1, L	1.72	47	+14
FEV_1/FVC	0.39		

Discussion. Algorithmic interpretation of the pulmonary function tests (see Fig. 44-8). The FEV_1/FVC ratio is reduced, indicating an obstructive defect. The FVC is also reduced, indicating the presence of a mixed disorder or an obstructive defect with gas trapping. These alternatives can be distinguished by measurement of TLC.

The TLC is slightly increased, indicating that there is **not** a reduction in the amount of air-containing lung. Therefore, the disorder is an **obstructive defect with gas trapping.** If lung volume measurements are not available, the chest x-ray can be used as a qualitative estimate of TLC.

The markedly reduced FEF_{25-75} does not add any additional diagnostic information. This test may be used to diagnose an obstructive defect in cases where the FEV_1/FVC is normal or borderline low. It cannot be relied upon in the presence of a low vital capacity since restrictive disorders produce proportionate reductions in lung volume and expiratory flow.

Following the administration of an inhaled bronchodilator aerosol there are significant increases in both the FVC and FEV_1. This response indicates the presence of bronchial smooth muscle constriction that contributes to airway narrowing and promotes gas trapping. A significant increase in FVC and FEV_1 following bronchodilator inhalation may occur in any airway disease, although large increases are most characteristic of asthma. The normalization of FVC after bronchodilator is further evidence that the cause of the pre-bronchodilator reduction in FVC is gas trapping.

Bibliography

Clausen JL (ed.). *Pulmonary Function Testing Guidelines and Controversies.* Orlando: Grune & Stratton, 1982. *A monograph from the California Thoracic Society covering technical aspects of pulmonary function testing and written by experts in the field. Includes lucid explanations of body plethysmography and inert gas dilution for measurement of lung volumes.*

Light RW. Mechanics of respiration. In George RB, Light RW, Matthay MA, and Matthay RA (eds.). *Chest Medicine.* Baltimore: Williams & Wilkins, 1990, pp. 39–56. *Excellent discussion of the effort-independence of forced expiratory flow including the equal pressure point and collapsible-segment concepts which have been advanced to explain this observation.*

Lung function testing: Selection of reference values and interpretative strategies. *Am Rev Respir Dis* 144: 1202–1218, 1991. *An official statement of the American Thoracic Society covering sources of variation in lung function testing, derivation of prediction equations, selection of reference values, and interpretation. An excellent resource with 249 references.*

Pride NB and Macklem PT. Lung mechanics in disease. In Fishman AP, Macklem PT and Mead J (eds.). *Handbook of Physiology — the Respiratory System III.* Bethesda, MD: American Physiological Society, 1986, pp. 659–692. *A scholarly and critical review of the effects of disease processes on lung mechanics. An outstanding resource with 303 references.*

Wilson, AF (ed.). *Pulmonary Function Testing Indications and Interpretations.* Orlando, FL: Grune & Stratton, 1985. *A companion to the Clausen reference covering all facets of pulmonary function testing including spirometry, bronchodilator response, and lung volumes.*

45 Control of Breathing

Barry A. Gray

Objectives

After completing this chapter, you should be able to

Explain the modification of the ventilatory responses to hypoxemia, metabolic acidosis, and metabolic alkalosis by CSF acid-base balance

Describe the subjective symptoms of acute altitude exposure and the process of acclimatization

Distinguish between abnormal ventilatory control and respiratory pump failure in the production of hypercapnia and respiratory acidosis

Characterize the control of breathing in COPD

Assess the relative importance of altered respiratory drive, abnormal lung function, and neuromuscular dysfunction in the patient with hypercapnia

Distinguish between the two major types of sleep apnea

Describe the factors, other than abnormal blood gases, involved in the production of dyspnea

---

Abnormalities in the control of breathing lead to disorders of carbon dioxide homeostasis, hypocapnia and hypercapnia, and to an abnormal sensation of air hunger, dyspnea, which may be totally unrelated to blood gas abnormalities. Normally alveolar ventilation is precisely matched to metabolic demands, resulting in a normal value for arterial PCO_2 (40 mm Hg). With exercise, O_2 consumption and CO_2 production can increase more than 20-fold (from 0.2 to 4 liters/minute). Despite these large changes in metabolic rate, arterial PO_2 and PCO_2 are maintained constant. The maintenance of normal PCO_2 depends both on the integrity of neural control mechanisms (which include the respiratory control center, the central chemoreceptors, the peripheral chemoreceptors, and a variety of mechanoreceptors) and on the integrity of the respiratory pump (which includes the lungs, chest wall, and muscles of respiration). Clinically, hypoventilation and hypercapnia are the most significant abnormalities in the control of breathing. They occur in a variety of diseases, usually as the result of abnormal function of the respiratory pump or, less frequently, as the result of abnormal function of neural control mechanisms. But abnormalities of both neural con-

trol mechanisms and the respiratory pump may occur together in some patients. Because of the frequency with which physicians must deal with hypercapnia in patients with chronic obstructive pulmonary disease (COPD) and because of the difficulty in sorting out the mechanisms of hypercapnia in these patients, this problem will be given special consideration.

Neural Mechanisms

The neural mechanisms for the control of ventilation include the respiratory center in the brain stem, the peripheral arterial chemoreceptors, the central chemoreceptors, and lung and chest wall receptors which respond to mechanical stress and noxious chemical irritants.

Respiratory Center

The rate and depth of breathing are subject to a number of neural controls. Clearly there is voluntary control exerted by the cerebral cortex. There is also coordination with speech, and swallowing. Underlying these higher controls, respiration is maintained by groups of cells in the brain stem which act together as a basic rhythm generator whose activity is modulated by afferent activity from the peripheral chemoreceptors, central chemoreceptor cells, sensory receptors in the airways, lung and chest wall, and other neural and humoral inputs which provide information necessary to match ventilation to metabolic demand during exercise.

Peripheral Chemoreceptors

There are two sets of peripheral chemoreceptors which are sensitive to changes in the PO_2 and pH of arterial blood. The carotid bodies, located at the bifurcation of the internal and external carotid arteries, have their afferent innervation by the carotid sinus branch of the glossopharyngeal nerve. The aortic bodies, located close to the arch of the aorta, have their afferent innervation by a branch of the vagus. The arterial chemoreceptors are not sensitive to molecular CO_2 per se, but only to the reduction in plasma pH produced by hypercapnia. They exhibit an equivalent response to reductions in blood pH during metabolic acidosis. The response to hypoxia is their primary function. There are no other neural mechanisms to increase respiratory drive in response to hypoxemia. The chemoreceptors also appear to be sensitive to changes in local blood flow mediated either by a reduction in blood pressure or activation of their efferent innervation from the cervical sympathetic chain as might occur with shock or sepsis.

Central Chemoreceptors

Groups of chemoreceptor cells sensitive to reductions in pH are located just beneath the ventral surface of the medulla oblongata close to the roots of cranial nerves VII through XI. These cells are distinct from the cells of the respiratory center which are inhibited by hypercapnia and acidosis. Although the central chemoreceptors are not sensitive to molecular CO_2 per se, their separation from the arterial blood by the blood-brain barrier can produce apparent sensitivity to CO_2 under some conditions. The pH in the vicinity of the central chemoreceptor depends on the ratio of local $[HCO_3^-]$ to PCO_2. Since the blood-brain barrier is far more permeable to CO_2 than the H^+ or HCO_3^- ion, increases in arterial PCO_2 produce greater increases in local H^+ and ventilatory drive than equivalent changes in blood pH associated with metabolic acidosis. Normally CSF $[HCO_3^-]$ is different from that in plasma due to active transport of HCO_3^- and CSF pH, 7.32, differs from plasma

pH, 7.40. With sustained changes in CSF acid-base balance, CSF pH is returned toward normal over a period of 24–48 hours by changes in the active transport and passive diffusion of HCO_3^-. These initial and subsequent changes in CSF acid-base balance play a fundamental role in the activity of the central chemoreceptor in metabolic acidosis and alkalosis as well as the responses to chronic hypercapnia and hypoxemia. There is no central chemoreceptor response to hypoxia.

Lung and Chest Wall Receptors

A variety of receptors sensitive to mechanical stress and chemical irritants influence the rate and depth of breathing. The major relevance of these receptors to pathophysiology stems from their potential ability to detect alterations in lung mechanics and the work of breathing and allow for load compensation. Receptors located in the airways and lung have afferent fibers in the vagus nerves. These include stretch receptors, which provide feedback to the respiratory centers in the brain stem regarding lung volume, the rate of inflation, and distortion of lung tissue such as would occur with atelectasis. There are also the J receptors, so named because of their juxtacapillary location in the pulmonary interstitium, which produce an increase in respiratory rate when stimulated by increases in pulmonary blood volume and interstitial edema. Some of the vagal receptors also elicit respiratory reflexes such as cough, laryngospasm, bronchospasm, and apnea.

Ventilatory Responses to Physiologic Stimuli

The normal responses to physiologic stimuli, which can be studied in the laboratory, are fundamental to an understanding of the pathophysiology of control of breathing in disease states.

Ventilatory Response to Hypercapnia

The ventilatory response to acute changes in $PaCO_2$ may be measured by having a subject rebreathe from a bag containing 7% CO_2 and 93% O_2 which will produce a gradual increase in $PaCO_2$. Over the range from 40 to 70 mm Hg there is a linear relationship between ventilation and $PaCO_2$. The normal slope is 3 liters/minute/mm Hg, but there is considerable variation between subjects (1–6 liters/minute/mm Hg). If the test is performed with a reduced PaO_2, two differences are seen. There is a higher ventilation for any given PCO$_2$ and the slope of the response is increased. The response to chronic hypercapnia is quite different. With chronic hypercapnia, mechanisms concerned with acid-base homeostasis in the CSF produce an increase in CSF [HCO$_3^-$]. As CSF pH is returned toward normal this reduces stimulation of the central chemoreceptor cells. In patients with lung disease and chronic hypercapnia these changes make the linkage between ventilation and arterial blood gases increasingly dependent on hypoxic drive.

Ventilatory Response to Hypoxemia

That there is hypoxic drive to ventilation under normal conditions (PaO$_2$ = 90 mm Hg) is evident from two types of observations. First, in experimental animals one can measure a decrease in carotid body sensory discharge when the inspired O$_2$ is changed from 21 to 100%. Second, in normal man a sudden increase from 21 to 100% O$_2$ produces a transient decrease in respiratory rate and tidal volume for several breaths followed by a return to a level of ventilation equal to or slightly greater than baseline. In contrast, the steady-state ventilatory response to hypoxemia at constant PaCO$_2$ shows little change in ventilation until PaO$_2$ is reduced below 50–55 mm Hg. The discrepancy between the transient response to hyperoxia and the steady-state response curve is not fully understood, but it probably involves changes in cerebral blood flow and brain tissue PCO$_2$.

Metabolic Acidosis and Alkalosis

With the acute onset of metabolic acidosis, the fall in plasma [HCO$_3^-$] is not immediately reflected by a decrease in CSF [HCO$_3^-$], but the decrease in arterial pH does produce an increase in arterial chemoreceptor activity which leads to an increase in alveolar ventilation and a decrease in arterial PCO$_2$. In the early stages of metabolic acidosis CSF may experience a paradoxical increase in pH due to the fall in arterial PCO$_2$. This alkalosis of the CSF inhibits central chemoreceptor activity and limits the immediate ventilatory response to metabolic acidosis. With time (24–48 hours) passive diffusion of HCO$_3^-$ and changes in active transport return CSF pH toward normal, allowing a more complete ventilatory compensation for metabolic acidosis. Whether CSF pH actually becomes acidotic ($\leq$ 7.32) during metabolic acidosis is a subject of debate. Similar transients occur when metabolic acidosis is rapidly corrected. Despite the increase in plasma pH and [HCO$_3^-$] there is a paradoxical acidosis of the CSF as the decrease

in peripheral chemoreceptor activity leads to a decrease in ventilation and an increase in PaCO$_2$. In this case the decrease in CSF pH sustains respiratory drive and retards the return of ventilation to normal.

In metabolic alkalosis the opposite sequence of events takes place. Peripheral chemoreceptor activity is diminished by the increase in plasma pH, ventilation decreases, and PCO$_2$ increases, but the full measure of accommodation is delayed by paradoxical CSF acidosis. Eventually, in 24–48 hours, when CSF acid-base balance is restored the increase in PCO$_2$ is about 1 mm Hg for each milliequivalent per liter change in plasma [HCO$_3^-$]. It is important to note that metabolic alkalosis produced by potassium depletion is not accompanied by the same degree of respiratory compensation as that produced by a simple excess of base.

Acclimatization to High Altitude

With ascent to high altitude there is a gradual reduction in barometric pressure (approximately 50% for each 6000 meters increase in altitude). At 6000 m above sea level (19,685 ft) barometric pressure (Bar) is equal to 380 mm Hg, and since O$_2$ concentration is still 21%, inspired PO$_2$ is 70 mm Hg.

$$P_IO_2 = F_IO_2 \times (Bar - PH_2O) = 0.21 \times (380 - 47)$$
$$= 69.7 \text{ mm Hg}$$

With no change in alveolar ventilation or PaCO$_2$, alveolar PO$_2$ (P$_A$O$_2$) would be 20 mm Hg.

$$P_AO_2 \approx P_IO_2 - \frac{PaCO_2}{R} = 70 - \frac{40}{0.8} = 20 \text{ mm Hg}$$

But ventilation does increase and if PaCO$_2$ decreases from 40 to 20, P$_A$O$_2$ becomes 45 mm Hg.

The symptoms described by normal man upon acute high altitude exposure are relevant to the interpretation of symptoms in patients with hypoxemic lung disease. The first symptom is a decrease in night vision which becomes apparent at 2000 m (Bar $\approx$ 600 mm Hg). At about 3000 m, (Bar $\approx$ 540 mm Hg) the first symptoms of central nervous system dysfunction appear: usually lightheadedness, euphoria, and unwarranted self-confidence not unlike alcoholic intoxication. With further increase in altitude there will be loss of short-term memory and impairment of fine motor movements. With sudden decompression in an airplane cabin at altitudes above 7000 m (Bar $\approx$ 340 mm Hg) there is a brief period of useful function of about 5 minutes before coma and death ensue. It should be noted that, despite reductions in alveolar PO_2 to values approaching 35 mm Hg, shortness of breath is not a symptom described. Patients with hypoxemic lung disease who experience a sudden discontinuation of oxygen therapy are at risk of a severe decrease in mental function before they realize their predicament. On the other hand when patients with lung disease and severe ventilatory impairment, but only mild hypoxemia ($PaO_2 \approx 50$ mm Hg), complain of shortness of breath and oxygen lack it should be recognized that factors related more to mechanical dysfunction of the respiratory system than hypoxemia may be responsible for this complaint.

When a healthy subject travels to high altitude the decrease in PaO_2 produces stimulation of the arterial chemoreceptors, an increase in alveolar ventilation, and a reduction in arterial PCO_2. The resulting alkalosis in plasma and CSF reduce respiratory drive and limit the magnitude of the initial ventilatory response to hypoxemia. Over the first few days the plasma pH returns toward normal as the result of the excretion of HCO_3^- by the kidneys. Three to four days are required for this process of renal compensation. The adjustment of CSF pH develops more rapidly. In 24–48 hours changes in HCO_3^- transport return CSF pH toward normal and allow further increases in ventilation and reductions in $PaCO_2$. In the fully acclimatized subject with normal CSF pH and reduced CSF $[HCO_3^-]$ there is increased sensitivity to changes in $PaCO_2$. If the hypoxic drive is suddenly removed by oxygen administration or return to sea level, increased ventilation continues for several days. The sustained hyperventilation occurs because with the reduction in hypoxic drive and initial decrease in alveolar ventilation the increase in $PaCO_2$ produces acidification of the CSF which sustains increased respiratory drive until CSF $[HCO_3^-]$ and sensitivity to PCO_2 are returned to normal. The time required for the CSF adjustment is again about 24–48 hours, and during the next 48–72 hours arterial blood gas measurements reveal decreased pH and $[HCO_3^-]$ suggestive of mild metabolic acidosis until renal compensation returns plasma $[HCO_3^-]$ to normal.

Accelerated erythropoiesis is another more slowly developing aspect of adaptation to the hypoxemia of high-altitude residence, which produces an increase in hemoglobin concentration and blood oxygen-carrying capacity. After three weeks at altitude the hemoglobin and hematocrit may increase by as much as 20% (increasing hemoglobin from 15 to 18 g/dl). Similar adaptive responses may be seen in patients with hypoxemic lung disease.

There are three disorders of altitude acclimatization which require brief discussion. **Acute mountain sickness,** which frequently occurs with rapid ascent to 3000–4000 m, is manifested by lassitude, decreased appetite, vomiting, and insomnia. These symptoms are thought to be due to acute alkalosis. They last only 2–3 days and can be ameliorated by prophylactic administration of the carbonic anhydrase inhibitor acetazolamide which hastens the alkaline diuresis normally associated with altitude adaptation. **Chronic mountain sickness** is an uncommon disorder of long-time residents at altitude which is manifested by cyanosis, fatigue, somnolence, decreased mental function, exaggerated erythrocytosis, and peripheral edema. This syndrome is thought to result from decreased hypoxic respiratory drive. The clinical analogy is cor pulmonale in the patient with hypoxemic lung disease which presents with many of the same signs and symptoms.

Alterations in Carbon Dioxide Homeostasis

Respiratory alkalosis with hypocapnia and respiratory acidosis with hypercapnia represent control system failures. In some cases the failure is intrinsic to the control system. In other cases it reflects inability of the system to compensate for unusual stresses.

Hypocapnia and Respiratory Alkalosis

By definition, hypocapnia indicates alveolar hyperventilation, i.e., ventilation in excess of metabolic requirements. The recognition of respiratory alkalosis is of importance primarily because it may be the first clue to a life-threatening medical problem. Some of the causes of hypocapnia are listed in Table 45-1. Notice that the list includes hypoxemia and metabolic acidosis as causes of hypocapnia. When these conditions are associated with hypocapnia their presence will be obvious from the arterial blood gas analysis which indicated hypocapnia. Some of the other causes of hypocapnia will be more difficult to identify unless there is some other clue to their existence. The presence of unexplained hypocapnia should alert the physician to the need for a detailed workup.

The complications which may result from severe respiratory alkalosis are listed in Table 45-2. In general, respiratory alkalosis is a benign condition which does not require specific treatment unless there is evidence of a serious complication. The treatment of respiratory alkalosis varies with its cause; basically, it is the treatment of the underlying medical problem.

Table 45-1. Causes of Hyperventilation and Hypocapnia

CENTRAL STIMULATION

Central neurogenic hyperventilation
Pregnancy
Thyrotoxicosis
Salicylate toxicity
Anxiety — pain

PERIPHERAL CHEMORECEPTOR STIMULATION

Hypoxemia ($PO_2 < 50$–55 mm Hg)
Metabolic acidosis
Thyrotoxicosis

STIMULATION OF PULMONARY MECHANORECEPTORS

Congestive heart failure
Asthma
Pulmonary fibrosis
Pneumonitis
Pulmonary embolism

UNKNOWN MECHANISM

Sepis
Hepatic encephalopathy

Table 45-2. Complications of Respiratory Alkalosis

Decreased cerebral blood flow
Decreased ionized calcium
Hypophosphatemia
Tetany
Seizures
Cardiovascular collapse (shock)

Table 45-3. Causes of Hypercapnia

DECREASED RESPIRATORY DRIVE

Depressed level of consciousness
    Narcotics, opiates, benzodiazepines
    Cerebral vascular accident
    Head injury
    Hypothyroidism (Myxedema)
Normal level of consciousness
    Primary alveolar hypoventilation

FAILURE OF THE RESPIRATORY PUMP

Increased mechanical loads
    Chronic obstructive pulmonary disease
    Upper airway obstruction
    Pulmonary edema
    Kyphoscoliosis
    Asthma (rare, but carries poor prognosis)
Ventilation perfusion mismatch
    Chronic obstructive pulmonary disease
    Pulmonary embolism (rare)
    Adult respiratory distress syndrome (rare)
Neuromuscular dysfunction
    Fatigue of the respiratory muscles
    Guillain-Barré syndrome
    Myasthenia gravis
    Toxic neuropathy (arsenic)
    Myopathy, muscular dystrophy, myotonic
    dystrophy
    Electrolyte depletion (potassium, phosphate)
    Acetylcholinesterase inhibitors: insecticides,
    nerve gas
    Hypothyroidism (myxedema)

Hypercapnia and Respiratory Acidosis

By definition, hypercapnia indicates reduced alveolar ventilation ($\dot{V}_A$), i.e., insufficient to meet metabolic requirements. Basically hypercapnia can occur as the result of decreased respiratory drive or failure of the respiratory pump (Table 45-3). Most patients with depressed respiratory drive will also have a depressed level of consciousness, but level of consciousness is not always a reliable guide to the cause of hypercapnia since severe hypercapnia from any cause may produce a reduction in the level of consciousness (this is known as CO_2 narcosis). While those abnormalities of respiratory control associated with depressed consciousness represent global dysfunction of the central nervous system, the abnormalities in respiratory control which may be associated with a normal level of consciousness represent more specific disorders. Pa-

tients with so-called **primary alveolar hypoventilation** have abnormal blood gases but normal ventilatory function and gas exchange, i.e., no evidence of ventilation perfusion mismatch. They have reduced ventilatory response to CO_2 and may also have a reduced response to hypoxemia. Some, but not all, have other manifestations of neurologic disease. These patients may appear otherwise normal or they may present with signs and symptoms similar to those seen in chronic mountain sickness (fatigue, somnolence, decreased mental function, secondary erythrocytosis, and peripheral edema).

Failure of the respiratory pump may result from increased mechanical loads, inefficient ventilation produced by ventilation-perfusion mismatch, or neuromuscular dysfunction. It should be noted that whereas the mechanical loading associated with increased airway resistance frequently produces hypercapnia, the loss of lung compliance in pulmonary fibrosis seldom produces hypercapnia except as a terminal event.

Ventilation-perfusion mismatch results in alveoli which have both low $\dot{V}/\dot{Q}$ ratios and high $\dot{V}/\dot{Q}$ ratios, but it is only the alveoli with high $\dot{V}/\dot{Q}$ ratios which produce physiologic deadspace and alveolar hypoventilation. Destruction or obliteration of alveolar capillaries is the cause of increased deadspace in COPD. While vascular obstruction causes increased deadspace in pulmonary embolism, the effect on arterial PCO_2 is usually determined by other factors which increase respiratory drive, resulting in alveolar hyperventilation and hypocapnia. Rarely vascular destruction and obstruction by micro-emboli are sufficient to produce hypercapnia in the adult respiratory distress syndrome. When increased physiologic deadspace (V_D) due to $\dot{V}/\dot{Q}$ mismatch is the primary mechanism of alveolar hypoventilation and hypercapnia, total expired ventilation ($\dot{V}_E$) is usually increased despite the decrease in alveolar ventilation ($\dot{V}_A$).

$$\dot{V}_E = \dot{V}_A + \dot{V}_D \qquad (45\text{-}1)$$

In contrast to hypercapnia due to decreased respiratory drive, which is not accompanied by evidence of air hunger, respiratory failure due to neuromuscular dysfunction is always accompanied by dyspnea.

While it is useful to classify the mechanisms of hypercapnia as illustrated in Table 45-3, it should be recognized that many patients with hypercapnia will have several mechanisms which operate to produce an increase in $PaCO_2$. For example, the deformation of the lungs and chest wall in kyphoscoliosis produce decreased lung compliance and increased airway resistance, but there is also evidence of decreased strength of the diaphragm in this disorder. Severe cardiogenic pulmonary edema presenting with hypercapnia represents a combination of increased airway resistance, and decreased lung compliance which is complicated by fatigue of the respiratory muscles due to inadequate perfusion and increased work of breathing. Hypothyroidism produces both decreased respiratory drive and muscular weakness.

Hypercapnia in Patients with COPD

Respiratory acidosis is often a primary feature of acute respiratory failure in patients with COPD. In patients with severe COPD, hypercapnia may also be present during periods of relative compensation and well-being. In these patients hypercapnia is a form of compensation for increased work of breathing and disordered gas exchange, and attempts to interfere with this compensation may be deleterious.

Mechanism of Hypercapnia

The relationship between arterial PCO_2, alveolar ventilation, and CO_2 production is essential to an understanding of hypercapnia in patients with lung disease.

$$PaCO_2 = k \times \frac{CO_2 \text{ production}}{\text{Alveolar ventilation}} \qquad (45\text{-}2)$$

Either an increase in CO_2 production or a decrease in alveolar ventilation can result in hypercapnia. In patients with abnormal lung function, CO_2 production should be thought of as the sum of basal metabolic rate plus the CO_2 produced by the respiratory muscles working against an increased mechanical load, and alveolar ventilation should be thought of as the difference between total ventilation and ventilation which is wasted due to increased physiologic deadspace.

$$PaCO_2 = k \times \frac{\text{Basal metabolism} + \text{Work of breathing}}{\text{Total ventilation} - \text{Wasted ventilation}} \qquad (45\text{-}3)$$

In patients with COPD, an increase in $PaCO_2$ occurs for two reasons. First, the wasted deadspace ventilation is increased by the obliteration of pulmonary capillaries and maldistribution of ventilation with respect to blood flow. As a result, alveolar ventilation is decreased, even though total minute ventilation may be normal or even increased. Second, the airway obstruction in these patients increases the work of breathing. In healthy subjects the O_2 consumed and the CO_2 produced by the respiratory muscles is less than 2% of total metabolic rate. In patients with lung disease the metabolism of the respiratory muscles may approach 20% of total metabolic rate. These two factors in CO_2 homeostasis are illustrated in Fig. 45-1.

When a healthy subject hyperventilates there is a reduction in arterial PCO_2 because the increase in alveolar ventilation is far greater than the increase in metabolism of the respiratory muscles. In the COPD patient with increased work of breathing and increased physiologic deadspace the patient will lose control over the $PaCO_2$. Hyperventilation may produce proportional increases in CO_2 production and alveolar ventilation, but no change in $PaCO_2$. Such a patient has no ventilatory reserve. The increase in CO_2 production associated with the minimal activities of

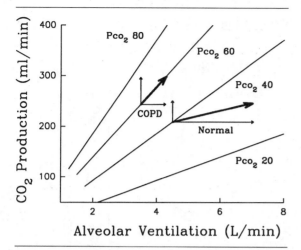

Fig. 45-1. CO_2 production ($\dot{V}CO_2$) and alveolar ventilation ($\dot{V}_A$) are plotted with PCO_2 isopleths. Along each diagonal line the ratio of $\dot{V}CO_2$ to $\dot{V}_A$, and therefore PCO_2, is constant. The relationship between $\dot{V}CO_2$ and $\dot{V}_A$ at rest and during voluntary hyperventilation are illustrated for a normal subject and COPD patient. At rest the COPD patient has a greater PCO_2 (60 mm Hg) than the normal subject (40 mm Hg) as the result of increased $\dot{V}CO_2$ due to the increased work of breathing and decreased $\dot{V}_A$ due to increased deadspace. During hyperventilation the change in PCO_2 is determined by the relative magnitudes of the change in $\dot{V}_A$ (horizontal arrows) and the change in $\dot{V}CO_2$ (vertical arrows) resulting from the increased metabolism of the respiratory muscles. In the normal subject the increase in $\dot{V}_A$ is relatively greater than the increase in $\dot{V}CO_2$ and the PCO_2 moves off the 40 mm Hg isopleth toward a lower value. In the COPD patient the increase in $\dot{V}_A$ is not as great due to mechanical limits on total ventilation and the increase in deadspace ventilation. This small increase in $\dot{V}_A$ is balanced by a large increase in $\dot{V}CO_2$ due to increased work of breathing. If the increase in $\dot{V}CO_2$ is proportional to the increase in $\dot{V}_A$ there will be no change in PCO_2. (Reprinted with permission from: Kaufman CE and Papper S (eds.). *Review of Pathophysiology.* Boston: Little, Brown, 1983, p. 416.)

daily life cannot be accommodated simply by an increase in ventilation. Each increase in metabolism must be accompanied by an increase in $PaCO_2$ which represents an unacceptable increase in respiratory drive. The patient has two alternatives. Either allow a gradual increase in $PaCO_2$ to accommodate increases in metabolic rate or curtail increases in metabolic rate. If the patient accepts an increase in $PaCO_2$, any level of metabolism can be accommodated at a lower rate of alveolar ventilation; for example, when

the $PaCO_2$ is 60, rearrangement of Eq. (3) predicts that the $\dot{V}_A$ needed to eliminate 200 ml of CO_2 is 2/3 of the $\dot{V}_A$ needed when $PaCO_2$ is 40 mm Hg.

$$\text{Alveolar ventilation} = k \times \frac{CO_2 \text{ production}}{PaCO_2} \qquad (45\text{-}4)$$

At the same time, the increase in $PaCO_2$ is accompanied by an increase in plasma and CSF $[HCO_3^-]$ which normalizes pH and decreases the sensitivity to changes in PCO_2. Increases in metabolic rate are easily accommodated with minimal increase in respiratory drive. This patient does not appear to be dyspneic, but clinical examination and arterial blood gas analysis reveal cyanosis and hypoxemia. With time the hypoxemia produces pulmonary hypertension, secondary erythrocytosis, and right ventricular failure manifested by peripheral edema (**blue bloater syndrome**). Other patients who cannot tolerate an increase in $PaCO_2$ struggle to breathe and maintain normal PCO_2, but are constantly plagued by shortness of breath. Because of normal alveolar PCO_2 and PO_2, oxygenation is reasonably well maintained and they are free of cyanosis, polycythemia, and edema, but constantly manifest tachypnea and shortness of breath (**pink puffer syndrome**). The factors which appear to determine whether a patient will become a "blue bloater" or "pink puffer" include the predominance of bronchitis versus emphysema in the underlying lung disease.

Ventilatory Control in COPD

For a number of years the prevailing concept was that patients with COPD had lazy respiratory centers. Work in many laboratories demonstrated that the slope of the standard CO_2 ventilatory response curve was markedly depressed in comparison to normal subjects. Consequently the use of respiratory stimulants was advocated for the correction of respiratory acidosis. More recently, there has been a change in point of view. As illustrated in Fig. 45-2, when the standard CO_2 ventilatory response curve is measured in normal subjects breathing through an external resistance to simulate the increased airway resistance of COPD, the ventilatory response measured as the change in $\dot{V}_E$ is diminished but the response expressed as inspiratory muscle work is not influenced by an increase in airway resistance. Thus the diminished ventilatory response to CO_2 in COPD patients does not mean that chemosensitivity and respiratory drive are necessarily abnormal.

At present the best method to assess respiratory drive in

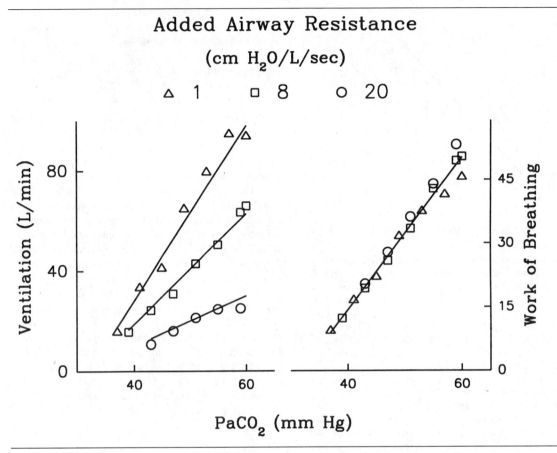

Fig. 45-2. Effect of increased airway resistance in normal man. Data plotted in the left panel show that an increase in PaCO$_2$ produced by breathing small concentrations of CO$_2$ leads to an increase in ventilation. However the increase is less and the rate of increase in ventilation is not so steep if the measurement is made with the subject breathing through an added airway resistance to simulate the situation which occurs in patients with COPD. The plot in the right panel uses work of breathing (more precisely inspiratory work rate) as the dependent variable and indicates that work is the same for any given PaCO$_2$. Thus decreased ventilatory response to CO$_2$ when airway resistance is increased by disease does not indicate abnormal control of breathing. (Reprinted with permission from: Kaufman CE and Papper S (eds.). *Review of Pathophysiology*. Boston: Little, Brown, 1983, p. 416. (Simulated data to illustrate the findings of Milic-Emili J and Tyler JM. *J Appl Physiol* 18:497–504, 1963.)

the presence of abnormal lung mechanics is the pressure generated by the inspiratory muscles during a brief occlusion of the airway using a mask and valve system. The subject, or patient, breathes through a mouthpiece which can be briefly occluded without the knowledge of the subject, and the pressure fall in the mouthpiece during the first 0.1 seconds is taken as a measure of respiratory drive (Fig. 45-3). This mouth occlusion pressure, usually referred to as the P$_{0.1}$ ("P point one"), averages 2 cm H$_2$O in healthy subjects and increases with exercise or any other respiratory stimulus. The best evidence that hypercapnia and respiratory acidosis are not the result of decreased respiratory

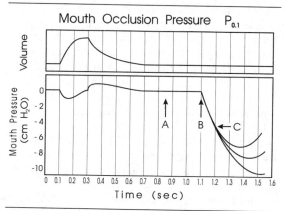

Fig. 45-3. Mouth occlusion pressure measurement. Volume is shown in the top panel with inspiration upward and mouthpiece pressure in the lower panel with inspiration downward (negative). At point A the mouthpiece is occluded after the end of a normal breath. At point B the subject initiates the next respiratory effort against the occluded airway, and at point C the $P_{0.1}$ is measured 0.1 second after the onset of the inspiratory effort. Several inspiratory efforts are superimposed to illustrate that approximately 0.2–0.3 seconds after the onset of the inspiratory effort reflex or volitional responses to the occlusion may either accelerate or diminish the pressure change, but the response is reproducible during the first 0.1 second. (Simulated tracings to illustrate the findings of Whitelaw WA, Derenne JP, and Milic-Emili J. *Respir Physiol* 23:181–199, 1975.)

drive in the patient with COPD comes from a study in which $P_{0.1}$ was measured during and after an acute episode of respiratory failure. These observations indicate that respiratory drive is increased fourfold in COPD patients with acute hypercapnic respiratory failure. When these patients were given supplemental oxygen, the $P_{0.1}$ fell but remained elevated about threefold. Following recovery from the episode of acute respiratory failure respiratory drive remained about twice normal, consistent with the abnormal lung mechanics and increased work of breathing that are present in these patients chronically. Of course these observations do not exclude the possibility that some patients with obstructive lung disease may have depressed respiratory drive which complicates their management. Respiratory drive is likely to be decreased by severe hypercapnia which impairs sensorium.

Complications of Hypercapnia

Values of $PaCO_2$ and pH which might be encountered under various conditions are listed in Table 45-4. The average values for the breaking point of a breath hold in normals are included to provide a sense of the respiratory drive associated with a mild level of acute respiratory acidosis. Notice that the distinction between acute and chronic respiratory acidosis is based on pH as an indicator of the increase in $[HCO_3^-]$ produced by renal compensation. The deleterious effects of hypercapnia result from two physiologic effects of increased PCO_2. First, carbon dioxide, like many other gases, exerts a narcotic effect on the central nervous system. The first signs of CO_2 narcosis are asterixis and subtle changes in mental status. With further elevation of $PaCO_2$ the patient becomes obtunded, and respiratory drive may be suppressed, eventually resulting in apnea and cardiac arrest. These effects of CO_2 on cellular function are reversible, provided the PCO_2 is returned to tolerable levels before cardiac arrest occurs. The second effect of elevated $PaCO_2$ results from a depression of alveolar and arterial oxygen tensions. At P_ACO_2 equal to 40 mm Hg, the P_AO_2 is 100. In a patient with lung disease, the alveolar-arterial oxygen gradient ($AaDO_2$) may be 40 mm Hg, leading to a PaO_2 equal to 60 mm Hg (oxygen saturation = 92%). If hypercapnia develops with $PaCO_2$ equal to 60, there will be a decrease in alveolar and arterial PO_2 equal to approximately 20 mm Hg, and the PaO_2 will be 40

Table 45-4. $PaCO_2$ and pH Values in Health and Respiratory Failure

$PaCO_2$ (mm Hg)	Arterial Blood pH	Condition
40	7.40	Normal
48	7.34	Breaking point of breath holding
70	7.20	Severe acute respiratory failure
70	7.30	Severe chronic respiratory failure
100	7.15	CO_2 narcosis, drowsiness and coma
		Compatible with survival only with oxygen supplementation

Modified from: Kaufman CE and Papper S (eds.). *Review of Pathophysiology.* Boston: Little, Brown, 1983, p. 415.

mm Hg (oxygen saturation = 75%), which represents severe arterial hypoxemia. Even with normal gas exchange $PaCO_2$ equal to 100 reduces P_AO_2 to 25 mm Hg ($0.21 \times (760 - 47) - 100/0.8$), which is compatible with survival only with O_2 supplementation.

Approach to the Patient with Hypercapnia

Hypercapnia and respiratory acidosis should be approached in terms of the physiologic mechanisms outlined in Table 45-3. First, is there evidence of increased or decreased respiratory drive? Usually respiratory rate will provide the best clue. The awake patient with $PaCO_2$ over 46 mm Hg and pH below 7.35 who has a respiratory rate below 20 has depressed respiratory drive. If the level of consciousness is depressed this could either be CO_2 narcosis, or central nervous system depression. In many cases it will be appropriate to administer an opiate antagonist to exclude the possibility of drug abuse or iatrogenic respiratory depression.

Patients who develop hypercapnia entirely from increased mechanical loads may have normal or decreased total ventilation but there should be evidence of increased work of breathing, i.e., intercostal retraction or use of the accessory muscles. There will also be evidence of increased airway resistance, i.e., inspiratory stridor (suggesting upper airway obstruction) or rhonchi and wheezes (suggesting intrathoracic airway obstruction), but with severe airflow obstruction there may be no auscultatory findings other than decreased air entry. When respiratory acidosis results from upper airway obstruction this represents a medical emergency requiring tracheal intubation or tracheostomy. The exception is in children with enlarged tonsils and adenoids, in whom the gradual onset of hypercapnia allows for compensation and the surgical management is less urgent. The asthmatic with respiratory acidosis requires intense therapy and close medical supervision. Some will require mechanical ventilation.

If ventilation appears to be increased, one should think of ventilation-perfusion mismatch due to pulmonary vascular abnormalities.

If ventilation is decreased despite increased respiratory rate and there is nothing to suggest airway obstruction or increased work of breathing, one should think of neuromuscular dysfunction. There will often be other clues such as decreased strength in the arms, legs, or muscles served by the cranial nerves.

The patient with hypoventilation and **acute** respiratory acidosis due to central nervous system depression or neuromuscular dysfunction will usually require tracheal intubation and mechanical ventilation because the process may progress to complete apnea. Respiratory acidosis due to primary hypoventilation is usually **chronic,** stable, and compensated. Emergency treatment is usually not required, but the patient should be evaluated for more severe hypoventilation and apnea during sleep.

In patients with chronic obstructive lung disease and hypercapnia, the increase in arterial PCO_2 must be viewed as a physiologic adaptation, rather than simply an abnormal laboratory result. Respiratory stimulants aimed at increasing ventilation may only complicate the problem by increasing the work of breathing. Instead, therapy should be directed at decreasing the work of breathing and improving the distribution of ventilation in the lung. Bronchodilators, antibiotics, and clearance of secretions to improve airway function and, in some patients, diuretics to reduce pulmonary vascular congestion should be employed. Of course, since alveolar PCO_2 is increased, alveolar PO_2 is decreased, and the careful administration of oxygen in a controlled fashion is necessary to alleviate the dangerous arterial hypoxemia that usually coexists with hypercapnia in patients with respiratory failure.

Oxygen-Induced Carbon Dioxide Retention

Early in the use of blood gas measurements to guide the treatment of patients with respiratory failure it became apparent that uncontrolled oxygen therapy could produce a worsening of hypercapnia, often resulting in CO_2 narcosis and coma. Initial insights suggested that this was the result of the loss of hypoxic respiratory drive due to the increase in PaO_2. More recent studies have suggested that the decrease in alveolar ventilation with O_2 therapy may be the result of an increase in physiologic deadspace due to changes in $\dot{V}_A/\dot{Q}$ distribution. Whatever the mechanism, oxygen-induced carbon dioxide retention can become a serious problem in the management of patients with hypercapnic respiratory failure because the process is not immediately reversible. The problem is illustrated in Table 45-5 with the possible course of events in a patient who presents with hypercapnic respiratory failure.

On admission to the hospital the blood gases show severe hypoxemia and combined acute and chronic respiratory acidosis. In response to therapy with 28% O_2 the PaO_2 increases, but it is still subtherapeutic, and there is a small progression of the respiratory acidosis. When 40% O_2 is

Table 45-5. Oxygen-Induced CO_2 Retention

Condition	$\%O_2$	pH	$PaCO_2$	PaO_2	P_AO_2	$A - aDO_2$
On admission	21	7.26	64	35	70	35
Initial therapy	28	7.23	68	45	116	71
Somnolent	40	7.18	85	55	182	127
Discontinue O_2	21	7.18	85	11	46	35

given the PaO_2 reaches a safe level, but there is a further progression of the hypercapnia and a change in sensorium suggesting the onset of CO_2 narcosis. At this point one might try to reverse the process by discontinuing O_2 therapy, but this could be very dangerous. The CNS depression can prevent the normal response to hypoxemia as O_2 is washed out of the lungs. On admission the alveolar to arterial O_2 gradient ($A - aDO_2$) was 35 mm Hg. If there were no increase in alveolar ventilation, the $PaCO_2$ would remain elevated at 85 mm Hg, at this $PaCO_2$ the P_AO_2 would be 46 mm Hg, and with an $A - aDO_2$ of 35 mm Hg the PaO_2 would be only 11 mm Hg. This level of hypoxemia would result in cardiac arrest. A safer approach is to produce a very gradual, stepwise reduction in the inspired O_2 concentration while using other forms of therapy, such as bronchodilators, to reduce the work of breathing and improve alveolar ventilation and $PaCO_2$. Most patients who develop O_2-induced CO_2 retention and CO_2 narcosis will require tracheal intubation and mechanical ventilation.

Sleep Apnea Syndromes

Sleep apnea can either be caused by intermittent upper airway obstruction (UAO) during sleep, called **obstructive sleep apnea,** or by periods of apnea with complete cessation of respiratory efforts, called **central sleep apnea.** Many patients with sleep apnea experience both obstructive and central apneas. Both represent disorders of respiratory control.

Healthy adults experience hypoventilation and an irregular respiratory pattern during sleep leading to an increase in $PaCO_2$ (4–8 mm Hg) and decrease in PaO_2 (3–10 mm Hg) and even brief (< 15 seconds) periods of central apnea during the rapid-eye-movement (REM) stage of sleep. During inspiration negative swings in airway pressure favor collapse of the upper airway, but this is prevented by phasic increases in the tone of certain muscle groups which maintain upper airway patency. During sleep there is progressive loss of inspiratory tone in these muscle groups,

which increases the likelihood of collapse and UAO. Patients with obstructive sleep apnea generally have predisposing anatomic characteristics such as morbid obesity with redundant pharyngeal soft tissue or reduced upper airway size due to enlarged lymphatic tissue. Patients with central sleep apnea generally have reduced respiratory drive which can be demonstrated by diminished ventilatory response to hypercapnia and hypoxemia while awake.

During both types of apnea, which may last for 60–90 seconds, there is a progressive increase in $PaCO_2$ and decrease in PaO_2 until the apnea is terminated by an arousal from sleep. Consequently the patients experience sleep deprivation and daytime hypersomnolence. They may report episodes of falling asleep while driving an automobile or carrying on a conversation. In the patient with obstructive sleep apnea, loud sonorous snoring punctuated by periods of apnea ending with a loud snort may sometimes be described by the bed partner. As the result of nocturnal hypoxemia both types of patients may present with the findings of chronic mountain sickness (fatigue, decreased mental function, secondary erythrocytosis, and peripheral edema). Other findings may include unexplained systemic hypertension and daytime hypercapnia.

Therapy depends on the predominant type of sleep apnea. The previous treatments for patients with obstructive apnea included tracheostomy or uvulopalatopharyngoplasty (UPP) to surgically correct the mechanism of airway obstruction. At present continuous positive airway pressure applied to the nose (nasal CPAP) is the favored form of therapy if it can be tolerated by the patient. By maintaining positive pressure in the upper airway, nasal CPAP prevents collapse during periods when there is loss of muscle tone. For central sleep apnea, central respiratory stimulants such as medroxyprogesterone, theophylline, and protriptyline have been tried with variable success. Sometimes nocturnal mechanical ventilation with a negative pressure ventilator or a rocking bed may be required. In both types of sleep apnea, oxygen administration may be of benefit by reducing the severity of hypoxemia during apneic episodes.

Mechanisms of Dyspnea

Dyspnea is a commonly encountered symptom for which the pathophysiology is poorly understood. Abnormalities in cardiopulmonary function leading to air hunger and the sensation of smothering are frequently accompanied by hypoxemia and hypercapnia, and the physician is tempted to attribute all dyspnea to the reduced arterial PO_2 or the increased PCO_2. When the dyspneic patient with normal or nearly normal arterial blood gas values is encountered, the symptom of dyspnea is written off as psychogenic or due to anxiety. Such thinking reveals an incomplete understanding of dyspnea and respiratory drive.

Investigations of dyspnea have been handicapped by its subjective nature, as well as by the difficulty of precisely reproducing the sensation of dyspnea experienced by patients in an experimental setting. In general, dyspnea is most closely related to the level of **efferent (motor) output from the respiratory center** to the inspiratory muscles, i.e., respiratory drive. Thus dyspnea is likely when an increase in respiratory drive is necessary to overcome abnormalities of lung mechanics. Dyspnea will also accompany respiratory muscle weakness since the impaired muscles must operate at a higher level of activation to maintain adequate ventilation. Increased minute ventilation — due to exertion, increased physiologic deadspace, or possibly hypoxemia — necessitates an increase in respiratory drive. In patients with obstructive disease, it has been found that the level of exertion sufficient to require a minute ventilation greater than one-third of the maximum voluntary ventilation is consistently associated with dyspnea. Respiratory drive may also be increased by afferent input from the various lung and chest wall receptors, and experimental observations indicate that stimulation of these afferent nerves may contribute to the sensation of dyspnea observed in breathholding. Although blood gas measurements provide clinically useful information when evaluating the dyspneic patient, it is important to remember that they do not provide the full explanation. Abnormalities in lung or chest wall mechanics can play an important role in creating the symptoms of dyspnea.

Clinical Example

1. A 62-year-old retired rodeo cowboy complains of longstanding dyspnea, cough, and sputum production. He has smoked two packs of Camels per day for 40 years. His dyspnea has worsened recently and he is now only able to walk about 20 ft. The patient is alert and oriented and in acute respiratory distress. There is mild cyanosis of the lips and extremities. He is using accessory muscles of respiration.

Physical Examination Results

Temperature	38.4°C
Blood pressure	135/85 mm Hg
Heart rate	105/min
Respiratory rate	38/min

Jugular venous distension is noted. Chest examination reveals increased anterior-posterior diameter with diffuse inspiratory and expiratory wheezes. Heart sounds are soft. Also noted is 2+ ankle edema. Chest x-ray reveals no acute disease. Electrocardiogram shows sinus tachycardia, p-pulmonale and possible old anteroseptal myocardial infarction.

Laboratory Results

Hemoglobin	16 g/dl
WBC	25.6×10^3
Na^+	136 meq/l
K^+	3.6 meq/l
Cl^-	92 meq/l
HCO_3	32 meq/l
BUN	24 mg/dl
Creatinine	1.6 mg/dl
Arterial blood gas on room air	pH 7.31
PCO_2	64 mm Hg
PO_2	39 mm Hg

O_2 was administered by nasal prongs at 2 liters/minute. Thirty minutes later the arterial blood gases were repeated with the following results:

On 2 liters O_2

pH	7.26
PCO_2	72 mm Hg
PO_2	46 mm Hg

O_2 flow was increased to 4 liters/minute.

Thirty minutes later, the patient was somnolent but arousable: BP 155/90, HR 123, RR 32. Asterixis was noted, and arterial blood gases were repeated.

On 4 liters O_2

pH	7.19
PCO_2	84 mm Hg
PO_2	55 mm Hg

O_2 was discontinued and blood gases ordered for 30 minutes later. While sample was being drawn patient developed bradycardia which progressed to asystole requiring cardiopulmonary resuscitation and mechanical ventilation.

Blood gases drawn just prior to cardiac arrest were

On air

pH   7.19
PCO_2 79 mm Hg
PO_2 22 mm Hg
$[HCO_3^-]$ 30 mm Hg

During an 8-day stay in the intensive care unit, ventilatory support was gradually withdrawn while the patient was being treated with antibiotics and bronchodilation.

Discussion.   The history and physical examination suggest severe COPD with signs of cor pulmonale. It is not unusual for the radiologist to find no evidence of acute disease in this setting. The white count suggests infection, probably acute or chronic bronchitis given the history of cough and sputum production. The blood gases indicate chronic respiratory acidosis with renal compensation and severe hypoxemia.

The initial administration of O_2 was appropriate, but 2 liters/minute did not allow PaO_2 to reach an adequate level. It was also appropriate to increase the O_2 flow rate. When the patient developed mental status changes with asterixis, however, the physician did not recognize this early sign of CO_2 narcosis. He did note that the O_2 therapy had induced further CO_2 retention and attempted to reverse this by discontinuing O_2. The course of events and subsequent blood gases drawn just prior to cardiac arrest indicate that the CNS depression induced by CO_2 narcosis did not allow the patient to respond to the fall in PaO_2 when O_2 was withdrawn.

Luckily, the patient suffered no serious sequelae from cardiac arrest resulting from the hypoxia. However, this potentially fatal course of events could have been avoided by electively instituting respiratory support with mechanical ventilation when progressive CO_2 narcosis was first recognized.

Bibliography

Aubier M, Murciano D, Fournier M, et al. Central respiratory drive in acute respiratory failure of patients with chronic obstructive pulmonary disease. *Am Rev Resp Dis* 122:191–199, 1980. *Clinical study which used $P_{0.1}$ to demonstrate increased respiratory drive in hypercapnic patients.*

Goldring RM, Cannon PJ, Heinemann HO, and Fishman AP. Respiratory adjustments to chronic metabolic alkalosis in man. *J Clin Invest* 47:188–202, 1968. *Carefully designed study in normals demonstrating the difference between the response to base excess and potassium depletion.*

Ingram RH Jr., Miller RB, and Tate LA. Ventilatory response to carbon dioxide and to exercise in relation to the pathophysiologic type of chronic obstructive pulmonary disease. *Am Rev Resp Dis* 105:541–551, 1972. *Classic study into the factors separating the "blue bloater" from the "pink puffer."*

Riley RL. The work of breathing and its relation to respiratory acidosis (editorial). *Ann Intern Med* 41:172–176, 1954. *The classic treatment of the problem.*

Tobin MJ. Dyspnea: pathophysiologic basis, clinical presentation, and management. *Arch Intern Med* 150:1604–1613. *Scholarly review of the literature on dyspnea.*

46 Diseases of Air Flow Limitation

David C. Levin

Objectives

After completing this chapter, you should be able to

List the three distinct mechanisms of air flow limitation

Know the clinical features and pathologic changes of chronic bronchitis

Recognize the three major kinds of emphysema and their relation to cigarette smoking

Understand the basic inflammatory nature of asthma

Be familiar with the most common types of inherited diseases of air flow limitation

---

Overview

Diseases Causing Air Flow Limitation

These include chronic bronchitis, emphysema, asthma, and mixtures of these three diagnoses, as well as cystic fibrosis and α_1-antitrypsin deficiency. These diseases, often referred to as chronic obstructive pulmonary diseases (COPD), represent the fifth leading cause of death in the United States and are associated with an increasing morbidity and mortality, especially in women.

Mechanisms of Air Flow Limitation

While these diseases exhibit a wide variation in risk factors, etiologies, prognosis, and pathologic findings, limitation of air flow as determined by simple spirometry (see Chap. 44) is a universal finding at some time in the course of each of them. There are three major changes in the lungs and connecting airways that account for the measurable decreases in air flow.

1. A bronchial component found primarily in chronic bronchitis, which consists of enlarged bronchial mucous glands with excess mucus production, some degree of inflammation, bronchial wall thickening, and smooth muscle hypertrophy.

2. Acinar enlargement characteristically seen in emphysema, likely the result of an imbalance in the protease-antiprotease levels found in the alveolar walls of smokers and patients with the inherited deficiency of α_1-antitrypsin.

3. A narrowing of small airways resulting from inflammation and fibrosis which cause an increase in airway resistance and decrease in air flow.

A summary of the pathophysiologic components common to the disease of air flow limitation are shown in Table 46-1.

Interrelationship Among Diseases of Air Flow Limitation

The complex, heterogenous overlapping of the three primary diagnoses included under diseases of air flow limitation is shown in Fig. 46-1. While air flow limitation is present during attacks in all asthmatics, it is totally reversible in most of them (subset 9, Fig. 46-1).

Role of Cigarette Smoking

Increases in cigarette smoking since the beginning of the twentieth century parallel marked increases in the prevalence of COPD in the United States.

The risk of developing COPD is 30 times higher in smokers than nonsmokers.

80–90% of deaths from COPD can be related to cigarette smoking.

Long-term studies on smokers have documented a dose-response relationship between cigarette smoking (number of pack-years) and the rate of decline in spirometric values.

Stopping smoking can result in improvements in pulmonary function, especially in early airway disease.

Chronic Bronchitis

Definition

The diagnosis of chronic bronchitis is based on the clinical history of chronic cough associated with sputum production for more than 90 days on two successive years, provided the patient does not have lung cancer, tuberculosis, or congestive heart failure. Abnormal pulmonary function or blood gas values, radiographic changes, and etiologic factors are not included in the definition of chronic bronchitis. Although cigarette smoking is the most common cause, occupational exposure and air pollution may contribute in some patients.

Anatomic Pathology

Although pathologic changes are not part of the diagnostic definition of chronic bronchitis, a number of structural findings are consistently noted.

Increase in Mucous Glands in Airways

There is enlargement in both size (hypertrophy) and number of the mucus-secreting elements found in the airways. The hypertrophy is exhibited as enlargement of the secretory cells as well as dilation of the ducts leading from the secretory glands. The Reid index, which measures the ratio of the bronchial gland thickness to the total bronchial wall thickness, is increased.

Mucus Accumulation in Small Airways

Post-mortem examinations in chronic bronchitis have documented a marked increase in mucus production, resulting in frequent obstruction of the airways.

Small (< 2 mm-Diameter) Airway Narrowing

Recurrent inflammation, infection, and subsequent scarring in the terminal airways results in a decrease in the average small airway diameter. This results in an increase in

Table 46-1. Pathophysiologic Components of the Diseases of Air Flow Limitation

Component	Chronic Bronchitis	Emphysema	Asthma
Bronchospasm	++	+/–	++++
Abnormal mucus	++++	+	++
Structural damage	+	++++	+/–
Inflammation	+++	+	++++
Hyperreactivity	++	–	++++
Infection	+++	+	–
Hypoxemia	+	+	–

Fig. 46-1. The interrelationship among the diseases of air flow limitation is demonstrated in this nonproportional Venn diagram. The three overlapping circles represent the primary diagnoses of chronic bronchitis, emphysema, and asthma. Subjects in black-banded area (subsets 1 through 8) have chronic obstructive pulmonary disease (COPD). True reversible asthmatics lie in area 9, while those with "asthmatic bronchitis" fall into areas 6 and 8. Subsets 1 and 2 have chronic bronchitis or emphysema, but do not have airflow limitation. Subset 10 represents patients with air flow limitation due to other diseases such as cystic fibrosis, bronchiectasis, or bronchiolitis obliterans. (Modified from: Snider GL, Faling J, and Rennard SI. Chronic bronchitis and emphysema. In Murray JF and Nadel JA (eds.). *Textbook of Respiratory Medicine* (2nd ed.). Philadelphia: Saunders, 1994, p. 1071.)

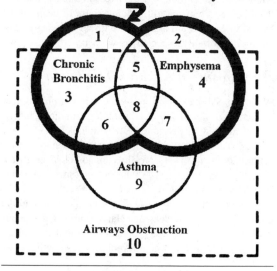

Chronic Obstructive Pulmonary Disease

airway resistance, contributing to the decrease in expiratory air flow seen in chronic bronchitis.

Clinical Features and Approach to Therapy

By definition, chronic bronchitis is a clinical diagnosis based on daily cough and expectoration of sputum. Bronchitic patients are often described as "blue bloaters" due to their tendency to exhibit both hypoxemia and right heart failure with peripheral edema in spite of only moderate obstructive changes on pulmonary function tests. Frequent exacerbations are common, precipitated by repeated infection (both viral and bacterial) and the copious mucoid sputum present in the airway. Such acute episodes result in marked hypoxemia (blueness) associated with an increase in pulmonary artery pressure, impairing right ventricular function, and significant jugular venous distension and ankle edema (bloated). Chest auscultation often demonstrates a mixture of coarse rhonchi and diffuse wheezing. Laboratory findings may show a slight leukocytosis associated with some degree of secondary erythrocytosis, due to long-standing hypoxemia. Arterial blood gases drawn during such an attack will often demonstrate an acute respiratory acidosis ($\downarrow$ pH and $\uparrow$ PaCO$_2$) associated with marked hypoxemia (PaO$_2$ < 50 mm Hg). Chest radiograph may show some degree of cardiomegaly, although frequently it is unchanged from prior films.

Treatment for chronic bronchitis includes both long- and short-term components. All patients should be strongly encouraged to quit smoking, as continued smoking further stimulates mucus production, worsening airway obstruction. In addition, the carbon monoxide associated with smoking binds to hemoglobin, lowering the oxygen-carrying capacity of the blood. Inhaled anticholineric bronchodilator (ipratropium bromide) has become the first line therapy for the bronchospasm associated with chronic bronchitis. In patients needing further therapy, the addition of β_2 adrenergic agonist (albuterol, pirabuterol, terbutaline) is often helpful in improving pulmonary function results and decreasing dyspnea. During mild exacerbations, the addition of a broad-spectrum antibiotic (amoxicillin, trimethoprim/sulfa, erythromycin) to decrease sputum colonization has been shown to decrease the need for hospitalization. During severe, acute exacerbations with hypoxemia, the delivery of low-flow oxygen (by nasal cannula or Venturi mask) is essential to decrease pulmonary hypertension and correct right heart failure (cor pulmonale). Some patients will require intubation and mechanical ventilation during an acute episode of respiratory failure. The use of cortico-steroids in such patients is frequent, but not fully supported in the literature. Long-term home oxygen therapy is recommended for those patients who cannot achieve PaO$_2$ greater than 55 mm Hg after maximum therapy.

Emphysema

Anatomic Pathology

Emphysema is characterized by permanent enlargement of the airspaces distal to the terminal bronchioles associated with destructive loss of the alveolar walls within the acinus without accompanying fibrosis. The acinus is the primary unit of the respiratory tissue of the lungs and consists of the respiratory airspaces arising from a single terminal bronchiole. Three distinctive pathologic patterns of alveolar destruction have been described, according to the portion of the acinus first involved with disease (Fig. 46-2).

Centrilobular (or Centriacinar) Emphysema

It is characterized by patchy involvement throughout the lungs, predominantly in the upper lobes and superior segments of the lower lobes (see Fig. 46-2A). Some lobules may be affected while adjacent ones in the same lobe are spared. The respiratory bronchioles are primarily affected in centrolobular emphysema and alveolar inflammation is not prominent. This pattern of emphysema is highly associated with smoking.

Panacinar (or Panlobular) Emphysema

It demonstrates involvement of the entire acinus, even in its earliest stages (Fig. 46-2B). This early diffuse destruction leads to loss of distinction between alveolar ducts and alveoli and ultimately total effacement of the alveolus with only strands of lung tissue remaining. Panacinar emphysema tends to be localized to the lower lobes and is uniquely associated with homozygous α_1-antitrypsin deficiency.

Distal Acinar (also Paraseptal, Periacinar, or Subpleural) Emphysema

It predominantly involves distal alveolar sacs and ducts, usually in the upper lobes and often subpleurally or along fibrous interlobular septa (Fig. 46-2C). The remainder of the lung is often spared so that air flow is not impaired and spirometry may be normal. This type of emphysema is typically seen in a young adult with a history of a spontaneous pneumothorax.

Pathogenesis

An imbalance between naturally occurring proteases and antiproteases is probably responsible for the development

A. Centrilobular Emphysema

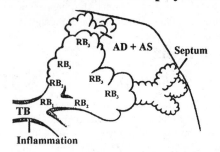

B. Panacinar Emphysema

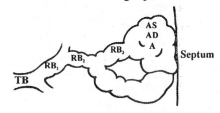

C. Distal Acinar Emphysema

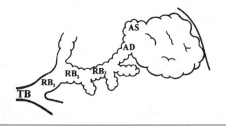

Fig. 46-2. Pathologic patterns of emphysema. (A) In centrilobular emphysema respiratory bronchioles are predominately involved. TB, terminal bronchiole; RB₁, RB₂, RB₃, respiratory bronchioles of the first, second, and third orders; AD, alveolar duct; AS, alveolar sac. (B) In panacinar emphysema the enlargement and destruction of the air spaces involve the acinus uniformly. A, alveolus; other abbreviations are as in Fig. 46-2A. (C) In distal acinar emphysema the peripheral portion of the acinus, the alveolar ducts and sacs, is selectively involved. Abbreviations are as in Fig. 46-2A. (Items A and B modified with permission from Thurlbeck WM, Dunnill MS, Hartung W, et al. A comparison of three methods of measuring emphysema. *Hum Pathol* 1:215–226, 1970. Item C reprinted from Thurlbeck WM. *Chronic Airflow Obstruction in Lung Disease.* Philadelphia: Saunders, 1976.)

of emphysema. According to this model, alveolar destruction occurs when the balance between lung matrix breakdown and defenses against lung breakdown is tipped in favor of destruction. Collagen breakdown by proteases is an ongoing process. The primary example of such an enzyme is neutrophil-derived elastase released from polymorphonuclear white cells. However, several circulating antiproteases are known. The lung is principally protected from elastolytic damage to the alveoli by α_1-antitrypsin, which inactivates neutrophil elastase by binding tightly with it, inactivating both proteins in the process. Normally, the antiprotease protection vastly exceeds the elastolytic threat to the lung and no alveolar damage occurs. This balance may be tipped in favor of alveolar destruction with either an increase in neutrophil elastase brought to the alveoli or when endogenous α_1-antitrypsin levels are inactivated. Cigarette smoke has been shown to do both, implicating it as the major stimulus to alveolar destruction found in emphysema.

Clinical Features and Approach to Therapy

As a group patients with emphysema are able to maintain a higher alveolar minute ventilation than those with chronic bronchitis. Thus they tend to have a higher PaO_2 and lower $PaCO_2$ and have classically been referred to as "pink puffers." This results in less pulmonary hypertension (or at least a delay in its development) and less peripheral edema than seen in the bronchitic "blue bloaters." Physical examination often reveals a thin, tachypneic patient using accessory muscles and pursed lips to facilitate respiration. The thorax is frequently barrel-shaped due to hyperinflation. This shape may initially improve ventilation by keeping open emphysematous terminal airways that have lost their elastic support. Ultimately, the chest wall can expand no further and this air-trapping leads to decreases in diaphragmatic and intercostal muscle efficiency and progressive respiratory failure. Chest auscultation reveals decreased breath sounds over large bullae and poor diaphragmatic movement due to hyperinflation. Chest radiographs classically demonstrate a small heart trapped in the midst of hyperinflated lungs with a flattened or inverted diaphragm. Very few patients have "pure" emphysema and most have various amounts of chronic bronchitis and bronchospasm as well. Therapy for these patients is nearly identical to those with chronic bronchitis, although right heart failure and the need for oxygen therapy are much later in the course of the disease.

Asthma

Definition

Asthma is a disease of reversible air flow obstruction manifested by wheezing and caused by a combination of airway mucosal edema and inflammation, increased secretions and smooth muscle constriction (see also Chap. 37). There is a new appreciation for the importance of inflammation in the airways of asthmatics. In addition, recognition of the associated airway hyperreactivity has dramatically altered therapy for these patients. Post-mortem examination of the lungs of patients dying with status asthmaticus have shown goblet cell hyperplasia, basement membrane thickening, epithelial denudation, eosinophil and neutrophil infiltration, smooth muscle and glandular hyperplasia, and signs of hypersecretion. These findings have strongly suggested the need for earlier and more prolonged use of both oral and inhaled corticosteroids in asthma therapy to combat the intense inflammatory response.

Inflammatory Mechanisms in Asthma

Specific inhaled antigen challenges have been used to better understand the pathophysiologic and immunologic mechanisms involved in the asthmatic airway response. There is always an immediate (< 15 minute) decrease in FEV_1 which is likely IgE associated. In addition, between one-third and one-half of the asthmatics show a dual response with a late (4–8 hours) bronchoconstriction following such allergen challenges. Figure 46-3 shows a typical dual asthmatic response to an antigen challenge. At present, the exact mechanisms involved in this late-phase reaction remains unclear. Multiple cells (macrophages, T-lymphocytes, eosinophils, and mast cells) and many mediators (cytokines, growth factors, enzymes, and superoxides) are involved following various airway challenges (antigens, chemical exposure, exercise). At least six separate steps in this complex chain of events have been identified.

Triggering

Specific allergens seem to trigger an attack through activation of a group of mast cells which have a number of high-affinity IgE receptors on their surface. Mediators of inflammation known to come from activated mast cells include tryptase, prostaglandin D_2, and leukotriene C_4 (LTC_4). Pretreatment with an antihistamine or sodium cromoglycate (a mast cell membrane stabilizer) blunts the releases of these mediators, giving further credence to the

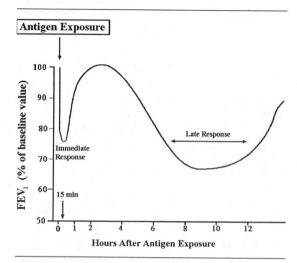

Fig. 46-3. Typical dual-phase asthmatic response to an antigen challenge demonstrating two distinct drops in FEV_1 over 8 hours. (Modified with permission from: Wenzel SE. Asthma as an inflammatory disease. *Seminars in Respiratory Medicine* 15:106–116, 1994, Thieme Medical Publishers, Inc.)

role of mast cell activation as the first step in the inflammatory process.

Signaling

After mast cell triggering, the inflammatory signal is passed along through the release of cytokines which activate T lymphocytes as intermediate messengers. Interleukin-2 (IL-2) receptor has been found in the airways of asthmatic patients and has been shown to correlate with asthmatic activity. In animal models, other cytokines (IL-3, IL-4, IL-5, IL-10, GM-CSF, and gamma-interferon) have very specific functions (induction of mast cell proliferation and maturation, increase eosinophil chemotaxis and activation, and up regulation of IgE production) that are likely to be involved in the human asthmatic response.

Migration

After the activation of triggering and signaling, cytokines stimulate the migration of neutrophils, eosinophils, lymphocytes, and monocytes to the area. These cells are likely involved in the last-phase portion of the dual asthmatic response, as well as the nocturnal asthma attacks seen in some patients. There are currently two possible explanations for the modulation of this inflammatory cell influx; either or both may be in effect.

Activated Signaling Cells. They may release mediators with chemoattractant properties, such as LTB$_4$, platelet-activating factor (PAF), IL-5, and IL-8.

Signaling Cells. These may release substances, such as IL-1 and tumor necrosis factor alpha (TNF-α), that leads to up-regulation of adhesion molecules (ELAM-1, ICAM-1, and Mac-1) expressed on epithelium, endothelium, and inflammatory cells. These molecules then serve as tethers to retain cells in an area of inflammation.

Inflammatory Cell Activation

The presence of inflammatory cells in the airway is not enough to produce an asthma attack, as eosinophils are recoverable from asthmatic airways most of the time and patients with eosinophilic pneumonia do not have wheezing. These cells must be activated by coming in contact with cytokines and activating compounds including IL-1, IL-5, TNF-α, and GM-CSF. Analysis of airway fluid from antigen-challenged subjects provides evidence for eosinophil activation in acute asthmatic inflammation. These samples contain large amounts of major basic protein, found in the eosinophil granule, as well as eosinophil cationic protein. Also recovered in these specimens is LTC$_4$, an important inflammatory activator and potent bronchoconstrictor, secretagogue, and inducer of permeability changes.

Inflammation Causes Bronchoconstriction

It is likely that the bronchoconstriction and airways hyperreactivity thought to be the hallmarks of asthma may actually be the result of epithelial cell damage from long-standing inflammation. The degree of bronchoconstriction could be influenced by a number of factors: increased glandular secretions; increased permeability, allowing greater access of bronchoconstrictors to nerves and smooth muscles; disruption of epithelium, allowing easier access of allergens to submucosal cells; and loss of specific bronchodilation substances produced in the epithelial cells, including nitrous oxide and PGE$_2$. New evidence has implicated the nonadrenergic, noncholinergic nervous system as an intermediary between the epithelium and bronchoconstriction.

Resolution

Although asthma is usually considered to be an episodic disease, fully reversible with periods of complete normalcy, chronic forms of the disease are becoming evident. It is uncertain if these chronic cases represent continuous stimulation by an antigen or an abnormality in the usual resolution processes seen in other types of inflammation. Of specific interest are those asthmatics with late-phase reactions because the antigen is often no longer present when the delayed response occurs. It is possible that the resolution process is inhibited in certain individuals, leading to a prolonged late-phase inflammatory response.

A summary of the cellular interaction in both the early- and late-phase asthmatic response is shown in Fig. 46-4.

For clinical features and approach to therapy, see Chap. 37.

Fig. 46-4. The mast cell plays a central role in initiating both the early-phase asthmatic response, which results only in bronchospasm, and the late-phase response, which results in inflammation and hyperresponsiveness as well as some chronic irreversible changes. (Modified from Lieberman P. Update on inflammation and hyperresponsiveness in asthma. *J Respir Dis* 15 (suppl): S15, 1994. Paul J. Singh-Roy, Medical Illustrator.)

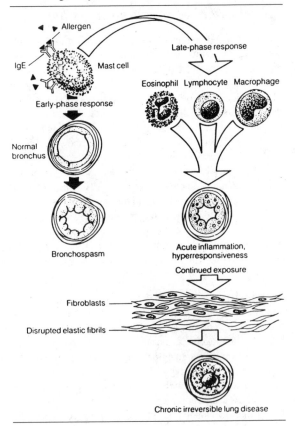

Cystic Fibrosis

Definition

Cystic fibrosis (CF), an autosomal recessive disease due to a defective gene on the long arm of chromosome 7, is inherited from asymptomatic, heterozygotic parents. Pulmonary disease, the most life-threatening aspect of CF, induces obstruction of the airways with thick, tenacious secretions and frequent respiratory infections resulting in bronchiectasis (dilation of the terminal bronchioles). Diagnosis of CF is based on a abnormally high sweat chloride test, although genetic analysis is now available. Once limited to childhood, patients with CF are now living into their fourth decade, causing physicians who deal with adults to become familiar with the disease.

Pathologic Mechanism

The primary problem causing the clinical manifestations in CF is a defect in chloride permeability at the bronchial cell luminal surface. Normally the epithelial cells allow for passive transport of chloride along an electrochemical gradient from the cytoplasm to the lumen. In CF patients, there is a defective response to cyclic AMP in these channels that prevents the normal secretion of chloride into the airway. In addition there is a threefold increase in reabsorption of sodium from the airway into the epithelial cell cytoplasm. This decrease in chloride secretion and increase in sodium reabsorption decreases airway water content, resulting in an increase in the viscosity and tenacity of airway secretions. Frequent infection of these thick CF secretions, especially by *Pseudomonas aeruginosa,* leads to multiple bouts of pneumonia, respiratory failure, bronchiectasis, and ultimately death.

Approach to Therapy

Traditional therapy for patients with CF includes improving bronchial hygiene to aid in clearance of secretions, antibiotics to decrease the number of pathogens, and bronchodilators to improve pulmonary function. Oxygen is given if hypoxemia ($PaO_2 < 55$ mm Hg) is present. Attempts to alter water content of bronchial secretions have not been successful. However, the latest therapy with nebulized human DNAase to degrade the macromolecules released in the airways from inflammatory cells in purulent secretions has produced 10–20% improvements in airflow measurements. Though this is a promising therapy, it is currently extremely expensive (~ $1000/month). While none of the current therapies address the basic genetic defect in patients with CF, attempts are underway to deliver normal genetic material to the airway to normalize the local electrolyte disorder that underlies this disease.

α_1-Antitrypsin Deficiency

Definition

As mentioned in the section on pathogenesis of emphysema, α_1-antitrypsin is a glycoprotein that functions in the lung as an antiprotease to inhibit neutrophil elastase and protect the connective tissue framework of the alveolar wall. α_1-Antitrypsin deficiency (AAT) is an autosomal disease in which decreased amounts of α_1-antitrypsin are produced, leading to the development of severe emphysema as early as the fourth decade of life or earlier in heavy smokers. More than 75 different alleles have been identified for the AAT gene.

Pathologic Mechanism

Increases in elastase (released from inflammatory cells) or decreases in α_1-antitrypsin (inactivated by cigarette smoke or congenitally absent) or both can lead to the development of panacinar emphysema. In normals, the MM phenotype consists of two codominantly inherited M alleles. The most important form of AAT deficiency is associated with the ZZ phenotype which produces less than 19% of the normal amount of the macromolecule, leaving the lung unprotected against protease activity.

Clinical Findings and Approaches to Therapy

Patients with ZZ type AAT develop emphysematous bulla, mostly in the lower lobes. Pulmonary function tests and arterial blood gases are similar to the "pink puffers" discussed above. In the past therapy has consisted of the usual array of bronchodilators, antibiotics, and oxygen. Recently attempts to stem the progression of AAT disease has led to liver transplantation in younger patients (to provide the missing α_1-antitrypsin) and also by weekly or monthly intravenous replacement of the α_1-antitrypsin protein that has now become commercially available. Long-term effectiveness of these therapies has not yet been reported and the expenses are great (> $100,000 for a liver transplant and ~ $1000/month for intravenous therapy).

Clinical Examples

1. A 19-year-old man came to the emergency department complaining of being unable to catch his breath and of his chest feeling tight. He had a 10-year history of periodic attacks of dyspnea and marked wheezing, occurring predominantly in the spring and summer. He has had eczema since infancy and hay fever from the age of seven. Physical examination revealed an increase in the anteroposterior diameter of his chest, which was hyperresonant; on auscultation diffuse, prolonged expiratory wheezes were easily heard. Examination of his sputum revealed numerous eosinophils; the peripheral white blood cell count had 12% eosinophils. Chest radiograph showed very large lung volumes and clear lung fields. Spirometry demonstrated an FVC of 3.4 liters (64% predicted) and an FEV_1/FVC = 0.47.

The patient was treated with a subcutaneous injection of epinephrine, albuterol by updraft nebulizer, and intravenous corticosteroids. Two hours later, repeat spirometry showed an FVC of 5.2 liters (98% of predicted), an FEV_1 of 3.6 liters (83% of predicted), and FEV_1/FVC = 0.69.

Discussion. This patient demonstrates an allergic-type asthma with a severe ventilatory defect and hyperinflation of the lung at a time of moderately severe bronchospasm. The prompt and dramatic response to bronchodilators (epinephrine, albuterol) is characteristic of the reversibility of airflow obstruction in asthma. The corticosteroids will help control inflammation and prevent a delayed response.

2. A 66-year-old white male carpenter was followed for 3 years in the chest clinic with shortness of breath on mild exertion and chronic cough productive of 1/4 cup of white sputum daily. He had smoked two packs of cigarettes per day for 35 years, but had cut back to one pack per day for the last two years (72 pack-years). During the week before his clinic visit he experienced increased dyspnea, increased cough productive of greenish yellow sputum, and persistent ankle edema, but denied hemoptysis, fever, chills, or night sweats. The patient's heart rate was 100/minute, respiratory rate 24/minute, blood pressure 105/80, and temperature 36.5°C (axillary). The neck veins were distended while the patient was lying at a 45-degree angle. There were diffuse bilateral rales and rhonchi, and slight end-expiratory wheezing. There was a faint fourth heart sound. The liver edge was palpable two fingerbreadths below the costal margin, and there was 2+ pretibial edema. Room air arterial blood gases showed a pH of 7.34, Pco_2 of 45 mm Hg, and Po_2 of 48 mm Hg. The chest radiography showed an increased anteroposterior diameter and retrosternal space. The heart size was slightly increased from previous films; there were no infiltrates or effusions. The ECG showed sinus tachycardia and tall P waves, the hematocrit was 56%, and the white blood cell count was 8.5×10^3/mm^3.

The patient improved after hospitalization and treatment with low-flow oxygen, bronchodilators, and antibiotics. A predischarge spirogram showed evidence of moderately severe airways obstruction consistent with the diagnosis of chronic bronchitis and emphysema.

Discussion. The patient's history of 72 pack-years of smoking and daily cough and sputum production indicate chronic bronchitis. The chest radiograph suggests elements of emphysema. The recent change in sputum is consistent with an exacerbation of bronchitis with worsening hypoxemia and pulmonary hypertension, leading to cor pulmonale (indicated by increased heart size, high venous pressure, and ankle edema). Pneumonia was not present (no change on the chest x-ray, normal white blood counts, no fever or chills). Hypoxemia was probably present for some period of time, as indicated by the increased hematocrit. The response to therapy is typical of patients with chronic bronchitis.

Bibliography

National Asthma Education Program: Guidelines for the Diagnosis and Management of Asthma. Bethesda: N.I.H., 1991 (DHMS publication No. (NIH) 91-3042). *An N.I.H. monograph sent to all physicians to alert them to the need for better diagnostic acumen and more aggressive corticosteroid therapy in asthma.*

Snider GL. State of the art: Emphysema: The first two centuries — and beyond; a historical overview, with suggestions for future research: Parts 1 & 2. *Am Rev Respir Rev* 146:1334–1344, 1615–1622, 1992. *A serious review of the pathology, epidemiology, and etiology of emphysema by a single author who has spent over 45 years in the field.*

Stoller JK and Wiedemann HP. Chronic obstructive lung diseases: Asthma, emphysema, chronic bronchitis, bronchiectasis, and related conditions. In George RB, Light RW, Matthay MA, et al. (eds.). *Chest Medicine.* Baltimore: Williams and Wilkins, 1990, pp. 161–204. *A thorough review of the basic chest diseases with emphasis on diagnostic problems and clinical impact.*

Thurlbeck WM. Pathophysiology of chronic obstructive pulmonary disease. *Clin Chest Med* 11:389–403, 1990.

The premier lung pathologist's views on the changes found in COPD.

Weinberger SE. Medical progress: Recent advances in pulmonary medicine (Part I). *N Engl J Med* 328:1389–1397, 1993. *An excellent review of the new clinical technologies used in chest diseases (high resolution CT,* pulse oximetry) and recent genetic advances, including 124 references.

Wenzel SE. Asthma as an inflammatory disease. *Sem Respir Crit Care Med* 15:106–116, 1994. *An excellent synthesis of the current understanding of the complex mechanisms involved in inflammation, including 92 references.*

47 Interstitial Lung Disease

Martin H. Welch

Objectives

After completing this chapter, you should be able to

Recognize the anatomic location of the interstitium in relation to the airways, alveoli, and vascular networks of the lung

Be familiar with the common features of pathogenesis of interstitial lung diseases subsequent to an injurious event

Describe characteristic pathologic features of common interstitial lung diseases

Describe the alterations in lung mechanics, respiratory gas exchange, and hemodynamics which characterize this group of diseases

Summarize characteristic clinical features which lead to recognition of interstitial lung disease

List the commonest diseases which affect the interstitium of the lung and those which are most important because of treatability

Outline a diagnostic approach to interstitial lung disease using common modalities with appropriate attention to cost-benefit relationships

List treatment approaches appropriate to the most common and most treatable interstitial lung diseases

There are a large number of diseases that affect the interstitium of the lung, causing a characteristic clinical syndrome. The lungs become shrunken and stiff, and oxygen uptake is impaired. The hypoxemia which results is worsened by exercise, but readily corrected by oxygen administration. Airflow is generally well preserved, and breathing is rapid and shallow. Carbon dioxide retention is usually not a problem except late in the course of disease. Pulmonary vascular resistance is increased and cardiac output is limited. This chapter will describe (1) the anatomic location of the interstitium, (2) some of the diseases that affect it, and (3) the pathogenesis and pathology of these diseases. Further, it will show how these pathologic changes affect the normal physiology of the lung and how, in turn, an appreciation of the pathophysiology contributes to an understanding of the clinical manifestations and management of interstitial lung disease.

Anatomic Location of the Interstitium of the Lung

The pulmonary interstitium is the connective tissue framework of the lung that surrounds blood vessels, alveoli, and the bronchial tree. It is present between the alveolar epithelium and capillary endothelium (Fig. 47-1), as well as surrounding the airways and vessels in the non-gas-exchanging portions of the lung (Fig. 47-2). Alternatively, the term *interstitium* refers to the potential space occupied by the connective tissue framework. It should be noted that many diffuse parenchymal lung diseases affect the alveolar epithelium and airspace as well as the interstitium, and to reflect this British physicians favor the terms *alveolitis* and *fibrosing alveolitis* over *interstitial lung disease* and *interstitial pulmonary fibrosis*.

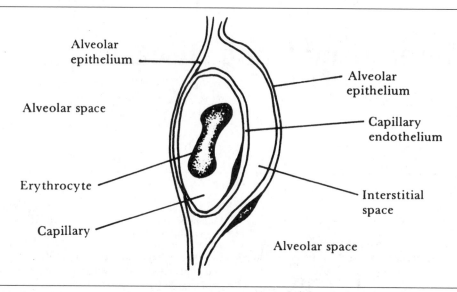

Fig. 47-1. The interstitial space, including capillary in cross-section with bordering alveoli. (From Kaufman CE and Papper S (eds.). *Review of Pathophysiology*. Boston: Little, Brown, 1983, p. 435.)

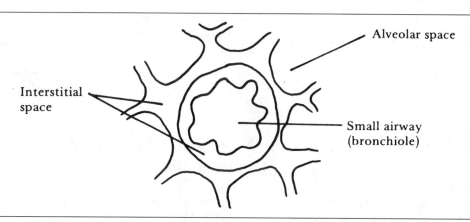

Fig. 47-2. The interstitial space, including a bronchiole and alveoli in cross-section. (From: Kaufman CE and Papper S (eds.). *Review of Pathophysiology*. Boston: Little, Brown, 1983, p. 435.)

Diseases Affecting the Interstitium

There are over 130 diseases that may affect the interstitial space (Table 47-1). Some, such as occupational diseases, have known etiologies (Table 47-1, bottom). This may have therapeutic implications; for example, stopping the occupational exposure may stop the disease process. Involvement of the interstitium of the lung may also be secondary to disease in other organ systems. For example, heart disease can lead to chronic pulmonary edema with involvement of the pulmonary interstitium.

Overall, the etiology can be determined in around 30%

Table 47-1. Interstitial Lung Disease

DISEASES WITH UNKNOWN ETIOLOGIES	DISEASES WITH KNOWN ETIOLOGIES
Idiopathic pulmonary fibrosis (IPF)	Occupational lung diseases
Diffuse interstitial fibrosis	Hypersensitivity alveolitis
Fibrosing alveolitis	Drug- and poison-induced lung diseases
Hamman-Rich syndrome (obsolete)	Radiation pneumonitis
Desquamative interstitial pneumonia (DIP)	Viral, parasitic, bacterial, mycobacterial, and fungal infections
(for the acute, reversible phase)	Chronic pulmonary edema
Usual interstitial pneumonia (UIP) (for the late,	Uremic pneumonitis
less reversible phase)	Lymphangitic carcinomatosis
Collagen vascular disease	
Sarcoidosis	
Vasculitides	
Lymphocytic infiltrative diseases	
Diffuse alveolar hemorrhage	
Eosinophilic granuloma	
Pulmonary veno-occlusive disease	
Lymphangioleiomyomatosis	
Diffuse amyloidosis	
Pulmonary alveolar proteinosis	

of patients presenting with interstitial disease. The rest will have interstitial involvement related to diseases of unknown etiology. The most frequent of these are idiopathic pulmonary fibrosis (sometimes called diffuse interstitial fibrosis, or fibrosing alveolitis), pulmonary fibrosis associated with collagen-vascular disorders, and sarcoidosis.

Pathogenesis of Interstitial Lung Disease

The remarkable thing about all these different diseases is that the interstitial involvement tends to be relatively similar, whatever the cause of the initial stimulus. Injury occurs initially to type I alveolar epithelial cells or to capillary endothelium, leading to edema and hemorrhage. Fibrin is deposited along alveolar walls, and is referred to as hyaline membrane. An inflammatory phase follows, with infiltration with neutrophils and subsequently macrophages and lymphocytes. The interactions among these inflammatory cells, mediated by humoral substances known as cytokines, appear to influence the subsequent intensity and duration of the disease process and the fibrosis and repair processes which follow. The details of these interactions are currently the subject of active investigation.

As the inflammatory process subsides, proliferation of type II alveolar cells and organization of the fibrinous exudate occur. Collagen is deposited, resulting in distortion of lung architecture and enlargement of alveolar air spaces follows. The degree to which reparative processes occur with restoration of gas exchange function, or fibrosis with irreparable loss of function, is variable. A goal of current research is to identify mediators and modulators of fibroblast proliferation so that new treatment approaches might be designed.

Although this process is initiated by an injurious agent, there is considerable evidence that the subsequent inflammatory process does much to promote lung damage. Therefore, present-day treatment approaches utilize antiinflammatory agents such as corticosteroids in attempts to arrest the process during the potentially reversible inflammatory or cellular stage. Unfortunately, this early stage of disease is often not apparent clinically, possibly because the acute process involves only a small portion of lung tissue at any one time and evolves slowly over months to years. Thus many patients present to a physician after the fibrotic process and distortion of lung architecture are well established, and response to therapy at this stage is quite poor. It is possible to characterize the cellular component of the disease process by a diagnostic technique called bronchoalveolar lavage, but clinical experience has shown that the ability to identify a reversible stage by this technique is imperfect.

Pathology of Interstitial Lung Disease

In normal lung, the alveolar septa are very thin and contain few cells. The cellular phase in the development of an interstitial lung disease is characterized by infiltration of these alveolar septa. This tends to destroy the capillaries in the alveolar septa early in the disease process. In addition, the interstitium surrounding the small airways may be involved by this cellular infiltrate. Thus the small airways can be occluded or partially occluded early in the development of this disease. If left unchecked, fibrosis and disorganization develop, with the almost complete destruction of the normal structures of the lung (end-stage fibrosis).

These pathologic changes are often reflected in the chest x-ray. Early in interstitial lung disease when there is histologic interstitial infiltrate, the chest x-ray may be completely normal. Computerized axial tomography (CAT scanning) is being utilized increasingly to detect interstitial disease in this early stage as well as aid in differential diagnosis by characterizing patterns of distribution of disease. As the disease progresses, more tissue and less air are present in the lung and a reticular, reticulonodular, or sometimes a nodular pattern develops. All these different patterns are seen in interstitial lung disease. End-stage fibrosis is often referred to as honeycomb lung; on the chest x-ray small cystic spaces that resemble a honeycomb are seen.

In summary, in interstitial lung disease there is obliteration of normal structure, especially the alveoli and capillaries, and marked alteration of the organization and components of the interstitium. There is destruction of normal alveoli, as well as infiltration of the interstitium of the airways and the alveolar capillary membranes.

Functional Consequences of Interstitial Lung Disease

Alterations in Lung Mechanics

Compliance Changes

These structural changes make the lung stiffer. For a relatively small change in the distending pressure of the normal lung, there is normally a large volume change. In interstitial disease, for the same change in pressure there is less change in volume: i.e., the lungs are less compliant. This is due to an alteration of the connective tissue present but is also due to destruction of the air-containing structures.

Changes in Lung Volumes

These pathologic changes will also affect the lung volumes. At functional residual capacity (FRC), the outward forces of the chest wall and the inward forces of the lung are in balance. In interstitial disease, a less compliant lung causes FRC to decrease. In attempting to take a deep breath to total lung capacity (TLC), one's inspiratory muscles will be unable to expand the lung as much as normal lung. Thus TLC is decreased. If one exhales down to residual volume (RV), the lung may contain a little less air than normal, due to both the decreased lung compliance and the fact that normal air-containing structures have been destroyed. Usually the decrease in TLC is more than the decrease in RV; thus the vital capacity (VC) is decreased in severe interstitial lung disease.

Maintenance of Expiratory Air Flow

One of the other hallmarks of interstitial lung disease is that expiratory air flow is well maintained despite the fact that lung volumes are decreased. Normally, most of the resistance to air flow is in the large airways. Radial tension by the normal lung tends to keep these airways open. In emphysema, the radial tension is decreased and the airways tend to collapse during exhalation. A person with interstitial lung disease is able to maintain air flow because the radial tension from the stiff (noncompliant) lungs tends to keep the airways open (Fig. 47-3).

Effects of these Changes on the Clinical Spirogram

Decreased lung volumes, with maintenance of flow, are evidenced in the restrictive pattern of spirometry seen in many people with interstitial lung disease. The vital capacity is often decreased; however, the percentage of air exhaled in 1 second (FEV_1/FVC) is normal (approximately 75% or greater).

Early in the course of interstitial lung disease spirometry may be normal. With progression of the disease the restrictive pattern often develops. It should be remembered that the restrictive pattern does not necessarily mean interstitial disease, since this pattern can also be caused by space-occupying lesions, pulmonary resection, pleural disease, chest-wall deformities, neuromuscular disease, and abdominal distention.

To summarize, the changes in lung mechanics are stiff lungs (decreased compliance) as well as decreased lung volumes and maintenance of airflow (FEV_1/FVC ratio is normal).

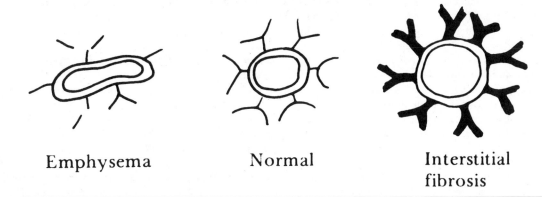

Emphysema   Normal   Interstitial
fibrosis

Fig. 47-3. Effect of radial tension of the lung on airway diameter in disease. (From: Interstitial Lung Disease. In Kaufman CE and Papper S (eds.). *Review of Pathophysiology*. Boston: Little, Brown, 1983, p. 437.)

Effects on Ventilation

How do these changes in lung mechanics affect the patient's ventilation? Total ventilation ($\dot{V}_E$), which is equal to breathing frequency (f) multiplied by tidal volume (V_T), is increased in patients with interstitial lung disease. Each tidal breath can be divided into a part that ventilates dead space (V_D), and does not participate in gas exchange, and the part that goes to the alveoli, where gas exchange occurs ($V_T - V_D$). V_D is increased in interstitial disease because of the mismatching of ventilation and perfusion. Thus for a given level of alveolar ventilation ($\dot{V}_A$), which is set by metabolic rate and arterial PCO_2 (see Chap. 45), $\dot{V}_E$ will be increased because of elevated V_D. The increase in $\dot{V}_E$ is accomplished by an increase in breathing frequency with a normal or slightly reduced V_T in patients with interstitial lung disease. Normal subjects and patients alike tend to choose a breathing pattern that minimizes the total amount of respiratory work, typically a respiratory rate of 10–15 breaths/minute and V_T of 450–500 ml in the absence of lung disease. Since the amount of elastic work is increased by stiff lungs in interstitial lung disease, respiratory work will be minimized by increasing breathing frequency (typically to a rate of 20–30 breaths/minute) rather than V_T. Despite the increase in wasted ventilation (f × V_D) at a more rapid respiratory rate, this pattern is preferred to deep slow breathing which would require stretching the stiff lungs and greatly increase the work of breathing. Similarly, during exercise patients with interstitial lung disease increase $\dot{V}_E$ by breathing faster with little change in V_T, in contrast to the normal subject who increases both f and V_T during exertion. Since V_D does not normally increase during exercise, the increased V_T makes breathing more efficient in a normal subject because a larger fraction of each breath participates in gas exchange. In contrast, efficiency does not improve during exercise in the interstitial lung disease patient because V_T and V_D remain about the same as resting values.

In summary, patients with interstitial lung disease have increased $\dot{V}_E$ and wasted ventilation and typically breathe with a faster frequency and normal or slightly reduced V_T compared to normal. The ventilatory pattern during exercise is abnormal with an increased breathing frequency but little change in V_T.

Gas Exchange in Interstitial Lung Disease

What are the effects on gas exchange (CO_2 elimination and oxygen uptake) and oxygenation of the arterial blood? Carbon dioxide elimination is not a problem in interstitial lung disease since this gas is readily diffusible and its excretion is ventilation-limited; oxygenation of the arterial blood does present a problem. Thickening of the alveolar interstitium, leading to a decrease in the rate at which oxygen can diffuse across this membrane into the blood, contributes little to hypoxemia at rest. With exercise, the blood has to go through the capillaries more rapidly, leaving less time for equilibrium with alveolar gas to occur. Thus, with exercise, diffusion limitation may make a small contribution to hypoxemia. Although a reduction in the diffusing capacity for carbon monoxide is one of the earliest and most consistent abnormalities in interstitial lung disease, this is explained by a reduced area of the alveolo-capillary membrane rather than a true "diffusion block." Shunting of pulmonary arterial blood into the systemic arterial blood may contribute to hypoxemia late in the disease; hypoxemia due to shunting does not correct with O_2 administration. The third and major cause of hypoxemia in interstitial disease is low ventilation/perfusion ($\dot{V}_A/\dot{Q}$) areas in which perfused portions of the lung are poorly ventilated, presumably due to patchy distribution of stiff, poorly compliant parenchyma and perhaps small airway obstruction from inflammatory and fibrotic infiltration. This has clinical significance, since hypoxemia due to low $\dot{V}_A/\dot{Q}$ areas responds to a small increase in inspired oxygen (low-flow oxygen).

In summary, low $\dot{V}_A/\dot{Q}$ areas are the number one cause of hypoxemia in people with interstitial lung disease. Shunt may be a late problem, and diffusion limitation makes a small contribution to hypoxemia during exercise. CO_2 elimination is not a problem except preterminally, when CO_2 retention may occur.

Hemodynamic Changes in Interstitial Lung Disease

Oxygenated blood must be delivered to the periphery. O_2 delivery is equal to cardiac output times O_2 content of blood. O_2 delivery may be low in interstitial disease because of decreased O_2 content; and in addition, cardiac output is limited by destruction of the pulmonary vascular bed with an increase in pulmonary vascular resistance. Early involvement of the capillaries decreases the cross-sectional area of the vascular bed. As a normal person exercises, the pulmonary artery pressure increases little. In severe interstitial lung disease, the restricted capillary bed leads to marked increase in the pressure in the pulmonary artery during exercise as the cardiac output increases. Due to this afterload, the right side of the heart is unable to attain a normal increase in cardiac output in response to exercise (Fig. 47-4).

Fig. 47-4. Effect of interstitial lung disease on pulmonary artery pressure in response to exercise. (From: Kaufman CE and Papper S (eds.). *Review of Pathophysiology*. Boston: Little, Brown, 1983, p. 439.)

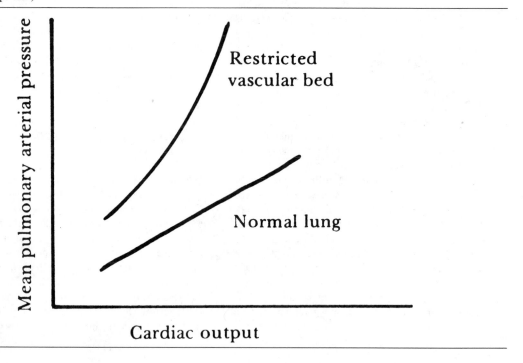

Thus destruction of the pulmonary vascular bed limits the cardiac output, limiting O_2 delivery.

Clinical Manifestations

Most patients with interstitial lung disease will complain of shortness of breath or dyspnea (Table 47-2). This symptom is primarily caused by increased work of breathing due to lung stiffness and wasted ventilation (hypoxemia contributes to dyspnea only when the PaO_2 is less than 60 mm Hg). In addition, patients quite commonly have a dry (nonproductive) cough due to stimulation of the irritant receptors that lie just under the bronchial epithelium in the large airways. The inflammation in the interstitium and traction due to abnormal mechanics of the lung can stimulate these receptors. Later in the disease, patients develop impaired clearance of bronchial secretions, leading to chronic bronchitis. Pneumonia is a common problem late in the course of this disease and is a frequent cause of death. Tachypnea is the most frequent clinical sign; the patient minimizes respiratory work by shallow, rapid breathing. In addition, crackles in the dependent portion of the lung are probably related to the involvement of the small airways by the interstitial inflammation. Clubbing is often seen; cyanosis is not a particularly sensitive or specific indicator of arterial hypoxemia but it is frequently seen. The right heart is under increased strain, since it must pump against increased pulmonary vascular resistance. As a result, it tends toward hypertrophy. Often one can palpate a left parasternal heave, and hear an increase in the intensity of the second heart sound. These are signs of cor pulmonale (pulmonary heart disease), which is hypertrophy or dilatation of the right ventricle from pulmonary disease.

Arterial blood gases often show an increased alveolar-arterial PO_2 difference early in the disease process, even before there is a restrictive pattern by spirometry or x-ray changes. The $PaCO_2$ may be normal or low, but just before death it may increase. Patients with interstitial disease generally do not have trouble eliminating CO_2; when given oxygen, they usually do not retain carbon dioxide readily. On the chest x-ray there is often an interstitial pattern.

Spirometry often reveals a restrictive pattern, that is, a decreased vital capacity with a normal or increased FEV_1/FVC ratio. Another of the earliest changes to occur in people with interstitial lung disease is a decrease in DLCO (diffusing capacity of the lung for carbon monoxide). This is a commonly used clinical test that is helpful in following these patients. The DLCO may be decreased in a wide variety of diseases and is not specific at all for interstitial lung disease. Why would interstitial lung disease affect this test? First, there is destruction of the capillaries of the lung, which decreases the surface area over which carbon monoxide can be taken up. Second, there is a decrease in the capillary blood volume in the lung, which would also decrease the amount of carbon monoxide that can be taken up into the red cells during the test.

Clinical Approach to Differential Diagnosis

When a patient presents with characteristic clinical, radiographic, and pathophysiologic findings of interstitial lung disease, an attempt to determine etiology is usually indicated. An exception might be the occasional patient in whom the disease can be determined to be of long duration and stable. In such a patient, the cause may be indeterminate, even with lung biopsy which will show nonspecific fibrotic changes, and treatment may be unnecessary or ineffective.

When progression is suggested by the clinical evaluation, treatment may be essential, and choice of therapy

Table 47-2. Clinical and Laboratory Manifestations of Interstitial Lung Disease

---

CLINICAL MANIFESTATIONS

Symptoms
    Dyspnea
    Cough
Signs
    Tachypnea
    Crackles
    Clubbing
    Cyanosis
    Cor pulmonale

LABORATORY DATA

Arterial blood gases
    Increased alveolar-arterial PO_2 difference (worse with exercise)
    Normal to low $PaCO_2$ (may increase late)
ECG — cor pulmonale
Chest x-ray — interstitial pattern
Spirometry — restrictive pattern
    Decreased vital capacity (VC)
    Normal FEV_1/FVC
Decreased DLCO (diffusing capacity of the lung for carbon monoxide)

Reprinted with permission from: Kaufman CE and Papper S (eds.). *Review of Pathophysiology.* Boston: Little, Brown, 1983, p. 439.

may be dependent upon etiology. Exposure to an injurious inhaled agent may be stopped, an infectious agent may be effectively treated with antibiotics, and steroids may be useful in halting or reversing lung injury in certain common diseases of uncertain etiology, especially in sarcoidosis and idiopathic pulmonary fibrosis.

Exposure to occupational and environmental inhalants can most often be determined readily from the clinical history. Workers in industries with heavy exposure to silica dust, asbestos particles, and welding fumes are generally well aware of the risks of their occupation. Farmer's lung as a prototype of hypersensitivity pneumonitis is well recognized as well, but there is a wide range of organic dusts which can produce a hypersensitivity response and in which the exposure may not be obvious. Heating and cooling systems, for instance, can be contaminated with microorganisms which can produce disease in predisposed individuals and the source of the injurious agent may not be readily apparent.

Infectious agents may occasionally be readily identified as the cause of interstitial lung disease when an acute febrile illness occurs within the framework of an epidemic, or with a characteristic rash, or in an immunocompromised host. Less often, fungal or mycobacterial agents produce a chronic illness with diffuse interstitial lung involvement. In either case, specific diagnosis is required to permit potentially curative antibiotic treatment, and avert use of an immunosuppressive agent which, when used alone, may accelerate the course of infectious disease.

Among the diseases of unknown etiology, sarcoidosis is one of the most common, which may present with interstitial infiltration of the lung. It is a multi-system granulomatous disease, and the pattern of organ system involvement may be so characteristic as to strongly suggest the diagnosis prior to confirmatory biopsy. It is especially common in the American black population, and often presents in young adults who may be relatively asymptomatic. It involves lymph nodes, salivary glands, and liver and may cause anterior or posterior uveitis. Association with erythema nodosum is characteristic when it occurs. Increase in calcium absorption may cause hypercalciuria or hypercalcemia. Indeed, any organ system may be involved with granulomatous inflammation in this disorder, and the clinical presentation may be confusing. But when a young, black adult presents with infiltrative lung disease and hilar adenopathy, with or without symptoms in other organ systems, sarcoidosis should come quickly to mind as a likely diagnosis. Biopsy evidence of granulomatous inflammation is usually sought, and infectious granulomatous disorders should be excluded. Some clinical presentations of sarcoidosis have a rate of spontaneous resolution so high that treatment is unnecessary, but progressive respiratory function deterioration or cardiac, ocular, or central nervous system involvement usually require corticosteroid treatment and often respond well.

Another common disorder involving the interstitium of the lung is idiopathic pulmonary fibrosis (IPF). This diagnosis is to some extent one of exclusion. Recognized causes of lung injury must be considered and discarded, involvement of other organ systems shown to be absent, and (perhaps most important) infectious agents sought and excluded. Lung biopsy should usually be performed, and a large specimen is useful not only to aid in excluding other diseases, but to help in predicting response to therapy by quantitating early, reversible inflammatory changes and chronic irreversible fibrosis. Histologic findings are rather nonspecific and must be interpreted in light of other clinical findings.

Terminology applied to IPF has varied over the years and from one region or country to another. The term diffuse "interstitial fibrosis" (DIF) is commonly applied in the United States. In Great Britain, "fibrosing alveolitis" is preferred. Influential American pathologist Averill Liebow constructed a system of terminology for interstitial pneumonias which included "desquamative interstitial pneumonia" (DIP) and "usual interstitial pneumonia" (UIP), which he considered to be distinct and separate entities. Currently, it is widely considered that DIP is an early, reversible stage and UIP a later, less treatment-responsive stage of idiopathic pulmonary fibrosis.

IPF often progresses over months to years to cause crippling and death. Corticosteroids are sometimes helpful, and can prolong life in patients who respond to them. Cyclophosphamide may be helpful in a subgroup of steroid-resistant patients.

Collagen vascular diseases, including rheumatoid arthritis and progressive systemic sclerosis, may produce a lung disease indistinguishable from IPF except by association. Treatment is similar as well.

Diagnostic Modalities

Serologic Tests

A variety of diagnostic tests may be helpful in selected patients, depending upon the etiology suspected from the clinical presentation. Antinuclear antigen determination may be indicated if collagen vascular disease is a possibility. Serum angiotensin-converting enzyme has some usefulness in sarcoidosis, and serum precipitins against a battery of antigens may be helpful in possible hypersensitivity alveolitis. Radiographic techniques and lung biopsy methods have application in most patients with interstitial lung disease, and warrant some general comments.

Radiographic Techniques

A conventional posteroanterior and lateral chest radiograph is a basic part of the initial evaluation, and may serve only to identify the presence of an interstitial infiltrate. Serial films may retrospectively or prospectively help to define stability or progression. Associated bilateral hilar adenopathy may point toward sarcoidosis, or less often toward neoplastic or infectious disease. Pleural involvement might suggest asbestosis, collagen vascular disease, or rarely

(in a woman of childbearing age) lymphangioleiomyomatosis. Occasionally, a normal radiograph is seen in a patient with symptoms and pulmonary function abnormalities of interstitial disease. Computerized axial tomography has increased sensitivity for visualizing interstitial infiltrates in such patients, especially with thin-section, high-resolution techniques (Fig. 47-5). Increasingly, CAT scanning is being utilized in attempts to identify patterns of distribution of disease which are characteristic of various etiologies.

Cytologic Studies and Tissue Biopsy

Microscopic examination of cells or tissue specimens is often necessary to establish a specific diagnosis and guide

Fig. 47-5. CAT scan of chest showing diffuse interstitial fibrosis which is most prominent in the left lung. (Scan provided courtesy of Tom Johnson, M.D.)

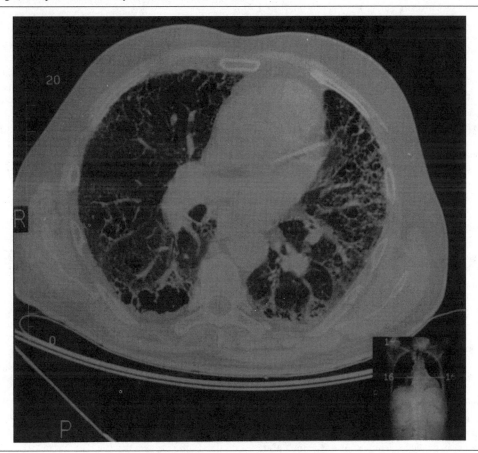

therapy. Techniques for obtaining specimens include bronchoalveolar lavage (BAL), transbronchial biopsy, and "open" (surgical) biopsy of the lung. BAL is carried out by instillation of saline into the lung through a fiberoptic bronchoscope, recovery of the lavage fluid and study of the cells washed out of the alveoli. A specific diagnosis is seldom made by this procedure, but different etiologies may be suggested by the observation of a predominately lymphocytic, granulocytic, or eosinophilic cell population. Transbronchial lung biopsy is carried out by passage of a small forceps via the fiberoptic bronchoscope, through the progressively smaller branches of the tracheobronchial tree to the periphery of the lung. Biopsies of lung parenchyma are obtained, usually under fluoroscopic guidance. The samples obtained are small and sampling error is a problem, but risks of the procedure are less than those of the more definitive surgical biopsy, which requires a thoracotomy. Small specimens are more likely to be adequate for diagnosis in the case of sarcoidosis, infectious diseases, and diffuse spread of carcinoma than in interstitial pneumonitis and fibrosis. Recently, the risks and morbidity associated with surgical biopsy have been reduced by development of video-assisted thoracoscopic techniques, so that large specimens can be obtained with small incisions. These techniques still require the use of operating rooms and general anesthetics, however.

Treatment Considerations

Treatment measures may include antibiotics in specific infectious diseases, avoidance of injurious inhaled agents in occupational diseases, and corticosteroids and other immunosuppressive agents in sarcoidosis and interstitial fibrosis.

Since low $\dot{V}_A/\dot{Q}$ is the major cause of hypoxemia and tends to respond to low-flow oxygen, one can often help the patient's symptoms and perhaps increase exercise tolerance by giving oxygen therapy. There is usually little danger of retaining carbon dioxide and developing CO_2 narcosis in response to oxygen (except in far advanced, preterminal stages of the disorder).

Clinical Examples

1. A 45-year-old man with idiopathic pulmonary fibrosis complained of progressive dyspnea on exertion over the past 6 months. He had a nonproductive chronic cough. Respiratory rate was 35 breaths/minute. His nails were clubbed, but not cyanotic. Chest examination revealed fine crackles, greater in the dependent portion of the lung. Cardiac examination revealed a parasternal heave and an increased intensity of P2. He had jugular venous distention.

Chest x-ray showed he had small lungs with increased interstitial markings. Spirogram results were FVC 2.8 liters (55% of predicted), FEV_1 2.1 liters (60% of predicted), and FEV_1/FVC 75% (normal). Arterial blood gases:

	Room air	Nasal O_2
PaO_2	45	60
$PaCO_2$	30	30
pH	7.43	7.44

Discussion. The patient had the typical restrictive pattern of spirometry seen in interstitial pulmonary disease with decreased FVC and FEV_1, but a normal FEV_1/FVC ratio, indicating that there was no obstruction to airflow.

On physical examination the patient had evidence of cor pulmonale with right ventricular heart failure. The increased pulmonary vascular resistance leads to pulmonary hypertension (increased P2), which contributes to hypertrophy of the right ventricle (parasternal heave). Eventually the systemic venous pressure increases as the right ventricle fails (jugular venous distention). Note also that cyanosis is not a reliable indicator of hypoxemia.

The patient's hypoxemia responds to low-flow oxygen, since most of the hypoxemia is due to ventilation-perfusion mismatching. Chronic oxygen therapy may improve the patient's dyspnea on exertion by increasing the O_2 content of the arterial blood and the cor pulmonale by partially reversing the hypoxic component of the increased pulmonary vascular resistance.

2. A 54-year-old white female secretary presented with arthralgias, uveitis, and Bell's palsy. Laboratory studies showed hypercalcemia and an elevated serum angiotensin-converting enzyme (SACE) level. Chest radiograph (Fig. 47-6) showed bilateral hilar adenopathy and a subtle reticulonodular infiltrate. Transbronchial biopsy was complicated by a small, transient pneumothorax, but was supportive of the diagnosis of sarcoidosis, showing noncaseating granulomas. Pulmonary function tests were normal.

Treatment with corticosteroids resolved her arthralgias, uveitis, and Bell's palsy, as well as clearing the radiographic abnormalities (Fig. 47-7).

Discussion. Clinical symptoms involving extrathoracic organs dominated the picture, and along with hilar adenopathy are characteristic of sarcoidosis. The charac-

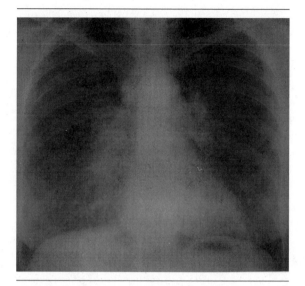

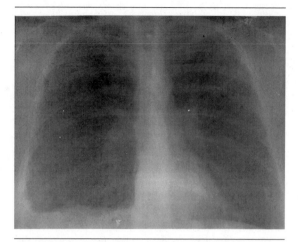

Fig. 47-8. Chest radiograph of 39-year-old white female with lymphangioleiomyomatosis, showing reticulonodular infiltrate and chronic pleural thickening.

Fig. 47-6. Chest radiograph of 54-year-old white female with sarcoidosis, showing bilateral hilar adenopathy and subtle reticulonodular infiltrate.

teristic functional abnormalities of interstitial lung disease are sometimes absent in sarcoidosis.

3. A 39-year-old white female smoker with asthma, COPD, and interstitial lung disease had a diagnosis of lymphangioleiomyomatosis (LAM) made by open lung biopsy. She had a history of recurrent pneumothorax, but not of chylothorax, which can complicate this disease.

Spirometry results were FVC 1.93 liters (58% of predicted), $FEV_{1.0}$ 0.76 liters (27% of predicted), and $FEV_{1.0}/FVC$ 39% (reduced). Chest radiograph showed a reticulonodular pattern with chronic pleural thickening (Fig. 47-8).

Her asthma and COPD showed some improvement with bronchodilators, but treatment of LAM with Provera produced little response.

Discussion.   Pleural thickening is rare in idiopathic pulmonary fibrosis, but may occur in LAM, asbestosis, and collagen vascular diseases. Open lung biopsy is usually necessary to confirm a diagnosis of LAM. Obstructive lung disease may coexist with interstitial lung disease and complicate the pulmonary function pattern.

Bibliography

Golden JA. Interstitial (diffuse parenchymal) lung disease: tissue diagnosis and therapy. In Baum GL and Wolinsky E (eds.). *Textbook of Pulmonary Diseases* (5th ed.). Boston/New York: Little, Brown, 1994, pp. 1067–96.

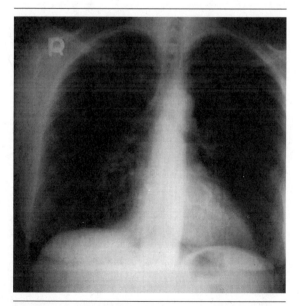

Fig. 47-7. Chest radiograph of 54-year-old white female with sarcoidosis after steroid treatment, showing clearing of hilar adenopathy and reticulonodular infiltrate seen in Fig. 47-6.

Summarizes invasive approaches to specific histologic diagnosis, relative merits, and significance of diagnosis in planning therapy. Other chapters in this textbook deal with etiology and physiology and with individual diseases.

Jackson LK and Fulmer JD. Structural-functional features of the interstitial lung diseases. In Fishman AP (ed.). *Pulmonary Diseases and Disorders* (2nd ed.). New York: McGraw-Hill, 1988. *Review of pathophysiology and pathology of this group of diseases. Other chapters in this textbook deal with individual disease entities.*

Schwarz MI and King TE Jr (eds.). *Interstitial Lung Disease.* (2nd ed.). St. Louis: Mosby, 1993. *Comprehensive coverage of pathology, pathogenesis, pathophysiology, and clinical aspects.*

Schwarz MI, King TE, and Cherniack RM. General principals and diagnostic approach to the interstitial lung diseases. In Murray JF and Nadel JA (eds.). *Textbook of Respiratory Medicine.* Philadelphia: Saunders, 1994, pp. 1803–1826. *Excellent clinically oriented summary of the initial approach to the patient with interstitial lung disease. Other chapters in this textbook deal in detail with features of individual diseases causing interstitial lung disease.*

48 Pulmonary Edema

Barry A. Gray

Objectives

After completing this chapter, you should be able to

Characterize the forces governing lung water balance

Characterize the membrane factors

Describe the effects of pulmonary edema on lung function

Distinguish between pulmonary edema due to increased filtration forces and edema due to altered permeability

Characterize the physiologic basis for treatment to (a) reduce pulmonary capillary pressure and (b) increase plasma protein osmotic pressure

---

We are born with fluid-filled lungs and, if we live long enough, we will likely die with fluid-filled lungs. Pulmonary edema occurs with left ventricular failure, mitral valve dysfunction, intravascular volume overload, and various forms of lung injury. This chapter will examine the pathophysiology of pulmonary edema and the physiologic mechanisms which keep the lungs dry.

Pulmonary edema can result from alterations either in the balance of forces which govern fluid filtration or in the permeability characteristics of the membranes which restrict fluid movement. The factors involved are listed in Table 48-1.

The Starling equation is useful for understanding the relationships between these factors as they relate to water balance in any tissue, including the lung:

$$F = K_F\left[\left(P_{CAP} - P_{ISF}\right) - \sigma\left(\pi_{CAP} - \pi_{ISF}\right)\right]$$

The equation states that there will be filtration out of the capillary whenever the difference between P_{CAP} and P_{ISF} is greater than the difference between π_{CAP} and π_{ISF} multiplied by σ. σ is the protein osmotic reflection coefficient of the endothelium, a function of endothelial permeability to protein (equal to 1 if the endothelium is perfectly semipermeable — i.e., impermeable to protein molecules — and 0 if the endothelium exerts no restraint on the diffusion of proteins in relation to H_2O). In other words the effectiveness of the oncotic pressure gradient, $\pi_{CAP} - \pi_{ISF}$ depends on the permeability to protein. When there is an unbalanced gradient for filtration the rate of fluid filtration from the capillary, F, depends on K_F, the filtration coefficient, which is equal to surface area A multiplied by the hydraulic conductivity Lp.

Classification of Pulmonary Edema

Pulmonary edema is generally classified according to the mechanism which produces the increase in fluid flux

Table 48-1. Factors Determining Lung Fluid Balance

INTRAVASCULAR FORCES

Capillary hydrostatic pressure, P_{CAP}
Plasma oncotic pressure, π_{CAP}

EXTRAVASCULAR FORCES

Interstitial fluid pressure, P_{ISF}
Interstitial fluid oncotic pressure, π_{ISF}

VASCULAR PERMEABILITY

To water — hydraulic filtration coefficient, $K_F = A \times Lp$
To proteins — osmotic reflection coefficient, σ

across the vascular endothelium. Thus the terms **high pressure, hydrostatic,** and **cardiogenic** pulmonary edema refer to conditions associated with elevated P_{CAP}, while the terms **low pressure, high permeability,** and **noncardiogenic** pulmonary edema refer to conditions in which K_F is elevated and σ is reduced.

Two aspects of the Starling equation deserve attention. First, if the hydraulic conductivity of the membrane is increased, fluid filtration will be more sensitive to small changes in the hydrostatic pressure gradient, ($P_{CAP} - P_{ISF}$). Second, as the membrane becomes more permeable to protein (σ approaches 0), the entire oncotic portion of the equation approaches zero and the hydrostatic pressure gradient assumes major importance. Thus the Starling relationship suggests that the distinction between high-pressure pulmonary edema and low-pressure pulmonary edema may not necessarily decide appropriate therapy. Whether the mechanism of pulmonary edema is increased pressure or increased permeability, the principle vehicle for therapeutic intervention might be a reduction in P_{CAP}.

Starling Forces

In clinical practice it is possible to estimate the intravascular Starling forces, P_{CAP} and π_{CAP}, but not the interstitial forces, P_{ISF} or π_{ISF}. The values for P_{ISF} and π_{ISF} can only be surmised from observations in experimental animals. Under normal conditions, when P_{CAP} is 10 mm Hg, π_{CAP} is 24 mm Hg and σ is close to one (0.9), the balance of intravascular forces should promote fluid absorption from the interstitial space, but this is not what is observed. Instead there is a continuous flow of lymph from the lung, indicating continuous filtration. The importance of the interstitial forces is demonstrated by the fact that the balance of intravascular and interstitial forces in fact favors filtration of fluid from the capillary into the interstitial space, where it is picked up and removed by the lymphatics. An accurate description of the intravascular and the interstitial forces is critical to an understanding of lung water homeostasis.

Capillary Hydrostatic Pressure

P_{CAP} is estimated from measurements of pulmonary artery pressure (P_{PA}) and left atrial pressure (P_{LA}) or pulmonary capillary wedge pressure (P_{PCW}). It must be emphasized that P_{CAP} is not equal to P_{PCW}, which is really just a means

to measure P_{LA} using right heart catheterization. P_{CAP} depends on the distribution of vascular resistance in the pulmonary circulation (Fig. 48-1).

Normally 60% of the resistance is upstream, between the pulmonary artery and capillary, and 40% is downstream, between the capillary and left atrium. Thus

$$P_{CAP} = P_{PCW} + 0.4 \left(P_{PA} - P_{PCW} \right)$$

Observations in patients and experimental animals indicate that the fraction of resistance located downstream is not always 40%, but can vary from 20% to 70% with some forms of lung disease and/or therapeutic intervention. This could be important when there are large elevations in P_{PA}, since P_{CAP} may be elevated even though P_{LA} or P_{PCW} is normal.

Capillary Oncotic Pressure

π_{CAP} can be estimated from measurement of plasma protein concentration (C);

$$\pi_{CAP} = 2.1C + 0.16C^2 + 0.009C^3$$

which evaluates to 24.50 mm Hg when total plasma protein is 6.8 g/dl. A pressure-measuring device with two chambers separated by a semipermeable membrane, known as an oncometer, can also be used to estimate π_{CAP}.

Fig. 48-1. Pulmonary capillary pressure (Pcap) is determined by pulmonary artery pressure (Ppa), left atrial pressure (P_{LA}) or pulmonary capillary wedge pressure (Ppcw) and the distribution of vascular resistances, between the arterial (Ra) and venous (Rv) sides of the pulmonary circulation.

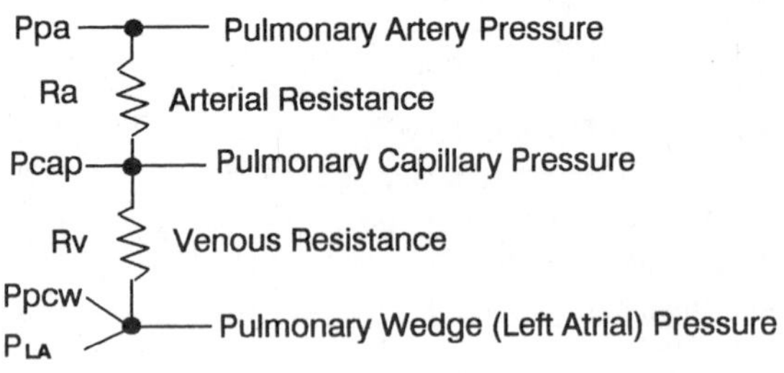

$$Pcap = Ppcw + \frac{Rv}{Ra + Rv} \times (Ppa - Ppcw)$$

Interstitial Fluid Pressure

There are three components to interstitial pressure in any tissue: total pressure, solid pressure, and fluid pressure;

total pressure = fluid pressure + solid pressure

P_{ISF} in the Starling equation refers only to the fluid component. Normally total pressure is close to zero and fluid pressure is negative. In a totally edematous tissue, fluid separates all the solid elements so that there is no solid-solid contact. Under this condition, solid pressure is zero, and total tissue pressure is equal to fluid pressure. As interstitial fluid is reabsorbed into the capillary, solid structures are pulled together to fill the space previously occupied by fluid. This removal of fluid and compaction of solids generates a positive solid tissue pressure. When solid tissue pressure is greater than total tissue pressure, fluid pressure becomes negative. This resists further resorption of tissue fluid into the capillary. The resulting pressure-volume curve (Fig. 48-2) is an important factor in lung water balance.

Normally P_{ISF} is negative and lies on the steep part of the curve where the accumulation of a small amount of fluid causes a relatively large increase in pressure (point A in Fig. 48-2). Thus with a modest increase in P_{CAP} only a small accumulation of fluid in the interstitial space will raise P_{ISF} steeply and restore the balance of forces governing fluid filtration. The limit to this homeostatic mechanism is reached when P_{ISF} reaches the flatter part of the curve where large volumes of fluid may accumulate with little further increase in pressure. This corresponds to the point at which solid-solid interaction is eliminated and P_{ISF} is equal to total pressure (point B in Fig. 48-2).

Pulmonary interstitial fluid pressure could be a central issue for respiratory therapy aimed at the treatment of pulmonary edema if increased airway pressure produced increased P_{ISF}. A great deal of research has been applied to this problem which has clarified the complexity of interstitial mechanics in the lung. As a result it is now known that increased airway pressure does not increase P_{ISF} nor does it reduce lung water accumulation. Any beneficial effect of increased airway pressure in pulmonary edema appears to be the result of increased lung volume and reversal of atelectasis.

Interstitial Fluid Oncotic Pressure

Measurement of protein in samples of pulmonary lymph indicate that π_{ISF} is about 75% of π_{CAP}. With an increase in

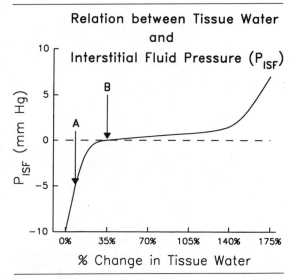

Fig. 48-2. Pressure-volume curve of the interstitial space. Normally P_{ISF} is negative and located on the steep phase of the curve (point A). With an increase in interstitial water P_{ISF} rises steeply until solid tissue pressure is zero (point B). At this point, with a 35% increase in water volume, fluid is confined to the interstitial space. Above this point, when P_{ISF} exceeds zero, alveolar flooding begins. Thereafter large increases in volume are accommodated with little change in P_{ISF} until the tissue volume approaches the maximum volume of the limiting structures. (Drawn to summarize the work of Guyton AC. *Circulation Res* 16:452, 1965.)

capillary pressure filtration and lymph flow increase and, at the same time, lymph protein concentration falls as the plasma ultrafiltrate appearing in the pulmonary interstitial space dilutes the existing protein (Fig. 48-3).

This **"washdown"** of interstitial protein decreases π_{ISF} and decreases the balance of forces favoring edema formation. In other words, there is a negative-feedback mechanism involving interstitial oncotic pressure, which tends to retard the rate of fluid filtration in edematous states. Notice that the decrease in π_{ISF} is approximately equal to 50% of the increase in P_{CAP}, so this mechanism is only a partial compensation for increases in P_{CAP}. This homeostatic mechanism operates only if endothelial permeability is normal and water is filtered faster than protein. When edema is caused by an increase in capillary permeability, as σ approaches zero the filtrate protein concentration approaches plasma protein concentration.

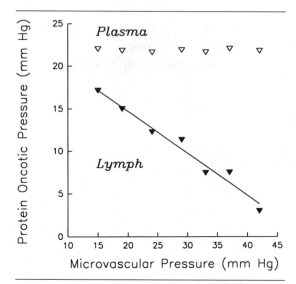

Fig. 48-3. Protein oncotic pressure in plasma and lung lymph from a sheep with a chronic lymph fistula and a balloon in the left atrium. Microvascular pressure has been calculated from pressures in the left atrium (P_{LA}) and pulmonary artery (P_{PA}) as $0.6P_{LA} + 0.4 P_{PA}$. With various elevations of P_{LA} produced by inflation of the left atrial balloon there is an increase in lymph flow and a decrease in lymph oncotic pressure. Assuming that $\pi_{Lymph} = \pi_{ISF}$, this interstitial protein washdown phenomenon would increase $\pi_{Plasma} - \pi_{ISF}$ and offset the increase in P_{CAP}. Estimates from several laboratories indicate that the increase in the $\pi_{Plasma} - \pi_{ISF}$ is equal to 50% of the increase in P_{CAP}. (Redrawn from: Erdmann AJ III, et al. Effect of increased vascular pressure on lung fluid balance in unanesthetized sheep. *Circulation Res* 37:271–284, 1975. Reproduced with permission. Circulation Research. Copyright 1975 American Heart Association.)

Lymphatic Drainage

Lymphatic drainage also plays an important role in protecting the lung from pulmonary edema. Animal studies have shown that (a) lymph flow is always present in the normal lung, (b) it is facilitated by respiratory movements, (c) lymphatic pumps can generate pressure gradients of at least 20 cm H_2O, (d) an acute increase in capillary filtration is accompanied by an increase in lymph flow, and (e) lymphatic hypertrophy occurs in states of chronic pulmonary vascular pressure elevation. This may be the explanation for the observation that patients with chronic

congestive heart failure may be relatively free of pulmonary edema at levels of left atrial pressure that would be expected to produce pulmonary edema in acute cardiac decompensation. There are three conditions in which alterations in lymphatic function promote the development of pulmonary edema. These include (a) immediately following lung transplantation, (b) radiation pneumonitis, and (c) right ventricular failure, in which increased right atrial pressure may impede the emptying of pulmonary lymphatics into the intrathoracic veins.

Vascular Permeability

This is an important determinant of pulmonary edema formation. An increase in vascular permeability can produce pulmonary edema at normal or reduced vascular pressures. The demonstration of continuous lymph flow indicates a balance of forces favoring fluid filtration in the lung under normal conditions, and any increase in the hydraulic filtration coefficient will cause increased filtration and pulmonary edema if the pumping capacity of the lymphatics is exceeded. Further, protein permeability usually increases at the same time, and the oncotic pressure of plasma proteins exerts little effect across the capillary endothelium.

Effects of Pulmonary Edema

The effect of pulmonary edema on lung function depends on whether the edema is cardiogenic or due to lung injury with increased vascular permeability. In the case of cardiogenic pulmonary edema there is also increased left atrial pressure and some of the physiologic alterations are the result of pulmonary vascular congestion.

Pulmonary Vascular Pressure and Volume

In cardiogenic pulmonary edema the increase in left atrial pressure is reflected passively in a retrograde direction to the pulmonary veins, capillaries, and arteries. This increase in pulmonary vascular pressure produces an increase in pulmonary blood volume. In permeability edema the passive increase in vascular volume is absent but the fundamental process of lung injury releases substances which may produce pulmonary vasoconstriction leading to increased pulmonary artery pressure despite normal left atrial pressure.

Pulmonary Blood Flow Redistribution

Cardiogenic pulmonary edema is associated with a redistribution of blood flow in the lung such that the lung bases, which normally receive the highest blood flow, experience a decrease in blood flow while the apices, which normally receive the least amount of flow, experience an increase in blood flow. For edema caused by increased permeability there are studies which indicate blood flow redistribution away from the most severely injured and edematous regions.

There are at least two areas in which perfusion redistribution in pulmonary edema may be relevant to clinical practice. First, perfusion redistribution in cardiogenic edema may be recognized on a perfusion lung scan if the injection of the radionuclide is made with the patient upright. It may also be detected in the upright chest film as distention of the upper lobe pulmonary vessels. In both cases cephalization of blood flow distribution provides a clue that left atrial pressure is elevated.

The second area in which perfusion redistribution becomes relevant is gas exchange. Perfusion of the pulmonary capillaries in an edema-filled alveolus has the effect of a right-to-left shunt since venous blood which is not exposed to alveolar air is admixed with oxygenated blood from nonedematous alveoli. If 50% of the alveoli are filled with edema fluid and these alveoli were perfused at the same rate as functioning alveoli the arterial blood PO_2 would be severely reduced just as it would be in the presence of a 50% shunt. On the other hand, perfusion redistribution limiting flow to the edematous alveoli to 30% of cardiac output would minimize the severity of arterial hypoxemia, making it equivalent to a 30% shunt. Vasodilator therapy for congestive heart failure, while improving cardiac function, usually increases the severity of hypoxemia by reversing pulmonary blood flow redistribution.

Lung Compliance

Interstitial edema produces a reduction in lung compliance which increases the elastic work the muscles must do to achieve a given tidal volume. In addition alveoli which are full of edema fluid do not participate in ventilation. Thus the remaining alveoli must each accommodate a larger fraction of the tidal volume and require greater distending pressures. Furthermore, even small amounts of edema fluid interfere with surfactant function, leading to increased surface tension at the air-liquid interface, alveolar instability, and alveolar collapse. In cardiogenic edema the increase in pulmonary blood volume causes a further increase in lung stiffness, but this effect is small in comparison to the effects of edema per se.

Lung Volume

Displacement of alveolar air with edema fluid, alveolar collapse, and the increase in lung recoil pressure (decreased compliance) all work in concert to produce a decrease in lung gas volume in both types of edema. In addition the increase in pulmonary blood volume in congestive heart failure tends to reduce lung gas volume for any given chest wall volume.

Airway Resistance

There are several factors which tend to increase airway resistance in pulmonary edema. First, a reduction in lung volume, for any reason, produces an increase in airway resistance. Second, edema in the bronchovascular sheath produces compression of small airways. Third, fluid in the airways combined with edema of the bronchial mucosa narrows the lumen and increases resistance to airflow.

The fourth and by far the most important source of increased airway resistance is reflex bronchospasm which occurs in some patients with congestive heart failure. In these patients the manifestations of left atrial hypertension may be indistinguishable from classic asthma. Not infrequently these patients with **"cardiac asthma"** may be misdiagnosed. The bronchospasm will respond to bronchodilator medication such as epinephrine, which can lead the physician on a therapeutic misadventure if the underlying cardiac problem is not recognized and addressed appropriately.

Oxygenation

As already mentioned, alveolar edema produces a physiologic right-to-left shunt, which has the same effect on arterial PO_2 as an anatomic shunt. In addition to fluid-filled alveoli, alveoli which are collapsed due to surfactant inactivation or to airway dysfunction also create shunting. The magnitude of the shunt effect depends on the fraction of cardiac output perfusing alveoli which are either edema filled or atelectatic. Interstitial edema-fluid accumulation in the bronchovascular sheath causes small airway dysfunction such that these airways tend to remain closed at all lung volumes except near the end of inspiration. Alveoli served by these airways develop low $\dot{V}_A/\dot{Q}$ ratios, which also produces hypoxemia. The relative importance of shunt and $\dot{V}/\dot{Q}$ mismatch depends on the amount of alveolar edema.

Acid-Base Balance

Mild forms of pulmonary edema stimulate interstitial "J" receptors in the lung, leading to hyperventilation and **respiratory alkalosis.** More severe forms of pulmonary edema by virtue of increasing the work of breathing lead to relative hypoventilation and **respiratory acidosis.** In cardiogenic pulmonary edema while the metabolism of the respiratory muscles is increased, cardiac dysfunction leads to decreased blood flow, resulting in reduced tissue PO_2, anaerobic metabolism, and **metabolic acidosis.**

Respiratory Failure

The combination of a failing heart, lungs full of edema fluid, refractory hypoxemia, respiratory acidosis, and metabolic acidosis make acute cardiogenic pulmonary edema one of the most challenging problems of acute care medicine. Ordinarily this combination of blood gas abnormalities would make the patient a candidate for mechanical ventilation, but there is convincing evidence that treatment directed at the cause of pulmonary edema will suffice in a significant proportion of the patients with cardiogenic edema. For patients with high-permeability edema the underlying lung injury is not as responsive to therapy and mechanical ventilation is almost always required. A full understanding of the pathophysiology is key to deciding which patients will require only pharmacologic support and which will require mechanical ventilation.

Diagnosis

The first step in the evaluation of patients with pulmonary edema is to determine the relative importance of alterations in hydrostatic pressure and vascular permeability for the increase in fluid filtration into the lung. Ninety percent of patients with high-pressure cardiogenic pulmonary edema will have ischemic heart disease and 30–40% will have had an acute myocardial infarction. Others will have valvular heart disease or cardiomyopathy. The prognosis for these patients largely depends on the successful management of the underlying cardiac disease.

Clinical examples of edema due to increased permeability include viral pneumonitis, "shock lung," fat embolism syndrome, gastric aspiration, and many others. Some au-

thorities group all of these under the broad classification of Adult Respiratory Distress Syndrome (ARDS), but use of this diagnosis does not bring one any closer to an understanding of the pathophysiology or treatment. There are also forms of pulmonary edema which appear to be a mixture of the two, i.e., evidence of increased pressure and increased permeability. Examples of the mixed type include high-altitude pulmonary edema and neurogenic pulmonary edema.

Measurement of Pulmonary Capillary Wedge Pressure

This is important in the management of any patient with unexplained pulmonary edema. Edema with a normal pulmonary capillary pressure suggests altered permeability. The relevance of changes in the post-capillary component of pulmonary vascular resistance will be more fully appreciated in the next few years as the result of emerging technologies for its measurement in critically ill patients. It should be remembered that an increase in post-capillary resistance could produce hydrostatic edema in the setting of pulmonary arterial hypertension with normal left atrial pressure.

Measurement of the Protein Concentration in Edema Fluid

This is another means to characterize the mechanism of pulmonary edema. In high-pressure pulmonary edema, the edema fluid protein concentration is usually less than 50% of the plasma protein concentration. In edema due to increased permeability, the protein concentration is greater than 50%, usually about 80% of the plasma protein concentration. Recently, active transport of fluid across the alveolar epithelium has been demonstrated to be an important mechanism for the clearance of pulmonary edema. Since the transport mechanism moves water and electrolytes, but not protein, the resolution of hydrostatic pulmonary edema will produce an increase in the protein concentration of alveolar fluid. This may confound the interpretation of edema fluid protein measurements during the resolution of cardiogenic edema.

Treatment

The treatment of patients with pulmonary edema is based on pathophysiologic consequences and on pathogenetic mechanisms.

Oxygen and Respiratory Support

The primary pathophysiologic consequences which must be addressed by therapy are hypoxemia and the increased work of breathing. Although hypoxemia due to the shunt effect of collapsed and fluid filled alveoli is relatively refractory to O_2 therapy, increases in the inspired O_2 concentration are routinely used. Most of the benefit from O_2 therapy is derived from the improved oxygenation in low $\dot{V}_A/\dot{Q}$ alveoli. Treatment directed at the reversal of atelectasis can be very effective. This can include encouragement of the patient to take deep breaths or positive-pressure breathing to increase lung volume. Positive-pressure breathing also reduces the work of breathing and by increasing pleural pressure may reduce venous return and left atrial pressure.

Acid-Base Balance

The metabolic acidosis of cardiogenic pulmonary edema is due to lactic acidosis which will be corrected as pulmonary edema resolves. The administration of $NaHCO_3$ is not recommended because the Na load increases intravascular volume and left atrial pressure. The respiratory acidosis will respond to therapy to reduce the work of breathing and does not require other specific treatment. Because it is due to increased work of breathing rather than an abnormality of respiratory drive, respiratory acidosis does not contraindicate the use of morphine, which is a mainstay of the treatment of cardiogenic edema. The beneficial effects of morphine are not completely understood, but probably derive from reduced venous return due to both dilatation of the large capacitance veins and decreased inspiratory efforts.

Reduce Pulmonary Capillary Pressure

Therapy which produces a reduction in P_{CAP} is effective in both types of pulmonary edema. In cardiogenic edema increased P_{CAP} is the primary pathogenetic mechanism. When edema is the result of increased permeability rather than increased pressure the hydraulic filtration coefficient (K_F) is increased, and the rate of fluid filtration is more sensitive to changes in capillary pressure than in the presence of high-pressure, cardiogenic pulmonary edema. Thus both types of pulmonary edema should respond to therapy that leads to a reduction in capillary pressure in the lung if it is possible to accomplish this while still providing adequate left atrial pressure to maintain cardiac output.

Increase Plasma Oncotic Pressure

Edema due to fluid overload with normal or low plasma protein concentration might respond to therapy that increases plasma oncotic pressure because the endothelial protein permeability is normal, but the benefits would be offset by any increase in P_{CAP} resulting from the infusion of colloid solutions. The limited benefit of therapy to increase π_{CAP} is derived from the fact that π_{ISF} is normally about 75% of π_{CAP}. So the patient with reduced π_{CAP} already has a reduced π_{ISF} and may have a normal transvascular oncotic pressure gradient. Furthermore, any benefit from therapy to increase the oncotic gradient will be short lived. It is known that labeled albumin infused into the vascular space equilibrates with interstitial albumin with a half-time of 1.5–4.0 hours. The rate of equilibration is increased if P_{CAP} is elevated or endothelial permeability is increased. Edema due to capillary injury, with high endothelial protein permeability and reduced σ, would not be expected to respond to any therapy which attempts to increase π_{CAP}.

Summary

Lung water balance is summarized in Figs. 48-4 through 48-7. Notice that the balance of forces in the normal lung produces continuous filtration of fluid into the interstitial space and the lung is maintained in a state of relative dryness by lymphatic clearance equal to the filtration rate (Fig. 48-4).

The lung has three mechanisms to protect against pulmonary edema with increases in pulmonary capillary pressure. First, because of the low compliance of the interstitial space, a small increase in interstitial fluid volume produces a sharp increase in interstitial fluid pressure, which opposes further fluid filtration. Second, the increase in interstitial fluid pressure increases the driving pressure for lymph flow. Third, the filtration of a plasma ultrafiltrate reduces interstitial fluid protein concentration and π_{ISF}, which also acts to reduce the net fluid filtration gradient.

These mechanisms operate in the patient with congestive heart failure (CHF) and interstitial edema produced by a moderate increase in P_{LA} (Fig. 48-5). Notice that a 10 mm Hg increase in P_{CAP} produces an increase in filtration across the capillary endothelium leading to an increase in P_{ISF} from −4 to −1, and a decrease in π_{ISF} from 18 to 13. Thus, while the 10 mm Hg increase in P_{LA} might have produced a 10 mm Hg increase in the filtration gradient, homeostatic mechanisms have limited the increase in gradient to only 2.5 mm Hg (11.1 − 8.6).

NORMAL

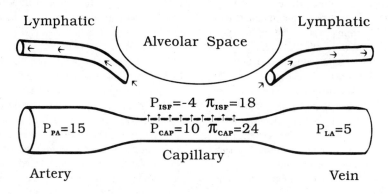

$$F = K_F[(P_{CAP} - P_{ISF}) - \sigma (\pi_{CAP} - \pi_{ISF})]$$

$$F = K_F[(10 - (-4)) - 0.9(24 - 18)] = K_F \times 8.6$$

Fig. 48-4. The normal balance of Starling forces produces a small amount of fluid filtration which is removed from the lung by lymphatic clearance.

CHF INTERSTITIAL EDEMA

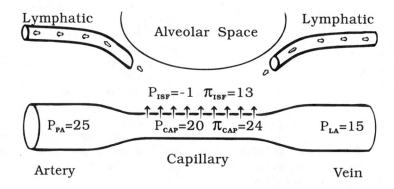

$$F = K_F[(P_{CAP} - P_{ISF}) - \sigma (\pi_{CAP} - \pi_{ISF})]$$

$$F = K_F[(20 - (-1)) - 0.9(24 - 13)] = K_F \times 11.1$$

Fig. 48-5. With a moderate increase in left atrial pressure there is an increase in filtration and lymph flow, but the size of these changes is restrained by adjustments in the interstitial forces. Notice that P_{ISF} has increased by 3 and π_{ISF} has decreased by 5 mm Hg, thus reducing the filtration gradient by $\approx$ 8 mm Hg.

HYDROSTATIC   EDEMA

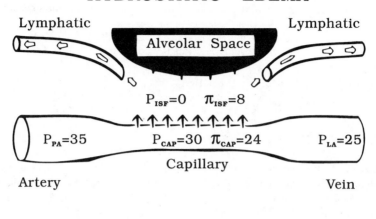

$$F = K_F[(P_{CAP} - P_{ISF}) - \sigma (\pi_{CAP} - \pi_{ISF})]$$

$$F = K_F[(30 - (0)) - 0.9(24 - 8)] = K_F \times 15.6$$

Fig. 48-6. With further increases in left atrial pressure there is a point at which the homeostatic mechanisms are overwhelmed and overt pulmonary edema develops. Notice that even under these circumstances the increase in filtration is restrained by adjustments in the interstitial forces.

PERMEABILITY   EDEMA

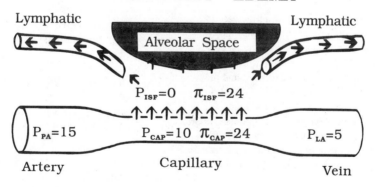

$$F = K_F[(P_{CAP} - P_{ISF}) - \sigma (\pi_{CAP} - \pi_{ISF})]$$

$$F = K_F[(10 - (0)) - 0 (24 - 24)] = K_F \times 10$$

Fig. 48-7. When pulmonary edema is produced by an increase in vascular permeability σ approaches 0 and π_{ISF} approaches π_{CAP}. The only forces which can produce a change in lung water balance are the hydrostatic pressures P_{CAP} and P_{ISF}.

Table 48-2. Diagnosis and Treatment of Pulmonary Edema

MECHANISM	CARDIOGENIC	HIGH PERMEABILITY
	Heart failure, mitral stenosis, volume overload	Injury to the capillary endothelium
DIAGNOSTIC FEATURES		
Pulmonary capillary wedge pressure	$\uparrow > 25$ mm Hg	Normal ≤ 12 mm Hg
Protein concentration		
Edema fluid/plasma	$< 50\%$	$> 50\%$
THERAPY	Reduce capillary pressure	Reduce capillary pressure

With further increases in left atrial pressure, the homeostatic mechanisms will eventually be overwhelmed, resulting in overt pulmonary edema with alveolar flooding (Fig. 48-6). Even with overt pulmonary edema the protective mechanisms provide for a prompt resolution of filtration with a small reduction in left atrial pressure. Notice that despite a 20 mm Hg increase in P_{LA} the pressure gradient for fluid filtration has only increased by 7 mm Hg (15.6 − 8.6).

The precise circumstances that trigger alveolar flooding are not yet understood, but the most attractive hypothesis is that the alveolar epithelium breaks down when P_{ISF} is equal to, or greater than, alveolar pressure because the alveolar surface lining cannot constrain a positive pressure. One problem with this hypothesis is the failure of continuous positive airway pressure ventilation to prevent pulmonary edema.

When filtration rate increases because of an increase in vascular permeability (Fig. 48-7), a critical defense mechanism is lost because the filtrate contains protein in a concentration that is higher than that in the interstitial space. As σ approaches zero π_{ISF} becomes equal to π_{CAP} and the only factor which determines changes in fluid filtration rate is the difference between capillary and interstitial pressures. Although the filtration pressure gradient is nearly normal the increase in K_F predicts an increase in filtration rate and only a reduction in P_{CAP} can reduce the rate of fluid filtration until permeability (K_F and σ) are restored to normal.

The diagnosis and treatment of the patient with pulmonary edema are summarized in Table 48-2.

Clinical Example

1. A 53-year-old man sustained multiple soft-tissue injuries in an automobile accident and required an emergency splenectomy. In the first 12 hours of hospitalization, he required fluid resuscitation, including four units of packed red blood cells, two units of plasma, and seven liters of Ringer's lactate solution. Surgery was without complication, and the patient appeared to be doing well until the second hospital day, when he became progressively short of breath. Past medical history includes a myocardial infarction.

Examination revealed: Temperature = 37.8°C, blood pressure = 130/70, respiratory rate = 48, with inspiratory rales in all lung fields, but no gallop on cardiac exam. A chest film revealed diffuse alveolar infiltrates in all lung fields. Blood gas results are listed in the accompanying tabulation. Mechanical ventilation was required, eventually with positive end-expiratory pressure (PEEP). A Swan-Ganz pulmonary artery catheter was inserted to measure wedge pressure and cardiac output.

Blood Gas Measurements	pH	PaCO$_2$	PaO$_2$
Nasal prongs, 3 liters/minute	7.52	28	42
High-flow O$_2$ by mask, 20 liters/minute	7.51	27	46
Mechanical ventilation, 100% O$_2$	7.48	32	55
100% O$_2$, 10 cm H$_2$O PEEP	7.46	36	80
60% O$_2$, 10 cm H$_2$O PEEP	7.47	35	60

Airway fluid protein was 4.2 g/dl and total serum protein was 4.8 g/dl. Hemodynamic data while briefly disconnected from ventilator showed pulmonary artery pressure (S/D) 35/17; wedge (indirect left atrial pressure) 11 mm Hg; and cardiac index 4 liters/minute/m^2.

Discussion. This patient has developed adult respiratory distress syndrome. The mechanism is low-pressure, high-permeability pulmonary edema with a normal (0–12 mm Hg) wedge pressure and cardiac index (3.2 ± 0.5 liters/minute/m^2). Given the past history of myocardial infarction and the large amount of fluid administered, cardiogenic pulmonary edema due to volume overload and left ventricular failure could also explain the clinical picture, but the normal hemodynamic data tend to exclude this, and suggest that the edema is due to increased permeability. This conclusion is further supported by the elevated airway fluid protein which is 88% of serum protein. Patients with ARDS have a 60–70% mortality. Fluid balance, colloid replacement therapy, and gas exchange are critical issues.

Despite the normal value for wedge pressure, it will be important to employ fluid restriction and diuretics. With injury to the pulmonary capillary endothelium and increased permeability, lung water balance is highly sensitive to small changes in capillary pressure. Those patients with ARDS who are able to achieve at least a 25% reduction in P_{PCW} in response to treatment enjoy a marked improvement in survival (25% mortality).

Serum protein is low, but we also know that σ of the pulmonary capillary endothelium must be reduced. Thus the infusion of a colloid such as albumin would be of no benefit. In fact if the endothelium of the systemic capillaries is intact the infusion of albumin would redistribute fluid from the peripheral extravascular space into the vascular space, producing an increase in P_{LA} and P_{CAP} in the lung and a consequent increase in pulmonary edema formation.

The poor response of arterial PO_2 to oxygen therapy is typical of the patient with shunting due to alveolar edema and atelectasis. The improved oxygenation with positive end-expiratory pressure is due to reversal of atelectasis. There is no evidence that PEEP reduces lung water.

Bibliography

Aberman A and Fulop M. The metabolic and respiratory acidosis of acute pulmonary edema. *Ann Int Med* 76:173, 1972. *Clinical study of gas exchange and clinical outcome in cardiogenic pulmonary edema.*

Eisenberg PR, Hansbrough JR, Anderson D, et al. A prospective study of lung water measurements during patient management in an intensive care unit. *Am Rev Resp Dis* 136:662, 1987. *First study to demonstrate the safety of negative fluid balance in ARDS.*

Gray BA, Hyde RW, Hodges M, et al. Alterations in lung volumes and pulmonary function in relation to hemodynamic changes in acute myocardial infarction. *Circulation* 59:551, 1979. *Clinical study of patients with various degrees of left ventricular failure.*

Humphrey H, Hall J, Sznajder I, et al. Improved survival in ARDS patients associated with a reduction in pulmonary capillary wedge pressure. *Chest* 97:1176, 1990. *Clinical study examining the importance of P_{CAP} in patients with low-pressure edema.*

Prewitt RM, McCarthy J, and Wood LDH. Treatment of acute low pressure pulmonary edema in dogs. *J Clin Invest* 67:409, 1981. *Classic study pointing to the importance of P_{CAP} in low-pressure edema.*

Simmons RS, Berdine GG, Seidenfield JJ, et al. Fluid balance and the adult respiratory distress syndrome. *Am Rev Respir Dis* 135:924, 1987. *One of the first clinical studies to call attention to the importance of fluid balance.*

Staub NC. The pathogenesis of pulmonary edema. *Prog Cardiovas Dis* 23:53,1980. *Classic review.*

49 Diseases of the Pleural Space

Gary T. Kinasewitz

Objectives

After completing this chapter, you should be able to

Recognize the similarities and differences in anatomical structure between parietal and visceral pleura

Describe how changes in the balance of hydrostatic and oncotic pressure affect the formation and reabsorption of pleural fluid

Understand how pleural pressure changes during respiration

Recognize the common symptoms and clinical signs of pleural effusion

Understand how the pathogenesis of transudative and exudative effusions differ

Identify the common causes of transudative effusions

Identify the common causes of exudative effusions

Understand why the treatments of transudative and exudative effusions differ

Functional Anatomy

The pleural cavity is the potential space between the membranes which cover the outer surface of the lung and the opposing aspects of the chest wall, mediastinum, and diaphragm. In health these pleural membranes are separated by a thin layer of fluid which in effect couples the chest wall to the lung and facilitates their expansion. However, the physiologic importance of this interaction is uncertain since obliteration of the pleural space has little demonstrable effect on pulmonary function.

The hallmark of pleural disease is an accumulation of excess fluid within the pleural space, a pleural effusion. This may occur as a response to local disease within the pleural membranes or the effusion may represent just one aspect of a systemic illness involving many organs. In the latter instance, examination of the pleural fluid may provide an important clue as to the nature of the underlying disorder. Pleural disease can produce distressing symptoms which are readily alleviated with appropriate treatment.

Functional Anatomy

The visceral pleural completely envelopes the lung except at the hilum where the bronchus, pulmonary vessels, and nerves enter the lung parenchyma. It covers the entire surface including the interlobar fissures, and reflections from the dorsal and ventral surface of the lung may persist to the level of the diaphragm as a double layer of mesothelial cells, the pulmonary ligament. The opposing parietal pleural membrane lines the inner surface of the chest wall, mediastinum, and diaphragm, merging with the visceral pleura at the hilum.

If one opens the pleural cavity and looks down upon the pleural membranes, they both have a similar smooth glistening semitransparent appearance. Each surface is covered by a single layer of mesothelial cells situated atop a submesothelial connective tissue layer containing abundant elastin and collagen fibers. The mesothelial cells form a flat to cuboidal epithelium with numerous microvilli upon their apical surface. The pleural surfaces are coated with a layer of glycoproteins rich in hyaluronic acid which facilitates respiratory movement by decreasing the friction between the lung and chest wall.

The mesothelium is metabolically active and helps maintain the integrity of the pleural cavity. The normal mesothelial surface is nonthrombotic because local production of plasminogen activators such as urokinase and tissue plasminogen activator prevent intrapleural thrombosis. The mesothelial cell is the principal source of the hyaluronic acid in pleural fluid. Mesothelial cell thromboxane and prostacyclin contribute to the local regulation of pleural blood flow. In addition, the mesothelium plays a central role in orchestrating the inflammatory response within the pleural cavity. Cytokines such as interleukin-1 and tumor necrosis factor stimulate mesothelial cell production of chemokines such as interleukin-8 and induce expression of leukocyte adhesion molecules such as ICAM-1 on the surface of the mesothelium. These same stimuli also induce mesothelial cell production of tissue factor and plasminogen activator inhibitors, leading to fibrin deposition and the development of loculation within the pleural cavity. By secreting collagen and elastin as well as metalloproteinases which are important in tissue remodeling, the mesothelium also plays a key role in restoring the normal architecture after pleural injury.

Beneath the mesothelium there are important anatomic differences between the visceral and parietal membranes. The submesothelial connective tissue layer of the parietal pleural is thicker than its visceral counterpart. In addition to containing blood vessels which originate from the intercostal and pericardiophrenic arteries, the parietal pleural is richly innervated with pain fibers. Stimulation of these fibers is responsible for the pleuritic pain characteristic of pleural disease. The visceral pleural lacks innervation and its blood supply is more complex. The bronchial arteries are the major source of the flow to the submesothelial capillaries but these capillaries drain into pulmonary rather than systemic veins. Therefore, the hydrostatic pressure within the visceral pleural microvessels is similar to that within the pulmonary capillaries and significantly lower than in the systemic capillaries within the parietal pleura.

The lymphatic networks within the visceral and parietal pleura also differ. Lymphatic vessels in the connective tissue layer beneath the visceral pleural mesothelium do not communicate with the pleural cavity and appear to function as part of the pulmonary lymphatic system. A rich lymphatic network within the parietal pleura provides the major route of lymphatic drainage from the pleural space. These parietal pleural lymphatics are connected to the pleural cavity via submesothelial lacunas or spaces which open to the pleural cavity via stoma in the mesothelial surface. These stoma are primarily located in the lower portion of the mediastinal and costal pleura and over the diaphragmatic portion of the parietal pleura. In addition to providing an important means of fluid removal, these lymphatics are the major route by which protein, cells, and particulate matter leave the pleural space. Efferent lymphatic vessels from the costal surface of the parietal pleura drain to parasternal and paraverbral nodes, whereas the lymphatics of the mediastinal surface of the parietal pleura drain into tracheobronchial nodes.

Pleural Fluid Dynamics

In health the parietal and visceral membranes are separated by a thin (10–30 μm) layer of fluid which is formed as an ultrafiltrate of plasma. The normal pleural fluid volume is 0.1–0.2 ml/kg or less than 15 ml in a 70-kg individual. Small molecules such as glucose have pleural fluid concentrations similar to that of plasma, whereas the concentrations of albumin and other macromolecules are considerably lower than in the blood (Table 49-1). Pleural fluid normally contains some mesothelial cells and macrophages but few lymphocytes and neutrophils. Despite the relatively small volume of fluid normally present in the pleural space, the rate of pleural fluid filtration and reabsorption may exceed 1 liter/day. The rate of pleural fluid efflux equals its rate of formation so that the pleural fluid volume remains minimal in a healthy individual.

As in other organs, the movement of fluid between the submesothelial capillaries within the pleural membranes and the pleural space is determined by the balance of hydrostatic and oncotic pressures between the microvasculature and the pleural cavity. The mesothelium is extremely permeable and offers little resistance to water and protein flux. Therefore, the primary barrier to fluid movement is the endothelium of the pleural capillaries. Fluid exchange across the pleural membranes can be described in terms of Starling's law of capillary exchange:

Table 49-1. Normal Pleural Fluid Values*

Volume	0.1–0.2 ml/kg
Cells/mm³	1000–5000
% mesothelial cells	3–70%
% monocytes	30–75%
% lymphocytes	2–30%
% granulocytes	10%
Protein	1–2 g/dl
% albumin	50–70%
Glucose	≈ plasma level
LDH	< 50% plasma level
pH	≥ plasma

* Data from humans and animals.

$$F = Lp \times A\left[\left(P_{cap} - P_{pl}\right) - \sigma\left(\pi_{cap} - \pi_{pl}\right)\right]$$

where F is the rate of fluid movement, P and π are the hydrostatic and oncotic pressures respectively within the capillaries (cap) and pleural space (pl), Lp is the hydraulic conductivity of the capillary endothelial-pleural mesothelial membrane, A is the surface area of the membrane, and σ is the osmotic reflection coefficient for protein.

The capillaries of the parietal pleura are derived from the systemic circulation, so the hydrostatic pressure within them is similar to that within other systemic capillaries, i.e., 25 mm Hg. Intrapleural pressure is slightly subatmospheric, about –3 mm Hg. Opposing this net hydrostatic pressure difference promoting fluid filtration is the oncotic pressure difference due to the higher concentration of protein in plasma (π_{cap} = 28 mm Hg) than in pleural fluid (π_{pl} = 5 mm Hg). The protein reflection coefficient of the pleural capillaries is similar to that observed in most other organs, approximately 0.9. Therefore the effective oncotic pressure difference opposing fluid efflux is 0.9 (28 mm Hg – 5 mm Hg) = 21 mm Hg. Thus the balance of Starling forces promotes the filtration of fluid from the parietal pleural capillary into the pleural space (Fig. 49-1).

There are two potential routes by which fluid can be reabsorbed from the pleural space, via the capillaries in the visceral pleura and via the lymphatics in the parietal pleura. The capillaries of the visceral pleura empty into the pulmonary veins and, because the resistance of these vessels is low, hydrostatic pressure within the visceral pleural capillaries is similar to that within the pulmonary capillaries, i.e., about 10 mm Hg. Thus the balance of Starling forces across the visceral pleura favors fluid reabsorption from the pleural cavity under physiologic conditions.

However, under physiologic conditions the most important route for pleural fluid reabsorption is the lymphatics of the parietal pleura. While the visceral pleural capillaries can reabsorb water from the pleural space, they are relatively impermeable to protein, so that the protein content of pleural fluid increases as fluid is reabsorbed. If the lymphatics did not remove protein from the pleural space, the oncotic gradient opposing fluid filtration would dissipate and fluid would accumulate. The bulk removal of fluid and protein by lymphatics is essential to maintain a normal oncotic gradient across the pleural membranes. Quantitatively lymphatic flow appears to be responsible for most of the fluid efflux and virtually all protein reabsorption from the pleural cavity under physiologic conditions.

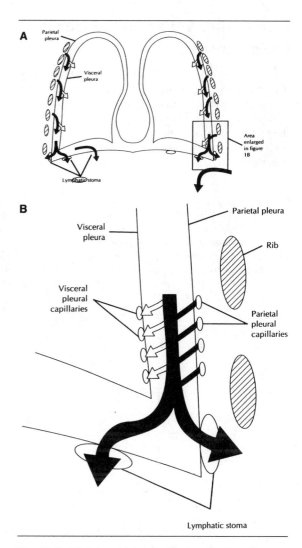

Fig. 49-1. (A) Schematic representation of pleural fluid flux within the pleural cavity under physiologic conditions. Fluid is filtered from the parietal membrane into the pleural cavity. Some fluid is reabsorbed across the visceral pleura (thin arrows) but the bulk of the fluid flows toward the dependent regions of the pleural cavity where it is removed by the lymphatics. (B) Insert illustrating the movement of fluid from the parietal pleural capillaries to the visceral pleural microvessels and parietal lymphatics in greater detail. (Reprinted with permission from: Kinasewitz GT. Pleuritis and pleural effusions. In Bone RC (ed.). *Pulmonary and Critical Care Medicine* (Vol. 2, Part O). St. Louis: Mosby-Year Book, 1993, pp. 1–22.)

Respiratory Variation in Pleural Fluid Pressures

The hydrostatic pressure within the pleural cavity is slightly negative (subatmospheric) at the end of expiration (functional residual capacity, FRC). This negative intrapleural pressure counterbalances the tendency of the chest wall to recoil outward and the lung to collapse.

Pleural pressure becomes even more negative during a spontaneous inspiration (Fig. 49-2). During active expiration pleural pressure may become positive during the expiratory phase of the respiratory cycle. In contrast, pleural pressure fluctuates in the opposite direction during positive pressure ventilation (IPPV). IPPV produces an inspiratory rise in pleural pressure which falls back to subatmospheric levels during expiration. However, when positive end expiratory pressure is utilized, the pleural pressure may be positive throughout the respiratory cycle. This positive intrapleural pressure can have profound effects on venous return and intravascular pressures.

Fig. 49-2. Respiratory variations in pleural pressure. (A) During spontaneous respiration pleural pressure is slightly subatmospheric at end-expiration (FRC). It decreases during inspiration and then returns to the end-expiratory level during quiet respiration. (B) Even while spontaneously breathing, active expiratory muscle contraction may produce positive pleural pressures during expiration. (C) Positive pressure ventilation (IPPV) reverses the pleural pressure changes during the respiratory cycle. Pleural pressure rises during inspiration and falls back to subatmospheric levels during expiration. (D) Applying positive end expiratory pressure (PEEP) during mechanical ventilation (IPPV) may result in a positive intrapleural pressure throughout the entire respiratory cycle. (Reprinted with permission from: Kinasewitz GT. Pleuritis and pleural effusions. In Bone RC (ed.). *Pulmonary and Critical Care Medicine* (Vol. 2, Part O). St. Louis: Mosby-Year Book, 1993, pp. 1–22.)

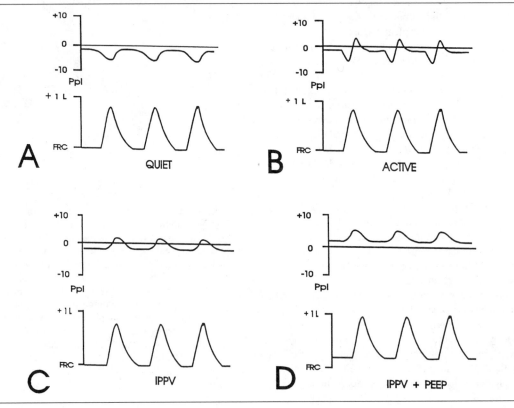

Consequences of Pleural Effusions

Patients with pleural effusions typically complain of chest pain, cough, and shortness of breath. Irritation of the nerve fibers within the parietal pleura causes pleuritic pain, i.e., pain which increases with respiration and may be localized to a specific area of the chest wall. When the diaphragmatic portion of the parietal pleura is involved, the pain may be referred to the ipsilateral shoulder. Nonproductive cough is due to reflex stimulation of receptors within the compressed lung. If the cough is productive, this suggests the presence of an infiltrate in the underlying lung parenchyma. Several factors contribute to the sensation of breathlessness or dyspnea produced by a pleural effusion. A large effusion acts as a space-occupying lesion, compressing the lung and producing a restrictive ventilatory impairment. The consequent ventilation-perfusion mismatching produces hypoxemia which is accentuated when the thorax with the effusion is dependent and receiving a greater fraction of the total pulmonary blood flow. In addition, a large effusion permits the chest wall to expand outward, thereby shortening the resting length of the inspiratory muscles. Removing a modest amount of fluid can produce dramatic symptomatic relief without significantly changing arterial oxygenation or vital capacity. This symptomatic improvement is thought to be due to a shift of the chest wall pressure-volume curve toward its normal position which enables the inspiratory muscles to contract from a more advantageous position on their length-tension curve.

Pathogenesis of Pleural Effusions

An accumulation of fluid in the pleural space is called pleural effusion. Pleural effusions develop whenever the rate of fluid entry into the pleural cavity exceeds its removal. The first step in establishing the cause of an effusion is to determine whether it is a transudate or an exudate. Effusions are classified as either transudates or exudates based on the protein and LDH concentrations in the fluid (Table 49-2). This classification has important im-

plications regarding the pathogenesis of the effusion. The protein content of a transudative effusion is low because the pleural capillary endothelium is intact and its ability to retain plasma proteins within the vascular compartment is preserved. The development of an exudative effusion implies a loss of the integrity of the pleural membrane or disruption of the normal lymphatic clearance mechanisms or both. The physiologic derangements are more severe and management will be correspondingly more difficult.

Transudates

Transudates develop whenever the balance in Starling forces is altered so that the rate of fluid filtration into the pleural space exceeds its rate of reabsorption. This most commonly occurs in a patient with congestive heart failure. The underlying mechanism is an increase in capillary hydrostatic pressure. Clinical studies have found that the development and size of the effusion is more closely correlated with increased left rather than right atrial pressure, suggesting that the effusion is a consequence of decreased reabsorption or increased filtration from the capillaries within the visceral pleura or both. Pleural effusions in patients with congestive heart failure are usually bilateral. However, unilateral effusions do occur, in which case they are more common on the right side.

Decreased plasma oncotic pressure due to hypoalbuminemia may also result in the development of a transudative effusion, especially in patients with hepatic cirrhosis or the nephrotic syndrome (Table 49-3). Fluid filtration due to the hydrostatic pressure within the microvasculature is normally opposed by the oncotic pressure of the plasma proteins. A reduction in plasma oncotic pressure changes the distribution of Starling forces to favor increased fluid formation and, if the pumping capacity of the lymphatics

Table 49-2. Transudative Versus Exudative Effusion

Criteria	Critical Value*
Pleural fluid to serum protein ratio	> 0.5
Pleural fluid LDH	> 200 IU/liter
Pleural fluid-to-serum LDH ratio	> 0.6

*If any one critical value is exceeded, the effusion is an exudate.

Table 49-3. Common Etiologies of Pleural Effusions

Transudates	Exudates
Increased venous pressure	Parapneumonic*
CHF*	Malignancy*
Constrictive pericarditis	Pulmonary embolism*
Hypoalbuminemic	Tuberculosis
Cirrhosis	Collagen vascular disease
Nephrosis	Abdominal disease
Malnutrition	Trauma
	Hemothorax

*These four entities account for 90% of all effusions.

within the parietal pleura is exceeded, pleural fluid will accumulate.

Decreased intrapleural pressure may be responsible for the abnormal accumulation of pleural fluid in patients with obstructing bronchial lesions, e.g., lung carcinomas, and in patients with postoperative atelectasis. Local collapse of the lung from the chest wall creates a more negative intrapleural pressure that augments the hydrostatic pressure gradient favoring fluid formation. Transudative effusions which develop in response to the lowering of intrapleural pressure are called ex vacuo effusions.

The transdiaphragmatic movement of ascitic fluid from the peritoneal to the pleural cavity can also result in the development of an effusion. The usual route is via microscopic pores in the diaphragm though macroscopic defects have been observed in some individuals. This typically occurs in a patient with portal hypertension in which case both the peritoneal and pleural fluid have the characteristics of a transudate. However, the effusion may have a high protein content if the ascitic fluid is inflammatory or malignant in origin. A similar mechanism accounts for the transudative effusions which occasionally develop in patients undergoing peritoneal dialysis; the pleural fluid resembles the dialysate with a low protein level (< 1.0 g/dl) and a markedly elevated glucose level (> 300 mg/dl).

Transudative effusions are managed by correcting the underlying problem. The pleural membranes per se are intact and, if a normal distribution of Starling forces can be restored, the effusion will be reabsorbed. On rare occasion a therapeutic thoracentesis may be indicated for the relief of symptoms. However, unless the underlying pathology is reversed, the fluid will reaccumulate. Diuretics are the mainstay of therapy because they reduce the intravascular hydrostatic pressure promoting fluid formation. Albumin infusion may be helpful in an occasional malnourished patient, but it rapidly escapes the vascular compartment in patients with cirrhosis and/or nephrotic syndrome and is not indicated for the treatment of pleural effusions in these individuals.

Exudates

In contrast to transudates, exudative effusions are characterized by high pleural fluid protein and LDH concentrations. Exudative effusions develop because the rate of protein entry into the pleural cavity is increased and/or the lymphatic mechanism for reabsorbing pleural fluid is impaired. Whenever the integrity of the pleural capillary is disrupted, e.g., in the presence of pleural inflammation, protein-rich fluid will extravasate into the pleural cavity.

Increased pleural membrane permeability is usually due to infection, pulmonary infarction, or neoplasm. Blockage of the parietal pleural lymphatic stoma or malignant invasion of the mediastinal lymph nodes can also result in the retention of protein-rich fluid within the pleural space. Malignant invasion of the mediastinal lymph nodes is the most common cause of lymphatic obstruction. However, in the presence of severe pleural inflammation, e.g., bacterial empyema, mesothelial cell swelling and the accumulation of cellular debris and fibrin may obstruct the parietal pleural stomata and impair the normal lymphatic drainage of the pleural space.

A parapneumonic effusion is one that develops in a patient with pneumonia. Fluid accumulates because the underlying parenchymal infection increases the permeability of the adjacent pleural vessels. Protein-rich fluid leaks into the pleural cavity. Initially the effusion is sterile but, if therapy is delayed and the pneumonia progresses to involve the pleural surface, bacterial invasion of the pleural cavity may occur. Once bacteria are within the pleural fluid, the infection may spread to involve the entire pleural surface. At this stage the infected pleural fluid is termed an empyema. The neutrophil concentration in the fluid increases and the fluid becomes frankly purulent. Fibrin deposition on the pleural surfaces may lead to loculations which makes treatment more difficult. Early antibiotic therapy to prevent infection of the parapneumonic effusion and drainage of infected empyema fluid are the mainstays of therapy.

Primary tumors of the pleura are rare but metastatic malignancy is a relatively common cause of an exudative effusion. The effusion may be a consequence of pleural invasion by tumor, in which case cytologic examination of the fluid may be diagnostic. In other patients the exudative effusion is due to mediastinal lymph node involvement. Endobronchial tumors can cause obstructive atelectasis leading to an ex vacuo effusion or predispose to the development of a pneumonia and associated parapneumonic effusion. In many patients more than one mechanism contributes to the development of the effusion. Pleural effusions usually develop late in the course of malignancy and they are difficult to treat. Removal of fluid by thoracentesis can provide symptomatic relief. Oftentimes sclerosing agents which produce intense inflammation and induce fibrosis are instilled in an attempt to obliterate the pleural cavity and prevent the reaccumulation of the effusion.

Pulmonary embolism is the third major cause of exudative pleural effusions. These effusions (which typically are small or moderate in size) develop within hours of the embolus as a consequence of local ischemia or pulmonary infarction which increases the permeability of the pleural capillaries. In addition to having elevated protein and LDH levels, the fluid usually contains an increased number of neutrophils and erythrocytes. Pleural effusions due to thromboemboli do not require specific therapy since they will resolve spontaneously if recurrent embolization is prevented.

Since the pathogenesis of an exudative effusion implies that the normal mechanisms governing pleural fluid filtration and reabsorption are deranged, one would expect that they would be more difficult to manage than a transudative effusion. In addition to treating the underlying disorder, local measures may be required for the control of the effusion and to restore the integrity of the pleural membranes. Whenever diagnostic thoracentesis confirms the presence of an exudative effusion, its etiology should be established so that proper therapy can be instituted. In all instances, treatment of the underlying disease is the preferred mode of therapy. Unfortunately, many diseases which produce exudative effusions may be refractory to therapy and pleural sclerosis may be required for the management of persistent or recurrent effusions which cause significant symptoms.

Clinical Example

1. A 55-year-old woman comes to the emergency room complaining of shortness of breath. She has had a nonproductive cough for several days but denies chest pain or fever. A chest radiograph reveals a large pleural effusion in the left hemithorax (Fig. 49-3). Thoracentesis obtains straw-colored pleural fluid with a protein of 4.2 g/dl and an LDH of 260 IU/liter. Simultaneously drawn serum values are 7.0 g/dl and 180 IU/liter respectively. She is then referred for further evaluation and management.

Discussion.   The initial step in evaluating an effusion is to determine if it is a transudate or an exudate. This patient's effusion has high protein and LDH levels relative to serum values, indicating it is an exudate.

The majority of exudative effusions are parapneumonic, malignant, or due to pulmonary thromboembolism. Additional testing can help distinguish among these possibilities. The absence of fever and sputum production makes it unlikely that the patient has an underlying pneumonia. A positive Gram's stain of the pleural fluid and/or bacterial culture would confirm the presence of a parapneumonic effusion but one would expect both tests to be negative in this patient. Pleural fluid cytology is an excellent method

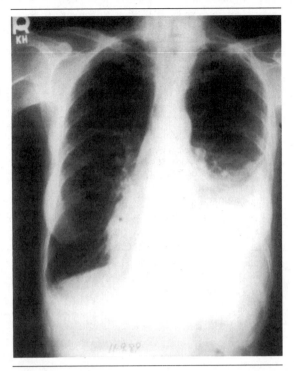

Fig. 49-3. Chest radiograph of patient revealing pleural effusion in the left hemithorax. Note widening of the left intercostal spaces indicating outward displacement of the chest wall.

of diagnosing malignant pleural disease. Unfortunately, a negative cytology does not absolutely exclude a malignant cause since, in the absence of malignant invasion of the pleura, the pleural fluid cytology will be negative. Bronchoscopy and other testing may be indicated to exclude malignancy with confidence. Pulmonary emboli usually arise from thrombi in the legs. As discussed in Chap. 50, venous studies and perfusion lung scanning can help establish or rule out this diagnosis. If these initial tests fail to suggest the cause of the effusion, additional tests for less common types of effusion will be necessary.

While the results of the pleural fluid testing are pending, consideration must be given to alleviating the patient's symptoms. Her dyspnea is probably multifactorial. Compression of the underlying lung causes a restrictive impairment while outward displacement of the chest wall forces the inspiratory muscles to operate at a mechanical disadvantage. The dyspnea could also be due to the underlying condition, e.g., malignancy or pneumonia, which is responsible for the exudative effusion. Nonproductive cough is oftentimes due to reflex stimulation of parenchymal receptors. Removing some of the effusion by thoracentesis may provide immediate relief of the patient's symptoms though the long-term management is directed toward treatment of the underlying disorder.

Bibliography

Agostoni E. Mechanics of the pleural space. In Fishman AP (ed.). *Handbook of Physiology: The Respiratory System* (Vol. 3, Part 2). Bethesda, MD: American Physiological Society, 1986, pp. 531–559. *Comprehensive review of the biology and physiology of the pleura.*

Bartlett JG and Finegold SM. Anaerobic infections of the lung and pleural space. *Am Rev Respir Dis* 110:56–77, 1974. *Describes the pathophysiology and clinical manifestations of pleural infection.*

Estenne M, Yernault J, and de Troyer A. Mechanism of relief of dyspnea after thoracentesis in patients with large pleural effusions. *Am J Med* 74:813–819, 1983. *Examines the causes of dyspnea in patients with pleural effusions.*

Kinasewitz GT and Fishman AP. Influence of alterations in Starling forces on visceral pleural fluid movement. *J Appl Physiol* 51:671–677, 1981. *Demonstrates that fluid movement across the pleural membranes is determined by the balance of Starling forces.*

Light RW. *Pleural Diseases* (2nd ed.). Philadelphia: Lea & Febiger, 1990. *Monograph which reviews the physiology of the pleural space and provides in-depth descriptions of the clinical aspects of pleural disease.*

Light RW, MacGregor MC, Luchsinger PC, et al. Pleural effusions: The diagnostic separation of transudates and exudates. *Ann Intern Med* 77:507–513, 1972. *Classic paper which describes how to distinguish transudates from exudates.*

Sahn SA. The pleura. *Am Rev Respir Dis* 138:184–234, 1988. *Comprehensive review of the many clinical disorders which produce pleural effusions.*

50 Venous Thromboembolism

Brent R. Brown

Objectives

After completing this chapter, you should be able to

Understand the meaning of the terms thromboembolism, superficial venous thrombosis, deep venous thrombosis, and pulmonary thromboembolism

Be familiar with the general incidence, morbidity, and mortality of venous thromboembolism

Know the risk factors for venous thromboembolism

Discuss the factors that lead to the formation of venous thrombi (Virchow's triad)

Understand the evolution of venous thrombi

Know the sequelae of venous thromboembolism

Be familiar with the pathophysiology of acute pulmonary thromboembolism

Understand the pathophysiology of chronic thromboembolic pulmonary hypertension

Know the clinical manifestations of venous thromboembolism

Know the general techniques for the prophylaxis and diagnosis of venous thromboembolism

---

An understanding of the pathophysiology of venous thromboembolism (VTE) requires familiarity with concepts derived from multiple medical disciplines including pulmonary medicine, cardiovascular medicine, and hematology. The term VTE includes both deep venous thrombosis (DVT) and pulmonary thromboembolism (PTE), emphasizing their common pathophysiologic basis and the concept that PTE is actually a sequela of DVT rather than a distinct disease entity. This chapter will discuss the significance and harm of VTE, the pathophysiology of both DVT and PTE, the clinical manifestations of VTE, and briefly review the diagnosis and treatment of VTE.

Key Concepts of VTE

VTE Defined

The term VTE includes superficial venous thrombosis, DVT, and the most serious complication of DVT, PTE. Superficial venous thrombosis is painful, but usually resolves

without serious consequences as long as thrombi do not propagate into the deep venous system. **The inclusive term VTE is justified because almost all pulmonary thromboemboli arise from deep venous thrombi and because PTE is very common in patients with DVT.** The last fact was confirmed by a study revealing that 40% of DVT patients suffered asymptomatic pulmonary emboli based on lung perfusion scans.

Significance and Consequences of VTE

VTE is a very common disorder. Precise figures do not exist, but it has been estimated that 5 million people in the U.S. develop venous thrombosis each year. Ten percent or 500,000 of these people will develop clinically significant PTE. Ten percent of these 500,000 cases, or 50,000, will prove fatal. Autopsy studies indicate that about 15% of acute-care hospital deaths are primarily caused by PTE. Recent data suggest the incidence of VTE may be increasing despite advances in its prevention and treatment. No data exist concerning the financial cost of the treatment of

VTE and loss of productivity caused by VTE, but the figure would prove enormous.

VTE Is Often Preventable

The risk factors for VTE are well known. Efficacious and cost-effective regimens for VTE prophylaxis have been widely published, but physician utilization of these preventive measures has been poor.

Accurate Diagnosis of VTE Is Difficult

Autopsy studies reveal 40–70% of major pulmonary thromboemboli were unsuspected prior to death. Clinicians must maintain a high index of suspicion for VTE which cannot be excluded by the history or examination alone. Suspected VTE must be confirmed or excluded by objective tests.

Deep Venous Thrombosis

Normal Venous Anatomy and Physiology

Familiarity with normal venous anatomy and physiology is helpful in understanding the pathophysiology of DVT. This information is reviewed in Chap. 13.

Risk Factors for DVT

A number of risk factors for DVT have been identified and are summarized in Table 50-1. Patients often have multiple risk factors which have additive effects. Some factors in-

Table 50-1. Risk Factors for Deep Venous Thrombosis

Lower extremity trauma/surgery
Advanced age
Immobilization
Cancer
Obesity
Inherited/acquired hyper-coagulability
Pregnancy/oral contraceptives
History of DVT
Intravenous devices (catheters, etc.)
Respiratory failure
Congestive heart failure/cor pulmonale
Myocardial infarction
Hemi/para/quadriplegia
Extensive burns
General anesthesia (> 30 minutes)

crease risk more than others. Conditions associated with a very high risk of DVT include surgery or fracture of the hip and acute hemiplegia, paraplegia, or quadriplegia.

Virchow's Triad

Abnormalities in venous blood flow, injury to the intima of the vein, and alterations in the blood remain the cornerstone to understanding the pathophysiology of DVT. Blood coagulation was not understood in Virchow's time, but the "alterations in the blood" he described are now known to be states of hyper-coagulability.

Abnormalities in Venous Blood Flow

Stasis is the primary alteration in venous blood flow that leads to DVT. Intermittent muscle contraction enhances flow through the deep venous system, and the loss of this "pumping" action accounts for the increased risk of DVT associated with immobilization and acute paralysis. Elevations in central venous pressure in CHF and cor pulmonale also result in altered venous flow. Patients with previous DVT may have incompetent venous valves or old organized thrombi which result in venous stasis predisposing to recurrent DVT.

Intimal Injury

The venous system is lined by a monolayer of endothelial cells that form a nonthrombogenic surface. Deep to this endothelial cell monolayer lie extracellular matrix proteins like collagen that can rapidly bind to and activate platelets. Additionally, perivascular fibroblasts deep to the endothelial cell monolayer express **tissue factor,** the principle activator of the extrinsic arm of the coagulation mechanism. The localization of tissue factor on perivascular cells forms a protective "extravascular envelope" capable of immediate activation of the clotting mechanism whenever integrity of the venous system is breached, thus providing hemostasis. Unfortunately, injury to the endothelial cell layer can occur from surgery or trauma to an extremity or from insertion of venous catheters. This exposes blood to the subendothelial collagens and tissue factor, resulting in platelet activation/aggregation and the initiation of coagulation. Significant venous thrombi may develop if not rapidly checked by anticoagulant and fibrinolytic mechanisms. In vitro, endothelial cells exposed to inflammatory cytokines will express tissue factor on their surfaces. It is possible that minor injuries to endothelial cells in vivo could also result in tissue factor expression, resulting in the activation of the clotting mechanism potentially leading to DVT.

Alterations in Blood Coagulability

The coagulation and fibrinolytic systems are reviewed in Chap. 34 and this information is useful in understanding how blood hyper-coagulability relates to DVT. Only a minority of patients with DVT have increased coagulability, making hyper-coagulability the least common of Virchow's three pathophysiologic mechanisms. Under normal conditions homeostasis exists between procoagulants, natural anticoagulants, activators of fibrinolysis, and the inhibitors of these activators. Perturbations in this homeostasis can lead to excessive bleeding or to thrombosis. Hemostatic abnormalities associated with VTE are listed in Table 50-2. Some of these disorders are genetic defects, others are acquired. Deficiency of anticoagulants like protein C and antithrombin III can lead to excessive thrombin generation. Fibrinolytic defects like decreased levels of plasminogen or tissue plasminogen activator or increased levels of plasminogen activator inhibitors may lead to excessive fibrin deposition. Each of these disorders can lead to DVT. Table 50-2 also mentions several disorders associated with hyper-coagulability that are incompletely understood.

Evolution of Venous Thrombi

Venous thrombi are rich in platelets, fibrin, and red blood cells. The initial aggregation of platelets and fibrin occurs at sites of reduced flow such as venous valves and side branches of veins as well as sites of endothelial injury (Fig. 50-1). The surfaces of aggregated, activated platelets greatly enhance the interaction of clotting factors accelerating the generation of thrombin and fibrin. Reductions in

Table 50-2. Hemostatic Abnormalities Associated with Venous Thromboembolism

Deficient anticoagulants
    Protein C
    Protein S
    Antithrombin III
Fibrinolytic defects
    Decreased plasminogen
    Decreased tissue plasminogen activator
    Increased plasminogen activator inhibitors
Miscellaneous disorders
    Antiphospholipid syndrome
    Nephrotic syndrome
    Polycythemia rubra vera
    Essential thrombocythemia
    Paroxysmal nocturnal hemoglobinuria

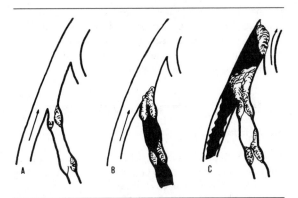

Fig. 50-1. Representation of the genesis of venous thrombi within the venous system. Initial aggregates of platelets and fibrin may be seen in three of the four depicted valve cusps in (A) but blood flow through the venous system remains uncompromised. More fibrin, platelets, and red blood cells have been deposited in (B) leading to thrombus propagation and stasis of blood flow (see dark regions) in a branch of the main vein. Further thrombus propagation has occurred in (C) leading to stasis in the main vein and risk of embolization. (Reproduced with permission from: Mammen EF. Pathogenesis of venous thrombosis. *Chest* 102:640S–644S, 1992.)

flow are important in thrombus propagation as activated coagulation factors remain in contact with the thrombus instead of being swept away by normal blood flow. There are three possible outcomes for small venous thrombi. The first and probably most common is either thrombolysis via the fibrinolytic system or the small thrombus is swept away, causing a clinically inapparent pulmonary embolus. A second possibility is thrombus propagation by alternating layers of fibrin and platelets resulting in partial venous obstruction. The third and least common possibility is explosive thrombus growth resulting in total venous occlusion. The last two possibilities may lead to clinically significant DVT and potential embolization.

Sequelae of Deep Venous Thrombus

Thrombi are dynamic structures modulated by both procoagulant and fibrinolytic processes. Some significant venous thrombi may undergo complete thrombolysis with a restoration of normal venous physiology. Often resolution is incomplete, although thrombus organization or thrombolytic recannulation through an extensive thrombus may partially restore blood flow. Venous valves are often left incompetent. These changes frequently lead to **chronic venous insufficiency,** an **increased risk of recurrent DVT,** and may result in the **post-phlebitic syndrome** (see Chap. 13). Thrombi can also break or dislodge, resulting in potentially fatal **pulmonary embolism.**

Pulmonary Thromboembolism

Key Concepts

Pulmonary thromboembolism (PTE) is not a distinct disease but rather the most serious complication of DVT. There has been past overemphasis on the diagnosis and treatment of PTE and underemphasis of the fact that **virtually all PTE can be avoided by preventing DVT.** An ounce of DVT prevention is worth a pound of PTE treatment.

Almost all pulmonary emboli arise from DVT. In 90% of the cases they arise from thrombi of the venous system of the lower extremities. There is a rising incidence of venous thrombosis of the subclavian and internal jugular veins related to intimal damage by central venous catheters. These catheter-related thrombi can cause PTE with occasional fatalities. A small number of PTE originate in pelvic or renal veins or from the right heart.

PTE is common in patients with DVT. Many of these embolic episodes are clinically apparent, many more are inapparent and undetected.

The consequences of PTE are determined by the extent of obstruction of the pulmonary vasculature and the presence or absence of underlying cardiopulmonary disease. The larger the embolus the more severe the disturbances in cardiovascular and pulmonary physiology. The morbidity and mortality of PTE is greater in individuals with significant heart or lung disease.

Most deaths due to PTE occur in the first few hours after embolization. Subsequent deaths in the first month following PTE are due either to **recurrent pulmonary embolism** or to **underlying disease. Immediate and adequate anticoagulation is paramount in preventing recurrent PTE.** Some patients with PTE later succumb to underlying diseases like cancer or heart failure which had predisposed them to the development of VTE. Mortality from PTE rises with advancing age. The **mortality of untreated symptomatic PTE is 30%.** This figure drops to **10% or less with appropriate treatment.**

Pathophysiology of Acute PTE

Hemodynamic Effects
The normal pulmonary circulation is characterized by low pressure (mean value 15 mm Hg) and low resistance. The pulmonary vasculature is highly distensible, allowing for increases in blood flow during periods of increased cardiac output without significant increases in pulmonary arterial pressure. In PTE, the embolized thrombus causes **mechanical obstruction** of portions of the pulmonary vasculature. Blood flow is diverted to patent vessels, with a resultant increase in pulmonary vascular resistance. If greater than 30% of the vasculature is obstructed an increase in pulmonary artery pressure often occurs. **In patients without preexistent pulmonary vascular disease, the pulmonary arterial pressure rises in proportion to the degree of embolic vascular obstruction** (Fig. 50-2). Further increases in resistance may occur from **vasoconstriction** of patent vessels by serotonin and thromboxane A_2 released by platelets in the embolus (see Table 50-3).

The increase in pulmonary vascular resistance and pressure increases the workload placed on the right ventricle. The load rises rapidly if greater than 50% of the pulmonary vasculature is obstructed. The normal right ventricle can not acutely generate pressures greater than a mean value of 40 mm Hg. In patients with chronic lung or vascular diseases causing pulmonary hypertension and

Fig. 50-2. Relationship between mean pulmonary arterial pressure and estimated percentage of pulmonary vascular obstruction following acute pulmonary embolus in patients without preexistent cardiopulmonary disease. (Reprinted with permission from: Sharma GVRK, McIntyre KM, et al. Clinical and hemodynamic correlates in pulmonary embolism. *Clin Chest Med* 5:421–437, 1984.)

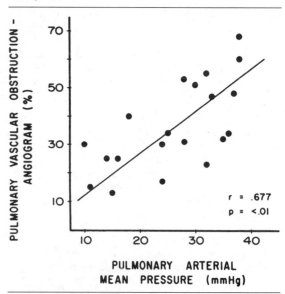

Table 50-3. Pulmonary Consequences of Acute
Pulmonary Thromboembolism

HEMODYNAMICS

Increased pulmonary vascular resistance
Increased right ventricular workload

GAS EXCHANGE

Increased physiologic dead space
Hypoxemia from shunt, low $\dot{V}/\dot{Q}$ areas

VENTILATORY CONTROL

Reflexive increase in respiratory drive

ATELECTASIS

Reduced surfactant, edema

PULMONARY INFARCTION

Compromised tissue oxygenation

COMPLIANCE

Reduced from edema, atelectasis, infarction

right ventricular hypertrophy, much higher pulmonary artery pressures can develop after acute PTE. If ventricular loading becomes severe the ventricle may begin to fail. Systemic arterial pressure will fall if the left ventricle receives an inadequate volume of blood from the failing right ventricle. Myocardial perfusion is reduced if aortic diastolic pressure falls, resulting in ischemia of both ventricles and possible ventricular tachycardia, fibrillation, or asystole.

Effects on Gas Exchange

When PTE occurs, some areas of lung receive **no perfusion** ($\dot{Q}$) but still receive ventilation ($\dot{V}$). Areas of lung that have $\dot{V}$ **without** $\dot{Q}$ are ineffective in gas exchange and are referred to as **dead space.** Other areas of lung have only **partial** embolic obstruction of their vascular supply, but normal $\dot{V}$, and are termed **high $\dot{V}/\dot{Q}$ areas.** The dead space and high $\dot{V}/\dot{Q}$ areas do not cause hypoxemia, but reduce lung efficiency in CO_2 elimination.

Most patients with PTE have hypoxemia. The hypoxemia can be severe. A few patients with PTE have totally normal oxygen tension and saturation. **In patients without underlying cardiopulmonary disease, the severity of hypoxemia correlates with extent of pulmonary vascular obstruction.** Hypoxemia is more severe in patients with preexistent heart or lung disease. One cause of hypoxemia in PTE is termed **shunt.** Shunt occurs when blood passes from the venous circulation into the arterial circulation without being exposed to alveolar gas. Large shunts cause profound hypoxemia. In PTE, shunt can occur through areas of atelectasis or areas of pulmonary infarc-

tion which receive **no ventilation** but are **still perfused.** Right atrial pressures may exceed left atrial pressures following PTE, and if a patent foramen ovale is present intracardiac shunting can occur. A second cause of hypoxemia after PTE is areas of **poor ventilation with normal or excessive perfusion.** These are termed **low $\dot{V}/\dot{Q}$ areas.** Emboli direct blood flow to nonobstructed vasculature, resulting in hyperperfusion of these areas. Blood flow rates through these hyperperfused areas may be greatly increased. The transit time of blood through these hyperperfused alveoli may be too brief to allow for adequate oxygen transfer from the alveoli to capillary blood. Reflex bronchoconstriction in areas adjacent to pulmonary emboli has also been implicated in causing low $\dot{V}/\dot{Q}$ areas in PTE.

Ventilatory Control

Hyperventilation is present in most patients with PTE. Increased respiratory drive is expected if severe hypoxemia is present, but often persists after correction of hypoxemia with supplemental oxygen. There is evidence that PTE results in stimulation of lung juxtacapillary receptors which in turn stimulate increased ventilatory drive in central nervous system centers of respiratory control.

Atelectasis

Alveolar surfactant is essential to maintain normal lung aeration. The effects of PTE can injure the type II pneumocytes which produce surfactant, resulting in areas of collapse or atelectasis.

Pulmonary Infarction

Infarction represents necrosis of the lung parenchyma and occurs only in a minority of patients with PTE. Infarction is unusual because the lung has a redundant supply of oxygen from the pulmonary arteries, bronchial arteries, and the airways. It is thought that two of these three supplies of oxygen must be compromised before infarction occurs. Infarction is more common if underlying heart or lung disease is present.

Compliance

Compliance can be defined as the amount of change in lung volume per unit of applied pressure (see Chap. 44 for more details on compliance). PTE may cause a reduction in lung compliance, particularly if atelectasis, edema, or infarction is present.

Sequelae of PTE

Many small pulmonary emboli presumably undergo complete thrombolysis with no acute or chronic effects. Larger clinically apparent emboli also often undergo complete thrombolysis, leaving no permanent pulmonary vascular abnormalities. Other emboli undergo partial thrombolysis and thrombus organization with eventual thrombus incorporation into the arterial wall covered by a new endothelial cell monolayer. Most thrombolysis occurs during the first week, but the process continues for up to 8 weeks. Thrombolysis is accelerated by the use of plasminogen-activating drugs like streptokinase, urokinase, and tissue plasminogen activator. Anticoagulation alone may also hasten thrombolysis by preventing new thrombus growth while natural fibrinolytic mechanisms work. **Clinically significant pulmonary emboli treated with appropriate medical therapy generally have minimal or no longterm health sequelae.**

A small minority of patients develop **chronic thromboembolic pulmonary hypertension following PTE.** They often present with progressive dyspnea or right heart failure without awareness of previous VTE. Angiography confirms the presence of large often multiple emboli involving the central pulmonary arteries and their principle branches. These thrombi are potentially removable via pulmonary thromboendarterectomy performed by an experienced surgeon (Fig. 50-3). This procedure may lessen pulmonary hypertension and dyspnea. **Chronic throm-**

Fig. 50-3. Large organized thromboemboli successfully removed from the right and left pulmonary arteries in a patient suffering from chronic thromboembolic pulmonary hypertension.

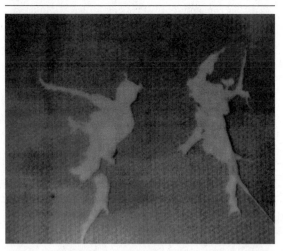

boembolic pulmonary hypertension is rare when VTE is diagnosed and treated appropriately.

Clinical Manifestations of VTE

The symptoms and signs of both DVT and PTE are very nonspecific, forcing the clinician to always remain on guard to the possibility of VTE.

Symptoms and Signs of DVT

Many patients with DVT are asymptomatic and patients hospitalized for surgery or other illnesses who develop DVT may overlook their symptoms. Patients who develop symptoms most commonly complain of pain and/or swelling of the involved extremity. Signs include tenderness, edema, increased circumference of the extremity, increased temperature of the extremity, and tender palpable cords. Less commonly, distended superficial veins, pallor, or cyanosis is seen. Homan's sign, the development of pain on dorsiflexion of the foot, is neither sensitive nor specific for DVT.

Symptoms and Signs of PTE

Many small pulmonary emboli are asymptomatic. Dyspnea and pleuritic chest pain are the most common symptoms noted. Anxiety, cough, nonpleuritic chest pain, diaphoresis, and syncope are other complaints. Hemoptysis is present in only 30% of patients with PTE. The most common signs are tachypnea and crackles on auscultation. The intensity of the second heart sound may be increased due to pulmonary hypertension. Tachycardia, fever, edema, and cyanosis can be seen. If right heart failure ensues jugular venous distention, a third heart sound, and hypotension may develop.

Diagnosis of VTE
Diagnosis of DVT

Because the history and physical examination and routine lab tests are neither specific nor sensitive in the diagnosis of VTE, other methods are used to establish or exclude its presence. The "gold standard" for the diagnosis of DVT is contrast venography. Venography is painful and can have complications, thus "noninvasive" tests like impedance plethysmography and compression ultrasonography are often used. The serial performance of these noninvasive tests accurately diagnoses or excludes DVT in outpatients presenting with symptoms suggestive of DVT. However, these noninvasive tests may be less sensitive in the diagnosis of DVT in hospitalized patients without symptoms of DVT, particularly when thrombi are confined to the iliac veins.

Diagnosis of PTE

There are several electrocardiographic patterns and chest x-ray findings suggestive of PTE, but they are present only in a small percentage of patients. Lung perfusion scanning is the most useful screening tool (Fig. 50-4). If perfusion defects are present, their size and location are compared with the chest x-ray or with a lung ventilation scan to ex-

clude the presence of corresponding radiographic or ventilation abnormalities.

A practical way to categorize perfusion scan results is normal, "high probability," or indeterminant. A normal scan excludes the presence of significant PTE. A high-probability scan shows two or more perfusion defects of significant size with no corresponding chest x-ray or ventilation scan abnormalities. A high-probability scan is considered diagnostic of PTE. Patients with indeterminant scans still have a 20–40% incidence of PTE and require further diagnostic tests. Pulmonary angiography is the definitive test for PTE (Fig. 50-5). The test is costly and uncomfortable but serious complications are uncommon. Most patients with indeterminant lung scans require angiography to exclude PTE.

Fig. 50-4. A normal lung perfusion scan is seen in (A). (B) depicts a pulmonary perfusion scan demonstrating large perfusion defects which appear as blank spaces due to the absence of perfusion.

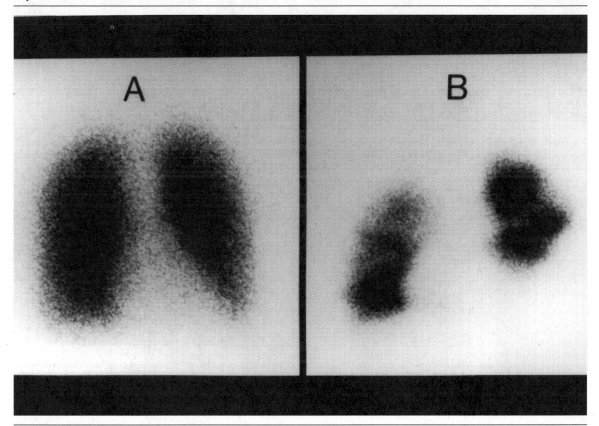

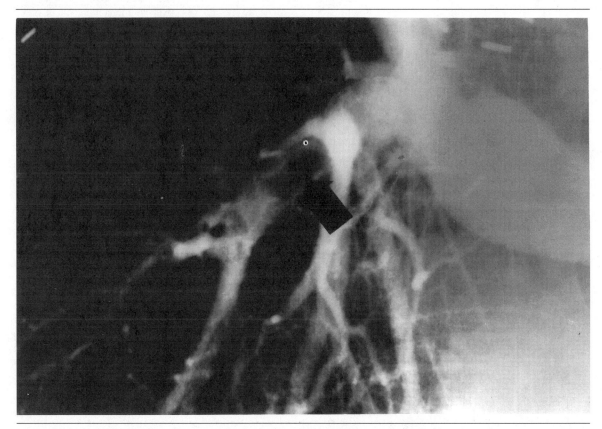

Fig. 50-5. A pulmonary angiogram showing a filling defect in a major branch of the right pulmonary artery due to a thromboembolus (see arrow).

Prophylaxis of VTE

The cost of VTE in terms of morbidity, mortality, and financial loss is tremendous. The risk factors for VTE are well known. Prophylactic measures include graduated compression stockings, subcutaneous heparin, and low-molecular-weight heparin. Consensus conference recommendations have been issued regarding appropriate prophylactic regimens for the various risk factors, but physician implementation of these preventative strategies needs improvement.

Treatment of VTE

DVT

Patients are immediately anticoagulated with a continuous infusion of intravenous heparin to achieve an activated partial probothastin time (APPT) of at least 1.5 times control values. Anticoagulation prevents further thrombus propagation, allowing unopposed thrombolysis to occur. Heparin is continued for 7–10 days. Oral anticoagulation is started with warfarin several days before the heparin is stopped and continued **for at least 3 months.** Patients with ongoing risks for VTE require longer oral anticoagulation.

PTE

Patients with PTE are also immediately anticoagulated with heparin. Patients who survive the first few hours after PTE and then succumb usually die from recurrent embolism. Anticoagulation prevents new thrombus propagation, lessening the chances of recurrent emboli. **Delays in achieving adequate APPT prolongation adversely affect outcome.** There is no good correlation between supratherapeutic APPT times during the first 48 hours and bleeding episodes. Thus when initiating heparin for PTE it is better to err on the side of excessive anticoagulation than to run the risk of inadequate anticoagulation. After several days of heparin treatment patients are started on warfarin for a minimum of 3 months. Patients with massive pulmonary emboli and resultant hypotension or severe hypoxemia are often treated with thrombolytic agents in addition to heparin to accelerate thrombolysis. The use of thrombolytic drugs in stable patients with PTE or in patients with DVT alone remains controversial.

Clinical Examples

1. A 70-year-old moderately obese female fell, suffering a fracture of the right femoral neck. She underwent an uneventful open reduction and internal fixation of the left hip and was fitted with sequential compression stockings for DVT prophylaxis. Two days later the left leg was noted to be edematous with tenderness on palpation of the leg musculature. Compression ultrasonography confirmed the presence of extensive proximal DVT. The patient had no chest pain or dyspnea and normal arterial blood gases.

Discussion.   This case illustrates a common presentation of DVT. There is no evidence of PTE, but inapparent emboli may have occurred. The risks of VTE are very high following fracture or surgery of the hip. Prophylaxis with compression stockings or subcutaneous heparin is inadequate in these patients and more potent preventative measures like low-molecular-weight heparin or warfarin are indicated.

2. A 39-year-old male with nephrotic syndrome developed a dry cough, dyspnea, and fevers. A chest x-ray revealed bilateral patchy shadows and his arterial oxygen tension was 60 mm Hg. He was admitted to the hospital with a diagnosis of pneumonia and treated with oxygen and broad spectrum antimicrobials. Extensive diagnostic tests for infectious etiologies were unrevealing. The patient developed progressive respiratory failure and was transferred to the Intensive Care Unit. Extreme hypoxemia prompted intubation and mechanical ventilation. A chest x-ray revealed bilateral pulmonary infiltrates. The patient was anticoagulated with heparin and a lung perfusion scan revealed multiple large perfusion defects. Compression ultrasonography confirmed extensive proximal DVT. Heparin anticoagulation was continued and an infusion of urokinase was given. The patient improved but 2 days later developed sudden hypotension and worsening hypoxemia.

There was no hemodynamic improvement with fluids or pressor agents and the patient expired. An autopsy revealed multiple pulmonary thromboemboli with varying degrees of organization and persistent DVT.

Discussion.   This case illustrates how VTE can resemble other diseases like pneumonia. There is an association between nephrotic syndrome and VTE. A key point is that although elevations in blood urea nitrogen (which were present in this case) adversely affect platelet function, they do not make patients immune to VTE. The use of urokinase is controversial in the absence of hypotension but was probably warranted by the severe hypoxemia and very high risk of **recurrent PTE.** Despite anticoagulation and thrombolytic treatment the probable cause of death was recurrent PTE.

3. A 79-year-old female with a history of polycythemia rubra vera complained of progressive dyspnea on exertion. She denied chest pain, leg pain, swelling, or known prior VTE. She had undergone repeated phlebotomies and had a hemoglobin of 14 g/dl. The examination revealed clear lung fields and a prominent second heart sound. A chest x-ray showed prominent central pulmonary vasculature and clear lung fields. An echocardiogram was normal. $\dot{V}/\dot{Q}$ scanning was indeterminant for the presence of PTE. Pulmonary angiography revealed several emboli involving the central pulmonary arteries. The mean pulmonary artery pressure was 60 mm Hg. The patient was treated with lifelong oral anticoagulation and periodic phlebotomies.

Discussion.   Chronic thromboembolic pulmonary hypertension is uncommon. Patients may present with dyspnea and no apparent evidence of past VTE. The patient suffered recurrent PTE despite appropriate treatment of her polycythemia rubra vera. The elevation of pulmonary artery pressure above 40 mm Hg indicates right ventricular hypertrophy compatible with recurrent embolic disease. The patient was not a candidate for pulmonary thromboendarterectomy due to advanced age but was treated with lifelong anticoagulation.

Bibliography

Andersons FA, Wheeler HB, and Goldberg RJ, et al. A population-based perspective of the hospital incidence and case-fatality rates of deep vein thrombosis and pulmonary embolism. *Arch Int Med* 151:993–938, 1991. *A recent study of the incidence and mortality of VTE in hospitalized patients. Reveals an exponential rise in VTE with age.*

Clagett GP, Anderson FA, Levine MN, et al. Prevention of venous thromboembolism. *Chest* 102:391S–407S, 1992. *Recommendations on prophylaxis for at-risk patients from a recent consensus conference.*

Diebold J and Lohrs U. Venous thrombosis and pulmonary embolism — a study of 5039 autopsies. *Path Res Pract* 187:260–266, 1991. *A large autopsy series showing a rising incidence of DVT and of catheter-related upper extremity DVT.*

Elliot CG. Pulmonary physiology during pulmonary embolism. *Chest* 101:163S–171S, 1992. *An excellent review of the pathophysiology of PTE.*

Goldhaber SZ and Morpurgo M. Diagnosis, treatment and prevention of pulmonary embolism. *JAMA* 268:1727–1733, 1991. *A review of the subject with emphasis on treatment and prophylaxis.*

Kinasewitz, GT. Thrombophlebitis and pulmonary embolism in the elderly patient. *Clin Chest Med* 14:523–536, 1993. *A comprehensive review of VTE with insight into the increased risk of VTE with age.*

Mammen, EF. Pathogenesis of venous thrombosis. *Chest* 102:640S–644S, 1992. *A cogent review of the genesis of venous thrombi.*

Moser KM. Venous thromboembolism. *Am Rev Respir Dis* 141:235–249, 1990. *A review by a leading authority emphasizing conceptual advances about VTE.*

Part VI Questions: Pulmonary Diseases

1. Which of the following situations will have the greatest effect on oxygen content?
   A. Transfusing a patient with a hemoglobin of 7 g/dl and a PaO_2 of 60 mm Hg to a hemoglobin of 10 g/dl with no change in the PaO_2
   B. Increasing the PaO_2 in a patient with a hemoglobin of 7 g/dl and a PaO_2 of 60 mm Hg to a PaO_2 of 100 mm Hg with no change in the hemoglobin
   C. Increasing the PaO_2 in a patient with a hemoglobin of 7 g/dl and a PaO_2 of 40 mm Hg to a PaO_2 of 60 mm Hg with no change in hemoglobin
   D. Tranfusing a patient with a hemoglobin of 7 g/dl to a hemoglobin of 9 g/dl and increasing the PaO_2 from 40 to 60 mm Hg
   E. Increasing the PaO_2 in a patient with a normal hemoglobin (15 g/dl) from 40 to 60 mm Hg

2. Which of the following is most consistent with a restrictive ventilatory defect?
   A. Reduced TLC and increased FEV_1/FVC ratio
   B. Reduced TLC and decreased FEV_1/FVC ratio
   C. Normal FVC and decreased FEV_1/FVC ratio
   D. A 15% increase in FEV_1 following an inhaled bronchodilator
   E. Normal FVC and FEV_1 and decreased FEF_{25-75}

3. A patient was evaluated (in Cleveland, Ohio, where barometric pressure is 747 mm Hg) for the complaint of dyspnea at rest. The respiratory rate was 35 breaths/minute. Auscultation of the chest revealed no wheezes or rales. Arterial blood was sampled, revealing a pH of 7.42; PCO_2 25 mm Hg; and PO_2 60 mm Hg (normal values: pH 7.35–7.45, PCO_2 38–42 mm Hg, PO_2 75–100 mm Hg). Which of the following statements about the patient is true?
   A. The hyperventilation and complaint of dyspnea are explained by anxiety, because there is no evidence of lung disease.
   B. The dyspnea and hyperventilation must be explained by something other than blood gas abnormalities, and there is evidence of lung disease.
   C. The dyspnea, tachypnea, and acute respiratory alkalosis are due to arterial hypoxemia.
   D. The presence or absence of a lung disorder cannot be determined from the information provided.
   E. None of the above.

4. Which of the following types of emphysema is seen in patients with homozygous α_1-antitrypsin deficiency?
   A. Centrilobular
   B. Distal acinar
   C. Panacinar
   D. Paraseptal
   E. Periacinar

5. In patients with interstitial lung disease, which makes the largest contribution to hypoxemia at rest?
   A. Diffusion abnormality
   B. Low ventilation/perfusion ($\dot{V}/\dot{Q}$) areas

6. The balance of transvascular filtration forces across the pulmonary capillary endothelium
   A. allows fluid filtration only when pulmonary capillary pressure is greater than plasma protein oncotic pressure.
   B. favors the reabsorption of fluid from the interstitial space under normal physiologic conditions.
   C. favors the filtration of fluid into the interstitial space under normal physiologic conditions.
   D. is in equilibrium (no net fluid filtration or reabsorption) under normal physiologic conditions.
   E. is reduced by positive pressure breathing leading to reduced fluid filtration.

7. Pleural effusions produce symptoms by all of the following mechanisms except
   A. compression of the lung which causes ventilation perfusion mismatching.
   B. outward displacement of the chest wall which shortens the resting position of the inspiratory muscles.
   C. stimulation of receptors in compressed lung which reflexively induce cough.
   D. stimulation of pain receptors in the parietal pleura.
   E. stimulation of pain receptors in the visceral pleura.

8. Which of the following is **not** true of venous thromboembolism (VTE)?
   A. Most pulmonary emboli arise from lower-extremity DVT.
   B. Asymptomatic pulmonary emboli are common in patients with DVT.
   C. The incidence of VTE is declining due to the use of prophylactic measures.
   D. 40–70% of pulmonary emboli noted at autopsy were unsuspected prior to death.
   E. Age is a risk factor for VTE.

VII Renal and Electrolyte Disorders

Part Editor

Chris E. Kaufman

51 Disorders of Sodium and Water Metabolism

Chris E. Kaufman

Objectives

After completing this chapter, you should be able to

Describe the volume and composition of the body fluid compartments

Predict changes in the volume and osmolality of the fluid compartments in response to gain or loss of water or saline

Explain the pathogenesis and consequences of sodium depletion

Explain the pathogenesis and consequence of excess total body sodium

Describe mechanisms which maintain normal water balance

Outline the ways in which a water deficit may occur

Explain the mechanism by which hypoosmolality may occur

Describe the consequences of hypo- and hyperosmolality

Volume and Composition of the Body Fluid Compartments

As shown in Fig. 51-1, total body water averages about 60% of body weight. Of this total, approximately two-thirds is confined to the intracellular space and one-third constitutes the extracellular compartment. The extracellular space consists of the interstitial compartment and the plasma. Sodium is the major cation and chloride and bicarbonate are the major anions in the extracellular compartment. Consequently, the concentration of sodium correlates closely with the osmolality of the extracellular fluid. The composition of the plasma and the interstitial fluid are virtually identical with the exception of the higher protein content of the plasma. In the intracellular water, potassium is the major cation and phosphate and proteins the major anions. Therefore, in the intracellular compartment, the osmolality will correspond to approximately twice the concentration of the potassium. Since cell membranes are freely permeable to water, the osmolality is

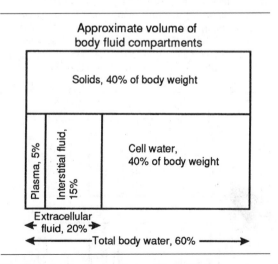

Fig. 51-1. Approximate volume of body fluid compartments in a normal adult, expressed as a percent of body weight. (Used with permission from: Kaufman CE and Papper S (eds). *Review of Pathophysiology.* Boston: Little, Brown, 1983, p. 248.)

identical (about 285 mOsm/kg) in the extracellular and the intracellular compartments.

Fluid Compartment Volume and Osmolar Changes

Understanding disorders of sodium and water metabolism depends on a clear concept of how the volume and osmolality of body fluid compartments change in response to loss or gain of sodium and water from the body (Fig. 51-2).

The addition of solute-free water to the extracellular space (Fig. 51-2A) lowers the osmolality and increases the volume of this compartment. Water then moves along an osmotic gradient into cells until the osmolality is equal in both compartments. Thus a new equilibrium is established whereby osmolality is decreased and the volume is increased in both compartments. The magnitude of these changes is proportional to the increase in total body water. Similarly, loss of solute-free water results in opposite

Fig. 51-2. Changes in volume and osmolal concentration of intracellular (I) and extracellular (E) fluids. (A) addition of water to the body; (B) addition of hypertonic salt solution; (C) addition of isotonic salt solution; and (D) loss of sodium chloride. Compartments enclosed by solid lines represent initial normal state; those enclosed by dashed lines represent the final experimental state. Height of compartment represents osmolal concentration; width represents volume. (From: Darrow DC and Yannet H. The changes in the distribution of body water accompanying increase and decrease in extracellular electrolyte. *J Clin Invest* 14:266–275, 1935. Reproduced from *The Journal of Clinical Investigation,* 1935, 14:266–275, by copyright permission of The American Society for Clinical Investigation.)

changes (decreased volume, increased osmolality) in both compartments.

The addition of a hypertonic sodium solution to the extracellular compartment (Fig. 51-2B) increases the osmolality of the extracellular fluid. Since sodium is confined to the extracellular space, water moves out of the cells along an osmotic gradient. Thus extracellular volume increases while intracellular volume decreases; both changes are proportional to the increase in osmolality of the body fluids.

When an isotonic sodium solution is added to the extracellular space (Fig. 51-2C), no osmotic gradient is generated between the extracellular and the intracellular fluid. Therefore, the increase in extracellular fluid volume is equal to the administered volume of isotonic saline. Likewise, loss of isotonic fluid from the extracellular space does not change volume or composition of the intracellular fluid compartment.

Loss of sodium without the net loss of water results in the changes depicted in Fig. 51-2D. Since sodium cannot be lost from the body without a concomitant loss of water, the changes in Fig. 51-2D generally result from the replacement of sodium-rich fluid losses with plain water. Figure 51-2D can be envisioned as the result of loss of isotonic saline (reverse of Fig. 51-2C) and the subsequent addition of an equal quantity of solute-free water (reverse of Fig. 51-2A). At equilibrium, the osmolality is decreased throughout body fluids, and the intracellular volume is increased to the same extent that extracellular volume is decreased. In effect, water moves from extracellular to intracellular compartments because of a net loss of extracellular solute (sodium).

Normal Regulation of Sodium Balance

The principal factor determining the extracellular fluid volume is the amount of sodium present in the body. Normally the extracellular fluid volume is closely regulated by the kidneys, and any tendency toward expansion of the extracellular space results in excretion of the excess sodium. Likewise, loss of sodium and contraction of the extracellular space promptly cause excretion of sodium-free urine. Since sodium is confined to the extracellular space, loss or gain of sodium will be reflected by contraction or expansion of the extracellular compartment. This occurs because change in sodium balance induces a secondary passive movement of water across cell membranes (Figs. 51-2B, 51-2D) and because of changes in total body water. As illustrated in Fig. 51-3, an increased amount of sodium in

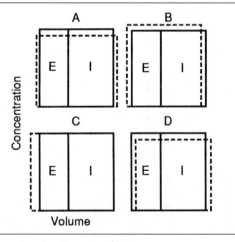

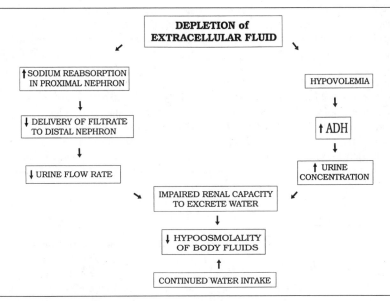

Fig. 51-3. The mechanisms by which sodium depletion and continued water intake may cause hypoosmolality of body fluids.

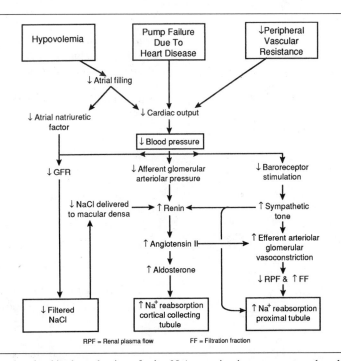

Fig. 51-4. The mechanisms involved in the reduction of urine Na⁺ excretion in response to reduced Na⁺ intake. (Reproduced with permission from: Abuelo JG. Review of normal renal physiology. In *Renal Pathophysiology — The Essentials.* Baltimore: Williams and Wilkins, 1989, p. 17.)

the extracellular space will result in positive water balance (increased total body water). This is because the increased osmolality that occurs stimulates both thirst and the secretion of antidiuretic hormone, resulting in greater water intake and less water loss.

Hence the sodium content determines the volume of the extracellular compartment, which in turn is the major factor influencing renal sodium excretion. The mechanisms by which a decrease in extracellular fluid volume leads to a reduction in renal sodium excretion are illustrated in Fig. 51-4. Alterations of these pathways are important in the pathogenesis of the abnormal sodium retention that occurs in some disease states.

Disorders of Extracellular Fluid Volume

Sodium Depletion (Contraction of Extracellular Volume)

The terms "sodium depletion" and "contraction of extracellular fluid volume" are virtually synonymous. They refer to a deficit of sodium and not to a decrease in the concentration of sodium (hyponatremia) in the extracellular field. A sodium deficit may or may not be associated with hyponatremia.

Pathogenesis
Sodium depletion results from abnormal loss of sodium-containing fluids. The potential mechanisms are listed in Table 51-1. The normal renal response to even mild sodium depletion is avid reabsorption of virtually all the filtered sodium (mechanisms outlined in Fig. 51-4). Since

Table 51-1. Mechanisms of Sodium Loss

Type	Mechanism
Urinary	Renal disease
	Diuretic therapy
	Osmotic diuresis
	Adrenal insufficiency
Gastrointestinal	Vomiting
	Diarrhea
	Drainage
Skin	Sweating
	Burns
Drainage of extracellular fluid	Peritoneal
	Pleural

normal fecal and sweat losses of sodium are minimal, inadequate sodium intake alone cannot result in significant sodium depletion. However, poor intake of salt may contribute to sodium depletion when excessive losses are also present.

Effects of Sodium Depletion
Contraction of the extracellular space results in proportional changes in the plasma and interstitial volume. The subsequent decrement in blood volume reduces cardiac output and may cause hypotension and impair tissue perfusion. The result is the constellation of hemodynamic and metabolic changes listed in Table 51-2. Of these, orthostatic hypotension and prerenal azotemia are usually the most reliable signs of a sodium deficit. It should be noted, however, that there are no specific indicators of sodium depletion. For example, orthostatic hypotension (a fall in systolic blood pressure exceeding 10 mm when changing from the supine to the standing position) may accompany any disease or drug effect which impairs the autonomic nervous system. Likewise, prerenal azotemia (an elevation of blood urea nitrogen [BUN] that is not secondary to renal disease or urinary obstruction) may result from any factor that reduces renal blood flow, including conditions as diverse as congestive heart failure and acute blood loss. The renal response is similar, regardless of the cause of renal hypoperfusion. When renal perfusion is severely impaired, the rate of glomerular filtration falls, resulting in an increase in serum creatinine concentration as well as the

Table 51-2. Effects of Sodium Depletion ($\downarrow$ Extracellular Volume)

$\downarrow$ PLASMA VOLUME $\rightarrow$ $\downarrow$ CARDIAC OUTPUT

Cardiovascular
  $\downarrow$ BP $\uparrow$ Pulse rate
  $\downarrow$ Pulse pressure
  Orthostatic hypotension
CNS: $\downarrow$ Cerebral function
Liver, muscle: "lactic acidosis"
Renal
  "Prerenal azotemia"
  $\downarrow$ Urine Na^+, volume
  $\uparrow$ Urine osmolality
  $\downarrow$ Diluting capacity ($\pm$ hyponatremia)

$\downarrow$ INTERSTITIAL VOLUME "POOR SKIN TURGOR"

HEMOCONCENTRATION

$\uparrow$ Hgb, Hct
$\uparrow$ Plasma protein concentration

BUN. Typically, however, BUN increases proportionately more than plasma creatinine as a result of the greatly enhanced tubular reabsorption of urea that occurs whenever renal perfusion is reduced. Since renal tubular sodium reabsorption is stimulated and vasopressin levels are usually high under these conditions, the normal response to depletion of the extracellular compartment (or any state of hypoperfusion) is the excretion of scanty, concentrated urine, virtually free of sodium.

An important consequence of the renal response to volume depletion is an inability to excrete a normal volume of dilute urine. Continued water intake, when coupled with this impaired water excretion, may result in dilution of body fluids and development of hyponatremia (Fig. 51-2D). However, since sodium depletion generally results from loss of hypotonic, sodium-rich fluids, hyponatremia is not a necessary feature of sodium depletion. (If net water losses exceed one liter for each 140 meq of sodium deficit, the concentration of plasma sodium will tend to rise.) Hence salt depletion can be accompanied by a normal, high or low serum sodium concentration, depending upon the patient's water balance.

Sodium Excess (Expansion of Extracellular Space)

Any tendency for expansion of the extracellular space normally results in excretion of the excess sodium via modulation of the renal control mechanisms outlined in Fig. 51-4. Failure of these mechanisms, which may result from conditions listed in Table 51-3, causes retention of sodium and water resulting in the formation of edema, which is the clinical hallmark of an expanded extracellular space.

In all of these disorders, edema results from an imbalance of the capillary Starling forces (Fig. 51-5). In renal or cardiac failure, edema results primarily from an increase in capillary hydrostatic pressure. Edema may also result from

Table 51-3. Causes of an Expanded Extracellular Space

Heart failure
Severe liver disease
Renal failure
Nephrotic syndrome

Fig. 51-5. Capillary Starling forces that influence fluid distribution between plasma and interstitial compartments. (Used with permission from: Schrier RS. *Renal and Electrolyte Disorders* (4th ed.). Boston: Little, Brown, 1992, p. 107.)

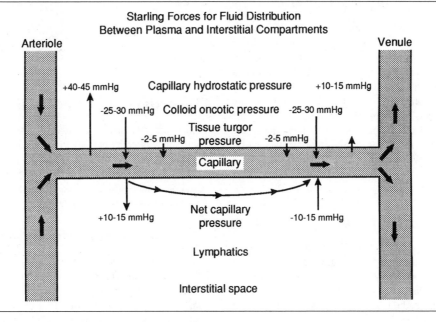

a reduced plasma oncotic pressure, (nephrotic syndrome, for example) or from the combined effects of increased hydrostatic and decreased oncotic pressure as occurs in decompensated cirrhosis. Occasionally, edema results from a damaged capillary endothelium, which leaks plasma proteins into the interstitital space (some examples of lung edema). Impairment of lymphatic drainage can also cause edema.

Normal Regulation of Water Balance

Water moves freely across cell membranes, quickly abolishing any osmotic gradient between the intracellular and the extracellular compartments. In health, the tonicity of body fluids is closely regulated to maintain a concentration of total solute of 280–290 mOsm/kg of water by adjustments in water intake (thirst) and excretion (urinary). Whereas sodium balance regulates the volume of the extracellular compartment, water balance is adjusted according to the osmolality of body fluids. The renal capacity to adjust body fluid tonicity is quite remarkable, in that normal kidneys can produce as little as 400 cc of concentrated urine or excrete as much as 10–20 liters of "solute-free water" each day as needed to regulate water balance.

Renal Concentrating Mechanism

Hypothalamic neurons secrete antidiuretic hormone (ADH) in response to elevation of body fluid osmolality or depletion of blood volume. As a result of the action of ADH, the permeability to water of the distal convoluted tubule and the collecting duct is markedly enhanced. This system provides the mechanism for water to diffuse into the hypertonic medullary interstitium as fluid traverses the distal convoluted tubule and collecting duct. Hence the presence of sufficient ADH permits normal kidneys to conserve water by excreting the daily solute load in as little as 400 ml of highly concentrated urine (up to 1200 mOsm/kg).

Renal Diluting Mechanisms

By contrast in the absence of ADH, a normal consequence of the hypotonic state, the distal tubule and collecting duct are rendered impermeable to water (Fig. 51-6). Therefore, water reaching the tip of Henle's loop does not "back-diffuse" into the medullary interstitium and is virtually all excreted in the urine. Hence water excretion can be adjusted to match intake by changes in ADH secretion.

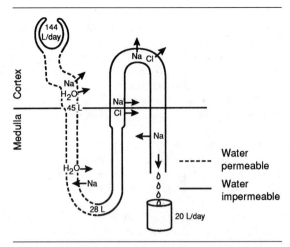

Fig. 51-6. Renal diluting mechanisms. The sites of sodium chloride and water reabsorption in the absence of antidiuretic hormone (ADH) are indicted in this composite nephron. With a glomerular filtration of 144 liters/day, approximately 45 liters of filtrate would remain at the end of the proximal tubule and 28 liters would remain at the tip of Henle's loop. In the absence of ADH very little water is reabsorbed beyond this point, and up to 20 liters of solute-free water can be excreted in the urine. (Used with permission from: Kaufman CE and Papper S (eds.). *Review of Pathophysiology.* Boston: Little, Brown, 1983, p 253.)

As noted earlier, if necessary up to 10–20 liters of solute-free water can be excreted each day to maintain water balance.

Disorders of Water Metabolism

Since water balance is normally adjusted to maintain a constant osmolality of body fluids, disorders of water metabolism are defined with reference to the osmolality. Therefore, two potential disorders exist: too much water in relation to solute (hypoosmolality) and too little water in relation to solute (hyperosmolality).

Hyperosmolality (Hypernatremia)

Since sodium is the predominant cation in the extracellular fluid, any significant increase in sodium concentration indicates hyperosmolality of the body fluids. Osmolality may also be increased owing to a high concentration of other solutes (i.e., glucose, mannitol, ethanol, etc.) in extracellular fluid. Under these circumstances, the serum sodium concentration is not necessarily increased and the hyperosmolar state must be detected by direct measurement of plasma osmolality. However, if glucose or urea are known to be the only solute present in excess, then plasma osmolality (P_{osm}) can be estimated from:

$$P_{osm} = 2 \times \text{Plasma} \left[Na^+\right] + \frac{\text{Glucose}}{18} + \frac{\text{BUN}}{2.8}$$

A distinction should be made between the effects of solutes such as sodium, mannitol, or glucose (which are confined to the extracellular spaces and therefore draw water from the cells) and urea or ethanol (which readily diffuse into cells). These diffusible solutes also raise osmolality but do not cause hypertonicity and cellular dessication.

Although hypernatremia is occasionally associated with an increased sodium content of the extracellular space, the sodium content is usually normal or low and the sodium concentration is high owing to a water deficit. Since intracellular solutes are not lost from most tissues (brain is an exception), hypernatremia causes cells to shrink (see Fig. 51-2B). Therefore, the hypernatremia state is invariably associated with a deficit of intracellular water. The total body water deficit can be estimated by assuming that the plasma sodium concentration (or osmolality) is increased in proportion to the deficit according to

$$\left[Na_{obs}\right] \times TBW_{obs} = \left[Na_N\right] \times TBW_N$$

where $[Na_{obs}]$ is observed sodium concentration, TBW_{obs} is observed total body water, $[Na_N]$ is normal sodium concentration, and TBW_N is normal total body water.

Rearranging this equation

$$TBW_{obs} = \frac{Na_N \times TBW_N}{Na_{obs}}$$

Water deficit = $TBW_N - TBW_{obs}$

Note that this method of estimating a "water deficit" does not account for sodium depletion which may coexist. Hence replacing the water deficit will correct the hypernatremia (and restore intracellular water) but repletion of extracellular volume will be incomplete if a sodium deficit is also present. (Correction of salt defects will require oral salt supplements or infusion of a quantity of isotonic saline which can only be judged by observing for the presence or absence of the items listed in Table 51-2.)

Example

Calculate the water deficit of a 70-kg man with a serum sodium = 170 meq/liter. Assume no evidence of sodium depletion. Na_N = 140 meq/liter.

$$TBW_N = 0.6 \times 70 \text{ kg} = 42 \text{ liters}$$
$$TBW_{obs} = \frac{140 \text{ meq/liter} \times 42 \text{ liters}}{170 \text{ meq/liter}} = 34.6 \text{ liters}$$

Water deficit = $42 - 34.6 = 7.4$ liters

It is apparent that since water is lost from the intracellular and extracellular spaces, the magnitude of the deficits may be substantial.

Pathogenesis of Hypernatremia

The mechanisms by which hypernatremia may occur are listed in Table 51-4. A water deficit may potentially develop from inadequate water intake or excessive water losses. Since a normal, alert adult will adjust water intake to match losses, hypernatremia (hyperosmolality) usually implies an impairment of water intake. In many patients with hypernatremia, both inadequate water intake and excessive loss are present. Hypernatremia can also result from the administration of a hypertonic sodium solution. However, since hypernatremia induces extreme thirst, the hypertonic state will not be sustained unless water intake is also impaired.

Effects of Hypernatremia

Since water is lost proportionally from all compartments and the blood volume normally constitutes one-twelfth of total body water, a pure water deficit will have little tendency to produce hypovolemia. For example, in a 70-kg man with a pure water deficit causing serum Na = 170 meq/liter, the blood volume would be reduced by 600 cc.

Calculation

To ta l H_2O deficit = 7.4 liters (see above)

$$\Delta \text{ Blood volume} = \left(\frac{1}{12}\right)(7.4) = 600 \text{cc}$$

Table 51-4. Mechanisms of Hypernatremia (Hyperosmolality)

Mechanism	Effect
Inadequate water intake	Impaired consciousness
	Impaired thirst
	Weakness, physical restraints, etc.
Excessive water (solute-free) loss	Renal losses (concentrating defect)
	Extrarenal, i.e., sweat, GI, respiratory
Addition of hypertonic sodium solution to the extracellular fluid	Hypertonic NaCl, or $NaHCO_3$
	Massive sodium ingestion

A reduction of the blood volume by 600 cc often will not be detected on clinical evaluation. Hence, with a pure water deficit, the features of a reduced blood volume (see Table 51-2) are not usually present. If these features are prominent, coexisting sodium depletion is likely.

The major consequences of water depletion are due to the effects of hypertonicity on brain function. Acute hypernatremia, whether due to addition of hypertonic saline or loss of water, results in cell shrinkage throughout the body, including the central nervous system (Fig. 51-2B).

In the brain, a change in cell size and tonicity is particularly disruptive. Not surprisingly, acute hypernatremia is often associated with encephalopathy. However, within 12–24 hours of the onset of hypernatremia, the brain can protect cell volume by generating new intracellular solute called "idiogenic osmoles" (Fig. 51-7). In experimental

Fig. 51-7. The brain in hypertonic states. In the top section, the dashed line separates the brain (exaggerated in its relative size) from the rest of the ICF. Early in hypertonic states, the brain shares the water loss incurred by the rest of ICF proportionately. Later (middle section), appearance of idiogenic osmoles (solid squares) causes the brain to expand toward its normal volume. Correction of hypertonicity by rapid replacement of water deficits (bottom section) results in brain swelling due to the extra solute. (Modified from: Feig PU. The hypertonic state. *New Engl J Med* 297:1445, 1977.)

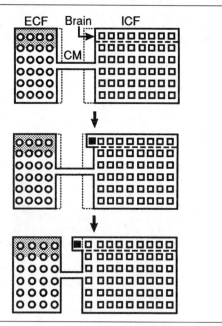

hypernatremia, this mechanism allows brain volume to return to normal within about 7 days. The development of idiogenic osmoles, although protective of cell volume during hypernatremia, will result in cell swelling if osmolality is rapidly returned toward normal. This may explain the neurologic deterioration that sometimes occurs during rapid correction of hypernatremia. These considerations suggest that in chronic hypernatremia, water replacement should be gradual, with correction in 48–72 hours.

Hypoosmolality (Hyponatremia)

Since sodium is the major cation in the extracellular fluid, hypoosmolality is invariably accompanied by hyponatremia. Although the osmolality of body fluids is usually reflected by the serum sodium concentration, one should be aware of "pseudo-hypoosmolality." This results when glucose, or any small-molecular-weight solute, is present in a high concentration in the extracellular compartment; water is drawn from the intracellular space, lowering the sodium concentration of the extracellular fluid. In this circumstance, there will be a significant discrepancy between the serum sodium concentration and the serum osmolality.

Pathogenesis of Hypoosmolality (Hyponatremia)

Hypoosmolality indicates excess water relative to the solute content of the fluid compartments. Since the intracellular solute content remains relatively constant, hyponatremia indicates generalized cell swelling. However, the volume of the extracellular space is subject to marked variation in the disease states associated with hyponatremia. Therefore, hyponatremia may be associated with an increased, decreased, or normal extracellular fluid volume and sodium content.

As described earlier (see Fig. 51-6) hypoosmolality should inhibit ADH secretion and induce renal excretion of the excess water. Therefore, the occurrence of hyponatremia implies impairment of the normal mechanisms for eliminating water. Hyponatremia will result whenever the intake of solute-free water exceeds the renal capacity to eliminate it. The disease states associated with impairment of water excretion are listed in Table 51-5.

A useful clinical approach is to classify causes of hyponatremia according to a clinical assessment of extracellular volume. All of the causes of either sodium depletion or volume expansion discussed above (Disorders of Extracellular Fluid Volume) may be associated with hyponatremia. Hyponatremia may also be associated with an approximately normal extracellular fluid volume (Table 51-6). In this circumstance, the total body sodium content

Table 51-5. Causes of Impaired Water Excretion

Hypovolemia (including sodium depletion)
Drugs (thiazide diuretics and many agents that affect CNS)
Endocrine disorders (deficiency of aldosterone, cortisol, or thyroxin)
Congestive heart failure
Hepatic cirrhosis
Renal failure
Emotional and physical stress
Positive pressure ventilation
Syndrome of inappropriate ADH secretion

Table 51-6. Causes of Hyponatremia with an Apparently Normal Extracellular Fluid Volume

Hypothyroidism
Drugs
Positive pressure ventilation
Pain, emotional stress
Syndrome of inappropriate ADH secretion

is also approximately normal. Therapy of hyponatremia follows logically. Sodium depletion requires repletion; otherwise, restriction of water intake and treatment of the underlying cause are the basic elements of management.

Effects of Hypoosmolality (Hyponatremia)

The effects of hyponatremia are due to the resultant increase in brain water. Acute hyponatremia, developing in hours, produces more severe brain swelling than does chronic hyponatremia. Animal experiments have shown that an adaptive loss of solute occurs in brain cells which are chronically exposed to a low osmolality. If solute loss is proportional to the fall in osmolality, little or no brain edema occurs. The major clinic features of hyponatremia are listed in Table 51-7. Most, if not all, can be attributed to the increased brain water.

Table 51-7. Effects of Hyponatremia

Nausea and vomiting
Confusion
Lethargy
Stupor
Coma
Seizures

Clinical Examples

1. A 72-year-old woman is brought to the hospital from a nursing home because she is lethargic and refused to drink fluids. On admission, her blood pressure is 100/60, the pulse is 110/minute, and her skin turgor is poor. Laboratory testing reveals BUN 100 mg/dl, sodium 170 meq/liter, potassium 4.0 meq/liter, Cl 124 meq/liter, CO_2 24 meq/liter, and serum creatinine 2.5 mg/dl. Urinalysis shows a specific gravity of 1.030; no protein, glucose, or acetone is present. Urine sodium is 5 meq/liter and urine osmolality 726 mOsm/kg. She weighs 60/kg.

Discussion. This patient demonstrates severe hyperosmolality of body fluids, due to inadequate water intake. The water deficit is approximately 6.4 liters. Of this deficit, approximately 1/3 or 2 liters were lost from the extracellular space, and 2/3 or 4 liters were lost from cell water.

$$TBW_N = 0.6\,(60kg) = 36 \text{ liters}$$
$$TBW_{obs} = \frac{140 \text{ meq/liter }(36 \text{ liters})}{170 \text{ meq/liter}} = 29.6 \text{ liters}$$
Water deficit = 36 liters = 6.4 liters

Since there was no evidence of expansion of extracellular fluid volume and no evidence of sodium loss, the sodium content of the extracellular space is probably close to normal. Furthermore, since about 2 liters of water was lost from the ECF (see above), significant sodium depletion is unlikely, because a further contraction of ECF volume would have induced circulatory collapse (shock).

2. A 42-year-old woman with chronic renal disease is seen on return to the Nephrology Clinic. She complains of nausea and vomiting for about one week. She appears chronically and acutely ill. Blood pressure is 118/90 supine, 90/60 standing. She weighs 64 kg. The neck veins are flat; there is no edema. The remainder of the physical exam is unremarkable. Review of the record reveals that 3 weeks previously she was feeling well. Her blood pressure then was 138/86 supine and 134/88 standing. She weighed 63 kg on that visit.

Blood Chemistries

	Three weeks ago	This visit
Na^+	139 meq/liter	116 meq/liter
K^+	5.5 meq/liter	3.9 meq/liter
HCO_3^-	20 meq/liter	15 meq/liter
Cl^-	105 meq/liter	94 meq/liter

BUN	29 mg/dl	56 mg/dl
Glucose	104 mg/dl	111 mg/dl
Hemoglobin	10.4 gm/dl	11.1 gm/dl

Discussion. The history of vomiting coupled with the reduction in blood pressure, orthostatic hypotension, and worsening azotemia indicated depletion of extracellular fluid volume. The presence of hypoosmolality indicates that continued water intake coupled with impairment of water excretion, from depletion of ECFV, resulted in dilution of body fluids. The increase in weight indicates an increase in total body water. Therefore, the decrease in extracellular volume must have been accompanied by a greater increase in intracellular fluid volume. (Figure 51-2D schematizes this situation.) Correction of the sodium depletion would best be achieved by an intravenous infusion of 0.9% sodium chloride (154 meq/liter). After sufficient saline is given, the signs of extracellular fluid volume depletion and the hyponatremia will resolve.

Bibliography

Bichet DG, Anderson RJ, and Schrier RW. Renal sodium excretion, edematous disorders, and diuretic use. In Schrier RW (ed.). *Renal and Electrolyte Disorders* (4th ed.). Boston: Little, Brown, 1992, pp. 89–160. *An insightful review of normal sodium homeostasis and disorders of sodium balance.*

Epstein M and Perez GO. Pathophysiology of the edema-forming states. In Narins RG (ed.). *Maxwell & Kleeman's Clinical Disorders of Fluid and Electrolyte Metabolism* (5th ed.). New York: McGraw-Hill, 1994, pp. 523–544. *A contemporary and comprehensive review of edematous disorders. This textbook is the ultimate source for disorders of fluid and electrolyte metabolism.*

Feig PU. The hypertonic state. *New Engl J Med* 297:1445, 1977. *The classic review article on hypertonicity.*

Rose BD. Introduction to renal function. In Rose BD (ed.). *Clinical Physiology of Acid-Base and Electrolyte Disorders* (4th ed.). New York: McGraw-Hill, 1994, Chap. 1, pp. 3–19. *A very complete and lucid description of normal and abnormal water homeostasis.*

Rose BD. *Clinical Physiology of Acid-Base and Electrolyte Disorders* (4th ed.). New York: McGraw-Hill, 1994. *This is an excellent source for explanation of any disorder of fluid-electrolyte homeostasis.*

52 Disorders of Potassium Homeostasis

Satish Kumar

Objectives

After completing this chapter, you should be able to

Understand normal regulation of potassium homeostasis

Define hypo- and hyperkalemia and distinguish each from changes in total body potassium

Outline potential mechanisms which may cause hypokalemia

Outline potential mechanisms of hyperkalemia

Describe the clinical and electrocardiographic consequences of hypokalemia and hyperkalemia

Explain the rationale and principles of treatment for hypo- and hyperkalemia

Background: Normal Physiology

Potassium Content and Distribution

Potassium is the most abundant cation in the human body. It is located predominantly inside the cells at a concentration of 150 meq/liter, while the extracellular and plasma concentration is 3.5–5.0 meq/liter. In a normal adult male, intracellular potassium content is 3500 meq and the extracellular content is only about 50 meq.

Function of Potassium

Potassium has several important functions in the body. The intracellular to extracellular potassium gradient is of major importance in maintenance of resting cell membrane potential, and is hence critical to cardiac and neuromuscular electrical activity. The abundant pool of intracellular potassium is necessary for maintenance of osmolality and hence the volume of body cells. In addition, optimal concentrations of potassium are essential for enzymatic reactions that regulate protein synthesis, growth, and metabolic processes in the cells. Hence it is important for the body to have

mechanisms to regulate potassium content in the body as a whole, and in both the extracellular and the intracellular compartments.

Potassium Homeostasis

Potassium homeostasis involves an external balance related to potassium intake and excretion and an internal balance related to distribution of potassium between the intracellular and extracellular compartments of the body.

External Balance
The average American adult ingests about 100 meq of potassium daily. In a steady state, an equal amount is excreted daily; 90 meq in the urine and 10 meq in the stool. In patients with renal failure, reduction in urinary excretion increases the importance of bowel excretion of potassium for the maintenance of the external balance (Fig. 52-1).

Renal Handling of Potassium.
Potassium is freely filtered at the glomerulus. The proximal tubule reabsorbs 50–60% of the filtered load of potassium passively via a

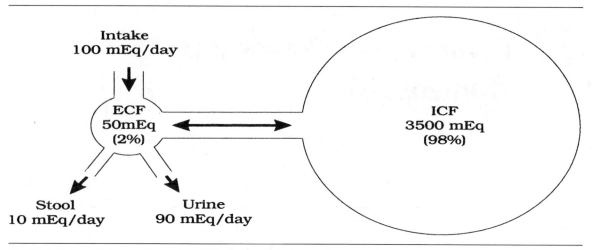

Fig. 52-1. External balance of potassium. ICF = intracellular fluid; ECF = extracellular fluid.

convective process driven by the active absorption of sodium, bicarbonate, glucose, and amino acids. Another 30–40% of the filtered potassium is reabsorbed in the loop of Henle by the Na-K-2Cl cotransporter in an energy-dependent process, and the remainder is reabsorbed in the distal convoluted tubule by H-K-ATPase in another energy-dependent mechanism. Tubular fluid reaching the collecting duct is essentially free of potassium and all the potassium that appears in urine is actually **secreted** in the collecting duct via potassium channels passively along its concentration gradient. The collecting duct is the major regulatory site of potassium excretion, and the major regulating factor is the hormone aldosterone.

Factors Affecting Renal Handling of Potassium

1. Intracellular potassium content. An increase in potassium concentration in the renal tubular cells results in increased potassium secretion. Conversely, a decrease in intracellular potassium concentration results in decreased potassium secretion. Factors that affect intracellular potassium concentration such as potassium intake, pH, catecholamines, and insulin are discussed below.
2. Urinary flow rate. Potassium secretion in the collecting duct varies directly with urinary flow rate. This phenomenon partially accounts for the increased potassium excretion seen with infusion of saline or with the use of diuretics that act proximal to the collecting duct.

3. Aldosterone. Aldosterone and other mineralocorticoids act on the distal convoluted tubule and the collecting duct to increase potassium excretion. Aldosterone acts by three mechanisms:
   a. It increases sodium channels in the luminal membrane, and hence stimulates sodium reabsorption and makes the lumen more electronegative.
   b. It activates Na-K-ATPase on the basolateral side of the cell and thereby increases intracellular potassium concentration.
   c. It increases the number of potassium channels in the luminal membrane.
4. Distal delivery of sodium. Potassium secretion is directly proportional to the distal delivery of sodium. This is an additional mechanism for the potassium excretion seen with diuretics in addition to the increase in urinary flow rate.

The above factors often act in combination to have additive or mutually opposing effects on net potassium excretion.

Internal Balance

The substantial potassium concentration gradient across the cell membrane is maintained largely by the action of the sodium-potassium pump (Na-K-ATPase). This enzyme is situated in the cell membrane and actively pumps potassium into the cell and sodium out of the cell in an energy-dependent process. Since the intracellular potassium concentration is several times higher than that in the extracellular fluid, factors that affect this equilibrium, even a little, can produce significant changes in the plasma concentration of potassium. These factors are not completely understood. They include the following.

Acid-Base Status.   In general, plasma potassium concentration rises with acidosis and falls with alkalosis. In acidemia, plasma H^+ concentration rises, H^+ ions move into cells, and K^+ moves out to maintain electroneutrality. A reverse process occurs in alkalosis. Transcellular shifts in potassium are less marked with organic acidosis than with mineral acidosis, with respiratory acidosis than with metabolic acidosis, and with chronic acidosis compared with acute acidosis.

Plasma Tonicity.   Increased tonicity of extracellular fluid increases plasma potassium concentration, probably because the increased tonicity pulls water out of cells and raises intracellular potassium concentration, causing passive diffusion of potassium out of cells.

Hormones

1. Insulin stimulates the activity of Na-K-ATPase and increases the uptake of potassium by muscle, liver, and fat cells.
2. Catecholamines: Alpha-adrenergic receptor stimulation causes release of potassium from cells and beta-adrenergic stimulation causes net influx into the cells via alterations in the activity of Na-K-ATPase. Beta-blockers, such as propranolol, impair cellular uptake of potassium and can contribute to hyperkalemia.
3. Glucagon, growth hormone, and glucocorticoids can affect potassium in pharmacologic doses but are not thought to have a major effect in physiologic concentrations.
4. Aldosterone stimulates potassium excretion in the distal nephron but also stimulates potassium influx into cells.
5. Exercise: Potassium moves out of cells in response to exercise. ATP depletion causes opening of ATP-dependent potassium channels and decreased activity of the Na-K-ATPase pump.

Hypokalemia

Definition

Hypokalemia is defined as a serum potassium less than 3.5 meq/liter. Hypokalemia usually occurs in concert with

potassium depletion but can occur even with normal total body potassium content due to excessive shift of potassium from extracellular to the intracellular compartment. Alternatively, serum potassium can remain normal or high in spite of total body potassium depletion due to shift of potassium out of the cells.

Causes of Hypokalemia

Potassium Redistribution

Potassium can be translocated into the cells without altering total body stores. Patients with severe alkalosis transfer H^+ out of cells as part of a buffering response to minimize the rise in extracellular pH; electroneutrality is then maintained in part by potassium entry into cells. When extreme stress is placed on the body, such as with acute myocardial infarction, a catecholamine surge ensues, which stimulates beta-adrenergic receptors and causes an intracellular shift of potassium. Insulin administration also causes an intracellular shift of potassium. These effects form the basis of treatment of **hyperkalemia** with intravenous sodium bicarbonate or insulin or with inhaled beta-adrenergic stimulants (Table 52-1). Rare causes of redistribution-induced hypokalemia include hypokalemic periodic paralysis (in

Table 52-1. Causes of Hypokalemia

POTASSIUM REDISTRIBUTION

Alkalosis
Insulin therapy
Beta-agonist therapy
Familial hypokalemic periodic paralysis
Treatment of megaloblastic anemia
Barium poisoning

POTASSIUM DEPLETION

Impaired potassium intake
Increased gastrointestinal loss
    Diarrhea
    Laxative abuse
Increased urinary loss
    Diuretics
    Vomiting
    Primary or secondary hyperaldosteronism
    Renal tubular acidosis
    Magnesium depletion
    Bartter's syndrome
    Polyuria

POTASSIUM DEPLETION WITHOUT HYPOKALEMIA

Diabetic ketoacidosis
Chronic renal failure

---

which a calcium channel is abnormally permeable to calcium and increased intracellular calcium secondarily decreases potassium efflux), treatment of megaloblastic anemia with vitamin B_{12} or folate (in which rapid production of new red cells results in the uptake of potassium from the extracellular fluids), and poisoning with barium salts (which blocks potassium channels in cell membranes).

Hypokalemia with Potassium Depletion

Poor Intake.   Poor dietary intake is only rarely the sole cause of hypokalemia but can occur in the setting of chronic starvation, for instance, anorexia nervosa, dementia, alcoholism, and fad diets. Common American diets contain about 100 meq potassium per day. The kidney has a good ability to conserve potassium. However, some losses of potassium continue even on a potassium-free diet (about 10–20 meq/day). Hence dietary deficiency of potassium can become clinically important if it is especially prolonged or if it is associated with abnormal potassium loss.

Gastrointestinal Loss.   All gastrointestinal secretions contain some potassium. Diarrhea can result in sufficient potassium loss to cause severe hypokalemia. With vomiting or nasogastric suction, direct potassium losses in the gastric juice are small but larger amounts of potassium are lost in urine due to the effect of alkalosis on renal potassium excretion. Alkalosis raises intracellular potassium and hence stimulates increased renal excretion in the collecting duct.

Renal Loss.   All the potassium appearing in the urine is secreted in the cortical collecting duct. This secretion is increased by increased sodium reabsorption, increased urinary flow rate, and increased aldosterone levels. The conditions that cause hypokalemia due to excessive urinary loss of potassium can be identified by measuring urine potassium. A urinary excretion of > 25 meq/day in the presence of hypokalemia suggests excessive urinary loss of potassium.

1. Diuretics. Diuretics are perhaps the most common cause of hypokalemia. All types of diuretics except potassium-sparing diuretics have been associated with hypokalemia. The hypokalemia associated with diuretics is due to several factors:
   a. increased delivery of sodium to the collecting duct
   b. hyperaldosteronism induced by volume depletion
   c. hypomagnesemia associated with loop diuretics (see below for mechanism of hypokalemia secondary to hypomagnesemia)

Urine potassium concentration is high immediately after the diuretic dose but may be low if measured several hours later, when the diuretic effect has worn off, due to the coincidental volume depletion and hypokalemia. Hypokalemia seen with diuretics is dose-dependent.

2. Other drugs causing urinary loss. A number of other drugs besides diuretics have been associated with hypokalemia. These include the penicillins (that act as osmotic diuretics and as nonreabsorbable anions stimulating potassium secretion in collecting duct), amphotericin, gentamicin, cisplatinum (hypokalemia partly due to the associated hypomagnesemia), levodopa, and lithium. The cellular mechanisms involved in these drug effects have not been studied extensively.

3. Mineralocorticoid excess. Aldosterone and other mineralocorticoids increase potassium secretion in the collecting duct by mechanisms described earlier. Both primary (adrenal adenoma or hyperplasia) and secondary (heart failure, hepatic cirrhosis, renovascular hypertension) causes of hyperaldosteronism can lead to hypokalemia (Table 52-2). Bartter's syndrome is an unusual condition in which the primary defect is lack of absorption of sodium and chloride in the thick ascending limb of Henle's loop. The resultant hypovolemia leads to hyperreninemia and to hyperaldosteronism.

4. Vomiting or nasogastric suction. Removal of gastric acid by vomiting or nasogastric suction leads to elevation of plasma bicarbonate and hence of the filtered bicarbonate load in the kidney. The excess bicarbonate acts as a nonreabsorbable anion in the collecting duct, making the lumen electronegative and stimulating increased secretion of potassium.

5. Hypomagnesemia. Hypomagnesemia is often associated with hypokalemia. Some conditions such as cisplatinum nephrotoxicity or hyperaldosteronism can cause

Table 52-2. Causes of Mineralocorticoid Excess

PRIMARY HYPERALDOSTERONISM
Adrenal adenoma
Bilateral adrenal hyperplasia
SECONDARY HYPERALDOSTERONISM
Congestive heart failure
Cirrhosis
Renovascular hypertension
CUSHING'S SYNDROME
EXOGENOUS MINERALOCORTICOID
Licorice ingestion

simultaneous loss of both potassium and magnesium. In addition, hypomagnesemia itself stimulates potassium secretion by stimulating aldosterone release and by directly activating potassium channels in the luminal membrane of the collecting duct.

6. Polyuria. The kidney's capacity to conserve potassium in face of hypokalemia is not perfect. Normal subjects, when kept on a potassium-free diet, continue to excrete about 5–10 mmol of potassium per liter of urine. These modest concentrations of potassium can add up to become substantial if the urine volume is very high, as in the polyuric states.

Potassium Depletion without Hypokalemia

In diabetic ketoacidosis and chronic renal failure, total body potassium depletion can exist with a normal or increased plasma potassium due to shift of potassium out of the cells.

Consequences of Hypokalemia

Major manifestations of hypokalemia involve the kidney and excitable tissues such as heart, nerves, and muscle.

Renal Effects

Hypokalemia typically causes loss of urine concentrating ability, increased ammonia generation, and increased excretion of hydrogen ions and phosphate. Severe chronic hypokalemia causes structural tubulointerstitial changes of vacuolization, disorganized cellular hypertrophy, and fibrosis.

Neuromuscular Effects

Hypokalemia increases the potassium concentration gradient across the cell membrane resulting initially in hyperpolarization of the cell membrane. The hyperpolarization opens sodium channels, leading to an influx of sodium into cells, causing net depolarization. These changes manifest clinically as weakness in skeletal muscles and adynamic ileus in the gastrointestinal tract.

Cardiovascular Effects

The cardiac effects of hypokalemia include delayed repolarization and rhythm disturbances. Supraventricular and ventricular tachyarrhythmias and ectopy are common (Fig. 52-2). The EKG may show flattening of the T-wave and prominence of U-waves, indicating disturbed repolarization. Myocardial contractility may also be decreased. Chronic severe hypokalemia may cause structural changes such as myocardial necrosis and fibrosis.

Metabolic Effects

Hypokalemia inhibits the release of insulin, resulting in glucose intolerance. Secretion of growth hormone, renin, and aldosterone is also inhibited by hypokalemia.

Estimation of Potassium Deficit

The severity of hypokalemia is roughly proportional to the degree of total body potassium deficit as shown in Table 52-3.

Diagnosis

In most patients the cause of hypokalemia is readily apparent from the history since the two most common causes of hypokalemia are diuretic usage and gastrointestinal loss from vomiting or diarrhea. Measurement of urinary potassium helps distinguish renal loss of potassium (> 25 meq/day) from extra-renal loss (< 25 meq/day).

Treatment

Hypokalemia usually develops slowly and, in the absence of life-threatening manifestations, can be treated by oral potassium supplements. Potassium chloride is generally more effective than other potassium salts such as bicarbonate, gluconate, citrate, or phosphate in replenishing potassium stores. This is because the common causes of hypokalemia — diuretic use, vomiting, and diarrhea — cause a simultaneous deficiency of chloride. Moreover, gluconate and citrate are metabolized to bicarbonate. Bicarbonate and phosphate can act as nonreabsorbable anions in the collecting duct, obligating more potassium secretion. In certain situations, however, when potassium deficiency is combined with deficiency of an anion other than chloride, potassium replacement can be advised with salts other than potassium chloride. For instance, in diabetic ketoacidosis, potassium phosphate may be used or, in renal tubular acidosis, potassium bicarbonate can be used. Fruits contain substantial quantities of potassium but the potassium in fruits is present in combination with organic anions that might function as nonreabsorbable anions in the collecting duct. Hence fruits might not be very effective in correcting hypokalemia. Salt substitutes contain substantial potassium (50–65 meq/teaspoon) and provide an effective, inexpensive option for preventing or correcting hypokalemia. Intravenous therapy is needed if oral replacement is not possible or if cardiac arrhythmias or neuromuscular paralysis exist. Intravenous potassium therapy carries a risk of hyperkalemia and of local phlebitis. Doses higher than 10 meq/hour require EKG monitoring and the use of a central vein for infusion. Saline solutions are preferred to dextrose because the latter stimulates insulin secretion that tends to shift potassium into the cell and can transiently worsen the hypokalemia.

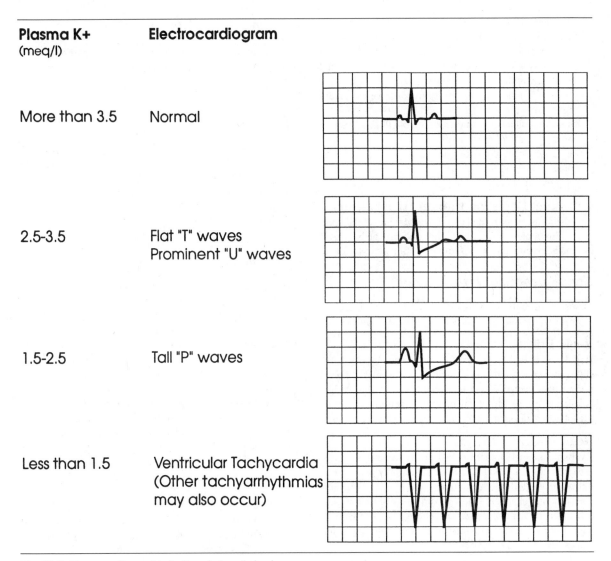

Plasma K+ (meq/l)	Electrocardiogram
More than 3.5	Normal
2.5–3.5	Flat "T" waves Prominent "U" waves
1.5–2.5	Tall "P" waves
Less than 1.5	Ventricular Tachycardia (Other tachyarrhythmias may also occur)

Fig. 52-2. Electrocardiographic findings in hypokalemia.

Table 52-3. Estimate of Potassium Deficit from Serum Potassium

Serum Potassium (meq/liter)	Total Body Potassium Deficit (meq)
3.0	100
2.5	300
2.0	500
1.5	700
1.0	1,000

Hyperkalemia

Definition

Hyperkalemia is defined as a serum potassium exceeding 5.5 meq/liter. Unless potassium is given very rapidly, the body has a fairly good capacity to handle a potassium load by shifting potassium into cells and by increasing potassium excretion in urine and stool. Hence hyperkalemia usually signifies rapid entry of potassium into the extracellular compartment and/or impaired excretion.

Causes of Hyperkalemia

Pseudohyperkalemia

Pseudohyperkalemia refers to those disorders in which a high serum potassium concentration is due to release of potassium from cells during or after drawing of the blood specimen (Table 52-4). Hemolysis due to traumatic blood drawing is the most frequent cause of this problem. Some potassium is also released from blood cells during the act of blood clotting. Hence serum potassium is usually slightly (0.1–0.5 meq/liter) higher than plasma potassium but this effect can be substantial if the white cell count is more than 100,000/mm^3 or if the platelet count is more than 400,000/mm^3. The diagnosis of pseudohyperkalemia in these settings can be made by demonstrating that the potassium concentration is normal in a nonhemolyzed plasma sample.

True Hyperkalemia

Redistribution.   Insulin and epinephrine promote the transfer of potassium into cells by stimulating the activity of Na-K-ATPase. Hence insulin deficiency or beta-blockade can lead to an increase in plasma potassium concentration. Hypertonicity and acute acidosis cause hyperkalemia by mechanisms mentioned earlier. Massive cell breakdown (as seen with rhabdomyolysis, trauma, or cell lysis follow-

Table 52-4. Causes of Hyperkalemia

PSEUDOHYPERKALEMIA
Hemolyzed blood specimen
Prolonged use of tourniquet
Leukocytosis
Thrombocytosis

TRUE HYPERKALEMIA
Redistribution
   Insulin deficiency
   Hypertonicity
   Drugs (beta-blockers, digitalis, succinylcholine)
   Acute metabolic acidosis
   Tissue/cell breakdown
   Exercise
   Hyperkalemic periodic paralysis
Increased potassium load
   Oral or intravenous
Decreased potassium secretion
   Renal failure
   Decreased mineralocorticoids
   Disorders of distal tubule
   Drugs: K-sparing diuretics

ing chemotherapy for leukemia and lymphoma) releases potassium from the damaged cells and can lead to acute, life-threatening hyperkalemia. Less commonly, hyperkalemia can be seen with prolonged exercise and certain drugs such as digitalis and succinylcholine that shift potassium out of cells. Hyperkalemic periodic paralysis is a rare condition in which the sodium channel is excessively permeable to sodium ions. Entry of sodium depolarizes the cell, leading to potassium efflux.

Increased Intake.   Hyperkalemia due to an intravenous or oral load is usually transient unless renal potassium excretion is concomitantly reduced. A rapid intravenous potassium load, however, can cause fatal hyperkalemia. Such hyperkalemia can occur in infants given a large intravenous dose of potassium-penicillin or exchange transfusion with stored blood.

Decreased Potassium Excretion.   The secretion of potassium in the collecting duct is dependent upon adequate delivery of fluid, availability of aldosterone, and normal functioning of collecting duct cells. Thus hyperkalemia from decreased urinary excretion can be caused by decreased flow rate, hypoaldosterone states, and almost any renal disease that impairs tubular function. Renal failure from any cause, especially if oliguric, may result in hyperkalemia directly from the reduced number of functioning nephrons. Hyperkalemia is common in acute renal failure. In chronic renal failure, however, there is compensatory increase in potassium excretion in the surviving nephrons and in the gut, and hyperkalemia is unusual till the glomerular filtration rate falls below 20 ml/minute. Aldosterone deficiency (Table 52-5) may result from direct impairment of aldosterone secretion such as in

Table 52-5. Causes of Hypoaldosteronism

Decreased renin-angiotensin activity (low renin, low aldosterone)
   Hyporeninemic hypoaldosteronism (type IV renal tubular acidosis)
   Drugs: NSAIDs, ACE inhibitors, beta-blockers, cyclosporine
Direct suppression of aldosterone synthesis (high renin, low aldosterone)
   Addison's disease
   Congenital adrenal hyperplasia
   Drugs: heparin
Aldosterone resistance (high renin, high aldosterone)
   Pseudohypoaldosteronism

Addison's disease (physical destruction of the adrenal gland) or in heparin-induced inhibition of aldosterone synthesis. Since aldosterone synthesis is stimulated by angiotensin, any of the causes of decreased renin-angiotensin activity such as hyporeninemic hypoaldosteronism (Type IV renal tubular acidosis), or drugs that suppress aldosterone synthesis (such as angiotensin-converting enzyme inhibitors, nonsteroidal anti-inflammatory drugs, cyclosporine, or beta-blockers) can contribute to hyperkalemia. Hyporeninemic hypoaldosteronism is said to account for 50–75% of initially unexplained hyperkalemia in adults. It is usually associated with diabetes mellitus or obstructive uropathy.

Pseudohypoaldosteronism is a syndrome in which aldosterone levels are normal but there is end-organ resistance to aldosterone due to tubular injury. This situation is seen primarily in tubulointerstitial diseases such as obstructive uropathy, interstitial nephritis, and amyloidosis. The aldosterone-antagonist spironolactone directly inhibits the actions of aldosterone. The other potassium-sparing diuretics (amiloride and triamterene) inhibit the sodium channel in the luminal membrane, leading to decreased sodium absorption and consequently decreased potassium secretion.

Clinical Features

Although hyperkalemia is defined as a serum potassium greater than 5.5 meq/liter, patients are usually asymptomatic until the plasma potassium concentration is above 6.5–7.0 meq/liter. Since the level of extracellular potassium is critical to maintaining the normal excitability of cell membranes, the major consequences of hyperkalemia are referable to excitable tissue such as myocardium and skeletal muscle.

Cardiovascular Effects. Cardiac arrhythmias are the most serious and life-threatening complication of hyperkalemia. Bradyarrhythmias are more common than tachyarrhythmias. Hyperkalemia induces distinct changes in the EKG (Fig. 52-3). The earliest change is the characteristic peaked T-wave. Other changes include flattening of P-waves, prolongation of the PR interval, and widening of the QRS complex. Ultimately, ventricular fibrillation or asystole may occur.

Muscle Weakness. Hyperkalemia decreases the potassium concentration gradient across the cell membrane, which tends to depolarize the membrane, but this small effect is offset by a larger hyperpolarization effect owing to inactivation of sodium channels. Muscle weakness becomes apparent only with severe hyperkalemia (> 8.0 meq/liter).

Metabolic Effects. Other effects of hyperkalemia include increased release of insulin, glucagon, aldosterone, and prostaglandins.

Diagnosis

Determining the cause of hyperkalemia in a given patient consists first of excluding pseudohyperkalemia from a hemolyzed blood specimen or from a very high white cell or platelet count. Conditions leading to excessive intake (enteral or intravenous) can usually be identified from the history and conditions causing shift of potassium should be apparent from the clinical setting. Once pseudohyperkalemia, excessive intake, and cellular shift are excluded, most cases of hyperkalemia are due to renal failure or reduced aldosterone effect. Renal failure is easily excluded by measuring plasma creatinine. Plasma renin and aldosterone levels can help distinguish various causes of reduced aldosterone effect (Table 52-5).

Treatment

Patients with mild hyperkalemia can be treated conservatively by reducing potassium intake and by discontinuing any drugs that may be interfering with potassium homeostasis (Table 52-6). More aggressive therapy should be initiated if plasma potassium concentration rises acutely above 6.0 meq/liter or if EKG changes are present. It should be remembered that fatal hyperkalemia can occur with a minimal or no elevation in total body potassium content. Drugs effective in hyperkalemia can act by three different mechanisms:

Antagonism of Effects of Potassium at Cell Membrane

Infusion of calcium opposes the effects of hyperkalemia on the myocardial cell membrane without changing the plasma potassium concentration. Calcium effect begins within minutes but persists only for 30–60 minutes after a single intravenous dose.

Transfer of Potassium into Cells

Sodium bicarbonate and insulin reduce hyperkalemia by causing movement of potassium into cells. Sodium bicarbonate acts via its ability to raise the blood pH, hence affecting the transcellular exchange of H^+ and K^+ ions. Insulin promotes potassium movement into cells by stimulating the Na-K-ATPase pump. It is usually necessary to administer glucose with the insulin to avoid hypoglycemia. A reduction in plasma potassium concentration is typically observed within 30–60 minutes and lasts 4–8 hours.

Plasma K+	Electrocardiogram	
Less than 5.5	Normal	
5.5 - 6.5	Peaked "T" waves	
6.5 - 8.0	Flat "P" waves Prolongs "PR" interval Widened "QRS" complex Deep "S" wave	
More than 8.0	Sine-wave (Proceeds to asystole)	

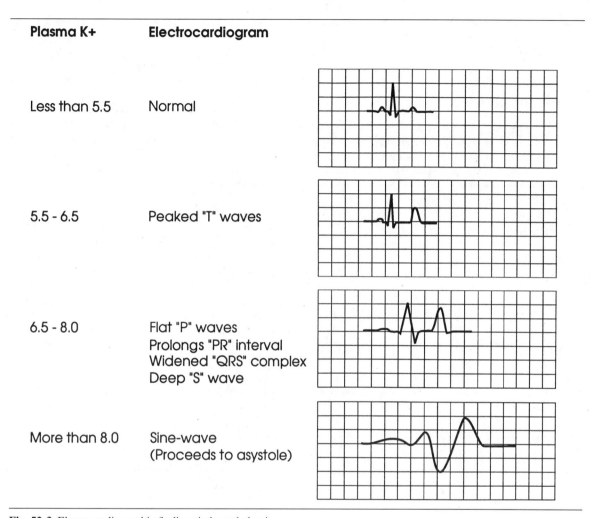

Fig. 52-3. Electrocardiographic findings in hyperkalemia.

Removal of Potassium from Body

The use of calcium, sodium bicarbonate, and insulin are only temporizing measures. Ultimately, potassium must be removed from the body to prevent return of the plasma potassium concentration to pretreatment levels. The kidney and gut are the only significant excretory pathways for potassium. Renal excretion of potassium can be increased by diuretics or mineralocorticoids. Many cases of hyperkalemia, however, occur in patients with complete renal failure; hence elimination of potassium through the kidney may not be possible. In such patients, potassium may be removed via the gut by using the sodium-potassium cation

Table 52-6. Treatment of Hyperkalemia

Disorder	Treatment
Membrane effects	Calcium
Potassium redistribution	Insulin
	Sodium bicarbonate
	Beta-adrenergic agents
	Diuretics
	Mineralocorticoids, e.g., fludrocortisone
Potassium removal	Cation exchange resins
	Dialysis

exchange resin "Kayexalate," given orally or as a retention enema. Alternatively, peritoneal- or hemo-dialysis can be performed to remove potassium.

Clinical Examples

1. A 25-year-old woman with no previous history of medical illness was brought to the emergency room by her husband. The patient had one-week history of weakness. She denied vomiting, diarrhea, or diuretic use. There was no history of fevers or chills.

Physical examination reveals a thin, white female.

Examination Results

Supine BP	110/80 mm Hg
Pulse	84/min
Standing BP	90/70 mm Hg
Pulse	120/min
Temp	37°C
Heart	Regular rhythm, normal heart sounds
Lungs	Clear
Abdomen	Normal
Extremities	No cyanosis, clubbing, or edema
Neurological examination	Weakness in both lower extremities

Laboratory Results

Serum sodium	138 meq/liter
Potassium	2.1 meq/liter
Chloride	85 meq/liter
Bicarbonate	41 meq/liter
Blood urea nitrogen	25 mg/dl
Creatinine	0.6 mg/dl
Arterial pH	7.54
pCO_2	50 mm Hg
pO_2	86 mm Hg
EKG	Sinus rhythm; rate of 110/min, flattened T-waves
Spot urine potassium	40 meq/liter

Discussion.   The patient has severe hypokalemia, which has caused flattening of T-waves on EKG and probably accounts for her weakness. The presence of metabolic alkalosis suggests that some of the hypokalemia could be due to redistribution. A large deficit, however, is also present. Urine potassium is high (more than 10–20 meq/liter) in spite of low serum potassium indicating renal potassium wasting. Many of the causes of renal potassium owing to mineralocorticoid excess, especially primary hyperaldo-

steronism, are associated with high blood pressure. In this patient, the blood pressure is normal to low, which excludes primary hyperaldosteronism and renovascular hypertension. The patient has orthostatic changes in pulse and blood pressure, findings consistent with diuretic abuse or vomiting. Although the patient did not volunteer this history, a urine test for diuretics was positive, indicating diuretic abuse as a cause of the hypokalemia and metabolic alkalosis. When hypokalemia is due to stool losses of potassium secondary to chronic diarrhea or laxative abuse, patients often present with a hyperchloremic metabolic acidosis and urine potassium concentration is low.

2. A 51-year-old white male with a history of chronic alcohol abuse was found unconscious by a friend who summoned an ambulance. History revealed that the patient may have been lying on the floor for at least 24 hours.

Physical examination revealed an elderly man responsive only to painful stimuli. Supine BP 110/60 mm Hg and pulse 60/minute, sitting BP 100/50 mm Hg and pulse 98/minute, temp 37.6°C. The remainder of physical exam was significant only for dry mucus membranes and for tenderness and swelling in the right thigh.

Laboratory Results

Serum sodium	148 meq/liter
Potassium	6.8 meq/liter
Chloride	115 meq/liter
Bicarbonate	15 meq/liter
Glucose	140 mg/dl
Blood urea nitrogen	34 mg/dl
Creatinine	5.4 mg/dl
Urinalysis:	
Color	Slightly pink
Specific gravity	1.010
Dipstick	
Protein	1+
Blood	3+
Glucose	Negative
Ketones	Trace
Microscopy	0–3 WBC/hpf, granular casts seen, no red cells present

Discussion.   This is a typical history and laboratory presentation for acute renal failure secondary to rhabdomyolysis. The history is significant for an unconscious patient with a tender leg, which is probably the leg that he compressed while unconscious. The discrepancy between the positive urine dipstick test for blood and absence of red cells on microscopy suggests that the urine might have contained myoglobin and would lead one toward the diagnosis of rhabdomyolysis. Measurement of plasma creatine kinase would help to confirm this possibility.

The cause of hyperkalemia in this disease is multifactorial. First, there is renal failure as evidenced by the elevated blood urea nitrogen and creatinine; this leads to a marked decrease in the renal excretory capacity of potassium. Second, there is a redistribution of potassium from the intracellular space to the extracellular space due to acute metabolic acidosis. Third, in rhabdomyolysis there is cellular injury with release of potassium from muscle cells.

Initial therapy in this case should be with sodium bicarbonate, insulin, and glucose which shift potassium into the cells. Potassium removal from the body could then be accomplished with dialysis. The cause of alteration in mental status also needs to be investigated.

Bibliography

Allon M, Dunley R, and Copkney T. Nebulized albuterol for acute hyperkalemia in patients on hemodialysis. *Ann Intern Med* 110:426–429, 1989. *A clinical study of the therapeutic effects of beta-adrenergic agents in hyperkalemia.*

Ptacek LJ, George AL, Griggs, RC, et al. Identification of a mutation in the gene causing hyperkalemic periodic paralysis. *Cell* 67:1021–1027, 1991. *Article describing the elucidation of the molecular basis of hyperkalemic periodic paralysis.*

Ptacek LJ, Tarvil R, Griggs RC, et al. Dihydropyridine receptor mutations cause hypokalemic periodic paralysis. *Cell* 77:863–868, 1994. *Paper on elucidation of the molecular basis of hypokalemic periodic paralysis.*

Rose BD. Disorders of Potassium Balance. In *Clinical Physiology of Acid-Base and Electrolyte Disorders* (4th ed.). New York: Little, Brown, 1994, pp. 763–862. *Comprehensive yet lucid review incorporating cellular mechanisms for most potassium disorders of clinical importance.*

Sterns RH and Narins RG. Disorders of Potassium Balance. In Stein JH (ed.). *Internal Medicine* (4th ed.). St. Louis: Mosby, 1994, pp. 2681–2693. *Concise review by two leading authorities in this area.*

53 Acid-Base Disturbances

James A. Pederson

Objectives

After completing this chapter, you should be able to

Discuss the meaning of acidemia, acidosis, alkalemia, and alkalosis

Define the roles played by the kidney, lung, and acid-base buffers in acid-base homeostasis

List the primary simple acid-base disturbances

Discuss the processes initiating and sustaining these simple acid-base disorders

Detect and classify simple acid-base disturbances utilizing clinical and laboratory data

Definitions

The following definitions are essential to any discussion of hydrogen ion homeostasis. **Acidemia** refers to an increase in plasma hydrogen ion concentration [H^+]. In man this occurs when the [H^+] exceeds 42 nanoequivalents per liter (nEq/liter) or the pH falls below 7.38. Conversely, **alkalemia** means that the plasma concentration of H^+ falls below 38 nEq/liter or the pH exceeds 7.42. **Acidosis** is a pathologic process which tends to acidify body fluids while alkalosis is a process which promotes alkalinization. **Hypercapnia** indicates that the partial pressure of carbon dioxide in arterial blood ($PaCO_2$) is increased while hypocapnia means a decreased $PaCO_2$. **Buffers** are substances which resist net changes in the free H^+ concentration of solutions by either binding or releasing H^+. **Compensation** is the term applied to the normal physiologic response by the kidney or lung which attempts to return an abnormal H^+ concentration toward a normal value.

Normal Physiology

As depicted in Fig. 53-1, acid-base homeostasis involves interactions between the lungs, kidneys, and a variety of cellular and extracellular buffers.

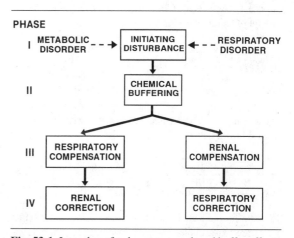

Fig. 53-1. Interplay of pulmonary, renal, and buffer effects during the evolution and resolution of acid-base disturbances.

Acid Generation

Metabolic processes generate acids. Carbonic acid (H_2CO_3), the so-called "volatile acid," is derived from hydration of carbon dioxide, according to the reaction $CO_2 + H_2O \rightarrow H_2CO_3$. The CO_2 results from the complete oxidation of carbohydrates, lipids, and certain amino acids. Once formed, H_2CO_3 dissociates to bicarbonate (HCO_3^-) and H^+. Some nonvolatile acids, e.g., H_2SO_4 and H_3PO_4, are normal products of the catabolism of phosphoesters and sulfur-containing amino acids. If oxidative metabolism of carbohydrate and fat is incomplete, nonvolatile organic acids are also formed. For example, beta-hydroxybutyric acid and acetoacetic acid are the result of incomplete oxidation of fat, and lactic acid is generated from incomplete oxidation of carbohydrate. Normally, these compounds are produced in small amounts, but in pathologic situations production rate may overwhelm the capacity of the kidney to compensate and metabolic acidosis will ensue.

Role of the Lungs

In health, alveolar ventilation adjusts CO_2 excretion to maintain a $PaCO_2 = 40$ mm Hg, despite wide fluctuations in CO_2 production rate. This function stabilizes the plasma H_2CO_3 concentration within narrow limits. With impaired ventilation, CO_2 is retained and the concentration of H_2CO_3 increases. The reverse occurs when alveolar ventilation is excessive (see Chap. 45 for a more complete discussion of CO_2 homeostasis).

Buffers

They minimize variations in H^+ concentration resulting from changes in acid-base balance. The numerous buffers involved in acid-base homeostasis exist as chemical pairs in equilibrium with one another.

$$\left[H^+\right] \sim \frac{H_2CO_3}{HCO_3^-} \sim \frac{H_2PO_4^-}{HPO_4^-} \sim \frac{H\,Hb}{Hb^-} \sim \frac{H\,protein}{Protein^-} \sim \frac{H\,apatite}{Apatite^-} \sim etc.$$

Some buffer pairs are intracellular, e.g., hemoglobin (Hb); others are extracellular, e.g., the calcium-phosphate crystals of the bone (apatite) and the bicarbonate-carbonic acid buffer pair. Among these buffers the bicarbonate-carbonic acid system is unique in three respects. First, the concentration of buffer acid (H_2CO_3) can be altered by changing $PaCO_2$ with adjustments in alveolar ventilation. Second, this buffer pair is also the major extracellular buffer (therefore, it is easily sampled). Finally, it is the only buffer pair for which mechanisms exist to replenish the buffer base (HCO_3^-) consumed in neutralizing metabolic acids. This task is accomplished by the kidneys.

Role of the Kidneys

Acid-base homeostasis requires that the concentration of bicarbonate in the extracellular fluid remains within narrow bounds (22–26 meq/liter). To accomplish this the kidneys must reclaim all bicarbonate filtered through the glomerulus and replenish the bicarbonate expended in buffering the nonvolatile acid products of metabolism. The net effect of these actions is reflected by the rate of urinary H^+ excretion as shown in

$$\text{Net } H^+_{exc} = \left[NH_4^+ + \text{Titratable acid}\right]_{urine} - HCO_3^-_{urine}$$

$$(53\text{-}1)$$

A brief summary of the mechanisms involved in Net H^+ excretion follows.

Following glomerular filtration, bicarbonate combines with H^+ secreted into the lumen of the proximal tubule by the tubular epithelial cells. This produces H_2CO_3 which dissociates to CO_2 and water. The process is accelerated enzymatically by carbonic anhydrase located on the luminal membrane of the epithelial cells in the proximal tubule. As the CO_2 forms, it freely diffuses from the lumen into the tubular cell cytoplasm, where it is hydrated to H_2CO_3 which dissociates to H^+ and HCO_3^-. The bicarbonate is then transferred into the plasma and the H^+ is secreted into the tubular fluid. About 90% of filtered bicarbonate is reabsorbed by the proximal tubule by this mechanism; the remainder is reabsorbed distally in a similar manner. The final urine is normally bicarbonate-free.

To replace bicarbonate consumed in buffering, the kidney excretes approximately 1 meq of H^+ per kilogram of body weight each day, and generates an equivalent amount of HCO_3^-. This process of HCO_3^- generation and H^+ secretion depends on buffering of H^+ within the nephron lumen by ammonia (NH_3) and acid-salt buffers to form ammonium (NH_4^+) and titratable acid salts, e.g., $H_2PO_4^-$.

The amount of NH_3 available for urinary buffering is influenced by several factors, including the acid load, potassium balance, and renal mass. Acid loading and hypokalemia increases NH_3 generation and therefore NH_4^+ excretion, whereas any disease which reduces renal tubular mass diminishes the kidneys' capacity to excrete NH_4^+. The ability of the kidneys to adjust NH_4^+ excretion in response to metabolic demands is crucial to maintaining bicarbonate and other buffer stores in health and disease.

Titratable acid excretion depends on both filtration of urinary buffer anions and H^+ secretion by the tubular epithelium. Due to continuing H^+ secretion, the pH of the luminal fluid would progressively decrease along the length of the nephron if not for urinary buffers (such as $HPO_4^=$) which are titrated to their more acidic forms ($H_2PO_4^-$). Most of the urinary buffering occurs distally where the luminal fluid pH is minimal. The buffer salts, together with the secreted H^+, are then excreted in the urine. A deficiency of buffer such as with phosphate depletion can occasionally limit excretion of titratable acid. However, a compensatory increase in ammoniagenesis will usually occur and prevent any decrease in total acid excretion under these conditions.

The H^+ which is excreted as titratable acid and NH_4^+ is derived from dissociation of intracellular H_2CO_3 to HCO_3^- and H^+. This newly formed bicarbonate together with sodium is then absorbed into the plasma. Under normal conditions the rate of formation of this new bicarbonate exactly matches the rate of bicarbonate consumption.

Disorders of Acid-Base Homeostasis

Definitions

The H^+ concentration in any solution can be related to the partial pressure of carbon dioxide ($PaCO_2$) and the concentration of HCO_3^-. This relationship, defined by Henderson, is shown in Eq. (53-2), where the value 24 equals the product of the solubility coefficient for CO_2 in plasma at body temperature (0.03 mmol/liter/mm Hg) and the dissociation constant (800 mmol/liter) for H_2CO_2, i.e., 0.03 × 800 = 24

$$\left[H^+\right] = 24 \times \frac{PaCO_2}{\left[HCO_3^-\right]} = 24 \times \frac{40 \text{ mm Hg}}{24 \text{ meq/liter}} = 24 \times 1.6 = 40 \text{ neq/liter}$$

$$(53\text{-}2)$$

If the H^+ is expressed as a negative logarithm, i.e., pH, the relationship becomes the Henderson-Hasselbach equation

$$pH = 6.1 + \log\frac{\left[HCO_3^-\right]}{\left[H_2CO_3\right]} = 6.1 + \log\frac{24 \text{ meq/liter}}{1.2 \text{ meq/liter}} \quad (53\text{-}3)$$
$$= 6.1 + \log 20 = 6.1 + 1.3 = 7.4$$

Since all acid-base disturbances stem from changes in $PaCO_2$ or $[HCO_3^-]$, four primary acid-base disturbances can be defined as outlined in Table 53-1. These are **metabolic acidosis,** initiated by reduction in plasma $[HCO_3^-]$;

Table 53-1. Arterial Blood Gas Changes in the Four Primary Acid-Base Disorders

Disorder	Primary Change	Secondary Response	Net Effect
Metabolic acidosis	↓↓ HCO_3^-	↓ $PaCO_2$	↓ pH
Metabolic alkalosis	↑↑ HCO_3^-	↑ $PaCO_2$	↑ pH
Respiratory acidosis	↑↑ $PaCO_2$	↑ HCO_3^-	↓ pH
Respiratory alkalosis	↓↓ $PaCO_2$	↓ HCO_3^-	↑ pH

metabolic alkalosis reflecting an increase in plasma $[HCO_3^-]$; **respiratory acidosis** resulting from an increase in $PaCO_2$, and **respiratory alkalosis** due to reduced $PaCO_2$. Mixtures of these primary acid-base disturbances also occur as a consequence of the simultaneous presence of two or more primary disturbances.

Diagnosis of Acid-Base Disturbances

Arterial Blood Gases

The concentration of H^+ and the $PaCO_2$ can be readily measured electrochemically in arterial or venous blood samples by most clinical laboratories. The normal range for arterial $[H^+]$, pH, and $PaCO_2$ are 43–37 neq/liter, 7.37–7.43 units, and 36–44 mm Hg respectively. Bicarbonate concentration in meq/liter can then be calculated from the H^+ concentration or pH and $PaCO_2$ using eq. (53-2) or a simple nomogram. Normal values for plasma $[HCO_3^-]$ range from 22 to 27 meq/liter. Table 53-1 summarizes the deviations expected in these parameters in the four primary acid-base disorders.

The expected compensatory response for each primary acid-base disturbance is illustrated in Fig. 53-2. This acid-base map depicts 95% confidence intervals for the relationships of pH or $[H^+]$ and $PaCO_2$ from observations in patients with a simple acid-base disturbance. Bicarbonate isopleths, derived from the Henderson-Hasselbach equation, are also included on the map. Several points need to be kept in mind about such acid-base maps. First, the more severe the primary disturbance, the more intense should be the compensatory response. Second, parameters that fall outside the confidence bands indicate that a mixed acid-base disturbance is present. However, it should be noted that parameters falling within a confidence band are compatible with but not diagnostic of single acid-base disorders. Thus a pH of 7.30 at $PaCO_2$ of 70 mm Hg is compatible with either a chronic respiratory acidosis or two

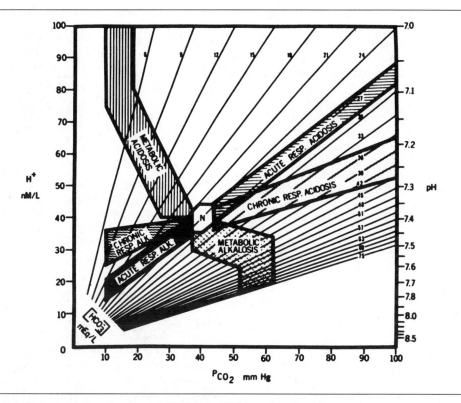

Fig. 53-2. An acid-base map based on arterial pH, [H⁺] and HCO₃⁻ values in patients with various acid-base disturbances. Normal values are defined in the area labeled N. (Used with permission from: Goldberg M, et al. Computer-based instruction and diagnosis of acid-base disorders. *JAMA* 223:269, 1973. Copyright 1973, American Medical Association.)

concurrent acid-base disturbances (acute respiratory acidosis and metabolic alkalosis).

Anion Gap

Measuring serum electrolytes (including sodium, chloride, potassium, and bicarbonate) is also useful in analysing acid-base disturbances. The difference between the sodium concentration and the sum of the bicarbonate and chloride concentrations is known as the "anion gap" [Eq. (53-4)]. This value represents anions not included in the routine electrolyte report, i.e., proteins, phosphates, sulfates, and organic acids. Potassium is usually ignored in the calculation because its concentration is low compared to the other elements of the electrolyte profile. The anion gap is normally 12 ± 4 meq/liter. Figure 53-3 compares the electrolyte compositions of normal plasma to plasma with an increased anion gap.

$$\text{Anion gap} = \left[Na^+ \right] - \left(\left[Cl^- \right] + \left[HCO_3^- \right] \right) \qquad (53\text{-}4)$$

Calculation of the anion gap is useful in the differential diagnosis of causes of metabolic acidosis. These can be divided into those associated with either a normal or a wide anion gap. The latter group can be further classified according to the serum potassium concentration (Table 53-2).

Metabolic Acid-Base Disorders

Metabolic Acidosis

Defined as an acid-base disturbance in which the primary or inciting event causes a fall in the plasma bicarbonate concentration, metabolic acidosis results in an increase in H⁺ concentration which is reflected by a decline in the

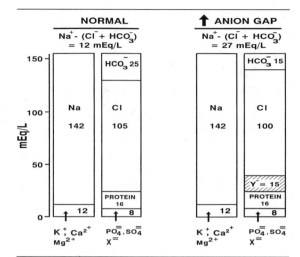

Fig. 53-3. Electrolyte composition of plasma with a normal and an increased anion gap. $X^=$ represents lactate and other unmentioned anions which are normally present in low concentrations. Y^- represents 15 meq of excess unmeasured anions. In each example the total anion gap represents the difference between the concentration of all anions and cations which are not measured on the routine electrolyte profile.

Table 53-2. Classifications of Metabolic Acidosis According to Anion Gap and Serum Potassium

Wide Anion Gap	Normal Anion Gap	
	Serum [K$^+$] Normal or ↓	Serum [K$^+$] Normal or ↑
Uremia	Diarrhea	Interstitial
Ketoacidosis	Pancreatic fistula	nephritis
Lactic acidosis	Ureteral diversion	Adrenal
Salicylate	Renal tubular	insufficiency
Methanol	acidosis	Hydronephrosis
Ethylene glycol	Post hypercapnia	NH$_4$Cl
	Diamox	Arginine HCl
	Sulfamylon	CaCl$_2$
	Post-ketoacidosis	Lysine HCl
		Cholestyramine

plasma pH. The acidemia initiates a compensatory increase in ventilation, which results in a reduction in PaCO$_2$ (see Fig. 53-2).

The mechanisms by which metabolic acidosis may develop are outlined in Table 53-3. The clinical features and

Table 53-3. Mechanisms of Metabolic Acidosis

Primary bicarbonate loss
  Gastrointestinal losses: diarrhea, fistulae, or ureterosigmoid anastomosis
  Renal losses: proximal renal tubular acidosis
Increased bicarbonate utilization (consumed in buffering)
  Ketoacidosis: diabetic, alcoholic, or starvation
  Lactic acidosis: tissue hypoxia, impaired oxygen utilization, severe liver dysfunction, and idiopathic
  Exogenous acid intake: ammonium chloride, salicylate, ethylene glycol, or methanol intoxication
Impaired renal bicarbonate generation: renal failure and distal renal tubular acidosis

therapy of metabolic acidosis depend on the underlying cause, its severity and duration, and the associated electrolyte abnormalities. The consequences of the resulting acidemia are outlined in Table 53-4.

Metabolic Alkalosis

It is the result of factors that initiate and then sustain an increase in the plasma bicarbonate concentration. The conditions which initiate metabolic alkalosis may differ from those which sustain it. The initial increase in the concentration of bicarbonate occurs through one or more of the factors listed in Table 53-5. Some of these conditions deserve comment regarding the mechanisms of plasma bicarbonate elevation. For example, how does a loss of H$^+$ in urine or gastric juice raise the plasma bicarbonate level? The key concept here is that H_2CO_3 is the source of H$^+$ secreted by either the renal tubular or gastric mucosal cells. In either organ, HCO_3^- is liberated and enters the extracellular fluid according to the following reaction: $H_2CO_3 \rightarrow H^+ + HCO_3^-$. The result is an increased quantity of HCO_3^- entering in the extracellular fluid whenever H$^+$ is transferred into the lumen. In contrast, contraction of the extracellular volume raises the concentration but not the quantity of HCO_3^- in the extracellular compartment.

In any of the situations listed in Table 53-5, metabolic alkalosis will persist only if excretion of the excess bicarbonate is prevented by factors which "maintain" the alkalosis. Normally the addition of alkali to the plasma is followed by transient expansion of the plasma volume, suppression of renal acid excretion, and a bicarbonate diuresis. This restores both extracellular volume and bicarbonate concentration to normal. A decrease in extracellular fluid volume is the most common factor involved in maintaining metabolic alkalosis. This is because volume depletion markedly enhance the renal tubular reabsorption of filtered sodium and available anions (HCO_3^- and Cl$^-$). Occasionally alkalo-

Table 53-4. Clinical Effects of Metabolic Acid-Base Disturbances

Metabolic Acidosis	Metabolic Alkalosis
Pulmonary: Hyperventilation **Heart:** Decreased contractility at pH < 7.20. Ventricular fibrillation potentiated. **Vascular:** Arterial vasodilatation and venous vasoconstriction which promotes central vasocongestion. **Neurohumoral:** Catecholamine release counteracts depressed myocardial contractility and causes arterial vasoconstriction. **Oxygen transport:** Acutely increases O_2 release from red cells. After 6–8 hours, 2-3-DPG decreases and O_2 dissociation curve shifts back to the left. **Other effects:** Nausea and vomiting are common. Potassium shifts out of the cells. Chronic acidosis increases calcium excretion and promotes bone demineralization.	**Pulmonary:** Hypoventilation, increases $PaCO_2$ and decreases PaO_2 **Heart:** Ventricular ectopy. Reduced fibrillation threshold. **Metabolic:** Potassium and phosphate shift into cells. Urinary excretion of potassium is increased. Ionized calcium and magnesium fall, owing to protein binding. **Oxygen transport:** Acutely oxyhemoglobin curve shifts left, impairing O_2 release. At 6–8 hours, 2-3-DPG increases and curve shifts back towards the right. **Central nervous system:** Confusion, agitation, disorientation, muscle tremors, and seizures.

Table 53-5. Mechanisms of Bicarbonate Generation in Metabolic Alkalosis

EXCESS BICARBONATE LOAD

Bicarbonate intake: parenteral or orally
Metabolism of bicarbonate precursors: lactate, acetate, citrate

NET LOSS OF HYDROGEN IONS (GENERATES BICARBONATE ENDOGENOUSLY)

Renal hydrogen loss
   Hyperaldosteronism: Cushing's syndrome, 1° Aldosteronism — Bartter's syndrome
   Thiazide and loop diuretics
   Post-hypercapnic alkalosis
Gastrointestinal hydrogen ion loss: vomiting or nasogastric suction
Movement of H^+ into cell (K^+ depletion)

CONTRACTION OF EXTRACELLULAR SPACE (LOSS OF NACL WITHOUT LOSS OF HCO_3^-)

Loop diuretics
Villous adenoma

sis will be sustained in the face of volume expansion. In such situations, renal failure, continued bicarbonate administration, or the presence of stimuli for sodium retention independent of volume such as primary hyperaldosteronism or congestive heart failure are usually involved.

Respiratory Disorders

The pathophysiology and clinical consequences of respiratory acidosis and alkalosis are discussed in detail in Chap.

45. The discussion which follows here will be limited to the clinical sequelae (Table 53-6) and the effects of these disorders on acid-base homeostasis.

Respiratory Acidosis

This results from an increase in $PaCO_2$ due to impaired alveolar ventilation relative to CO_2 production. Rapid titration by tissue buffers produces a small increase in plasma bicarbonate concentrations. If the hypercapnia is sustained, renal acid excretion increases the plasma bicarbonate further. In acute respiratory acidosis buffer responses produce up to a 3–4 meq/liter increase in the plasma bicarbonate concentration. This response begins within 5–10 minutes of the onset of hypercapnia. Renal response to acute hypercapnia include a decrease in urine pH, increased ammonium excretion, increased bicarbonate reabsorption, and a fall in urinary potassium excretion.

Chronic respiratory acidosis stimulates renal tubular bicarbonate reabsorption as well as generation of new bicarbonate. Plasma bicarbonate increases until a new steady state is achieved. The rise in bicarbonate is accompanied by a fall in the plasma chloride due to renal loss. As shown in Fig. 53-2, the plasma hydrogen ion increase is less than that noted in acute respiratory acidosis with similar $PaCO_2$ values.

Respiratory Alkalosis

It results from a reduction in $PaCO_2$ due to alveolar hyperventilation. In acute respiratory alkalosis, buffer responses of tissues and blood produce up to 2–4 meq/liter decrease in the plasma bicarbonate level. A new steady state is reached in about 15 minutes and is maintained for 2–5

Table 53-6. Clinical Effects of Respiratory Acid-Base Disturbances

Respiratory Acidosis	Respiratory Alkalosis
CENTRAL NERVOUS SYSTEM	**CENTRAL NERVOUS SYSTEM**
Acute: Anxiety, dyspnea, disorientation, confusion, EEG abnormalities, altered reflexes, headache and papilledema. Coma at a PaCO$_2$ > 60 mm Hg. **Chronic:** Effects minimal, but muscle drowsiness and disturbed sleep patterns.	**Acute:** Dizziness, confusion, seizures. Cerebral vascular resistance increases. Cerebral blood flow & oxygen delivery fall.
CARDIOVASCULAR	**CARDIOVASCULAR**
Acute: Vasodilatation and sympathetic stimulation. If not hypoxic or in CHF, skin is warm, flushed & diaphoretic. Bounding pulse, increased cardiac output & blood pressure. **Chronic:** Cardiac output is normal.	Initially heart rate increases but stroke volume decreases. After 12 hours cardiac output increases, peripheral resistance falls, and stroke volume returns to normal. After 2–3 days cardiac output becomes normal and pulse rate remains elevated.
	METABOLIC
	Increased plasma lactic acid, shift of potassium and phosphate into cells, and a decrease in ionized calcium.

hours if PaCO$_2$ remains unchanged. The renal responses to acute hypocapnia include a rise in the urine pH due to a bicarbonate diuresis and a decrease in ammonium excretion. These changes are detectable within 30 minutes of a decrease in PaCO$_2$ but add little to the initial decline in the bicarbonate concentration effected by tissue buffering. In chronic respiratory alkalosis 36–72 hours are required for the renal responses to become maximum. Diminished renal H$^+$ excretion is the major factor that determines further decreases in plasma bicarbonate. In the chronic state, the renal response reduces plasma bicarbonate level about 5 meq/liter for each 10 mm Hg fall in PaCO$_2$. Despite this renal compensation, H$^+$ concentration decreases linearly with the PaCO$_2$ (see Fig. 53-2).

Clinical Examples

1. A 36-year-old man was hospitalized with a 3-day history of fever and watery diarrhea. He was acutely ill with a blood pressure of 90/60 mm Hg, a pulse of 112/minute, a respiratory rate of 24/minute, and a temperature of 37.5°C. The abdomen was distended, hyperresonant on percussion, and diffusely tender. On auscultation rushes of bowel sounds were heard. The following laboratory results were obtained.

Venous blood	Arterial blood	Urine
Na$^+$ 135 meq/liter	pH 7.21	Specific
K$^+$ 2.0 meq/liter	H$^+$ 62 neq/liter	gravity
Cl$^-$ 110 meq/liter	PaCO$_2$ 26 mm Hg	1.028
HCO$_3^-$ 12 meq/liter	PaO$_2$ 108 mm Hg	pH 5.0
		Na$^+$ 2.0 meq/liter

Discussion. The patient's problems include extracellular volume depletion, metabolic acidosis, and hypokalemia. The initiating disturbance is diarrhea. This results in the loss of isotonic fluid, which may contain large amounts of bicarbonate (e.g., 40–80 meq/liter) and potassium. The loss of bicarbonate would reduce the blood pH dramatically, but this effect is minimized by chemical buffering. A rise in blood H$^+$ stimulates ventilation, which further limits the increase in the hydrogen ion concentration. This patient has an appropriate respiratory response for the decrease in blood bicarbonate level (see Fig. 53-2). The renal response is slower; the maximum renal response may not occur until 5 days after the onset of the acid-base disturbance. The expected renal response would be the formation of an acid urine that contains no bicarbonate and has an increased amount of titratable acid and markedly increased amounts of ammonium. The increased renal hydrogen ion excretion generates bicarbonate, which is added to the extracellular fluid. If bicarbonate generation equaled bicarbonate loss, there would be no change in plasma bicarbonate concentration. In this patient, bicarbonate loss exceeded the rate of renal generation of bicarbonate, resulting in the development of metabolic acidosis. When the diarrhea ceases, the kidneys will reconstitute buffer stores.

2. A 32-year-old male presented with vomiting of one week's duration. On examination, he appeared apathetic and had a supine blood pressure of 90/60 mm Hg and a pulse of 116/minute. See the laboratory results on page 576.

Discussion. This patient demonstrates moderately severe metabolic alkalosis (Fig. 53-4). Respiratory compensation is appropriate. There is also evidence of decreased extracellular fluid volume, e.g., hypotension, tachycardia, a

Venous blood	Arterial blood	Urine
Na$^+$ 143 meq/liter	pH 7.55	Specific
K$^+$ 2.7 meq/liter	H$^+$ 28 neq/liter	gravity
Cl$^-$ 93 meq/liter	PaCO$_2$ 46 mm Hg	1.028
HCO$_3^-$ 39 meq/liter	H$^+$ 28 neq/liter	pH 5.0
	PaCO$_2$ 46 mm Hg	Na$^+$ 5
	PaO$_2$ 90 mm Hg	meq/liter
		K$^+$ 46
		meq/liter

urine specific gravity of 1.028, and urine sodium of 5 meq/liter. Vomiting is associated with the loss of water, hydrogen ion, chloride, and small amounts of sodium and potassium. The source of the hydrogen ion is the gastric parietal cell, which dissociates carbonic acid to hydrogen ion and bicarbonate. The hydrogen ion is secreted into the gastric lumen and lost with the vomitus. For each H$^+$ lost a bicarbonate ion is added to the extracellular fluid, resulting in alkalemia. Initially, HCO$_3^-$ appears in the urine with its attendant cations, sodium and potassium. The decrease in blood H$^+$ initiates chemical buffering and induces hypoventilation so that PaCO$_2$ increases. These adjustments limit the decrease in the plasma H$^+$ concentration. The kidneys maintain the metabolic alkalosis because decreased

Fig. 53-4. The pathophysiology of metabolic alkalosis associated with vomiting (see text for explanation).

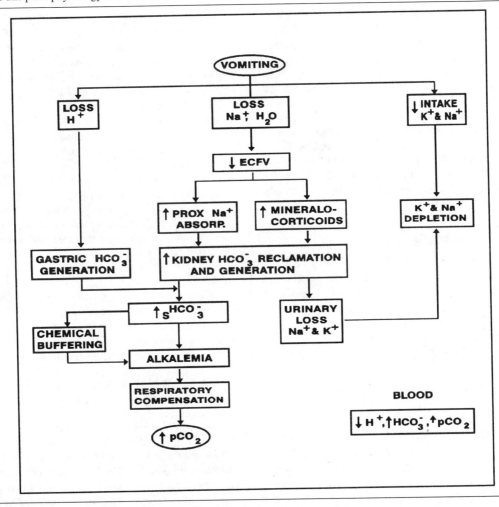

extracellular fluid volume and potassium depletion enhance renal tubular reabsorption of bicarbonate and prevent its excretion. The decreased extracellular volume results from loss of water and sodium in the vomitus, as well as a urinary loss of sodium during an initial period of bicarbonate diuresis. The potassium depletion stems from the small loss of potassium in the vomitus and a much larger cumulative loss of potassium in the urine that is enhanced by secondary hyperaldosteronism. Thus the kidney is pivotal in the maintenance of the metabolic alkalosis. Renal correction of metabolic alkalosis cannot occur until the factors maintaining increased bicarbonate generation and reclamation are corrected. The excess bicarbonate will then be excreted. During the period when all the filtered bicarbonate is being reabsorbed, the urine will be acidic despite systemic alkalemia (paradoxical aciduria).

3. A 58-year-old man is brought to the hospital after choking during dinner. He is in moderate respiratory distress. Stridor is heard over both lung fields. Supplemental oxygen is administered. The laboratory data are as follows.

Venous blood		Arterial blood	
Na^+	142 meq/liter	pH	7.24
K^+	4.9 meq/liter	PaO_2	122 mm Hg
Cl^-	100 meq/liter	$PaCO_2$	64 mm Hg
HCO_3^-	27 meq/liter	H^+ ion	56 neq/liter

Discussion. The presence of acidemia and hypercapnia indicate respiratory acidosis (Fig. 53-5). Partial tracheal obstruction has caused an abrupt increase in $PaCO_2$ to 64 mm Hg. The fact that the serum $[HCO_3^-]$ has increased by only 3 meq/liter supports a clinical diagnosis of acute hypercapnia. Serum bicarbonate values exceeding 29 meq/liter or less than 24 meq/liter would suggest a complicating metabolic acid-base disturbance or a chronic respiratory disorder. Alveolar hypoventilation would be expected to produce hypoxemia but administration of supplemental oxygen prevented this from occurring.

4. A 52-year-old man with chronic obstructive lung disease is admitted to the hospital with worsening dyspnea. He appears cyanotic and in respiratory distress. The laboratory data follow.

Venous blood		Arterial blood	
Na^+	136 meq/liter	pH	7.34
K^+	4.9 meq/liter	$PaCO_2$	60 mm Hg
Cl^-	96 meq/liter	H^+	46 neq/liter
HCO_3^-	31 meq/liter	PaO_2	50 mm Hg

Discussion. This man also has respiratory acidosis but the history and the elevated plasma HCO_3^- point to a chronic condition (Fig. 53-6). Note that the arterial pH is almost normal despite an increase in $PaCO_2$ which is of a magnitude similar to that occurring in the previous case. What do you expect the urine pH to be in a patient like this? Why?

5. A 32-year-old woman is admitted to the hospital in a confused state, complaining of flank pain and chills. She is febrile, and has a respiratory rate of 28/minute. The blood pressure is 100/60 mm Hg and the heart rate is 120/minute. The urine contains large numbers of white cells, white cell casts, and gram-negative rod-shaped bacteria. Blood urea nitrogen and serum creatinine are normal. The laboratory data follow.

Venous blood		Arterial blood	
Na^+	136 meq/liter	pH	7.59
K^+	3.5 meq/liter	$PaCO_2$	20 mm Hg
Cl^-	100 meq/liter	H^+	25 neq/liter
HCO_3^-	19 meq/liter	PaO_2	100 mm Hg

Discussion. The presence of hypocapnia and alkalemia indicate respiratory alkalosis (see Fig. 53-6). The history and laboratory data point to an illness, probably urosepsis, of short duration. The serum bicarbonate has dropped by 5 meq/liter partially due to tissue buffering. The anion gap is slightly increased, probably due to increased lactic acid production as a result of alkalemia and possibly sepsis. The serum potassium concentration is slightly low. This is probably the result of an intracellular potassium shift. As is usually the case with respiratory alkalosis, this acid-base disorder should respond to treatment of the underlying cause, i.e., sepsis.

6. A 24-year-old man has been hospitalized for one week with seizures and meningitis. Laboratory data reveal:

Venous blood		Arterial blood	
Na^+	143 meq/liter	pH	7.45
K^+	4.0 meq/liter	$PaCO_2$	25 mm Hg
Cl^-	111 meq/liter	H^+	35 neq/liter
HCO_3^-	16 meq/liter	PaO_2	95 mm Hg

Discussion. Marked hypocapnia with a mildly elevated pH suggests a diagnosis of chronic respiratory alkalosis (see Fig. 53-6). Another possibility is a mixed disorder, e.g., metabolic acidosis and acute respiratory alkalosis. The first alternative is more likely with meningitis as the

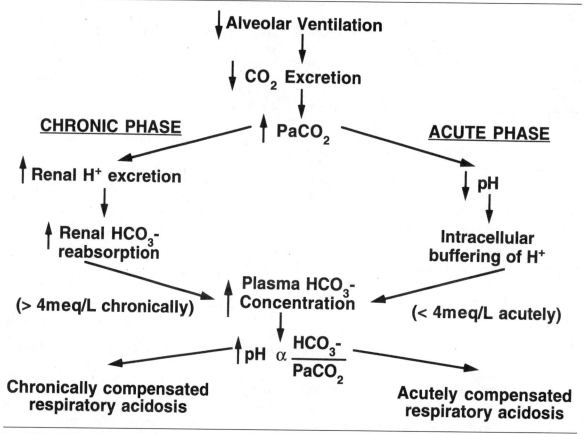

Fig. 53-5. Compensatory pathways initiated in acute and chronic respiratory acidosis. Elevations in $PaCO_2$ promote processes which raise plasma HCO_3^- concentration and thus return the pH back toward normal. (Used with permission from: Humes HD. Simple and mixed acid-base disorders. In Humes HD (ed.). *Pathophysiology of Electrolyte and Renal Disorders,* Churchill Livingston, New York, 1986, p. 96.)

probable explanation for the increased respiratory drive. Note that chloride retention compensates for most of the decrease in the bicarbonate concentration. In this case the serum chloride has increased about 5 meq/liter. The remainder of the anion gap is made up of organic acids which have increased the concentration of unmeasured anions to the upper limit of normal.

Bibliography

Clark DD. Acid-Base Disorders. In Abuelo JG (ed.). *Renal Pathophysiology — the Essentials.* Baltimore: Williams & Wilkins, 1989. *A concise summary of acid-base physiology and the disorders. Includes some interesting clinical acid-base problems.*

Emmett M and Narins RG. Clinical use of the anion gap. *Medicine* 56(1):38–54, 1977. *Classic description of the conceptual basis and clinical utility of the anion gap.*

Narins RG and Emmett M. Simple and mixed acid-base disorders: A practical approach. *Medicine* 59(3):161–187, 1980. *The fundamental concepts underlying simple acid-base disorders are elucidated. Mixed disorders are then explained and illustrated. This article is a must for those wanting a better understanding of mixed acid-base disorders.*

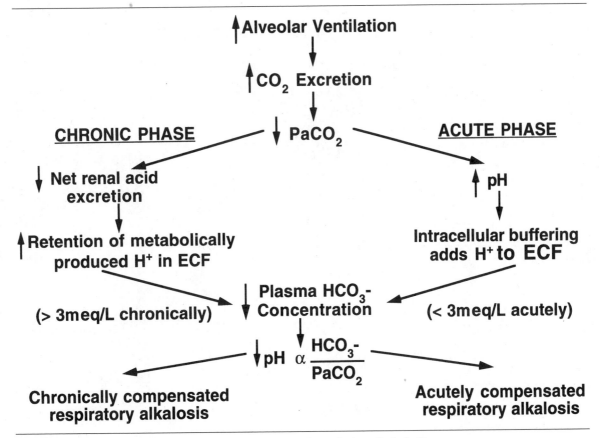

Fig. 53-6. Compensatory pathways initiated in acute and chronic respiratory alkalosis. Declines in $PaCO_2$ promote processes which lower plasma HCO_3^- concentration and thus return the pH back toward normal. (Used with permission from: Humes HD. Simple and mixed acid-base disorders. In Humes HD (ed.). *Pathophysiology of Electrolyte and Renal Disorders*, Churchill Livingston, New York, 1986, p. 89.)

Rose BD. *Clinical Physiology of Acid-Base and Electrolyte Disorders* (4th ed.). New York and St. Louis: McGraw-Hill, 1994. *This excellent book includes chapters on each of the cardinal acid-base disorders.*

Schrier RW (ed.). *Renal and Electrolyte Disorders* (4th ed.). Boston: Little, Brown, 1992. *An excellent reference with up-to-date chapters on simple and mixed acid-base disorders.*

54 Disorders of Calcium, Phosphate, and Magnesium

James E. Bourdeau

Objectives

After completing this chapter, you should be able to

Understand the physical chemistry of plasma calcium and its relationship to biologic activity

Discuss the endocrine regulation of calcium homeostasis

Explain the pathophysiology of hypocalcemia and hypercalcemia

Understand the metabolism of phosphorus and its regulation

Describe the pathophysiology of hypophosphatemia and hyperphosphatemia

Discuss the metabolism of magnesium and its regulation

Outline the pathophysiology of hypomagnesemia and hypermagnesemia

---

Calcium (Ca)

Bodily Content and Distribution

In normal humans, ~99% of bodily Ca is in bone. In a 70-kg adult male ~1300 g of Ca are in the skeleton, 7 g in teeth, 7 g in soft tissues, 700 mg in extravascular fluid, and 350 mg in plasma. Most of the skeletal Ca is unavailable for day-to-day regulation of extracellular fluid Ca concentration ([Ca]), serving primarily to provide structural support.

Homeostasis

The focal point for the endocrine regulation of Ca homeostasis is the plasma ionized Ca (Ca^{2+}) concentration. The plasma total [Ca] of adult humans is 2.10–2.60 mmol/liter (8.4–10.4 mg/dl) (Fig. 54-1). Of the total, ~40% is bound to serum proteins, primarily albumin. This fraction is not ultrafiltrable at the renal corpuscles. The ~60% of plasma total Ca that is ultrafiltrable consists of low-molecular-weight Ca complexes and Ca^{2+}. In descending order of concentration, the former include Ca bicarbonate, Ca citrate, Ca phosphate, Ca lactate, and Ca sulfate. Most of the plasma ultrafiltrable Ca is ionized, comprising ~50% of the plasma total [Ca]. Ca^{2+} is the biologically active component of the extracellular fluid Ca with respect to myocardial contractility, neuromuscular activity, and blood coagulation. In normal humans, the plasma [Ca^{2+}] ranges between 1.12 and 1.23 mmol/liter. Clinically, both serum total [Ca] and plasma [Ca^{2+}] are readily measurable. Although algorithms have been devised for the calculation of plasma [Ca^{2+}] based on the serum albumin concentration and blood pH, it is generally accepted that the [Ca^{2+}] should be measured directly using Ca^{2+}-sensitive electrodes.

The extracellular fluid [Ca^{2+}] is regulated by the actions of parathyroid hormone (PTH), calcitonin, and 1α,25-dihydroxyvitamin D_3 (calcitriol) on the organ systems that interface with the extracellular fluid, namely the intestines, the kidneys, and the skeleton (Fig. 54-2). PTH is synthesized and secreted by cells of the parathyroid glands, which detect small changes in plasma [Ca^{2+}] by means of a specific Ca^{2+} sensor. PTH release is stimulated by small

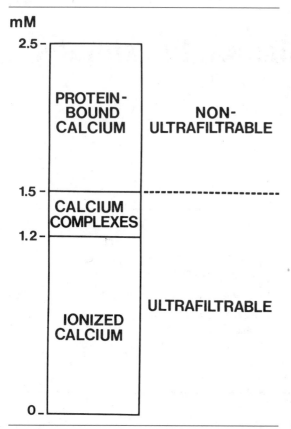

Fig. 54-1. Typical distribution of the components of plasma total Ca concentration in normal adult humans. Values may be converted from millimoles per liter (mM) to milligrams per deciliter (mg/dl) by multiplying the former by 4. (The atomic weight of Ca is 40.08 grams per mole.) (Reproduced with permission from: Bourdeau JE and Attie MF. Calcium metabolism. In Narins RG (ed.). *Maxwell & Kleeman's Clinical Disorders of Fluid and Electrolyte Metabolism* (5th ed.). New York: McGraw-Hill, 1994, pp. 243–306.)

decrements in plasma [Ca²⁺] and inhibited by small increments. These changes occur within minutes. In contrast, calcitriol regulates PTH biosynthesis and secretion over a period of hours to days. High plasma calcitriol concentrations suppress PTH biosynthesis and secretion, whereas low calcitriol levels have the opposite effect. Accordingly, negative feedback loops exist between serum [PTH] and both plasma Ca^{2+} and calcitriol concentrations. PTH increases the fluxes of Ca into the extracellular fluid from bone and kidney, thereby raising plasma [Ca²⁺]. It acts on the cellular elements of bone to stimulate resorption of both Ca and phosphate (P_i) from the surface layer of mineral and acts on the thick ascending limb of Henle's loop and distal convoluted tubule of the nephron to stimulate Ca reabsorption. PTH also stimulates the biosynthesis of calcitriol in the mitochondria of the proximal tubules of the kidneys. Calcitonin stimulates both deposition of Ca within bone and tubular Ca reabsorption at the same sites of action as PTH. In the nephron, both PTH and calcitonin increase Ca absorption by stimulating adenylate cyclase. After its synthesis in the kidneys, calcitriol is transported in the circulation by a 58-kDa vitamin D-binding protein. Calcitriol acts on the duodenum to promote active Ca absorption. During states of Ca deprivation, plasma [calcitriol] is increased, and calcitriol-stimulated Ca absorption occurs in the colon as well as the duodenum. Calcitriol acts on the skeleton to release Ca and P_i into the extracellular fluid, an action that is additive or synergistic with PTH.

Balance

Approximately 20 mmol (800 mg) of Ca are ingested in the diet each day. Milk (which contains 1.37 mg of Ca per ml) and other dairy products are the major source of dietary Ca. Exclusion of dairy products from the diet reduces daily intake to approximately 5 mmol (200 mg). Approximately 20–30% of ingested Ca is absorbed in the intestines, the remainder appearing in the feces. In addition to calcitriol-regulated transcellular absorption (described above), Ca absorption also occurs by paracellular diffusion. This process is driven by the chemical concentration difference between Ca^{2+} in the lumen of the gut and the extracellular fluid. By raising the luminal [Ca²⁺] in the gut above that in the extracellular fluid, it is possible to effect Ca absorption even in the absence of calcitriol. The molecular mechanisms by which calcitriol increases intestinal Ca absorption remain to be fully elucidated, but probably involve stimulation of Ca^{2+} entry across the luminal cell membrane, facilitation of Ca^{2+} diffusion through the cytosol of duodenal enterocytes by calbindin-D_{28k}, and increased activity and/or number of the high-affinity calcium and magnesium-dependent-ATPase (Ca,Mg-ATPase) pumps located in the basolateral cell membranes of the duodenal enterocytes. Intestinal Ca absorption changes in response to dietary Ca intake. There is a reciprocal relationship between the latter and fractional intestinal Ca absorption, which is homeostatically appropriate. This adaptation is in large part, if not entirely, mediated through the actions of calcitriol.

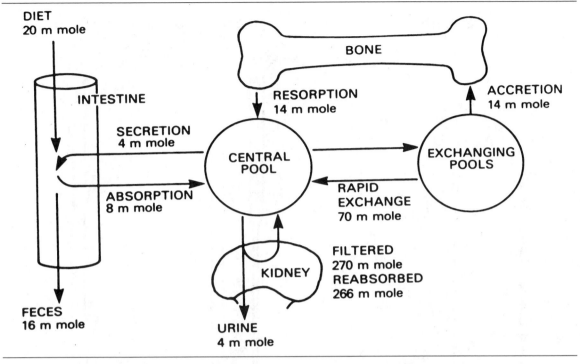

Fig. 54-2. Ca fluxes between body pools for a 70-kg adult with unchanging total body Ca (i.e., in external balance for Ca). All fluxes are in millimoles per day. (Reproduced with permission from: Bourdeau JE and Attie MF. Calcium metabolism. In Narins RG (ed.). *Maxwell & Kleeman's Clinical Disorders of Fluid and Electrolyte Metabolism* (5th ed.). New York: McGraw-Hill, 1994, pp. 243–306.)

Approximately 270 mmol of Ca are filtered at the glomeruli each day, of which 266 mmol are reabsorbed by the kidney tubules (Fig. 54-3). Accordingly, urinary Ca excretion is ~4 mmol (160 mg) per day. Both PTH and calcitonin stimulate tubular reabsorption of Ca. The role, if any, of calcitriol in stimulating renal tubular Ca absorption is uncertain. In healthy, adult males, administration of physiologic concentrations of calcitriol causes hypercalciuria. Under these circumstances, the increase in filtered Ca load (brought about by an elevated plasma [Ca²⁺] from the actions of calcitriol on the gut and skeleton) exceeds any increase in tubular reabsorption of Ca that may be present. In a normal individual in external Ca balance, net intestinal absorption of Ca equals urinary Ca excretion. For example, in an individual consuming 20 mmol of Ca daily, 4 mmol are absorbed from the intestines into the extracellular fluid and 4 mmol are excreted in the urine. In healthy adults, there is a direct relationship between dietary Ca in-

take and urinary Ca excretion (Fig. 54-4). For typical dietary Ca intakes in the United States, urinary Ca excretion ranges between 2.5 and 7.5 mmol/day (100–300 mg/day). Thiazide diuretics increase, whereas loop-acting diuretics decrease renal tubular Ca absorption.

Hypercalcemia

Causes

Hyperparathyroidism. Primary hyperparathyroidism is the most common cause of hypercalcemia. It is diagnosed most commonly between 40 and 70 years of age, but it can be seen at earlier ages. The fundamental abnormality is an excessive, unregulated secretion of PTH by either four hyperplastic glands, a single adenoma, or an adenocarcinoma. By stimulating resorption of mineral from bone, tubular reabsorption of Ca from the glomerular fil-

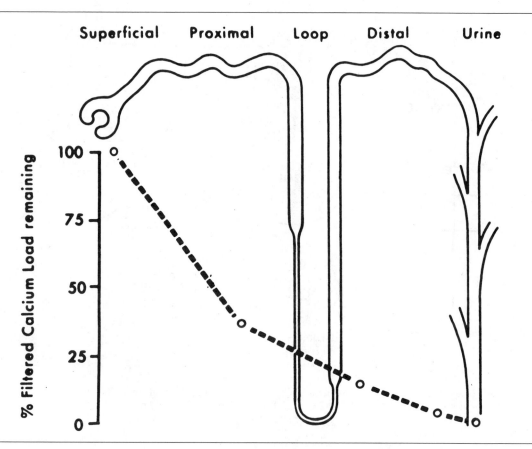

Fig. 54-3. Sites of Ca absorption along the nephron. (Reproduced with permission from: Sutton RAL and Dirks JH. Renal handling of calcium and phosphate. In Brenner BM and Rector FC (eds.). *The Kidney* (2nd ed.). Philadelphia: W. B. Saunders, 1981, pp. 551–618.)

trate, and (via calcitriol) increased intestinal absorption of Ca, the high circulating levels of PTH cause hypercalcemia. Although tubular reabsorption of Ca is augmented by the high plasma [PTH], urinary Ca excretion usually is increased because the elevated filtered load of Ca exceeds the rate of tubular Ca absorption (Fig. 54-5).

Malignancy.   The second most common cause of hypercalcemia in the general population and the most common cause among hospitalized patients is neoplastic disease. For several decades the hypercalcemia associated with malignancy was believed to be the result of destructive bony lesions caused by metastases. However, the lack of correlation between skeletal involvement by neoplastic cells and the serum [Ca] questioned this explanation. In the past decade, a novel PTH-related protein (PTH-rp) has been

isolated from tumors of patients with the humoral hypercalcemia of malignancy. The gene encoding this protein is a complex transcriptional unit that by alternative splicing gives rise to messenger RNAs that encode three related PTH-rps. These proteins interact with the PTH receptors found in the cellular elements of the skeleton and the renal tubule and mimic the actions of PTH. In addition to the release of PTH-rps, certain malignancies also can produce prostaglandin-stimulating bone-resorbing factors. Such factors also may play an important role in the hypercalcemia of certain malignancies.

Other Causes.   Lithium therapy of chronic manic-depressive illness and familial hypocalciuric hypercalcemia are both PTH-related causes of hypercalcemia distinct from primary hyperparathyroidism. Hypercal-

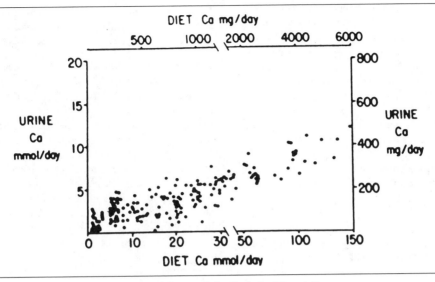

Fig. 54-4. Urinary Ca excretion as a function of dietary Ca intake in healthy adults. (Reprinted by permission of the *New England Journal of Medicine* 301:535–541, 1979.)

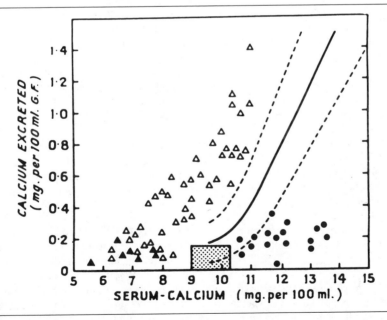

Fig. 54-5. Relationship between serum [Ca] and urinary Ca excretion (expressed as Ca excreted = [Ca]$_{urine}$ × [creatinine]$_{serum}$/[creatinine]$_{urine}$) during Ca-loading experiments in humans. The stippled rectangle represents the normal ranges in euparathyroid individuals. The solid line surrounded by broken lines indicates the mean ± 2 SD for normal subjects. The triangles indicate values for hypoparathyroid individuals and the closed circles represent values for hyperparathyroid individuals. (Reproduced with permission from: Nordin BEC and Peacock M. Role of the kidney in regulation of plasma calcium. *Lancet* 2:1280–1283, 1969; © by The Lancet Ltd., 1969.)

cemia also may result from inappropriately high plasma calcitriol levels, as occurs with vitamin D intoxication, excessive production of endogenous calcitriol by the macrophages in the granulomata of sarcoidosis (and other granulomatous diseases), and the idiopathic hypercalcemia of infancy. Hypercalcemia is also associated with states of high bone turnover, including hyperthyroidism, immobilization, and vitamin A intoxication. Reduced urinary excretion of Ca, as occurs with thiazide diuretics or early renal failure in association with the milk-alkali syndrome, can cause hypercalcemia. Finally, patients recovering from acute rhabdomyolysis-induced acute renal failure may become hypercalcemic, especially if they have been supplemented with parenteral Ca during the acute phase of their renal failure. This form of hypercalcemia results from mobilization of Ca-P_i precipitates within damaged soft tissues as the latter repair themselves and by unusually high levels of PTH and calcitriol, both of which are inappropriate for the high serum [Ca] during recovery from acute renal failure.

Consequences

Neurologic.   High serum [Ca]s have a depressive effect on both the central and peripheral nervous systems. With modest hypercalcemia, patients demonstrate apathy, lack of energy and spontaneity, anxiety, and depression. With severe hypercalcemia, there may be mental confusion with disorientation, memory loss, bizarre behavior, psychosis, and coma. Peripherally, patients demonstrate muscle weakness and depressed deep tendon reflexes.

Cardiovascular.   With moderate to severe hypercalcemia, the QT-interval of the electrocardiogram is shortened, patients demonstrate increased susceptibility to digitalis-induced arrhythmias, and hypertension is frequently present. The latter can occur in the presence of normal renal function, suggesting that increased peripheral arterial resistance caused by the hypercalcemia and increased cardiac output caused by the positive inotropic effect of Ca are important factors in its genesis.

Renal.   Hypercalcemia reduces renal blood flow and, when severe, may cause acute renal failure. Chronic hypercalcemia causes a reduction in glomerular filtration rate and a loss of urinary concentrating and diluting ability. Chronic hypercalcemia also can be associated with the deposition of Ca-P_i within the renal parenchyma, resulting in inflammation and fibrosis, which can ultimately lead to chronic renal failure.

Gastrointestinal.   Anorexia, nausea, vomiting, and constipation are commonly present with hypercalcemia. Pancreatitis and duodenal peptic ulcer disease occur on occasion.

Soft Tissue Calcification.   In the presence of a normal or elevated serum [P], hypercalcemia may cause metastatic calcification of soft tissues. Calcification occurs most readily in regions of an alkaline pH, where Ca-P_i salts readily precipitate. These include the blood side of the gastric mucosa, the peritubular aspect of acid-secreting segments of the nephron, and the lung alveoli. Periarticular soft tissues are also common sites of metastatic calcification. On physical examination, metastatic calcification may be detected in the cornea of the eye, where Ca-P_i crystals may be visible by slit-lamp examination. With chronic hypercalcemia, a band keratopathy along the lateral margin of the cornea may be visible to the naked eye.

Hypocalcemia

Causes

Parathyroid Deficiency or Absence.   PTH deficiency causes a reduction of the bone turnover that normally sustains the serum [Ca]. In addition, it results in decreased renal tubular Ca reabsorption. Together, these cause hypocalcemia. Finally, because PTH deficiency is frequently associated with hyperphosphatemia, which itself suppresses calcitriol synthesis, low circulating levels of calcitriol cause reduced intestinal absorption of Ca, which also contributes to the hypocalcemia. Idiopathic forms of PTH deficiency in adults include the autoimmune polyglandular syndrome and isolated late-onset hypoparathyroidism. Acquired forms of hypoparathyroidism include surgical removal of the parathyroid glands, radiation damage, neoplastic infiltration, and other miscellaneous pathologic processes. Finally, severe hypomagnesemia associated with substantial Mg depletion reduces PTH secretion.

Resistance to PTH Action.   Renal failure and pseudohypoparathyroidism are two conditions in which elevated plasma [PTH]s fail to maintain normal plasma [Ca^{2+}]s. In the former, PTH fails to stimulate resorption of mineral from the bones, resulting in hypocalcemia. An important component of this resistance may be the absence or a low plasma [calcitriol]. As discussed above, under normal circumstances PTH and calcitriol act additively or synergistically to stimulate release of both Ca and P_i from the skeleton. With pseudoparathyroidism, PTH fails to stimulate the generation of cyclic AMP in either renal tubular cells or in cells surrounding the skeleton. Consequently, bone turnover is slowed and renal tubular absorption of Ca is diminished. These actions result in hypocalcemia.

Vitamin D Deficiency.   Historically, vitamin D deficiency was the primary cause of nutritional rickets. Nowadays, rickets is rarely seen but vitamin D deficiency can result in hypocalcemia. In all forms of vitamin D deficiency the plasma calcifediol concentration, which is the most accurate indicator of bodily vitamin D stores, is low. Consequently, plasma [calcitriol]s are low, resulting in reduced intestinal absorption of Ca. Examples of vitamin D deficiency include decreased intake of dietary vitamin D, inadequate exposure to sunlight, malabsorption syndromes with steatorrhea, and administration of the cholesterol-binding agent cholestyramine.

Abnormal Metabolism of Calcifediol.   Vitamin D_3 is hydroxylated to 25-hydroxyvitamin D_3 in the liver. Production of this calcitriol precursor is reduced in diffuse parenchymal liver disease and abnormalities of the biliary tract. Under these circumstances, low plasma [calcifediol]s have been observed. Reduced hepatic production of calcifediol plays a role in these disorders, but abnormal intestinal absorption of vitamin D may also be involved. The prolonged administration of anticonvulsant drugs may cause hypocalcemia and osteomalacia because they induce hepatic microsomal enzyme activity which accelerates degradation of calcitriol.

Reduced Production of Calcitriol.   Patients with chronic renal failure have reduced plasma calcitriols. Because the kidneys are the major site of calcitriol synthesis, chronic renal failure is associated with reduced production of this metabolite. The latter results in decreased intestinal Ca absorption and skeletal resistance to the calcemic actions of PTH. Decreased production of calcitriol has also been observed in patients with proximal tubular dysfunction, such as the Fanconi Syndrome.

Hyperphosphatemia.   In adult humans, variations in dietary P intake that produce changes in serum [P] within the physiologic range regulate proximal tubular production of calcitriol. Hyperphosphatemia suppresses, whereas hypophosphatemia stimulates, calcitriol production. Thus, in addition to its physical chemical effect to depress plasma $[Ca^{2+}]$, hyperphosphatemia reduces plasma [calcitriol]. Hyperphosphatemia is most commonly seen in chronic renal failure, but is also observed in the therapy for neoplasms such as acute leukemia and lymphoma.

Other.   Because severe Mg depletion suppresses PTH secretion and causes resistance to the calcemic action of PTH on bone, it can cause hypocalcemia. Acute pancreatitis can cause hypocalcemia by an unknown mechanism. It has been speculated that the liberation of fatty acids during the inflammation of the pancreas may bind Ca from the extracellular fluid. Finally, several drugs cause hypocalcemia. These include plicamycin, calcitonin, colchicine, intravenous citrate, Ca-free albumin, and furosemide, among others.

Consequences

Neurologic.   Clinical symptoms and signs of hypocalcemia are more dramatic than those of hypercalcemia. Early symptoms include paresthesias, depression, emotional instability, confusion, and anxiety. Early physical signs include Parkinsonian-like tremors and positive Chvostek's and Trousseau's signs. Chvostek's sign is spasm of the muscles innervated by the facial nerve, which is elicited by tapping the supramandibular portion of the parotid gland with the finger. Trousseau's sign is carpal spasm occurring within three minutes of inflating a sphygmomanometer around the upper arm. The carpal spasm results in flexion contracture of the wrist and the metacarpal-phalangeal joints, with the fingers held straight and grouped with the tips together (Fig. 54-6). The test is considered negative if

Fig. 54-6. Trousseau's sign. (Reproduced with permission from: Ganong WF. Hormonal control of calcium metabolism & the physiology of bone. In *Review of Medical Physiology* (17th ed.). East Norwalk: Appleton and Lange, 1995, Chap. 21, p. 361.)

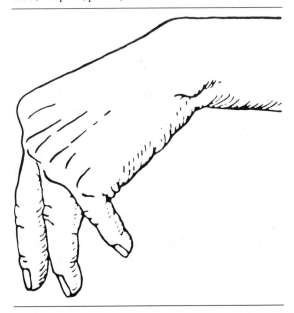

carpal spasm does not develop within 3 minutes. With severe hypocalcemia more dramatic signs ensue. Specifically, patients may experience muscle cramps followed by tetany and then seizures. Tetany may be life-threatening if either the pharyngeal or the respiratory muscles are affected.

Cardiovascular.   Reductions in cardiac index and stroke volume and congestive heart failure have been observed with prolonged hypocalcemia. In the intensive care unit, an association has been demonstrated between arterial hypotension and hypocalcemia. On the electrocardiogram the QT-interval is prolonged.

Other.   With chronic hypocalcemia, dry skin and eczema, hair loss, brittle nails, moniliasis, and cataracts have been observed.

Phosphorus (P)

Bodily Content and Distribution

A 70-kg adult male contains ~700 g of elemental P. Approximately 600 g are in bone, 3 g in teeth, 100 g in soft tissues, 0.20 g in extravascular fluid, and 0.17 g in plasma. In contrast to Ca, P is widely distributed in nonosseous tissues, both in inorganic forms as well as a component of phospholipids, phosphoproteins, nucleic acids, and the intermediates of carbohydrate metabolism. The inorganic P within bone exists primarily as Ca hydroxyapatite, but there is also a nontrivial component of amorphous Ca-P_i.

Homeostasis

Serum [P] is regulated, though much less closely than [Ca]. In adult humans, it varies between 0.8 and 1.4 mmol/liter (2.5–4.5 mg/dl) (Fig. 54-7); 85% is free, whereas 15% is protein-bound. At the physiologic pH of 7.40, HPO_4^{2-} + $NaHPO_4^-$ account for 85% of the free P_i, whereas $H_2PO_4^-$ accounts for 15%. The serum $[P_i]$ may vary by as much as 50% within a single day, and is set by the balance between intestinal absorption and renal excretion. Absorption occurs transcellularly, primarily in the jejunum. The first step is sodium-dependent P_i uptake across the luminal cell membrane. Elevated plasma [calcitriol]s augment intestinal P_i absorption, whereas decreased concentrations diminish it. Following a meal, serum [P] rises significantly. Excess P_i is excreted by the kidneys under the influence of PTH. The latter inhibits sodium-dependent P_i uptake

across the luminal cell membrane of the proximal tubules, thereby increasing urinary P_i excretion. In states of dietary P deprivation, urinary P excretion is nil and fractional intestinal P absorption is maximized.

Balance

Approximately 850 mg of elemental P are ingested per day, primarily in the form of dairy products, cereals, and animal proteins. Approximately 50–60% of dietary P is absorbed in the intestines. Although P absorption is augmented by calcitriol, it is not strictly dependent upon this hormone. For example, in patients with chronic renal failure who have nondetectable plasma [calcitriol]s, intestinal P absorption continues at a significant rate. Approximately 300 mg of P are eliminated in the feces each day, and 550 mg are excreted in the urine. The tubular reabsorption of P under normal circumstances is equal to or greater than 85% of the filtered load. The P_i is reabsorbed primarily by the proximal tubules via a sodium-dependent P_i cotransporter in the luminal cell membranes. This process is regulated by PTH, which inhibits reabsorption of P_i. Phosphaturia occurs within minutes after elevation of serum [PTH]. There may be a site of P_i absorption in the distal nephron that is also regulated by PTH, but its role is small compared to that of the proximal tubules. The importance of the kidneys in regulating serum [P] is demonstrated by the observation that patients with renal failure who are not treated develop significant hyperphosphatemia as glomerular filtration rate falls.

Hyperphosphatemia

Causes

Renal Failure.   The most common causes of hyperphosphatemia are acute and chronic renal failure. Under these circumstances, intestinal P absorption outstrips urinary excretion, thereby elevating serum [P]. In some patients with secondary hyperparathyroidism, the release of skeletal P resulting from dissolution of bone mineral by the action of PTH may also contribute to the severe hyperphosphatemia.

Increased P_i Entry into Extracellular Fluid.   This can occur endogenously or exogenously. Excessive influx of P_i from the intestines to the extracellular fluid may occur with oral ingestion of P_i-containing compounds (for example, P_i supplements), vitamin D intoxication (which increases intestinal P absorption), or the use of P_i-containing laxatives or enemas. Hyperphosphatemia can also result

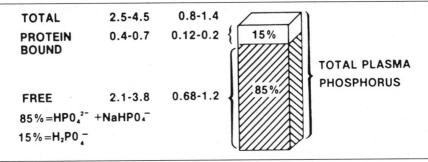

Fig. 54-7. Distribution of plasma total [P] in normal adult humans. Values in the left column are mg/dl, whereas values in the right column are mmol/liter. (Reproduced with permission from: Arnaud CD. Mineral and bone homeostasis. In Wyngaarden J, et al. (ed.). *Cecil Textbook of Medicine* (17th ed.). Philadelphia: W. B. Saunders, 1985, Chap. 243, pp. 1415–1423.)

from the parenteral administration of P_i supplements, the transfusion of old blood, or the use of lipid emulsions for total parenteral nutrition. Patients who have suffered white P burns can also become hyperphosphatemic.

In addition to entry of P_i into the extracellular fluid from exogenous sources, there may be redistribution of P between the intracellular and extracellular compartments. This occurs in respiratory acidosis, diabetic ketoacidosis, and lactic acidosis with tissue ischemia. There is also a redistribution when cells are destroyed. Examples of the latter include rhabdomyolysis, malignant hyperpyrexia, cytotoxic therapy for neoplastic disease, and hemolysis. Very high ambient temperatures also can produce hyperphosphatemia.

Consequences

Severe acute hyperphosphatemia may cause acute hypocalcemia with tetany and/or convulsions. More commonly, metastatic calcification in the form of amorphous $Ca-P_i$ precipitation in the kidneys, Purkinje fibers in myocardium, alveolar membranes of the lungs, subcutaneous tissues, conjunctivae, the gastrointestinal tract, and the small arteries and veins is observed. As a result of metastatic calcification, cardiac conduction disturbances with arrhythmias may develop. In some patients cardiac failure leading to hypotension and shock has been observed. Oliguric acute renal failure has been documented with acute hyperphosphatemia. An acute polyarticular joint pain syndrome may result from metastatic calcification. Haziness of the corneas with conjunctivitis and ischemic necrosis of the fingertips and toes can occur because of $Ca-P_i$ precipitation in the cornea and in the small blood vessels of the digits, respectively.

Hypophosphatemia

Causes

Hypophosphatemia results from either a decreased entry of P_i from the intestinal tract to the extracellular fluid, a transcellular shift from the extracellular fluid to within the cells, or increased P_i loss via the intestines or the kidneys. Given the ubiquity of P in commonly ingested foods, decreased intake is rarely a cause of hypophosphatemia. However, with starvation, the malabsorption syndrome, or vigorous use of P_i-binding antacids, notably aluminum hydroxide or aluminum carbonate, P depletion can occur. P_i shifts from the extracellular fluid into cells are common. They are related to the formation of P_i-containing intermediates of glycolytic metabolism. These include glucose-6-phosphate, 1,3-diphosphoglycerate, and high-energy P_i compounds such as adenosine triphosphate. Movement of P_i from the extracellular to the intracellular compartment plays a major role in the hypophosphatemia of intravenous hyperalimentation, respiratory alkalosis, the treatment of diabetic ketoacidosis, and the response of alcoholic individuals to infusions of intravenous dextrose in the absence of P_i supplementation. P_i loss from the intestinal tract can cause hypophosphatemia. Not only do aluminum-containing antacids bind dietary P, thereby blocking their intestinal absorption, but they also can remove endogenous P_i that is secreted by the small intestine during the absorptive process. P_i losses from the intestinal tract can also occur with the malabsorption syndrome. Renal losses of P_i can also cause hypophosphatemia. These include the Fanconi syndrome, X-linked hypophosphatemic rickets, and severe hypomagnesemia. Finally, elevated plasma [PTH], by inhibiting proximal tubular P_i absorption, can also cause hypophosphatemia.

Consequences

There are both short- and long-term consequences of severe hypophosphatemia. Acutely, there is red cell dysfunction, sometimes eventuating in hemolysis. Depletion of intracellular 2,3-diphosphoglycerate and ATP are most important. 2,3-diphosphoglycerate normally shifts the oxyhemoglobin dissociation curve in a direction that enhances tissue availability of oxygen. Lowering 2,3-diphosphoglycerate within red blood cells impairs oxygen delivery to peripheral tissues. When ATP levels within the erythrocyte fall to very low levels, they may be inadequate to maintain the structure of the cell membrane, resulting in hemolysis. Studies in experimental animals have shown that P depletion impairs chemotaxis, phagocytosis, and bacteriocidal function. Patients may develop muscle weakness with severe hypophosphatemia, which can involve the diaphragm and thereby cause respiratory failure. Rarely, rhabdomyolysis occurs. Severe P depletion can also cause congestive cardiac failure, which reverses on P_i repletion, and central nervous system dysfunction. Symptoms and signs include irritability, weakness, and paresthesias, which may progress to obtundation, seizures, and coma.

Magnesium (Mg)

Bodily Content and Distribution

A 70-kg adult male contains ~1.1 mol (27 g) of elemental Mg. Of this total, 14 g are located within bone, 12 g within soft tissues, 170 mg within the extracellular fluid, and 60 mg within the plasma. The normal plasma [Mg] varies between 0.8 and 1.0 mmol/liter (Fig. 54-8). Ionized Mg (Mg^{2+}) comprises 55% of the total, protein-bound Mg 32%, and Mg complexes 13%. Mg is an essential cofactor of ~300 different enzymes, including transphosphorylation reactions involving adenosine triphosphate. Thus it is central to cellular energy metabolism and the synthesis of macromolecules. Mg also plays a structural role in bone crystals.

Homeostasis

In a given individual, plasma total [Mg] is tightly controlled, deviations from the mean rarely exceeding 15%. Similar to serum [P], no one hormone is known to primarily regulate serum [Mg]. Calcitriol does augment intestinal Mg absorption, and PTH stimulates tubular absorption of Mg in the thick ascending limb of Henle's loop, the major site of Mg reabsorption within the nephron. In response to dietary Mg deprivation, urinary Mg excretion diminishes to virtually undetectable levels.

Balance

Typically, 12.5 mmol of Mg are ingested daily by individuals living within the United States. Since Mg is an integral part of chlorophyll, leafy green vegetables are the most abundant source of Mg in the North American diet. Additionally, Mg is present in meats, grains, seafood, and coconuts. Fractional absorption of Mg varies inversely with dietary intake. For example, in one study dietary Mg content was increased in a stepwise fashion from 0.95 to 10 to 23.5 mmol/day. The corresponding values of the fractional absorption of Mg were 76, 44, and 24%. Qualitatively, this adaptation is quite similar to what is seen with dietary Ca deprivation. When in Mg balance, individuals excrete in their urine the amount of Mg that they absorb in their intestines. Urinary Mg excretion is the difference between its glomerular filtration and tubular reabsorption. The thick ascending limb of Henle's loop accounts for 60–70% of the latter. Urinary Mg excretion is increased by extracellular fluid volume expansion, by dilation of the renal blood vessels, by osmotic diuresis, by alcohol, and by loop-acting diuretics, such as furosemide.

Hypermagnesemia

Because normal kidneys have a large capacity to excrete Mg, significant hypermagnesemia is rarely seen in individuals with normal renal function. Intravenous infusion of $MgSO_4$ is used in the treatment of pre-eclampsia and eclampsia in pregnant women. Under these circumstances, symptomatic hypermagnesemia may develop. Elevated ionized Mg (Mg^{2+}) concentrations depress the central nervous system and exert a curarelike effect on neuromuscular junctions. Hypermagnesemia causes peripheral vasodilatation resulting in hypotension. In addition, hypermagnesemia depresses the cardiac conduction system, causes bradyarrhythmias, and can cause asystole with cardiac arrest during diastole. In patients with renal insufficiency, excessive use of Mg-containing antacids can cause clinically significant hypermagnesemia.

Hypomagnesemia

Causes

Hypomagnesemia may be caused by decreased Mg absorption from dietary sources or increased loss of Mg from the body. Decreased absorption of dietary Mg occurs most frequently in alcoholics, who typically have a diet that is poor

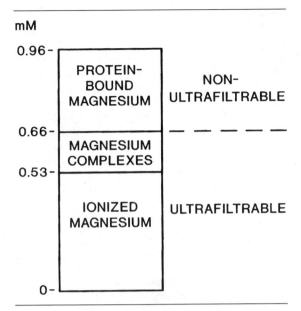

Fig. 54-8. Typical distribution of the components of plasma total [Mg] in normal adult humans. Values may be converted from mM to mg/dl by multiplying the former by 2.43. (The atomic weight of Mg is 24.305 g/mol.)

in Mg. Frequently, they show some degree of malabsorption because of chronic pancreatitis, thereby aggravating this problem. There is some evidence that ethanol has a direct suppressive effect on intestinal Mg absorption. This combination of poor intake combined with suboptimal absorption can lead to hypomagnesemia. Loss of Mg from the body can occur via the gastrointestinal tract. Specifically, chronic vomiting, diarrhea, fistulas, and/or nasogastric suction can produce Mg depletion. Urinary Mg losses also can produce hypomagnesemia. Loop-acting diuretics and certain antibiotics are the most common causes of renal magnesium wasting. The former include furosemide, bumetanide, and piretanide, and the latter include gentamicin and amphotericin B. Cisplatin, an antineoplastic agent, is also a well-known renal Mg-wasting agent. Magnesuria has been observed during the treatment of diabetic ketoacidosis. Rarely, breast feeding can cause lactation hypomagnesemia.

Consequences

Because hypomagnesemia rarely occurs as an isolated entity, it is difficult to distinguish symptoms and signs related to a low serum [Mg] alone. Three clinically significant syndromes are associated with Mg depletion. First, hypocalcemia is one of the most consistent and important findings in Mg deficiency with hypomagnesemia. The causes of the hypocalcemia are twofold. Severe Mg depletion blocks PTH secretion without blunting its synthesis, and there appears to be end-organ resistance to the action of PTH on bone. Typically, patients afflicted with this syndrome are alcoholics who present with lethargy, weakness, fatigue, poor mentation, paresthesias, tremors, muscle fasciculations, and occasionally tetany. Chvostek's and Trousseau's signs may be positive. These patients do not respond symptomatically to parenteral Ca administration, but their hypocalcemia and associated symptoms respond within minutes to parenteral Mg replacement, which is accompanied by a rise in plasma [PTH]. A second syndrome frequently associated with Mg depletion is that of hypokalemia secondary to urinary potassium wasting. With severe Mg depletion, hypokalemia cannot be corrected with potassium replacements alone. Although loop diuretics produce potassium depletion directly by increasing urinary potassium excretion, they may also increase urinary potassium excretion secondarily by causing Mg depletion. Correction of this form of hypokalemia requires the replacement of Mg prior to treatment of the hypokalemia with potassium supplements. The mechanism by which Mg depletion prevents repletion of body potassium is unknown. Finally, hypomagnesemia can cause cardiac arrhythmias and an increased sensitivity to digitalis glycosides. The former can include ventricular premature beats, ventricular tachycardia, or ventricular fibrillation.

Clinical Examples

1. A 40-year-old white woman discovered that she had an elevated blood pressure during a hypertension-screening session in a shopping mall near her home. She made an appointment with an internist, who found that she had passed a kidney stone 6 months previously. In the doctor's office her blood pressure was 150/105 mm Hg. She was prescribed hydrochlorothiazide, 100 mg daily. One and one-half years after starting the diuretic, her serum [Ca] and [P] were 11.8 and 2.1 mg/dl, respectively. Her physician requested that she discontinue the hydrochlorothiazide and return in one month with a 24-hour urine collection.

Laboratory Results

(Serum) sodium	138 meq/liter
Potassium	3.6 meq/liter
Chloride	114 meq/liter
Bicarbonate	21 meq/liter
Ca	11.9 mg/dl
P	2.0 mg/dl
Creatinine	1.0 mg/dl

24-hour urine

Ca	350 mg/24 hours
P	800 mg/24 hours
Creatinine	1,330 mg/24 hours

Discussion.   This patient most likely has primary hyperparathyroidism. Findings that support this diagnosis are (1) hypercalcemia, (2) hypophosphatemia, (3) hypercalciuria, (4) hyperphosphaturia, and (5) hyperchloremia combined with hypobicarbonatemia. Diagnostic tests that might prove useful in this patient's case include measurements of the serum [PTH], measurement of 24-hour urinary cyclic AMP excretion, and an ultrasound examination of the neck looking for a parathyroid adenoma. Ca-containing kidney stones are quite common in primary hyperparathyroidism. Elevated serum [PTH] increases plasma [calcitriol], resulting in increased intestinal Ca absorption as well as increased mobilization of Ca from bone. Although PTH increases Ca reabsorption by the renal tubules, hypercalciuria is present in hyperparathyroidism because of the high filtered load of Ca. The hypercalciuria is believed to be the major cause of the Ca-containing kidney stones. Hydrochlorothiazide was stopped because the thiazide-class of diuretics can cause hypercalcemia in the setting of hyperparathyroidism. By stimulating Ca absorption in the distal convoluted tubule, thiazides decrease its urinary excretion. However, in the absence of other predisposing causes, thiazides rarely cause an elevation in plasma [Ca] above 11 mg/dl. In part, the patient's hypertension may relate to her hypercalcemia because the latter constricts the major peripheral vascular resistance vessels. Hypophosphatemia results because the elevated serum [PTH] causes a significant phosphaturia. The tubular reabsorption of P is calculated as follows: TRP (%) = (1 − phosphate clearance ÷ creatinine clearance) × 100. When the tubular reabsorption of P is less than 85%, serum [PTH] is frequently elevated, especially when renal function is normal. What is the tubular reabsorption of P for this patient?

2. A 56-year-old white man was admitted to the hospital complaining of low back pain radiating down his right leg for 3 months. The pain was evoked by moving from the sitting to the standing position and was relieved by lying down. He also complained of losing 25 lb. (from 165 to 140 lb.) over 4 months and of frequent urination (including nocturia) and excessive thirst for 2 months. Finally, he suffered from constipation, ringing in his ears, and poor appetite for several weeks. He had smoked one package of cigarettes per day for 40 years and was producing one tablespoon of gray sputum per day without hemoptysis at the time of ad-

mission. Physical examination revealed a weight of 140 lb. His pulse was 104 and 144 bpm in the supine and upright positions, respectively. His corresponding blood pressures were 150/78 and 132/85 mm Hg. He had a 2.5-cm (in diameter) fixed hard mass at the sternal angle, and there was severe pain with straight leg raising on the right at 30°. There was no pain on the left, even when the leg was raised to 75 deg. A chest x-ray revealed a mass in the left upper lobe of the lung which measured 4 cm × 3 cm. Sputum cytology and bronchoscopy washings were consistent with squamous cell carcinoma. Bone scan was negative.

Laboratory Results

(Serum) sodium	136 meq/liter
Potassium	4.3 meq/liter
Chloride	43 meq/liter
Bicarbonate	26 meq/liter
Ca	17.4 mg/dl
P	2.1 mg/dl
Creatinine	0.9 mg/dl

Discussion.   The most likely diagnosis in this patient is the syndrome of humoral hypercalcemia of malignancy associated with squamous cell carcinoma of the lung. These neoplasms may produce a PTH-rp which occupies the PTH receptor in cells of the skeleton and the kidney tubules. The physiologic actions of the PTH-rp are virtually identical to those of PTH, although this peptide is antigenically and structurally distinct. Serum [PTH] is suppressed in these patients by the high plasma [Ca^{2+}]. The patients develop hypercalcemia because of the combined actions of the PTH-rp on the cells surrounding bone that cause its demineralization and by increased renal tubular absorption of Ca by the action of the PTH-rp on the kidney tubules. Similar to PTH, the PTH-rp increases urinary P excretion by inhibiting proximal tubule P_i absorption. PTH-rp also may be elevated with renal cell carcinoma and other neoplasms. The patient had symptoms and signs of extracellular fluid volume contraction, resulting from the actions of hypercalcemia on the kidney. Hypercalcemia causes increased salt wasting by the kidney and a vasopressin-resistant form of diabetes insipidus.

3. A 56-year-old Afro-American female nursing assistant complained to her physician of shortness of breath, nasal congestion, and painful elevated red skin over her shins for 6 months. Her physical examination was unremarkable with the exceptions of moderately enlarged lymph nodes diffusely and of two distinct lesions of erythema nodosum

over her shins. Chest x-rays showed bilateral hilar lymphadenopathy, but the pulmonary parenchyma was normal. Serum [Ca] was 12.3 mg/dl, serum [P] was 4.3 mg/dl, serum [creatinine] was 1.0 mg/dl, and serum [PTH] was below the lower limits of normal. Tomograms of the chest revealed hilar and paratracheal adenopathy.

Discussion.   This patient presents with the classic features of sarcoidosis. Ten percent of patients with normal renal function and sarcoidosis demonstrate hypercalcemia. In these patients, elevated plasma [calcitriol]s correlate directly with plasma [calcifediol]s, unlike normal individuals in whom plasma [calcitriol]s are independent of the precursor. The cause of the elevated plasma [calcitriol]s in patients with sarcoidosis is unregulated biosynthesis of calcitriol by the granulomata. A combination of the elevated plasma [Ca^{2+}] and plasma [calcitriol] suppress PTH biosynthesis and secretion, leading to a low serum [PTH]. Unlike the hypercalcemia of malignancy, serum [P] is normal. Prednisone is useful in treating the hypercalcemia of sarcoidosis because it inhibits the production of calcitriol by the granulomatous tissue.

Bibliography

Agus ZS and Massry SG. Hypomagnesemia and hypermagnesemia. In Narins RG (ed.). *Maxwell & Kleeman's Clinical Disorders of Fluid and Electrolyte Metabolism* (5th ed.). New York: McGraw-Hill, 1994, Chap. 34, pp. 1099–1119. *Contemporary view of the disorders of magnesium metabolism.*

Benabe JE and Martínez-Maldonado M. Disorders of calcium metabolism. In Narins RG (ed.). *Maxwell & Kleeman's Clinical Disorders of Fluid and Electrolyte Metabolism* (5th ed.). New York: McGraw-Hill, 1994, pp. 1009–1044. *Contemporary view of the disorders of calcium metabolism.*

Bourdeau JE and Attie MF. Calcium metabolism. In Narins RG (ed.). *Maxwell & Kleeman's Clinical Disorders of Fluid and Electrolyte Metabolism* (5th ed.). New York: McGraw-Hill, 1994, Chap. 11, pp. 243–306. *Contemporary view of normal calcium metabolism and homeostasis.*

Favus MJ (ed.). *Primer on the Metabolic Bone Diseases and Disorders of Mineral Metabolism* (2nd ed.). New York: Raven, 1993. *Concise, but authoritative, treatise on the physiology and pathophysiology of bone and mineral metabolism.*

Levin BS and Kleeman CR. Hypophosphatemia and hyperphosphatemia: Clinical and pathophysiologic aspects. In Narins RG (ed.). *Maxwell & Kleeman's Clinical Disorders of Fluid and Electrolyte Metabolism* (5th ed.). New York: McGraw-Hill, 1994, Chap. 33, pp. 1045–1097. *Contemporary view of the disorders of phosphorus metabolism.*

Quamme GA and Dirks JH. Magnesium metabolism. In Narins RG (ed.). *Maxwell & Kleeman's Clinical Disorders of Fluid and Electrolyte Metabolism* (5th ed.). New York: McGraw-Hill, 1994, Chap. 13, pp. 373–397. *Contemporary view of normal magnesium metabolism and homeostasis.*

Yanagawa N, Nakhoul F, Kurokawa K, and Lee DBN. Physiology of phosphorus metabolism. In Narins RG (ed.). *Maxwell & Kleeman's Clinical Disorders of Fluid and Electrolyte Metabolism* (5th ed.). New York: McGraw-Hill, 1994, pp. 307–371. *Contemporary view of normal phosphorus metabolism and homeostasis.*

55 Glomerular Disorders

Sudhir K. Khanna

Objectives

After completing this chapter, you should be able to

Describe normal glomerular structure and function

Outline current understanding of potential mechanisms of glomerular injury

Explain how physicians identify the presence of a glomerular disorder

Define seven clinical syndromes which may result from glomerular disorders

Explain the mechanisms of edema formation related to glomerular disease

List the common systemic diseases which may be associated with glomerular damage

List the four most common primary renal disorders causing nephrotic syndrome

---

Renal diseases which initially or primarily involve the glomeruli are considered in this chapter. Classification of glomerular disorders currently represents a mixture of clinical findings, histologic appearances, pathogenic mechanisms, and etiology. The kidney can only respond in a limited number of ways to a variety of pathogenic stimuli and therefore clinical presentation often does not predict the underlying histologic appearance, etiology, or pathogenesis. For example, patients with proliferative glomerulonephritis can present with either hematuria or hematuria and proteinuria with or without azotemia, while the nephrotic syndrome may be due to several histologic lesions of various etiologies and pathogenesis.

Glomerular disorders are conveniently divided into primary and secondary types. **Primary disorders** affect only the kidney, although there can be some systemic effects of the renal disease. In **secondary disorders** glomeruli are involved as part and parcel of more widespread systemic disease. A useful clinical approach is to consider glomerular disorders as follows:

Clinical syndromes, e.g., nephritic or nephrotic syndrome or rapidly progressive glomerulonephritis.

Histologic diagnosis, based on light microscopy, immunofluorescence, and electron microscopy.

Pathogenic mechanisms.

Etiology, which for most conditions is still unknown.

This detailed analysis helps in prognostication and establishing a long-term treatment and followup plan.

Glomerular Anatomy

The glomerulus is essentially a tuft of capillaries interposed between two resistance vessels, the afferent and efferent arterioles (Fig. 55-1). This unique arrangement provides a mechanism to control the glomerular capillary hydraulic pressure within a narrow range, despite wide fluctuations in the systemic blood pressure. Bowman's capsule surrounds this capillary network and is lined by a monolayer of epithelial cells.

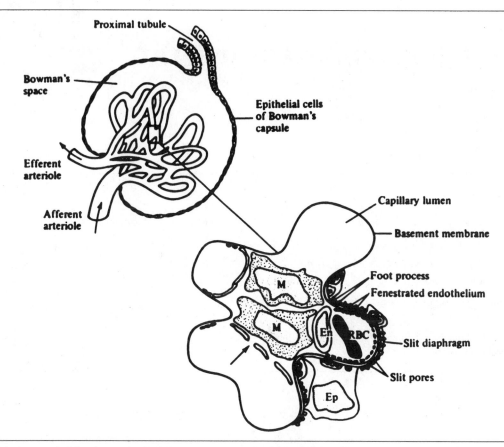

Fig. 55-1. Anatomy of the glomerulus and diagram of part of capillary tuft with mesangial cells (M). (Modified from: Rose D. *Clinical Physiology of Acid-Base and Electrolyte Disorders* (4th ed.). New York: McGraw-Hill, 1994.)

Glomerular Capillary Wall Has Three Layers

Endothelial Cells

Glomerular capillaries are lined by this layer of cells containing pores or fenestra ranging from 70 to 100 nm in diameter. The surface of these cells is negatively charged.

Glomerular Basement Membrane

GBM is composed of three layers, lamina rara externa, a central dense layer, and the lamina rara interna. The main component of the GBM is type IV collagen. The GBM is also negatively charged and is the principal structure responsible for permeability properties of the glomerulus.

Epithelial Cell Layer

This outermost layer is composed of cells called podocytes. These cells have interdigitating foot processes and the space between them is called the filtration slit or slit-pore. The epithelial cell plasma membrane is negatively charged, which is important for maintenance of the filtration barrier.

Mesangium

Composed of mesangial cells and the surrounding matrix (Fig. 55-1), mesangium is located between the capillary loops. Mesangials cells are specialized pericytes and have functional properties of smooth muscle cell. They respond to vasoactive hormones and prostaglandins and regulate the capillary surface area and glomerular blood flow.

Glomerular Physiology

The first step in the process of urine formation is passage of a cell- and protein-free ultrafiltrate of plasma which contains small solutes (such as urea, creatinine, sodium, potassium, and uric acid) and water. Solutes up to the size of inulin (MW 5200) are freely filtered, while albumin (MW 69,000) and globulins are filtered in very small amounts. This is achieved by both size and charge selectivity properties of the capillary membrane. Since albumin is a polyanion at physiologic pH, electrostatic repulsion by anion sites in the filtration barrier is the major factor which prevents albumin from crossing the capillary wall.

The main determinant of the ultrafiltration rate is the difference between transcapillary hydraulic pressure gradient (ΔP) and the colloid osmotic pressure gradient ($\Delta\pi$) across the glomerular capillaries. This can be expressed by the following equation:

$$J_v = K(\Delta P - \Delta\pi)$$
$$= K\left[\left(P_{gc} - P_t\right) - \left(\pi_{gc} - \pi_t\right)\right]$$

where J_v is fluid movement, K is effective hydraulic permeability of capillary wall, P_{gc} and π_{gc} are hydraulic and osmotic pressure in glomerular capillaries, and P_t and π_t are hydraulic and osmotic pressure in tubules.

Normal glomerular filtration rate (GFR) in humans is 100–125 ml/minute or 180 liters/day. GFR can be accurately estimated by measuring the clearance of an inert substance like inulin, which is freely filtered but is neither metabolized nor reabsorbed or secreted by the tubules. Creatinine clearance is easier to measure but, because of variable secretion of creatinine in the proximal tubule, it may overestimate the GFR by approximately 10–30%.

Mechanism of Glomerular Injury

The two major mechanisms of glomerular injury are **inflammation** and **hemodynamic** injury. Both inflammatory and hemodynamic injury cause glomerular sclerosis, which may lead to progression of renal failure, despite the primary initiating event being in some cases inactive. Mechanisms of glomerular injury as listed in Table 55-1 are discussed below.

Table 55-1. Mechanisms of Glomerular Injury

INFLAMMATORY
Immunologic injury
    Anti-GBM disease
    Immune complex disease
    Alternate complement pathway activation
    Cell-mediated injury
Vascular disorders
    Systemic vasculitis
    Thrombotic microangiopathies
    Cholesterol embolization
Metabolic or toxic damage
    Diabetes mellitus
    Amyloidosis
    Drugs and toxins
Idiopathic
HEMODYNAMIC FACTORS

Inflammatory Mechanisms of Glomerular Injury

The mechanisms initiating inflammatory injury include immunologic damage to glomeruli and chemical mediators liberated by glomerular and inflammatory cells in response to nonimmune disorders. Immune mechanisms are responsible for a majority of glomerular diseases. Recently some "idiopathic" conditions have also been associated with immunologic markers, e.g., antineutrophil cytoplasmic antibodies (ANCA).

Immunologic Injury

Antigen can be either endogenous (e.g., glomerular basement membrane) or exogenous (e.g., drugs and infectious agents). Humoral and cell-mediated immunity and the complement cascade may be involved.

Antibodies Directed Against GBM. This is a rare condition accounting for < 5% of human glomerulonephritis. It may be associated with Goodpasture's syndrome, which typically presents with pulmonary hemorrhage and crescentic glomerular nephritis (Fig. 55-2). Some patients may only have isolated renal involvement. The experimental counterpart of anti-GBM disease in rats is called Masugi Nephritis and is produced by injecting antibodies prepared in rabbits by immunization with rat GBM. Once antibodies bind to GBM, injury is initiated by activation of humoral and cellular pathways of inflammation. On immunofluorescent microscopy these antibodies show a characteristic linear staining pattern (Plate 5).

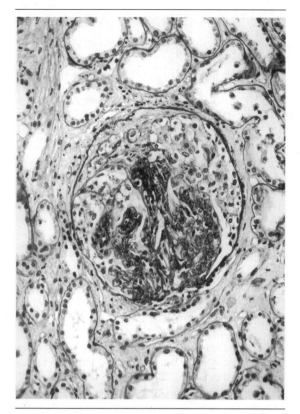

Fig. 55-2. Crescentic glomerulonephritis. An epithelial crescent has compressed the glomerular tuft. (Jones-Methanamine: silver, original magnification 250×). (Courtesy of K. Min, M.D.)

Immune Complex Disease.   This can occur either by deposition of preformed antigen-antibody complexes which get trapped in the glomerular capillaries or by in situ formation of antigen-antibody complexes. The immune complex mechanism is responsible for the majority of glomerulonephritis in humans. Antigens can be endogenous (systemic lupus or tumors) or exogenous (hepatitis B, streptococci, and treponema). Ag-Ab complexes get deposited in the capillary wall (mostly subendothelial) and mesangium and appear as granular deposits on immunofluorescence microscopy (Plate 6). Size and electrical charge on the complexes determine whether glomerular trapping will take place.

Heymann nephritis, an experimental model of membranous nephropathy, is an example of in situ immune complex formation. In this model antibodies leave the circulation, cross the GBM, and bind with epithelial cell antigens. No circulating immune complexes are detected, but on im-

munofluorescence and electron microscopy subepithelial deposits are identified.

Alternate Pathway Activation of Complement System.   These patients usually have membranoproliferative glomerulonephritis, and typically have C_3 nephritic factor ($C_3 N_e F$) in their serum. This antibody acts at the same step as properdin and helps in cleavage of C_3 to C_3b. Since C_3N_ef is an IgG, this is really an autoimmune disease.

Cell-Mediated Injury.   The role of cells in initiating glomerular injury is not well defined, although monocytes and T lymphocytes are present in glomeruli in several types of glomerulonephritis. It has been hypothesized that in minimal change disease, cytokins released by T lymphocytes are responsible for increased capillary permeability leading to proteinuria.

Irrespective of the initial events, further injury depends on the interaction of cellular and humoral mediators. Neutrophils and monocytes infiltrate from the circulation and adhere to the glomerular capillaries. This cellular adhesion occurs by receptor ligand interactions involving adhesion molecules (LCAM-1, ELAM-1, ICAM-1) which are unregulated during inflammation. Activated neutrophils and monocytes release enzymes, toxic metabolites, and cytokines which destroy GBM (causing proteinuria and hematuria) and growth factors like TGFβ which cause glomerular proliferation and increased mesangial matrix causing sclerosis. Endogenous glomerular cells also participate and release substances like endothelin and thromboxane, which reduce glomerular blood flow and promote capillary thrombosis.

Vascular Disorders

The glomerulus, being a capillary network, is affected by many disorders which involve blood vessels. Some of the important ones are:

Vasculitis.   Inflammation of the blood vessels may be confined to the kidneys or be part of a systemic disorder. The major renal syndromes in this group are pauci-immune necrotizing glomerulonephritis and hypersensitivity vasculitis.

Pauci-immune necrotizing glomerulonephritis manifests clinically as rapidly progressive glomerulonephritis. Previously most of these patients were classified as idiopathic crescentic glomerulonephritis, but recently antineutrophil cytoplasmic antibody (ANCA) has been found in the serum of these patients. Renal biopsy findings include glomerular crescents (Fig. 55-2) and the absence of immune deposits. A pathogenic role of these antibodies is not clearly defined, although ANCA can activate neutrophils and monocytes, which then can release toxic metabolites and lytic enzymes causing inflammation and necrotizing lesions. ANCA can be of two types based on staining characteristics. In microscopic polyarteritis, the staining pattern is perinuclear (P-ANCA), while in Wegener's granulomatosis the staining pattern is cytoplasmic (C-ANCA).

Hypersensitivity vasculitis is a heterogenous group of diseases, characterized by inflammation of arterioles, capillaries, and venules often seen in association with use of certain drugs like penicillin, sulfonamides, thiazide diuretics, and allopurinol. It causes focal necrotizing glomerulonephritis, and there may be crescent formation. Immune mechanisms may be involved since immunoglobulins and complement are usually identified in the renal tissue.

Thrombotic Microangiopathies. Thrombosis of glomerular capillaries and arterioles and a microangiopathic hemolytic anemia are the characteristic features of these disorders. The pathogenesis involves endothelial injury from varied causes like bacterial toxins (*E. coli* verotoxin), drugs (cyclosporin, mitomycin), and autoantibodies (anti-cardiolipin). Injury to the endothelium predisposes to thrombus formation and increases transudation of plasma into the subendothelial compartment. The thrombotic microangiopathies include hemolytic uremic syndrome (HUS), thrombotic thrombocytopenic purpura (TTP), malignant hypertension, renal crisis of progressive systemic sclerosis, and preeclampsia. Patients usually present with acute renal failure and evidence of a micro-angiopathic hemolytic anemia. Treatment depends on the underlying cause.

Cholesterol Embolization. This syndrome occurs mostly in elderly patients with aortic atherosclerosis, after they undergo arterial surgery or angiography. Occlusion of small blood vessels by embolized cholesterol particles causes ischemia and biconvex "cholesterol clefts" can often be identified in the tissues. Renal failure can be acute or progressive over several weeks depending upon the extent of the embolization. These patients also have eosinophilia, low C_3 complement levels, livedo reticularis of skin, abdominal pain, microscopic hematuria, and focal digital ischemia. Treatment is supportive and renal function may recover after weeks to months.

Metabolic and Toxic

A variety of these conditions can cause glomerular damage. Examples include diabetes mellitus, amyloidosis, and drugs.

Diabetes Mellitus. This is the single biggest cause of end-stage renal disease (ESRD) in the U.S.A. It occurs commonly in patients with insulin-dependent diabetes mellitus (IDDM) and in some patients with non-insulin-dependent diabetes (NIDDM). Persistent microalbuminuria (urine albumin excretion of 20–200 mcg/minute) has been identified to be a marker for development of nephropathy in IDDM. Treatment at this early stage with tight control of hyperglycemia and hypertension may postpone onset of the overt nephropathy. Some 10–15 years after the onset of IDDM and at variable time intervals in NIDDM, patients develop overt proteinuria and hypertension, which over several years progresses to renal insufficiency and ESRD. The glomerular lesions are characterized by thickening of GBM, increase mesangial matrix, and glomerulosclerosis. In the initial stages, glomerular filtration rate (GFR) increases above normal, but subsequently declines. Angiotensin-converting enzyme inhibitors have been shown to reduce the raised intraglomerular pressure and may be more effective than other antihypertensive agents in slowing progression of this disorder. (Diabetic nephropathy is also discussed in Chap. 24.)

Amyloidosis. Renal involvement is seen in approximately 80% of patients with amyloidosis. Amyloid protein is deposited in capillary walls and mesangium, causing proteinuria, nephrotic syndrome, and progressive renal insufficiency. Prognosis is poor unless the underlying cause of the amyloidosis can be effectively treated.

Drugs and Toxins. A large number of drugs — including captopril, gold, antibiotics (cephalosporins, penicillin), and penicillamine — can cause glomerulonephritis. Mechanisms are largely unknown but immunologic pathways are probably involved. (For example, captopril and penicillamine induced membranous glomerulonephritis.) The renal disease is mostly reversible if the offending agent is withdrawn early.

Idiopathic. The pathogenesis of focal segmental glomerulosclerosis is unknown. However, immune mechanisms may play a part, as shown by abnormal T lymphocyte function and presence of immune complexes in serum of some of these patients. Hemodynamic mechanisms may also be important.

Hemodynamic Mechanisms of Glomerular Injury

In rats after five-sixths nephrectomy, progressive focal and segmental glomerulosclerosis develops in association with proteinuria, hypertension, and progressive renal insufficiency. These rats demonstrate glomerular hypertrophy and increased single nephron GFR (overall GFR is reduced) in response to the increased functional demand. This so-called **hyperfiltration** is caused by increased glomerular plasma flow and capillary pressure resulting from disproportionately greater afferent than efferent arteriolar dilatation. Similar lesions are seen in human focal segmental glomerulosclerosis and similar alteration in glomerular hemodynamics occurs in sickle cell nephropathy and experimental diabetes mellitus. Angiotensin-converting enzyme inhibitors slow progression of glomerulosclerosis and reduce proteinuria, presumably by reversing the altered glomerular hemodynamics.

Clinical Manifestations of Glomerular Diseases

The kidney can only respond in a few ways, despite the numerous diseases affecting it. The hallmarks of glomerular diseases are proteinuria, hematuria, hypertension, and disturbance of excretory function. Usually it is difficult to predict the underlying pathologic condition without a kidney biopsy, because similar presentations can happen with several different diseases. A number of clinical syndromes are known, but these syndromes describe only the clinical features and are not diagnostic of histopathology or pathogenesis.

Proteinuria

Normally 25–150 mg of protein is excreted per day in the urine. This is composed of 20% albumin (filtered by glomerulus), 40% other plasma proteins (immunoglobulins), and 40% tubular proteins (mainly Tamm-Horsfall protein and some secretory IgA, lysozyme, and urokinase). Total 24-hour urine albumin excretion is normally < 20 mg/day.

Dipstick urine testing, a semiquantitative test, is a good screening procedure for proteinuria. It detects negatively charged proteins such as albumin, but does not detect positively charged proteins like immunoglobulin light chains (myeloma protein). This method usually detects albuminuria greater than 60 mg/24 hours, but if the urine is dilute it may not show positive. A 24-hour urine protein estimation should be performed in any patient suspected of having renal disease. Excessive proteinuria can be due to one or more of the mechanisms listed in Table 55-2.

When evaluating the etiology and significance of proteinuria, the following questions need to be answered: What is the composition of the urinary protein? What is the rate of a urine protein excretion? Are other renal and/or systemic abnormalities present? Does the patient have the nephrotic syndrome?

Table 55-2. Mechanisms of Proteinuria

Presence of an abnormal plasma protein (e.g., immunoglobulin light changes in myeloma).
Increased glomerular permeability due to altered barrier size or charge selectivity.
Defective tubular function or saturated tubular capacity for reabsorption of filtered proteins.
Increased secretion of tubular or lower urinary tract proteins.

Asymptomatic Proteinuria

This usually is detected during screening, commonly in young adults having an examination for insurance or employment purposes. Urine protein excretion is usually less than 3.0 g/day. It may or may not indicate renal disease. For example, proteinuria can be induced by vigorous exercise. Sometimes in young adults proteinuria may be present during upright posture which will disappear during supine posture. This is referred to as "orthostatic proteinuria" and is usually less than 1.0 g/day. The mechanism of this kind of proteinuria is not clear. If the proteinuria is persistent and is not related to exercise and posture, it is likely to be indicative of underlying glomerular disease, especially if most of the protein is albumin.

Nephrotic Syndrome

The nephrotic syndrome is characterized by proteinuria greater than 3.5 g/day, hypoalbuminemia, and edema. Hyperlipidemia is a usual accompaniment and in some patients hypercoagulability is also present. The fundamental defect is increased glomerular permeability to plasma proteins. Tubular capacity to reabsorb the protein load presented by glomerular filtration is limited and gets saturated very quickly. The extra protein which is not reabsorbed will appear in the urine. Protein reabsorbed by the tubules is catabolized; therefore net loss of protein is always more than the amount of protein present in the urine.

Hypoalbuminemia.   It results from a combination of albuminuria and tubular catabolism of protein despite increased compensatory albumin synthesis. Low plasma albumin levels reduce oncotic pressure, causing edema. The correlation between serum albumin concentration and edema is poor, but edema will be present in most patients when serum albumin is less than 3.0 gm/dl.

Edema.   Although usually dependent in location, in children facial edema is often noted. In severe cases massive generalized swelling may be present. Edema formation is classically attributed to a reduced plasma oncotic pressure causing transudation of fluid from vessels into the interstitium and renal salt and water retention owing to the resulting reduction in plasma volume. This explanation has recently been challenged with the discovery that most nephrotic patients have normal or increased blood volume. Also activity of the renin-angiotensin system is not increased in most patients with nephrotic syndrome. Hence the mechanisms of the increased sodium and water retention are not fully defined.

Hyperlipidemia.   It is due to a combination of increased production and diminished clearance of plasma lipoproteins. Characteristically, LDL and VLDL cholesterol are increased and HDL cholesterol levels are variable. The clinical consequences of these changes in lipid profile in nephrotic patients are not well described possibly because of the long time period involved in development of atherosclerosis. Animal experiments show that hyperlipidemia may accelerate progression of glomerulosclerosis, but the relevance of these findings to human disease is unknown.

Other Features of Nephrotic Syndrome.   Venous and arterial thrombosis are reported in 2–50% of patients with nephrotic syndrome. A common site is the renal veins, especially in membranous nephropathy. The underlying mechanism(s) of the hypercoagulability are not well defined but low concentrations of antithrombin III and free protein S, altered platelet function, and hyperfibrinogenimia may play a role.

Other aspects of the nephrotic syndrome include muscle wasting due to increased protein catabolism needed to maintain plasma protein levels. Infection is common but the mechanisms are not well understood. Hypocalcemia occurs owing to reduced protein availability to bind calcium as well as loss of 25-hydroxycholecalciferol in the urine.

The causes of nephrotic syndrome are listed in Table 55-3. An effort should always be made to exclude a secondary condition, because treatment of underlying cause may lead to remission of nephrotic syndrome. A renal biopsy may be needed to define the histology and determine the therapy and prognosis. Management includes controlling hypertension, relieving edema, and maintaining adequate nutrition. Dietary sodium intake should be lowered, hyperlipidemia treated and potential complications should be anticipated and treated as they arise.

Hematuria

Hematuria is a common finding in glomerular disorders but the workup should take into account the many and diverse causes of this condition. A positive dipstick test may

Table 55-3. Causes of Nephrotic Syndrome

Primary glomerular diseases
  Minimal change disease
  Membranous nephropathy
  Mesangial proliferative glomerulonephritis
  Focal and segmental glomerulosclerosis
  Membranoproliferative glomerulonephritis
Secondary causes
  Infections: hepatitis B and C, HIV, endocarditis, streptococcal infection
  Neoplasms: lymphomas, leukemias, carcinoma
  Drugs: gold, penicillamine, captopril, heroin
  Systemic diseases: systemic lupus erythematosus, amyloidosis, diabetes mellitus
  Hereditary and familial diseases: Alport's syndrome, sickle cell disease
  Miscellaneous: obesity, pre-eclampsia, chronic kidney allograft rejection.

occur from myoglobin, free hemoglobin, or RBCs in the urine. True hematuria may be from glomerular disease, renal neoplasia, lower urinary tract disorders, or coagulation disturbances. Glomerular hematuria is indicated by presence of dysmorphic RBCs and red cell casts. The presence of proteinuria also points towards a glomerular etiology for hematuria.

Recurrent gross hematuria with or without persistent microscopic hematuria occurring hours to days after an upper respiratory tract infection is likely secondary to an IgA nephropathy. This condition is characterized by mesangial proliferation with IgA deposits and usually presents in young males between ages 15 and 25. Other glomerular conditions causing persistent hematuria include hereditary nephritis and basement membrane disorders. It is important to exclude urologic causes of hematuria by appropriate investigations, especially in elderly patients.

Nephritic Syndrome

Nephritic syndrome is characterized by acute onset of hematuria, proteinuria, hypertension, and renal insufficiency. All or some of these features may be present in any given patient. Urinary RBCs are usually dysmorphic, and red cell casts (Plate 7) are often noted. This often happens in post-infective glomerulonephritis when, 10–20 days after streptococcal infection, patient presents with signs of the nephritic syndrome. The pathogenesis involves antigen-stimulated antibody formation and then immune complex disease involving complement system and other mediators of inflammation. Other causes of acute nephritic syndrome are listed in Table 55-4. The nephritic syndrome may be self-limiting or chronic and progressive (e.g., vasculitis, systemic lupus, or Wegener's granulomatosis). Clinical and serologic information in conjunction with renal histology are crucial in making an early diagnosis and initiating appropriate therapy.

Hypertension

Sometimes patients present with hypertension and are found to have features of glomerular disease. Most of these patients will have a primary glomerulopathy.

Rapidly Progressive Glomerulonephritis

In contrast to acute renal failure, the glomerular filtration rate falls over a period of weeks rather than days. Usually crescentic glomerulonephritis is the underlying pathologic lesion. These conditions usually do not recover spontaneously. Common causes are infections, drugs (penicillamine, allopurinol), multi-system diseases (Goodpasture's syndrome, systemic necrotizing vasculitis), and pauci-immune glomerulonephritis. Treatment involves glucocorticoids, cytotoxic agents, and treatment of infection or withdrawal of offending drug(s) if indicated. Prognosis for recovery of renal function depends on the underlying cause and the timeliness of appropriate therapy.

Chronic Renal Failure

A significant number of patients presenting with chronic renal failure are found to have features of a glomerulopathy, including proteinuria, hematuria, and hypertension. There may not be a history of renal disease in the past. Renal parenchyma is usually shrunken and a biopsy is usually not done because kidney tissue is fibrosed and scarred. Many of the conditions which cause the nephrotic or

Table 55-4. Causes of Nephritic Syndrome

Primary glomerular diseases
  Mesangial proliferative and membrano-proliferative
    glomerulonephritis, IgA nephropathy
Infections
  Post streptococcal, infective endocarditis
Multisystem diseases
  Goodpasture's syndrome, systemic lupus, vasculitis,
    cryoglobulinemia, thrombotic microangiopathy
Miscellaneous
  Serum sickness, cholesterol embolization

nephritic syndrome can present in this manner. Most of these patients progress to end-stage renal disease.

Clinical Examples

1. A 35-year-old black male presented with a 4-week history of recurrent abdominal pain, generalized joint pain, low grade fever, and fatigue. He had also noted a skin rash involving the bridge of nose, both ears, cheeks, and chin. He denied any urinary symptoms. Physical examination revealed a 160-lb. male who appeared uncomfortable. Blood pressure was 180/110 mm Hg, pulse 90 beats/minute, temperature 37.5°C. He had a raised discrete patchy rash all over his body including both palms and feet. The rash was scaly with well defined margins. He had mild diffuse abdominal tenderness and bowel sounds were hypoactive. Joint movements were painful, but there were no effusions. He had bilateral lower-extremity pitting edema. Urinalysis revealed pH 6.0, protein 3+, and blood 2+. Microscopic examination showed lots of RBCs and few RBC casts. Urine protein excretion was 3.5 g/day. ANA was positive in 1:2500 and anti-DNA was 1:2000, and C_3 and C_4 were both low. Serum BUN was 50 mg/dl and serum creatinine 2.5 mg/dl.

Discussion.   This patient presents with a disease process which involves multiple organs. The renal involvement includes proteinuria of 3.5 g/day, microscopic hematuria with RBC casts, hypertension, and renal impairment. He has gastrointestinal, musculoskeletal, and dermatologic involvement along with serologic findings typical of systemic lupus erythematosus. A kidney biopsy was performed and it revealed a diffuse proliferative glomerulonephritis. Immunofluorescent microscopy demonstrated "lumpy, bumpy" deposition of immunoglobulins, complement, and fibrin in glomerular tufts and mesangium, which again is characteristic of systemic lupus. This disease will require aggressive immunosuppressive therapy to prevent complete destruction of the kidneys.

2. A 45-year-old white male presented with a history of swelling of the ankles for about 3 months. He denied hematuria, exposure to drugs, or medications or any other symptoms. Physical examination revealed a well developed male. Blood pressure was 130/70 mm Hg and heart rate 76 beats/minute. He had 3+ dependent edema and the rest of the examination was normal.

Urinalysis showed 4+ protein, but was negative for blood; microscopy showed no casts, cells, or crystals. Serum urea nitrogen was 18 mg/dl, creatinine 1.1 mg/dl, and serum albumin 1.8 g/dl. Serum cholesterol until 3 months ago was 180 mg/dl, but a recent one was 325 mg/dl. Urine protein excretion was 9 g/day.

Discussion.   This patient is normotensive with normal renal functions but has nephrotic syndrome. There are no features suggestive of an underlying cause. Urinalysis is "bland." These features indicate a primary glomerulopathy and a renal biopsy is indicated to delineate type, estimate the prognosis, and guide therapy. A kidney biopsy was performed which showed membranous nephropathy. The treatment of this condition is controversial partially because only about one-third of these patients develop progressive renal failure. However, some patients respond favorably to immunosuppressive therapy.

Bibliography

Cotran RS, Kumar V, and Robbins SL. *Pathologic Basis of Disease* (5th ed.). Philadelphia: Saunders, 1994. *Excellent review of the pathogenic mechanisms of immuno- logic glomerular injury with helpful diagrams of each histologic type.*

Glassock RJI, Adler SG, Ward HJ, et al. Primary Glomeru- lar Diseases. In Brenner BM and Rector FC (eds.). *The Kidney* (4th ed.). Philadelphia: Saunders, 1991, pp. 1082– 1279. *Detailed discussion of glomerular diseases.*

Kaysen GA, Myers BD, Couser WG, et al. Mechanisms and consequences of proteinuria. *Lab Invest* 54:479–98, 1986. *A good review of the pathophysiology of protein leak from the glomerulus and mechanisms of edema in nephrotic syndrome.*

Olson JL and Heptinstall RH. Non-immunologic mecha- nisms of glomerular injury. *Lab Invest* 59:564–578, 1988. *Discussion of dietary, hormonal, and hemody- namic factors in progression of glomerular injury and chronic renal failure.*

Pusey CD and Peters DK. Immunopathology of Glomerular and Interstitial disease. In Schrier RW and Gottschalk CW (eds.). *Diseases of the Kidney* (5th ed.). Boston: Little, Brown, 1993, pp. 1647–1680. *Excellent discus- sion of immune mechanisms causing renal injury.*

56 Acute Renal Failure

Laura I. Rankin

Objectives

After completing this chapter, you should be able to

Describe mechanisms which control glomerular filtration and renal blood flow in normal kidneys

Define acute renal failure

Outline three major types of acute renal failure and describe the clinical and laboratory characteristics of each

Explain the mechanisms of prerenal azotemia

List the types of renal disease which can cause acute renal failure and describe the clinical and laboratory characteristics of each type

List the causes of renal failure due to obstruction

Explain current understanding of the pathogenesis of acute tubular necrosis

Discuss the principles of management of acute renal failure

Acute renal failure is defined as the sudden decrease in glomerular filtration rate, resulting in an increase in the plasma concentration of waste products normally excreted by the kidneys. The wastes that are used to define renal failure are urea (blood urea nitrogen, BUN) and creatinine. Other compounds also accumulate because of decreased renal function; these include uric acid, phosphate, and sulfates. Acute renal failure may be observed in patients with previously normal renal function or patients whose prior renal function was impaired but stable. Some patients will be anuric (less than 100 cc/day), some will be oliguric (less than 400 cc/day), and some will have normal urine output or polyuria (more than 3 liters/day). The diagnosis of acute renal failure is made in 2–5% of hospital inpatients and accounts for at least one-third of the consultations requested of hospital nephrologists. Knowledge of the factors which control renal blood flow and glomerular filtration rate is central to the understanding of acute renal failure, its pathogenesis, and prognosis.

Normal Renal Hemodynamics

Under basal conditions, the kidneys receive 20–25% of the cardiac output. The renal blood flow is 1.0–1.2 liters/minute,

with a renal plasma flow of 650–750 ml/minute. Although the kidneys are metabolically quite active, the large requirement for blood flow is not primarily for tissue oxygenation. The major need is to sustain the glomerular filtration rate. Changes in systemic blood pressure could cause large changes in renal perfusion and glomerular filtration if not for autoregulation which is accomplished by the two arteriolar beds, between which the glomerular capillaries exist. Changes in vasomotor tone in the afferent and efferent arterioles protect the glomerulus from high perfusion pressure and maintain filtration pressure when renal perfusion pressure decreases. This function is referred to as "autoregulation."

Autoregulation of Renal Blood Flow and Glomerular Filtration

The afferent and efferent arterioles are responsive to changes in perfusion pressure, neural stimulation, drugs, hormones, and perhaps other influences. The vascular tone of the two arterioles is regulated under most circumstances, to ensure a normal filtration pressure. An increase in systemic blood pressure could damage the delicate capillary wall or excessively increase blood flow and filtration rate. To prevent this, the afferent arteriole constricts, modulating the pressure head and blood flow in the capillaries. Conversely, if the systemic blood pressure decreases, the afferent arteriole dilates in order to allow adequate blood flow and pressure to be transmitted to the glomerular capillaries. The efferent arteriole also constricts in response to hypotension, which helps to maintain pressure in the capillary bed. Several theories exist to explain autoregulation.

Myogenic Theory

This theory hold that arteriolar smooth muscle contracts in response to an increase in vascular wall tension. Thus the radius of the afferent arteriole would diminish in response to higher perfusion pressure.

Metabolic Theory

Changes in renal perfusion pressure could alter tissue oxygen tension, pH, and local concentrations of metabolites. A decrease in blood pressure would decrease blood flow, allowing the accumulation of metabolites which would then cause vasodilatation. This theory does not explain how the tone in the efferent and afferent arterioles could be selectively regulated.

Humoral Factors

Angiotensin II. With elevated systemic levels of this hormone, blood pressure increases and vasoconstriction of both afferent and efferent arterioles occurs. If the increased renal perfusion pressure is prevented by aortic constriction, vasoconstriction of the afferent arteriole is attenuated. Thus the primary site of action of angiotensin II is the efferent arteriole, where an increase in tone tends to maintain glomerular filtration. However, angiotensin II also causes mesangial contraction and thus a decrease in K_f, the glomerular ultrafiltration coefficient. (The K_f is an index of the permeability of the glomerular membrane. It is determined by the porosity and the surface area of the capillary membrane.) The changes in blood flow, efferent arteriolar tone, and K_f induced by angiotensin II are attenuated by calcium entry antagonists.

Norepinephrine. The actions of this hormone are to induce vasoconstriction of both the afferent and efferent arteriole. Norepinephrine also causes mesangial contraction and thus a decrease in K_f. Calcium entry blockers also inhibit the changes seen with norepinephrine stimulation.

Prostaglandins. Thromboxane A_2 is a potent renal vasoconstricting agent. It is produced in response to obstruction of urine flow. This effect may help explain the decreased glomerular filtration seen with partial urinary obstruction.

Prostaglandins of the E and F series are vasodilators of the afferent and efferent arterioles, especially the former. The role of prostaglandins in the maintenance of glomerular filtration and renal blood flow under normal circumstances is not defined. However, in disease states prostaglandin production is increased whenever renal vasoconstriction occurs. Consequently, inhibition of prostaglandin synthesis by nonsteroidal antiinflammatory drugs (NSAIDs) results in a further decrease in renal blood flow and glomerular filtration whenever norepinephrine or angiotensin II levels are elevated.

Atrial Natriuretic Peptide (ANP). This hormone causes afferent arteriolar vasodilatation and efferent arteriolar vasoconstriction and an increase in K_f. The net effect is an increased glomerular filtration rate.

Renal Nerves

Adrenergic nerves extend along the afferent and efferent arterioles and into the juxtaglomerular complex. The primary effect of renal nerve stimulation is vascular smooth muscle constriction, resulting in a decrease in renal blood flow. Neural stimulation also redistributes blood flow from the outer cortex to the inner cortex and medulla and enhances tubular reabsorption of sodium. However, renal autoregulation occurs even in denervated kidneys; therefore, the precise role of the renal nerves is not clear.

Tubuloglomerular Feedback

An increased concentration of chloride in the distal tubular fluid decreases glomerular filtration. The mechanism is thought to involve sensing by the juxtaglomerular apparatus and local activation of the renin-angiotensin system.

Medullary Blood Flow

In contrast to glomerular blood flow, the blood flow to the medulla is not autoregulated. Consequently, low perfusion of the medulla may compromise cellular function especially in the thick ascending limb which requires a lot of oxygen to energize NaCl transport. Tubular injury may then result and eventuate in a decrease in the glomerular filtration. This phenomenon may be relevant in the pathogenesis of acute tubular necrosis.

Mechanisms of Acute Renal Failure

The causes of acute renal failure are varied and yet treatment depends on identifying the mechanisms involved. A useful approach is to evaluate the patient for clues to three broad categories of mechanisms: prerenal, postrenal, and intrinsic renal disease. Table 56-1 compares these categories with respect to features of the urinary output, physical examination, urinalysis, and laboratory parameters which are helpful in this diagnostic process.

Prerenal Azotemia

When renal blood flow is sufficiently decreased, autoregulation begins to fail and the glomerular filtration rate decreases. However, tubular functions remain intact. Because the tubules perceive a low perfusion state, they avidly reabsorb water and sodium, resulting in a low volume of concentrated urine containing very little sodium. In this setting the urine flow is slow, allowing reabsorption of urea nitrogen back into the blood. This results in a proportionally greater increase in BUN compared to serum creatinine. The causes of this state are outlined in Table 56-2.

Fluid losses from the gastrointestinal tract, urine or sweat, or sequestration of fluid into damaged tissues or the peritoneal cavity as well as bleeding will reduce blood volume and may cause prerenal azotemia. Likewise the "effective volume" may be decreased, without a change in the actual blood volume. In this situation, blood flow to the kidneys may be compromised despite the presence of edema or high central venous or pulmonary capillary wedge pres-

sure. Examples include congestive heart failure, cirrhosis (with maldistribution of blood flow), and sepsis (when venodilatation compromises return of blood to the heart).

It should be remembered that occasionally a patient is not oliguric but still has prerenal azotemia. This can occur whenever the urinary concentrating mechanism is impaired (e.g., diabetes incipidus, osmotic diuresis, interstitial nephritis), and when volume depletion is due to renal salt and water losses (e.g., adrenal insufficiency, diuretic therapy, salt-losing nephropathy).

Therapy for prerenal azotemia is directed at correcting the underlying cause. If hypovolemia is present, colloids and/or blood products should be administered. If blood volume is normal or increased, poor cardiac output or maldistribution should be addressed. Therapy must be timely as some cases of prerenal azotemia, left untreated, will progress to acute tubular necrosis.

Postrenal Azotemia

Obstruction of urine flow results in increased intratubular pressure. Tubuloglomerular feedback and local thromboxane A_2 production then play a role in decreasing the glomerular filtration rate. Initially, the laboratory parameters may resemble prerenal azotemia. However, as obstruction continues, the tubules lose their ability to concentrate the urine and conserve sodium. Causes of this type of renal failure are displayed in Table 56-3. Keep in mind that

Table 56-1. Differential Diagnosis of Acute Renal Failure

Variable	Prerenal	Renal	Postrenal
Urine output	Decreased unless renal losses are excessive	Variable, occasionally anuric or polyuric	Variable; must rule out if anuria or wide fluctuations are noted
Blood pressure	Often low or orthostatic drop	Normal, low, or high	Normal or high
Microscopic urinalysis	No cells; hyaline and granular casts	Brown granular casts if ATN; RBC casts if GN	Normal; WBCs if infected
BUN: creatinine ratio	> 14:1	approx. 10:1	> 14:1 if acute 10:1 if chronic
Urine osmolality (mOsm/kg)	> 400	< 350 in ATN > 400 early in GN	> 400 if acute < 350 if chronic
Urine Na concentration (meq/L)	< 20 unless renal salt & water losses are excessive	> 40 if ATN < 20 early in GN	variable
FE_{Na}	< 1% unless renal salt & water losses are excessive	> 1% if ATN < 1% early in GN	< 1% if acute > 2% if chronic

ATN = acute tubular necrosis; GN = glomerulonephritis; RBC = red blood cells; WBC = white blood cells; BUN = blood urine nitrogen; FE_{Na}, = fractional sodium excretion.
Calculation of $FE_{Na} = (U_{Na}/P_{Na})/(U_{Cr}/P_{Cr}) \times 100$, where U_{Na} is the urinary sodium concentration, P_{Na} is the plasma sodium concentration, U_{Cr} is the urinary creatinine concentration, and P_{Cr} is the plasma creatinine concentration.

Table 56-2. Causes of Prerenal Azotemia

HYPOVOLEMIA

Hemorrhage
Gastrointestinal fluid losses (vomiting, diarrhea)
Renal salt & water losses (diuretics, salt wasting,
    Addison's disease)
Third space losses (burns, pancreatitis, peritonitis)

DECREASED "EFFECTIVE VOLUME"

Congestive heart failure
Cirrhosis
Peripheral vasodilation (sepsis, antihypertensives,
    anesthetics)

REDUCED CARDIAC OUTPUT

Myocardial infarction
Pericardial tamponade or constrictive pericarditis
Acute pulmonary embolism

VASCULAR OBSTRUCTION

Bilateral renal artery occlusion
Dissecting aortic aneurysm

Table 56-3. Causes of Postrenal (Obstructive) Azotemia

URETHRA

Strictures

BLADDER NECK

Prostatic hypertrophy or cancer
Tumor at bladder neck
Neurogenic bladder (neurologic disease or drugs)

INTRA-URETERAL*

Stones
Necrotic papillae
Blood clots
Crystals or sludge
Edema from ureteral instrumentation
Tumor

EXTRA-URETERAL*

Retroperitoneal fibrosis
    Idiopathic
    Drug-induced
    Aortic aneurysm or aortic graft
Para-aortic lymphadenopathy (lymphoma, testicular
    cancer)
Local spread of cancer of cervix or prostate
Surgical ligature

---

*Obstruction must be bilateral or involve a single functioning kid-
ney to cause renal failure.

ureteral obstruction must be bilateral or involve a single functioning kidney to cause azotemia.

The possibility of obstruction should always be considered in patients with renal failure, as continued obstruction results in progressive loss of renal tissue. The history and physical examination may provide useful clues, but the diagnosis is usually indicated by ultrasonography, which shows dilatation of the renal pelvis and calyces in the vast majority of patients. Relief of the obstruction usually leads to prompt return of renal function. The osmotic effect of increased BUN and creatinine concentrations, volume expansion, and unresponsiveness of the tubules to aldosterone and antidiuretic hormone combine to cause a temporary diuresis in many patients after the obstruction is relieved. During this time of "postobstructive diuresis," appropriate fluids should be given to prevent sodium and water depletion, with resultant prerenal azotemia.

Intrinsic Renal Disease

The causes of acute renal failure owing to intrinsic renal disease are diverse and may present in a variety of different ways. These numerous conditions listed in Table 56-4 can be divided into four groups, based upon the substructure of the kidney which is primarily involved: glomeruli, vessels, interstitium, or tubules. The urinalysis is the cornerstone of the diagnostic evaluation.

Glomerulonephritis

These patients usually have hypertension and it may be severe. They often have peripheral edema. The urinalysis is typically notable for the presence of proteinuria and hematuria (either gross or microscopic), and may reveal red blood cell casts. White blood cells and WBC casts are also seen. Initially the urinary chemistry parameters are similar to prerenal azotemia; however, later these indices resemble those of acute tubular necrosis. Glomerulonephritis is discussed in greater detail in Chap. 55.

Vasculitis

These patients present much like those with glomerulonephritis, except that hypertension may be more severe. Hematuria, RBC casts, and WBC casts are also seen in this group of diseases. A systemic disease process is generally identified and therapy is based upon the specific diagnosis.

Tubulointerstitial Nephritis

The presence of white blood cells and WBC casts, with fewer RBCs and little protein, should suggest this category. Pyelonephritis should be suspected if flank pain,

Table 56-4. Parenchymal Cause of Acute Renal Failure

GLOMERULONEPHRITIS

Postinfectious
Rapidly progressive glomerulonephritis
Systemic disease (Lupus, Wegener's, Goodpasture's, polyarteritis, . . .)

VASCULOPATHIES

Bilateral renal artery occlusion (thrombosis/emboli)
Bilateral renal vein thrombosis (acute)
Cholesterol emboli
Malignant hypertension
Scleroderma
Vasculitis

TUBULOINTERSTITIAL NEPHROPATHIES

Pyelonephritis
Allergic (penicillins, phenytoin, diuretics, rifampin)
Infiltrative (myeloma, leukemia)
Uric acid nephropathy
Hypercalcemia
Infections (Legionnaire's, Rocky Mountain Spotted Fever)

ACUTE TUBULAR NECROSIS

Ischemic (trauma, surgery, hemorrhage, volume depletion, obstetrical catastrophe, cardiac arrest, . . .)
Nephrotoxin (radiocontrast dye, aminoglycoside; amphotericin B, methanol, ethylene glycol, heavy metals incl. cisplatin, myoglobin, hemoglobin, pesticides, . . .)

fever, and bacteriuria are present. Careful review of recent medications may suggest allergic interstitial nephritis (penicillins or sulfonamides are often implicated). Similarly, the patient may have an immunologic type of disease which involves the renal interstitium. Uric acid nephropathy is seen in patients with malignancy and severe hyperuricemia, usually in response to a large cell kill owing to chemotherapy. This diagnosis is confirmed by finding a urinary uric acid:creatinine ratio of greater than 1. Hypercalcemia causes acute renal failure by causing renal vasoconstriction (decreasing renal blood flow) and by precipitation of calcium in the tubules and interstitium. Treatment of these forms of acute renal failure is directed at the causative factor.

Acute Tubular Necrosis (ATN)

This form of acute intrinsic renal failure accounts for approximately 75% of the cases. Despite its name, morphologic changes may be minor or in fact absent. Inciting events include a variety of ischemic and nephrotoxic in-

sults, as seen in Table 56-4. Hypoperfusion may be accompanied by hypotension or the body may maintain blood pressure by activation of neurohumoral responses which compromise renal blood flow. It should also be recognized that there is a wide range in the susceptibility of patients to seemingly identical insults.

Three phases are recognized: the initiation phase, during which the insults occur, but therapeutic interventions may prevent the development of established ATN; the maintenance phase, when renal function is impaired or absent and interventions may optimize the ability of the patient to survive but will not reverse the renal failure; and the recovery phase, when the kidneys gradually regain function, generally returning to baseline function, within several days to a few weeks after the insult.

Pathogenesis. Several theories have been advanced to explain the loss of renal function in ATN (Fig. 56-1). However, no one theory explains all forms of ATN, nor is a single etiology explained fully by only one theory.

One theory is that of afferent arteriolar constriction. Despite normal cardiac output and blood pressure, renal cortical blood flow is invariably decreased in ATN and remains so for at least 24 for 48 hours after the initial insult. Since the glomeruli are located in the cortex, afferent arteriolar constriction results in cortical ischemia which could explain the markedly decreased glomerular filtration despite only a modest decrease in renal blood flow. Acute renal failure can be induced experimentally by intrarenal infusion of angiotensin II or norepinephrine, both of which induce afferent arteriolar constriction.

A second theory is that of decreased glomerular permeability (K_f). Abnormalities in surface area or the intrinsic permeability of the glomerular capillary membrane could account for decreased glomerular filtration rate. These changes have been demonstrated in models of ischemic ATN and when ATN is induced by angiotensin II or norepinephrine infusions and with some nephrotoxins.

A third theory is backleak of ultrafiltrate. Loss of functional integrity of the tubular cells could allow the passive reabsorption of tubular fluid into the peritubular vessels. (With this theory, glomerular filtration could either be normal or decreased.) The net effect would be a lack of clearance of waste products. Although this theory can be supported in some experimental models of acute tubular necrosis, it is less clearly defined in human disease.

A fourth theory is tubular obstruction. Precipitation of nephrotoxins (including uric acid, myoglobin, hemoglobin or oxalate) may plug the tubules. Alternatively, congealed

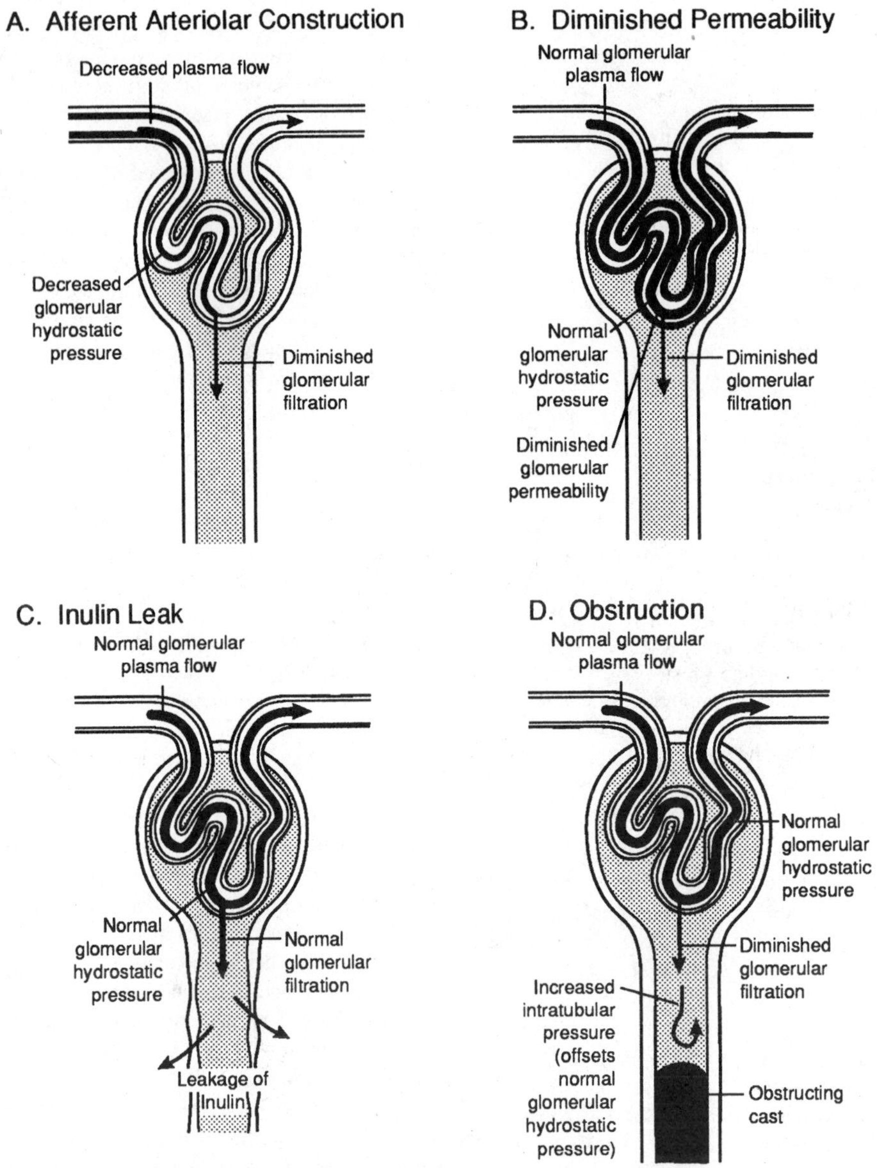

A. Afferent Arteriolar Constriction

Decreased plasma flow

Decreased glomerular hydrostatic pressure

Diminished glomerular filtration

B. Diminished Permeability

Normal glomerular plasma flow

Normal glomerular hydrostatic pressure

Diminished glomerular filtration

Diminished glomerular permeability

C. Inulin Leak

Normal glomerular plasma flow

Normal glomerular hydrostatic pressure

Normal glomerular filtration

Leakage of Inulin

D. Obstruction

Normal glomerular plasma flow

Normal glomerular hydrostatic pressure

Diminished glomerular filtration

Increased intratubular pressure (offsets normal glomerular hydrostatic pressure)

Obstructing cast

Fig. 56-1. Four theories of acute renal failure. A. Afferent arteriolar constriction decreases blood flow to the glomerulus, with a fall in glomerular filtration pressure and thus decreased glomerular filtration. B. Decreased glomerular permeability may diminish glomerular filtration even if glomerular filtration pressure and blood flow are kept constant. C. Because of backleak of filtrate through damaged tubular epithelium, the clearance of creatinine or inulin underestimates GFR and azotemia results. D. Casts lodge in lumina and increase intratubular pressure so that net glomerular filtration pressure (glomerular pressure minus intratubular pressure) is near zero. (Modified from: Schrier RW. Acute renal failure: Pathogenesis, diagnosis, and management. *Hosp Practice* 16:94, 1981.)

protein in the form of casts, sloughed cells, cellular debris, or simply cells swollen from ischemia could block urine flow. Intratubular pressure would then increase and be reflected as increased pressure in Bowman's space. If the pressure in Bowman's is high enough, filtration would cease. However, in the experimental models which support this theory, intratubular pressures do not approach this level. Additionally, intratubular pressures generally return to normal within 24–48 hours, but renal function does not improve at the same time.

Thromboxane A_2, endothelin, adenosine, nitric oxide, platelet-activating factor, and epidermal growth factor are currently being investigated for their roles in the induction and maintenance of acute tubular necrosis.

The four major theories undoubtedly assume varying importance in different types of acute tubular necrosis. For example, myoglobinuric ATN is generally associated with hypotension and with a markedly decreased renal blood flow. The pigment is also a direct tubular toxin, especially in cells already compromised by ischemia. In contrast, "pure" ischemic ATN may be primarily explained by tubular obstruction and backleak of ultrafiltrate whereas aminoglycoside (an antibiotic) causes a marked decrease in K_f and direct tubular injury.

Clinical Course and Therapy.   Therapy of acute tubular necrosis is supportive. Maintenance of optimal blood volume, avoidance of fluid overload, management of acid-base and electrolyte disorders, and adjustment of medications for renal function are essential. Nutritional support may be required. One must be vigilant for gastrointestinal bleeding and infection, addressing these complications promptly if they occur. Dialysis is indicated for fluid overload, severe acidosis or hyperkalemia, and to maintain plasma urea and creatinine concentrations at acceptable levels, in order to avert uremic symptoms, maintain platelet function, and optimize wound healing and white blood cell functions. Despite major advances in dialytic therapy and medical care in general, the mortality associated with ATN remains approximately 50%. The deaths are related primarily to the condition causing the renal failure and to infections.

Clinical Examples

1. A 52-year-old woman has been referred to the Gynecology service for staging and treatment of newly diagnosed cancer of the cervix. Her past health has been good and she is taking no medications. Her initial physical examination is entirely normal except for the presence of a fungating lesion of the cervix. Laboratory studies reveal a BUN of 25 mg/dl and a serum creatinine level of 1.4 mg/dl. She has several tests done over the next 2 weeks, including a contrast-enhanced CT scan of the abdomen and pelvis. Her family then brings her into the emergency room because of weakness, nausea, vomiting, and a decrease in mental alertness. Her blood pressure is 152/88 supine and standing with no change in heart rate. She has scattered rales in the lung bases, but they clear with coughing. The heart has an S4 gallop and there is 1+ edema in the lower legs and over the sacrum. Bladder catheterization reveals 50 cc urine, which is sent for testing. The urinary sodium is 56 meq/liter, the urine creatinine is 133 mg/dl, and microscopic urinalysis shows occasional red and white cells, but no casts. There is 1+ proteinuria. The BUN is now 142 mg/dl, the serum creatinine concentration is 10.6 mg/dl, the potassium level 6.9 meq/liter, and the serum bicarbonate 12 meq/liter. The electrocardiogram shows tall peaked T-waves and barely discernible P-waves. She is rapidly admitted and emergently hemodialyzed for hyperkalemia. Ultrasonography reveals two kidneys and a suggestion of hydronephrosis bilaterally. The CT scan is reviewed; it reveals extensive retroperitoneal lymphadenopathy. A urologic consultant performs retrograde pyelography with placement of stents (tubes going from the renal pelvis to the bladder) bilaterally. Urine flow promptly resumes, at first at 800 ml/hour but gradually decreasing to 1500–2500 ml/day. The BUN and creatinine concentrations decrease rapidly to 13 and 0.9 mg/dl. She is then transferred back to the Gynecology service for hysterectomy and further oncologic care.

Discussion.   The initial renal function was abnormal since the usual serum creatinine concentration for a woman with normal renal function is about 0.7 mg/dl. The presenting symptoms of nausea, vomiting, and decreased mentation are due to uremia. Weakness is explained by hyperkalemia as well. Mild fluid overload was present because of continued intake in the absence of urine production. A mechanism for ureteral obstruction was suggested by the clinical setting and CT scan. The urinary indices are consistent with either obstruction or ATN (What is the fractional excretion of sodium?). The urinary sediment is more compatible with obstruction. Radiocontrast-dye-induced ATN is a possibility, but the prompt return of renal function with stent placement indicates obstruction to urine flow as the cause of the acute renal failure.

2. A 32-year-old man was admitted to the oncology service for therapy of recently diagnosed testicular cancer.

His health previously had been good; however, he had lost 20 lb. in the last two months, due to surgery and the anorexia of metastatic cancer. He was receiving no medications. Physical examination revealed a thin man with a blood pressure of 120/76 supine and standing. He had inguinal lymphadenopathy and no edema. Laboratory studies showed normal electrolytes, BUN 10 mg/dl, and serum creatinine 1.0 mg/dl. The uric acid was 13.5 mg/dl (normal less than 6) and phosphate 5.0 mg/dl (normal 2.5–4.5). The chest x-ray revealed 25 to 50 metastatic nodules of varying sizes. Urinalysis was reported as normal with no protein. He was admitted, begun on allopurinol 300 mg/day, and the next day a cisplatin chemotherapy protocol was begun. The patient was given saline before and after the chemotherapy, but had intractable vomiting. The vomiting continued through the next day. On the following day, his weight had decreased 3.5 kg, his BP was 100/60 supine and 80/50 sitting, and he had no edema. He insisted upon a bedside commode because "the bathroom is too far away." Laboratory studies showed a BUN of 55 mg/dl, creatinine 3.4 mg/dl, sodium 136 meq/liter and potassium 6.9 meq/ liter, uric acid 25 mg/dl, and phosphate 17 mg/dl. Urinalysis now showed much amorphous crystalline material and many hyaline and granular casts. Urine chemistries showed a sodium 30 meq/liter, creatinine 22 mg/dl (what is the fractional excretion of sodium?), and uric acid 46 mg/dl. Because of hyperkalemia and hyperuricemia, he underwent emergency hemodialysis. Three liters of saline were given before he went to the dialysis unit. The potassium and uric acid levels were 3.9 meq/liter and 10 mg/dl, respectively, immediately after dialysis. An ultrasound examination of the kidneys and retrograde dye studies of the ureters showed no obstruction. However, hyperkalemia and hyperuricemia recurred and required daily hemodialysis for two more days. Thereafter, he continued to need thrice-weekly dialysis for control of the BUN level. Thrombocytopenia and leukopenia ensued from the chemotherapy. Gastrointestinal bleeding, nosebleeds, and skin oozing occurred, and were treated with antacids, H_2 blocker, and transfusions of blood and platelets. Pneumonia due to *Klebsiella pneumoniae* was treated with acephalosporin and tobramycin, with dosages adjusted for absent renal function. Due to his inability to eat, hyperalimentation was begun through a central venous catheter. Daily increases in BUN and creatinine levels began to lessen and dialysis was discontinued. Urine output was 1000 cc/day 16 days after admission and still increasing. Suddenly his temperature rose to 40°C and hypotension ensued. Despite administration of antibiotics, fluids, and pressor drugs, he had irreversible septic shock and a cardiac arrest. The autopsy demonstrated no evidence of residual metastatic disease. *Candida* species and *Serratia marcescens* were cultured from blood and the tip of the central venous catheter used for hyperalimentation. The kidneys showed focal areas of regenerating tubular epithelium.

Discussion.   Based upon the history, physical examination, and some initial laboratory results, prerenal, renal parenchymal, and postrenal causes of this man's acute renal failure were considered. Depletion of extracellular fluid volume (as indicated by vomiting, weight loss, and orthostatic hypotension) was certainly present. Although the BUN-creatinine ratio was 14 and not suggestive of prerenal azotemia, the BUN might be relatively low because of poor dietary protein intake. Hyaline and granular casts could be seen with either prerenal or intrinsic renal problems. However, the high urinary sodium concentration and the FEN_{Na} of 3.4% suggest that ATN or obstruction were present in addition to renal hypoperfusion. Obstruction was a definite possibility, either from uric acid crystal formation in the renal tubules or from ureteral compression by enlarged lymph nodes. The former possibility is strongly suggested by the high urine urate-creatinine ratio and the high serum uric acid and phosphate levels. The possibility of cisplatin-induced ATN also deserves consideration, especially since coexisting volume depletion predisposes to virtually all types of nephrotoxicity.

Several strategies could have been better employed to avert the development of acute renal failure. Vigorous hydration prior to the chemotherapy might have inhibited the renin-angiotensin system and decreased the serum urate level. Increasing the urine flow rate would also have reduced the urine uric acid concentrations, decreasing the risk of precipitation. A delay in the chemotherapy administration until allopurinol more completely blocked the production of uric acid would have blunted the hyperuricemia and hyperuricosuria. In addition, either successful antiemetic therapy or hydration sufficient to prevent weight loss would have prevented the renal ischemia which resulted from sodium and water depletion. Lastly, although the mechanism is unclear, the toxicity of cisplantinim and most other nephrotoxins is decreased by vigorous hydration before and after the drug is given.

The patient's clinical course was complicated by electrolyte problems, gastrointestinal bleeding, and infection. Typical of the 40–60% patients dying with acute renal failure, the death was caused not by renal failure but by infection, bleeding, or a complication of the underlying disease or its therapy.

Bibliography

Anderson RJ and Schrier RW. Acute tubular necrosis. In Schrier RW and Gottschalk CW (eds.). *Diseases of the Kidney* (5th ed.). Boston: Little, Brown, 1993. Vol. 2, pp. 1287–1318. *A detailed and scholarly review of all aspects of the subject.*

Rose BD and Rennke HG. *Renal Pathophysiology — The Essentials.* Baltimore: Williams & Wilkins, 1994. *This book is aimed at the early medical student and provides an excellent discussion of acute renal failure and electrolyte problems.*

Rotellar Carlos. *Acute Renal Insufficiency Made Ridiculously Simple.* Miami: MedMaster, 1988. *An enjoyable small text summarizing basic and practical aspects of acute renal failure.*

57 Chronic Renal Failure

James E. Bourdeau and Chris E. Kaufman

Objectives

After completing this chapter, you should be able to

Define chronic renal failure and distinguish it from end-stage renal disease

Explain the functional adaptations which occur in patients with progressive chronic renal disease

Outline the cardiovascular, skeletal, and neurologic sequelae of chronic renal failure

Explain the pathophysiologic principles of management for chronic renal failure

Explain why NSAIDs may be deleterious in patients with chronic renal failure

Definitions

Homeostasis

Homeostasis is the tendency toward maintenance of a stable internal environment in higher animals through a series of interacting physiologic processes. Examples of organ systems and vital substances in part regulated homeostatically by the kidneys are shown in Table 57-1. In health, the capacity of the kidneys to regulate H_2O, Na^+, K^+, Ca^{2+}, P_i, or H^+ is so large that their intakes can vary widely without causing detectable metabolic disturbances. Chronic renal failure narrows the limits of the range within which the intake of vital substances can be safely varied.

Chronic Renal Failure

This is a syndrome of impaired homeostasis owing to structural damage of the kidneys. The most common causes in order of decreasing frequency are diabetes mellitus, hypertension, glomerulonephritis, cystic diseases, and tubulo-interstitial nephropathies. Chronic renal disease is often progressive, eventually resulting in end-stage renal failure. The terms chronic renal insufficiency, chronic renal failure and uremia are used to encompass a spectrum of kidney dysfunction from minimal impairment to the functionally anephric state, as shown in Fig. 57-1. In end-stage renal failure, homeostatic mechanisms are insufficient to preserve life, necessitating some form of kidney replacement therapy.

Table 57-1. Homeostatic Regulation by the Kidneys

Organ System	Regulated Parameter	Controlling Factor(s)	Role of the Kidney
Body water	Serum osmolality	Antidiuretic hormone	Water excretion
Body sodium	ECF volume	GFR; tubular Na absorption	Sodium excretion
Body potassium	Plasma $[K^+]$	Aldosterone; tubular K^+ secretion	Potassium excretion
Bone marrow	Hematocrit (RBC mass)	Erythropoietin	Synthesis of erythropoietin
Calcium balance	Plasma $[Ca^{2+}]$	1α, 25-dihydroxyvitamin D_3	Synthesis of 1,25-$(OH)_2$-D_3
Phosphate balance	Plasma $[P_i]$	Parathyroid hormone	Inorganic P excretion
Hydrogen ion balance	Arterial pH	H^+ secretion; NH_4^+ production	Proton excretion

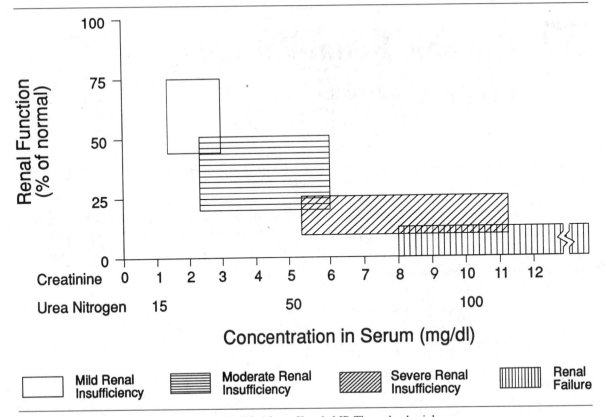

Fig. 57-1. Staging of chronic renal disease. (Modified from: Knochel JP. The pathophysiology of uremia. *Hosp Practice* 16(11):65–76, 1981. Original illustration by Albert Miller, p. 67.)

Diagnosis

The best single indicator of overall kidney function is glomerular filtration rate (GFR). Clinically, GFR is estimated by the creatinine clearance (C_{Cr}), calculated from a timed urine collection using the formula $C_{Cr} = U_{Cr} \cdot V/S_{Cr}$, where U_{Cr} is the urine Cr concentration, V is the urine flow rate, and S_{Cr} is the serum creatinine concentration. The relationship between GFR and S_{Cr} is a rectangular hyperbola (Fig. 57-2). Thus an increase in S_{Cr} from 1.0 to 2.0 mg/dl represents a 50% decline in GFR, whereas an increase in S_{Cr} from 4.0 to 5.0 mg/dl only represents a decline in GFR from 25% to 20% of normal.

Persistently elevated serum concentrations of creatinine or serum urea nitrogen (BUN) are the usual initial findings in chronic renal insufficiency. A $S_{Cr} > 1.4$ mg/dl and a BUN > 21 mg/dl are abnormal. Many patients are asymptomatic when their kidney dysfunction is discovered, usually as a result of blood chemistry testing. However, by the time that S_{Cr} is frankly elevated, GFR may be only 35% of normal in some individuals. Often patients will not seek medical attention until they have developed symptoms related to advanced chronic renal failure, including anorexia, nausea, vomiting, fatigue, weakness, restlessness, difficulty concentrating mentally, or somnolence, among others. This constellation of findings is known as the uremic syndrome.

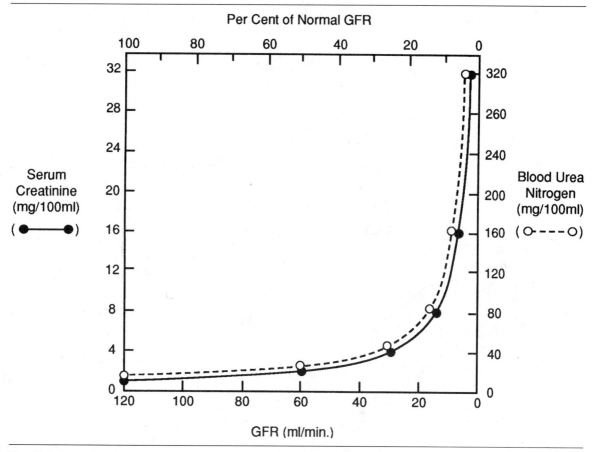

Fig. 57-2. Approximation of the steady-state relation between serum creatinine, blood urea nitrogen (BUN), and glomerular filtration rate (GFR). (Adapted from: Kassirer JP. Clinical evaluation of kidney function: Glomerular function. *N Engl J Med,* 1971, 285:385–389. Copyright 1971, Massachusetts Medical Society. All rights reserved.)

Progression to End-stage Renal Disease

Regardless of cause, chronic renal disease often progresses. For an individual in whom acute insults to renal function are avoided (e.g., severe hypertension, nephrotoxic antibiotics, nonsteroidal anti-inflammatory agents, intravenous radiocontrast dye), the rate of progression from mild renal insufficiency to end-stage renal failure is usually linear (Fig. 57-3). Chronic dialysis or kidney transplantation are typically required when C_{Cr} is below 10 ml/minute in nondiabetic and somewhat earlier in diabetic patients. At this stage, features of the uremic syndrome begin to appear and will become debilitating if renal replacement therapy is delayed. Of course, renal function may deteriorate more rapidly when acute insults to kidney function are superimposed on chronic renal insufficiency.

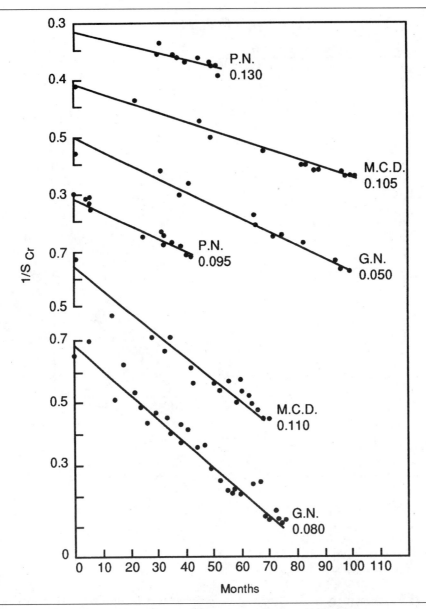

Fig. 57-3. Progression of renal insufficiency plotted as the reciprocal of the serum creatinine concentration ($1/S_{Cr}$) as a function of time in months for individual patients. The numerical values are the slopes of the lines describing $1/S_{Cr}$ versus time. (Reproduced with permission from: Mitch WE, Walser M, Buffington GA, and Lemann J, et al. A simple method of estimating progression of chronic renal failure. *Lancet* 2:1326–1328, 1976, © by *The Lancet Ltd.* 1976.)

Adaptations

In the 1960s, Dr. Neal S. Bricker formulated the "intact nephron hypothesis" to explain many of the adaptations observed in chronic renal failure. This theory, which has been validated by experimental studies, states that as nephrons are destroyed the remaining functional counterparts adapt in a physiologically appropriate way to carry out the excretory functions of the kidneys. The adaptations involve changes in both glomerular and tubular functions.

Glomerular Hyperfiltration

A combination of markedly decreased afferent arteriolar and modestly decreased efferent arteriolar tone increases glomerular capillary blood flow, pressure, and filtration in surviving renal corpuscles (Fig. 57-4). When the number of functional nephrons is sufficiently reduced, total renal blood flow and GFR fall despite this adaptation at the single nephron level. Studies in experimental animals indicate that the high intracapillary pressure and blood flow cause structural damage to the remaining functional glomeruli, thereby perpetuating nephron loss and perhaps explaining the inexorable loss of kidney function.

Renal Tubular Adaptations

Isosthenuria

The excretion of urine which has an osmolality that is relatively invariable and comparable to that of the plasma (approximately 300 mOsm/kg H_2O or a specific gravity of 1.010), isosthenuria results from the increased solute excretion per surviving nephron. Isosthenuria implies a decreased ability to concentrate or dilute the urine (Fig. 57-5). Clinical consequences include nocturia and susceptibility to dehydration or water retention if fluid intake is not optimal.

Sodium

With normal kidney function, greater than 99% of the sodium filtered at the glomeruli is reabsorbed by the tubules, and less than 1% is excreted in the urine. When sodium intake remains constant but GFR is reduced, sodium balance is maintained by reductions in tubular absorption. For example, in a normal person ingesting four grams (174 meq) of sodium daily, approximately 171 meq are absorbed from the gastrointestinal tract and three meq are eliminated in the feces. Of the 171 meq that enter the body, only three meq are lost via sweat and the remaining 168 meq in the

Fig. 57-4. Glomerular hemodynamic changes associated with hyperfiltration. Glomerular blood flow is increased owing to relaxation of both afferent and efferent arterioles. Capillary hydraulic pressure increases because the decrease in resistance is greatest in afferent arterioles. Q = glomerular blood flow, ΔP = net transcapillary pressure, R_A = afferent arteriolar resistance, R_E = efferent arteriolar resistance. (Original illustration by M. Rodriguez, M.D.)

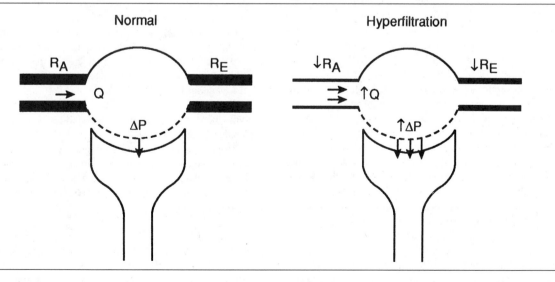

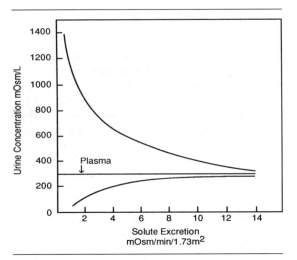

Fig. 57-5. Maximum concentration and dilution of the urine during solute diuresis in normal subjects. Note that an increase in solute excretion limits the maximum urine concentration and the ability to dilute the urine. (Reproduced with permission from: Seldin DW, Carter NW, and Rector FC. Consequences of renal failure and their management. In Strauss MB and Welt LG (eds.). *Diseases of the Kidney* (2nd ed.). Boston: Little, Brown, 1971, pp. 211–272.)

urine. Each day 24,192 meq (120 ml/min × 1,440 min/day × meq sodium/liter) of sodium are filtered at the glomeruli. The tubules absorb 24,024 meq/day or 99.3% (24,024 meq/24,192 meq × 100) of the filtered load, whereas 0.7% (168 meq/24,192 meq × 100) of the filtered load is excreted in the urine. When GFR is reduced to 25% of normal, the filtered load of sodium is reduced to 6,048 meq/day. The fractional excretion of sodium is increased to 2.8% of the filtered load (168 meq/6,048 meq × 100), whereas the fractional absorption is decreased to 97.2%. The mechanisms by which tubular absorption of sodium is decreased in chronic renal insufficiency are not well understood. Changes in plasma aldosterone concentrations are unlikely to provide a sole explanation. Increases in atrial natriuretic peptide (ANP) levels probably help maintain sodium balance but other natriuretic hormones may also be involved. In normal individuals, removal of sodium from the diet promptly results in elimination of nearly all sodium from the urine. Conversely, urinary sodium excretion promptly rises to values in excess of 500 meq/day to match high dietary salt intake. In contrast, individuals with chronic renal failure have obligatory urinary sodium losses of at least 25 meq/day and may not be able to excrete more than 200 meq/day.

Potassium

Plasma potassium concentration is normally maintained between 3.5 and 5.1 meq/liter. Of the 75 meq of potassium typically ingested by a healthy individual, 70 meq are excreted in the urine and the remainder in the feces. In health, potassium balance is maintained over a range of intake varying from virtually nil to greater than 200 meq/day. In most patients with chronic renal disease potassium balance is usually maintained until the end stages of renal failure. This is achieved primarily by an increased secretory capacity of the remaining distal nephrons. Potassium secretion from the extracellular fluid to the tubular urine is a two-step process. First, potassium is taken into the cells of the connecting tubules and cortical collecting ducts by the Na-K dependent ATPase located on the basolateral plasmalemma of these cells. This potassium "pump" raises intracellular potassium concentrations to values of ~160 meq/liter. Secondly, potassium diffuses from the cytoplasm of these cells into the tubular lumen via an apical cell-membrane potassium channel. This process depends on several factors, including cell-to-lumen potassium concentration and electrical potential differences. The latter driving force depends on entry of sodium ions from the tubular lumen into the cells through an electrogenic channel which generates the lumen-negative voltage. In chronic renal failure the number of potassium pumps is increased, in part owing to elevated plasma aldosterone levels and in part through undefined mechanisms. This augments uptake of potassium from the extracellular fluid into tubular cells. Also, the movement of potassium from the cells into the tubular fluid is enhanced by the increased fractional excretion of sodium discussed above. Because of the large capacity of these adaptations, maintenance of normal plasma potassium concentrations usually persists until near end-stage renal failure unless other factors supervene (see Chap. 52 for a discussion of factors which impair potassium excretion).

An interesting nonrenal adaptation that aids disposal of bodily potassium in chronic renal failure is augmented colonic secretion owing to increased numbers of Na,K-ATPase pumps in the colonic epithelial cells. Whereas the normal colon excretes no more than 10% of ingested potassium, the colon of individuals with chronic renal failure may dispose of up to 50% of daily potassium intake by this mechanism.

Phosphate

In health serum phosphorus concentration ranges between 2.7 and 4.5 mg/dl. Phosphorus intake in normal humans varies between 1,000 and 2,000 mg/day. Phosphorus, in the form of inorganic phosphate, is freely filtered at the glomeruli and 85% is normally reabsorbed by the kidney tubules. Urinary phosphate excretion is regulated primarily by the action of parathyroid hormone (PTH) on the cells of the proximal tubule. Occupancy of the PTH receptor on the peritubular membrane activates both protein kinases A and C, which in turn inhibit sodium-dependent phosphate uptake at the apical plasmalemma. Consequently, urinary phosphate excretion is increased.

In mild renal insufficiency, plasma phosphorus levels are normal or slightly low, because PTH levels are increased owing to low circulating calcitriol concentrations. In moderate renal insufficiency normal serum phosphorus concentrations are maintained at the expense of greater elevations of parathyroid hormone levels. As severe renal failure ensues, with GFRs falling below 20 ml/minute, serum phosphorus concentration rises above normal because the diseased kidneys' capacity to excrete phosphate is exceeded, despite markedly elevated PTH levels. Phosphorus balance is now maintained at the expense of elevated concentrations of both plasma phosphorus and PTH.

There are several adverse consequences of chronically elevated PTH. One is dissolution of the skeleton by osteoclastic resorption of bone mineral or, in other words, renal osteodystrophy. Secondly, in the presence of a high calcium-phosphorus product (e.g., > 60 mg^2/dl^2) ectopic calcification of vital soft tissues (including the blood vessels, myocardium, lungs, and kidneys) may occur.

Calcium

In normal individuals total serum calcium concentration is between 8.4 and 10.2 mg/dl (Fig. 57-6). Typically, 800 mg of calcium is ingested daily, of which 160 mg is absorbed in the intestines and appears in the urine. However, as PTH levels increase in chronic renal insufficiency, urinary calcium excretion falls to as low as 50 mg/day because this hormone increases calcium absorption in the distal segments of remaining intact nephrons. With severe renal insufficiency hypocalcemia typically develops. This occurs for at least three reasons. First, elevated inorganic phosphorus complexes with calcium. Secondly, reduced production of calcitriol by the kidneys results in diminished intestinal absorption of calcium. Thirdly, skeletal resistance to the calcium-mobilizing action of PTH occurs due in part to low circulating calcitriol concentrations and in part to hyperphosphatemia. In response to hypocalcemia, parathyroid glands synthesize and release PTH into the circulation, resulting in secondary hyperparathyroidism.

Fig. 57-6. Disordered calcium metabolism and hyperparathyroidism in chronic renal failure. (Modified from: Coles G. Chronic renal failure. In Williams JD, et al. (eds.). *Clinical Atlas of the Kidney.* New York: Gower, 1992, pp. 12.1–12.24.)

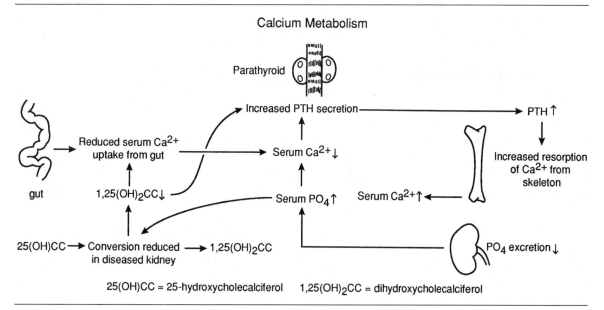

The very high PTH levels which result prevent ionized calcium concentration from falling below mild hypocalcemic levels in most patients. Hence symptomatic hypocalcemia is rarely encountered in chronic renal failure.

Hydrogen Ions

Under normal circumstances, plasma pH is maintained between 7.37 and 7.42 by the lungs, which regulate carbon dioxide excretion, and kidneys, which produce bicarbonate and excrete acids in the urine. In the United States, where meat constitutes a significant portion of the diet, 40–60 meq of sulfuric and phosphoric acids are produced daily by metabolism. The protons generated by these processes are excreted in the urine, primarily in the form of ammonium and titratable acid. Ammonia (NH_3) is produced within the proximal tubules by phosphate-dependent glutaminase and is converted to ammonium (NH_4^+) within the lumen of the collecting ducts, where it is trapped for excretion in the urine. With moderate renal insufficiency, proximal tubular production of ammonia falls, resulting in consumption of extracellular fluid bicarbonate, owing to inadequate H^+ excretion. With severe renal insufficiency, metabolic acidosis worsens with serum bicarbonate concentrations typically falling to values of 14–16 meq/liter. Urinary pH may reach minimal values of 4.5 to 5.0, but because of reduced ammonium excretion insufficient bicarbonate is generated. Finally, in advanced chronic renal failure, retained protons are buffered by the hydroxyapatite of bone. Although this reaction serves to maintain the serum bicarbonate concentration between 12 and 15 meq/liter, it does so at the expense of dissolution of bone mineral, which contribute to osteomalacia.

Endocrine Dysfunction

Anemia

In health the kidneys produce a 165-amino acid glycoprotein hormone erythropoietin, which binds to erythrocyte precursors within the bone marrow and increases the production of circulating red blood cells. Peritubular capillary endothelial cells are believed to respond to decrements in oxygen tension or delivery by increasing synthesis and release of erythropoietin into the blood. When GFR falls below 40 ml/minute, reflecting destruction of sufficient renal parenchyma, patients typically develop anemia, owing to reduced circulating erythropoietin levels. The anemia is usually normocytic and normochromic, and the hematocrit usually varies between 22 and 35% depending on the severity of the renal disorder. Other factors may contribute to anemia in chronic renal failure, such as decreased ery-

throcyte survival and inhibitors of erythropoietin action on the bone marrow. However, restoration of the hematocrit to normal is usually achievable by administration of exogenous recombinant human erythropoietin provided that tissue iron stores are adequate.

Hyperparathyroidism

The production of calcitriol, the active metabolite of vitamin D, is regulated by circulating PTH and inorganic phosphate. Increased levels of PTH stimulate calcitriol synthesis and release. In contrast, there is an inverse relationship between serum phosphorus levels and calcitriol production. An early abnormality in the calcium-phosphorus-PTH-vitamin D axis is a fall in circulating calcitriol concentration. This typically occurs at a GFR ~40 ml/minute and results from a decrease in renal parenchyma. The low circulating calcitriol level releases the parathyroid gland from inhibition of PTH biosynthesis and secretion, resulting in elevated PTH concentrations. When serum phosphorus concentrations become elevated later in the course of chronic renal insufficiency, calcitriol secretion is further suppressed, resulting in greater elevations in PTH secretion. In addition, plasma ionized calcium concentrations fall, and this second stimulus to PTH biosynthesis and release further elevates PTH levels. The final consequence of markedly elevated serum PTH levels is hyperparathyroid bone disease with resulting skeletal pain and fractures (see Chap. 28).

Gastrointestinal Symptoms

Anorexia, nausea, and vomiting are often the reason that patients with chronic renal failure seek medical attention. The upper gastrointestinal tract may appear anatomically normal or gastritis may be observed endoscopically. Restriction of dietary protein intake and/ or institution of regular dialysis will usually alleviate these symptoms, suggesting that these gastrointestinal consequences of renal failure are due to the accumulation of toxic products of protein catabolism. However, the specific toxic compounds have not been identified.

Cardiovascular Complications

Systemic Arterial Hypertension

An almost universal feature of progressive renal disease, it results primarily from expansion of extracellular volume owing to impairment of salt and water excretion. Activation of both the renin-angiotensin systems and the adrenergic nervous system occur to a variable extent in patients with chronic renal failure. (See Chap. 12 for discussion of these mechanisms.) Hypertension contributes importantly to the cardiac complications of renal failure as well as accelerating progression of the renal disease.

Myocardial Complications

Congestive heart failure and myocardial ischemia are commonly encountered in patients with progressive renal failure and constitute the most frequent cause of death in this population. Coronary artery atherosclerosis occurs at an accelerated rate, as a consequence of long-standing hypertension and hyperlipidemia owing to the renal disease. Obstruction to coronary artery flow is the major reason for myocardial ischemia. However, volume overload, anemia, hypertension, and left ventricular hypertrophy also contribute to the imbalance of myocardial oxygen supply and demand. The mechanisms leading to congestive heart failure are complex and not fully understood. Diastolic dysfunction owing primarily to left ventricular hypertrophy is an important factor in many patients. Systolic dysfunction is common but more difficult to explain. It often results from multiple factors including myocardial calcification and ischemia (or infarction) and myocardial damage from long-standing pressure and volume overload. Severe secondary hyperparathyroidism, poor nutrition, hypocalcemia, and uremic myocardial toxins may further depress myocardial contractility. The result is more difficult to treat than to prevent but both can be achieved by careful attention to controlling each of the pathogenic factors discussed above. Angiotensin-converting enzyme inhibitors are also appropriate in patients with systolic myocardial failure.

Pericarditis

It is a common feature of advanced renal failure and a clear indication to initiate regular dialysis treatments. The clinical features include precordial pain, fever, and a pericardial friction rub. An effusion may be present, and acute pericardial tamponade may result if adequate dialysis is not promptly instituted. (See Chap. 8 for a more complete discussion of pericarditis.)

Neurologic Disturbances

Advanced renal failure is associated with disturbances of cerebral and peripheral nerve function. The encephalopathy is manifested by lethargy, impaired cognition, and insomnia which may progress to stupor and coma. Diffuse myoclonic jerking and seizures may occur with severe azotemia. (BUN and serum creatinine exceeding 100 and 10 mg/dl, respectively). As a rule, all but the most subtle neuropsychological deficits clear promptly with adequate dialysis therapy.

A progressive sensory-motor polyneuropathy may result from long-standing chronic renal failure. Loss of vibratory sense and stretch reflexes are early features which may be followed by progressive muscle weakness and generalized sensory loss. The lower extremities are most severely affected. The accumulation of neurotoxic metabolites is thought to be responsible for this syndrome and some improvement may be observed with institution of regular dialysis therapy. However, in some patients the process can only be halted by successful renal transplantation.

Approach to Patients with Chronic Renal Failure

When evaluating a patient with renal failure, it is important to ascertain whether the dysfunction is acute, chronic, or a superimposition of an acute insult on chronic dysfunction. Historical information is the most valuable, especially the presence of subtle symptoms such as nocturia (reflecting isosthenuria), fatigue, anorexia, and malaise. These clues suggesting chronic renal failure can often be corroborated by records indicating prior elevation of the serum creatinine concentration or perhaps the presence of hypertension or anemia. As a rule, the presence of mild symptoms despite severe azotemia indicates chronic renal failure; patients do not tolerate acute renal failure nearly as well. Many factors can acutely aggravate chronic renal insufficiency. These may include extracellular fluid volume depletion (e.g., from diarrhea, vomiting, or overzealous use of diuretics), drugs (e.g., nonsteroidal antiinflammatory agents, angiotensin-converting enzyme inhibitors, aminoglycoside antibiotics, radiocontrast dye), obstruction, infection, hypertensive crisis, congestive heart failure, and arterial hypotension. It is important to evaluate each patient for factors such as these, which when reversed can lead to improved renal function. After a careful history and physical examination, routine laboratory testing including a CBC, chemistry profile, chest x-ray, electrocardiogram, and urinalysis should be done. Renal ultrasonography is often useful in elucidating the cause (obstruction or polycystic kidneys) and chronicity of renal failure. Highly echogenic small kidneys (< 9 cm in length) indicate chronic renal disease for which renal biopsy is not needed, because the disease process is too far advanced to be treatable.

Principles of Management

While the disease process causing chronic renal failure is often not treatable, the functional derangements which occur can often be effectively controlled with proper diet and medication. The goals of this therapy are to retard progression of the renal disease and to minimize damage to other organs, especially the cardiovascular system.

Diet

Dietary protein restriction by reducing glomerular hyperfiltration may slow the progression of chronic renal failure. This effect is probably related to the protein, per se, although phosphorus intake is also diminished whenever dietary protein is restricted. Restricting the ingestion of milk products and other phosphorus-rich foods is also advisable in order to help prevent hyperphosphatemia and its associated sequelae (soft tissue calcifications, hyperparathyroidism). Sodium intake should be limited when signs of extracellular volume expansion including hypertension are noted. There is rarely a need to restrict fluid intake in patients with chronic renal disease; since the diseased kidney cannot concentrate the urine, most patients will need to take in enough fluids to produce at least 2–3 liters of urine each day for optimal renal function.

Treatment of Arterial Hypertension

Clinical studies have shown that treatment of arterial hypertension slows the rate of decline in GFR in patients with diabetic nephropathy (Fig. 57-7) and other forms of chronic renal disease. Careful control of hypertension is also essential to minimize development of future cardiovascular events.

Prevention of Secondary Hyperparathyroidism

There are two important elements of this therapy. The first is reduction in intestinal absorption of phosphorus to prevent elevations in serum phosphorus concentration. In conjunction with reduced dietary phosphorus intake, patients usually need to take oral calcium carbonate or calcium acetate with each meal as an intestinal phosphorus binder. The goal of these measures is to maintain the serum calcium concentration between 10 and 10.5 mg/dl and to keep the serum phosphorus concentration ≤ 4.5 mg/dl. The second element is exogenous replenishment of calcitriol. If the serum PTH concentration can be maintained no higher

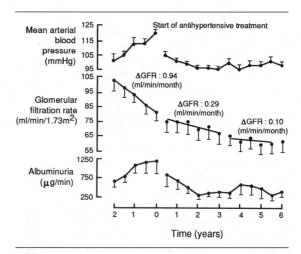

Fig. 57-7. Effect of treating arterial hypertension on the progression of chronic renal insufficiency in patients with diabetic nephropathy. (Modified from: Coles G. Chronic renal failure. In Williams JD, et al. (eds.). *Clinical Atlas of the Kidney.* New York: Gower, 1992, pp. 12.1–12.24.)

than twice the upper limits of normal with dietary phosphorus restriction and oral calcium supplements alone, oral calcitriol is usually unnecessary. However, if a patient remains hypocalcemic or if the serum PTH level is progressively increasing despite a normal serum phosphorus, then calcitriol supplementation should be administered.

Treatment of Metabolic Acidosis

When the serum bicarbonate concentration falls below 16 meq/liter, patients should receive supplemental sodium bicarbonate in order to minimize skeletal dissolution. One must be mindful of the extracellular fluid volume expansion that may be engendered by the additional sodium load and be prepared to use loop-acting diuretics to maintain extracellular fluid volume balance.

Control of Extracellular Fluid Volume

For those individuals who retain excessive sodium chloride and water, loop-acting diuretics (e.g., furosemide, bumetanide) may be useful. In patients refractory to maximal doses of the above, addition of metolazone or a thiazide diuretic (which act in the distal convoluted tubule) may dramatically enhance the effectiveness of the loop diuretic. Potassium-sparing diuretics should be avoided in patients with chronic renal failure.

Correction of Anemia

One of the payoffs of recombinant DNA technology is the availability of human erythropoietin for replacement therapy. Proper use of this hormone will correct the anemia of chronic renal disease, with resulting improvement in appetite, exercise tolerance, and general well-being. A tendency for blood pressure to rise with the increase in hemoglobin concentration is the only adverse effect.

Decisions Regarding Renal Replacement Therapy

When individuals with advanced chronic renal failure develop troublesome symptoms or can no longer control extracellular fluid volume excess, some form of renal function replacement therapy is necessary. The available options include hemodialysis, peritoneal dialysis, and renal transplantation. The morbidity and mortality of these therapies is substantial, so it behooves physicians and patients to optimize dietary and drug modalities in order to delay the onset of end-stage renal failure.

Clinical Examples

1. A 30-year-old man with membranoproliferative glomerulonephritis comes to see you after a long respite from physician visits. His major complaints include fatigue and dyspnea on exertion which are limiting his ability to work as a mail carrier. He fears losing his job and his health insurance program. He is taking no medications and is following an "ad lib" diet. Medical records show that 4 years ago his serum urea nitrogen and creatinine levels were 28 and 2.8 mg/dl respectively. Blood pressure then averaged about 150/100 mm Hg.

Physical examination now reveals a chronically ill-appearing man who appears depressed. Blood pressure is 160/108 mm Hg, pulse 94 beats/minute, sitting. The remainder of the physical examination is unremarkable except for slight bilateral ankle edema. The hemoglobin concentration is 8 gm/dl.

Serum Chemistries

BUN	50 mg/dl
Creatinine	5.4 mg/dl
Sodium	140 meq/liter
Potassium	5.0 meq/liter
Chloride	104 meq/liter
Bicarbonate	17 meq/liter
Calcium	8.4 mg/dl
Phosphorus	6.1 mg/dl
Albumin	3.2 gm/dl

Urinalysis reveals 4+ protein, specific gravity 1.010, granular casts, and numerous red blood cells. Chest x-ray shows mild cardiomegaly but is otherwise normal. An arterial blood sample reveals pH 7.34, $PaCO_2 = 30$ mm Hg, $PaO_2 = 104$ mm Hg.

Discussion.   This patient demonstrates many of the typical features of chronic renal failure including fatigue and dyspnea which are largely explained by the anemia. Hypertension, azotemia, metabolic acidosis, and disordered calcium and phosphorus homeostasis are also present. The cardiomegaly is probably related to volume loading, owing to anemia and salt and water retention but systolic dysfunction must be ruled out.

This patient's disease will progress to end-stage renal failure; however, with appropriate care he should be able to continue to work and feel much better than he currently does. His therapy should include dietary counseling, antihypertensive drugs (including a loop diuretic to decrease extracellular volume), a phosphate binder, and regular erythropoietin injections. When his endogenous creatinine clearance is less than 10 ml/minute he should benefit from renal transplantation. He will probably require a period of regular dialysis until a suitable renal allograft can be procured.

2. A 56-year-old man presents to the emergency department with complaints of nausea, vomiting, and weakness of one-week duration. He has not felt well for about 6 months but his current problems began about a week after he started taking ibuprofen for a nagging pain in his right flank. Physical examination reveals a middle-aged man who is retching repeatedly. His blood pressure is 110/70 supine and 70/40 standing. The remainder of the examination is nonrevealing except for a slightly tender mass in the right flank.

Serum Chemistries

Hemoglobin	14.6 gm/dl
BUN	142 mg/dl
Creatinine	8.4 mg/dl
Sodium	140 meq/liter
Potassium	3.0 meq/liter
Chloride	92 meq/liter
Bicarbonate	26 meq/liter
Total calcium	10.4 mg/dl
Phosphorus	5.6 mg/dl

The urinalysis revealed 1+ protein, pH 5.5, occasional red blood cells and white blood cells and numerous granular casts.

Discussion.   This patient probably has chronic renal failure, owing to polycystic kidney disease or obstructive uropathy, either of which could explain the pain and palpable mass in the right flank. Undoubtedly, his current renal function is not a good reflection of his "baseline status" for at least two reasons. First, his extracellular fluid compartment is markedly depleted from the combined effects of vomiting, poor intake, and ongoing urinary losses of salt and water. Secondly, he has been taking ibuprofen, a nonsteroidal antiinflammatory drug (NSAID). By blocking cyclo-oxygenase these agents impair renal synthesis of vasodilating prostaglandins. In the presence of chronic renal insufficiency, the result is often an abrupt decline in renal blood flow and glomerular filtration. In addition, the NSAIDs may be responsible for his initial vomiting (from gastritis). The azotemia is another possible reason for his nausea and vomiting.

Appropriate management should include intravenous saline to correct volume depletion, avoidance of NSAIDs, and abdominal ultrasonography to confirm or refute the clinical impression. These measures may be rewarded by marked improvement in renal function and symptomatology. It should be noted that in this patient an anemia may be masked by some degree of hemoconcentration. However, patients with polycystic kidney disease often do not have anemia despite the presence of severe renal failure. Alternatively, he might have acute renal failure, which is also often not associated with anemia. However, this would not explain his chronic symptoms nor the palpable mass.

Bibliography

Ardaillou R and Dussaule JC. Role of atria natriuretic peptide in the control of sodium balance in chronic renal failure. *Nephron* 66:249–257, 1994. *Contemporary editorial review of the role of ANF in maintaining sodium balance in chronic renal failure.*

Espinel CH. Diagnosis of acute and chronic renal failure. *Clin Lab Med* 13:89–102, 1993. *Discussion of the laboratory methods that are useful in the diagnosis of chronic renal failure.*

Fine LG, Kurtz I, Woolf AS, et al. Pathophysiology and nephron adaptation in chronic renal failure. In Schrier RW and Gottschalk CW (eds.). *Diseases of the Kidney* (5th ed.). Boston: Little, Brown, 1993, Vol. III, pp. 2703–2742. *Detailed examination of the nephronal adaptations that are operative in chronic renal failure.*

Tuso PJ, Nissenson AR, and Danovitch GM. Electrolyte disorders in chronic renal failure. In Narins RG (ed.). *Maxwell & Kleeman's Clinical Disorders of Fluid & Electrolyte Metabolism* (5th ed.). New York: McGraw-Hill, 1994, Chap. 39, pp. 1195–1212. *Concise, but thorough, discussion of disorders of water, sodium, potassium, and hydrogen ion homeostasis in chronic renal failure.*

Valtin H. *Renal Dysfunction: Mechanisms Involved in Fluid and Solute Imbalance.* Boston: Little, Brown, 1979. *Lucid, 500-page examination of the adaptations, both renal and nonrenal, occurring in response to chronic renal insufficiency and failure.*

58 Tubulointerstitial Disorders

Sudhir K. Khanna

Objectives

After completing this chapter, you should be able to

Briefly outline the normal function of each major segment of the nephron

Describe how to identify proximal tubular dysfunction

Define renal tubular acidosis and explain the differences between the three major types

Outline mechanisms which impair urinary concentration

Discuss acute tubulointerstitial nephritis with regard to pathogenesis and clinical course

List the major causes of chronic tubulointerstitial nephropathy

Discuss the clinical and laboratory features which help distinguish glomerular from tubulointerstitial disorders

---

This diverse group of conditions predominantly involve the renal tubules and the space between the tubules (interstitium), causing histologic and functional abnormalities. In some conditions (e.g., multiple myeloma), there may be associated glomerular and/or vascular involvement, but the tubulointerstitial compartment is most severely affected. Approximately 25% of all the cases of chronic renal failure are from tubulointerstitial diseases, and these disorders are also a common cause of acute renal failure. These nephropathies can be caused by drugs, autoimmune diseases, infections, hypersensitivity reactions, and metabolic conditions.

Normal Renal Tubular Function

Glomerular filtrate is modified in different segments of the tubules (Fig. 58-1). In the proximal tubule most of the filtered amino acids, organic acids, glucose, phosphate, sodium, chloride, and bicarbonate are reabsorbed. Water moves passively out of the proximal tubule along the osmotic gradients set up by active solute transport. Therefore, the fluid remaining at the end of proximal tubule is iso-osmotic to plasma, even after 60–70% of the filtered water has been reabsorbed.

The Loop of Henle dips deeply into the medulla and, because of its permeability characteristics, works as a countercurrent multiplier. This produces a graded increase in the osmolality of the interstitial fluid, which at the tip of the papillae is $\approx$ 1200 mOsm/kg. However, the tubular fluid at the end of the ascending limb of the loop of Henle is hypotonic to plasma because of the active transport of sodium and chloride out of the lumen.

The distal tubule which lies in the cortex is a site of potassium and hydrogen ion secretion. Most of the filtered potassium is reabsorbed in the proximal tubule; hence potassium excreted in the final urine comes largely from secretion in this segment and more distal sites in the nephron.

The collecting duct has cortical and medullary portions. The medullary portion is the primary site of action of antidiuretic hormone (ADH), which increases the permeability to water by inserting water channels in the luminal membrane. In the presence of ADH approximately 10% of the filtered water is reabsorbed in the cortical collecting duct, rendering the tubular fluid iso-osmotic to plasma. The medullary interstitium is hypertonic and in the presence of ADH is the site of further water reabsorption. Hence the final urine osmolality can vary from 30 to 1200 mOsm/kg, depending upon the permeability of the distal tubule and collecting duct.

627

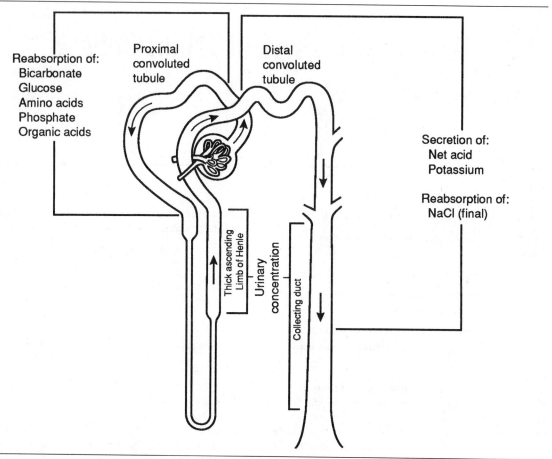

Fig. 58-1. Segmental physiologic aspects of nephron function. (Modified from: Cogan MC. Tubulo-interstitial nephropathies: A pathophysiologic approach. *Western J Med,* 132:134–140, 1980.)

The renal tubules play a major role in acid-base homeostasis, being responsible for hydrogen ion excretion and maintenance of bicarbonate stores in the extracellular fluid. Normally 85% of the filtered bicarbonate is reclaimed in the proximal tubule. Hydrogen is secreted into the lumen, where it binds with bicarbonate to form H_2CO_3. In presence of carbonic anhydrase, water and CO_2 are formed and absorbed into the cell. In the distal nephron hydrogen ion secretion occurs in the cortical and medullary collecting duct by virtue of a H^+ ATPase pump. Hydrogen ion in the lumen binds with bicarbonate to reclaim it as in the proximal tubule; additional H^+ binds to the urinary buffers and ammonia present in the lumen. During metabolic aci-

dosis NH_3 production can increase 6–8 fold to facilitate excretion of hydrogen ions. The rate-limiting factors for H^+ secretion in the distal tubule are luminal pH, which cannot go below 4.5, and the rate of NH_3 production.

Tubulointerstitial Disorders

Different tubulointerstitial disorders affect different segments of the nephron, causing the functional syndromes and structural disorders outlined in Table 58-1. The latter are classified as either acute or chronic nephropathies, reflecting somewhat different etiologies and prognosis.

Table 58-1. Tubulointerstitial Disorders

FUNCTIONAL SYNDROMES

Proximal nephron dysfunction
Distal nephron dysfunction
   Distal (type 1) renal tubular acidosis
   Type IV renal tubular acidosis
   Nephrogenic diabetes insipidus

TUBULOINTERSTITIAL NEPHROPATHIES

Acute tubulointerstitial nephritis
Chronic tubulointerstitial nephropathy

Functional Disorders

There are a number of conditions which disturb the function of the tubular epithelium without producing prominent structural changes in the nephron or renal interstitium. As a rule, glomerular filtration is well preserved and renal failure occurs only after many years, if at all. These disorders are classified according to whether the major features reflect proximal or distal nephron dysfunction.

Proximal Nephron Dysfunction

Dysfunction of this portion of the tubule causes variable urinary losses of sodium, bicarbonate, phosphate, uric acid, glucose, amino acids, and tubular proteins. The term "Fanconi syndrome" is applied when multiple defects are present. When bicarbonate wasting occurs plasma bicarbonate level is reduced, leading to metabolic acidosis. This syndrome is called Type II or proximal renal tubular acidosis (RTA). It is usually associated with other signs of proximal tubular dysfunction but may occur in isolation. Proximal RTA may be accompanied by a urine pH < 5.5, which helps to distinguish it from the distal variety (see below).

Distal Nephron Dysfunction

The distal portions of the nephron are responsible for secretion of potassium and hydrogen ions and production of a concentrated urine. Therefore, dysfunction of these segments typically causes urinary concentrating defects, metabolic acidosis, and disturbances of potassium homeostasis.

Type I Renal Tubular Acidosis.
In this disorder inadequate H^+ excretion leads to impairment of bicarbonate regeneration, resulting in hyperchloremic metabolic acidosis. The acidification defect may be directly due to impaired hydrogen ion secretion or possibly a "back leak" of hydrogen ion into the tubular cells. The net result is that urine pH cannot be reduced below 5.5 despite metabolic acidosis. These patients invariably have a low rate of ammonium excretion, which has been attributed to the inability to lower urine pH. The causes of distal RTA are shown in Table 58-2.

Clinical features of distal RTA reflect disturbances of calcium metabolism, the effects of renal potassium wasting, and direct consequences of metabolic acidosis per se (Chap. 53). The latter is largely responsible for the leaching of skeletal calcium and contributes to the hypercalciuria and osteomalacia which typically occur. In children growth retardation is common. At any age skeletal pain and fractures may result from the osteomalacia. Nephrolithiases and nephrocalcinosis are additional features of distal RTA. Pathogenesis of the stone disease is multifactorial, including hypercalciuria, decreased urinary citrate excretion, and the high urine pH.

Type IV Renal Tubular Acidosis.
Aldosterone stimulates distal acidification by inserting sodium channels in the luminal side of the membrane and stimulating the H^+ ATPase pump, which cause H^+ and K^+ secretion in exchange for sodium. Hence deficiency of aldosterone or resistance to its action leads to hyperkalemia and mild metabolic acidosis. This syndrome is termed Type IV RTA. In addition to the direct effect of inadequate aldosterone action on H^+ secretion, hyperkalemia impairs NH_4^+ excretion which contributes to the metabolic acidosis. Since NH_3 synthesis (from glutamine) is low, urine pH often is < 5.5 owing to lack of this important urinary buffer. Causes of Type IV RTA include hyporeninemic hypoaldosteronism secondary to diabetes mellitus or any of the tubulointerstitial diseases discussed below. Drugs which impair aldosterone secretion or action can cause similar manifestations. These include spironolactone, angiotensin-converting enzyme inhibitors, nonsteroidal antiinflammatory drugs, and heparin. Patients with Type IV RTA are treated with a combination of low K^+ diet, loop diuretics, and fludrocortisone (mineralocorticoid replacement).

Table 58-2. Causes of Distal Renal Tubular Acidosis

Hereditary
Autoimmune diseases: SLE, chronic active hepatitis, Sjögren's syndrome
Drugs and toxins: Amphotericin B, Lithium
Calcium disorders: Idiopathic hypercalciuria, primary hyperparathyroidism
Idiopathic

Disorders of Urinary Concentration. Water reabsorption in the distal nephron requires three prerequisites: a hypertonic medullary interstitium, presence of ADH, and a responsive distal tubule and collecting duct. Dysfunction of any of these steps would cause passage of inappropriately dilute urine, resulting in an inability to conserve water. This condition is termed **diabetes insipidus** (DI). When it results from inadequate ADH it is called central DI (discussed in Chap. 26).

Nephrogenic DI may result from hypercalcemia, severe hypokalemia, and drugs like lithium and demeclocycline. Other causes include the rare X-linked congenital variety, sickle cell anemia, and amyloidosis. Affected patients have polyuria, nocturia, and polydipsia. Hypernatremia only occurs if the patient is deprived of access to water. Many of these patients have an incomplete syndrome and do not require specific therapy. Those who have marked polyuria may be helped by a thiazide diuretic and a low-sodium, low-protein diet. A low-sodium diet and thiazide diuretics cause mild volume depletion, which causes increased proximal absorption of salt and water, leading to a decrease in urine volume. Low protein intake reduces solute load and therefore urine volume.

Tubulointerstitial Nephropathies

These disorders are classified according to the tempo of the illness as acute or chronic nephropathies, reflecting different etiologies and prognosis.

Acute Tubulointerstitial Nephritis (TIN)

As the name implies, the inflammatory reaction evolves over a period of a few days to weeks. Typically, mononuclear cells infiltrate the interstitium, but in drug-related acute TIN, eosinophils and neutrophiles may be present. Acute TIN is underdiagnosed and by some estimates accounts for 15% of all cases of acute renal failure. Drugs and infections are common causes but immune, toxic, and metabolic causes also occur. Many drugs can cause acute TIN but beta lactam antibiotics, nonsteroidal antiinflammatory drugs (NSAIDs), allopurinol, and diuretics are most frequently incriminated. Patients present with various combinations of fever, rash, eosinophilia, hematuria, proteinuria, pyuria, and azotemia. Drug-induced acute TIN typically develops 10–14 days or more after starting the medication. Eosinophilia and skin rash are common except when an NSAID is the cause. In this situation acute renal failure and nephrotic syndrome occur simultaneously. Diagnosis is made by the clinical and laboratory findings. If doubts exists a renal biopsy can be done which will show of cellular infiltrate,

interstitial edema, and some tubular necrosis (Plate 8). Withdrawal of the offending agent or treatment of infection (acute pyelonephritis) is all that is required for most of these patients. Some patients may need temporary dialysis to control uremia. Steroid treatment may hasten recovery in patients with an allergic-type acute TIN syndrome.

Chronic Tubulointerstitial Nephropathies

These conditions are caused by even more disparate diseases than acute TIN (Table 58-3). Most of these conditions appear similar pathologically and are characterized by interstitial fibrosis and tubular atrophy. There is generally a patchy chronic inflammatory cell infiltrate. Glomeruli appear normal in the early stages. Chronic TIN may result from progression of acute TIN or may evolve insidiously from a chronic insult.

These patients usually present with chronic renal insufficiency and may also demonstrate one or more of the functional syndromes described above. Some of the underlying conditions like myeloma, chronic analgesic abuse, and polycystic disease have characteristic features which help in making a diagnosis. In some conditions like systemic lupus erythematosus and amyloidosis, glomerular involvement may predominate. Chronic tubulointerstitial nephropathy owing to analgesic abuse was until recently quite common in certain parts of the United States. Analgesic compounds containing aspirin, phenacetin, and caffeine taken in large quantities over many years have been clearly incriminated. It is believed that acetaminophen or NSAIDs can cause similar chronic renal damage when taken in excess. Management of chronic tubulointerstitial nephropathies is determined by the underlying cause. Avoidance of offending agent wherever possible, treatment of infections, control of hypertension, and treatment of acid-base

Table 58-3. Causes of Chronic Tubulointerstitial Nephropathy

Progression of acute tubulointerstitial nephropathies
Drugs: analgesics, lithium
Infections: chronic bacterial and tubercular infection
Metabolic: hypercalcemia, hyperuricemia
Metals: lead, cadmium
Immunological: systemic lupus erythematosus, primary
    biliary cirrhosis, transplant
Chronic urinary tract obstruction
Neoplasms: multiple myeloma, leukemia, lymphoma
Cystic diseases: polycystic kidney disease
Miscellaneous: amyloidosis, sickle cell disease, radiation,
    sarcoidosis

Table 58-4. Differentiating Features of Glomerular and Tubulointerstitial Disorders

Feature	Glomerular	Tubulointerstitial
Proteinuria	Often > 3 g/24 hr, containing mostly albumin	< 2.0 g/24 hr containing tubular proteins
Sediment	Red cell casts, dysmorphic RBCs	White cell casts, RBCs
Sodium handling	Retention	Sodium wasting may occur
Anemia	Moderate	Severe
Hypertension	Frequent	Less frequent because of salt wasting
Acidosis	Late, anion gap type	Early and hyperchloremic
Urine volume	Normal	High because of medullary dysfunction

Fig. 58-2. Obstructive nephropathy. Real-time ultrasound scan of kidney showing markedly dilated pelvicalyceal system. (Courtesy of D. Nguyen, M.D.)

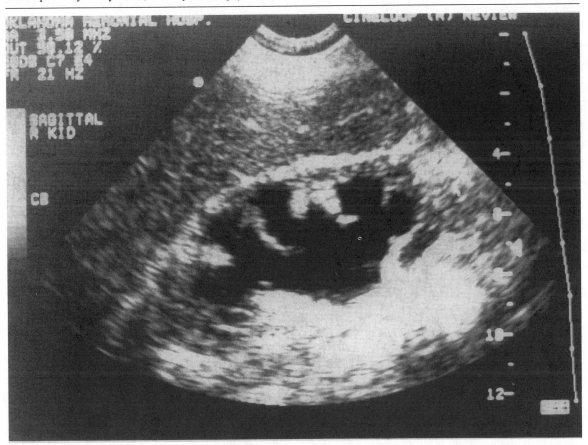

and electrolyte disorders should be done as appropriate. Progression to chronic renal failure is not uncommon.

Features Differentiating Glomerular and Tubulointerstitial Diseases

Certain features are quite characteristic of tubulointerstitial disorders and help distinguish them from glomerular disorders (Table 58-4). In glomerular disorders, proteinuria (especially albuminuria) is a prominent finding owing to leakage of albumin from the damaged filtration barrier. In tubulointerstitial disorders proteinuria consists of tubular proteins like Tamm-Horsfall protein, β_2 microglobulin, immunoglobulins, and lysozyme. Total protein excretion rarely exceeds 1–2 g/day in the tubulointerstitial diseases.

Urinary sediments also can be helpful. In glomerular disorders red blood cells and red blood casts may be present, while in tubulointerstitial disorders white blood cells and white blood cell casts are characteristic findings.

Patients with glomerular disorders often have salt and water retention, causing hypertension and edema early in the course of illness, while patients with tubulointerstitial disorders do not and may even require NaCl supplements because of salt wasting.

Other features like hyperchloremic metabolic acidosis and urine concentration defects are often seen early in the course of chronic tubulointerstitial nephropathy. In contrast patients with glomerular disorders typically have a wide anion gap metabolic acidosis but only with advanced renal failure.

Clinical Examples

1. A 62-year-old white male presents with progressive decrease in urinary stream and difficulty starting micturition. The blood pressure is 160/100. The rest of the physical examination is unremarkable except for a prostatic enlargement found on rectal examination and a large, slightly tender bladder.

Laboratory Results

Sodium	132 meq/liter
Chloride	114 meq/liter
Potassium	6.1 meq/liter
Bicarbonate	14 meq/liter
Creatinine	3.5 mg/dl
Blood urea nitrogen	41 mg/dl

A twenty-four-hour urine collection shows: volume of 2.1 liters, protein excretion 532 mg, and creatinine clearance 32 ml/minute. Urine pH is 6.1 and urine sediment shows 5–6 white blood cells, 2–3 red blood cells, and occasional granular casts. The ultrasound of the kidney demonstrates dilatation of the pyelocalyceal system in both kidneys (Fig. 58-2). Shortly after admission a foley catheter is placed and urine output during the following 12 hours was 3.5 liters. Renal function and laboratory abnormalities improved over a period of a few weeks after the obstruction was relieved, and serum creatinine came down to 1.3 mg/dl.

Discussion.   The symptoms and physical findings were strongly suggestive of obstructive nephropathy. However, in contrast with acute urinary obstruction, patients with chronic obstruction may present with minimal symptoms, and urine output may be decreased, increased, or normal. Renal ultrasound is usually diagnostic because chronic obstruction of the urinary flow increases the intratubular pressure and produces dilatation of the pyelocalyceal system. The glomerular filtration rate decreases as a direct consequence of the elevation of intratubular pressure which eventually also damages the tubules. If obstruction is not relieved the damage is progressive, causing irreversible tubular atrophy and interstitial fibrosis. The decrease in serum bicarbonate with an elevation in serum chloride and inappropriately elevated urinary pH suggest renal tubular acidosis. This is a common electrolyte pattern in obstructive nephropathy. Whereas "classical" distal renal tubular acidosis is associated with hypokalemia, chronic obstructive nephropathy impairs the ability of the tubule to secrete potassium, thus leading to hyperkalemia. However, after obstruction is released a diuresis may occur and the urine loss of potassium may cause hypokalemia. This "post-obstructive polyuria" is due to filtration of retained solutes and defective reabsorption of sodium and water by the damaged tubules. When the latter is prominent the patient may become depleted of salt and water if replacement is inadequate.

2. A 42-year-old woman presents with complaints of dysuria (pain with urination), flank pain, anorexia, and fever. The past medical history includes frequent urinary tract infections and persistent headaches for the past 20 years for which she takes large doses of over-the-counter analgesics.

Physical exam shows pale skin and conjunctiva. Blood pressure is 115/75 mm Hg, pulse 105 bpm supine and 93/70 mm Hg, pulse 120 bpm in the upright position. The remainder of the physical exam is normal.

Laboratory Results

Sodium	135 meq/liter
Chloride	85 meq/liter
Potassium	6.2 meq/liter
Bicarbonate	13 meq/liter
Creatinine	3.1 mg/dl
Blood urea nitrogen	67 mg/dl
Hematocrit	26%
Hemoglobin	8.3 gm/dl

The urine sediment reveals many white blood cells, 5–7 red blood cells, 4–6 granular casts. The urine specific gravity is 1.010. The urine culture is positive for *E. coli*. An intravenous pyelogram is suggestive of papillary necrosis.

Discussion. This patient represents a typical case of chronic tubulointerstitial nephropathy most likely due to analgesic abuse. This typically occurs in middle-aged women with a psychoneurosis who take excessive amounts of analgesic for back pain and/or headache. After several years they develop renal disease primarily affecting the medulla. Analgesics such as aspirin, phenacetin, and caffeine (particularly when taken in combination) are capable of directly producing oxidative cellular injury. These compounds are concentrated in the medulla, resulting in more severe damage there. Papillary necrosis is frequently the result. Urinary tract infections are common in this setting but even more common is pyuria with a negative urine culture. Anemia is due to the decrease in erythropoietin production and gastrointestinal bleeding caused by the analgesics.

In addition to having a decrease in glomerular filtration, patients with analgesic abuse nephropathy commonly present with features of distal tubular disorder and medullary dysfunction. When the tubular component of a nephron is severely affected and fibrosis occurs, the corresponding glomerulus becomes sclerotic. When this process is widespread, overall filtration decreases and serum creatinine rises. In this patient the blood urea nitrogen is excessively high for the increment in serum creatinine. This suggests renal underperfusion as a result of extracellular fluid volume depletion. The finding of an orthostatic fall in blood pressure supports this hypothesis. Patients with distal tubular dysfunction may not be able to reabsorb all of the sodium that is delivered there, resulting in urinary salt wasting. When the patient is anorexic and salt intake is low, sodium depletion commonly occurs. In this situation the patient should improve with the administration of saline. Another frequent problem with medullary dysfunction is that the ability to conserve water is impaired. Nocturia is a typical symptom of this inability to concentrate the urine.

3. A 40-year-old white male presents with gross hematuria and flank pain. The patient reports having nocturia for several years. He has taken antibiotics in the past for urinary tract infection, and has been diagnosed as having hypertension.

Positive findings in the physical exam include a blood pressure of 165/97 and enlarged kidneys. Ultrasound shows enlargement of both kidneys with multiple cysts.

Laboratory Results

Sodium	139 meq/liter
Potassium	4.7 meq/liter
Chloride	100 meq/liter
Bicarbonate	21 meq/liter
Creatinine	3.2 mg/dl
BUN	40 mg/dl
Hematocrit	45%
Hemoglobin	13.5 gm/dl

Urine sediment shows numerous red blood cells, white blood cells and occasional granular casts. Protein excretion is 600 mg/24 hours.

Discussion. Polycystic kidney disease is a frequent cause of chronic renal failure. This is a genetic disease (autosomal dominant trait) that result in cysts formation in medullary collecting ducts causing tubular dysfunction and progressive loss of nephrons. The kidneys become enlarged and when the disease is advanced they are often easily palpable. Ultrasound or computed tomographic scanning typically demonstrate renal enlargement and innumerable cysts in both kidneys. Patients often have urinary tract infection, and cysts may become infected or disrupted, causing pain and hematuria. The blood pressure is usually increased, perhaps due to compression of renal tissue by the cysts, causing increase in renin secretion. Excessive salt loss in the urine may occur owing to inability of the distal tubule to conserve sodium. However, this is not common and when renal function declines, patients typically retain sodium, causing expansion of the extracellular volume.

Typically, the hematocrit and hemoglobin are not decreased as one would expect in patients with renal failure of other etiologies. Perhaps this is because compression by the cyst produces relative ischemia of the renal interstitium leading to an increase in erythropoietin production.

The renal function continues to deteriorate over a period

of years; so, if the patient lives long enough, he will eventually require dialysis or renal transplant therapy.

Bibliography

Brenner BM and Rector FC. *The Kidney* (4th ed.). London: Saunders, 1991. *Especially see Chap. 25: Wilson CB. The renal response to immunologic injury (pp. 1062–1181) and Chap. 29: Bennett WM, Elzinga LW, and Porter GA. Tubulointerstitial disease and toxic nephropathy (pp. 1430–1496). These chapters provide detailed descriptions of tubulointerstitial disorders.*

Davison AM. Tubulointerstitial Disorders. In *Nephrology* (1st ed.). London: Saunders, 1988, pp. 336–347. *Good review of tubulointerstitial disorders.*

Klemkhect D, Vanhille PH, Morel-Maroger L, et al. Acute interstitial nephritis due to drug hypersensitivity. *Adv Nephron* 12:227–308, 1983. *Discussion of drugs and kidney diseases.*

Perneger, TV, Whelton PK, and Klaf MJ. Risk of kidney failure associated with use of acetaminophen, aspirin, and nonsteroidal noninflammatory drugs. *N Engl J Med* 331:1675–1679, 1994. *Epidemiologic study of risk of kidney failure from individual analgesics.*

Ronco PM and Flahault A. Drug-induced end stage renal disease. *New Engl J Med* 331:1711–1712, 1994. *Description of drugs implicated in causations of renal disease.*

Part VII Questions: Renal and Electrolyte Disorders

1. Sodium depletion is virtually always associated with
   A. hyponatremia.
   B. contraction of the intracellular space.
   C. contraction of the extracellular space.
   D. expansion of the extracellular space.
   E. expansion of intracellular space.

2. A person on a low potassium diet for three weeks will show lower than normal urinary excretion of potassium, primarily because
   A. filtered load of potassium is decreased.
   B. plasma concentration of aldosterone is increased.
   C. reabsorption of potassium in the proximal renal tubule is increased.
   D. secretion of potassium in the collecting duct is decreased.
   E. secretion of potassium in proximal renal tubule is decreased.

3. Match laboratory data sample number with the acid-base disturbance.

	Serum				Arterial			
Sample	Na^+	Cl^-	HCO_3^-	K^+	Anion Gap	pH	pCO_2	H^+
i	140	100	15	5.0	25	7.10	50	79
ii	140	90	25	4.0	25	7.40	40	40
iii	140	100	27	3.0	13	7.60	26	25
iv	140	114	6	5.0	20	7.16	18	70
v	140	105	8	4.0	27	7.46	15	35
vi	140	95	33	3.0	12	7.40	58	40

Disturbance
   A. Metabolic acidosis and metabolic alkalosis
   B. Metabolic acidosis and respiratory acidosis
   C. Metabolic alkalosis and respiratory acidosis
   D. Respiratory alkalosis and metabolic acidosis
   E. Metabolic acidosis with appropriate respiratory compensation
   F. Acute respiratory acidosis and metabolic alkalosis

4. Urinary Mg-wasting would be expected with
   A. diarrhea.
   B. dietary Mg deprivation.
   C. nasogastric suction.
   D. bumetanide.
   E. hyperphosphatemia.

5. A 40-year-old male who has 25 g proteinuria per day owing to nephrotic syndrome presents with worsening of the edema. Serum creatinine is 1.3 mg/dl. Previous renal biopsy showed membranous nephropathy. He is at risk of which one of the following complications?
   A. Hypocalcemic tetany
   B. Congestive heart failure
   C. Rapidly progressive uremia
   D. Renal vein thrombosis
   E. Hypothyroidism

6. A patient with severe congestive heart failure will typically have all of the following except
   A. BUN 48 mg/dl, creatinine 1.5 mg/dl.
   B. urinary sodium concentration 8 mEq/liter.
   C. urine output 600 cc/day.
   D. fractional sodium excretion 2.5%.
   E. hyaline casts in the urinary sediment.

7. The acidosis of chronic renal failure is characterized by
   A. normal arterial PCO_2.
   B. low serum chloride concentration.
   C. increased renal production of ammonia.
   D. high urinary pH.
   E. decreased serum bicarbonate concentration.

8. Which finding is not typically present in tubulointerstitial nephropathy?
   A. Non-anion gap metabolic acidosis
   B. Decrease in glomerular filtration rate
   C. Increase in fractional excretion of sodium
   D. Decreased ability to concentrate the urine
   E. Proteinuria exceeding 3 g/24 hr

VIII Neurologic Diseases and Special Senses

Part Editor

Peggy J. Wisdom

59 Disorders of Consciousness and Cognition

Peggy J. Wisdom

Objectives

After completing this chapter, you should be able to

Understand the functions of the reticular activating system and cortical areas concerned with consciousness and cognition

Develop concepts of localization of lesions which result in disorders of consciousness

Develop concepts of localization of lesions which result in disorders of cognition

Develop concepts regarding diseases which result in disorders of consciousness and cognition

---

Consciousness and cognition are the result of complex linkages between the brainstem, thalamus, and cortex. These linkages allow the individual to arouse and attend to important stimuli, process and synthesize stimuli, and respond. Lesions in the components of this system, or lesions which disconnect the components of this system, result in disorders of consciousness, attention, or cognition.

Anatomy and Physiology Related to Consciousness and Cognition

The brain receives many stimuli from the external and internal environment but the individual responds to only those stimuli that are relevant. The neural mechanism which allows the individual to respond to only relevant stimuli consists of reciprocal linkages between the ascending reticular activating system (ARAS), the thalamus, and the cortex (Fig. 59-1).

Ascending Reticular Activating System

The ARAS is a system of neurons in the rostral pontine tegmentum and periventricular midbrain which project to the cortex through the hypothalamus and thalamus. The ARAS is activated by a sensory stimulus to mediate arousal. In the normal state, the ARAS influences shifting from sleep to wakefulness. Preceding wakefulness, ARAS neurons increase firing rate which is associated with desynchronization on the electroencephalogram (EEG) and behavioral evidence of arousal. Prior to sleep, ARAS neurons decrease rate of firing which is associated with slowing on the EEG and behavioral evidence of sleep. During wakefulness, the rate of firing of ARAS neurons varies, suggesting that the ARAS influences the degree of vigilance in the waking state. Destructive and compressive lesions which specifically involve the ARAS result in coma and confusion.

Thalamus

Thalamic nuclei relay information to and from the cortex.

Thalamic Nuclei

Those that relay information in a specific modality to and from a specific area of the cortex are the primary relay nuclei: ventroposterior lateral (VPL) and ventroposterior medial (VPM) nuclei link to parietal lobe to relay somatosensory information; lateral geniculate (LG) nucleus

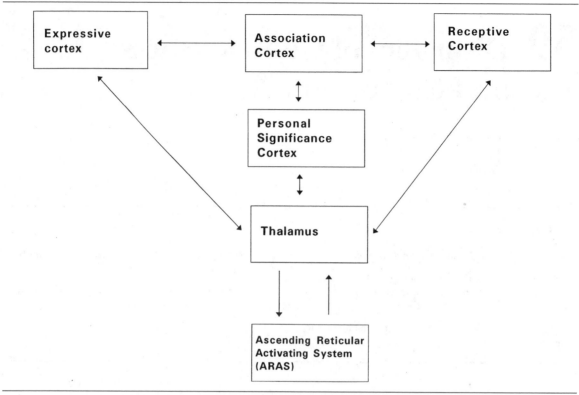

Fig. 59-1. Diagrammatic representation of the ARAS-thalamic-cortical system. The ARAS modulates arousal based on input from internal and external stimuli and cortical projections. The thalamus is a relay. The cortex provides synthesis; attachment of meaning and personal significance to the stimulus; and plans, organizes, and mediates a response.

links to occipital lobe to relay visual information; medial geniculate (MG) nucleus links to temporal lobe to relay auditory information; and ventral lateral (VL) nucleus links to the frontal lobe to relay motor information. Lesions involving modality-specific thalamic nuclei, like lesions in the cortical areas they reciprocate with, result in modality-specific impairments.

Reticular and Intralaminar Nuclei of Thalamus

These nuclei surround the primary thalamic relay nuclei. Unlike the primary thalamic relay nuclei, the reticular and intralaminar nuclei have diffuse projections to other thalamic nuclei and the reticular activating system.

Arousal and attention require interaction between the ARAS and the cortex. The thalamus serves to reciprocally relay information between the ARAS and the cortex. While modality-specific sensory information is relayed from the periphery to specific receptive areas of the cortex, via specific thalamic nuclei, the reticular nuclei of the thalamus plays a role in controlling input from these specific thalamic nuclei to the cortex. The thalamic reticular nuclei are modulated by the cortex and the ARAS to either inhibit or facilitate transmission of sensory information from the thalamus to the cortex.

Lesions of the thalamus that involve the reticular nuclei are associated with disorders of consciousness.

Cerebral Cortex

The cerebral cortex is divided into hemispheres which are subdivided into lobes which have specific functions (Fig. 59-2). The left hemisphere specializes in language functions and the right hemisphere specializes in visuospatial

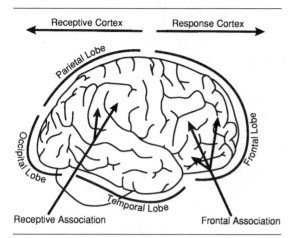

Fig. 59-2. Organization of the cerebral cortex. The cortex is organized in such a way that stimuli from the environment are transmitted to the lobes posterior to the Rolandic fissure. This receptive cortex is divided into the parietal lobe (which processes somatosensory information), the occipital lobe (which processes visual information), and the temporal lobe (which processes auditory information). The area anterior to the Rolandic fissure is the response cortex (frontal lobe) which receives information from the receptive cortex in order to plan, organize, and initiate a response to the stimulus.

The receptive and response cortex have association areas to inter-relate information received from the environment and to organize, plan, and initiate responses which are relevant to the individual.

and directed attentional functions. The cortex posterior to the Rolandic fissure receives information (receptive cortex) from the internal and external environment. The cortex anterior to the Rolandic fissure is concerned with output of information (response cortex).

Association Cortex

While a simple sensory input and response system would be suitable for an organism with one type of sensory receptor, the human has multiple types of sensory receptors which transmit information to the cortex. The association cortex serves to inter-relate information by receiving information from each primary receptive area as well as the limbic cortex. Association cortex has the ability to analyze stimuli from all receptive modes and access information stored in limbic structures to determine relevance based on past experience and motivation, thus allowing the individual to plan and initiate behavior in response to relevant stimuli.

Association cortex is located in the inferior parietal lobule which is strategically placed to receive sensory information from the somatosensory cortex, visual cortex, auditory cortex, and the limbic system. Association cortex is also located in the frontal lobe to mediate behavioral responses (Fig. 59-3). As determination of stimulus significance is a cortical phenomenon, the inferior parietal lobule and prefrontal lobe, particularly of the right hemisphere, function to enhance and maintain arousal and attention through linkage to the ascending reticular activating system when relevant stimuli are being processed (Fig. 59-4).

Lesions of the unimodal cortex result in the inability to receive and interpret unimodal information but preservation of the ability to receive and interpret information in other modalities. Word blindness (alexia), word deafness, and inability to recognize objects by touch (astereognosia) are examples. Lesions of the association cortex result in multimodal language disorders when the left hemisphere is involved, for example, Wernicke's aphasia which is characterized by the inability to interpret words that are written or presented auditorially. Lesions of the right hemisphere result in the neglect syndrome, which is characterized by multimodality inattention to left sided stimuli.

Specialized Anatomy of Left Hemisphere. Language functions are localized to the left hemisphere. This is true for 98% of right handers and 60% of left handers. In the left hemisphere receptive aspects of language are located posterior to the Rolandic fissure and expressive aspects of language are located anterior to the Rolandic fissure (Fig. 59-5). Heschl's gyrus (transverse superior temporal gyrus), Wernicke's area (posterior superior temporal gyrus), and Gerstmann's area (inferior parietal lobule) are the three prominent cortical areas of the left

Fig. 59-3. The association cortex of each hemisphere inter-relates information. The inferior parietal lobule inter-relates all receptive modalities and the prefrontal cortex inter-relates behavior responses.

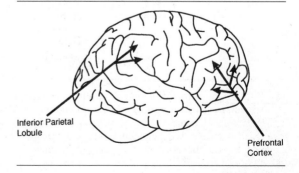

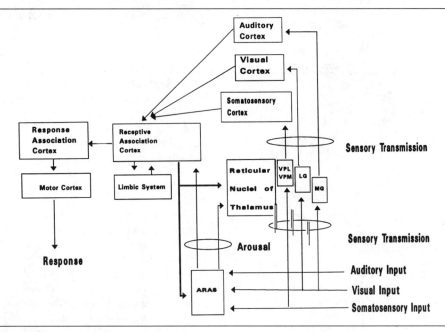

Fig. 59-4. ARAS-thalamic-cortical linkage for consciousness and cognition. The receptive cortex receives stimuli from the periphery via modality-specific thalamic nuclei (VPL, ventroposterior lateral; VPM, ventroposterior medial; LG, lateral geniculate; MG, medial geniculate). Arousal to a relevant stimulus is determined by the significance of the stimulus when processed by the receptive association and limbic cortices. This information in turn feeds back to the ARAS (ascending reticular activating system) to enhance arousal to that particular stimulus. Once a relevant stimulus is processed, a behavior response is planned, organized, and implemented by the response association and motor cortices. (Adapted from: Heilman KM, et al. Neglect and related disorders. *Seminars Neurol* 4:209–219, 1984.)

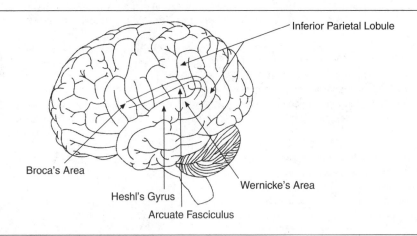

Fig. 59-5. Language representation of the left hemisphere. Heshl's gyrus and Wernicke's area receive auditory language information. The inferior parietal lobule in addition to Wernicke's area is important for determining the meaning of incoming language information. Once meaning/significance is determined, language information is conveyed to Broca's area via the arcuate fasciculus for encoding of language expression.

hemisphere concerned with analysis and processing of language information. Broca's area (inferior frontal operculum) is the prominent cortical area concerned with formulation and expression of language.

Specialized Anatomy of Right Hemisphere. The right hemisphere has traditionally been associated with spatial functions which include topographic localization, constructional capacity, and depth perception. However, the right hemisphere also specializes in regulation of attention. Lesions of association cortex of the right hemisphere (inferior parietal lobule and dorsolateral frontal lobe) are associated with the neglect syndrome. Association cortex of the right hemisphere detects stimuli which are relevant to the individual, directs analysis and responses of both hemispheres, and influences generalized arousal by feedback to the ARAS.

Disorders of Consciousness and Cognition

Disorders of Consciousness

Consciousness is defined as a state of wakefulness (arousal), awareness of self and environment (ability to perceive and interpret stimuli), and responsiveness. Disorders of consciousness are manifested by a spectrum of degrees of impairment in arousal and attention: coma, stupor, lethargy, alert, and hyperalert. Consciousness is comprised of an arousal component and a content component. The arousal component is mediated predominantly by the ARAS and the content component is mediated predominantly by the cerebral hemispheres. Both components are dependent upon the linkage between the ARAS, thalamus, and cerebral hemispheres for normal consciousness. If the arousal component is impaired, the individual will have impaired wakefulness which ranges from coma (the absence of wakefulness and meaningful response to a stimulus) to lethargy (sleepiness and inconsistent responses to a stimulus). In this circumstance, the individual cannot be aroused sufficiently to perceive a stimulus and therefore cannot respond. If the linkage between the ARAS-thalamus-cortex is involved, the individual will also have impaired arousal or attention. When there is impairment of attention, information from peripheral receptors is misinterpreted and responses are incorrectly planned and executed. This results in the presentation of confusion (encephalopathy).

There are three broad categories of pathophysiologic mechanisms which result in disorders of consciousness and attention:

Metabolic-Toxic Mechanisms

All neurons depend upon a continuous supply of substrates and a normal chemical environment to maintain functional integrity, maintain synaptic connections, and synthesize and release neurotransmitters. Any condition which depletes substrates or results in accumulation of endogenous or exogenous toxins disrupting the ARAS-thalamic-cortical neurons can impair consciousness. In general, metabolic and toxic mechanisms are reversed when substrates are repleted or toxins are removed as long as the degree of insult does not produce neuronal death.

Unlike other pathophysiologic mechanisms, metabolic and toxic insults are not associated with focal neurologic signs which localize lesions to one specific area of the brain. A patient who is comatose from a metabolic or toxic insult will have abnormal arousal implying neuronal dysfunction of the ARAS-thalamic-cortical system but the brainstem functions which can be evaluated are preserved (pupillary light responses, reflex extraocular movements, and blink reflexes to corneal stimulation).

Etiologies of coma related to metabolic and toxic insults can be broken down into four broad categories: (a) substrate depletion, (b) endogenous toxins, (c) exogenous toxins, and (d) fluid and electrolyte imbalance. Common examples of each are outlined in Table 59-1.

Destructive Mechanisms

Lesions which destroy neurons or connections of the ARAS-thalamic-cortical system will result in coma or confusional states. Unlike metabolic and toxic causes, destructive lesions are often associated with neurologic signs which localize the site of the destructive process and, in general, destructive lesions are irreversible.

As the ARAS-thalamic-cortical system that controls consciousness begins in the rostral brainstem and extends to the thalamus and cortex, destructive lesions can be localized by assessing pupil size, pupillary light reflex, reflex extraocular movements, and motor function.

Pupillary Signs of Destructive Lesions. Pupillary dilation is controlled by the sympathetics, and pupillary constriction is controlled by the parasympathetics. The sympathetics follow the descending sympathetic pathways from the hypothalamus to the gray matter of the thoracic cord. A destructive lesion along this pathway results in a small but reactive pupil. The parasympathetics originate in the oculomotor nuclear complex in the midbrain and follow the course of cranial nerve III. A destructive lesion will result in ipsilateral dilation and the pupillary light reflex will be slow or absent.

Table 59-1. Metabolic-Toxic Causes of Disorders of Arousal-Attention

SUBSTRATE DEPLETION

Hypoxia
Ischemia
Hypoglycemia
Cofactor depletion
    Thiamine
    Niacin
    Pyridoxine
    Cyanocobalamin

DISRUPTION OF INTERNAL MILIEU

Hypo- or hyperthermia
Fluid-electrolyte imbalance
    Hypo- or hypernatremia
    Hypo- or hyperosmolar state
    Hypercalcemia
    Hypomagnesemia
Endocrine abnormalities
    Hypo- or hyperthyroidism
    Hypo- or hypercortisolism
Seizures
    Partial complex status epilepticus
    Postictal state
Infection
    Meningitis
    Encephalitis

ENDOGENOUS TOXINS

Hepatic failure
Uremia
Hypercarbia
Acute intermittent porphyria
Sepsis
Intracranial hemorrhage
D-lactic acidosis

EXOGENOUS TOXINS

Medication overdosage or side effect
    Sedative drugs
    Tricyclic antidepressants
    Anticholinergic drugs
    Anticonvulsants
    Lithium
    Neuroleptics
    Salicylates
    Cardiac glycosides
    Cimetidine
Drugs of abuse
    Opiates
    Ethanol
    Amphetamines
    Phencyclidine

Table 59-1. (continued)

    LSD, mescaline
    Toluene
Nonmedicinal toxins
    Methyl alcohol
    Ethylene glycol
    Heavy metals
    Organic phosphates
    Cyanide

Used with permission from: Saper CB, Plum F. Disorders of consciousness. In Vinken PJ, Bruyn GW, Klawans HL, and Frederiks JAM (eds.). *Handbook of Clinical Neurology.* Vol. 45, Revised Series 1, Clinical Neuropsychology. Amsterdam: Elsevier, 1985, p. 122.

Reflex Extraocular Movement Signs of Destructive Lesions. The paramedian pontine reticular formation (PPRF) of the pons coordinates conjugate lateral eye movement to the ipsilateral side through connections with the ipsilateral cranial nerve VI and contralateral cranial nerve III. A lesion of one PPRF will result in the inability to move the eyes to the ipsilateral side with passive movement of the head (oculocephalic reflexes) or vestibular stimulation (oculovestibular reflexes). Bilateral involvement of the PPRF will result in the inability to move both eyes to either side.

The midbrain is the site of the nucleus and origin of fibers of cranial nerve III. Cranial nerve III innervates the medial rectus in addition to vertical eye muscles. Lesions which involve cranial nerve III result in inability to adduct the eye medially by oculocephalic or oculovestibular reflexes.

Lesions which disconnect the frontal eye fields from the brainstem PPRF will result in conjugate eye deviation to the side of the lesion. Like all upper motor neuron lesions, reflex movements will be intact (oculocephalic and oculovestibular reflexes).

Motor Signs in Destructive Lesions. While a hemiparesis is noted contralateral to destructive lesions which involve the motor pathways, two patterns of reflex motor response can be seen: decorticate rigidity and decerebrate rigidity. Decorticate rigidity is characterized by flexion of the upper extremities and extension of the lower extremities. This form of rigidity is seen with lesions which disconnect the cortex from the diencephalon and is most often seen with lesions of the frontal lobe and thalamus. Decerebrate rigidity is characterized by extension of the upper extremities and lower extremities. This form of rigidity is seen with lesions which disconnect the cerebrum from the brainstem (midbrain and pons).

Table 59-2 outlines the pattern of neurologic impairments associated with destructive lesions of the brainstem, thalamus, and cortex.

Compressive Mechanism

Mass lesions of the cerebrum can compress or distort brain tissue and arteries, resulting in shifting or herniation of brain tissue from one compartment to another. Herniation results in necrosis or ischemia of brain tissue distant from the site of the mass. When necrosis and ischemia involve the ARAS-thalamic-cortical system, coma results.

Herniation syndromes are important to recognize as early therapy can prevent irreversible tissue necrosis and ischemia. Four herniation syndromes are recognized: cingulate herniation, central herniation, uncal herniation, and tonsillar herniation. Anatomy and clinical characteristics are depicted and outlined in Fig. 59-6.

Disorders of Language

Aphasia is a disturbance of one or more aspects of the complex process of comprehending and formulating word messages and is the result of lesions which involve language areas of the left hemisphere. An aphasia must be distinguished from nonlinguistic disorders of speech. For example, weakness or incoordination of muscles that control vocalization result in disturbances of articulation (dysarthria). Signs of aphasia include disturbances of comprehension or expression of spoken and written language and disturbances of repetition. By evaluating these parameters, the clinician can localize lesions within the left hemisphere which result in aphasia.

Localization Rules of Aphasia

Three rules can be used in localization of lesions causing aphasia.

Anterior-Posterior Rule. Lesions anterior to the Rolandic fissure result in nonfluent aphasias and lesions posterior to the Rolandic fissure result in fluent aphasias. Nonfluent aphasias are characterized by effortful and sparse output and short or incomplete phrases (output is like a telegraphic message). Fluent aphasias are characterized by normal effort and increased rate and phrase length.

Perisylvian Rule. Lesions which involve the perisylvian area result in repetition disturbances.

Posterior Hemisphere Rule. Lesions which involve the area posterior to the Rolandic fissure result in disturbances of comprehension of spoken and/or written language.

Table 59-3 outlines the characteristics of common aphasias.

Types of Lesions Associated with Aphasia

Aphasias are the result of focal lesions of the left hemisphere. Disease states which result in focal lesions of the left hemisphere include cerebrovascular disease, neoplastic disease, traumatic diseases, and some infections. The most common cause of aphasia is cerebrovascular disease. As most of the language areas are located in the lateral aspect of the left hemisphere, cerebrovascular disease which involves the distribution of left middle cerebral artery is often to be associated with aphasia.

Disorders of Directed Attention

The neglect syndrome may result from right hemisphere lesions. The neglect syndrome is characterized by the inability to orient, report, or respond to a stimulus in the left hemispace. Patients behave as though the left personal and extrapersonal space is nonexistent. For example, the patient will fail to groom the left side of the body, fail to read the left half of a sentence, or fail to eat food on the left side of a plate.

Like aphasia, neglect syndrome is associated with dis-

Table 59-2. Localization of Destructive Lesions Producing Coma

Lesion Site	Pupil Size	Pupillary Light Reflex	Reflex Extraocular Movement	Motor Pattern
Cortex	Normal	Intact	Intact	Decorticate rigidity
Thalamus	Small	Intact	Intact	Decorticate rigidity
Midbrain	Dilated	Nonreactive	Cranial nerve III paralysis	Decerebrate rigidity
Pons	Pinpoint	Intact	Paralysis of lateral eye movements	Decerebrate rigidity

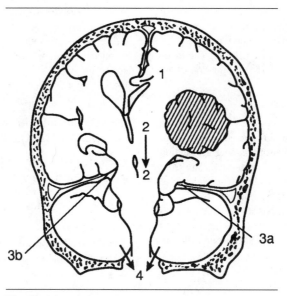

Fig. 59-6. Herniation syndromes are depicted in the figure with clinical characteristics described in the table. (Adapted from: Plum F and Posner JB (eds.). *Diagnosis of Stupor and Coma.* Philadelphia: Davis, 1972.)

Herniation Syndromes

Mass Locations	Structures Involved	Pupil	Reflex Extraocular Movement	Motor
Cingulate supratentorial (1)	Cingulate gyrus herniates under falx	Intact	Intact	Contralateral followed by ipsilateral leg paralysis
Central supratentorial (2)	Diencephalon, herniates the tentorium	Pupils dilated and nonreactive	Bilateral cranial nerve III paralysis	Decorticate rigidity
Uncal supratentorial (3)	Uncus of mesial temporal lobe herniates through tentorium	Pupil ipsilateral is dilated and nonreactive	Ipsilateral cranial nerve III paralysis	(3a) Contralateral decerebration if uncus compresses ipsilateral peduncle (3b) Ipsilateral decerbration if contralateral peduncle is compressed
Tonsillar subtentorial (4)	Cerebellar tonsils herniate through foramen magnum	Pinpoint and reactive pupils	Paralysis lateral eye movements	Decerebrate rigidity followed by flaccidity

ease states which produce focal lesions. As the inferior parietal lobule and dorsolateral frontal cortex are on the lateral aspect of the hemisphere, cerebrovascular disease which involves the distribution of the right middle cerebral artery is likely to be associated with the neglect syndrome.

Dementia

Dementia is a disorder characterized by the acquired loss of intellectual function which is of sufficient severity to interfere with the individual's social and vocational functions. Diagnostic criteria for dementia include the presence

Table 59-3. Clinical Characteristics of Language Disorders

	Fluency of Language	Repetition of Phrases	Comprehension of Language	Lesion Site
Broca's aphasia	Nonfluent	Impaired	Intact	Perisylvian aspect of the frontal lobe
Conduction aphasia	Fluent	Impaired	Intact	Supramarginal gyrus and arcuate fasciculus
Wernicke's aphasia	Fluent	Impaired	Impaired	Perisylvian aspect of the superior temporal lobe
Transcortical motor aphasia	Nonfluent	Intact	Intact	Frontal lobe
Transcortical sensory aphasia	Fluent	Intact	Impaired	Angular gyrus

of clear consciousness, memory loss, and cognitive and behavioral impairments. Cognitive impairments can include impairment in executive function (planning, organization, problem solving) and impairment in language or spatial/perceptual skills. Behavioral impairments range from apathy to impulsivity. Dementia is therefore not an isolated loss of cognitive function which can be localized to one area such as an aphasia, neglect syndrome, or amnesia. Dementia is the result of diffuse or multifocal lesions involving the cerebral hemispheres.

There are many diseases that can either produce dementia as an isolated syndrome or dementia as one of the clinical manifestations of the disease (Table 59-4). Clues to the etiology of dementia are found in the mode of onset, the rate of progression, and the pattern of symptom development. The patient's past history (which may extend back to the perinatal period) will provide clues to the patient's risk for dementia. A careful history and exam should include a search for symptoms and signs to consider a broad range of pathophysiologic categories as dementia can be associated with virtually all of them, as outlined in Table 59-4. Most common causes of dementia will fall in the degenerative category, with Alzheimer's disease being the most common. However, without a conscientious history and examination, treatable and potentially reversible causes may not be recognized.

Alzheimer's Disease

Alzheimer's disease is a cortical dementia which involves cortical structures concerned with cognition and spares sensorimotor and special sensory cortex. The disease is the most common single entity causing dementia, accounting for 40% of the causes in combined reports. The annual in-

Table 59-4. Etiologies of Dementia

CORTICAL DEMENTIAS (MANIFEST BY PREDOMINANTLY COGNITIVE OR BEHAVIORAL IMPAIRMENTS
Degenerative
    Alzheimer's disease
    Pick's disease
SUBCORTICAL DEMENTIAS (ASSOCIATED WITH EXTRAPYRAMIDAL, MOTOR, AND CEREBELLAR IMPAIRMENTS)
Degenerative
    Huntington's disease
    Parkinson's disease
    Progressive supranuclear palsy
Demyelinating disease
Hydrocephalus
Infections
    Creutzfeldt Jacob disease
    HIV and HIV-related infections
    Syphilis
Metabolic
    Post-anoxia
    Endocrinopathies
    Neuronal storage disease
    Vitamin deficiencies
    Wilson's disease
Neoplasia
    Primary brain tumors
    Metastatic brain tumors
    Meningeal carcinomatosis
Toxins
    Alcohol
    Carbon monoxide
    Heavy metal poisoning
    Polysubstance abuse
Vascular

cidence is 1.4%; however the prevalence increases with age, with 22% of the population past 80 years effected.

Clinical Features. Clinically, the disease is characterized by insidious and progressive intellectual disorientation. The pattern of clinical progression provides a clue to the diagnosis. Typically, the onset of the disease is tied to progressive memory loss which, while most prominently involving the acquisition of new memory, also effects remote or past memory. Visuospatial disturbances (such as spatial disorientation) and getting lost and language impairment (which resembles a transcortical sensory aphasia) are often identifiable by the second year. Personality changes which significantly impact function (apathy, paranoia, disturbances of affect) follow the onset of memory, language, and visuospatial disturbances. Late in the course of the disease, motor disturbances are noted.

Pathology. Neuropathologically, there is atrophy most prominent in the temporal, inferior parietal, and prefrontal cortex. Histologically, neuronal loss is prominent not only in cortical areas, which are grossly involved, but also subcortical neurons, particularly nuclear basalis of Meynert and septal nuclei which are cholinergic. Senile (neuritic) plaques (degenerating nerve terminals around a core of amyloid protein) and neurofibrillary tangles (neurons filled with paired helical filaments) are noted in the cortex.

The observation of significant neuronal loss in cholinergic neurons has led to the investigation of pharmacologic treatment of Alzheimer's disease with cholinergic agonists (lecithin, physostigmine, tetrahydroaminoacridine). The results of investigation into the efficacy of drug therapy have been generally disappointing.

With the identification of amyloid deposition in senile plaques and cerebral vessels, research efforts are now focused on the association of amyloid deposition and Alzheimer's disease. While some cases are familial and have been associated with chromosome 14 or 19, the etiology remains uncertain and may be related to multiple factors.

Management. Management of Alzheimer's disease remains problematic. Symptoms such as disturbances of affect, sleep disturbance, and agitation may be managed with psychopharmaceuticals. However, little can be done to enhance memory, language, and visuospatial skills lost by the disease. Avoidance of excessive sedation and anticholinergic drugs, close monitoring to prevent or treat intercurrent illness, and family education on care and behavioral management are the most important aspects of care.

Clinical Examples

1. A 64-year-old male with longstanding hypertension presented with the sudden onset of weakness of the right limbs and difficulty communicating. On examination, his blood pressure was 190/110. He was awake and attentive to the examiner, but unable to formulate words and sentences. He could not repeat the phrase, "The President lives in Washington." His comprehension assessed by his ability to follow a three-part command was intact. His right lower face drooped. He was unable to move his arm, and his leg was weak, but he could move it on command. A right Babinski sign was noted.

He was admitted with the diagnosis of a stroke. His blood pressure was treated with oral agents but remained severely elevated and labile. Over the first 6 hours after admission, he gradually became sleepy, then hard to arouse. When he was reexamined, several new findings were noted. His pupils were small and briskly reactive. While his gaze was fixed to the left, oculocephalic reflexes were noted to be intact. On painful stimulation, decortication was noted on the right. A Babinski sign was now present on the left.

Discussion. The patient presented with a right hemiparesis and a nonfluent aphasia. Given the anterior-posterior rule of aphasia, the lesion is anterior to the Rolandic fissure encompassing the inferior frontal operculum (to explain the aphasia) and the motor strip on the left (to explain the hemiparesis).

The sudden onset of neurologic impairments suggest cerebrovascular disease. Based on the history of hypertension and the course of rapid deterioration, an intracerebral hematoma with mass effect is most likely.

The development of an arousal disorder certainly suggests the presence of a compressive lesion. Based on the finding of a left Babinski sign on the later exam, cingulate herniation is suggested. A CT scan would be indicated to confirm a left-to-right shift of midline structures under the falx in support of the diagnosis.

Evacuation of the hematoma would reduce the volume inside the cranial cavity. Medical measures such as administration of hyperosmolar Mannitol and hyperventilation through assisted ventilation would be employed to reduce the intracranial pressure and decrease volume in the cranial cavity until surgical evacuation of the hematoma was completed.

2. A 70-year-old woman was brought to the hospital following the sudden onset of coma. Coma was preceded by a

2-week history of brief episodes of double vision, slurred speech, and generalized weakness. There was no past history of medical illness. On examination, she was comatose with no eye opening to any type of stimulation. Pupils were pinpoint and reactive. Oculocephalic and oculovestibular maneuvers elicited no eye movement to either side. She demonstrated decerebrate posturing with painful stimulation.

Discussion.   The history of diplopia, dysarthria, and ataxia suggest a lesion in the posterior fossa, and the findings of pinpoint pupils, ophthalmoplegia (paralysis of lateral eye movement), and decerebration indicate that the lesion is in the pons.

The finding on neurologic exam and the rapidity of onset suggest a destructive lesion of the pons. The transient symptoms which preceded the coma suggest transient ischemia in the distribution of the basilar artery. This is a strong clue to the ischemic nature of this stroke.

If this had been a compressive lesion, the symptoms would have been subtle at first and progressive over time.

3. A 64-year-old man was brought in by his family for evaluation of memory loss. For 2 years he had been forgetful, but over the past 6 months memory loss had worsened. Recently, he had started a fire in the kitchen after he left pots cooking on the stove overnight. He got lost for 2 days on his way to his daughter's home 20 miles from his home, and his home had been burglarized several times as he left without locking up. The family noted his communication skills were poor as he didn't seem to understand instructions and frequently misnamed things.

He had been in good health except for hypertension, which was easily controlled. His mother died at age 70 of senility in a nursing home. His father died at age 40 of a heart attack. He had no headaches, loss of vision, weakness, numbness, or poor coordination.

Physical examination revealed a blood pressure of 150/90, pulse 80, temperature 37°C. He had no carotid bruits. Cardiac exam revealed no murmurs. The remainder of the general medical exam was normal.

The patient was unable to give the date and did not recall a list of words after 5 minutes. He was not able to follow simple verbal or written requests and used incorrect names of objects. He was unable to draw or copy geometric structures. The patient's gait was normal. Strength and muscle stretch reflexes were normal. There were no Babinski signs. Coordination was intact. Sensory exam was not reliable.

Discussion.   The patient has memory loss which localizes to the limbic system, geographic localization and constructional apraxia impairments which localize to the right temporal lobe, and auditory and written comprehension impairments which localize to the left posterior temporal lobe. Progressive cognitive symptoms and signs which localize to bilateral inferior parietal and temporal cortex suggest Alzheimer's disease.

A brain biopsy which demonstrated neuronal loss with senile plaques and neurofibrillary tangles would confirm a diagnosis of Alzheimer's disease. However, this is not appropriate because the risks of biopsy outweigh the benefit of absolute confirmation of diagnosis.

A reasonable evaluation in this patient would be undertaken to exclude conditions which could mimic Alzheimer's disease. These include multiple strokes or metastatic disease which spare the motor/sensory cortex. Magnetic resonance imaging with a contrast agent would exclude strokes and neoplastic disease.

Bibliography

Cummings JL and Benson DF (eds.). *Dementia: A Clinical Approach.* Boston: Butterworths, 1983. *A comprehensive review of the clinical features of dementia and the broad categories of diseases which are commonly associated with dementia.*

Heilman KM. Neglect and related disorders. In Heilman KM and Valensteen E (eds.). *Clinical Neuropsychology.* New York: Oxford University Press, 1979, pp. 268–307. *A discussion of the clinical features and mechanisms underlying the neglect syndrome.*

Mesalam MM (ed.). *Principles of Behavioral Neurology.* Philadelphia: FA Davis, 1985. *A comprehensive review of neuroanatomy of consciousness and cognition and description of disorders of consciousness and cognition.*

Saper CB and Plum F. Disorders of consciousness. In Vinken PJ, Bruyn GW, Klawans HL, and Frederiks JAM (eds.). *Handbook of Clinical Neurology.* Volume 45: Revised Series 1, Clinical Neuropsychology. Amsterdam: Elsevier, 1985, pp. 109–122. *A comprehensive review of the pathophysiology of disorders of consciousness.*

60 The Motor System

Farhat Husain and Julie T. Parke

Objectives

After completing this chapter, you should be able to

Understand the anatomy of the upper and lower motor neuron systems

Understand the principles of localization of lesions of the motor system

Understand the concepts of localization of lesions involving the upper motor neurons

Understand the concepts of localization of lesions which involve the lower motor unit: anterior horn cell, ventral root, peripheral nerve, neuromuscular junction, and muscle

Develop concepts regarding the diseases which involve the motor system

Movement is a very complex function which requires dynamic interaction between the somatosensory, special sensory, extrapyramidal, and motor systems. Movement is organized in a hierarchial manner: reflex movement is controlled at the spinal level (withdrawal to a pain stimulus); stereotyped movement is controlled by neural networks in the diencephalon, brainstem, and spinal cord (walking); and goal-directed movement is initiated by the motor cortex in response to a stimulus (articulating a response to a question). The higher levels influence the lower levels to adjust the function of the lower levels. The motor system is the final pathway for movement and its action reflects the integrated activities of these other systems.

Anatomy and Physiology of Motor System

The motor system has two divisions: the upper motor neuron (which is comprised of the sensorimotor cortex and corticospinal and corticobulbar tracts) and the lower motor unit (which is comprised of the lower motor neuron, neuromuscular junction, and muscle).

Upper Motor Neuron

Sensorimotor Cortex, Corticospinal Tract, and Corticobulbar Tract

The sensorimotor cortex gives rise to the pyramidal system, which includes the corticospinal and corticobulbar tracts. The majority of fibers originate from the precentral gyrus of the frontal lobe (the motor cortex) and terminate in the ventral horn of the spinal cord. These are concerned with voluntary motor control. Some fibers originate from the parietal lobe and terminate in the dorsal horn. These are concerned more with modulation of movement.

The corticospinal tract descends ipsilaterally through the internal capsule, the cerebral peduncle of the midbrain, and the basis pontis to the medulla. At the level of the cervicomedullary junction, the majority of the corticospinal fibers decussate to form the lateral corticospinal tract, which descends now contralaterally to synapse on the appropriate motor neuron pool in the ventral horn. While about 10% of the corticospinal tract fibers remain ipsilateral to form the ventral corticospinal tract, the majority of these fibers finally decussate contralaterally at the level of the appropriate motor neuron pool.

Corticobulbar fibers are those fibers which innervate the face, tongue, pharynx, and larynx. These axons originate in the lateral aspect of the frontal and parietal lobes and descend ipsilaterally along with corticospinal fibers. However, they will synapse on motor neurons of the appropriate cranial nerve in the brainstem. Corticobulbar fibers are directed toward ipsilateral as well as contralateral motor neurons of the cranial nerves. So in essence there is bilateral innervation. The only exception is the facial expression, where corticobulbar fibers directed towards motor neurons which supply musculature to the lower face originate mainly from the contralateral hemisphere. This is why a unilateral corticobulbar lesion results only in weakness of the contralateral lower face, which is designated as a central seventh paralysis.

The cerebral cortex and the corticospinal tract fibers are somatotopically organized (Fig. 60-1). A lesion of the cerebral hemisphere which involves the frontal cortex or the posterior limb of the internal capsule will result in weakness of the contralateral limbs and contralateral lower face as will a lesion of one cerebral peduncle or one side of the basis pontis (if the lesion is above the facial nucleus at the pontomedullary junction). However, a lesion of the lateral corticospinal tract in the spinal cord will result in weakness of the ipsilateral arm and leg if the lesion is in the cervical cord and ipsilateral weakness of the leg if the lesion is in the thoracic cord. The face will not be affected, as corticobulbar fibers only descend to the level of the brainstem.

Associated Pathways

The pathways that are important for modulation of movement are the vestibulospinal tract (which arises from the vestibular nuclei), reticulospinal tract (which arises from the reticular formation of the brainstem), tectospinal tract (which arises from the tectum of the midbrain), rubrospinal tract (which arises from the red nucleus), and aminergic system (which arises from the locus ceruleus and median raphe nuclei). These pathways originate in the brainstem and descend in the lateral and ventral columns of the spinal cord. Little is known about the physiology of these pathways; however, they modulate movement.

Lower Motor Neuron

The lower motor neuron is part of the lower motor unit which is comprised of the motor neuron and its axon, neuromuscular junction, and muscle (Fig. 60-2). Each pool of motor neurons innervates a specific myotome (the group of muscles innervated by a pool of motor neurons).

Motor Neuron

The motor neurons are located in the ventral horn (anterior horn) of the spinal cord and cranial nuclei of the brainstem. In the spinal cord, the motor neurons in the cervical cord innervate muscles of the arms, motor neurons in thoracic cord innervate muscles in the chest and abdomen, and motor neurons in the lumbar cord innervate the legs. In the brainstem, motor neurons in the midbrain innervate extraocular muscles (cranial nerves III and IV). In the pons muscles of mastication (cranial nerve V), at the pontomedullary junction muscles of facial expression (cranial nerve VII) and extraocular movement (cranial nerve VI), and in the medulla muscles of swallowing and talking (cranial nerves IX, X, XII) and neck and shoulder movement (cranial nerve XI) all have pools of motor neurons.

Lesions involving any motor neuron pool will result in the loss of ability to move the muscles of the ipsilateral myotome. Therefore, motor neuron lesions in either the spinal cord or brainstem result in ipsilateral weakness.

Axon of the Motor Neuron

The axon of a motor neuron is a large-diameter myelinated structure which innervates the muscle. Its proximal segment is designated as the ventral root and the distal segment is designated as the nerve.

The Root.   The nerve root exits the spinal cord and courses ipsilaterally to the intervertebral foramen, where it exits. Motor roots exit ventrally and sensory roots enter dorsally. The ventral roots exit between two vertebra of the corresponding level. Therefore lesions which involve the ventral root will result in ipsilateral weakness of the myotome effected by the nerve root.

In the brainstem, the proximal motor axon is termed the fasciculus while it courses through the brainstem until it exits in a ventro-median position as the cranial nerve. Consequently, lesions which involve the medial brainstem will generally result in ipsilateral paralysis of the muscles innervated by a motor cranial nerve and contralateral hemiparesis from medial placed corticospinal fibers (syndrome of crossed plegia). The exception is cranial nerve IV, which exits at the pontomesencephalic junction dorsally and is crossed.

The Nerve.   The distal axons group together to form the motor component of peripheral nerves which usually contain both sensory and motor fibers. As such, most lesions which involve a nerve will result in both sensory loss and weakness. Table 60-1 outlines the characteristics of important nerves.

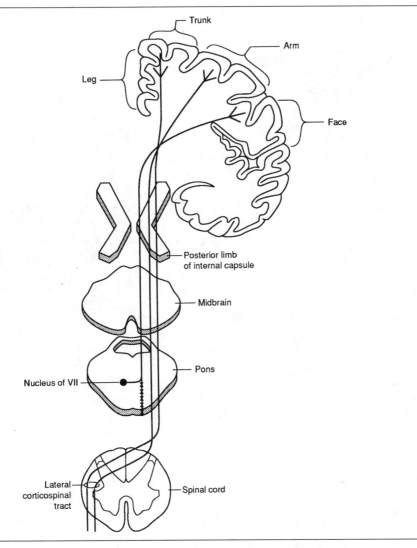

Fig. 60-1. Somatotopic organization of the cortex and corticospinal and corticobulbar tracts. In the frontal cortex neurons whose axons will synapse on motor neurons which supply the face and head are located in the lateral aspect of the hemisphere near the Sylvian fissure and descend via corticobulbar fibers to the genu (knee) of the posterior limb of the internal capsule, the medial aspect of the cerebral peduncle, the medial aspect of the basis pontis, and the medial aspect of the medullary pyramid. Fibers innervate the motor neuron pools at the appropriate brainstem level. Neurons which control movement of the hand and arm are located in the superior aspect of the lateral hemisphere and descend via corticospinal tract to the internal capsule (posterior to the genu) and then descend in the medial cerebral peduncle, basis pontis, and pyramid. After they decussate in the cervicomedullary junction, they assume a medial position in the cervical cord until they innervate the appropriate motor neuron pool. Analogous neurons for the leg are located in the medial aspect of the hemisphere and descend in the corticospinal tract posterior to the arm fibers in the internal capsule and then assume a lateral position in the cerebral peduncle, basis pontis, and pyramid. After these fibers decussate, they assume a lateral position in the lateral corticospinal tract. (Redrawn from: Netter FH in collaboration with Peterson BW. Physiology and functional neuroanatomy. In Brass A and Dingle RV (eds.). *The CIBA Collection of Medical Illustrations.* Vol. 1, Part l, Sec. 3, p. 197, Plate No. 44. CIBA Pharmaceutical Company, 1983.)

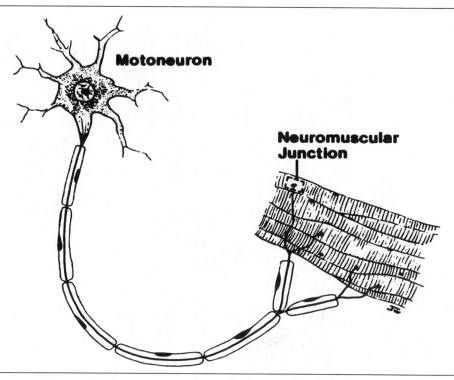

Fig. 60-2. The motor unit. It consists of the motor neuron, its axon, and the population of muscle fibers that it innervates. (Used with permission from: Maclean IC. Neuromuscular junction. In Johnson EW (ed.). *Practical Electromyography* (4th ed.). Baltimore/London: Williams and Wilkins, 1980, pp. 73–90.)

Table 60-1. Characteristics of Selected Nerves

Motor Neuron Pool and Root	Nerve	Muscles Innervated
C5	Dorsal scapular	Rhomboid
C5–6	Suprascapular	Supra and infraspinatus
	Axillary	Deltoid
	Musculocutaneous	Biceps
	Radial	Brachioradialis
C6–7	Radial (triceps branch)	Triceps
C6–7–8	Radial	Extensor carpi radialis and extensor indices
C8–T1	Ulnar	Dorsal interossei (first dorsal interosseus, abductor digiti quinti)
	Median	Thenar muscles (abductor pollicis brevis, opponens)
L2–3–4	Femoral	Quadriceps
L4–5–S1	Sciatic	Hamstrings
	Peroneal	Foot dorsiflexors (tibialis anterior, peroneus longus and brevis)
	Posterior tibial	Foot extensors (gastrocnemius and posterior tibial)

Neuromuscular Junction

The neuromuscular junction consists of the terminal portion of the motor nerve, the synaptic cleft, and the end-plate region of the muscle. The nerve action potential originates in the motor neuron of the spinal cord and is propagated down the axon of the motor nerve. When the terminal portion of the nerve is depolarized, calcium channels are opened, causing the release of acetylcholine into the synaptic cleft.

Synthesis and Release of Acetylcholine

Synthesis of acetylcholine occurs in the nerve terminal from acetyl coenzyme A and choline. It is then packaged in small vesicles. When the action potential reaches the terminal filaments of the axon, vesicles (quanta) of acetylcholine are released by exocytosis from sites in the presynaptic region at the axon terminal. Release of the vesicles into the synaptic cleft allows the acetylcholine molecules to interact with the acetylcholine receptors on the muscle end-plate, causing localized depolarization of the end-plate. Spontaneously released vesicles induce localized end-plate depolarization. However, when a nerve action potential reaches the presynaptic area, 100 to 200 vesicles are released simultaneously. The summation of the depolarization potentials reaches the threshold potential for the excitable muscle membrane, and a muscle action potential is generated (Fig. 60-3).

Excitation-Contraction Coupling

When the threshold potential is achieved, a muscle action potential is generated which is propagated along the muscle plasma membrane and into the interior of the muscle fiber by the T tubules, formed by minute invaginations of the muscle membrane. The spreading depolarization causes the release of calcium from the sarcoplasmic reticulum into the intracellular space of the muscle fiber, which contains the actin and myosin filaments. In the presence of calcium, cross-bridges form between the thick (myosin) and thin (actin) filaments. Repetitive attachment and detachment of the cross-bridges causes muscle contraction. Acetylcholine acts at the postsynaptic membrane for only a brief period before it is broken down by an enzyme, acetylcholinesterase, into two inactive components, choline and acetic acid. The choline is taken up by the presynaptic nerve terminal, where choline acetyltransferase catalyzes the resynthesis of acetylcholine.

Muscle

Skeletal muscle is composed of elongated, multinucleated cells arranged in fascicles. The fibers range in diameter

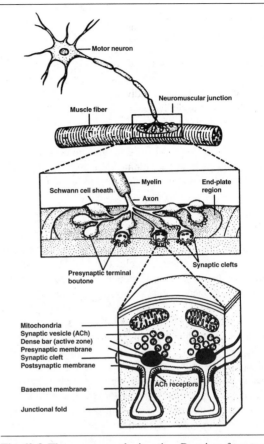

Fig. 60-3. The neuromuscular junction. Drawings from top to bottom show progressive enlargements of segments of a neuromuscular junction. The presynaptic terminals consist of multiple swellings or varicosities called synaptic boutons or terminals covered by a thin layer of Schwann cells. The boutons are separated from the postsynaptic cell by the synaptic cleft, which is about 50 nm wide. Directly apposed to the motor neuron terminals is the end-plate, a specialized region of the muscle fiber membrane. Junctional folds in the end-plate contain a high density of ACh receptors. Lying over the muscle fiber is a layer of connective tissue called the basement membrane (basal lamina), which contains acetylcholinesterase, the enzyme that breaks down ACh. Each presynaptic bouton contains mitochondria and synaptic vesicles clustered around dense bars or active zones that are the site of release of the ACh transmitter. (Adapted in part from McMahan UH and Kuffler SW. Visual identification of synaptic boutons on living ganglion cells. *Proc R Soc Lond* (Biol) 177:485–508, 1971. From: Kandel ER and Siegelbaum SA. Directly gated transmission at the nerve-muscle synapse. In Kandel ER, Schwartz JH, and Jessell TM (eds.). *Principles of Neural Science* (3rd ed.). Norwalk, CT: Appleton & Lange, 1991, p. 136. With permission.)

from 30 to 90 microns in the adult, with an average diameter of about 60 microns. The muscle fiber is enclosed in a cell membrane, or sarcolemma. The nuclei are peripheral in location, just under the sarcolemma. The cytoplasm (sarcoplasm) of the muscle cell contains myofibrils, which are composed of longitudinally oriented, interdigitating filaments of contractile proteins.

Within any muscle, there are metabolic and physiologic differences between fibers. All muscle fibers in the same motor unit have the same histochemical properties. The muscle fibers belonging to a motor unit are widely distributed within each muscle. Individual muscles contain different proportions of different motor unit types.

Disorders of Motor System

The key symptom and sign of disorders of motor system is weakness whether the lesion involves the upper motor neuron or the lower motor neuron, neuromuscular junction or muscle. If there is total paralysis, the term "plegia" is used, and if there is weakness, the term "paresis" is used. In the evaluation of persons with disorders of the motor system, it is first important to establish the localization of the lesion before one can develop a hypothesis about the pathophysiologic mechanism to explain the cause of the weakness. Table 60-2 outlines the clinical characteristics of upper motor neuron, lower motor neuron, neuromuscular junction, and muscle lesions. In general, upper motor neuron lesion patterns of weakness localize to the cerebral cortex or corticospinal or corticobulbar tracts. Unlike patterns of weakness in lower motor unit lesions, the weakness involves all of the muscles of one or more limbs (hemiparesis involves the arm and leg on the same side, monoparesis involves one limb, paraparesis involves both lower limbs, quadriparesis involves all four limbs). Since lesions of the upper motor neuron result in loss of descending influence or control of the lower motor neuron, there is associated hyperreflexia, clonus, and spasticity in the distribution of the upper motor neuron lesion and an extensor plantar response. The extensor toe sign (extensor plantar response) is the most reliable sign of an upper motor neuron lesion, which is characterized by extension of the great toe when a stimulus is applied to the dermatome of the first sacral segment (S_1). When the great toe extends when the lateral aspect of the sole is stroked, it is designated as the Babinski sign. Localization of lesions involving the upper motor neuron is detailed in Table 60-3.

In general, lower motor neuron lesions result in patterns of weakness that represent the distribution of a motor neuron(s), a motor root(s), or a peripheral nerve(s). Since the lesion involves the final common pathway for movement and interrupts the motor output of the monosynaptic reflex Fig. 60-4), there is associated hyporeflexia and atrophy because the muscle which is innervated by the motor neuron pool, root, or nerve is now denervated.

Disorders Involving Upper Motor Neuron

Generalized Upper Motor Neuron Disorders
There are a few diseases which can diffusely involve the upper motor neuron system. The most common is amyotrophic lateral sclerosis, which is discussed in more detail under disorders of the motor neuron.

Focal Upper Motor Neuron Disorders
All diseases which result in focal lesions can involve the upper motor neuron if the lesion involves the sensorimotor cortex, the corticospinal tract, or the corticobulbar tract. These include cerebrovascular (ischemic or focal hemor-

Table 60-2. Clinical Manifestations of Motor System Disorders

Type of Lesion	Pattern of Weakness	Muscle Stretch Reflex	Babinski Sign Response	Atrophy	Tone
Upper motor neuron	Hemiparesis	↑	+	−	Spasticity
	Monoparesis	↑	+	−	Spasticity
	Paraparesis	↑	+	−	Spasticity
	Quadriparesis	↑	+	−	Spasticity
Lower motor neuron					
Motor neuron	Segmental	↓	−	+	Hypotonia
Root	Segmental	↓	−	+	Hypotonia
Nerve	Multiple segments	↓	−	+	Hypotonia
Neuromuscular junction	Proximal	N	−	−	Normal
Muscle	Proximal	↓ (Late)	−	+	Normal

Table 60-3. Localization of Upper Motor Neuron Lesions by Pattern of Motor Signs

Pattern of Upper Motor Neuron Involvement	Localization of Lesion
HEMIPARESIS	
With central VII	Cerebral hemisphere
	Lesion contralateral in sensorimotor cortex
	Lesion contralateral in internal capsule
	Brainstem
	Lesion contralateral in cerebral peduncle
	Lesion contralateral in basis pontis
Crossed plegia	Brainstem
Ipsilateral III, contralateral hemiparesis	Lesion ipsilateral to cranial nerve III in midbrain
Ipsilateral VI, VII, contralateral hemiparesis	Lesion ipsilateral to cranial nerve VI or VII in pons
Ipsilateral XII, contralateral hemiparesis	Lesion ipsilateral to cranial nerve XII in medulla
Without central VII	Brainstem
	Lesion contralateral in medulla (above the decussation)
	Spinal cord
	Lesion ipsilateral in cervical cord
QUADRIPARESIS	
Bilateral corticobulbar involvement (pseudobulbar palsy)	Cerebral hemisphere
	Bilateral sensorimotor cortex
	Bilateral internal capsule
With bilateral cranial neuropathy	Brainstem
Bilateral III	Bilateral cerebral peduncle
Bilateral VI, VII	Bilateral basis pontis
Bilateral XII	Bilateral medullary pyramid
Without cranial neuropathy	Spinal cord
	Bilateral cervical cord
PARAPARESIS	
	Cerebral hemisphere
	Bilateral medial sensorimotor cortex
	Spinal cord
	Thoracic cord

rhagic), traumatic, autoimmune (demyelinating), mass lesions (infectious, neoplastic, benign tumors, etc.) Table 60-4 outlines focal upper motor neuron lesions and common pathophysiologic mechanism to consider.

Disorders of Lower Motor Neuron

Motor Neuron Disorders (Neuronopathies)

These are a heterogenous group of diseases that affect the motor neurons in the spinal cord and in the brainstem. They produce weakness and atrophy of skeletal muscles and fasciculations which represent signs of denervation. Disorders which involve the motor neuron include spinal muscular atrophies (SMA), amyotrophic lateral sclerosis, poliomyelitis, and some systemic diseases to include paraproteinemia.

Acute Infantile Type of SMA (Werdnig-Hoffmann Disease).   Werdnig-Hoffmann disease is inherited in the autosomal recessive form. Incidence is 1 : 15,000. Fetal movements may be diminished during pregnancy and the disease manifests itself by 3 months of age. The clinical findings include weakness and hypotonia. Difficulty in breathing and feeding are common, presenting manifestations and reflect involvement of bulbar and respiratory motor neurons. Death usually occurs by the age of 3 years.

Amyotrophic Lateral Sclerosis (ALS).   ALS in common usage is synonymous with motor neuron disease. This is a progressive disease of adulthood characterized by both upper and lower motor neuron lesions. It may start as the **bulbar** form with dysphagia and dysarthria (motor neurons of cranial nerves IX, X, XII). Ultimately, the

The Monosynaptic Reflex

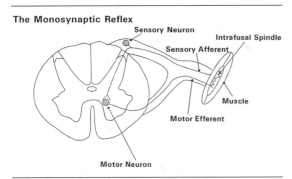

Fig. 60-4. The monosynaptic reflex is comprised of specialized intrafusal spindles (sensory receptors within the muscle) which detect information on length of muscle fiber, a sensory afferent axon which conveys information to the spinal cord via the dorsal root and horn to end monosynaptically on the motor neuron, and a motor axon which conveys information to the muscle. This reflex results in muscle contraction and is the anatomic representation of the muscle stretch reflex. While also referred to as the deep tendon reflex, the muscle stretch reflex is the correct clinico-anatomic term. A lesion which involves any of the components of the monosynaptic reflex will result in loss of the muscle stretch reflex. The monosynaptic reflex, in addition to being a segmental loop, is under the control of descending fibers from higher centers which provides the basis for maintenance of posture.

symptoms become generalized. The diagnosis of ALS is made by the clinical picture and electromyography (EMG) which shows generalized fibrillations, fasciculations, and large motor units.

The mean age of onset of ALS is 56 years. It is usually sporadic in occurrence but 8–10% of cases are familial. The most common clinical presentation is bilateral but asymmetric weakness, wasting, and fasciculations representing lower motor neuron involvement and hyperreflexia, spasticity, and Babinski signs representing upper motor neuron involvement. Cramps are a common presenting complaint. The course is relentlessly progressive with death in about 3 years on average.

The pathogenesis of ALS remains uncertain but theories include autoimmune, infectious, and toxic factors.

Disorders of Nerve Roots (Radiculopathy)

Focal lesions involving motor roots are characterized by segmental weakness, atrophy, and loss of reflexes. Sensory root involvement is characterized by radicular pain (pain which radiates down a dermatome) and dermatomal sen-

sory loss. Lesions which compress or inflame the nerve root are the most common etiologies. Compressive lesions include herniated nucleus pulposus, osteophytes, metastatic neoplasms, and benign tumors of the root (neurofibroma).

Inflammatory lesions include infections like shingles (herpes zoster) and Lyme disease, which can involve either the motor or sensory root or both and acute demyelinating polyradiculoneuropathy (Guillain-Barré syndrome), which has a predilection for the motor root.

Disorders of Nerve (Neuropathy)

Peripheral neuropathy is defined as the disorder in which there is altered function and structure of peripheral motor, sensory, or autonomic nerves. Neuropathies are classified as to whether there is generalized involvement of nerves (polyneuropathy) or focal involvement of a nerve (mononeuropathy). Subclassification of neuropathies is dependent on whether the myelin sheath, axon, or neuron is primarily involved as outlined in Table 60-5.

Neuronopathy. This involves primary loss of nerve cell bodies accompanied by degeneration of entire peripheral and central processes. Technically, motor neuron diseases are motor neuronopathies as they involve the cell body. Sensory neuronopathies are those which involve the dorsal root ganglion cells, in which there is striking sensory loss, diffuse areflexia, and "sensory ataxia." These will be discussed in Chap. 61.

Axonal Polyneuropathies. These are the result of degeneration of the distal axon. Presumably, the axon transport system is affected by metabolic or toxic factors which results in distal axonal degeneration (dying back neuropathy). These neuropathies present with a symmetrical, distal loss of sensory and motor function. Sensory loss is in a stocking-glove distribution, muscle weakness is predominantly distal and usually associated with atrophy, and muscle stretch reflexes are lost early particularly if the disease involves large fibers which contribute to the monosynaptic reflex. Electrodiagnostic studies show low-amplitude response and mild slowing of nerve conduction velocities. The cerebrospinal fluid (CSF) is normal. Etiologies to be considered include metabolic and toxic factors outlined in Table 60-5.

Demyelinating Polyneuropathies. These may be inherited or acquired. Injury occurs to the myelin sheath or the myelin-producing Schwann cells with relative sparing of axons. Clinically, these present as motor weakness with mild sensory loss and early generalized loss of muscle

Table 60-4. Characteristics of Diseases Associated with Focal Upper Motor Lesions

		Maximal Deficit at Onset	Maximal Deficit Over Hours to Days	Maximal Deficit Over Days to Weeks to Months

CEREBRAL		**TRAUMATIC**
		Contusion
		Intracranial hematoma
		VASCULAR
		Ischemic
		  Arterial
		    Anterior cerebral artery
		    Middle cerebral artery
		    Internal carotid artery
		    Basilar artery
		  Venous
		    Sagittal sinus thrombosis
		  Hemorrhagic
		    Intracerebral hematoma
			AUTOIMMUNE
			Multiple sclerosis
			INFECTION
				MASS
				Metastatic neoplasm
				Metastatic neoplasm
				  Glioma
				  Meningioma
				  Ependymoma
				Non-tumorous masses
				  Cysts
				Hydrocephalus
				INFECTION
				  Abscess
				  Empyema
				INFECTION
				Viral
				  Progressive multifocal
				    leukoencephalopathy

SPINAL CORD		**TRAUMATIC**
		Physical distortion
		Contusion
		Hematomyelia
		VASCULAR
		Anterior spinal artery
			AUTOIMMUNE
			Multiple sclerosis
			Transverse myelitis
			  Lupus
			  Collagen disease
			INFECTION
			Viral
				MASS
				Metastatic neoplasm
				Primary neoplasm
				  Intramedullary
				    Ependymoma
				    Glioma
				  Extramedullary
				    Meningioma
				    Neurofibroma
				Epidural empyema granuloma
				Non-tumor masses
				  Osteophyte
				  Herniated disc
				SYRINGOMYELIA
				INFECTION
				Syphilis
				Viral
				  HIV infection

stretch reflexes. In general, hereditary, inborn errors of the metabolism, and immunologic diseases should be considered in the differential diagnosis as outlined in Table 60-5.

Guillain-Barré syndrome (GBS), also known as inflammatory polyradiculoneuropathy, is the most notable example. There is commonly a preceding event like an upper respiratory tract infection which suggests an immunologic pathogenesis. Symptoms consist predominantly of weakness with mild paresthesias which develop subacutely over days or a few weeks.

The weakness is usually symmetrical and ascending in character. It may be mild or very severe. Hyporeflexia or areflexia are invariably present. Cranial nerve involvement, usually of facial nerves bilaterally, is present in at least 50% of cases. Objective sensory loss is not commonly found. Autonomic dysfunction is often seen and can lead to cardiac arrhythmias. In severe cases, respiratory failure may occur. The diagnosis is supported by a CSF examination which reveals elevated protein levels with normal cell count. In most cases, nerve conduction studies show slowing of velocities.

About 80% of patients have almost complete functional

Table 60-5. Classification of Peripheral Neuropathies

Classification	Etiology	Predominant Type of Involvement			
		Motor	Sensory	Sensorimotor	Autonomic
GENERALIZED POLYNEUROPATHY					
Neuronopathy (ganglionopathy)	Degenerative				
	Hereditary sensory neuropathy		√		
	Motor neuron disease	√			
	Spinal muscular atrophies	√			
	Immune mediated				
	Sjögren's syndrome		√		
	Infectious				
	Lyme disease		√		
	Poliomyelitis	√			
	Shingles (herpes zoster)		√		
	Malignancy				
	Carcinomatous		√		
Myelinopathy	Hereditary				
	Charcot-Marie-Tooth	√			
	Immune mediated				
	Acute (Guillain-Barré syndrome)	√			
	Relapsing polyradiculoneuropathy	√			
	Chronic polyradiculoneuropathy	√			
	Metabolic				
	Krabbe's disease			√	
	Metachromatic leukodystrophy			√	
	Refsum's disease			√	
Distal axonopathy	Hereditary				
	Hereditary amyloid		√		√
	Nutritional				
	B_{12} (dorsal column involvement)		√		
	Niacin			√	
	Pyridoxine		√		
	Thiamine			√	
	Systemic diseases				
	Diabetes	√		√	√
	Hepatic neuropathy			√	
	Porphyria	√			
	Uremia			√	
	Toxins				
	Alcohol			√	
	Drugs				
	Antibodies			√	
	Antiepileptic drugs			√	
	Chemotherapy			√	
	Industrial solvents			√	
	Heavy metals			√	
	Lead	√			

Table 60-5. (continued)

Classification	Etiology	Predominant Type of Involvement			
		Motor	Sensory	Sensorimotor	Autonomic
FOCAL NEUROPATHIES					
Mononeuropathy	Infiltrative				
	Amyloid			√	
	Hypothyroid			√	
	Physical injury (crush, compression, traction)			√	
	Tumor				
	Neurofibroma			√	
	Lymphoma			√	
Multiple Mononeuropathy	Immune mediated				
	Polyarteritis nodosa			√	
	Rheumatoid arthritis			√	
	Sarcoid			√	
	Infectious				
	Lyme disease		√		
	Leprosy		√		
	Vasculopathy				
	Diabetes			√	

recovery. However, attention should be given to potentially fatal but treatable complications which include respiratory and autonomic dysfunction. Plasma exchange or intravenous immune globulin is utilized in selected cases.

Mononeuropathies. They are characterized by symptoms and signs in the distribution of one or more individual nerves. Trauma and mechanical distortion due to entrapment, ischemia, and neoplastic infiltration may play a part in the pathogenesis. The term "multiple mononeuropathy" (mononeuritis multiplex) is used if several noncontiguous nerves are involved. Nerve conduction studies show abnormalities only in the affected nerves.

Disorders of the Neuromuscular Junction

A number of different conditions may interfere with the transmission of the electrical impulse across the neuromuscular junction (Table 60-6). A common feature of all of the disorders is fluctuating or episodic weakness. Weakness is usually exacerbated by exercise and improved by rest. Defects in neuromuscular transmission can be documented by pharmacologic tests and by electrophysiologic studies, including repetitive nerve stimulation and single-fiber electromyography.

Table 60-6. Disorders of Neuromuscular Transmission

PRESYNAPTIC

Botulism
Lambert-Eaton syndrome
Hypermagnesemia
Hypocalcemia
Snake bite
Antibiotics
Congenital myasthenia gravis
?Tick paralysis

INHIBITION OR DEFICIENCY OF ACETYLCHOLINESTERASE

Organophosphates
Congenital myasthenia gravis

POSTSYNAPTIC

Autoimmune myasthenia gravis
Curare (d-tubocurarine)
Alpha-bungarotoxin
Congenital myasthenia gravis

Used with permission from Parke JT. Diseases of the neuromuscular junction. In Oski FA, DeAngelis CD, Feigin RD, et al. (eds.). *Principles and Practice of Pediatrics.* Philadelphia: Lippincott, 1994, p. 2077.

Myasthenia Gravis (MG)

Myasthenia gravis is an autoimmune disorder in which antibodies are produced against the acetylcholine receptor in the muscle membrane. Circulating antibodies bind to the receptor on the muscle end-plate, reducing the number of functional receptors by impeding the interaction of ACh with the receptors, thus interfering with synaptic transmission.

The cardinal feature of the disease is easy fatigability. Symptoms are most apparent in the evening when the patient is tired. There is weakness of cranial muscles as well as extremity muscles. The most common presentation is ptosis or diplopia. As in myopathies, the proximal muscles are more affected than distal ones. There are few physical findings other than weakness. Muscle stretch reflexes are typically well preserved. Thymic tumors occur in approximately 10% of patients. Thyroid disorders occur in approximately 60% of patients and may contribute to weakness. Other autoimmune diseases occur with increased frequency in patients with MG.

The diagnosis of MG may be confirmed by pharmacologic tests. A small dose of an anticholinesterase, such as edrophonium chloride (Tensilon), blocks the degradation of acetylcholine, producing a dramatic improvement in strength. Electrophysiologic studies are helpful in documenting transmission failure at the neuromuscular junction. Antibodies to the human muscle acetylcholine receptor are found in the serum of up to 90% of patients.

A number of different therapeutic modalities are available for the treatment of MG. Cholinesterase inhibitors, thymectomy, corticosteroid therapy, immunosuppressive agents, and plasmapheresis are useful in treatment of MG. Spontaneous remissions may occur, particularly in the early years of the disease. Fatalities in severe, generalized disease are mainly related to respiratory complications.

Botulism

The exotoxin of *Clostridium botulinum* is one of the most potent neurotoxins known. The toxin irreversibly blocks acetylcholine release from the presynaptic nerve terminals. Recovery occurs by sprouting of terminal motor neurons and formation of new motor end-plates. Poisoning may occur following ingestion of the toxin in inadequately cooked or improperly canned food or from infection of wounds.

Early symptoms include blurred vision, diplopia, dizziness, dysarthria, and dysphagia. Weakness may occur rapidly, causing a flaccid paralysis and respiratory failure.

A third type of botulism, infant botulism, is due to ingestion of the spores of *C. botulinum.* The ingested spores colonize the intestinal tract and produce the botulinum toxin. Symptoms include constipation followed by listlessness, weakness, difficulty feeding, and a weak cry. Respiratory arrest may occur abruptly in patients with severe disease.

Lambert-Eaton Syndrome (Myasthenic-Myopathic Syndrome)

This myasthenic syndrome is associated with neoplasms, particularly oat-cell carcinoma of the lung in about 50% of the cases. This is a presynaptic disorder with a defect in the release of acetylcholine from the nerve terminals. No receptor antibody is present.

The muscles most involved are the shoulder girdle, pelvic girdle, lower extremities, and muscles of the trunk. Patients often complain of paresthesias, aching pain, and autonomic disturbances, such as dryness of the mouth, constipation, difficulty with micturition, and impotence. The onset is usually subacute. Symptoms may precede diagnosis of the tumor by months or years.

The response to pyridostigmine is variable. Electrodiagnostic studies show a low-amplitude muscle action potential which increases in amplitude with rapid repetitive stimulation.

Patients with the Lambert-Eaton syndrome should be carefully evaluated for occult tumor. Treatment of an underlying tumor may result in improvement of the neurologic syndrome. Guanidine hydrochloride, prednisone, and plasmapheresis are effective in some patients. The response to treatment is slow, taking months to a year.

Disorders of Muscle (Myopathies)

Myopathies may be inherited or acquired. The initial complaint is usually weakness. The family history is of utmost importance in diagnosis. Family members may have very mild symptoms in dominantly inherited diseases. Specific findings important in the physical examination include atrophy or hypertrophy of muscles, muscle weakness and its distribution, and evidence of myotonia (delayed relaxation of a muscle after contraction). Weakness in myopathies is usually more severe in the proximal muscles. A Gower's maneuver (inability to get up without using the arms to pull oneself up from a sitting position) is usually present because of pelvic girdle weakness. Reflexes are usually preserved unless the muscle weakness is severe. Ptosis and weakness of the extraocular muscles may be seen in ocular dystrophies and myotonic dystrophies but are more typical of disorders of the neuromuscular junction than myopathies. Facial and bulbar muscles may be involved in some myopathies.

Laboratory tests for the evaluation of a possible myopathy include measurement of muscle enzymes, EMG, and muscle biopsy. The EMG is usually nonspecific but may be very helpful in excluding other disorders of the motor unit. Specific diagnoses can often be made by muscle biopsy.

Muscular Dystrophies

The muscular dystrophies are a group of inherited muscle diseases which are progressive and degenerative. They are characterized by their clinical presentation and pattern of muscle involvement.

Duchenne Muscular Dystrophy (DMD). Duchenne muscular dystrophy is the most severe form of muscular dystrophy. It affects approximately 1 in 3000 males, and one-third of cases represent a new mutation. Recent work has identified the genetic defect at Xp21 and the gene product dystrophin.

Weakness usually becomes clinically evident between ages 3 and 5 years, and progresses over the next two decades. The gait is characterized by pelvic waddling, a wide base, toe walking, and lumbar lordosis. Enlargement or "pseudohypertrophy" of muscles, particularly the gas-

trocnemius muscles, is characteristic. Proximal arm weakness becomes more noticeable as the child grows older. Most boys become wheelchair-dependent between ages 10 and 12, and death usually occurs by the late second decade, usually due to respiratory compromise. Patients frequently have associated mild mental retardation or learning problems. Becker dystrophy is similar to DMD; however, the age of onset is later and progression is slower.

Myotonic Dystrophy (MyD). Myotonic dystrophy is an autosomal dominant condition. Gene mapping studies have localized the defect to an abnormal triplicate repeat in the proximal portion of the short (p) arm of chromosome 19. The molecular basis for the myotonia appears to involve abnormal sodium channel function. The disorder is a systemic disorder, characterized by gonadal atrophy, diabetes mellitus, gallbladder dysfunction, cataracts, mental retardation, early baldness, and cardiac conduction defects.

The presenting symptom of MyD is usually weakness, which, unlike other myopathies, is distal in distribution. There is usually facial weakness with a typical phenotypic appearance of slender facies, temporal hollowing, and

Fig. 60-5. Rapid firing of potentials with waxing and waning of motor unit firing is characteristic of a myotonic discharge. The discharge sounds like a dive bomber when heard.

MOTOR UNIT POTENTIAL

Normal

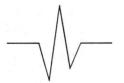

Myotonic Discharge:

Producing waxing and waning causing dive-bombing effect.

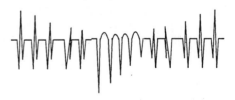

0.5 mv

50 ms

open mouth. The myotonia can be elicited by percussion or activation of muscles and is characterized by delayed relaxation after contraction. Infants with MyD present with severe hypotonia and developmental delay. Diagnosis of MyD relies heavily on the EMG examination which shows myotonic discharges (Fig. 60-5).

Hereditary Myopathies

Congenital Myopathies.   These are a group of disorders that present in early infancy and are recognized by distinctive histochemical abnormalities of skeletal muscle. They are usually, but not invariably, nonprogressive. In addition to weakness and hypotonia, these patients frequently have orthopedic deformities such as congenital hip dislocation and kyphoscoliosis. Diagnosis is usually made by muscle biopsy.

Metabolic Myopathies.   These myopathies derive from defects in energy production, including abnormalities in glycogen and lipid metabolism and abnormalities in respiratory chain function. Clinical manifestations vary from exercise intolerance and cramps with little weakness to severe weakness.

Acquired Myopathies

Acquired myopathies tend to be subacute in presentation and are rarely the cause of an acute paralytic state.

Inflammatory Myopathies.   Infectious agents known to cause myopathy include viruses, bacteria, fungi, and parasites. Bacterial infections are less common and more localized than viral infections. Idiopathic inflammatory myopathies are much more common, and include dermatomyositis and polymyositis. If the skin is involved as well as striated muscle, the disease is dermatomyositis (DM). If restricted to muscle, the disease is polymyositis (PM). Approximately 10–15% will have carcinoma at the time of diagnosis or will develop carcinoma within one year.

Endocrine Myopathies.   Muscle weakness may accompany several endocrinopathies including Cushing's syndrome, parathyroid, and thyroid disorders. Weakness usually resolves in these disorders when hormonal balance is achieved. Proximal weakness may also occur as a result of corticosteroid therapy.

Clinical Examples

1. A 50-year-old woman presented with a 3-month history of progressive difficulty swallowing and slurring of speech. This was followed by weakness on the left side.

The symptoms slowly progressed and are now associated with a dull occipital headache.

On examination, the funduscopic examination showed loss of venous pulsations. Palatal movements were decreased bilaterally. Speech was dysarthric. Patient was unable to protrude the tongue, which was atrophic. There was weakness in the left upper and lower limbs. Reflexes were brisk on both sides and Babinski signs were present bilaterally.

Discussion.   The difficulty with speech, decreased palatal movements, and inability to protrude tongue signifies involvement of cranial nerves IX, X, and XII bilaterally. Bilateral but asymmetrical corticospinal tract involvement is suggested by left-sided weakness and bilateral hyperreflexia and Babinski signs. As cranial nerves IX, X, and XII are associated with the medulla and the descending corticospinal fibers are involved, the lesion is localized to the ventral medulla. The onset of headache later in the course and the finding of papilledema signifies raised intracranial pressure.

Since the onset was gradual and the course was progressive, a mass lesion compressing the ventral medulla and obstructing the fourth ventricle would be the first concern. MRI of the brain and cervicomedullary junction would be the most useful test for detecting a lesion in the posterior fossa. Etiologies to consider would be an extra-axial neoplasm (meningioma and metastatic neoplasm). Treatment would depend upon the nature of the lesion.

2. A 25-year-old man presented with one-week history of distal paresthesias in the legs associated with progressive weakness. This started in the lower limbs and ascended to involve all four limbs. The patient complained of difficulty in breathing. There was a history of a vague viral illness preceding the problem.

On examination, the patient had severe generalized weakness in all four limbs associated with hypotonia and areflexia. Plantar responses were flexor. Sensory examination was normal.

Discussion.   Profound generalized weakness, absent muscle stretch reflexes, and the absence of Babinski signs suggest a lesion in the lower motor unit. However, the most important alternative consideration in the clinical setting would be to consider an acute spinal cord syndrome presenting in the spinal shock phase (paralysis, hypotonia, and absence of reflexes).

The localization of the lesion to the lower motor unit plus the complaint of distal paresthesias (even in the absence of sensory findings on examination) suggest that the lesion involves the peripheral nerve. A predominantly motor polyneuropathy combined with the subacute onset and the history of a preceding viral illness suggest an acute inflammatory condition like Guillain-Barré syndrome. The diagnosis would be confirmed by the demonstration of an elevated protein and the absence of cells in the spinal fluid and slowing of nerve conduction velocities. In similar cases where the sensory symptoms or findings are less prominent, one would have to consider and pursue the possibility of other lesions involving the motor neuron (poliomyelitis), the neuromuscular junction (myasthenia gravis or botulism), and the muscle.

3. A 5-year-old boy was referred to his pediatrician by his pre-school teacher for evaluation of clumsiness. He was the product of a normal pregnancy and delivery. He began to walk at 18 months but never was able to run. He had difficulty climbing stairs and when rising from a sitting to standing position. He had to pull himself up with his arms. His teacher also noted that he had difficulty learning letters and had a poor attention span.

On examination, he was clumsy and had a wide-based gait with a tendency to toe walk. He could not raise his arms over his head or rise from a chair. The gastrocnemius muscles were enlarged and firm to palpation. Sensory examination was normal. Laboratory studies demonstrated a serum creatine phosphokinase of 11,000 IU/liter.

Discussion. Proximal weakness with normal sensation suggests a myopathy. Progressive myopathy and pseudohypertrophy in a young boy would suggest Duchenne muscular dystrophy. Weakness progresses relentlessly and death usually occurs by the late second decade, most commonly due to respiratory failure.

DMD is inherited as an X-linked recessive trait. The genetic defect has been localized to Xp21 and the gene product dystrophin (a protein important in maintaining the structural integrity of muscle) has been identified.

Bibliography

Adams RD and Victor M. The muscular dystrophies. In *Principles of Neurology.* New York: McGraw-Hill, 1993, pp. 1215–1232. *A review of classification and clinical features of the muscular dystrophies.*

Adams RD and Victor M. Myasthenia gravis and episodic forms of muscular weakness. In *Principles of Neurology.* New York: McGraw-Hill, 1993, pp. 1252–1270. *A clinical review of myasthenia gravis and myasthenic syndromes.*

Ghez Claude. The Control of Movement. In Kandel ER, Schwartz JH, and Jessell TM (eds.). *Principles of Neural Science.* New York: Elsevier, 1991, pp. 534–547. *Review of upper motor neuron disorders.*

Rowland LP. Diseases of the motor unit. In Kandel ER, Schwartz JH, and Jessell TM (eds.). *Principles of Neural Science.* New York: Elsevier, 1991, pp. 244–257. *A review of disorders affecting the cell body and axon of the motor neuron and the muscle cell; includes discussion of molecular genetics of X-linked muscular dystrophies.*

Rowland LP. Diseases of Chemical Transmission at the Nerve-Muscle Synapse: Myasthenia Gravis. In Kandel ER, Schwartz JH, and Jessell TM (eds.). *Principles of Neural Science.* New York: Elsevier, 1991, pp. 235–243. *A comprehensive review of myasthenia gravis.*

Schaumberg H. Anatomic Classification of Peripheral Neuropathy. In Schaumberg H, Spencer P, and Thomas PK (eds.). *Disorders of Peripheral Nerve.* Philadelphia: Davis, 1983, pp. 9–23. *Classification of peripheral nerve disorders.*

61 The Sensory System

Osvaldo H. Perurena

Objectives

After completing this chapter, you should be able to

Understand the anatomic pathways of the sensory system from receptors to the cortex

Understand the function of the spinothalamic and proprioceptive system

Understand the function of the parietal cortex

Localize lesions which involve the sensory system

Identify pathophysiologic mechanisms which give rise to sensory system lesions

---

Somatosensory information is transmitted from the periphery to the parietal lobe by a three-neuron pathway: the first neuron located in the dorsal root ganglia receives information from the ipsilateral sensory receptor, the second neuron crosses to convey information to the thalamus, and the third neuron conveys information to the parietal lobe. There are two types of sensory systems which convey somatosensory information to the parietal lobe: the spinothalamic system (which conveys pain and temperature sensation) and the dorsal column system (which conveys proprioception and vibration). Lesions in either of these systems produce modality-specific abnormalities which specifically localize to the system involved. However, since the parietal cortex functions to synthesize and interpret modality-specific sensory information, lesions in the parietal cortex result in the inability to attach meaning and significance to the stimulus (agnosia).

Anatomy and Physiology of Somatosensory System

Peripheral Sensory System

The primary sensory modalities are touch, proprioception, vibration, pain, and temperature. Each modality has a specialized receptor which detects a specific stimulus (Fig. 61-1). The stimulus is then transmitted to the dorsal root ganglion by a peripheral nerve. The diameter and degree of myelination of the nerve fiber influence the speed of conduction, with large myelinated fibers conducting the fastest and small unmyelinated fibers conducting the slowest.

Large Fiber System

Proprioception (perception of body position and movement) and vibration are somatosensory functions conveyed by large myelinated fibers.

Proprioception. Proprioception is generated by mechanoreceptors in the muscle spindle, the joint capsule, and connective tissue, all which inform limb position and movement. Proprioception is explored by examination of position sensation (which evaluates the ability to recognize position of body parts) and the Romberg (sway) test (which evaluates perception of body position). The Romberg test is done by observing the change of the balance of a subject standing with his eyes closed as compared to eyes opened. To maintain an erect posture, we depend on visual cues and proprioceptive information (both inform us of the position of the body in space) and, to a lesser extent, from the vestibular apparatus and cerebellum. Normally, there may be only a slight sway with eyes closed. When the visual information is removed, if the proprioception is impaired the subject will sway and possibly fall (positive Romberg test). A person with vestibular or cerebellar disease will sway proportionally with the eyes opened or closed.

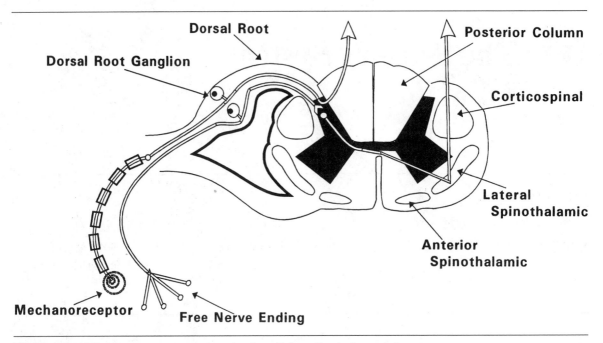

Fig. 61-1. Specialized sensory receptors transmit sensory information to the central nervous system. The large fiber system is comprised of mechanoreceptors which transmit proprioceptive information to the dorsal columns. The small fiber system is comprised of free nerve endings which transmit pain and thermal information to the spinothalamic tract.

Vibration.   Vibration is generated by touch and proprioceptive mechanoreceptors located in the subcutaneous tissues which are sensitive to minimal skin distortions at high frequencies (up to 500 Hz). Vibration is tested by evaluating the subject's ability to discriminate between the vibrating and nonvibrating surface of a 256-Hz tuning fork placed on a distal bony prominence.

Light Touch.   Light discriminative touch is conveyed by cutaneous and subcutaneous mechanoreceptors that transmit sustained or variable pressure and flutter (the sensation associated with low-frequency oscillation). It is tested by contacting the skin lightly with a cotton swab and asking the patient to acknowledge the touch and describe its localization on the skin.

Small Fiber System
The small fiber system transmits sensory information concerning pain and temperature from free nerve endings which detect mechanical and thermal stimulation. Pain is tested with an ad hoc point made from a broken tongue depressor. It is crucial to discard the instrument after finishing the examination. Appreciation of pain is evaluated by

asking the subject to discriminate between the sharp point or the blunt point of the instrument but without detail and localization.

Temperature.   Temperature is detected by receptors which discriminate between warm (33–47°C) and cool (12–40°C) stimuli. Temperature is evaluated by asking the subject to differentiate warm and cold objects within an innocuous range of temperature.

For the screening of all somatosensory function, symmetrical areas in the face and extremities (both proximal and distal sites) are examined to determine the patient's ability to perceive the stimulus. Examination is tailored to identify patterns of sensory loss that suggest a specific nerve, sensory root, or sensory tract pattern of abnormalities which have localizing value.

Central Sensory Pathways

Sensory information ascends in the spinal cord to the thalamus, then on to the parietal lobe for synthesis and interpretation as depicted in Fig. 61-2.

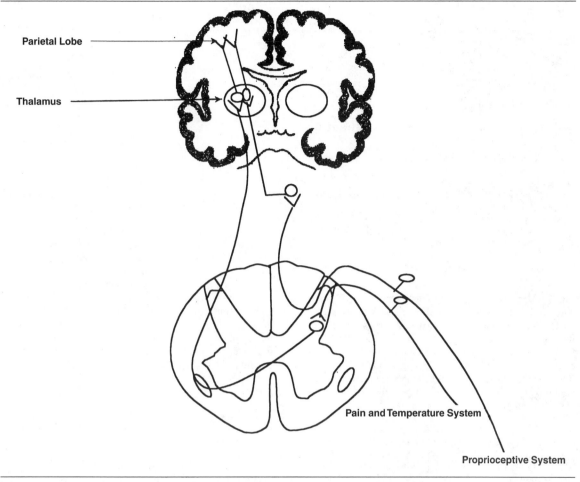

Fig. 61-2. Sensory pathways. Pain and temperature fibers enter the dorsal horn and synapse in the dorsal horn. Fibers then cross to the lateral spinothalamic tract and ascend to the thalamus. In the ventral posterior lateral nucleus fibers synapse on the third-order neuron to project through the internal capsule to the parietal cortex. Proprioceptive fibers enter through the dorsal horn. Unlike the pain and temperature fibers, they do not synapse but travel ipsilaterally through the dorsal column to the medulla, where they synapse on the nucleus cuneatus or gracilis. At this point, fibers decussate to project to the thalamus where they synapse on neurons of the ventral posterior dorsal nucleus and then project to the parietal cortex.

Anterolateral Spinothalamic System (Small Fiber Sensory Modalities)

Pain, temperature, and crude touch are conducted by small myelinated and unmyelinated fibers which have their first-order neuron in the dorsal root ganglia. The central branches enter in the spinal cord and synapse with the second neuron in the dorsal horn in the same side. The ascending axons of the second neuron decussate in the white matter ventral to the central canal over a rostrocaudal length of three spinal cord segments (Fig. 61-3A). These fibers now ascend in the anterolateral portion of the contralateral spinal cord (lateral spinothalamic tract and anterior spinothalamic tract), through the lateral brainstem to terminate in the ventral posterolateral thalamic nucleus (third-order neuron) (Fig. 61-4). From there, the spinothalamic system projects to the post-central gyrus (parietal

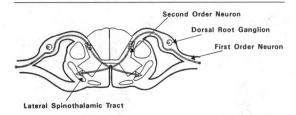

A. Pain and Temperature Sensation

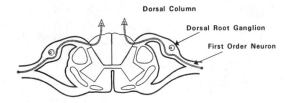

B. Proprioceptive Sensation

Fig. 61-3. Pathways for somatosensory system. A. Spinal cord level: Pain and temperature sensation is transmitted via the dorsal root ganglia to the dorsal horn where the first-order neuron synapses. The second-order neuron fibers then decussate in the central cord to the lateral spinothalamic tract. B. Proprioceptive sensation is transmitted via the dorsal root ganglia to the ipsilateral dorsal column. The first-order neuron synapses in the nucleus cuneatus and gracilis.

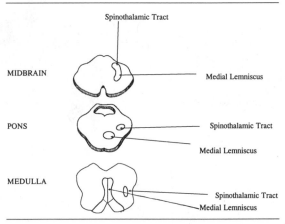

Fig. 61-4. Sensory tracts in the brainstem. Pain and temperature sensation is transmitted through the brainstem in the lateral spinothalamic tract which is laterally placed in the medulla, pons, and midbrain. Proprioceptive sensation ascends in the dorsal column ipsilaterally until the first-order neuron synapses on the second-order neuron in the medulla (nucleus gracilis and cuneatus). At this time, fiber decussates to form the medial lemniscus, which assumes a medial position in the medulla and pons. At the level of the midbrain, the medial lemniscus assumes a lateral position adjacent to the lateral spinothalamic tract.

lobe) via the posterior limb of the internal capsule and the corona radiata.

There are four features of the spinothalamic tract relevant in the understanding of the pain and temperature deficits found in spinal cord lesion. These features are (a) the spinothalamic tract is somatotopically organized; (b) the spinothalamic tract ascends contralaterally from the origin of the small fiber system; (c) the spinothalamic tract decussates in the center of the cord; and (d) lesions of the ascending or decussating spinothalamic fibers produce a circumferential limit around the trunk between normal and abnormal sensory perception referred to as a "sensory level." A sensory level is pathognomonic of a spinal cord lesion.

Somatotopic Organization of Spinothalamic System.   The spinothalamic tract is somatotopically organized with the pain and temperature fibers arranged in layers (Fig. 61-5). Fibers conveying somatosensory information from the sacral region and lower limb lie more su-

perficially and those for the trunk, arm, and neck (in that order) lie more deeply inside the substance of the cord.

Pathways of Spinothalamic System.   The spinothalamic tract ascends contralaterally from the body part. A lesion of the spinothalamic tract of one side will produce a sensory deficit in the contralateral limbs. If the compression of the cord is from the outside (extramedullary mass) the earliest deficit will be contralateral in the sacral area (early sacral deficit). As the lesion progresses, the more deeply located fibers are affected and the dermatomes of the abdomen and chest become affected. The sensory level clinically "ascends" toward the level of the compression.

Decussation of Spinothalamic System.   The spinothalamic tract decussates in the center of the cord. If the lesion is centrally located in the cervical cord, it will disrupt the crossing fibers coming from both sides, producing loss of pain and temperature in a bilateral dermatomal pattern in a form of a "suspended band" or "vestlike" distribution. The deficit will be "dissociated," that is, it will affect pain and temperature but not proprioception and discriminative

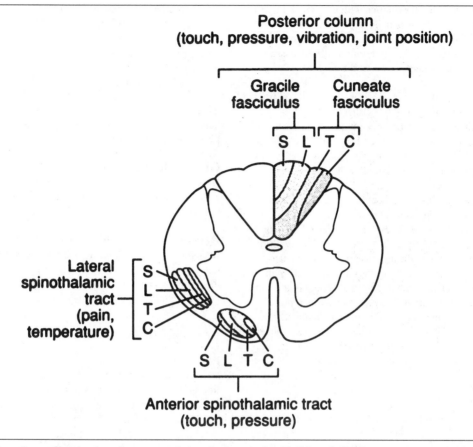

Fig. 61-5. Location and lamination of sensory pathways in the spinal cord. C (cervical), T (thoracic), L (lumbar), and S (sacral) indicate the level of origin of fibers within each tract. (Used with permission from: Greenberg DA, Aminoff MJ, and Simon RP. *Clinical Neurology* (2nd ed.). Norwalk, Conn.: Appleton & Lange, 1993.)

touch. As the lesion expands outwards and longitudinally, the anterior horn cells, the pyramidal tract, and the ascending fibers of the spinothalamic tract and posterior columns will be affected. As a rule the sacral fibers of the spinothalamic tract placed outermost in the cord will be affected last, resulting in the finding of relative preservation of the sacral sensation up to the final stages of so-called "sacral sparing."

Sensory Level. A sensory level is a sensory deficit found on the trunk which designates the level of the spinal cord lesion. Sensory levels are produced by a lesion which interrupts the sensory tracts of the cervical and thoracic cord. Sensory levels affect all sensory modalities but they are more clinically evident by testing pain and from the practical standpoint are usually described with this sensory modality. The dermatomes that mark the passage between normal and abnormal sensation are used to describe the limit or limits of the level. Most commonly the sensory loss may affect the entire body below the level; in that case the dermatome which marks the upper level of the loss will point to the approximate area of the cord where the lesion is localized.

In other cases the sensory loss occurs in a form of a

band around or across the midline with a horizontal upper and lower limit beyond which the sensation is normal (suspended sensory level). "Suspended" sensory levels are pathognomonic of a lesion interrupting the decussating spinothalamic fibers in the center of the cord.

Dorsal Column — Medial Lemniscal System (Large Fiber Sensory Modalities)

Discriminative touch and proprioception are conducted by intermediate and large myelinated fibers which have their first-order neuron in the dorsal root ganglia. The central branches of the dorsal root ganglia cells ascend ipsilaterally in the dorsal columns (Fig. 61-3B). The medial fibers of the dorsal columns carry input from the legs and lower trunk (gracile fasciculus) and the lateral fibers carry input from the upper trunk, arms, and neck (cuneate fasciculus). The ascending fibers of the first neuron synapse with the second-order neuron in the nucleus gracile and cuneate situated also ipsilaterally in the posterior medulla. The fibers from these nuclei cross the midline and ascend in the contralateral side of the brainstem as the medial lemniscus to terminate in the ventral posterior lateral thalamic nucleus. Tertiary fibers originate in the thalamus and are projected to the postcentral gyrus via the posterior limb of the internal capsule and corona radiata.

Parietal Lobe

The parietal cortex synthesizes and integrates the data of the primary sensory modalities into the perception of the object or meaning of the stimulus. Such synthesis involves discrimination in space and time of the primary sensory input.

Recognition of the object implies also comparison with past memories (associative functions). Parietal lobe cortical lesions produce an impairment of the cortical modalities with relative preservation of the primary modalities. The cortical modalities tested in routine examination are stereognosis, graphesthesia, and recognition of simultaneous stimulation of homologous areas.

Stereognosis

Stereognosis is the ability to recognize the nature of an object placed in the hand through its shape, texture, weight, etc.

Graphesthesia

Graphesthesia is the ability to recognize letters or numbers written on the patient's skin (usually the digits of the fingers).

Recognition of Double Simultaneous Stimuli

Recognition of simultaneous stimuli applied to homologous areas of the body is a cortical function. Extinction of the stimulus contralateral to the parietal lesion is a phenomenon indicative of a cortical lesion.

Concepts of Localization

Localization and the cause of a lesion responsible for a sensory problem is determined by the anatomic distribution of the sensory abnormality, the sensory modalities affected, and the associated neurologic abnormalities (motor, extrapyramidal, cerebellar), in addition to the mode of onset and course of the symptoms. The anatomic distribution of a sensory deficit may follow characteristic patterns which suggests a specific localization as outlined in Table 61-1. Clinical terminology of sensory abnormalities associated with the sensory system are outlined in Table 61-2.

Table 61-1. Patterns of Sensory Abnormalities Associated with Lesions of the Sensory System

Localization	Distribution of Sensory Loss
Cutaneous nerve	Area of distribution of the specific cutaneous nerve
Root	Dermatome
Cord	
Central cord (intramedullary)	Bilateral suspended sensory deficit (pain and temperature dissociated from proprioception)
Transection	Sensory level (all modalities)
Hemisection	Ipsilateral proprioceptive loss, contralateral pain, and temperature loss
Brainstem	Crossed sensory (ipsilateral face, contralateral limbs)
Thalamus: internal capsule	Contralateral face, arm, leg (all modalities)
Parietal	Contralateral face, arm, leg (cortical modalities)

Table 61-2. Clinical Terminology of Sensory Abnormalities

Allodynia	Painful sensation abnormally induced by an ordinarily nonpainful stimulus.
Anesthesia	Absence of sensation of any primary sensory modality.
Dermatome	Area of skin innervated by the axons of a single root.
Hyperalgesia	Exaggerated painful perception of a low-level painful stimulation.
Hypothesia	Decreased sensitivity to any given primary sensory modality.
Numbness	Conscious perception of sensory loss in a body part. May also be used by the patient to describe paresthesias, motor weakness, or clumsiness.
Paresthesia	Abnormal, spontaneous sensation experienced without external stimulation (burning, prickling, tingling, or formication).
Sensory ataxia	Clumsiness of gait related to loss of proprioception.
Suspended anesthesia	Band or vestlike distribution of anesthesia commonly associated with intramedullary cord lesions.

Disorders of Sensory System

Disorders that effect the sensory system are classified into peripheral sensory disorders (neuropathies and radiculopathies) and central disorders (spinal cord, brainstem, and cerebral hemisphere).

Peripheral Sensory Disorders

Diseases which involve the nerves and roots are discussed in more detail in Chap. 60. However, notable diseases which predominantly involve the peripheral sensory system are radiculopathies and neuronopathies, which involve the dorsal root ganglia (ganglionopathies).

Herpes Zoster

Herpes Zoster (shingles) presents with vesicular eruptions along a sensory dermatome. The dermatomes of thoracic nerves and trigeminal nerves are most commonly involved. Post-herpetic neuralgia occurs in 20% of cases. The dorsal root ganglia is the site of cellular infiltration with inclusion bodies seen in the ganglion cells.

Sensory Neuropathy Associated with Malignancy

Neuropathies occur in 1–5% of patients with malignancy most commonly involving the lung, breast, colon, and stomach and may precede the diagnosis of malignancy up to 3 years. While the majority of patients develop a distal axonal sensorimotor neuropathy, 20% are associated with a progressive sensory neuropathy characterized by numbness, paresthesias, and sensory ataxia (loss of proprioception resulting in gait imbalance) from involvement of proprioceptive fibers in the dorsal root ganglia.

Hereditary Sensory Neuropathies

Sensory neuropathies may be inherited in dominant or recessive patterns. The neurons of cutaneous unmyelinated and small myelinated fibers are involved. Progressive loss of pain appreciation results in numbness and cutaneous ulcers.

Central Sensory Disorders

Central sensory disorders are associated with diseases which result in focal lesions to include traumatic, vascular, autoimmune, infectious, and neoplastic etiologies. The diseases which result in disorders of the central sensory system are similar to focal upper motor neuron lesions as outlined in Chap. 60 and Table 60-4. Specific sensory syndromes which have localizing value (Fig. 61-6) are discussed below.

Spinal Cord Syndromes

Spinal Cord Transection. Transection of the spinal cord (Fig. 61-6A) results in cessation of function below the level of transection (Table 61-3). All sensory modalities are lost below the level of transection. Since transection involves both ascending and descending white matter tracts, there is also a paralysis indicative of bilateral corticospinal tract involvement. At the level of the lesion which involves the ventral horn and ventral root, there is also evidence of lower motor neuron dysfunction. This finding in addition to the sensory level localizes the site of the transection.

Spinal cord transection is most commonly seen in the setting of trauma. However, rapidly expanding mass lesions and myelitis from infections and immunologic dis-

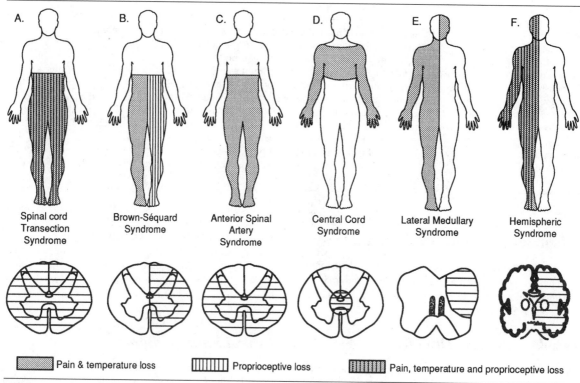

Fig. 61-6. Sensory syndromes and clinicoanatomic correlation. The distribution of proprioceptive loss is represented by areas of parallel vertical lines on each figure and the distribution of pain and temperature loss is represented by the solid shaded areas. The hatched areas in each corresponding anatomic section (spinal cord, brain stem, or cerebral) represent the side and/or location of each corresponding lesion. (A) Spinal cord transection: paralysis and anesthesia below the level of the lesion. (B) Brown-Séquard syndrome: proprioceptive loss and weakness ipsilateral to the lesion; pain and temperature loss contralateral to the lesion. (C) Anterior spinal artery syndrome (anterior two-thirds syndrome): loss of pain and temperature and weakness in legs with preservation of posterior column below the level of the lesion. (D) Central cord syndrome: loss of pain and temperature in a suspended sensory pattern. (E) Lateral medullary syndrome: loss of pain and temperature on the ipsilateral face and contralateral body. (F) Hemispheric syndrome: loss of pain, temperature, and proprioception contralateral to the lesion.

eases should be considered as causes of transection in the absence of a history of trauma.

Brown-Séquard Syndrome (Lateral Hemisection of Spinal Cord).   Depicted in Fig. 61-6B, hemisection of the spinal cord is clinically characterized by ipsilateral loss of proprioception (uncrossed fibers in dorsal column), contralateral loss of pain and temperature (crossed fibers in lateral spinothalamic tract), and ipsilateral upper motor neuron signs.

Extramedullary (extrinsic to cord) mass lesion which compresses the cord laterally and myelitis from infections and immunologic diseases are the most common causes of the Brown-Séquard syndrome. A history of ascending numbness with early sacral involvement should suggest an extramedullary mass process (meningioma, metastatic neoplasm, epidural abscess, and herniated disc).

Anterior Spinal Artery Syndrome.   This disorder, also known as the anterior two-thirds syndrome, is depicted in Fig. 61-6C. The anterior two-thirds of the spinal cord is supplied by the anterior spinal artery which runs

Table 61-3. Localization of the Level of Spinal Cord Transection

Level of Lesions	Sensory Level	Lower Motor Neuron Signs	Upper Motor Neuron Signs
Cord segment C4	Below base of neck	Diaphragmatic paralysis	Quadriparesis and hyper-reflexia below C4
Cord segment C5–6	Below shoulder and lateral arm	Shoulder girdle (spinatus, deltoid, biceps, brachioradialis) weakness and atrophy, loss of biceps, and brachioradialis reflex	Quadriparesis and hyper-reflexia below C5–6
Cord segment C7	Below medial arm	Arm extensor (triceps) weakness and atrophy, loss of triceps reflex	Quadriparesis, hyperreflexia below C7
Cord segment C8–T1	Below medial arm	Hand weakness and atrophy	Paraparesis and hyperreflexia below C8 and T1
Cord segment T8–10	Below upper abdomen	Weakness of superior rectus abdominus	Paraparesis and hyperreflexia below T10
Cord segment T10–12	Below the umbilicus	Weakness of inferior rectus abdominus	Paraparesis and hyperreflexia below T12
Cord segment L2–3–4	Below hips	Weakness and atrophy of quadriceps and loss of quadriceps reflex	Weakness of extensors and flexors of foot, hyper-reflexia below L2–3–4
Cord segment L5–S1		Weakness and atrophy of extensors and flexors of feet and loss of Achilles reflex	None

the length of the spinal cord to perfuse the anterior and lateral columns. The vascular supply of the posterior one-third comes from two paired posterior spiral arteries. All three arteries arise from radicular arteries that are branches of the vertebral arteries and aorta.

The presence of a sensory level and bilateral upper motor neuron signs with sparing of proprioception represents the anterior two-thirds syndrome. Ischemia from thrombotic and embolic events involving the spinal cord is not as common as cerebral ischemia although the mechanism is the same (thrombosis due to atherosclerosis and nonatherosclerotic conditions such as arteritis or aortic dissection and embolism). Vascular malformation, trauma, and blood dyscrasia are the most common factors in hemorrhagic spinal cord lesions.

Central Cord Syndrome. The central cord syndrome is the result of a lesion which involves decussating fibers of the spinothalamic tract resulting in a "suspended band" of anesthesia with preservation of proprioception (dissociation of sensory loss) (Fig. 61-6D). With expansion of the lesion, the ventral horn is involved, resulting in bilateral segmental weakness, atrophy, and loss of muscle stretch reflexes.

Central cord syndromes are the result of disease pro-

cesses which are intramedullary (intrinsic to cord) and include syringomyelia (cavitation of the cord often associated with congenital anomalies), hematomyelia (hemorrhage into the cord), and intramedullary masses (ependymoma, glioma, or granuloma).

Posterior and Lateral Column Syndrome. Involvement of the dorsal (posterior) columns and lateral columns results in bilateral loss of proprioception and bilateral upper motor neuron signs. The occurrence of this pattern is typical of Vitamin B_{12} deficiency (subacute combined degeneration) and syphilis but can also be associated with other infections (HIV, HTLV-1) and immune-mediated diseases (multiple sclerosis).

Brainstem Syndromes

The spinothalamic tract assumes a lateral position in the medulla, pons, and midbrain on its ascent to the thalamus. The proprioceptive fibers in the dorsal columns cross in the medulla to form the medial lemniscus, which assumes a medial position in the medulla and pons until it assumes a more lateral position ventral to the spinothalamic tract in the midbrain (see Fig. 61-4). At this level and above, a contralateral hemisensory deficit involving face, arm, and leg and all modalities is expected.

Lateral Brainstem Syndrome.   A lesion of the lateral medulla and pons will involve the spinothalamic tract along with the laterally placed spinal tract and nucleus of cranial nerve V. This will result in ipsilateral loss of pain and temperature of the face and contralateral loss of pain and temperature of the limbs (lateral medullary syndrome) as depicted in Fig. 61-6E. The lateral syndrome is commonly associated with ischemic lesions involving the posterior inferior cerebellar artery or the anterior inferior cerebellar artery.

Medial Brainstem Syndrome.   A lesion in the medial medulla and pons will involve the medial lemniscus and result in contralateral loss of proprioception in the limbs. Since the medial lemniscus is near the descending corticospinal fibers, a contralateral hemiparesis also occurs. Depending on mode of onset, the differential diagnosis of medial brainstem syndromes include vascular, infectious, autoimmune, and mass lesions.

Thalamic Syndromes

At the level of the thalamus, all sensory modalities have crossed; therefore, lesions of the thalamus result in contralateral hemisensory abnormalities involving the face, arm, and leg (hemispheric syndrome) as depicted in Fig. 61-6F.

One of the most troublesome disorders, the thalamic pain syndrome (Dejérine-Roussy syndrome), which is excruciatingly painful paresthesias, hyperalgesia, and allodynia involving the contralateral limbs and face. This syndrome generally follows the occurrence of sensory loss from an acute lesion in the posterolateral thalamus. Ischemic or hemorrhagic lesion involving the thalamic perforating branches of the posterior cerebral artery are the most common causes.

Lesions Involving Parietal Lobe

Somatosensory information is analyzed in the parietal lobe, which is essential for localization and determination of the stimulus intensity, shape, size, and texture. Lesions of the parietal lobe may result in astereognosis, agraphesthesia, and extinction as defined earlier in this chapter.

Clinical Examples

1. A 20-year-old woman presented with a 2-year history of brief episodes of numbness of her right foot. The episodes lasted 2–3 minutes and would result in a fall if she were walking. On one occasion, she was noted to have a convulsion which was preceded by a prolonged episode of numbness of her right foot. She had no history of injury or CNS infection and had no risk factors for stroke.

On examination, her strength was normal as were her muscle stretch reflexes. She could appreciate pain, temperature, vibration, and joint movement in all extremities; however, she could not recognize numbers written on her right foot.

Discussion.   The episodes of numbness of the right foot suggest a lesion in the sensory system. As her symptoms involved the right foot, a thorough examination of the sensory system identified agraphesthesia of the right foot which localized the lesion to the left medial parietal cortex, not the peripheral sensory system. The episodic nature of the numbness suggested a localized seizure phenomenon which was further supported by the occurrence of one episode before a convulsion.

The occurrence of a localized seizure phenomenon in a young woman who has a parietal lobe deficit by examination would suggest a focal disease process. In the absence of a prior history of trauma, CNS infection, or ischemia, MRI would be the most appropriate diagnostic tool to evaluate the left parietal lobe for the presence of a mass.

2. A 30-year-old man known to have an Arnold-Chiari malformation (hindbrain anomaly with chronic tonsillar herniation) presented with progressive numbness of the hands which resulted in burns as he could not detect water temperature. This was followed by weakness and wasting of the hands.

On examination, he had anesthesia to pain and temperature of the medial aspect of both arms but proprioception was intact. There was marked atrophy and weakness of the intrinsic muscles of the hands. The muscle stretch reflexes were normal. There were no Babinski signs.

Discussion.   The weakness and atrophy of the hands suggests a lower motor neuron lesion which, combined with a sensory loss which conforms to the C8 dermatome, localizes the lesion to the central cord. While a combined sensory and motor loss could also suggest a lesion of the sensory and motor roots of C8–T1, or the median and ulnar nerves, the symmetry of the problem (which suggests a suspended sensory deficit) and the sensory loss (which spares proprioception: dissociation of sensory deficit) indicate a central cord syndrome.

The progressive nature suggests a mass process, which in this case would be cavitation of the spinal cord (syringomyelia) which is often associated with hindbrain anomalies.

Bibliography

Adams AD and Victor M. Cerebrovascular Diseases. In Adams AD and Victor M (eds.). *Principles of Neurology* (5th ed.), Part IV. St. Louis: McGraw-Hill, 1993, pp. 669–748. *A comprehensive review of the relationship between vascular lesions of the brain and its sensory manifestations.*

Adams AD and Victor M. Diseases of the Spinal Cord. In Adams AD and Victor M (eds.). *Principles of Neurology* (5th ed.), Part V. St. Louis: McGraw-Hill, 1993, pp. 1078–1116. *A comprehensive review of the clinical features of spinal cord diseases relating the clinical manifestations to specific disease processes.*

Adams AD and Victor M. Pain and Other Disorders of Somatic Sensation, Headache, and Backache. In Adams AD and Victor M (eds.). *Principles of Neurology* (5th ed.), Part II, Sec. 2. St. Louis: McGraw-Hill, 1993, pp. 111–196. *A comprehensive review of the pathophysiology of sensory complaints.*

Kandel ER, Schwartz JH, and Jessell TM. Sensory Systems of the Brain: Sensation and Perception. In Kandel ER, Schwartz JH and Jessell TM (eds.). *Principles of Neural Science* (3rd ed.), Part 5. New York: Elsevier, 1991, pp. 329–399. *A comprehensive review of the anatomy and physiology of the sensory pathways.*

62 The Extrapyramidal System

Gary B. Bobele

Objectives

After completing this chapter, you should be able to

Understand the functions of the extrapyramidal system

Develop an understanding of the broad classification of extrapyramidal movement disorders: hypokinetic movement disorders and hyperkinetic movement disorders

Understand clinical characteristics and pathogenesis of hypokinetic movement disorders

Understand clinical characteristics and pathogenesis of hyperkinetic movement disorders

---

The basal ganglia, along with the cerebellum, brain stem motor nuclei, and deep cerebral nuclei, make up the *extrapyramidal motor system*. The purposes of the extrapyramidal system are to maintain posture and tone in the motor system and to organize patterns of voluntary and involuntary movement.

Anatomy and Physiology of Extrapyramidal System

Anatomy of Basal Ganglia

The basal ganglia are part of a group of CNS structures collectively called "the deep cerebral nuclei." The other structures in this loose grouping include thalamic nuclei, substantia nigra, medial and lateral geniculate bodies, claustrum, subthalamic nucleus, and nucleus accumbens. The basal ganglia consist of the caudate nucleus, putamen, and globus pallidus (Fig. 62-1).

Cytologically, the caudate and putamen are identical, with irregularly and densely packed small neurons and large multipolar ("spiny") neurons. The globus pallidus, which appears paler grossly than the putamen because of the large number of myelinated fibers traversing it, consists of a medial and a lateral component, both containing large polygonal neurons with long dendrites.

The striatum (caudate and putamen) receives afferents

from the cerebral cortex, the thalamus, the substantia nigra, and the median raphe nucleus in the brainstem and projects efferents to the globus pallidus and the substantia nigra.

The globus pallidus receives afferents from the corpus striatum and from the medial two-thirds of the subthalamic nucleus. Efferents from the globus pallidus project to the thalamic nuclei, to the subthalamic nucleus, and the substantia nigra.

Physiology of Basal Ganglia

The striatum receives information from the sensory association cortex and from peripheral sensory systems. Information is projected and feedback received from the substantia nigra. The striatum primarily projects to the globus pallidus, which then projects to the thalamus and the brainstem tegmentum and subthalamic nucleus. Thalamocortical fibers project to the motor cortex to modify motor activity initiated in the motor cortex. The motor cortex in turn projects to the brain stem and to the spinal cord. The alpha and gamma motor neurons in the spinal cord terminate on intrafusal and extrafusal muscle fibers. The muscles and tendons, by means of muscle spindles and Golgi tendon organs, convey information about muscle tone, posture, and movement back to the thalamus and sensory association cortex and thus back to the striatum.

This system sets up a feedback loop for the modulation

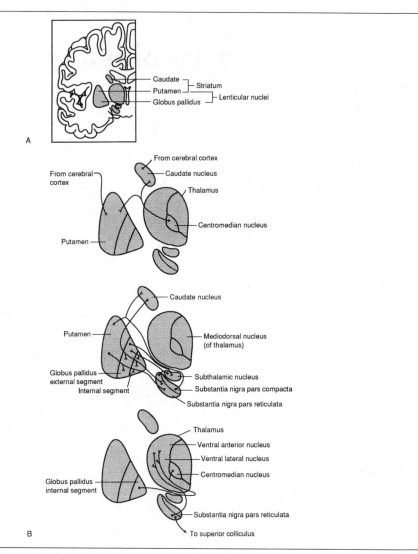

Fig. 62-1. Anatomy of the basal ganglia. A. The caudate and putamen are collectively called the corpus striatum (or simply the striatum) because of the striations in the internal capsule caused by fibers going between the caudate and putamen. The putamen and globus pallidus are collectively referred to as the lenticular nuclei because they physically resemble the shape of a magnifying lens.

The caudate is a long, comet-shaped nucleus whose medial extent is on the lateral border of the lateral ventricle; its lateral boundary is the internal capsule. The globus pallidus is bounded medially by the internal capsule and laterally by the putamen. The putamen is bounded medially by the globus pallidus and laterally by the external capsule. B. Major anatomical connections of the basal ganglia. Afferent connection: The caudate nucleus and putamen receive almost all afferent input to the basal ganglia. Connections among basal ganglia: The internuclear connections include topographically organized connections between all of the nuclei of the basal ganglia. Efferent connections: The principal target of efferent connections from the basal ganglia is the thalamus. (Adapted from: Côté L and Crutcher MD. The basal ganglia. In Kandel ER, Schwartz JH, and Jessell TM (eds.). *Principles of Neural Science.* Norwalk, Conn.: Appleton & Lange, 1991, pp. 649.)

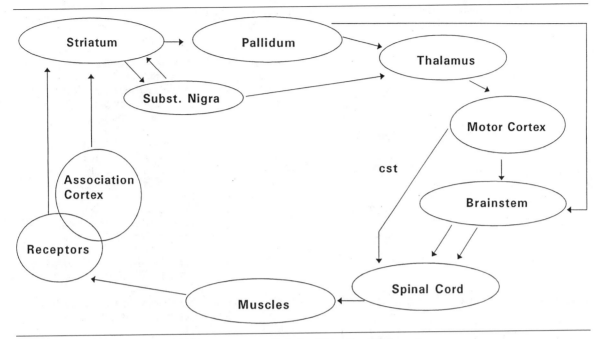

Fig. 62-2. Afferent, efferent, and intrinsic connections of the basal ganglia with the motor system. (Adapted from: Schmidt RF. Motor systems. In Schmidt RF (ed.). *Fundamentals of Neurophysiology.* New York: Springer, 1985, p. 192.)

and monitoring of muscle tone, posture, and position to allow organization of patterns of movement (Fig. 62-2). Input into this feedback system is also received from the prefrontal cortex (for voluntary movement), from the subthalamic nucleus, from the median raphe nuclei, from the cerebellum, and from the reticular activating system.

Afferents to the striatum from the cortex, thalamus, and substantia nigra appear to be excitatory, whereas fibers projecting from the striatum to the substantia nigra and globus pallidus are predominantly inhibitory.

Neurochemistry of Basal Ganglia

Striatal afferents from the substantia nigra appear to be predominantly **dopaminergic.** Afferents from the cerebral cortex to the striatum utilize **glutamate.** Fibers from the median raphe nuclei to the striatum contain **serotonin.** These neurotransmitters are usually **excitatory.** Cholinergic interneurons in the striatum also appear to be excitatory.

The striatal efferents to the globus pallidus contain **gamma-amino-butyric acid (GABA)** as the main transmitter. Striatal efferents to the substantia nigra contain both GABA and **substance P.** These are **inhibitory** neurotransmitters.

The output of the globus pallidus is inhibitory, and it is in turn under inhibition from the striatum. Input into the striatum will excite striatal neurons, which will in turn inhibit pallidal neurons, which are inhibitory on their thalamic and brainstem projections.

Disorders of Extrapyramidal System

Disorders of the basal ganglia and extrapyramidal motor system lead to abnormalities of **tone** (dystonia, rigidity, cogwheeling, gegenhalten, asterixis) and **posture** (flexion of trunk and neck, falling, tilting), **difficulty initiating movement** (bradykinesia, akinesia, hypokinesia, hypomimia, festination), and **involuntary movements** (tremor, chorea, athetosis, tics, and ballismus). The definitions of these various movement disorders are outlined in Table 62-1.

Disorders of the basal ganglia can be divided into two

Table 62-1. Categories and Clinical Characteristics of Extrapyramidal Movement Disorders

Category	Sign	Definition
Disorders of tone	Dystonia	A sustained abnormal posture or abnormal tone from sustained muscle contraction
	Rigidity	Increased muscle tone throughout the range of motion of the muscle ("lead-pipe" rigidity). Occasional lapses in tone can sometimes be felt as the muscle is stretched ("cogwheeling").
	Gegenhalten	Apparent active resistance to passive range of motion when patient has been asked, and is trying, to relax.
	Asterixis	Momentary losses of postural stability and tone, usually seen in the outstretched hands, and usually in the context of a metabolic (such as hepatic) encephalopathy.
Disorders of initiation of movement (hypokinesia)	Hypomimia	Reduced facial expression due to reduced voluntary motor activity to muscles of facial expression ("masked facies").
	Akinesia	Inability to engage in motor activity not due to paralysis or weakness.
	Bradykinesia	Reduced speed of motor activity or reduced ability to initiate and terminate motor activity (inability to terminate gait to come to a stop is a festinating gait).
Disorders of excessive movement (hyperkinesia)	Chorea	Rapid, nonstereotypic, and nonrhythmic, jerky, discrete movements of the muscles of the face, head, trunk, or limbs.
	Athetosis	Slow, writhing, twisting movements of the head, trunk, or limbs, usually around the long axis of the limb or trunk. Usually more pronounced in digits and head and face.
	Tics	Rapid, nonrhythmic but usually stereotypic, jerky, discrete movements of head, face, or limbs. Movements are faster than chorea but usually more limited in distribution (most often involving head, face, or shoulders).
	Myoclonus	Very rapid, "lightninglike" contractions of isolated muscles or muscle groups. A relatively common form is the "sleep jerks" many humans and their canine/feline friends have as they fall asleep.
	Ballismus	Rapid, large, "flinging" movements of limbs in which the motor activity appears to be initially "launched" and then the limb is flying on its own inertia ("ballistic"). Due to a lesion in the contralateral subthalamic nucleus.
	Tremor	Involuntary, rhythmic, oscillating activity which has the same amplitude and velocity in each direction of movement. The activity results from either sequential or simultaneous contraction of agonist and antagonist muscles.

broad categories: the **hyperkinetic** movement disorders and the **hypokinetic** movement disorders, depending on whether excessive movement or reduced movement is the dominant clinical feature. Etiologies associated with these disorders are outlined in Table 62-2.

Parkinson's disease as an example of a hypokinetic disorder and Huntington's disease as an example of a hyper-

kinetic disorder will be discussed. However, it is important to remember that many of the movement disorders overlap, having elements of both hyperkinesis and hypokinesis (such as dystonia and choreatheosis); the above assignment of a particular condition as hyperkinetic or hypokinetic is therefore somewhat arbitrary and is based on the predominant symptoms and signs of each disorder.

Table 62-2. Etiologies Associated with Hypokinetic and Hyperkinetic Movement Disorders

Hypokinetic Movement Disorders	Hyperkinetic Movement Disorders
DEGENERATIVE	**DEGENERATIVE**
Parkinson's disease	Huntington's disease
Parkinsonian syndrome	Senile chorea
Progressive supranuclear palsy (Steele-Richardson- Olszewski syndrome)	**INFECTIOUS**
Striatonigral degeneration	Sydenham's chorea
Dystonia musculorum deformans	Encephalitis
INFECTIOUS	**METABOLIC**
Post-encephalitic parkinsonism	Lafora body disease
METABOLIC	Lesch-Nyhan syndrome
Fahr's syndrome	Neuronal ceroid lipofuscinosis
Hallervorden-Spatz disease	Porphyria
Wilson's disease	Thyrotoxicosis
TOXINS	Wilson's disease
Anoxia	**TOXINS (AND MEDICATION)**
Carbon monoxide poisoning	Anticholinergic drugs
Manganese	Antiepileptic drugs
MPTP poisoning	Dopaminergic drugs
Neuroleptics	Levodopa
Reserpine	Methylphenidate
	Tricyclic antidepressants
	Neuroleptics
	Oral contraceptives
	MPTP
	VASCULAR
	Systemic lupus erythematosis
	Infarction
	Polycythemia rubra vera
	OTHER
	Essential (familial) tremor
	Gilles de la Tourette syndrome
	Paroxysmal choreoathetosis/dystonia

Hypokinetic Movement Disorders

Parkinson's Disease (PD)

This disorder was first described by James Parkinson in 1817 and today remains one of the leading causes of neurologic disability in the elderly. Parkinson's disease has a prevalence of 100–150/100,000 and an incidence of 20/100,000/year. Parkinson's disease usually appears after age 60 but cases as young as 40 have been described. The etiology is unknown but much current opinion and research are directed at the hypothesis that PD is a mitochondrial disorder.

Clinical Features. The clinical features of PD are those of a **tremor** present at rest, described as a "pill-rolling" tremor with a frequency of 4–8 Hz; **rigidity; bradykinesia;** and **postural instability,** characterized by stooped posture and festinating gait (Fig. 62-3). In the early phases of the disorder, symptoms and signs may be relatively nonspecific, such as loss in the volume of the voice, fatigue, and apathy. As the disorder progresses, difficulty with gait or the appearance of the typical tremor is often the first clear indication of PD.

The gait of people with PD shows a variety of abnormalities. They may have hypokinesia and difficulty getting

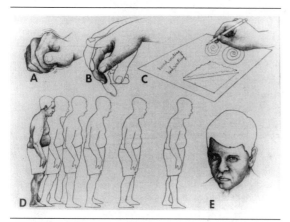

Fig. 62-3. Features of Parkinson's disease. A. The "pill-rolling" tremor. B. Tremor that may become worse with emotional stress. C. Handwriting abnormalities, which include micrographia. D. Typical posture and gait, which becomes faster (festination). E. Lack of facial expression as well as "stare" from decreased blinking. (Reproduced with permission from: Olson WH, Brumback RA, Gascon G, et al. *Handbook of Symptom Oriented Neurology.* Chicago: Year Book Medical Publishers, 1989, p. 97.)

started when starting to walk, with a shuffling of their feet in small steps on initiation of the gait ("marche a petit pas"). Once in motion, it may be difficult for them to stop or change direction, and they may run into walls or furniture (festinating gait). When changing direction, they often turn their whole body as a unit, "en bloc," rather than a fluid turn. At times they may be totally unable to initiate voluntary movement and appear to be "frozen" and immobile due to akinesia. Their posture becomes stooped and the center of gravity is thus moved anteriorly, leading to problems with balance when erect and the tendency for the gait to become propulsive.

The tremor of PD is reasonably distinctive and is the initial symptom in 70% of people with PD. It may begin unilaterally but eventually spreads. It is often the least disabling symptom but the most upsetting to patients because of its visibility. It uncommonly affects the head.

Rigidity of the lead-pipe type, often with cogwheeling, is present in nearly all people with PD. In early stages of PD, the rigidity may only be appreciated by having the contralateral limb perform active movements while the ipsilateral limb is passively moved. Rigidity and the akinesia are the problems producing most of the disability from PD.

Another problem seen with PD is hypokinesia of facial expression, leading to a face that demonstrates little emotional expression and evokes little empathy from others. Eye-blinking frequency is also reduced. Autonomic features such as hyperhidrosis, hypotension, poor bladder and bowel emptying, and thermal paresthesias due to peripheral vasomotor instability are common.

People with PD often become completely disabled in 5 to 10 years after symptom onset, regardless of therapy.

Pathogenesis.   The fundamental pathologic change in PD is the loss of pigmented neurons (which are the dopaminergic neurons projecting to the striatum). There is also loss of pigmented neurons which produce norepinephrine in the locus ceruleus. On gross examination of the midbrain, the substantia nigra appears pale. Loss of these pigmented neurons appears to be a feature of aging and normally progresses at a slow but linear rate. The rate of loss of these neurons appears to be accelerated in PD. In animal experiments, the greater the loss of neurons in the substantia nigra, the lower the concentration of dopamine in the striatum and the more severe the clinical features of Parkinsonism. The cause of this neuronal loss in humans remains unknown.

Treatment.   Pharmacologic treatment of PD is based on the presumption that most of the symptoms of PD are due to relative deficiency of dopamine in the striatum as compared to cholinergic activity.

Early in the course of PD, anticholinergic medications may be of benefit especially in reducing the symptom of tremor. Appropriate precautions should be taken in those with glaucoma, prostatic hypertrophy, or other conditions which might be affected by anticholinergic drugs. Mental confusion may occur with high doses.

Other strategies in treatment of PD involve either the replacement of dopamine or the stimulation of dopamine secretion. L-dopa, given in sufficient quantities, will cross the blood-brain barrier and be active in the central nervous system. Unfortunately, much of this L-dopa will be degraded systemically by dopamine decarboxylase, making the doses required to get adequate levels in the CNS so high that peripheral side effects occur. Consequently, L-dopa is usually given with carbidopa, an analogue that inhibits peripheral dopamine decarboxylase and allows lower doses of L-dopa to be used. Another strategy for elevating dopaminergic activity is the use of bromocriptine, apomorphine, or pergolide, which are dopamine agonists (at D2 receptors) and directly stimulate dopamine receptors in the CNS. Dopaminergic agents are of value in controlling the akinetic and bradykinetic symptoms of PD.

As more becomes known about the different types of dopamine receptors in the CNS, more "tailored" agents for the treatment of PD should become available. It is worth remembering that even with the use of the above agents, PD is a progressive disease; the natural history of the disorder will eventually overwhelm any palliative effect of the above agents on restoring dopaminergic activity.

Other Types of Parkinsonism

Cerebrovascular disease with an infarction in the basal ganglia obliterating the nigrostriatal tract can produce features of PD which are typically unilateral. Additional causes include viral encephalitis (encephalitis lethargica), poisoning by carbon monoxide or manganese, toxicity from MPTP (a byproduct in the manufacture of synthetic meperidine analogues in illicit labs), and anoxia. We usually call these "Parkinsonlike states" or parkinsonian syndrome to distinguish these from idiopathic Parkinson's disease.

Hyperkinetic Movement Disorders

Huntington's Disease (Huntington's Chorea)

Huntington's disease (HD) was probably first described by Charles Waters in 1841 but was not widely recognized until George Huntington published a paper describing several families on Long Island, NY. The prevalence of HD in North America is between 4 and 10 per 100,000. Geographic clusters (such as in Wales and in Lake Maracaibo, Venezuela) are known to occur. HD is an autosomal dominant disorder with complete penetrance.

Clinical Features.   HD is characterized by the occurrence of chorea, dementia, and personality disturbance. The clinical features can occur in any order, and some patients are followed for some years for a psychiatric disorder before other symptoms appear. The clinical symptoms usually appear at 35–40 years of age, although onset in old age or adolescence is not uncommon.

The dementia presents with memory loss (particularly antegrade), slowed mental processing, apathy, emotional lability, and eventual inattention to personal hygiene. These all reflect a "subcortical" type of dementia. The personality disturbances seen in people with HD are manifested by easy irritability ("short temper"), impulsiveness, depression, violence, and psychosis. A history of infractions of the law early in the course of HD is not unusual. As the disease progresses, these personality disturbances may require institutionalization, as might the dementia and the chorea. The chorea in HD may be of any grade of severity

and may affect any part of the body. The chorea may increase in severity early in the course of disease and then plateau in severity. Like most movement disorders, the chorea of HD disappears during sleep. Other motor disturbances, such as rigidity, dystonia, bradykinesia, akinesia, and impaired ocular saccades are common in HD. Other features of HD include dysphagia, dysarthria, cachexia, disturbed sleep, epilepsy, and incontinence. In children and adolescents with HD, rigidity and epilepsy appear to dominate the clinical picture rather than chorea and dementia. Regardless of the age of onset, HD appears to run a progressive course of debilitation and dementia leading to death approximately 15 years from the time of symptom onset.

Pathogenesis.   The fundamental pathologic change seen in the central nervous system in people with HD is atrophy of the caudate nucleus and, to a similar extent, the putamen. This leads to compensatory dilation of the lateral ventricles ("box-car" ventricles), which can be seen on neuroimaging studies. Much of the neuronal loss appears to be of the spiny neurons in the striatum, which are the GABA-ergic (inhibitory) efferent neurons from the striatum. Thus there is atrophy of the striatopallidal and striatonigral tracts. Diffuse cerebral atrophy and loss of neurons in layer 3 of the cortex also occur.

HD is an autosomal dominant disorder with complete penetrance. Thus an individual who inherits the gene is doomed to get the disorder. The genetic defect causing HD has been localized to the short arm of chromosome 4. DNA probes adjacent to this site, and linked to it, have been used to ascertain the status of offspring of affected people to aid in genetic counseling, although some ethical problems have surfaced with this practice (some people, on being told they had inherited the gene, have committed suicide).

In 1993, the underlying defect causing HD was found to be an expanded trinucleotide repeat sequence, similar to the defect in myotonic dystrophy and spinobulbar atrophy. The exact mechanism by which this impairs transcription and the protein product which is affected in HD have not yet been identified.

Clinical Management.   Much of the management of HD is supportive, with institutionalization when appropriate, family and genetic counseling, and home health care. Pharmacologic agents can be of benefit in controlling the chorea, especially early in the course. The most useful drugs are those which are dopamine antagonists such as the phenothiazines, haloperidol, pimozide (not an approved use), reserpine, and tetrabenazine. Benzodiazepines may be of use in controlling agitation and aiding sleep, both of which will reduce chorea. Antidepressants are sometimes necessary to treat concomitant personality disorders and depression.

Other Movement Disorders

Essential Tremor

There are three basic types of tremor: cerebellar, Parkinson, and essential. Table 62-3 illustrates the differentiation among these three tremors according to clinical features of each. Parkinsonism has been discussed earlier and cerebellar tremor is covered in Chap. 63. Essential tremor is the most common of the three. This disorder usually presents in the adult years with a symmetric, slow tremor (2–8 Hz) in the upper limbs. It is very common for essential tremor to involve the head. When the disorder affects the lower limbs, a tremor while standing can be seen (orthostatic tremor). When essential tremor presents after age 60, it is called senile tremor. Patients with essential tremor often report improvement of the tremor for several hours after drinking alcoholic beverages. Essential tremor is usually inherited in an autosomal dominant fashion; when a positive family history can be elicited, the term "familial tremor" is appropriate. Essential tremor is one of the more common movement disorders and in its severe form can be disabling. There is an increased incidence of PD in individuals with essential tremor, but it is unclear whether essential tremor is a precursor to or precipitator of PD. The tremor is ameliorated by ethanol and can be treated with propranolol, primidone, or valproic acid. However, these drugs are effective in only half of patients with essential tremor.

Table 62-3. Clinical Features of the Different Tremors

Feature	Parkinson	Cerebellar	Essential
Present at rest	Yes	No	Yes
Tone	Increased	Decreased	Normal
Abnormal posture	Yes	Yes	No
Head involvement	Occasionally	Yes	Yes
Intentional components	No	Yes	Yes
Incoordination	No	Yes	No

Used with permission from: Olson WH, Brumback RA, Gascon G, et al. *Handbook of Symptom Oriented Neurology.* Chicago: Year Book Medical Publishers, 1989, p. 95.

Gilles de la Tourette Syndrome

This syndrome is a chronic movement disorder presenting in early childhood with tics and outbursts of noises (usually grunts, sniffing, barking, or other sounds but there may be vocal utterances which can in some cases be obscene). Compulsive behaviors, learning disabilities, and attention deficit disorder are also frequently seen in this disorder, and these problems as well as a history of tics can often be found in close relatives. The tics can be functionally disabling when severe and may also lead to social ostracization. The comorbid problems of learning disabilities and attention deficit disorder are a cause of significant academic difficulty for the child in school. Treatment is with dopamine antagonists such as haloperidol or pimozide or with clonidine. Behavioral management, psychotherapy, supplemental academic tutoring, and family support may be needed in an individual situation.

Wilson's Disease (Hepatolenticular Degeneration)

This is a disorder of copper metabolism, leading to copper deposition in the hepatocytes of the liver and in the basal ganglia and other gray matter. The abnormality appears to be an ineffective binding of intestinally absorbed copper to serum ceruloplasmin in the liver. Wilson's disease is autosomal recessive and the locus is on chromosome 13. The clinical features begin in childhood and consist of dystonias, rigidity, involuntary "wing-beating" movements, psychiatric disturbances, deposition of copper in Descemet's membrane of the cornea (Kayser-Fleischer ring), hepatic disease, and hemolytic anemia. Specific therapy is aimed at leaching the copper out of tissues with chelating agents such as D-penicillamine. About 50% of patients with neurologic involvement will respond well to such therapy.

Sydenham's Chorea (St. Vitus' Dance)

An unusual movement disorder characterized by the acute appearance of chorea following streptococcal infection (usually pharyngitis), Sydenham's chorea typically occurs in the school-age child and there is no sex predilection. Many of the children affected will also have other manifestations of rheumatic fever. (Chorea is one of the major Jones criteria for the diagnosis of acute rheumatic fever.) The chorea is self-limited and symptoms usually abate within 2 or 3 months after onset but may recur months or years later. The chorea can be managed with sedating drugs such as benzodiazepines or barbiturates plus dopamine antagonist agents such as haloperidol or phenothiazines.

Tardive Dyskinesia

This is an iatrogenic movement disorder produced by the long-term use of phenothiazines or butyrophenones. The abnormal involuntary movements typically involve the face and mouth, producing chewing, grimacing, and tongue protrusion. Tardive dyskinesia usually occurs as a delayed (hence "tardive") side effect of the use of neuroleptic medications and may not be apparent until the dosage of medication is reduced or discontinued. Tardive dyskinesia is more common in elderly patients and more common with high-dose or long-duration treatment with the offending agents. Affected patients may also exhibit akathisia, rocking the body forward and backward when seated, or walking in place when standing. Unlike some of the acute extrapyramidal side effects of antipsychotic agents, tardive dyskinesia may be permanent. Elimination of neuroleptic agents may reduce symptoms and the use of reserpine to deplete dopamine from dopaminergic nerve endings may also be helpful.

Clinical Examples

1. A 69-year-old man was brought for evaluation by his wife, who reported he was "having trouble getting around." She reported that he has been having trouble walking and "could not get going." He was apt to run into things when walking and appeared to be unable to stop. He had shaking of his right hand for about 7 months, chronic constipation for about a year, and trouble sleeping for about 6 months.

On examination, the patient had a stooped posture and very little spontaneous movement. At rest, there was a rhythmic shaking of the right hand at about 6 Hz. There was resistance to movement of all limbs to passive range of motion but more obviously on the right, and the resistance did not appear to change through the excursion of the joint. When asked to ambulate, the patient began with small-excursion steps and took several seconds to achieve a more normal gait and gait velocity. When asked to turn suddenly while walking, the patient began to turn his whole body as a unit and then lost his balance and fell.

Discussion.   The abnormalities of posture and tone, the difficulty initiating movement, and the presence of involuntary movements (tremor) suggest a lesion in the basal ganglia.

The lack of spontaneous movement in the patient points to the presence of a hypokinetic movement disorder, which could result from a lack of inhibitory input from the striatum to the globus pallidus (GABA-ergic) or from a lack of excitation of the striatum by projections from the substan-

tia nigra (dopaminergic), cerebral cortex (glutaminergic), or median raphe (serotoninergic).

The most likely cause is Parkinson's disease. Other considerations should include parkinsonian syndrome from infarcts of the basal ganglia due to cerebrovascular disease, post-encephalitic parkinsonism, or the residua of carbon monoxide poisoning or anoxia. It seems unlikely that this elderly gentleman has been using designer drugs and has MPTP poisoning.

2. A 45-year-old woman was sent for evaluation by her psychologist. The woman's son related that his mother had "been getting weird." She had become forgetful, was easily angered, and was becoming isolated from her family and friends. She was sent to a psychologist after being arrested for shoplifting; she had no prior problems with the law and had the money in her purse to pay for the items she took. The woman's father died in a mental institution at age 60.

On examination, the patient had a flat affect, was somewhat unkempt (her hair is not combed and there is dirt under her fingernails), and took longer than usual to answer questions or execute commands. She was unable to do simple arithmetic in her head. When observed at rest, fine, rapid, irregular twitches of the corners of her eyes and mouth as well as of her outstretched hands were seen. When asked to visually track, the eyes followed jerkily after the moving target rather than displaying a smooth pursuit.

Discussion.   The presence of involuntary movements suggests a disorder in the basal ganglia. In addition, the findings of slowed mental processing, flat affect, and inattention to personal hygiene suggest a coexisting dementia of the subcortical type.

The involuntary movements suggest a hyperkinetic movement disorder. The age of the patient and combination of involuntary, chorealike movements, dementia, and personality change strongly suggest the possibility of Huntington's disease. The hospitalization of her father in a mental institution is supportive, but further details of his illness would be needed. Although uncommon at her age, Sydenham's chorea can occur in adults. A history of treatment with neuroleptic medications should be sought to ensure that the problem is not a thought disorder now presenting with a complication of treatment (tardive dyskinesia). A history of current oral contraceptive use or other medications should also be sought. The eyes should be carefully examined for the presence of Kayser-Fleischer rings, which would suggest Wilson's disease. The presence of a rash over the malar regions or a history of hematuria might suggest a collagen-vascular disorder such as systemic lupus, which can also cause chorea.

3. A 10-year-old boy was sent by his school principal for being disruptive in class. According to the note sent by his teacher, the boy was constantly making faces at the other children and squirming and fidgeting in his chair. This had been going on since school began 4 months ago, but similar behaviors had been noted by his second- and third-grade teachers. He also had been taking things that did not belong to him. The problems escalated 2 months ago when he began repeatedly clearing his throat or burping in class, to the amusement of his classmates. The teacher had disciplined him for this "attention-seeking behavior" to no avail.

Examination was perfectly normal except that, during portions of the interview and examination, the child was noted to close his eyes in a forceful fashion for one to two seconds and, when holding his fingers outstretched, he had faint flickering movements of the digits.

Discussion.   The presence of involuntary movements suggests a lesion in the basal ganglia. The involuntary movements suggest a hyperkinetic movement disorder.

The combination of involuntary movements (tics) and vocal utterances (in this case, clearing the throat and eructating) suggests the probable diagnosis of Tourette's syndrome. Other possibilities to consider in this child are Sydenham's chorea, hyperthyroidism, and Wilson's disease. Vocal manifestations in these disorders is unusual. The child might be taking neuroleptic medication surreptitiously. If there were a family history, the child might have Huntington's disease of juvenile onset.

Bibliography

Carpenter MB and Sutin J. *Human Neuroanatomy* (8th ed.). Baltimore: Williams and Wilkins, 1983, pp. 579–611. *An authoritative, comprehensive, and detailed review of the anatomy of the basal ganglia.*

Fahn S. In Rowland LP (ed.). *Merritt's Textbook of Neurology* (8th ed.). Philadelphia: Lea & Febiger, 1989, pp. 48–50. *One of the definitive texts on clinical neurology. This chapter provides an overview of involuntary movements.*

Harper PS (ed.). *Huntington's Disease.* Philadelphia: Saunders, 1991. *A comprehensive monograph reviewing the history, epidemiology, clinical features, genetics, and management of Huntington's disease.*

Nutt JG, Hammerstad JP, and Gancher ST. *Parkinson's Disease: 100 Maxims.* St. Louis: Mosby Year Book, 1992. *A review of various aspects of Parkinson's disease, presented as a series of "clinical pearls." More useful for the somewhat experienced clinician.*

Olson WH, Brumback RA, Gascon G, and Iyer V. *Symptom Oriented Neurology.* Chicago: Year Book Medical Publishers, 1989, pp. 92–109. *A well-written and well-illustrated introduction to clinical neurology.*

Schmidt RF. *Fundamentals of Neurophysiology* (3rd ed.). New York: Springer, 1985, pp. 155–200. *A broad overview of concepts of physiologic organization of extrapyramidal motor control, with an emphasis on feedback mechanisms.*

Yahr MD. In Rowland LP (ed.). *Merritt's Textbook of Neurology* (8th ed.). Philadelphia: Lea & Febiger, 1989, pp. 658–671. *A comprehensive review of Parkinson's disease and Parkinson-like syndromes, emphasizing clinical features and discussing pathology and management.*

63 The Cerebellar System

Sanford Schneider

Objectives

After completing this chapter, you should be able to

Understand the anatomic organization of the cerebellum

Understand the function of the cerebellum

Develop concepts regarding clinicoanatomic localization of lesions involving the cerebellum

Develop concepts regarding diseases which involve the cerebellum

---

Motor movements are regulated and coordinated by the cerebellum. The cerebellum receives afferents from the special sensory system (vestibular, auditory, visual), somatosensory system and motor system. Cerebellar output is directed towards the motor cortex, the axial motor neurons and the vestibular nuclei. The cerebellum coordinates the smooth and continuous execution of motor movements and truncal (axial) balance. Cerebellar failure results in primarily three dysfunctions: (1) loss of equilibrium, stance, and balance, (2) ataxia (incoordination) of volitional movement, and (3) decrease in muscle tone (hypotonia).

Anatomy

The cerebellum ("little brain"), a rotund structure the size of a navel orange, resides in the skull's posterior fossa and is separated from the cortex by an incomplete tough fibrous membrane, the tentorium. The cerebellum comprises 10% of the brain's volume but 50% of its neurons.

The cerebellum consists of two paired hemispheres each divided into three lobes (Fig. 63-1). A large fissure divides each hemisphere into a smaller anterior lobe and a posterior lobe. The posterior lateral fissure, nearly hidden from direct view, separates a small flocculonodular from the posterior lobe. The inferior portion of the posterior lobes are known as the cerebellar tonsils. Following massive brain swelling the tonsils can herniate through the foramen magnum producing an acute syndrome of increased intracranial pressure and brain stem compression (tonsillar herniation).

Interposed between the hemispheres is the midline vermis, while deep within the hemispheres are paired gray matter structures, the dentate, globus, and fastigial nuclei. The input of the cerebellum is through the paired inferior and middle cerebellar peduncles and the output is through the superior cerebellar peduncles (Table 63-1).

The vascular supply to the cerebellum is via paired posterior inferior cerebellar arteries and the paired circumferential branches of the basilar artery (anterior inferior cerebellar arteries, superior cerebellar arteries).

The cerebellar cortex contains five cell types (Purkinje, Golgi, stellate, basket, and granule cells) which are organized in three layers: granular layer, Purkinje cell layer, and molecular cell layer. Input to the cerebellar cortex is from two projection systems which are excitatory (mossy fiber system and climbing fiber system) to the cerebellar cortex and deep cerebellar nuclei (Fig. 63-2). Output of the cerebellar cortex is inhibitory through synapses formed between the Purkinje cell and the deep cerebellar nuclei.

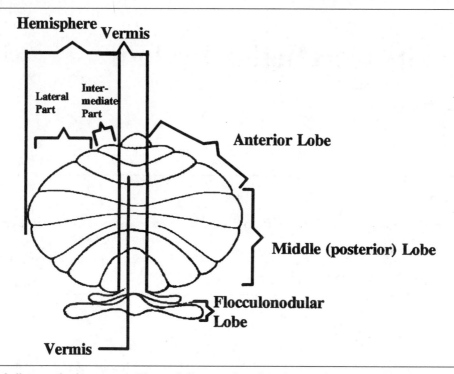

Fig. 63-1. Cerebellar organization anatomy. The cerebellum consists of the flocculonodular lobe, the vermis, and the lateral hemisphere.

Table 63-1. Cerebellar Pathways and Function

Cerebellar Region	Input	Output	Function
Medial			
Flocculonodular	Vestibular	Axial motor neurons	Balance and trunk control
Vermis	Vestibular system	Vestibular system	Trunk and proximal limb coordination
	Visual system	Reticular formation	
	Auditory system	Motor cortex	
	Trigeminal system		
Intermedial portions	Spinal afferents	Red nucleus	Fine motor coordination
of hemisphere		Motor cortex	
Lateral hemisphere	Cerebellar cortex	Red nucleus	Modulate limb coordination
		Premotor cortex	

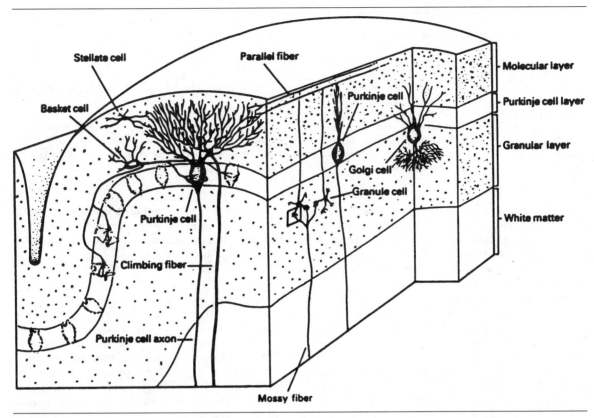

Fig. 63-2. The cerebellar cortex is organized into three layers and contains five types of neurons. This vertical section of a single cerebellar folium, in both longitudinal and transverse planes, illustrates the general organization of the cerebellar cortex. Mossy fibers arise from the spinal cord (dorsal and ventral spinocerebellar) and brainstem nuclei (vestibular, reticular, and pontine) to terminate in the granular cell layer. The granule cells (excitatory neurons) send axons into the molecular layer to form excitatory synapses on dendrites of the Purkinje cells and also synapse on interneurons in the molecular layer (basket cells, golgi cells, and stellate cells). These interneurons form inhibitory synapses with either the Purkinje cells or granule cells. The other excitatory input is from the inferior olive and is designated as the climbing fiber system which terminate on Purkinje cells. The Purkinje cell is the primary output of the cerebellum, which sends axons to the deep nuclei of the cerebellum where inhibitory synapses are formed. (Used with permission from: Ghez C. The cerebellum. Kandel ER, Schwartz JH, Jessell TM (eds.) *Principles of Neural Science* (3rd ed.). New York: Elsevier, 1991, p. 630.)

Assessment of Cerebellar Function

This is accomplished by examination of the fluidity and quality of motor movements. The quality of cerebellar function is established by careful and systematic observation of organized motor activity. Cerebellar deficits can be mimicked by sensory deficits involving the proprioceptive system (large myelinated nerve fibers, posterior columns and medial lemniscus), weakness and vestibular dysfunction. The clinical features and signs of cerebellar lesions are summarized in Table 63-2, but in general represent excess of movement as demonstrated by dysmetria, intention tremor, loss of control of axial muscles (titubations), and hypotonia.

Table 63-2. Clinical Features and Signs of Cerebellar Lesions

Symptom	Clinical Evaluation
Ataxia	Irregularly performed motor actions
Gait ataxia	Wide-based unsteady gait
Dysmetria	Inability to smoothly pursue object by reach. Examine by asking the subject to touch finger to nose or heel to shin.
Intention (action) tremor	Involuntary upper extremity tremor intensified by voluntary movement
Dysdiadochokinesia	Decomposition of smooth rapid alternations during forearm supination and pronation
Hypotonia	Reduced resistance to passive movement of limbs
Titubation	Inability to maintain truncal control resulting in continuous involuntary attempts to correct axial posture

Afferents to the vermis and flocculonodular lobe are from the brain stem and spinal cord and efferents ascend to the cerebral cortex, and descend in the vestibulospinal and reticulospinal tracts. As such, the predominant function of this system is for involuntary control of balance. The intermediate zone efferents are from the ipsilateral descending rubrospinal tracts. The function of this system is fine motor coordination of ipsilateral limb. The lateral cerebellar hemisphere whose afferents are from the corticopontine fibers and feeds back to the cerebral cortex to modulate limb coordination.

Although cerebellar connections are complex they can be simplified for practical purposes (Table 63-3). Deficits to midline cerebellar structures appear as midline loss of truncal balance (titubation), widening of gait (ataxia), and lateral gaze nystagmus. Midzone dysfunction causes dysmetria (past pointing) and intention tremor. Damage to either system can cause hypotonia. Alteration of the lateral cerebellar hemispheres distorts motor coordination and timing (dysdiadochokinesia and synkinesia).

Cerebellar hemisphere lesions produce ipsilateral deficits due to the crossing output of the superior cerebellar peduncle and the recrossing of the higher cortical pathways returning to the *same* side as the lesion.

Table 63-3. Pattern of Clinical Signs Associated with Cerebellar Lesion

Site of Lesion	Pattern of Deficit
Midline cerebellar lesion	Gait ataxia
	Truncal imbalance
	Hypotonia
Hemispheric cerebellar lesion	Limb ataxia
	Loss of fine motor control

In summary, midline cerebellar lesions produce titubation, ataxia, nystagmus, and hypotonia; lateral lesions produce past pointing, intention tremor, and coordinative dysfunction on the *same* side as the lesion.

Disorders of Cerebellum

Disease states originating in the cerebellum have etiologies similar to other regions of the central nervous system. Characterization includes vascular, neoplastic, degenerative (genetic or acquired), demyelinating, or embryonic malformation. The site of origin, midline or hemispheric, frequently separates these disorders into typical presentation syndromes.

Lateral (Hemispheric) Cerebellar Disorders

Vascular

Arterial blood supply can be interrupted by embolus, thrombus, or hemorrhage. Ischemia in the distribution of anterior inferior cerebellar artery or posterior inferior cerebellar artery results in ipsilateral ataxia, from involvement of the cerebellar peduncle, crossed sensory deficit from involvement of the lateral brainstem and variable dysfunction involving the nuclei of cranial nerves VIII, IX, and X. Cerebellar infarction or hemorrhage can be difficult to recognize clinically as symptoms are non-specific (acute onset dizziness, poor balance, nausea, and headache) and may not be associated with the classic ipsilateral ataxia one would expect. The importance of early recognition of cerebellar infarction or hemorrhage is that it may be followed by cerebellar edema and ultimately tonsillar herniation.

Demyelinating Disorders

Include those disorders in which there is reduced or abnormal production of myelin (leukodystrophies) and immunologic or infectious diseases which involve the destruction of myelin.

Multiple Sclerosis.   MS is a recurrent, relapsing, and occasionally remitting disorder which may be confined to the white matter of cerebellum. MS may present either acutely or subacutely with the onset of limb ataxia and loss of balance which reflects demyelination of cerebellar white matter. The disease is diagnosed by the clinical documentation of symptoms with signs which represent multiple white matter lesions and a course which reflects exacerbation and remissions of the lesions.

Acute Disseminated Encephalomyelitis.   This is an uncommon disorder of children that presents acutely as a diffuse cerebellar demyelinating syndrome several weeks after a viral illness, especially varicella (chicken pox).

Neoplasia

Primary neoplastic disease of the pons or cerebellum can occur at any age. Tumors affect the nervous system either by tissue destruction or by enlarging to a size which disrupts spinal fluid mechanics resulting in increased intracranial pressure. The most common cerebellar hemispheric tumor is the cerebellar astrocytoma which usually presents insidiously with minimal cerebellar dysfunction before the onset of acute hydrocephalus.

Midline Cerebellar Disorders

Midline cerebellar disorders are characterized by gait ataxia and titubation. In general, metabolic disorders, toxic exposures and midline tumors are the primary causes of midline dysfunction.

Toxic Exposures

Alcoholic cerebellar degeneration is believed to result from the toxic effects of ethanol and associated thiamine deficiency. Cerebellar manifestations include the gradual development of ataxia of gait, truncal titubation, and leg ataxia. This is frequently accompanied by a sensorimotor polyneuropathy. Pathologic changes in the cerebellum consist of selective Purkinje cell destruction as well as diffuse degeneration.

Neoplasia

Neoplasms that arise in the midline cerebellar structures disrupt the efferent output. The most frequent midline tumor of childhood is a **primary neuroectodermal tumor (PNECT),** formerly known as a medulloblastoma, which produces gait ataxia often associated with increased intracranial pressure.

Brainstem gliomas tend to simultaneously interrupt cerebellar outflow, descending corticospinal tract(s), and cranial nerve nuclei (usually seventh) producing progressive weakness, hyperreflexia; Babinski sign (corticospinal); facial lower motor neuron weakness (seventh nerve); and gait ataxia (cerebellar).

Other Disorders Involving the Cerebellum

Cerebellar Malformations

Malformations which represent failure of normal embryogenesis of the posterior fossa can result in several syndromes that are compatible with long-term survival.

Arnold-Chiari Malformation.   This consists of four different entities (Types I, II, III, IV). Type I is a "low-lying" cerebellar medullary malformation with the cerebellar tonsils below the foramen magnum. If the defect is associated with meningomyelocele and hydrocephalus it is classified as Type II. (Type III is an occipital/cervical encephalocele and Type IV is cerebellar/brainstem hypoplasia). When the anomaly is expressed with meningomyelocele or encephalocele, the diagnosis is made by observation. When occult, the anomaly may present with progressive dysfunction of the medulla (dysphagia, dysarthria, and stridor), ataxia, and pyramidal dysfunction (spasticity and weakness) which localizes to the cervicomedullary junction.

Dandy-Walker Cyst.   This is due to partial failure of midline cerebellar fusion resulting in a posterior fossa cyst which usually communicates with the fourth ventricle. Clinical presentation is usually a combination of a large head, ataxia, and occasionally, increased intracranial pressure.

Hereditary Disorders

Ataxia is a prominent feature of many hereditary disorders designated as spinocerebellar atrophies, olivopontocerebellar atrophies, ataxic myoclonus, and cerebellar atrophies which involve degeneration of spinal cord, brainstem, and/or the cerebellum. These disorders are inherited and characterized by progressive ataxia as the most notable clinical feature.

Spinocerebellar Atrophies.   These are disorders associated with ataxia, areflexia, and hypotonia. Seven genotypes (similar phenotypes) are presently known. The most common example of progressive ataxia is **Friedreich's ataxia,** which initially presents before puberty with progressive ataxia, dysarthria, loss of proprioception, and loss of deep tendon reflexes usually accompanied by skeletal abnormalities (scoliosis, hammer toes) and cardiomyopathy. Although commonly discussed as a cerebellar disorder, ataxia is due to loss of proprioception from involvement of the dorsal root, dorsal root ganglion, and dorsal column.

Olivopontocerebellar Atrophies. These are disorders which present with progressive ataxia associated with extrapyramidal and pyramidal findings. In some cases, autonomic dysfunction is a prominent feature. The most constant pathologic features are atrophy of the inferior olive, basis pontis, and cerebellum.

Ataxic Myoclonias. These are a group of inherited disorders characterized by progressive ataxia and myoclonus. However, similar presentations can be seen with metabolic and mitochondrial disorders.

Cerebellar Atrophies. They are characterized by progressive ataxia without involvement of other neural systems. As with ataxic myoclonias, metabolic and toxic disorders, particularly remote effects of carcinoma and alcoholic cerebellar degeneration must be considered.

Clinical Examples

1. A 6-year-old boy was noted by his teacher to have progressive difficulty while running. He was described as awkward when he walked and fell excessively on the playground. The symptoms have been noted for 2 months and have become progressively worse. Neurologic examination demonstrated mild weakness of the entire left side of his face, a right Babinski sign, a wide-based gait, and awkwardness in changing direction while running.

Discussion. The combination of ataxia of gait, right lower motor neuron, seventh nerve paresis, and corticospinal tract dysfunction (left Babinski sign) would place the lesion in the right side of the pons at the level of the seventh nerve nucleus disrupting the descending corticospinal tract (which will cross in the medulla) and the crossing pontocerebellar fibers.

The symptoms have progressed over several months which suggests an infiltrating mass. The most likely diagnosis is a brainstem glioma.

Visualization of the pons by MRI would be the most appropriate test to confirm the diagnosis. Brain biopsy may not be possible because of the location of the lesion. The child would then be treated with radiation therapy (infants less than 4 years old are usually treated with chemotherapy because of risk of long term radiation damage to the developing nervous system).

2. A 20-year-old woman presented with the onset of poor coordination of her left limbs which developed insidiously over 3 days and has persisted for one week. She reported a previous episode of blindness in her left eye 2 years ago which resolved over 6 months to normal vision. On examination, she had dysmetria of the left limbs, but no weakness or sensory loss. Cranial nerve exam revealed no abnormalities.

Discussion. The left dysmetria suggests a disease process in the left cerebellar hemisphere. The subacute onset of symptoms over several days, combined with a prior history suggesting an optic nerve lesion (monocular blindness), would suggest a demyelinating disorder. Vascular, infectious, and mass lesions would also be considered in this case but the most likely etiology is multiple sclerosis.

Bibliography

Adams RD and Victor M. *Principles of Neurology* (5th ed.). New York: McGraw-Hill, 1993, pp. 74–82; pp. 669–748. *A clinical text emphasizing pathophysiology.*

Kandel ER, Schwartz JH, and Jessell TM (eds.). *Principles of Neural Science* (3rd ed.). New York: Elsevier, 1991, pp. 626–646; pp. 711–730. *An excellent and highly recommended comprehensive review of neurophysiology and the mechanisms of neurologic dysfunction.*

64 The Special Senses and Oculomotor System

Bradley K. Farris, Keith F. Clark, and Gary W. Harris

Objectives

After completing this chapter, you should be able to

Develop an understanding of the anatomy of the visual and oculomotor systems and the auditory and vestibular systems

Assess the function of the visual, oculomotor, auditory, and vestibular systems

Develop concepts regarding localization of lesions which involve the visual, oculomotor, auditory, and vestibular systems

Develop concepts concerning the pathophysiologic mechanisms which result in lesions of the visual, oculomotor, auditory, and vestibular systems

---

The special senses are essential for accurate perception of our environment. In addition, the special senses interact with other systems to provide information which is important for optimal arousal, meaningful cognition, and precise behavioral and motor responses.

Anatomy and Physiology

Visual System

The Eye

The human adult eye is almost spherical with a diameter of about 25 mm. Myopic (near-sighted) eyes tend to be longer than hyperopic (far-sighted) eyes. The eye functions to gather light and convert light energy to an electrical current which is transmitted through the optic nerves and visual pathways to the visual cortex of the occipital lobes where electrical signals are interpreted as vision. Light rays entering the eye pass through the cornea, anterior chamber, lens, vitreous, and sensory retina. The central ray of light (axial ray) passes through the refractive media of the eye undeviated while the other rays are refracted varying amounts. In the normal eye, the central rays focus at a single point on the retina. Glasses and/or contact lenses help to focus the light in myopic or hyperopic eyes. The cornea is the strongest refracting surface, followed by the lens.

The cornea is the clear, front surface of the eye which is moist and crystal clear. Light rays pass through the cornea and anterior chamber and enter the crystalline lens, a clear, biconvex structure that measures about 10 mm in diameter and 4 mm in thickness at the center. The light rays then pass through the clear vitreous body which fills the cavity of the eye, and are received by the retina.

The retina is composed of a pigment epithelial layer which absorbs light after it has passed through the entire sensory retinal layer. The layers, from anterior (inside) to posterior (outside) are (1) inner limiting membrane, (2) nerve fiber layer (axons of the ganglion cells), (3) ganglion cell layer, (4) inner plexiform layer, (5) inner nuclear layer, (6) outer plexiform layer, (7) outer nuclear layer, (8) external limiting membrane, (9) rod and cone layer, and (10) the pigment epithelium. The rods function in low light (scotopic vision) and the cones in bright light (photopic vision). Color vision is a cone function and night vision is a rod function.

The central retina (macula lutea) measures about 6 mm in diameter and lies temporal to the optic nerve head. The macula lutea is characterized by a yellow pigment which is visible by using the "red-free" light of the direct ophthalmoscope. At the very center of the macula lutea lies the fovea centralis and at the center of the fovea centralis lies the foveola. The axial ray and central rays of light focus on the foveola. Only cone receptors are present in the foveola and this area functions for central vision (sharp vision), color vision, and photopic vision.

Optic Nerve, Neural Pathways of Visual System, and Occipital Lobe

The axons of the ganglion cells exit the back of the eye through the ipsilateral optic nerve. The **optic nerves** are divided anatomically into four sections: (1) the intraocular portion, (2) the intraorbital portion, (3) the intracanalicular portion, and (4) the intracranial portion. The two optic nerves join above the pituitary gland to form the **optic chiasm.** The optic chiasm is an important neuro-ophthalmologic structure because the nasal retinal fibers from each eye cross to join the uncrossed temporal retinal fibers of each eye to form each **optic tract.** Fibers from each optic tract enter the ipsilateral **lateral geniculate body** (LGB). Visual fibers from each LGB then pass to the ipsilateral **occipital cortex** through the **optic radiation.** Visual fibers maintain a superior and inferior retinal orientation in the optic nerve and chiasm. Within the optic tract, the superior retinal fibers pass through the parietal lobe of the brain while the inferior retinal fibers pass through the temporal lobe. Visual fibers maintain a superior and inferior retinal orientation in the occipital cortex, the superior retinal fibers terminating above the calcarine fissure and the inferior retinal fibers below the fissure.

Oculomotor System

There are two primary gaze centers which control conjugate movement of eyes as depicted in Fig. 64-1.

Frontal Lobe Gaze Center

Located in each frontal lobe, the center drives the eyes symmetrically to the **contralateral** side.

Brainstem Gaze Center and Medial Longitudinal Fasciculus (MLF)

The second gaze center lies within the pons, specifically the paramedian pontine reticular formation (PPRF). The PPRF controls horizontal gaze to the **ipsilateral side.** The MLF, comprised of myelinated nerve fibers, extends from the pons to the midbrain to interconnect the ipsilateral sixth with the contralateral third nerve nucleus for conjugate gaze.

Cranial Nerves

Oculomotor Nerve (CN III). CN III has **somatic motor fibers** that innervate the ipsilateral superior, medial, and inferior rectus muscles, the ipsilateral inferior oblique muscle, and the ipsilateral levator palpebrae suprioris muscle. The oculomotor nerve also contains **visceral motor fibers** (parasympathetic) to the sphincter pupillae and ciliary muscles. These muscles control constriction of the pupil and accommodation.

The oculomotor nerve nucleus is located in the midbrain at the level of the superior colliculus. Efferent fibers exit the midbrain ventrally, passing between the superior cerebellar and posterior cerebral arteries. CN III passes forward and lies very close to the posterior communicating artery. The nerve enters and passes through the ipsilateral cavernous sinus. CN III divides into a superior division (to innervate the ipsilateral superior rectus and levator superioris muscles) and an inferior division (to innervate the ipsilateral medial rectus, inferior rectus, and inferior oblique muscles) before it enters the orbit through the superior orbital fissure. The parasympathetic visceral motor component to CN III has its origin in the Edinger-Westphal nucleus and courses to the eye along the surface of CN III, following the inferior division to the pupil.

Trochlear Nerve (CN IV). CN IV contains only somatic motor fibers that innervate the contralateral superior oblique muscle. The nucleus is located in the midbrain at the level of the inferior colliculus. Efferent fibers leave the nucleus, decussate within the superior medullary velum, and exit the dorsal midbrain. The nerve courses around the cerebral peduncles, through the ipsilateral cavernous sinus, and enters the orbit through the superior orbital fissure. It is the only cranial nerve that exits the dorsal brainstem and the only cranial nerve in which all of the axons are crossed.

Abducens Nerve (CN VI). CN VI contains only somatic motor fibers that innervate the ipsilateral lateral rectus muscle. The nucleus of CN VI is located in the pons. Efferent fibers leave the brainstem at the pontomedullary junction and pass forward to enter the posterior cavernous sinus. It passes through the cavernous sinus (near the intracavernous portion of the carotid artery) to enter the ipsilateral orbit through the superior orbital fissure.

Auditory System

Our dynamic range for hearing, or range of sound intensities from the lowest sound barely perceived to the loudest sound which is just painful, is 120 decibels. We enjoy a

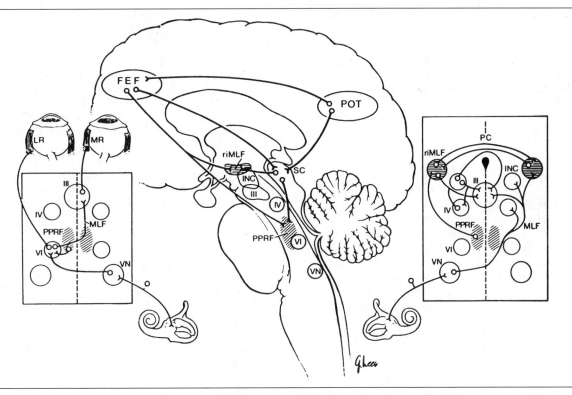

Fig. 64-1. Summary of eye movement control. The center figure shows the supranuclear connections from the frontal eye fields (FEF) and the parieto-occipital-temporal junction (POT) region to the superior colliculus (SC), rostral interstitial nucleus of the medial longitudinal fasciculus (riMLF), and the paramedian pontine reticular formation (PPRF). The FEF and SC are involved in the production of saccades, while the POT is thought to be important in the production of pursuit. The schematic drawing on the left shows the brainstem pathways for horizontal gaze. Axons from the cell bodies located in the PPRF travel to the ipsilateral abducens nucleus (VI), where they synapse with abducens motoneurons whose axons travel to the ipsilateral lateral rectus muscle (LR) and with abducens internuclear neurons whose axons cross midline and travel in the medial longitudinal fasciculus (MLF) to the portion(s) of the oculomotor nucleus (III) concerned with medial rectus (MR) function (in the contralateral eye). The schematic drawing on the right shows the brainstem pathways for vertical gaze. Important structures include the riMLF, PPRF, the interstitial nucleus Cajal (INC), and the posterior commissure (PC). Note that axons from cell bodies located in the vestibular nuclei (VN) travel directly to the abducens nuclei and, most via the MLF, to the oculomotor nuclei. (Used with permission from: Miller NR. *Walsh and Hoyt's Clinical Neuro-Ophthalmology* (4th ed.). Baltimore: Williams and Wilkins, 1985.)

very wide dynamic range of hearing yet, at the same time, we can recognize very small frequency differences across the entire range of frequencies, as measured by Hertz (cycles per second or Hz) and intensities, as measured by the decibel. We are able to hear frequencies as low as 20 Hz up to those near 20,000 Hz but are most sensitive at 4000 Hz.

The decibel scale (dB) is a logarithmic measure of sound intensity or sound pressure. The ratio between sound intensities of painful and barely audible sounds is about 10^{12} or 120 dB (the roar of a crowd at a football game or headphones of a stereo system). During a normal conversation, a 70-dB sound level may be measured. Since the dB scale is logarithmic, one cannot describe a percentage of hearing loss! Our ability to detect, discriminate, and identify sounds requires the structures of the external, middle, and inner ear along with the central nervous system connections.

External Ear

The external portion includes the pinna and ear canal. A blockage due to cerumen (wax) impaction, foreign bodies, or infection (external otitis or swimmer's ear) will result in conductive hearing loss.

Middle Ear

The middle ear allows sound transmission from the air into the fluid of the inner ear. Without the tympanic membrane and ossicles of the middle ear, 99.9% of the sound energy would be reflected from the inner ear fluid. The middle ear is connected to the nasopharynx by the eustachian tube. The middle ear must be air filled in order for sound to vibrate the tympanic membrane and pass sound energy along the ossicles to the inner ear. Poor function or blockage of the eustachian tube leads to a fluid-filled middle ear with a conductive hearing loss, as seen in children with otitis media with effusion or adults with a tumor obstructing the eustachian tube in the nasopharynx.

Tympanic Membrane (TM).   Any hole in the TM can cause a hearing loss. A pantympanic perforation (tympanic membrane missing) causes a significant conductive hearing loss. In this case a small amount of sound is transmitted directly down the exposed malleus. Since the TM is missing, some sound can also travel directly to the stapes footplate and into the inner ear. However, more than 99.9% of the sound reaching the stapes footplate directly through the hole in the TM is reflected, producing a loss of 34 dB.

Ossicles.   The three middle ear ossicles attach the TM to the inner ear. The malleus is connected to the TM, and the incus is between the malleus and the stapes. The stapes completes the ossicular chain with its footplate in the oval window.

The handle of the malleus is 1.3 times longer than the long process of the incus (lever ratio), and the area of the TM is 17 times larger than the area of the stapes footplate (area ratio). The total sound pressure increase from TM to stapes footplate due to the lever and area ratios is over 20-fold or approximately 30 dB. One can appreciate that a 30-dB hearing loss could result if the entire TM were lost.

Immobility of any of the ossicles (traumatic dislocation or otosclerosis) will impair sound conduction. A gradual loss (from chronic middle ear disease) of the portion of the incus which articulates with the head of the stapes will re-

sult in a disconnection of the ossicles and a "maximum conductive hearing loss." The maximum conductive hearing loss possible (60 dB) is produced when the TM is intact (without holes) and the ossicles are disconnected. In this instance, the sound is prevented from reaching the middle ear and is reflected by the TM. Adding a cerumen impaction blocking the external canal or filling the middle ear with fluid will not increase the conductive loss! When the loudness of a sound reaches 60 dB, it begins to vibrate the skull directly and travels through the skull to the inner ear. Once a rock concert reaches a sound level of 60 dB or greater, the music begins to vibrate the skull directly, allowing us to hear the music (and possibly cause noise damage) despite ear plugs.

Stapedius Muscle.   The stapedius muscle (whose nerve supply comes from the facial nerve) attaches to the stapes. Contraction of this muscle provides a sound-dampening mechanism for sounds louder than 90 dB. The acoustic reflex seen during impedance tympanometry is caused by contraction of the stapedius muscle. This reflex is useful in site of lesion testing for facial nerve lesions and diagnosis of an acoustic neuroma. Facial nerve paralysis proximal to the stapedius nerve or an acoustic neuroma (benign tumor) of the eighth nerve can lead to a loss of the stapedius reflex by interfering with stapedius muscle innervation from cranial nerve VII.

Inner Ear

The inner ear contains the cochlea (the hearing end-organ) and the vestibular labyrinth, a group of end-organs specialized for sensation of movement.

The cochlea is a tubelike structure which spirals through two and one-half turns inside the temporal bone. Vibration of the stapes footplate causes movement of the oval window membrane and corresponding fluid waves which travel along the cochlear partition and stimulate cochlear hair cells (receptors).

The turn closest to the stapes footplate is called the basal turn (responsible for high frequencies) and the top of the cochlea is the apex (responsible for low frequencies). This orderly representation of frequency (tonotopic organization) is preserved in the anatomic organization of the central auditory pathways as well. The internal membrane of the cochlea (basilar membrane) is narrow and stiff near the basilar turn (better for high-frequency vibration) and wide and more supple near the apical end (better for low-frequency vibration). Ototoxic drugs (drugs which damage auditory or vestibular neuroepithelium) and very loud sounds are more likely to damage hair cells sitting on the basilar membrane at the basal turn and cause a high-frequency sensorineural hearing loss.

Within the cochlea are three fluid-filled compartments: the scala vestibuli is superior, scala media is in the middle, and scala tympani is lowest. Perilymph, a fluid similar to cerebrospinal fluid, fills the scala vestibuli and scala tympani. Endolymph (which fills the scala media) has a high potassium concentration and a high electrical potential as compared with the perilymph in the other two compartments. This potential is important for depolarization and release of excitatory neurotransmitters by the hair cells of the cochlea. Hearing loss will occur if either of the membranes surrounding the scala media rupture or the perilymph and endolymph are allowed to mix. A perilymphatic fistula may arise during barotrauma (rapid pressure changes from scuba diving or altitude changes when flying) or intense straining when inner ear fluid from the scala vestibuli leaks around the stapes footplate into the middle ear. Patients with this problem experience fluctuating hearing loss and imbalance. Fortunately, these leaks can be patched surgically if discovered.

The organ of Corti lies along the entire length of the basilar membrane. The auditory neuroepithelium of the organ of Corti along with the supporting structures transforms the movement of the inner ear fluids into electrical signals in the auditory nerve. The cilia of the hair cells are key players in hearing. The hair cells are organized in three rows of outer hair cells and one row of inner hair cells. They are bent as the basilar membrane moves up and down. When the cilia of the hair cells are bent, K^+ channels open and ultimately action potentials arise in the afferent neuron. The inner hair cells are actually the "true" receptor cells and receive most of the afferent fibers of the auditory nerve. The cell bodies of these afferent fibers lie in the spiral ganglion. The outer hair cells receive a few afferent fibers but receive all of the efferent fibers. Outer hair cells have been shown to have contractile properties which may allow tuning of the basilar membrane or may change the sensitivity of inner hair cells. The fact that the ototoxic drugs and noise cause damage to the outer hair cells is supportive evidence for the idea that outer hair cell function is important. Noise-induced hearing loss causes clumping and loss of the cilia.

Vestibular System

The vestibular system is largely responsible for stable head positioning, stabilization of the visual image on the retina during head movement, and adjustment of posture during body movements. Much of the work of the vestibular system goes unrecognized by the individual; however, malfunctions in the system can become especially symptomatic. Vestibular symptoms range from a mild queasiness to profuse sweating with violent vomiting and severe hallucinations of movement called vertigo. The person who has labyrinthine hypofunction will feel unsteady and must grab for the wall when walking. Symptoms are worse at night since visual cues are absent. While riding in a car the scenery bounces all around (ossillopsia). If peripheral labyrinths are unequally affected, motion sickness is experienced unless the eyes are closed.

Peripheral Vestibular Apparatus

The vestibular labyrinth consists of the semicircular canals, the utricle, and the saccule. The utricle and saccule are known as the otolith organs. The hair cells (sensory receptor) in the vestibular apparatus (which bond with movement of fluid from head movement) transform movement into electrical activity in much the same way that the cochlea transforms sound.

Semicircular Canals (Angular Accelerometers).

The semicircular canals are stimulated by rotational accelerations of the head. The orientation of the canals in the temporal bone determines how head movement affects endolymph movement and deflection of hair cells. Each of the three canals (lateral, superior, and posterior) has a specific orientation of the cilia relative to the ampullary end of the canal and has specific neural connections to eye muscles. Ampulopetal (toward the ampulla) movement of fluid in the lateral canal causes excitation (stereocilia toward kinocilium) and ampulofugal (away from the ampulla) movement in the other two canals causes excitation. For example, excitation of the lateral (horizontal) canal produces a slow deviation of the eyes away from the affected side by stimulating contraction of the ipsilateral medial rectus and contralateral lateral rectus muscles of the eye. At the same time, the antagonistic muscle is being inhibited.

Each canal produces a tonic neural activity balanced by an opposite tonic activity from the counterpart canal in the opposite ear. If both ears are healthy, there is no eye movement. Almost all labyrinthine disorders produce a weakness of canal function. When one side becomes weak, the tonic activity from the opposite side produces a slow movement of the eyes toward the weak side. Simply remember that the intact lateral canal produces a tonic slow conjugate movement of the eyes away from that side. When the eyes deviate due to weakness of a canal, the reticular formation causes a rapid movement of the eyes in the opposite direction. This slow eye movement followed by a rapid movement in the opposite direction is called **nystagmus.** The direction of nystagmus is defined by the direction of the fast (nonlabyrinthine) component since it is the easiest for an examiner to see. Nystagmus can be horizontal, vertical, or rotatory depending on the labyrinthine canal producing the movement and is considered a sign of vestibular system dysfunction.

A patient with a right acute labyrinthine hypofunction will have a slow deviation of the eyes to the right, toward the weak labyrinth (tonic activity of the normal left side overpowers the weak, right side.) The quick component is to the left so the nystagmus produced is described as left beating. The patient feels the **vertigo** (the hallucination of movement) as movement in the same direction as the slow component, to the right. If asked to stand on one foot with eyes closed, the patient will fall to the right.

Saccule and Utricle (Linear Accelerometers).
The hair cells of the otolith organs, the saccule and utricle, are embedded in a gelatinous substance covered with calcium carbonate particles called otoliths. The utricle and saccule detect maintained tilts of the head. When the head is held tilted, a constant deflection of the gelatinous substance occurs as gravity pulls on the otoliths. Sometimes head trauma causes the otoliths to become dislodged, float away from the utricle, and land on the membrane of the horizontal canal, where they (we think) cause benign positional paroxysmal vertigo. These patients have vertigo usually when rolling over to one side in bed. The vertigo has some latency (delay in onset for less than 10 seconds), reoccurs when the position is assumed again, and is fatigable (becomes less after repeated occurrences).

Central Vestibular Processing and Vestibular Reflexes
Unlike other sensory modalities, there are sparse connections from the vestibular system to the thalamus and the cortex. The major projections from the vestibular system are to the oculomotor system, cerebellum, and spinal cord.

Vestibulo-Ocular Reflex (VOR).
The vestibulo-ocular connections to the abducens, trochlear, and oculomotor extraocular muscle motor nuclei are involved in adjustments of the eyes to head movement detected by the canals. Specific canals are connected through the vestibular nuclei to specific extraocular muscles through the medial longitudinal fasciculus and ascending tract of Deiters. The effect of all of the vestibulo-ocular pathways acting together is to produce compensatory eye movements for any direction of head rotation so that the direction of the gaze does not change.

Other Vestibular Reflexes.
Vestibular connections to the motor (vestibulo-colic reflex) nuclei of the neck muscles provide a system for compensatory adjustments of head position in much the same way as described for the VOR. Vestibular pathways to the spinal cord (vestibulospinal reflex) serve the limb and axial muscles during reflexive posturing movements during walking, standing, etc. The vestibular system is helped by the vestibulocerebellum (flocculus) by facilitating the rapid modification of the various reflexes. This is especially important for adjustment to various neurologic, optical, and other insults. Cerebellar compensation provides us with the ability to recover from the symptoms of nausea and vertigo after labyrinthine injuries. The older patient with poor cerebellar function may never adjust to the loss of one labyrinth.

Disorders of Special Senses and Ocular Systems
Disorders of Visual System

Normal binocular vision requires that the central rays of light be focused precisely in each foveola. This requires clear corneas, aqueous fluid, lenses, and vitreous. It requires coordination of the extraocular muscles through normal cranial nerve function, gaze centers in the frontal lobes and brainstem, vestibular centers, and occipital lobes, and it requires normal accommodation and pupillary function through the sympathetic and parasympathetic nervous systems.

"Poor vision" may be the result of any lesion along the visual pathway and requires evaluation of visual acuity, visual fields, pupillary reflexes, extraocular movements, as well as examination of the eye. It is very important, especially following trauma, to document the visual acuity of each eye in the patient's records, which is done using a Snellen eye chart or newsprint. Table 64-1 outlines clinical characterizations of lesions along the visual pathway.

It is not uncommon to have an entirely normal eye and neurologic examination in a patient with poor vision. The term **amblyopia** describes a condition of poor vision without apparent organic disease. It develops owing to a problem in childhood that prevented the normal development of the visual system. The eye may have been hyperopic and/or crossed (esotropia). If the central rays of light are not focused on the foveola, an infant will see double and therefore suppress the image from one eye. If the eye is suppressed long enough, it will become amblyopic or "lazy." This refers to an eye with poor vision rather than an

Table 64-1. Clinical Characteristics of Lesions of the Visual System

Lesion Site	Pain	Visual Acuity	Visual Field	Ophthalmoscopy	Pupil
Cornea	+	Decreased	Normal	Normal	Normal
Retina	–	Decreased	Central scotoma	Abnormal macula	Normal
Optic nerve	+/–	Decreased	Arcuate scotoma	Atrophic or swollen disc	+ APD*
Optic chiasm	–	Normal	Bitemporal hemianopsia	Normal or atrophic disc	Normal
Optic radiation	–	Normal	Homonymous hemianopsia	Normal disc	Normal

*APD indicates afferent pupillary defect.

eye that is crossed. Although both may be present, amblyopia may be present in an eye that is not deviated. Patching the good eye prior to age 6 years, thereby forcing the child to use the amblyopic eye, may reverse the suppression.

The differential diagnosis of transient visual loss should be addressed from a time-interval perspective. Visual loss lasting only a few seconds at a time in one or both eyes suggests either a dry eye syndrome or papilledema (transient obscurations of vision), from 3 to 5 minutes suggests transient ischemic attacks (TIA) resulting in **amaurosis fugax** (fleeting blindness), and 15 to 45 minutes of visual disturbance suggests migraine.

Functional visual loss is also associated with normal ocular exam, although tunnel visual fields are also typical. Depression, conversion reactions, and malingering can present with functional visual loss.

Cornea, Lens, Vitreous, and Refractive Problems

Decreased vision may be the result of any condition that impedes the light rays after they enter the eye or prevents precise focus of light on the retina. Refraction problems are the most common. A myopic eye will focus the light rays in front of the retina, while a hyperopic eye will focus the light rays behind the eye (Fig. 64-2). Corneal scars from injury or infection may be so faint or small that they are only seen with magnification but may still cause blurred vision or monocular diplopia (double vision

Fig. 64-2. Light rays are focused in front of the retina in a myopic eye, behind the retina in a hyperopic eye, and on the retina in an emmetropic eye.

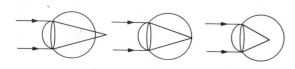

through one eye). Lens opacities (cataracts) may also cause blurred vision or monocular diplopia. Hemorrhage, infection, or inflammation of the vitreous will impede light rays as well. The three most common causes of monocular diplopia are refractive error, dry eye, or cataract.

Retinal and Vascular Disorders

Retinal scars from injury, diabetes mellitus, macular degeneration, congenital lesions (coloboma), or inflammation may prevent precise focusing of the light on the retina. Central visual acuity is typically impaired, with a central scotoma present in the affected eye. Macular pigmentation or hemorrhage may be noted on direct ophthalmoscopy.

Central Retinal Artery Occlusion. A history of sudden loss of vision in one or both eyes suggests a vascular event. The cause may be thrombus, embolus, or vasospasm. An embolus might be cholesterol or fibrin-platelet aggregates breaking away from an atheromatous plaque within the ipsilateral carotid artery or embolic material from the heart. If the embolus reaches the central retinal artery and does not break up or pass to a distal artery, the patient will be found to have a **central retinal artery occlusion (CRAO).** An acute CRAO has two characteristic signs: the "cherry red spot" in the macula produced by the normal red-orange color of the choroid contrasted against a background of ischemic pale retina and "box-caring" within the retinal vessels produced by clumping of blood cells. The visual loss with a CRAO is acute and painless.

Optic Nerve

Disease processes that involve the optic nerve will produce findings in that eye only. If both optic nerves are involved the findings are usually asymmetric. An arcuate scotoma (an area of visual loss connected to the physiologic blind spot) is the result of a lesion or disease involving the optic nerve. An afferent pupillary defect (a normal consensual response with little or no response to direct light) is the hallmark of optic nerve disease. Visual acuity is frequently significantly decreased, with a pale or swollen optic nerve noted on direct ophthalmoscopy. Flame hemorrhages or cotton-wool spots may be present, depicting an ischemia process. Acute optic nerve disease with sudden visual loss is likely vascular in origin (**ischemic optic neuropathy**), whereas insidious visual loss over days is more suggestive of inflammatory disease (**optic neuritis**). Multiple sclerosis may present as optic neuritis with a central scotoma (the blind area involves the central fixation point) and pain on movement of the eye. Visual loss that is gradual and progressive over weeks to months is highly suspicious for compressive disease (optic nerve meningioma, giant aneurysm). Glaucoma causes progressive visual loss over years, with pronounced optic nerve cupping owing to increased intraocular pressure.

Visual Pathways

The chiasm, optic tract, and radiations comprise the visual pathways to the occipital lobe. Visual field defects are characteristic signs of lesions involving the visual pathways. Fig. 64-3 depicts the classic visual field defects associated with lesions along the pathway.

Fig. 64-3. Illustration of visual field defects that follow damage to different levels of the optic pathways. (Used with permission from: Newell FW. *Ophthalmology Principles and Concepts* (6th ed.). St. Louis: Mosby Year Book, 1986, p. 56.)

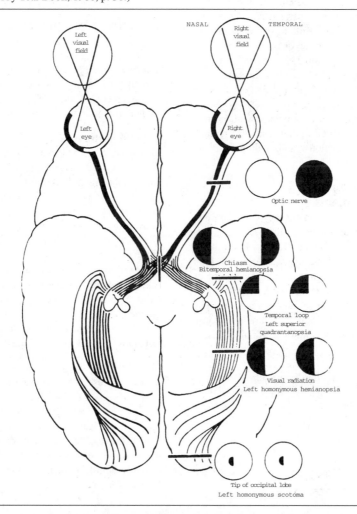

Optic Chiasm. Lesions that involve the pathways from the optic chiasm to the occipital lobes will produce visual field defects in both eyes. These visual defects will respect the vertical meridian of the visual field. A **bitemporal hemianopsia** describes a loss of vision in the temporal half of each eye. To produce this type of visual field defect, the lesion must involve the optic chiasm. What appears at first to be a unilateral field defect may in fact represent a **junctional scotoma.** A junctional scotoma consists of a central scotoma and a superior temporal visual field defect in the contralateral eye. These findings are the result of a lesion compressing one optic nerve (central scotoma) and extending posteriorly to compress the chiasm and involve the crossing lower nasal retinal fibers from the contralateral eye (superior temporal visual field defect). The most characteristic lesions involving the chiasm are masses that include pituitary tumor, craniopharyngioma, meningioma, or aneurysm. Special studies such as magnetic resonance imaging (MRI) of the brain and arteriography might be needed to make the correct diagnosis.

Optic Tract. Optic tract lesions are most often iatrogenic, resulting from neurosurgical intervention, although they can occur from trauma or tumor. Tract lesions result in complete contralateral homonymous hemianopsia.

Temporal Lobe, Parietal Lobe, and Occipital Lobe. Lesions involving the optic radiations or occipital lobes will produce **homonymous** field defects (vertical midline defects that involve the same area of each visual field). A left homonymous **hemianopsia** involves the left half of both visual fields and would localize to the right visual pathways. A right inferior homonymous **quadrantanopsia** signifies a lesion in the left superior occipital lobe and involves the right inferior quadrant of each visual field. Temporal lobe lesions may produce a contralateral **incongruous** (unequal) superior sector defect ("pie in the sky" visual field defect), usually accompanied by other neurologic findings such as temporal lobe seizures. Parietal lobe lesions will result in a contralateral incongruous homonymous hemianopsia more pronounced inferiorly ("pie on the floor" visual field defect). These patients will have an accompanying contralateral hemiparesis and are usually found in the neurology ward rather than in the ophthalmology clinic. A lesion involving an occipital lobe will produce a contralateral homonymous hemianopsia. Within the occipital lobe, a lesion of the inferior calcarine strip will produce a superior quadrantanopsia on the contralateral side and a lesion of the superior calcarine strip will produce a contralateral inferior quadrantanopsia. Occipital lobe lesions with visual field defects may present without other lateralizing signs or symptoms. Diseases which produce localized lesions should be considered in the differential diagnosis when the visual pathways are involved. Common lesions are vascular events involving the middle cerebral artery or posterior cerebral artery distribution, and occasional masses that include neoplasm, infections (abscesses), and arteriovenous malformations. It must be emphasized that lesions involving the visual pathways from the optic tract to the occipital lobes will produce homonymous field defects, with the field defects becoming more congruous (similar) the further posterior the lesion.

Disorders of Oculomotor System

Normal binocular vision requires that the movement of the eyes be perfectly coordinated. **Esotropia, exotropia, hypertrophia,** and **hypotropia** are terms used to describe an eye that is turned in, out, up, or down respectively. Movement of one eye is described by the term **duction. Abduction** is a movement toward the ipsilateral ear. **Adduction** is a movement toward the nose. **Version** movements describe the simultaneous movement of both eyes in the same direction. **Dextroversion** is movement of both eyes to the right and **levoversion** to the left. A version movement requires the action of "yoked" muscles. For example, movement of the eyes to the right requires the yoked simultaneous contraction of the left medial rectus muscle and the right lateral rectus muscle. Movement of the eyes in opposite directions is described by the term **vergence. Convergence** requires the contraction of both medial rectus muscles and **divergence** requires the simultaneous contraction of the lateral rectus muscles. Eye movement may be compromised by disease involving the nerves (neuropathy), muscles (myopathy), or the myoneural junction.

Brainstem Lesions Involving CN III, IV, and VI

Involvement of specific brainstem structures along with one or more cranial nerves may produce characteristic neurologic defects that localize the lesion. Some are labeled by names of the person who first described them but are probably better described by the structures affected as outlined in Table 64-2.

Isolated CN III, IV, and VI Lesions

Neuropathy. The most common cause of isolated CN III, IV, and VI palsies is trauma, followed by ischemia, compression, and inflammatory disorders (autoimmune and infectious). Meningeal carcinomatosus presents with progressive CN palsies developing over days to weeks. The occurrence of a pupil-sparing CN III is suggestive of

Table 64-2. Nuclear/Fasicular Lesions Involving Cranial Nerves III, IV, and VI

WEBER'S SYNDROME
Ipsilateral CN III
Contralateral hemiparesis

BENEDIKT'S SYNDROME
Ipsilateral CN III
Contralateral hemitremor (red nucleus)

RAYMOND'S SYNDROME
Ipsilateral CN VI
Contralateral hemiparesis

FOVILLE'S SYNDROME
Ipsilateral CN V, VII, VIII
Horizontal gaze palsy
Ipsilateral Horner's

MILLARD-GUBLER SYNDROME
Ipsilateral CN VI
Ipsilateral CN VII
Contralateral hemiparesis

ischemia and is not uncommon in diabetes. The occurrence of CN III palsy with pupillary involvement suggests a compressive lesion such as an aneurysm.

Myopathy.   Restrictive myopathy that results in progressive diplopia can be the result of an orbital floor fracture or thyroid eye disease. Thyroid eye disease (Graves' disease) is usually (but not always) accompanied by hyperthyroidism and is usually associated with lid retraction and proptosis.

Neuromuscular Junction.   Intermittent extraocular muscle palsies that do not follow a cranial nerve pattern and are associated with ptosis may indicate systemic or ocular myasthenia gravis. A positive edrophonium (**Tensilon**) test is diagnostic of myasthenia gravis.

Combined Extraocular Muscle Palsies

Cavernous Sinus.   Lesions within the cavernous sinus may involve cranial nerves III, IV, and VI, along with the first and second divisions of the trigeminal nerve (CN V). The optic nerve is typically not involved and vision is therefore spared. Lesions can be the result of infections which commonly result in cavernous sinus thrombosis, carotid-cavernous fistulas, intracavernous aneurysms, and tumors such as meningiomas.

Orbital Apex (Superior Orbital Fissure).   Lesions at the apex of the orbit may also involve CN III, IV, VI, and the first division of V. The optic nerve may also be in-

volved at this site and the visual acuity decreased. Disease processes which involve the superior orbital fissure are trauma, inflammation (**orbital pseudotumor**), neoplasia (**meningioma**), or infections extending from the ethmoid sinus (**mucormycoses**).

Pupillary Disturbances

Parasympathetic.   These fibers of CN III constrict the pupil. Lesions of CN III will result in a dilated and nonreactive pupil. A dilated and fixed pupil is present when the ipsilateral oculomotor nerve is compressed by a mass such as an aneurysm of the posterior communicating artery or descent of the uncus through the tentorium. Any patient in whom increased intracranial pressure is suspected that presents with a dilated pupil must be assumed to have neurosurgical emergency until proven otherwise.

Sympathetic.   Horner's syndrome results from interruption of the sympathetic nerves to the eye. Clinical findings are an ipsilateral miosis (small pupil), ptosis, anhidrosis, and apparent enophthalmos. Since Horner's syndrome results from an interruption of sympathetic pathways, the lesion may be in the brainstem (lateral reticular nucleus of the brainstem), low cervical cord (intermedial gray column), apex of the chest (cervical sympathetic chain), the common carotid, the cavernous sinus, or the orbit. It is important to consider all of these sites in a patient with Horner's syndrome. A chest x-ray in a patient who develops an isolated Horner's syndrome is recommended because this may be the presenting sign of an apical bronchogenic carcinoma.

Supranuclear and Nuclear Gaze Disorders

Gaze palsy denotes a clinical condition which is characterized by the inability to move either eye symmetrically in a direction of gaze. If a lesion involves the supranuclear pathways of the frontal lobe horizontal gaze center, the patient will have eye deviation towards the side of the lesion, but (as with all upper motor neuron lesions) the cranial nerves and muscles will be able to be moved by reflex with passive rotation of the head (the "doll's eye" maneuver) or caloric testing. If the lesion involves the pontine horizontal gaze center (PPRF), the patient will have eye deviation away from the side of the lesion. If the PPRF or CN III, IV, or VI nerves are involved, the muscles cannot be moved either voluntarily or by reflex.

Vascular lesions are the most common cause that are associated with gaze palsies. However, any disease process which results in localized (focal) lesions should be considered in the differential diagnosis (vascular, trauma, demyelinating, mass).

Internuclear Gaze Disorders

An internuclear ophthalmoplegia (INO) is manifest by decreased *ad*duction of the ipsilateral eye and nystagmus (involuntary to and fro movement) of the *ab*ducting eye. The lesion can only be in the median longitudinal fasciculus (MLF) on the same side as the adduction paresis. The MLF is a large myelinated tract, and is commonly affected in demyelinating disease. Therefore a unilateral or bilateral INO is commonly seen in multiple sclerosis as an isolated finding. As the MLF is located in the median position of the pons and midbrain, and is supplied by the distal segment of perpendicular penetrating branches of the basilar artery, ischemic vascular disease is a common cause of INO in persons who have risk factors for stroke.

Auditory System Disorders

Tinnitis

A ringing or buzzing noise in the ear which can be extremely aggravating to the patient, tinnitus can be subjective — which means the patient is the only one who can hear it. Objective tinnitus can be heard by both the examiner and the patient. Tinnitus can be caused by any lesion along the auditory pathway from the external ear to central pathways. However, any lesion resulting in sensorineural hearing loss is the most common cause of tinnitus. The pitch of the tinnitus can be predicted from the audiogram by noting that the tinnitus matches the frequency where the hearing drops off. Pulsatile tinnitus is suggestive of vascular sounds being transmitted from the carotid bulb to the middle ear. Venous hums can be blocked by pressure over the jugular system. Both types of vascular tinnitus may be auscultated with a stethoscope.

Hearing Loss

There are two categories of hearing loss, conductive and sensorineural.

Conductive Hearing Loss.   Conductive hearing losses are caused by problems in the external canal or middle ear

(Table 64-3). Most common causes of conductive losses are related to trauma or infection resulting in cerumen impaction, perforation of the TM, fluid in the middle ear, ossicular fixation, or discontinuity. Fortunately, most of these problems can be corrected. Otosclerosis (bony fixation of the stapes footplate) can be fixed by stapedectomy. In this operation, the stapes is removed and replaced by a prosthesis.

Sensorineural Hearing Loss.   Sensorineural hearing loss is caused by changes in the auditory pathways proximal to the conducting system, including the cochlea, auditory nerve, and central pathways (Table 64-4). The loss can be stable or progressive. The vast majority of sensorineural hearing losses are due to presbycusis or heredity, and are characterized by bilateral symmetric high-frequency loss. Little can be done to prevent the progression. Noise-induced hearing loss is also common. A characteristic notch is seen at 4 kHz on the audiogram (Fig. 64-4). Guidelines have been established which describe the safe number of hours of exposure per day to specific decibel levels of noise. A progressive hearing loss may be due to congenital anatomic abnormality, ototoxic drugs, or a mass compressing the nerve such as an acoustic neuroma. Each of these causes is treatable if the diagnosis can be made!

Mixed Hearing Loss.   A patient may present with both a conductive and a sensorineural hearing loss (see Fig. 64-4). These losses can be caused by independent processes or be produced by a single disease. Otosclerosis causes a conductive hearing loss due to stapes fixation and may occasionally be associated with a progressive sensorineural loss from toxins thought to be released from the overgrowth of bone in the oval window.

Central Processing Disorders

A poorly understood type of hearing loss involves problems in the central auditory pathways which lead to central processing disorders. Cochlear pathology causes loss of hearing for pure tones but no loss of understanding of the

Table 64-3. Causes of Conductive Hearing Loss

Disorder	Site	Treatment	Amount of Hearing Loss
Cerumen impaction	Ear canal	Removal	Usually 0 dB
Tympanic membrane perforation	Tympanic membrane	Surgery	0–45 dB
Fluid	Middle ear	Time vs. myringotomy and tube	0–30 dB
Eustachian tube obstruction	Eustachian tube	Examine nasopharynx	0–35 dB
Otosclerosis	Fixed stapes footplate	Stapedectomy	5–60 dB
Ossicular discontinuity	Displaced incus or stapes	Surgery	60 dB

Table 64-4. Causes of Sensorineural Hearing Loss

Disorder	Site	Special Circumstances	Treatment
Hereditary	Cochlea		None
Presbycusis (aging)	Cochlea		None
Noise trauma	Cochlea hair cells	4-kHz hearing loss	Noise protection
Ototoxicity	Cochlea	Aminoglycosides, furosemide, ethachrinic acid, aspirin, cis-platinum	None
Meniere's disease	Cochlea	Fluctuating hearing, ear fullness, dizziness, less than 24-hour duration	Low-salt diet, diuretics, possibly surgery
Acoustic neuroma	Eighth nerve at the cerebellopontine angle	Hearing loss, vertigo, discrimination problems	Surgical removal
Sudden sensorineural hearing loss	Internal cochlear membrane rupture	Barotrauma, heaving, straining	Rule out perilymph fistula

Fig. 64-4. An audiogram showing a mixed conductive and sensorineural loss on the left and noise-induced hearing loss on the right. The brackets depict bone conduction with the opposite ear masked. Masking prevents sounds being presented to the test ear from being heard by the nontest ear. The masked hearing level indicates bone conduction hearing level or the degree of sensorineural hearing. The connected circles indicate the hearing level with sound presented through the air to the ear canal and tests both the conductive component and the sensorineural component. This patient has a mixed hearing loss with both a sensorineural component and a conductive component. The sensorineural component is the difference between the masked bone level and normal, while the conductive component is the difference between the masked level and the air level or the level between the brackets and the circles.

The right panel depicts an audiogram from a 45-year-old musician with noise-induced hearing loss. The audiogram shows the characteristic drop in threshold at 4000 Hz due to noise. In this audiogram notice that the bone conduction and air conduction are the same as would be expected in a patient with a sensorineural loss without a conductive component. Xs indicate air conduction threshold, and brackets indicate bone conduction threshold.

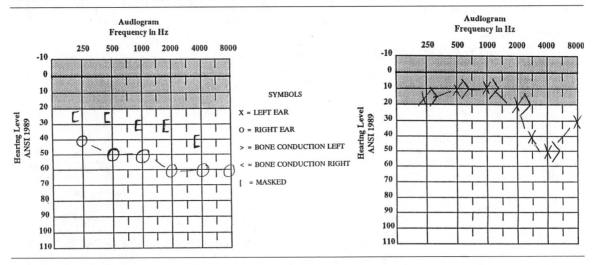

SYMBOLS

X = LEFT EAR
O = RIGHT EAR
> = BONE CONDUCTION LEFT
< = BONE CONDUCTION RIGHT
[= MASKED

words presented at an intensity above threshold. Sensorineural losses with good understanding of pure tones and poor understanding of language (poor discrimination) suggests retrocochlear disease. A retrocochlear lesion might involve the brainstem, thalamus, or temporal cortex and would be associated with other neurologic symptoms and signs. Audiologic testing to include ABR are used to localize the site and to focus the neurodiagnostic evaluation.

Evaluation of Auditory System

Tuning Fork Tests.   Tuning fork tests are very useful and can actually be done to verify that the audiometer is functioning correctly! The tuning fork is available in 256, 500, and 1024 Hz. The Weber Test is done to determine which ear hears the tone better when the handle of the tuning fork is placed on the bridge of the nose or a tooth. Equal hearing is assumed if the tone is heard in the middle of the head. Lateralization of the tone is due to a conductive hearing loss on the side of lateralization or a sensorineural loss opposite the side to which the sound lateralizes. A patient with a conductive loss at a specific frequency will hear that frequency better when the tuning fork is placed on the skull as compared to being placed in the air next to the ear. This is called the Rinne Test. A patient with a conductive hearing loss hears "by bone" better at the frequency of the tuning fork than "by air." The 500-Hz tuning fork is the most useful and will be heard better by bone than by air with a 25–30 dB conductive hearing loss or greater.

Audiometry.   The audiogram determines the threshold for hearing frequencies from 256 to 8000 Hz (8 kHz) (see Fig. 64-4). Air level hearing is tested with headphones which broadcast pure tones to one ear at a time. The patient indicates when the tone is heard. The conducting system is included in the test since sound is passed through the air in the air canal. Bone level testing is done by sending the tones directly to the skull, bypassing the TM and middle ear ossicles.

Tympanometry can determine if there is negative pressure or fluid in the middle ear. It can also measure the stapedius reflex. The test takes advantage of the fact that the TM and ossicles absorb and reflect a certain amount of sound. To perform the test, a probe is seated tightly in the ear canal. A tone is broadcast into the ear canal from a speaker on the end of the probe. The amount of sound reflected back is measured as a range of positive and negative pressures that are exerted to the ear canal. When the pressure in the middle ear and ear canal are equal, the amount of sound reflected will be least. (Fig. 64-5).

Acoustic Brainstem Response Audiometry (ABR). The ABR could be thought of as the EEG (electroencephalogram) of the auditory system and is one of the family of evoked response tests. During the ABR, electrodes placed on the skull pick up electrical activity (action potentials) arising in the cochlea and along the auditory nerve while tones or clicks are played to the ears through headphones. The test is very useful in determining hearing thresholds in patients, such as children or incapacitated

Fig. 64-5. When the compliance of the tympanic membrane and middle ear conducting system is normal, the tympanogram tracing falls within the inverted "V" as shown on panel A. If the middle ear is filled with fluid, the tympanogram will be flat, as seen in panel B. If there is negative middle ear pressure, the tympanogram peak will be shifted to the left, as in panel C.

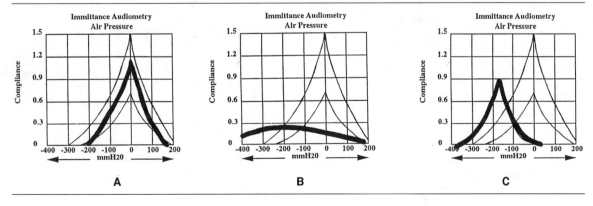

Table 64-5. Dizziness

Disorder	Site	Special Circumstances	Treatment
Viral labyrinthitis	Labyrinth	Vertigo, nausea, and vomiting with viral illness, day's duration	Time, supportive care
Meniere's disease	Endolymphatic hydrops	Fluctuating hearing, ear fullness, less than 24-hour duration	Low-salt diet, diuretics, possible surgery
Benign paroxysmal positional vertigo	Otoliths	History of head trauma, occurs while rolling over in bed	Head-positioning maneuvers
Cervical vertigo	Vestibulo-spinal reflexes?	Occurs with tilting head back	Anti-inflammatory, cervical collar
Ototoxic drugs	Labyrinth		Aminoglycosides

adults, who are unable to cooperate for standard audiometry. ABR can also be done during general anesthesia, making it useful for monitoring the integrity of the nerve as dissections at the internal auditory canal or middle cranial fossa are done. The ABR is an excellent test to screen for acoustic neuroma, a benign tumor of the eighth nerve. These patients often present with the complaint that they cannot use the affected ear to talk on the telephone. They may have problems understanding what is being said and sometimes have dizziness. The ABR shows a delay in the appearance of action potentials as the impulse travels from the cochlea to the brainstem. An MRI of the internal auditory canal will show the acoustic neuroma, which must be removed surgically.

Disorders of Vestibular System

Disorders of the vestibular system result in dizziness, vertigo, and loss of balance. The presence of nystagmus on examination suggests a vestibular system lesion. Electronystagmography (ENG) is the most direct test available for labyrinthine function. However, other findings on neurologic examination may have more specific localizing value as any lesion along the vestibular system may produce dizziness, vertigo, and/or nystagmus.

Specific problems and diseases are outlined in Table 64-5. However, a few of the most common disorders are discussed below in more detail.

Motion Sickness

Caused by an overstimulation of the labyrinthine system by motion, as one experiences on a boat or amusement ride, motion sickness is usually temporary but can be debilitating. Treatment with central depressants is effective (scopolamine patches, antihistamines, and benzodiazepines).

Meniere's Disease

It produces vertigo which reoccurs. This vertigo lasts up to one day and is associated with transient ear fullness, hearing loss, tinnitus, and nausea. The condition may progress to permanent hearing loss and vestibular dysfunction. The etiology is thought to be internal membrane rupture due to excess endolymphatic fluid. Medical treatment is aimed at reducing this excess fluid and includes a low salt diet and diuretics. Surgical therapies may also be employed.

Vestibular Neuronitis

Viral labyrinthitis causes vertigo, nausea, and vomiting which can be severely debilitating and last for days to over a week. The neurologic examination may reveal nystagmus; however, other brainstem functions are intact, including hearing. Treatment is mainly supportive and directed at symptoms. The presence of fever, nuchal rigidity, or neurologic signs other than nystagmus suggests problems other than vestibular neuronitis to include infections, mass, vascular and inflammatory lesions involving the brainstem, or vestibular pathways.

Clinical Examples

1. A 34-year-old woman accountant was referred to an ophthalmologist for evaluation of visual hallucinations. The patient reported brief episodes of stereotyped visual hallucinations which have occurred 2 times weekly for 2 months. Associated with the hallucinations were mild headaches relieved with aspirin. For the past month, she had progressive difficulty computing tax returns and understanding complex conversations with her clients. She had no complaint of weakness or sensory loss.

Her visual acuity was 20/15 in each eye without correction. The pupils measured 5 mm in each eye and there was no afferent pupillary defect. Extraocular movements were normal. There was no evidence of papilledema by ophthalmoscopic examination. Visual field examination by confrontation revealed a suggestion of a superior field defect on the right and tangent screen testing confirmed the presence of a right superior homonymous incongruous sector field defect.

She expressed herself well but had difficulty naming objects, performing complex commands, and calculating simple mathematical computations.

Discussion. Formed visual hallucination and receptive language problems suggest a lesion posterior to the Rolandic fissure within the temporal lobe. Even though the visual acuity is normal because the central visual fibers are not involved, the presence of a right superior homonymous incongruous section ("pie in the sky") field defect along with the language disorder localizes the lesion to the left temporal lobe. A lesion of the left occipital lobe lingula will produce a similar visual field defect although congruous, but the other findings will not be present.

The history of progressive symptoms along with focal signs suggest a mass process. The most likely cause would be a temporal lobe glioma, although other causes of a mass lesion should be considered to include metastatic disease, arteriovenous malformation, and abscess.

2. A 52-year-old man presented with a chief complaint of double vision of 2 days' duration. There was a history of progressive redness of the left eye, and his wife commented that the left eye appeared to be bulging. He has had trouble sleeping because of a noise in his head. His double vision was both horizontal and vertical.

Examination revealed 20/20 vision in both eyes. There was 4 mm of proptosis on the left. The conjunctival blood vessels are large, prominent, and tortuous. Cranial nerve examination revealed decreased corneal sensation on the left, decreased sensation to pinprick over the left forehead and cheek, and partial CN III, IV, and VI palsies. A loud bruit was heard over the left eye and head.

Discussion. This patient presents with multiple cranial nerve palsies. Cranial nerves III, IV, and VI can be involved together at two locations, the cavernous sinus and orbital apex. Other possibilities are a neuromuscular junction problem (myasthenia gravis) or restrictive myopathy (thyroid myopathy). Lesions in the orbital apex or cavernous sinus and thyroid myopathy may produce orbital congestion and proptosis but myasthenia gravis will not. Decreased corneal sensation and decreased sensation over

the forehead mean that there is involvement of the first division of the trigeminal nerve (V^1 division) and decreased sensation over the cheek means that there is involvement of the second division of the trigeminal nerve (V^2 division). The presence of trigeminal nerve involvement excludes neuromuscular junction and myopathy causes. The normal vision implies that the optic nerve is not involved, so the lesion must be in the *left cavernous sinus.*

The progressive and localized problem involving the cavernous sinus suggests either a mass process or inflammation. The bruit is characteristic of a direct carotid-cavernous fistula. An intracavernous aneurysm or meningioma might produce all of this man's signs and symptoms except the bruit. Septic thrombosis of the cavernous sinus is rare without fever.

3. A 23-year-old man was evaluated for the sudden onset of vertigo, nausea, and vomiting which began after a jump from a helicopter into a lake. While climbing into the boat, he experienced intense vertigo as though he was spinning, nausea and vomiting, and loss of balance. Every time he stood up, he fell to the left. He had not been feeling well for 2 days prior to the onset of symptoms, stating he felt like he was coming down with the flu. On his exam his blood pressure was 120/74 and his heart rate was 110. He had a temperature of 37°C. He was pale and ill appearing. His pupils were 4 mm on the right and 2 mm on the left. Both reacted to light. Extraocular movements were normal but there was right-beating nystagmus. His left face was numb to touch. The rest of the cranial nerves were intact. Strength was normal, but there was reduced pain sensation of the right limbs. He past pointed on left finger-to-nose maneuver.

Discussion. The complaints of vertigo associated with nausea and vomiting suggests a lesion involving the vestibular system to include the peripheral vestibular apparatus, the vestibular nucleus of the medulla, and the vestibular pathways of the brainstem. The presence of right-beating nystagmus suggests a left vestibular labyrinth, nerve, or nuclear lesion. However, the finding of the left Horner's syndrome, a left trigeminal sensory deficit, left ataxia, and a right hemisensory deficit together with the vestibular lesion localize to the left lateral medulla.

The acute onset of symptoms which localize to the lateral medulla, which is supplied by the posterior inferior cerebellar artery (a branch of the vertebral artery), would suggest a vascular etiology. The dive may have resulted in direct trauma or vasospasm to the vertebral artery with hyperextension or flexion of the neck related to the jump. An intracerebral hematoma from trauma might also be considered.

While the flulike illness prior to the onset of the vertigo might suggest an infectious cause, the highly localized findings within a specific vascular territory point to a vascular pathogenesis.

4. A 45-year-old woman presented with a chief complaint of gradually progressive hearing loss in the right ear. She had not been exposed to ototoxic medication, noise, head trauma, nor had she any family history of hearing loss. She had no symptoms of vertigo, nausea, or loss of balance. Upon further questioning, she admitted to tinnitus in the involved ear and difficulty understanding when someone talked into the affected ear. She was otherwise healthy, was not taking any medications, and had no other medical illness. Her biggest problem was the fact that she had to shift the telephone receiver to the opposite ear because of the difficulty in hearing when on the telephone.

Her physical exam was normal. Examination revealed clear ear canals with normal tympanic membrane and no fluid in the middle ear space, nor perforation in the eardrum. Her Weber lateralized to the left ear and the Rinne revealed air conduction better than bone conduction bilaterally. There was no nystagmus. Facial nerve function was intact.

An audiogram showed a sensorineural hearing loss in the right ear.

Discussion.   Any patient who presents with a unilateral sensorineural hearing loss should be evaluated for the possibility of an acoustic neuroma. An acoustic neuroma can present as a sudden sensorineural hearing loss in a small number of cases, but usually presents as a gradually progressive unilateral sensorineural loss. In this case, there are no other contributing factors and the findings on physical exam of a normal canal, tympanic membrane, and middle ear exclude other pathologies. Sensorineural loss as demonstrated by Weber and Rinne and audiometric tests along with poor discrimination or understanding of speech indicate retrocochlear pathology and are consistent with an

acoustic neuroma. Patients with cochlear hearing loss have good understanding of speech as long as the volume is turned up.

The most accurate test for the diagnosis in this patient would be an MRI scan with gadolinium which can identify very small acoustic neuromas within the internal auditory canal. One might also consider acoustic brainstem responses (ABR) which would indicate delays in neural transmission along the eighth nerve consistent with acoustic neuroma, but in a small number of cases can be falsely negative.

This patient had a small internal auditory canal acoustic neuroma and underwent surgical removal. Post-operatively, she experienced a transient facial nerve paralysis and a significant worsening of her sensorineural hearing loss.

Bibliography

Britton BH. *Common Problems in Otology.* St. Louis: Mosby Year Book, 1991. *This is a clinical, case-oriented approach to common otologic problems and is of interest to all physicians who treat ear diseases. It covers topics related to hearing and vertigo.*

Farris BK. *The Basics of Neuro-ophthalmology.* St. Louis: Mosby Year Book, 1991. *Basic overview of neuro-ophthalmology.*

Hart, Jr, WM (ed.). *Adler's Physiology of the Eye* (9th ed.). St. Louis: Mosby Year Book, 1992. *Basic pathophysiology of visual system.*

Miller NR. *Walsh and Hoyt's Clinical Neuro-ophthalmology* (4th ed.), Vol. 1. Baltimore: Williams and Wilkins, 1982. *The best comprehensive neuro-ophthalmology reference.*

Patton HD, Fuchs HF, Hill B, et al. *Textbook of Physiology. Excitable Cells and Neurophysiology.* Philadelphia: Saunders, 1989. *This is an outstanding physiology textbook with excellent chapters on the physiology of hearing and balance.*

Schuknecht HF. *Pathology of the Ear* (2nd ed.). Philadelphia: Lea & Febiger, 1993. *This is a classic reference with no equal.*

65 Disorders of Cerebrospinal Fluid and Intracranial Pressure

Mary K. Gumerlock

Objectives

After completing this chapter, you should be able to

Understand the formation, composition, and function of cerebrospinal fluid

Understand the physiology of intracranial pressure and the relationship of intracranial pressure to intracranial volume

Describe the factors which alter intracranial pressure: cerebrospinal fluid volume and blood volume

Describe the symptoms and signs of increased intracranial pressure

Cerebrospinal Fluid

Function and Formation

The normal adult brain weighs approximately 1500 g. It resides in the cranial vault which has a normal volume of approximately 1900 ml. Approximately 150 ml of this volume is cerebrospinal fluid (CSF). Of this volume, 20–30 ml is found within the ventricular system. The remainder (major portion) fills the subarachnoid space of the cranium and spinal canal. The CSF serves four main functions. It provides physical support for the brain and spinal cord; the buoyancy is protective. It serves an excretory role for removal of the products of brain metabolism, important with the absence of a lymphatic system in the brain, and it provides ready removal by rapid diffusion and bulk flow (sink action or sump effect). The CSF also plays an important role in intracerebral transport, particularly of the neuropeptides. Finally it serves a buffering role to control the chemical environment of the central nervous system.

CSF is formed at a rate of 0.35 ml/minute or ~500 ml/day. Given the fact that the system holds 150 ml, one immediately realizes that the CSF therefore turns over approximately three times per day. Eighty percent is produced in the choroid plexus, while the remainder is produced directly from the brain interstitial space. In general, CSF production is independent of intracranial pressure (ICP) until the ICP becomes so high that cerebral blood flow (CBF) is reduced. CSF formation is related to cerebral metabolic rate.

Pharmacologic manipulation of CSF production is possible, but the effect in man is slight. Acetazolamide, a carbonic anhydrase inhibitor, decreases CSF production at the level of the choroid plexus. Furosemide also has some effect on decreasing CSF production. Experimental work continues with other agents, such as spironolactone and vasopressin, on the inhibitory effect of CSF production. Cholera toxin and adrenergic stimulation act via adenylate cyclase to increase CSF formation by increasing cyclic adenosine monophosphate (cAMP). Few if any drugs are known to increase CSF resorption other than perhaps isosorbide.

CSF Composition

Experimental work continues, but at this point most consider that CSF is formed approximately 50% by active secretion and 50% as a dialysate of blood (plasma ultrafiltrate); it is essentially 99% water. CSF sodium concentration is similar to that of plasma, as are the bicarbonate concentration and osmolality. CSF contains higher concentrations of magnesium and chloride than plasma; it contains a lower concentration of glucose, proteins, calcium, and potassium. The glucose concentration is approximately 60 mg/dl, or about 60% of the serum glucose. This 60% does taper off in the diabetic patient such that in situations of hyperglycemia CSF glucose may be elevated, but still not reflect quite 60% of the serum glucose because glucose transport across the blood-brain barrier is a limited process.

Protein concentration in the CSF varies from 5 to 45 mg/dl. In the ventricles, normal protein concentration ranges from 5 to 15 mg/dl. Cisternal fluid at the level of the cisterna magna has a protein concentration of 15–25 mg/dl and CSF obtained at the lumbar level has a protein concentration of 15–45 mg/dl.

Normally, CSF is clear, colorless, and without cellular components. There should be no red blood cells and only a few (< 5, lymphocytes) white blood cells in the CSF. Turbidity increases with the presence of cells, and increased viscosity results from elevated CSF protein. Yellow color (xanthochromia) results from elevated protein, bilirubin, or other pigments derived from red blood cells.

Circulation and Absorption

CSF is formed within the choroid plexus of the lateral, third, and fourth ventricles. It exits the ventricular system through the foramina of Magendie and Luschka to circulate in the basal cisterns and along the spinal cord. It descends dorsal to the spinal cord and ascends ventrally. CSF then travels up the convexity of the cerebral hemispheres to be absorbed by the arachnoid villi, which lie in proximity to the major venous sinuses. These arachnoid villi can be considered microscopic valves which open at a pressure of 5 mm Hg. CSF resorption through these arachnoid villi does increase with increasing intracranial pressure. The anatomy of these arachnoid villi is such that there is essentially a one-way valve with fluid passing only from CSF to the venous sinus. Finally, there is some CSF absorption around the spinal nerve roots.

Intracranial Pressure

Intracranial Contents

Over a hundred years ago, neurophysiologists realized that the volume of the intracranial contents was constant. This has been described as the Monro-Kellie hypothesis, and

may be expressed by the equation $K_{ICV} = V_{CSF} + V_{blood} + V_{brain}$, where K is a constant, ICV is volume of intracranial contents, V_{CSF} is CSF volume, V_{brain} is brain volume, and V_{blood} is intracranial blood volume. This hypothesis simply states that an alteration in the volume of one of the three compartments is accompanied by alterations in one or more of the other compartments, such that intracranial pressure remains within the normal range. The intracranial space is connected to atmospheric pressure via the venous system, and small volume changes occur within the spinal dural sac and spinal epidural venous plexus.

Normal Intracranial Pressure

ICP as usually measured is pulsatile, varying both with respiration and with cardiac cycles (Fig. 65-1). Generally the respiratory oscillations are greater than the cardiac ones, but as cranial tightness increases the respiratory fluctuations are less obvious and the arterial pulsations become of greater amplitude.

The normal ICP is considered to be ≤ 180 mm H_2O or 15 mm Hg; pressures > 200 mm H_2O are considered abnormal. Elevations of intracranial pressure can occur normally with coughing, sneezing, straining, and standing on one's head. Such normal elevations are tolerated without any apparent neurophysiologic effect. Pressure values are usually measured from the level of the lateral ventricle when the head is level with the heart. In the recumbent position, intraventricular pressure and lumbar pressure will be equal. In the erect position, therefore, the ventricular pressure will be negative with reference to the heart while the lumbar pressure may be some 30 mm Hg increased, depending on the height of the patient. Under normal conditions the pressure in the lumbar space in the erect position rises to the mid-cervical level, and approximates venous pressures if related to the heart level.

Intracranial Pressure — Volume Relationships

Modifying the Monro-Kellie hypothesis, we have

$$V_{CSF} + V_{blood} + V_{brain} + V_{other} = K_{ICV}$$

where V_{other} is the volume of an additional component such as tumor, cyst, abscess, or hematoma. Again a change in volume within one compartment is offset by changes in one or more other compartments. For example, with tumor growth intracranially, an equal volume of either blood or CSF will be displaced. If the equation were completely ac-

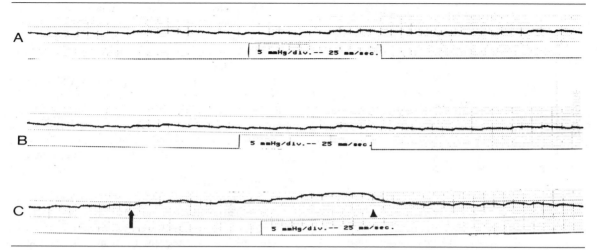

Fig. 65-1. A. Intracranial pressure tracing shows variation with cardiac cycle and more subtle changes with respiratory cycle. B. Same patient as in A after hyperventilation (pCO$_2$ decreases), shows a decline in ICP from 15–20 to 5–10 mm Hg. C. Same patient as in A and B now with jugular compression (arrow) by Queckenstedt maneuver (impedes cerebral venous outflow) shows an increase in ICP followed by a rapid decline after removal of compression (arrowhead).

curate and if the brain were incompressible and the cranium inexpandable, then the addition of volume to the intracranial space would lead to a theoretical pressure-volume curve as shown in (Fig. 65-2A).

The curve shows that as the volume is increased an equal volume is displaced, so that no change in pressure occurs. However, once all available compensation of blood, brain, and CSF has occurred, any further small increase in volume will result in a large rise in intracranial pressure. At the inflection point of the volume-pressure curve, the residual displaceable volume is significantly exhausted, so that relatively small further changes in volume will lead to large increases in pressure. The initial rather flat portion of the curve is related mainly to CSF buffering. As volume changes continue, CSF buffering becomes exhausted and the elastic properties of the cerebral substance and blood vessels play the major buffering role. These elastic properties can be described graphically (see Fig. 65-2). The term "elastance" describes the various portions of the curve and is determined by

$$\text{Elastance} = \frac{\text{Increase in pressure}}{\text{Increase in volume}} = \frac{\Delta P}{\Delta V}$$

To define the relative tightness of the intracranial space it is important to measure not only ICP but also to estimate elastance or compliance (the reciprocal of elastance). As can also be determined by the curve (Fig. 65-2B), the tightness of the neural axis increases with increasing ICP. The shape of the volume-pressure curve is influenced by the type of lesion causing the volumetric increase and by the rate of the increase in volume. Slower rates of increase are likely to be better tolerated and to elicit different compensatory mechanisms. Thus a slow-growing tumor or hematoma will be better tolerated to a larger volume than a more rapidly expansile mass lesion of similar or smaller volume.

Factors That Alter ICP

CSF Volume

Increases in CSF volume are due to either increased production or decreased absorption. A choroid plexus papilloma is known to increase CSF production. Otherwise, there are no other known clinical states in which CSF production is increased. Therefore, decreased absorption is the primary cause of increased CSF volume (hydrocephalus). Hydrocephalus may be either communicating (ventricular system open) or noncommunicating (a block within the ventricular system itself).

Communicating hydrocephalus occurs when CSF can exit the ventricular system, but either cannot reach the ab-

INTRACRANIAL PRESSURE–VOLUME CURVES

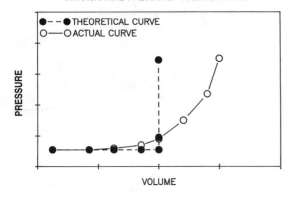

INTRACRANIAL PRESSURE–VOLUME CURVE

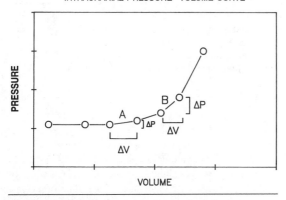

Fig. 65-2. Top: Theoretical pressure-volume curve generated under the assumption that the modified Monro-Kellie hypothesis is strictly true. Actual pressure-volume curve reveals an exponential curve with the flat portion not completely horizontal and the steep portion not perfectly vertical as a result of CSF buffering and some brain compressibility. Bottom: At point A, a change in volume causes only a small change in pressure, thus indicating low elastance (good compliance). At point B, the elastance is high (poor compliance) and the same or smaller volume change causes a much greater change in pressure.

sorption sites of the arachnoid villi or absorption at the arachnoid villi is decreased. This latter condition is largely due to widespread obstruction throughout the subarachnoid space, such as inflammation secondary to meningitis. Meningitis (an increase in CSF leukocytes) may be the result of an infection (bacterial or fungal) or of a subarach-

noid hemorrhage. A third condition, high protein content of any etiology, may also obstruct arachnoid villi absorption of CSF. A rare condition, congenital failure of arachnoid villi development, has also been described to cause hydrocephalus.

In noncommunicating hydrocephalus, the CSF is unable to exit the ventricular system. Blockage may occur at the level of the foramina of Monro, the aqueduct of Sylvius, or at the foraminal outlets of the fourth ventricle. This is most commonly due to blood or a tumor in the ventricular system or a congenital stenosis of the aqueduct of Sylvius.

Blood Volume

Cranial blood volume is confined to two compartments with 75% in the venous system and 25% in the arterial system. While these two systems are obviously connected across the capillary bed, the reaction to disease and intracranial pressure are such that they function almost independently. Arterial blood volume depends on autoregulation and remains relatively constant, independent of mean systemic arterial pressure. Outside of the range of autoregulation, as in severe disease such as trauma, CBF and therefore cerebral blood volume (CBV) become dependent upon mean systemic arterial pressure resulting in vascular congestion and an increased diffuse "mass" effect.

Other factors influencing cerebral arterial blood volume are chemical or metabolic. CBV is particularly sensitive to carbon dioxide levels (pCO_2). An increase in pCO_2 results in vasodilation of cerebral vessels and subsequent increase in ICP, again due to the increase in intracranial vascular volume; hypocapnia has the opposite effect (see Fig. 65-1). The magnitude of ICP change depends on brain compliance.

When the pO_2 falls below 54 mm Hg, cerebral blood flow and volume increase, with potential increase in ICP. Such may occur not only in pathologic conditions resulting in hypoxia, but also at high elevations. Because the pO_2 is less at altitudes above 10,000 feet, such hypoxia contributes to the increased intracranial pressure syndrome known as "altitude sickness."

The volume of the venous system is determined by the influx of blood from the arterial system. Venous drainage is passive with no valves, and the blood drains extracranially into the chest with the rate dependent on hydrostatic and intrathoracic pressures. Increased thoracic pressure, as with a tension pneumothorax, or Valsalva's maneuver will impede venous drainage. Any condition that increases central venous pressure (right heart failure, elevated positive end expiratory pressure, etc.) will impede cerebral venous drainage and thus increase intracranial pressure (Fig. 65-1).

Brain Volume

Brain volume can be divided into extracellular and intracellular volumes. It represents approximately 80% of the intracranial volume (blood 10%, CSF 10%, extracellular brain 15%, intracellular brain 65%). The brain is greater than 90% water. Normally, brain water changes less than 1% per day; however, in disease states, this water change plays a major role. An increase in brain water content is termed cerebral edema. Hypo-osmotic conditions, such as the syndrome of inappropriate antidiuretic hormone secretion or water intoxication, will increase brain water content. Most other pathologic conditions, such as tumors, infarction, hemorrhage, and infection, also result in cerebral edema and a secondary increase in intracranial pressure. By decreasing the water content of brain tissue with induced hyperosmolar states (mannitol, glycerol, urea), one can decrease intracranial pressure. Water deprivation can result in brain dehydration.

Pathophysiology of Increased Intracranial Pressure

Cerebral Edema

Brain edema is defined as a net increase in the water content of cerebral tissue which then leads to an increase in overall brain mass. It is useful to consider the brain in three compartments when discussing the anatomic and functional aspects of brain edema: the vascular compartment (arteries, capillaries, veins), the cellular compartment, and the extracellular compartment composed of the CSF and interstitial fluid spaces.

Vasogenic Edema

The most common type of cerebral edema is vasogenic edema, the result of movement of the liquid portion of blood across the blood-brain barrier (BBB) which is located at the cerebral capillary. Unlike capillaries elsewhere in the body, there are tight junctions between adjacent cerebral capillary endothelial cells. Normally these junctions prevent or markedly restrict the movement of plasma proteins and a wide range of molecules from entering the extracellular space of the brain. Trauma, hypoxia, ischemia, neoplasia, and infection can lead to the breakdown of the BBB. The hydrostatic gradient of the arterial system provides the force to drive the fluid into the extracellular space of the brain, where it spreads from the site of the BBB breakdown.

Cytotoxic Edema

This form of edema is less common, usually the result of hypoxia and cardiac arrest, but also seen after heavy metal poisoning. It represents an increase in cellular volume due to depletion of cellular energy with the subsequent failure of the sodium/potassium ATPase pump. When this occurs, intracellular sodium increases and water moves into the cell down an osmotic gradient.

Osmotic Edema

When the blood osmolality falls rapidly, an osmotic gradient develops between the blood and the extracellular space of the brain (brain > blood). Under these conditions water enters across the intact BBB and expands both the intracellular and extracellular compartments of the brain.

Hydrostatic or Hydrocephalic Edema

This type of edema is seen in acute obstruction of the cerebral subarachnoid space or ventricular system. This obstruction can be due to subarachnoid hemorrhage, meningitis, or obstructing mass lesion. The excess accumulation of fluid within the cerebral ventricles enters the extracellular space adjacent to the cerebral ventricles (transependymal absorption) and expands the extracellular space of the brain.

Signs and Symptoms of Increased Intracranial Pressure

Patients present variably with signs and symptoms of increased ICP. Some patients will display a gradual progression of all the symptoms and signs advancing to herniation. Others may present suddenly with intracranial pressure greater than mean systemic arterial pressure (i.e., CBF = 0) in full cardiorespiratory arrest. Some of the common symptoms and signs of increased intracranial pressure (intracranial hypertension) are listed in Table 65-1.

The combination of bradycardia and hypertension (Cushing reflex) is thought to be related to distortion of the brainstem with traction and compression of perforating arterioles. The respiratory disturbances also relate to compression of the brainstem and follow a specific pattern during herniation. Although not common, pulmonary interstitial edema may occur with acutely increased ICP.

Brain herniation may occur along three routes: (1) subfalcine: under the falx, (2) transtentorial: through the tentorial notch, and/or (3) tonsillar: cerebellar tonsils through

Table 65-1. Signs and Symptoms of Intracranial Hypertension

Headache
Vomiting (may not have accompanying nausea)
Diplopia (may be secondary to third- or sixth-nerve compression)
Slowing of mentation
Decreased vision or episodic blindness (transient obscurations of vision)
Papilledema
Alterations in vital signs (bradycardia, hypertension, and/or bradypnea)

the foramen magnum. Of the various types, transtentorial is clinically the most critical and yields the most diagnostic signs. These represent a progressive picture of neurologic deterioration and are well described in Chap. 59.

Clinical Example

1. A 40-year-old woman presented to the hospital for evaluation of progressively severe and more constant headaches of some 6 months' duration. The headaches were severe in the morning and improved during the day. There was occasional nausea and vomiting associated with the headaches.

On exam, the patient was lethargic but was arousable. Papilledema was noted bilaterally. There was a mild left hemiparesis associated with increased muscle stretch reflexes and an extensor plantar response (Babinski sign) on the left. The right pupil was 3 mm larger than the left and was poorly responsive to light.

A computerized tomography (CT) scan of the head showed a round lesion in the right frontotemporal area which was seen much better (enhanced) following an intravenous infusion of an iodinated radiocontrast agent (Fig. 65-3). There was significant surrounding edema especially above the mass, and the brain midline was shifted from right to left with partial collapse of the right lateral ventricle.

Discussion.   The clinical presentation of morning headaches is common in patients with increased intracranial pressure. During sleep, most people are recumbent (decreased venous drainage) and tend to hypoventilate (pCO_2 increases) compared to the awake state. In the upright position, the patient has improved venous outflow and a shift of CSF from the cranial to the spinal subarachnoid space.

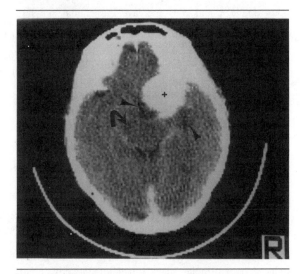

Fig. 65-3. Contrast-enhanced CT scan shows a large frontotemporal mass (+) with surrounding edema (arrowheads). Obliteration of the right incisural cistern in comparison with that on the left (curved arrow) is consistent with uncal herniation.

Both events decrease the intracranial volume. Some headache from tumors (masses) may result from traction on the dura or the large basal arteries.

The weakness of the opposite side of the body from the lesion is due to the mass effect on the motor cortex and or its projecting fibers. The increase in reflexes on the weak side and the pathological reflex (plantar extensor response) is part of the upper motor neuron syndrome.

The decrease in the state of consciousness (wakefulness) is a general effect of diffuse increased intracranial pressure presumably affecting the brainstem reticular activating system. This, along with the pupillary dilation, suggests early transtentorial herniation from a supratentorial mass in the right hemisphere.

The most likely etiology is a tumor, as suggested by the enhancing lesion on CT scan. The penetration of the normally excluded iodinated compound (intact BBB) into the tumor leads to an increase in the density of the tumor and its enhanced recognition over adjacent brain. This occurs in pathologic states which disrupt the BBB, such as within the tumor.

The patient was given an intravenous infusion of hypertonic mannitol and dexamethasone, with improvement of the left-sided weakness and other symptoms. This occurred because the blood became hyperosmotic to the brain and resulted in a movement of water from brain to blood. The dexamethasone was effective in decreasing the tumor-associated vasogenic edema. Subsequently, surgical removal of the tumor resulted in almost complete resolution of adjacent cerebral edema with improvement in the state of wakefulness and resolution of limb weakness.

Bibliography

Bruce DA. *The Pathophysiology of Increased Intracranial Pressure.* Upjohn Scope Publication, 1978. *An excellent discussion of ICP principles, equations, waveforms, and monitoring.*

Fishman RA. *Cerebrospinal Fluid in Diseases of the Nervous System* (2nd ed.). Philadelphia: Saunders, 1992. *A definitive, yet readable, treatise on CSF, a classic.*

Goldstein GW, Betz AL. The blood-brain barrier. *Sci Am* 255:74–83, 1986. *This article is a well-illustrated, thorough, basic introduction.*

Gumerlock MK. Blood-Brain Barrier and Cerebral Edema. In Tindall G, Cooper P, and Barrow D (eds.). *The Practice of Neurosurgery.* Baltimore: Williams and Wilkins, 1995. *An expanded discussion of cerebral edema in the context of the blood-brain barrier; good supplement.*

Milhorat TH. *Hydrocephalus and the Cerebrospinal Fluid.* Baltimore: Williams and Wilkins, 1972. *A very readable classic in neurosurgery.*

Milhorat TH. Classification of the cerebral edemas with reference to hydrocephalus and pseudotumor cerebri. *Childs Nerv Syst* 8:301–306, 1992. *Updates the previous reference and presents a new look at cerebral edema, evolving from that presented in Milhorat's earlier work and the work of Fishman cited above.*

66 Seizures and Epilepsy

Jeanne A. King

Objectives

After completing this chapter, you should be able to

Understand the pathogenesis of seizures

Learn the clinical criteria for the diagnosis of seizures

Develop concepts regarding the classification of seizures

Develop concepts regarding diseases that result in seizures

Epilepsy is the name given to a group of disorders of the central nervous system that cause a person to have recurrent, unprovoked seizures. A **seizure** is the subjective or objective behavioral manifestation of an abnormal excessive discharge of electricity from brain cells and its propagation in the brain. A seizure tends to be abrupt and result in alteration of cerebral function in the form of changes in sensation, motor activity, memory, and awareness or consciousness.

Neuroanatomy, Neurophysiology, and Neurochemistry of Epilepsy

Seizures result from an abnormal hypersynchronized electrical activation of a large group of neurons in the brain, either in one localized area or in multiple areas simultaneously. Even though this potential is always present, a given patient experiences seizures only occasionally. The medical profession has tried for years to explain the mystery of how a clinical seizure evolves. By understanding the mechanism by which seizures occur, we can better develop new, more effective treatments. Sometimes we learn in the reverse order; the treatment is found first and, in the study of how the treatment works, we learn more about the function of the brain.

It is possible that there may be more than one cellular

mechanism involved in the causation of seizures, especially seizures of different types.

Cellular Anatomy and Physiology

Neurons vary in size and shape, but the basic structure is the same for all. The cell body or soma contains the nucleus, Golgi apparatus, and Nissl substance (ribonucleic acid, RNA). Dendrites arise from the soma, branch repeatedly, and receive inputs from other nerve cells through numerous synaptic connections. Axons send impulses from the soma to other nerve cells by finely dividing and forming synapses on the soma, dendrites, or axons of other cells. Synapses are specialized interfaces between two nerve cells whose membranes are separated by a narrow cleft.

Any population of neurons, but especially the pyramidal cells, is capable of spontaneously discharging and resulting in a clinical seizure. Certain areas such as the temporal lobe are especially epileptogenic.

Normal Neuronal Electrical Activity
The excitability of the neuronal cell membrane depends on the maintenance of an electrical charge, or potential difference, between the intracellular and extracellular space. This resting membrane potential is a consequence of differences of ion concentrations (primarily sodium and potas-

sium) inside and outside the cell. However, nerve cell membranes of the central nervous system are continuously influenced by activity arising from other neurons and are never completely at rest. The action potential is a transient disturbance of the resting potential, which is then propagated, transmitting information. This phenomenon occurs at the synapse, where a presynaptic neurotransmitter substance evokes a change in the permeability of the postsynaptic membrane. Specialization of the postsynaptic junction in the form of various special receptor sites determines whether the induced permeability change will be excitatory or inhibitory.

Abnormal Neuronal Electrical Activity

The breakdown of normal inhibitory synaptic forces in patients with epilepsy can allow excess excitability to propagate via normal pathways to previously uninvolved brain structures. When this aberrant discharge reaches certain areas of the brain with sufficient intensity, it results in the behavioral manifestation of the seizure.

The normal action potential results from shifts in membrane potential from the resting polarized state. Depolarization occurs when the permeability of the membrane changes to allow the positive sodium ions to flow into the cell via the voltage-gated sodium channel, eliminating the potential difference. Pathologic sustained repetitive firing of action potentials may lead to propagation of seizures through brain pathways. Drugs such as phenytoin work by decreasing sustained repetitive firing at the level of the voltage-dependent sodium channel, the same channel that underlies generation of the normal single-action potential. Repolarization occurs via opening of the voltage-gated potassium channel. Whether the action potential will fire is determined by an interplay between excitatory and inhibitory forces.

Inhibitory Postsynaptic Potentials (IPSPs).   These potentials are caused by the inhibitory neurotransmitters, primarily **gamma-aminobutyric acid** (GABA) and **glycine.** These substances result in hyperpolarization of the membrane by either moving potassium out of the cell or chloride into the cell and therefore make rapid depolarization less likely. The chloride ion channel is critical. Its opening and closing is regulated by a number of receptors, and it is physically surrounded by these, including binding sites for GABA, benzodiazepines, steroids, barbiturates, and picrotoxin. There are two types of GABA receptors, type A and type B. The GABA A receptor actually forms the chloride channel. Some of the most effective drugs for epilepsy bind at these receptors, and presumably work by enhancing chloride ion flow and therefore inhibition. Picrotoxin

antagonizes chloride flow, reduces the seizure threshold, and thus causes seizures (Fig. 66-1).

Excitatory Postsynaptic Potentials (EPSPs).   These potentials are caused by excitatory neurotransmitters, which include the excitatory amino acids **glutamate** and **aspartate** as well as **acetylcholine.** These substances enhance depolarization by reducing the potential difference across the membrane by their effects primarily on sodium or calcium channels, making it easier to depolarize. An important subtype of glutamate receptor is the N-methyl-D-aspartate (NMDA) receptor; its activation allows an influx of sodium and calcium which will result in depolarization of the cell. Excess influx of calcium can lead to cell injury and death. The NMDA receptor is very complex, much like the GABA A receptor, and has various binding sites that allow it to be regulated by other substances such as magnesium, which blocks it, and glycine, which is necessary for its function (see Fig. 66-1).

NMDA receptor antagonists are being looked at in clinical trials for treatment of epilepsy. These receptors may be important in mediating the cell injury that may occur with a seizure discharge, perhaps due to the excess calcium entry into the cell in much the same way that calcium entry can cause injury in ischemia.

Calcium Channels.   These are also uniquely important in some forms of epilepsy. For example, low-threshold calcium current is thought to be responsible for the spike-wave activity generated by thalamic neurons in absence epilepsy; ethosuximide, a very effective drug for this condition, appears to act specifically on this current.

Electrical Activity Detected by Electroencephalography

Using an array of electrodes attached to the scalp which are then connected to a battery of powerful amplifiers (electroencephalograph), a record of electrical activity originating from the underlying cortex (electroencephalogram, EEG) can be made. This surface activity is believed to represent summated excitatory and inhibitory synaptic potentials generated along the apical dendrite of the pyramidal cells of the cerebral cortex located only 1–4 mm from the surface. Normal EEG patterns vary with the age of the patient and are different during wakefulness and sleep.

Epileptiform spikes and sharp waves have a high degree of correlation with the presence of clinical seizures. Other interictal EEG patterns do not. The EEG may provide a clue to the area of onset or to the type of clinical seizure. Techniques such as sleep deprivation, photic stimulation,

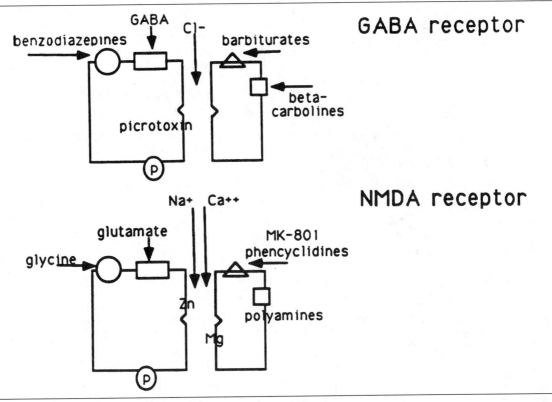

Fig. 66-1. Schematic diagrams of GABA A and NMDA receptors, simplified to exaggerate the similarities and parallels between these major inhibitory and excitatory receptor types. Each receptor has several binding sites for agents that can modulate the efficacy of the primary ligand (GABA and glutamate, respectively). GABA A: Benzodiazepines and barbiturates enhance the ability of GABA to open the chloride channel (through different mechanisms). A site within the channel (binding picrotoxin) blocks chloride flux. The beta-carboline site may be agonistic or antagonistic. NMDA: Glycine enhances the action of glutamate at the NMDA receptor. A phencyclidine binding site provides for noncompetitive inhibition of glutamate action, and a polyamine binding site may be agonistic or antagonistic. Magnesium (Mg) within the channel normally blocks significant ion-sodium (Na^+) and calcium (Ca^{++})-flux, but can be displaced with membrane depolarization. Zinc (Zn) also has a channel-blocking effect. Both GABA A and NMDA channels must be phosphorylated (P) for efficient function. (Used with permission from: Schwartzkroin PA. Basic mechanisms of epileptogenesis. In Wyllie E (ed.). *The Treatment of Epilepsy: Principles and Practice*. Philadelphia: Lea & Febiger, 1993, pp. 83–98.)

and hyperventilation are often used to provoke abnormalities. Recording the EEG during a clinical seizure and simultaneously video recording the seizure are occasionally necessary for accurate diagnosis.

The interictal spike discharge as depicted in Fig. 66-2 is the traditional electroencephalographic marker for a hyperexcitable area of the cortex with a high epileptogenic potential. Its basis is the paroxysmal depolarization shift.

During the interictal discharge, thousands of neurons in a small area of the cortex synchronously undergo an unusually large depolarization (called the depolarizing shift) on which a burst of action potentials is superimposed. The depolarizing shift is followed by a hyperpolarizing potential and neuronal inhibition. It appears to be generated by a combination of excitatory synaptic currents and intrinsic voltage-dependent membrane currents (Fig. 66-3).

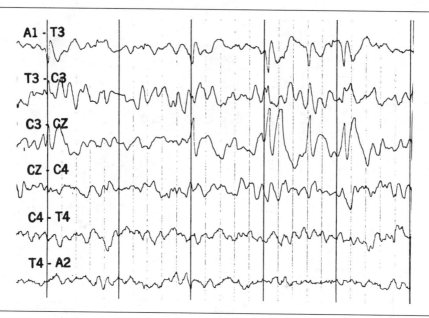

Fig. 66-2. Electroencephalogram. Left-sided spike focus. Note: Odd numbers indicate left-electrode placement and even numbers designate right-electrode placement. This pattern is indicative of seizures that are partial (focal) in onset.

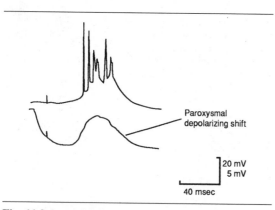

Fig. 66-3. Interictal discharges occur spontaneously in the in vitro hippocampus when the GABA blocking agent bicuculline is applied to the fluid bathing the tissue slice. Large-amplitude action potentials from the cell body and the dendrites (top trace) are superimposed upon the paroxysmal depolarization, a slow depolarization that is revealed when the neuron is hyperpolarized (bottom trace). (From: Wong RKS, Miles R, and Traub RD. Local circuit interactions in synchronization of cortical neurones. *J Exp Biol* 112:169–179, 1984. With permission of publisher, Company of Biologists Limited, England.)

Subsets of neurons with endogenous bursting characteristics may act as "pacemakers" in the generation of the depolarizing shift. These neurons are present in the pyramidal cells of the CA2 and CA3 segments of the hippocampus and layer 4 and superficial layer 5 of the neocortex. Their presence is not mandatory for the generation of epileptiform "spike" discharges, but may be facilitatory; CNS regions containing them seem to have a particularly high epileptogenic potential.

Symptoms and Signs

Everyone has the potential to have a seizure if the circumstances are conducive. Typical examples of this are alcohol-withdrawal seizures or hypoglycemia-induced seizures. These are secondary seizures: The term "epilepsy" is not used in these conditions, even when the seizures are occasionally recurrent, as these events are *provoked*. Sometimes epilepsy results from a disease process, such as a brain tumor, in which case the term "symptomatic" is prefixed. In most cases the cause is never identified; the term "primary" or idiopathic is then used.

Terminology

There are several terms specific to epilepsy that need to be defined.

The ictus is the seizure itself.
The clonic phase of a seizure is that portion in which there is alternate contraction and relaxation of skeletal muscles (often described as "jerking" by the witness).
The tonic phase is that portion in which there is sustained steady contraction of muscle (often described as "stiffening" by the witness).
The aura, although it has been considered a premonition of the coming seizure, is rather the very first phase of the ictus and implies a focal onset. Frequently the nature of the aura provides a clue to the seizure focus.
The postictal phase is the period immediately following the seizure.

Clinical Features

What a seizure looks like clinically depends upon which neurons in the brain are discharging. In other words, the symptoms of any particular attack depend on the function of the area of the brain that is being interrupted by the excessive neuronal discharge. If all the neurons are firing at the same time in a generalized fashion, then the term "generalized" seizure is used, but if only the neurons in one location are firing, then the term "partial" is used. One will also hear the term "focal." Deciding whether a seizure is partial or generalized in onset is an important task facing the physician who is treating a patient with epilepsy. It is important because different drugs are used depending on whether the seizure is partial or generalized in onset; the diagnostic evaluation is also different.

Generalized seizures are often genetic in origin or are more likely to be caused by diffuse processes such as metabolic or toxic derangements. The workup would focus on ruling out such things as hyponatremia, hypocalcemia, hypoglycemia, drug withdrawal, or drug intoxications. On the other hand, partial seizures are much more likely to be caused by structural lesions such as brain tumors and other mass lesions, glial scars, infarcts, etc., and imaging studies such as computerized tomography and magnetic resonance imaging are utilized early in the evaluation. Causes of seizures fall into many categories, including congenital malformations, degenerative, genetic, infectious, metabolic, neoplastic, perinatal or gestational insult, toxic, traumatic, and vascular.

Classification of Epileptic Seizures

The numerous types of epileptic seizures are recognized and classified according to clinical and electroencephalographic features.

Clinical

The most important means is clinical. This is done by acquiring a description of the seizure. In the ideal circumstance, this is accomplished by witnessing one personally. This, of course, happens uncommonly. The next best approach is to obtain a description from an eyewitness who is a reliable observer. The third source is the patient himself/herself, who frequently knows very little (because he/she may be amnestic/unconscious at the time) or knows only what others have told him/her about the event.

Electroencephalograms (EEG)

Once the clinical description has been acquired, one may have a good idea what type seizure one is dealing with, but the diagnosis can be supported by use of the EEG. An example of this is that not every staring spell may be absence (or petit mal). Sometimes staring spells can be partial complex seizures (temporal lobe or psychomotor seizures) and the EEG can differentiate between the two. Absence spells will be associated with a generalized 3-Hz EEG spike-wave abnormality as shown in Fig. 66-4 and partial complex seizures may be associated with a focal temporal lobe spike abnormality (see Fig. 66-2). This differentiation may not be so easily determined even by watching the seizure. Absence seizures are a form of generalized epilepsy and consequently the EEG pattern is generalized. In other words, the electrical abnormality is seen bilaterally and synchronously over the head. With partial complex seizures, the electrical abnormality is unilateral, usually in the temporal lobe.

Though the EEG can be useful in classifying a seizure disorder and guiding the selection of medications, the diagnosis is a clinical one no matter what the interictal EEG shows. The interictal EEG shows only what is happening electrically in the brain between seizures; many people with epilepsy have normal EEGs between seizures. Also normal people without epilepsy occasionally can have abnormal EEGs.

International Classification

A classification system for seizures has been developed through the years by an international team of epilepsy specialists (Table 66-1).

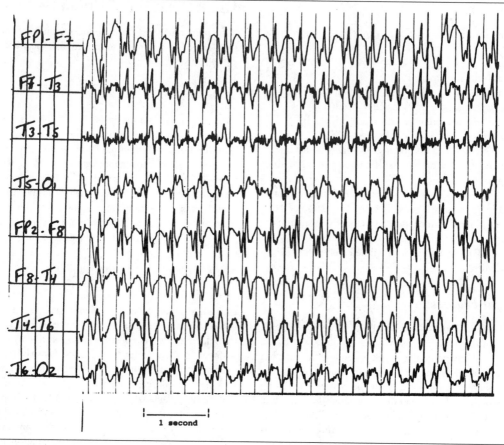

Fig. 66-4. Classic 3-Hz spike and wave discharges are seen in association with childhood absence. The seizures are brief (seconds) in duration and may have associated rhythmic eye blinking. The EEG background is normal and the epileptic discharges are generalized at 3 Hz frequently and provoked by hyperventilation.

Partial Seizures

Partial seizures are those seizures that begin focally. They are divided into two categories, those without alteration of consciousness with simple symptomatology such as motor jerking of one side of the body (i.e., **simple partial**) and those *with* alteration of consciousness (a better term would be *cognition*) and complex symptomatology (i.e., **complex partial**). This does not mean loss of consciousness as in a fainting spell, but only an impaired awareness or cognitive function. Simple partial seizures can begin anywhere in the brain; the symptom will reflect the origin of the focus. For example, if the origin of the seizure is the primary motor cortex, the seizure would manifest itself as motor activity of the contralateral body. Complex partial seizures often originate in the temporal or frontal lobe. When these seizures have onset in adulthood there is a correlation with the development of temporal lobe gliomas, particularly if the seizure is associated with a sensation of disagreeable odor. Both types of partial seizures may secondarily generalize if the electrical discharge spreads to involve the entire brain. If the generalization occurs rapidly, the clinical signs of the focal onset may not be evident, but the EEG may help locate the site of origin.

The duration can be quite variable for a simple partial seizure. A complex partial seizure will usually last from 30 seconds to 2 minutes. Postictal confusion is common after

Table 66-1. International Classification of Epileptic Seizures

---

PARTIAL (FOCAL, LOCAL) SEIZURES

Simple partial seizures
 With motor signs
 With somatosensory or special sensory symptoms
 With autonomic symptoms or signs
 With psychic symptoms
Complex partial seizures
 Simple partial onset followed by impairment of consciousness
 With impairment of consciousness at onset
Partial seizures evolving to secondarily generalized seizures
 Simple partial seizures evolving to generalized seizures
 Complex partial seizures evolving to generalized seizures
 Simple partial seizures evolving to complex partial seizures evolving to generalized seizures

**GENERALIZED SEIZURES (CONVULSIVE
OR NONCONVULSIVE)**

Absence seizures
 Typical absences
 Atypical absences
Myoclonic seizures
Clonic seizures
Tonic seizures
Tonic-clonic seizures
Atonic seizures

UNCLASSIFIED EPILEPTIC SEIZURES

Used with permission from: Commission on Classification and Terminology of the International League Against Epilepsy. Proposal for clinical and electrographic classification of epileptic seizures. *Epilepsia* 22:489–501, 1981.

a complex partial event but not common after a simple partial seizure unless there has been secondary generalization.

Generalized Seizures (Bilaterally Symmetric without Focal Onset)

Absence. These were formerly called petit mal and are characterized by episodes of brief staring, often with eye blinking and sometimes with loss of postural tone. Automatic motor movements or autonomic changes may occur if the episode is very prolonged. These are usually quite brief and may last only 5–15 seconds. They also tend to be quite frequent and may occur hundreds of times per day. There is no postictal state. These often occur in an autosomal dominantly inherited syndrome.

Tonic-Clonic Seizures. Formerly called grand mal seizures, these are characterized by bilateral tonic and clonic movements with loss of consciousness and often tongue biting and urinary incontinence. They typically last for 1–5 minutes and are associated with a postictal state.

Miscellaneous. A variety of other generalized seizures occur; these include infantile spasms, atonic seizures, akinetic seizures, tonic seizures, clonic seizures, etc.

Epileptic Syndromes

They are also classified based on age of onset, clinical profile, etiology, and prognosis. In general, primary epilepsy syndromes are those in which the patient has recurrent seizures, onset in childhood or adolescence, a family history of seizures, and no preexisting condition which would increase the risk of epilepsy (trauma, infection, tumor, etc.). It is important to recognize these syndromes as the seizures often respond well to specific antiepileptic drugs. On the other hand, symptomatic epilepsies are characterized by recurrent seizures in which there is a history of preexisting conditions (trauma, infection, etc.) or the presence of structural lesions that predispose to the development of epilepsy. While seizures associated with symptomatic epilepsy are responsive to many antiepileptic drugs, the prognosis for complete control is not as good as in the primary epilepsy syndromes.

Efforts to Treat Epilepsy
Drug Therapy

Our efforts to understand the cellular basis of epilepsy began *after* our early efforts to treat epilepsy with medication. Potassium bromide was first used to treat epilepsy in 1857 based on empirical observations. Phenobarbital came into use in 1912, but at that time there was no fundamental understanding of the epileptic process.

Beginning with the introduction of phenytoin in 1938, drugs were developed using screening techniques based on animal models. This was followed by trimethadione (1946), primidone (1954), ethosuximide (1960), diazepam (1968), carbamazepine (1974), valproic acid (1978), felbamate (1993), gabapentin (1994), and lamotrigine (1995).

Screening drugs with animal models currently remains the method of choice for developing antiepileptic drugs. Nonetheless, new understanding of the cellular and molecular mechanisms that underlie seizure activity is now being applied to the development of drugs that act on specific epileptogenic mechanisms.

In the last 10–15 years, neurotransmitter pharmacology has become better understood, and drug testing has centered on modifying specific synaptic systems to produce consistent antiepileptic effects (Table 66-2).

Although many classical neurotransmitter systems have been looked at, most interest has centered on drugs that are active at GABA-mediated inhibitory systems. Gabapentin was developed to mimic GABA, but instead works by a totally unknown mechanism. Likewise, felbamate also works by unknown mechanisms. Current areas of great interest in the investigation of the pathogenesis of epilepsy are glutamate (excitatory neurotransmitters), intrinsic voltage-dependent channels, calcium channels (especially in some of the primary generalized epilepsies), and neuromodulatory agents (including purines, peptides, cytokines, and some of the steroid hormones), and adenosine. These investigations may yet assume greater value as more is learned about neuropharmacology and as clinical syndromes are more systematically delineated.

Role of Antiepileptic Drugs

Treatment should be started with one drug only (monotherapy). Sometimes it is necessary to use two drugs simultaneously for control. The initial choice of drug should match the seizure type. Carbamazepine, phenytoin, and sometimes phenobarbital are used for focal or generalized tonic-clonic seizures. Valproic acid and ethosuximide are

Table 66-2. Anticonvulsant Drugs: Mechanisms of Action

Drug	Na$^+$ Channel[a]	Ca^{2+} Channel[b]	GABA[c]	Glutamate[d]
Phenytoin	++			
Carbamazepine	++			
Valproate	++			
Ethosuximide	–	++		
Phenobarbitone	+	–	+	+
Diazepam, clonazepam	+		++	
Vigabatrin			(++)	

+ +, strong action at clinically relevant concentration; +, action of possible significance; –, no action.
[a] Prolonged inactivation of the voltage-dependent Na$^+$ channel.
[b] Blockade of the T calcium current.
[c] Enhancement of GABA-mediated inhibition (by inhibition of GABA-transaminase in the case of vigabatrin).
[d] Antagonist action at the NMDA receptor.
Used with permission from: Meldrum B. Epileptic Seizures. In Siegel GJ et al. (eds.). *Basic Neurochemistry* (5th ed.). New York: Raven, 1994, pp. 885–897.

used in the treatment of absence seizures. Serum antiepileptic drug level determinations should be used to monitor drug treatment. Two new medications have been approved by the FDA and recently marketed: Felbamate appears to be useful in both partial and generalized epilepsies; however, because of recent concerns over its potential to cause aplastic anemia and hepatic failure, its future in the treatment of epilepsy is uncertain. Gabapentin is approved for adjunctive use in partial epilepsies. Both of these drugs are so new that their role in the treatment of epilepsy is still evolving.

Surgery Therapy

Surgery for epilepsy has also been used for more than 30 years. It is done

to remove pathological lesions.
to interrupt the CNS pathways by which seizures are thought to spread, or
to remove areas without gross lesions but with a clearly defined focal epileptogenic focus.

In general, surgery is recommended only after conventional medications fail to adequately control seizures unless there is an underlying lesion that requires treatment on its own merit.

Clinical Examples

1. A 32-year-old man began to have episodes in which he would suddenly begin to look about in a bewildered manner while fumbling aimlessly at his clothes, smacking his lips, and drooling saliva. The episodes lasted only 30 seconds, and the patient was unaware of their occurrence afterward. Neurologic examination was normal and EEG revealed a spike focus over the left anterior temporal region. An MRI scan revealed a mass lesion in the left anterior temporal region. The patient was placed on the antiepileptic drug carbamazepine at a dosage sufficient to achieve therapeutic drug levels. Surgical exploration was undertaken, revealing a meningioma over the left temporal area of the cortex.

Discussion.   The patient's symptomatology was consistent with complex partial seizure activity primarily manifested by psychomotor phenomena suggesting a focal process in one of the temporal lobes of the cortex. A search was made for an etiology utilizing careful neurologic examination, EEG, and MRI. A mass lesion was found. Antiepileptic drug therapy was begun and surgical exploration was carried out to determine whether the mass lesion was resectable. Fortunately, this was the case.

2. An 8-year-old girl was noted to be having staring spells in school, which were interfering with her studies. The episodes lasted from 1 to 20 seconds and were sometimes accompanied by blinking of the eyes. Neurologic examination was normal. A typical episode was reproduced by having the patient hyperventilate. The patient was noted to stop hyperventilation and stare blankly for approximately 10 seconds with some blinking of the eyes. She was unable to repeat numbers said to her at that time. An EEG revealed three-per-second, generalized spike-wave activity typical of absence seizures (petit mal). The patient was placed on ethosuximide, a drug often helpful in absence seizures and the episodes stopped.

Discussion. This description of staring episodes in an 8-year-old girl who is otherwise normal is strongly suggestive of seizure activity of the so-called absence type, particularly since there are no automatisms and the spells are very short.

An electroencephalogram revealed features classic for absence seizures (petit mal).

This is known to be a benign, hereditary seizure syndrome, so no further workup is necessary unless her course does not evolve as predicted.

Treatment with one of the drugs usually effective in the control of absence seizures was undertaken and was successful. Another drug considered by many to be the drug of choice in this condition is valproic acid.

Bibliography

Commission on Classification and Terminology of the International League Against Epilepsy. Proposal for revised classification of epilepsies and epileptic syndromes. *Epilepsia* 30:389–399, 1989. *This is the original description of The International Classification of Epileptic Syndromes.*

Engel J, Jr (ed.). *Seizures and Epilepsy.* Philadelphia: Davis, 1989, pp. 41–70. *This is a comprehensive text. The chapter entitled Mechanisms of Neuronal Excitation and Synchronization is particularly good for pathophysiology of epilepsy.*

Siegel GJ, Agranoff BW, Albers RW, et al. (eds.). *Basic Neurochemistry* (5th ed.). New York: Raven, 1994. *Recently revised edition of an excellent textbook on the subject.*

Wyllie E (ed.). *The Treatment of Epilepsy: Principles and Practice.* Philadelphia, PA: Lea & Febiger, 1993. *This is another excellent comprehensive text.*

67 Head Pain and Cranial Neuralgia

James R. Couch, Jr.

Objectives

After completing this chapter, you should be able to

Understand the basis for organization and classification of headache disorders

Develop concepts regarding classification of headache disorders

Learn how to approach headache patients and their problems

Develop concepts regarding the pathogenesis of the more common headaches

Headache has been called the most common symptom which is manifested by patients. In a large study of apparently normal subjects, 90% had had a headache in the previous year. Of this same group, some 50% had had a headache intense enough to be rated as severe to disabling. In another study, 25% of the patients who came to a primary care physician's office were noted to have headache

Table 67-1. Approach to the Patient with Headache or Facial Pain

Establish a profile of the headache.
    Determine the frequency of the pain or headache.
    Determine the duration of the pain or headache.
    Determine the intensity of the pain or headache.
    With the elements of frequency, intensity, and duration, a profile of headache at this time can be constructed.
Determine the nonpain symptoms associated with the headache (i.e., gastrointestinal, neurologic, etc.)
Determine the past history of the headache or facial pain and whether the patient has suffered the present pain at any time in the past. That is, did the patient have similar headaches or facial pains 1, 5, 10, 20, 30, 40 years ago? Were the frequency, duration, and intensity the same? Has the pain been present essentially most of the time since the onset or have there been cycles of occurrence of the pain or headache?
Determine the precipitating factors.
Carry out a physical and neurologic examination.

as either a primary or secondary complaint. Finally, one need only look at the frequency with which headache remedies are advertised to ascertain that the headache is a common problem for many people.

In this chapter, an approach to the headache patient will be presented along with an explanation and description of the more common headache problems. The approach to the headache patient is shown in Table 67-1. This should be kept in mind while reading the remaining material.

Pain-Sensitive Structures in the Head

Pain sensitive structures in the head are conveniently classified as intracranial or extracranial in location.

Extracranial Sources of Pain

For the extracranial space, virtually all structures are innervated with pain fibers and pain localization is accurate and dependable (Fig. 67-1). The head has a much higher density of sensory innervation than any other part of the body except for the tips of the digits. Pain-sensitive epidermal structures include the skin and all of the mucous membranes. These epidermal-derived coverings are exquisitely sensitive and heavily innervated. The only exception is the lining of the sinuses themselves, which is sparsely inner-

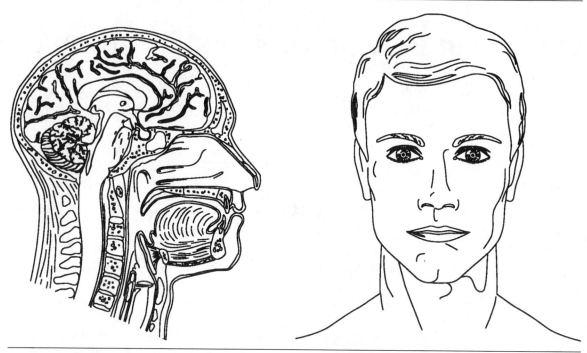

Fig. 67-1. Extracranial pain-sensitive structures include the skin, muscles, ligaments, periosteum, mucous membranes, eyes, and teeth. Intracranial pain sensitive structures include arteries, veins, venous sinuses, meninges, and sensory cranial nerves.

vated. However, the area around the ostium of each sinus is heavily innervated and highly pain sensitive. Consequently, in the typical "sinus" headache, pain is usually produced by irritation of the nasal mucosa around the ostium draining the sinus and not so much by irritation of the sinus itself.

The middle ear cavity represents another exquisitely pain-sensitive structure which is embryologically related to the nasopharynx and is connected to it by the eustachian tube. Irritation of the middle ear linings can produce severe pain in the ear and its surrounding area, including the nearby suboccipital and mastoid region.

The teeth are also subject to pain produced by caries, pulp abscesses, and tooth fractures.

The eye and the orbit may also be a source of pain. The conjunctiva over the eye is exquisitely sensitive to chemical or mechanical irritation. The muscles of the eye and the structures at the back of the eye including the meninges covering the optic nerve are quite pain sensitive. In patients with optic neuritis, movement of the eye will usually produce pain. The globe itself is very sensitive to pressure. Patients with glaucoma due to poor drainage of fluid from the anterior chamber, and resultant increased pressure in the eye, will often have severe pain.

The mesodermal structures in the head including arteries and muscles (masseter, temporalis, occipital frontalis) are also very pain sensitive; with increased contraction, these may provide the source of tension headache.

Finally, while the bones themselves are not innervated, the periosteum is very sensitive. The upper cervical spine may be subject to arthritis in the cranio-spinal or spino-spinal joints and the pain that is generated may be referred to the suboccipital region or to the retro-orbital region producing headache.

Intracranial Sources of Pain

These are primarily the meninges and blood vessels in the subarachnoid space. The parenchyma of the brain and intra-parenchymal blood vessels are not pain sensitive.

Pain related to stimulation of the meninges can be referred quite widely. For example, stimulation of the posterior fossa meninges refers pain to the retro-orbital region; stimulation of the area around the pituitary fossa refers pain to the vertex and stimulation of the frontal meninges refers pain to the suboccipital region.

A good deal of the pain referral results from the neural connections of the medullospinal junction as depicted in Fig. 67-2. At the medullospinal junction, there is a mixture of second-order neurons of the spinal V nucleus (spinal trigeminal nucleus) and those of the substantia gelatinosa whose input is from the C2 and C3 dermatomes with second-order neurons feeding into the lateral spinothalamic tract. It is thought this intermingling permits referred pain in both distributions. Hence pain generated from the retro-orbital region could be referred to the suboccipital region and pain generated in the C2 or C3 dermatomes could be referred to the retro-orbital region.

Fig. 67-2. Spinal trigeminal (spinal V) tract, where the first synapse of trigeminal nerve fibers occurs, courses down the brainstem from the main nucleus of the V nerve in the upper pons to the lower medulla. The spinal V tract then becomes contiguous with and intermingles with the Substantia Gelatinosa of Rolando in the dorsal horn of the spinal cord gray matter at the medullospinal junction. The termination of the spinal V tract neurons is arranged in a rostro-caudal fashion with lower branches terminating more rostrally and upper branches more caudally. The second-order neurons project rostrally in the trigeminal lemniscus to the posterior ventral medial nucleus of the thalamus. The mandibular branch input synapses most rostrally in the pons; the maxillary branch input synapses in the lower pons and upper medulla and the ophthalmic branch synapses in the lower medulla extending down to the medullospinal junction and even to the C3, C4 spinal level. For these axons, the second order neuron projects rostrally in the spinothalamic tract instead of the trigeminal lemniscus.

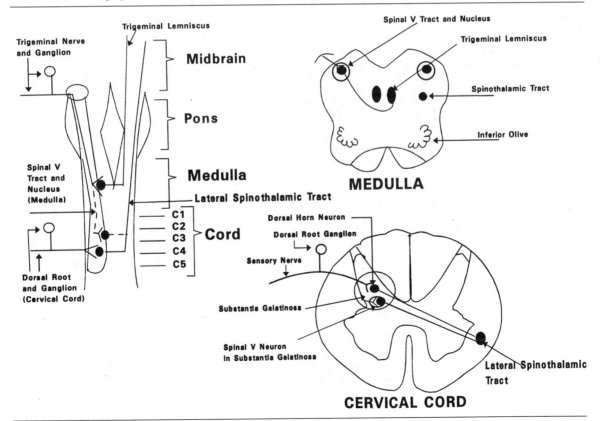

Headache

The types of headache can be broadly divided into the primary or functional and the secondary or organic types. Functional (primary or idiopathic) headaches are those for which we cannot identify a definite cause and organic (secondary) headaches are those for which some type of underlying etiology can be found. Secondary headaches can be broadly divided into headaches associated with toxic/metabolic disorders, vascular, or inflammatory problems, mass lesions, head or neck trauma, and "other." A decision algorithm for approaching the headache patient is presented in Fig. 67-3.

Functional Headaches

The major functional headaches are migraine, cluster, and tension type.

Migraine Headache

The migraine syndrome is very common. It is estimated that migraine occurs in between 15 and 30% of women and 3 to 13% of men. The onset of the migraine syndrome usually occurs at younger ages. 70% of patients with migraine headache will have onset before age 30 and approximately 95% will have onset before age 60. Approximately 5% of prepubertal children will have migraine type of headaches and in the prepubertal period the male-female incidence is equal.

Clinical Features.   The migraine syndrome has a number of prominent features that can be divided into five broad areas. (1) pain, (2) general symptoms that are difficult to localize — photophobia, phonophobia, (3) gastrointestinal and other autonomic symptoms, (4) neurologic symptoms, and (5) mood changes. Table 67-2 reviews the symptoms associated with the migraine syndrome.

The pain of migraine is classically described as a throbbing, pounding type of pain. In fact, the pain may be either throbbing or steady. It may be either unilateral or bilateral. It may be frontal, retro-orbital, vertex, suboccipital, or any combination of the above. As a rule, the characteristics of the pain are less important than the symptoms associated with the pain. Movement usually makes migraine worse.

Fig. 67-3. Clinical characteristics of organic and functional headaches are outlined. In general, headaches of organic etiology are of recent onset, are associated with reproduction pain or facial tenderness, and have symptoms or signs.

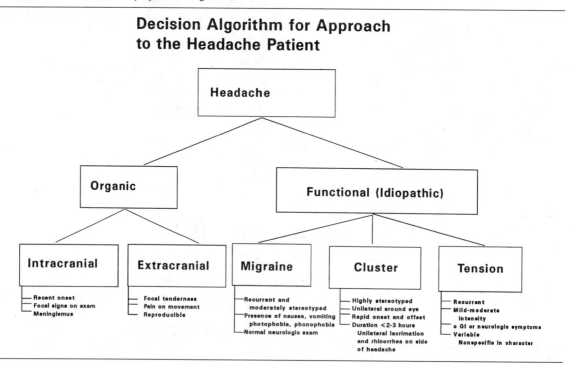

Table 67-2. Frequency of Migraine-Associated Symptoms and Clinical Features

Symptoms	Couch et al. (1991) 793 Subjects
LOCATION OF HEADACHE	
Unilateral only	48%
Bilateral or mixed (unilateral/ bilateral)	52%
NONPAIN SYMPTOMS	
General symptoms	
Nausea	92%
Vomiting	57%
Diarrhea	14%
Photophobia	79%
Phonophobia	62%
Neurologic symptoms	
Visual symptoms	57%
Positive visual symptoms	37%
Negative visual symptoms	20%
Blurred vision	30%
Mono- or hemiparesis	8%
Mono- or hemisensory loss	17%
4-limb weakness	8%
4-limb sensory loss	8%
Aphasia	18%
Dizziness (giddiness)	25%
True vertigo	11%
Loss or alteration of consciousness	17%
Confusional state only	9%

Modified from: Couch JR, Bearss CM, Kolm P, and Verhulst S. Migraine: a single entity or multiple syndromes? *Cephalalgia* 11(Suppl. II):91–92, 1991, by permission of Scandinavian University Press.

Therefore, most patients find that by lying down in a dark room produces some relief.

The origin of photophobia and phonophobia, or sensitivity to light and noise, is unknown. These are common symptoms and add significantly to the discomfort. The combination of nausea, photophobia, and phonophobia without meningismus and with a normal neurologic examination is the usual picture of migraine.

The incidence of neurologic symptoms outlined in Table 67-2 represents lifetime occurrences. These symptoms do not necessarily occur with every headache. The visual symptoms are the most common occurring in approximately 50% of patients. For the most part, these are usually unformed flashes of light, collections of "stars," or

black spots. Less often, the classical arcuate (C-shaped) scotoma or the fortification spectra of zig-zag lines are seen. The migraine-associated visual symptoms, whether positive (stars) or negative (spots), usually have a sensation of movement. If the visual phenomena are stationary, they are less likely to be migrainous in origin. Occipital lobe seizures (which constitute only 1–2% of all seizures) may produce visual phenomena very similar to those of migraine and should be ruled out in cases of visual aura related to migraine.

Other neurologic phenomena include cortical symptoms of transient hemiparesis, hemisensory loss, or aphasia and brainstem symptoms of quadraparesis, bilateral sensory loss, or vertigo. Loss of consciousness can be seen in patients with migraine headache, and periods of confusion or disorientation are not uncommon.

Visual and other neurologic symptoms may occur before or during a headache. These phenomena may occur in the absence of a headache, a condition termed migraine-sans-migraine.

Mood changes are also fairly common before or after a migraine. The most common mood change is that the patient will feel slowed down or depressed for a period of a few hours up to 24 hours after the migraine headache has remitted. Patients will often describe this as having a "hangover" after their headache. Patients often will attribute this to having taking medication for a headache, but the same phenomenon can be seen in patients who do not take medication. Depression may also occur in the period of up to 24 hours before a headache as a prodromal sign. Occasionally, patients will have a hypomanic phase of elevated energy before or after the migraine.

Pathogenesis. A combination of central nervous system and craniovascular system disturbances are postulated to explain the migraine headache. The CNS manifestations such as the visual symptoms, hemiparesis, aphasia, and hemisensory loss are thought to be related to the neurophysiologic phenomenon of "spreading depression." The theory suggests that spreading depression is initiated in the cerebral cortex at the onset of the migraine headache. As the spreading depression moves across the cortex, it produces the neurologic symptomatology.

The pain of migraine is postulated to be related to the trigeminal innervation of the cranial vascular system. Trigeminal afferent nerve endings on blood vessels can release neurotransmitters including substance P, neurokinin, calcitonin gene-related peptide, and possibly other compounds, including serotonin, onto the blood vessel wall. These neurotransmitters then produce sterile inflammation and pain. It would appear that these transmitters are released through an axon reflex type of mechanism. This is the same mechanism which produces the wheel and flare when one scratches the skin. This sterile inflammation in turn produces pain and swelling in the area of the artery.

The origin of the autonomic symptoms, the mood changes, and the photophobia and phonophobia is unclear. There must be multiple mechanisms to account for the five major areas of the migraine syndrome noted above.

Cluster Headaches

The cluster headache is seen in males at a frequency of 4–5:1 over females. The onset is usually in the 20s or 30s but may have onset as late as the 60s. Patients will often have the cycles of headache about the same time every year or every other year. However, the cycles may vary in their frequency from twice a year to as little as once every 8–10 years.

Clinical Features.   Cluster headache has a highly stereotyped pattern. The headache is always unilateral and located around the eye. It may be located in the eye or above or to the side or below, but the eye is virtually always involved. At times the pain may spread to the suboccipital region or even to the shoulder.

The patient with a cluster headache notes a rapid onset of pain over a few minutes with ascension of the pain to a plateau of great intensity which lasts for 10–120 minutes. During this time, the patient will usually note that being up and moving about will produce some relief from the pain as opposed to the migraine patient, who wants to be lying very still and not moving. After a period of 10–120 minutes, the pain will remit very rapidly. The patient will then have no residual pain until the next headache occurs. The "cluster headache" generally does occur in clusters. The patient will note onset of the first headache and then a gradually increasing frequency of headaches over a period of a week or so with a peak frequency of 1 to 3 headaches per day. The upside of the cycle will last for up to 12 weeks and then the headaches will remit. The headache will always remain on the same side during a bout of cluster headaches. Symptoms noted with the headache include nausea and vomiting in approximately 25–30%. Patient will often note unilateral photophobia on the side of the headache. Lacrimation and rhinorrhea on the side of the headache are very common symptoms with cluster headache. Occasionally the patient will have only a stuffy nose on the side of the headache. About 10% will have a partial Horner's syndrome characterized by miosis and ptosis.

Pathogenesis.   The etiology of the cluster headache is entirely unknown. The syndrome may be related to the petrosal ganglion which is located close to the mucosa of the nose in the lateral recess behind the middle turbinate bone. Indeed, cocaine applied to this area with its local anesthetic effect may relieve cluster headache in a significant number of patients, although this is not a generally recommended treatment. Patients with cluster headache have alterations of cerebral blood flow on the side of the headache and will also have loss of autoregulation of cerebral blood flow during the cluster headache.

Cluster headaches can be precipitated by alcohol during the period in which the patient is having the cluster. When the patients are out of the so-called cluster, they may drink heavily and have no difficulty with headache. The mechanism of this intermittent alcohol sensitivity is unknown.

Tension Headache

Tension headache is the most common type of headache and probably the least well understood. As a broad generality, when one has ruled out organic headaches, migraine headaches, and cluster headaches, one is left with the entity of tension headache. The tension headache probably occurs in most individuals at some time or other. It occurs equally in males and females and may occur essentially anytime throughout life.

Clinical Features.   The tension headache is usually described as a steady, aching pain which is bandlike about the head or feels like a skullcap that is too tight. In some the headache may be associated with suboccipital pain and even pain in the back of the neck. It is unclear, however, whether the neck pain is part of the tension headache syndrome or secondary to tensing up the neck muscles in association with the headache. Similar neck pain can be observed in the migraine syndrome.

Tension headache may be associated with some degree of photophobia or phonophobia, but these symptoms are usually mild. Nausea, vomiting, diarrhea, or anorexia do not occur nor is the headache associated with visual or neurologic symptoms.

The tension headache may last for a variable period of time, ranging from minutes to hours to days to years. The headache is usually bilateral but may be unilateral. It may be localized primarily to the front or the back of the head and it may vary in its location from time to time. The tension headache may respond to simple analgesics. If analgesics are overused, however, the headache may develop into a rebound type of headache related to withdrawal of the analgesic or sedative-tranquilizer or muscle relaxant medication used to treat the headache.

Pathogenesis.   The mechanism of generation of the tension headache is unknown. There have been many theories which, in general, have postulated that there is muscle contraction in response to psychological stress. Recent studies have demonstrated that patients with tension headache have alteration in "the exteroceptive mandibular response." This response is elicited by tapping on the masseter muscle and recording the electrical activity of the contraction response. The afferent limb is through the trigeminal sensory fibers and the efferent through the trigeminal motor fibers going to the masseter. Alteration in this reflex is thought to represent brainstem dysfunction in the tension headache patient.

Tension-Migraine Headache and Chronic Daily Headache

Patients who have frequent migraine headaches may develop intermittent tension headaches along with their frequent migraine headaches. Likewise, patients with frequent tension headaches may have migraine symptoms with their more severe headaches, suggesting that a migraine-type headache has started to occur in conjunction with the tension headache.

The patient with combination tension and migraine headache may develop a syndrome of daily or almost daily occurrence of headache which has come to be known as the "chronic daily headache." This is a descriptive term that only refers to the persistence of occurrence of headache and not to any etiologic mechanism. These patients typically complain of a daily headache of moderate or less intensity with characteristics of a tension headache. Superimposed on the daily tension headache the patient will have intermittent, more severe headaches which will fit a description of migraine.

This is an important entity for the physician to recognize. These patients often will have associated psychiatric problems of depression, anxiety, or both. Excessive use of analgesics, minor narcotics, barbiturates, benzodiazepines, or ergotamine may result in a rebound-withdrawal or habituation-withdrawal headache pattern. Here the patient habituates to the medication and withdrawal or nonuse precipitates a headache. The treatment includes withdrawal of such symptomatic medication.

Organic Headache

Seven basic categories of disease which may cause headache are listed in Table 67-3.

Toxic Headache

There is an extremely wide variety of environmental and other toxins which can cause headaches. Generally, these can be broken down into inorganic compounds, organic compounds, and gases. The usual inorganic compounds in-

Table 67-3. Etiologic Categories for Organic Headaches

Toxic
Metabolic
Vascular
Tumor
Trauma

clude lead, mercury, and arsenic. Cadmium, thallium, and other trace elements can cause headache in specific situations. Headache usually results when there is a low-level chronic or acute toxicity. In acute overwhelming intoxications, the patient usually develops an encephalopathy very rapidly, becomes unconscious, and does not complain of headache.

Headache-producing organic compounds include most of the organic solvents as well as a large number of other compounds that may appear in industrial processes ranging from herbicides and insecticides to aniline dyes. Again, exposure and dose are key elements. The headache associated with both inorganic and organic solvents is usually a nonspecific steady holocranial pain of modest intensity. The headache is seldom associated with neurologic manifestations until late in the course. Gastrointestinal manifestations may be due to a direct effect of the toxic agent.

The toxic headache is best typified by that of carbon monoxide intoxication. Carbon monoxide produces carboxyhemoglobin (CXHB) which is ineffective for oxygen transport; the result is tissue hypoxia. At CXHB levels of 5–10%, the patient usually notes a low-grade headache. At 20–30%, the patient notes a moderate to severe headache and at levels above 30% the patient continues to note a severe headache but begins to get confused. Above 40% the patient becomes more confused and encephalopathic with decreasing complaint of headache. Coma and death ensue at CXHB levels exceeding 50–60%.

This example illustrates some general principles of the toxic/metabolic headache. In general, the headache is holocranial and increases in severity with increasing exposure up to a point. Then the patient becomes confused and encephalopathic, and complaints of headache diminish. Finally, of course, comatose patients don't complain of headache or any other symptoms.

Metabolic Headache

Headaches are sometimes associated with hepatic or renal disease. Hypoglycemia and hyponatremia often produce headache. Endocrinopathies including hypothyroidism, hypoadrenalism, and (rarely) hypopituitarism may occasionally produce a headache of mild to moderate intensity.

Vascular Headache

Headaches of vascular origin include those of subarachnoid hemorrhage owing to ruptured aneurysms or arteriovenous malformations. The headache of subarachnoid hemorrhage is usually of sudden onset, holocranial, and very intense. The patient generally will have meningismus (nuchal rigidity). Patients with ruptured aneurysms often will have focal neurologic signs relating to the adjacent cranial nerves, usually III, IV, VI, or occasionally V. If the ruptured aneurysm causes brain parenchymal destruction or there is an intraparenchymal hematoma from an arteriovenous malformation, focal neurologic signs result and will reflect the area of brain damage.

Headaches may also be associated with vasculitis in and around the cranium. An important form of arteritis to recognize is temporal arteritis, which is characterized by occurrence of unilateral headaches in the older person with visual impairment accompanied by an elevated erythrocyte sedimentation rate. The condition can progress to irreversible blindness from ischemia to the optic nerve.

One-third of strokes are associated with headaches. Also headaches of a migraine-tension type may occur following endarterectomy. The cause of these headaches is unknown.

Tumors

They usually cause headaches by causing increased intracranial pressure. (The pathophysiology of intracranial pressure is detailed in Chap. 65.) However, Fig. 67-4 summarizes the relationship of intracranial pressure to the headache. With the above in mind, headache is usually a late manifestation of intracranial tumors. An exception to this generality occurs if the tumor involves a pain-sensitive structure early in its course.

Fig. 67-4. Schematic presentation of relation of size of an intracranial mass lesion to change in intracranial pressure (ICP). There is capacitance within the cranial space for accommodating to increase in lesion size by having lesion expand into ventricular, subarachnoid, or venous space.

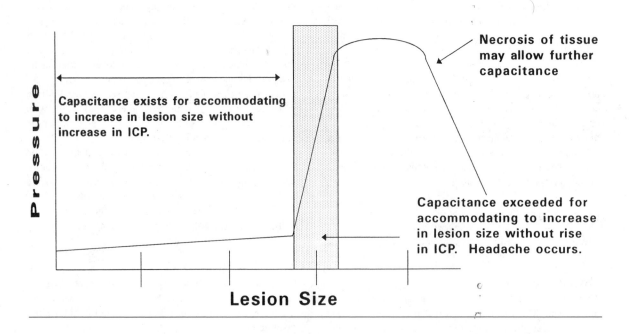

Trauma

Subdural and epidermal hematoma usually produce focal headaches in the region of the hematoma. The meninges are very pain sensitive and disruption of them by the hematoma will usually produce a headache early in the course. In addition, the patient may develop the increased intracranial pressure headache noted above.

Cranial Neuralgias

The cranial neuralgias constitute a particular type of pain which is very characteristic if not unmistakable. Neuralgias result when there is damage to a nerve resulting in ephaptic (nonsynaptic) conduction between nerve fibers, creating a short circuit. The area of ephaptic conduction may be in the nerve itself or in the central connections of the nerve. There are, of course, many aspects of this situation that are not understood. The most common types of neuralgic pain are trigeminal neuralgia and glossopharyngeal neuralgia.

Trigeminal Neuralgia

Usually of unknown etiology, it generally tends to occur in older individuals and is characterized by lancinating pains occurring in the distribution of one or (rarely) two divisions of the trigeminal nerve. Usually the mandibular or maxillary branches are involved, but occasionally the ophthalmic branch may be the source of the neuralgic pain. Patients with multiple sclerosis occasionally develop trigeminal neuralgia.

The lancinating pain is a brief, extremely intense lightninglike pain which seems to shoot into the area subserved by the nerve. The pain is usually triggerable by light touch to a trigger zone. Firm pressure to the trigger zone will usually not result in the lancinating pain, but light touch will often trigger the pain. Patient will usually have a normal neurologic examination with no indication of abnormality in the area of the nerve involved. The patient, however, will live in fear of the next lancinating pain. The trigger zones are often around or inside the mouth and patients may lose weight because eating provokes the pains.

Glossopharyngeal Neuralgia

This is a similar situation relating to the ninth cranial nerve, which has a small sensory representation in the oropharynx. In glossopharyngeal neuralgia, the patient has an intense lancinating pain in the throat triggered by swallowing. The pain will be felt on one side of the oropharynx. Again, the patient may be reluctant to eat because of the pain.

Clinical Examples

1. A 28-year-old woman is evaluated for intermittent headaches. She noted that for the last 6 months she has had a headache once per month. The headaches typically occurred one to two days before her menstrual period and would last for 24 hours. Approximately 30 minutes before the headache, the patient would note a sensation of twinkling stars in the upper right visual field. The stars would "swim" around. This sensation lasted 5–10 minutes and would remit; 10–20 minutes later the patient would note the onset of a pain in her right temple. The pain would escalate in intensity over the next hour and remain very intense over the next 3–6 hours. During this time, the patient would note photophobia, phonophobia, nausea, and vomiting. She would occasionally have 2–3 loose stools during the headache. After 3–6 hours the pain would begin to ease but the headache would often last for 12–24 hours. Typically, the patient would note that if she can get to sleep the headache would be gone when she awakens.

She had occasionally observed a sensation of numbness in her right hand during a headache. Occasionally at the peak of the headache the patient would have difficulty talking and would get words mixed up. The patient was taking birth control pills which she began 6 months ago and was on a cycle with 21 days on the pill and 7 days off.

The patient recalled having occasional severe headaches in junior high and high school which required her to go home or to the nurse's office. She recalled no details except that she did have nausea and vomiting with these headaches. Intermittent recurrent headaches occurred in her mother and maternal grandmother. The patient's general physical and neurologic examinations are normal.

Discussion.   The headache occurs intermittently and appears to be precipitated by the menstrual cycle. The duration of the headache is fairly stereotyped at 12–24 hours. The patient has visual symptoms that are compatible with migraine. She also has aphasia and a transient right hemiparesis. These are all features which can be associated with classic migraine headache. The history of headaches going back as far as junior high would strongly favor this being one of the functional varieties of headache and not a headache secondary to some organic etiology.

2. A 56-year-old man presented for evaluation of facial pain. For the last 6–8 months he had been having intermittent pains in his right upper jaw. The pain was characterized as a sharp, stabbing, lightninglike pain that was very brief in duration but of very high intensity. The pain seemed to shoot into the right maxillary region and right upper lip. Initially he had minimal difficulty with pain and it would occur only occasionally; however, the pain had become more frequent. The pain was triggered by touching the gum around the right upper canine tooth and he found it almost impossible to eat without triggering the pain. Over the last month, he had lost 15 pounds as a result of not eating. The patient recalled a similar pain which occurred for a brief period a few years ago.

General physical and neurologic examination was normal except for an appearance of recent weight loss. Stimulation of the gum around the first canine tooth would trigger the sharp shooting pain but there was no sensory loss in this area. Patient was treated with carbamazepine with complete remission of the pain while he was taking the medication. If he missed a dose of the carbamazepine, however, the pain would recur.

Discussion.   This patient has lancinating pains in the right upper jaw, which are very intense, brief, and triggerable. The pain follows the distribution of the maxillary branch of trigeminal nerve. The most likely etiology is idiopathic trigeminal neuralgia. However, an MRI was done to evaluate the course of the trigeminal nerve from its exit in the pons, to the trigeminal ganglion in the petrous bone, through the cavernous sinus, and to its exit from the cranium via the foramen rotundum to the facial structures. With a structural lesion along the course of the trigeminal excluded, treatment was initiated with carbamazepine to suppress pain.

Bibliography

Ad hoc Committee on Classification of Headache. Classification of Headache. *JAMA* 179:717–718, 1962. *The classification of headache outlines types of headache and clinical criteria.*

Cady RK and Fox AW. *Treating the Headache Patient.* New York: Dekker, 1995. *This is the newest reference on headache. It was written for the primary care physician and provides a good review of many aspects of headache. Especially recommended is Chap. 2: Couch, J. Complexities of Presentation and Pathogenesis of Migraine Headache, pp. 15–40.*

Couch JR, Bearss CM, Kolm P, and Verhulst S. Migraine: a single entity or multiple syndromes? *Cephalalgia* 11(Suppl. II):91–92, 1991. *Study which defines characteristics of migraine patients.*

Dalessio DJ. *Wolff's Headache and Other Head Pain* (5th ed.). New York: Oxford University Press, 1987. *This is a classic book on headache which has been recently updated.*

Olesen J, Tfelt-Hansen P, and Welch KMA. *The Headaches.* New York: Raven, 1993. *This is the most complete reference on headache available today. The book contains a number of thoughtful and well-written chapters giving highly developed references on many aspects of headache.*

Tollison CD and Kunkel RS. *Headache: Diagnosis and Treatment.* Baltimore: Williams and Wilkins, 1993. *Good reference book on headache. Especially recommended is Chap. 18: Couch J. Medical Management of Recurrent Tension-Type Headache, pp. 151–162.*

68 Cerebrovascular Disorders

Michael R. Hahn and L. Philip Carter

Objectives

After completing this chapter, you should be able to

Develop an understanding of cerebrovascular anatomy

Localize vascular lesions to an anatomic distribution

Develop concepts regarding ischemic cerebrovascular dis-

ease which will allow for a diagnostic and therapeutic plan

Develop concepts regarding hemorrhagic cerebrovascular disease which will allow for a diagnostic and therapeutic plan

---

Cerebrovascular disease is characterized by either an ischemic or hemorrhagic pathogenesis related to lesions involving the arterial or venous system. Ischemic lesions are localized to an arterial or venous distribution and are the result of thrombotic or embolic occlusions. Hemorrhagic lesions have a more heterogenous pathogenesis. Clinical diagnosis of cerebrovascular disease is dependent upon an understanding of the arterial and venous supply of the central nervous system, and the pathogenesis of ischemic and hemorrhagic lesions.

Cerebrovascular Anatomy and Localization of Occlusive Lesions

Arterial

The brain requires a near constant supply of nutrients to function and survive. The four arteries that supply the brain are the paired carotid and vertebral arteries.

Carotid Arteries

The common carotids are derived from the brachiocephalic artery on the right and the aortic arch on the left, but there are many variations in this anatomy. Branching into the internal and external carotid occurs at the level of the hyoid bone (Fig. 68-1). The first branch from the intracranial internal carotid is the ophthalmic artery which occa-

sionally provides an anastomotic pathway from the external to internal circulation in times of need. The internal carotid artery divides to become the anterior cerebral and the middle cerebral arteries. The middle cerebral artery behaves as a continuation of the internal carotid and carries approximately 80% of the blood flow entering the anterior circulation. Embolization occurs in this distribution most frequently. The middle cerebral artery emerges from the Sylvian fissure to nourish the lateral portion of the frontal, temporal, and parietal lobes (Fig. 68-2). The anterior cerebral arteries supply the brain bordering in the interhemispheric fissure from the frontal lobe to the precuneus in the parietal lobe (Fig. 68-3).

Symptoms of anterior circulation disease are those that reflect its distribution. Monocular blindness may occur from occlusion of the ophthalmic artery. Occlusion of an anterior cerebral artery would typically result in a sensorimotor deficit of the contralateral foot and leg with a lesser deficit to the arm. Sensation and movement of the face is generally spared. With bilateral involvement, the patient may develop bilateral leg weakness, urinary incontinence, and abulia (blunting of initiative). Occlusion of the middle cerebral artery will usually cause a dense sensorimotor deficit of the contralateral face, arm, with varying degrees of leg deficit. If the dominant hemisphere is affected, aphasia is likely. A homonymous hemianopsia or quadrantanopsia is possible if the blood supply to the visual pathway is affected.

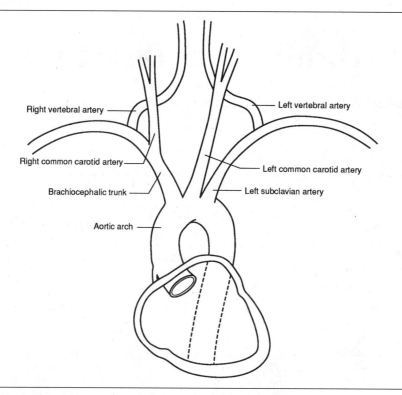

Fig. 68-1. Normal morphology of the common carotid and vertebral arteries.

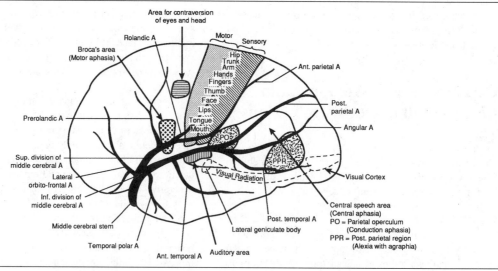

Fig. 68-2. The middle cerebral arteries supply: the lateral aspect of the frontal, parietal, and temporal lobes. (Used with permission from Adams RD and Victor M. *Principles of Neurology* (5th ed.). New York: McGraw-Hill, 1993, p. 677.)

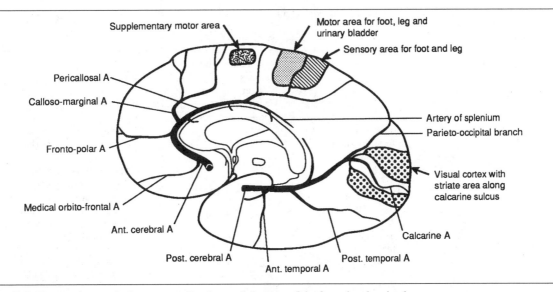

Fig. 68-3. The anterior cerebral artery supplies the medial aspect of the frontal and parietal lobes, while the posterior cerebral artery supplies the medial aspect of the occipital lobe. (Used with permission from: Adams RD and Victor M. *Principles of Neurology* (5th ed.). New York: McGraw-Hill, 1993, p. 680.)

Vertebral Arteries

The vertebral arteries usually originate from the subclavian arteries bilaterally. Entering the sixth vertebral body's foramina, they continue cephalad entering the skull through the foramen magnum. Once intracranial, the vertebral arteries give off the posterior inferior cerebellar arteries. The vertebrals then merge on the ventral portion of the brainstem at the level of the pontomedullary junction to form the basilar artery. The anterior inferior cerebellar arteries are the next significant branches, followed by the superior cerebellar arteries. Multiple small perforating vessels originate from the basilar artery along its course to provide blood to the brainstem. The median perforating branches supply the medial brainstem (motor cranial nerves and corticospinal tracts) and the lateral or circumferential branches supply the lateral brainstem (sensory cranial nerves, cerebellar peduncles, and spinothalamic tracts). The posterior cerebral arteries are formed from the terminal bifurcation of the basilar artery and supply the thalamus, splenium of the corpus callosum, midbrain, inferior temporal, superomedial parietal, and occipital lobes. Sustained primarily from the vertebrobasilar system, these structures are quite vulnerable to vascular occlusion (see Fig. 68-3).

A variety of neurologic syndromes may result from occlusions in the vertebrobasilar systems affecting the brainstem and cerebellum. Common symptoms to suggest vertebrobasilar disease include diplopia, vertigo, tinnitus, and poor coordination from involvement of cranial nerves and cerebellar peduncles. Specific syndromes are outlined in Table 68-1. A key feature of brainstem lesions is ipsilateral cranial nerve dysfunction in the setting of contralateral extremity weakness, contralateral sensory abnormalities of limbs, or ipsilateral ataxia.

Anastomotic Circle of Willis

The anterior communicating artery connects the two anterior cerebral arteries while the posterior communicating arteries connect the internal carotid arteries to the posterior cerebral arteries. This creates an anatomic anastomosis known as the Circle of Willis (Fig. 68-4). When patent, this structure provides a margin of safety against vascular accidents involving the major tributaries. However, a complete and patent anastomotic arterial circle occurs in only 20–70% of the population. The most common anomalies are a hypoplastic artery, absence of a vessel, or vessel duplication.

A watershed zone is created between the distal tributaries of the major cerebral vessels. This area is the first to be compromised when there is a decrease in global or regional blood flow.

Table 68-1. Clinical Symptoms and Signs of Ischemic Cerebrovascular Disease

Primary Artery	Secondary Artery	Symptoms	Signs
Carotid		Monocular blindness Aphasia Neglect syndrome Hemiparesis (face, arm, leg) Hemisensory deficit	
	Middle cerebral artery: proximal		Hemiparesis (face, arm, leg) Hemisensory loss (face, arm, leg) Homonymous hemianopsia Aphasia or neglect syndrome
	Middle cerebral artery: distal		Monoparesis (face and arm) Sensory loss (face and arm) Homonymous hemianopsia
	Anterior cerebral artery		Monoparesis (leg) Sensory loss (leg)
Basilar-vertebral		Bilateral visual loss Dizziness-vertigo Diplopia Poor coordination	Crossed plegia Crossed sensory deficit
	Posterior inferior cerebellar artery		Ipsilateral CRN V, Horner's, CRN IX, CRN X, and ataxia Contralateral hemisensory deficit
	Anterior inferior cerebellar artery		Ipsilateral CRN V, Horner's, CRN VIII, and ataxia Contralateral hemisensory deficit
	Superior cerebellar artery		Ipsilateral ataxia
	Posterior cerebral artery		Homonymous hemianopsia (alexia without agraphia with dominant occipital lesion)
	Basilar penetrators (medial)		Crossed plegia (ipsilateral CRN III, VI, VII, or XII and contralateral hemiparesis)

Venous System

The venous system is not as consistent in anatomic arrangement as the arterial system. However, certain venous circuits remain relatively constant. The superior sagittal sinus is created by the dural falx cerebri and its intersection with the dura overlying the cerebral cortex. This provides the drainage for the outer cortical mantle. The hydrostatic pressure is low in this structure and can sometimes be negative when compared with the outside environment. When a direct communication with atmospheric air is present, as in the case of penetrating trauma or by surgical entry, air can be drawn in and sent detrimentally to the heart. The anterior one-third of the superior sagittal sinus may be sacrificed without precipitating venous congestion. Acute occlusion of the posterior two-thirds, however, has an attendant great risk of producing cerebral infarction. However, slow occlusion via tumor or other compressive process may allow sufficient time for collateral venous circulation to develop. The sagittal sinus intersects the straight sinus posteriorly and creates the anatomic sinus confluens, also known as the torcular Herophili. A

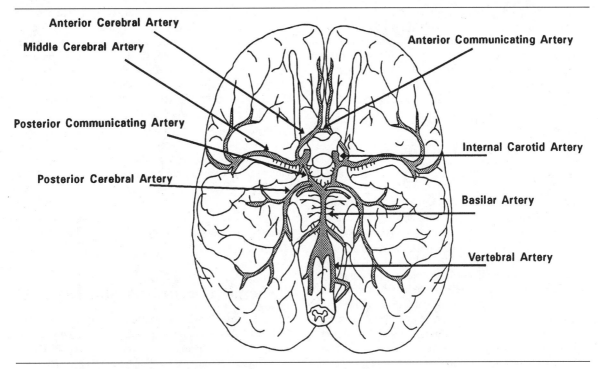

Fig. 68-4. The circle of Willis is comprised of the anterior communicating artery which provides an anastomosis between both anterior cerebral arteries; the posterior communicating arteries provide an anastomosis between the internal cerebral and posterior cerebral arteries.

bifurcation occurs creating the transverse sinuses, the right being dominant in most cases. Sigmoid sinuses are created at the floor of the posterior fossa as the venous channels make their exitus from the skull to create the internal jugular veins. There is venous drainage from non-nervous tissue, the scalp for example, inward towards these great sinuses from emissary veins. Bidirectional flow may occur because the veins of the central nervous system possess no valves. This may allow external infections to gain access to the cerebral venous system.

The signs and symptoms of venous occlusion are less well defined compared to the arterial system owing to the many variations of venous anatomy. Notable exceptions are occlusive lesions of the sagittal sinus and the cavernous sinus.

Saggital Sinus Occlusion

Occlusion of the sagittal sinus is typically associated with headaches, paraplegia, and seizures. Increased intracranial pressure from obstruction of venous return and hydrocephalus from decreased cerebrospinal fluid absorption are potential complications of sagittal sinus thrombosis. The somatosensory cortex lies under the sagittal sinus; therefore, motor and sensory function of the lower extremities would be impaired with thrombosis of the sagittal sinus.

Cavernous Sinus Occlusion

Cranial nerves to extraocular muscles (III, IV, VI) and the ophthalmic and maxillary branches of the trigeminal travel through the cavernous sinus. An injury or infection of the cavernous sinus may cause ipsilateral ophthalmoplegia and sensory loss on the upper half of the face. The cavernous sinus may have contributions from emissary veins from the nasal sinuses which may allow an ascending infection to enter the cavernous sinus. Any condition of the cavernous sinus may involve any structures surrounding or traversing this venous sinus.

Microvasculature

Arterioles provide most of the resistance to the cerebral vascular system with regional blood flow being controlled by the precapillary sphincter. The cerebral blood vessels are composed of an outer adventitia and media which is generally thinner and less pronounced than the systemic blood vessels. The intima with its inner elastic membrane is similar in structure and form to the systemic counterpart. The endothelial cells of the cerebral capillaries are tightly joined together which prevent the passage of most substances, as compared with the systemic capillaries. This creates the blood-brain barrier.

Cerebrovascular Physiology

Autoregulation

The cerebral blood vessels have a unique ability to control (autoregulate) the amount of blood the brain receives within a range of 50–150 mm Hg mean arterial blood pressure. There are several different mechanisms involved, including changes in arterial blood gases. Hypoxia will increase blood flow to maintain the strict aerobic metabolism of the brain. Increased carbon dioxide in the arterial circulation ($PaCO_2$) is a potent vasodilator. Contrarily, a decrease in $PaCO_2$ will produce vasoconstriction of the intracranial blood vessels, decreasing the amount of blood perfusing the brain which subsequently will decrease intracranial volume. Thus hyperventilation is the most rapid method of decreasing intracranial pressure.

High blood pressures in the systemic circulation will cause constriction of the cerebral arterioles. This protective mechanism ensures that the brain receives a near constant blood flow even when mean systemic blood pressure is as high as 160 mm Hg. Chronic hypertension will eventually raise the level of autoregulation, so cerebral blood flow remains constant at even higher blood pressures. Hypotension in the normotensive patient causes dilation of the cerebral arterioles. This protective mechanism (which occurs to a mean pressure of 50 mm Hg) ensures that the brain has adequate cerebral perfusion despite hypotension. This lower limit of effective autoregulation is elevated in individuals with severe chronic hypertension. In this setting, an acute reduction in blood pressure can impair cerebral perfusion at blood pressure levels that would be well tolerated in a normal individual. Also flow-limiting lesions, such as atheromatous plaques, may decrease the available pressure to the cerebral vessels such that a higher systemic blood pressure is required for adequate perfusion of the affected region.

Metabolic Requirements

Different regions of the brain receive differing amounts of blood. The grey matter secures approximately 70–80 ml of blood per 100 g of tissue per minute while the white matter uses approximately one-third that amount. Globally, each 100 g of brain tissue extracts 3.5 ml of oxygen from 50 ml of blood flow each minute. Cerebral perfusion pressure (CPP) is calculated by subtracting the intracranial pressure (ICP) from the mean arterial pressure (MAP) according to this formula: CPP = MAP – ICP. Generally, 70 mm Hg provides adequate cerebral perfusion pressure blood flow.

Neuronal tissue injury induces edema and swelling which, if significant, will cause an increase in intracranial pressure. By the above equation, an increase in intracranial pressure without a concomitant increase in the mean arterial pressure may cause a critical decrease in the cerebral perfusion pressure. When the CPP is below 60 mm Hg, the brain is at risk of ischemic damage which may lead to infarction. The pathophysiology and control of ICP are discussed in Chap. 65.

Ischemic Cerebrovascular Disease

Stroke and cerebrovascular accident are colloquial terms and are used synonymously to indicate an irreversible neurologic injury owing to interruption of cerebral blood flow or spontaneous intraparenchymal hemorrhage. Of these two basic mechanisms, ischemia is the more common and will be covered first followed by a discussion of cerebral hemorrhage.

Pathogenic Mechanisms

Thrombosis
Simply defined: a blood clot that obstructs a blood vessel or develops in a cavity of the heart. A thrombus may originate anywhere in the cardiovascular system. It often occurs when there is vessel wall injury with subsequent platelet aggregation. The obstruction may be asymptomatic, may cause limitation in flow, or may result in complete occlusion. If adequate collateral circulation is not present, the tissue downstream is at risk of ischemia or infarction.

Atherosclerosis.   There are many causes of ischemia and infarction and yet most are caused by two mechanisms: atherosclerosis and embolic events. Atherosclerosis tends to form where large and medium blood vessels divide and occurs in the same fashion as atherosclerosis in the systemic circulation. Atherosclerotic disease of the carotid and vertebral arteries generally occurs one to two decades after the onset of aortic and coronary disease. Hypertension, smoking, diabetes, and a familial history are known risk factors for significant cerebrovascular atherosclerosis. It can occur anywhere from the origin of the carotids to distal cerebral vessels. Most commonly, critical occlusion takes place at the bifurcation of the internal and external carotid artery, followed by the bifurcation of the subclavian and brachiocephalic arteries into the common carotid. The arthroma of atherosclerosis is caused by vascular injury with deposition of lipids, cholesterol, cellular debris, and fibrin. A stenosis of 60% or greater of the vessel lumen is considered significant in inhibiting blood flow.

Nonatherosclerotic Causes of Thrombosis. Nonatherosclerotic causes of thrombosis include fibromuscular dysplasia, arteritis from inflammatory and infectious disease, physical injury to vessels (trauma and radiation), "hypercoaguable states," and vasculopathies associated with amyloid. However, any vascular injury may promote clot formation and subsequent thrombosis.

1. Fibromuscular dysplasia. Fibromuscular dysplasia is a systemic affliction which most commonly affects large arteries such as the aorta, renal arteries, and carotid arteries. Occasionally the vertebral and intracranial vessels may be involved. Focal aneurysms along the vessel with lumenal narrowing occur from a fibroproliferative reaction of the media in the vessel wall. Diagnosis is most commonly made by angiography, which demonstrates a "string of pearls" appearance. Pathologic specimens will reveal replacement of smooth muscle by fibroproliferative tissue.

2. Hypercoagulable states. Conditions that cause hyperviscosity and hypercoagulability include dehydration, multiple myeloma and other dysproteinemias, anti-phospholipid antibodies, paraneoplastic conditions, and polycythemia. A "sludging effect" occurs which prevents adequate oxygenation of the cerebral parenchyma or thrombosis. Protein C, protein S, and antithrombin III deficiencies are usually associated with venous thrombosis but have also been implicated in arterial occlusion. Approximately 15% of patients with homozygous sickle cell anemia will have an occlusive cerebrovascular incident.

Embolism

Occlusive embolization occurs when any material travels intravascularly to cause obstruction at a site removed from its origin. Emboli are most commonly dislodged thrombi, but air, fat, bone marrow, and iatrogenically introduced material may also embolize.

Cardiogenic Embolism. The most common source of cerebral thromboembolism is the left side of the heart. Mural thrombi may form in response to endothelial injury from myocardial infarction or from the left atrium owing to atrial fibrillation. Also, injured or infected cardiac valves

may allow vegetations to form, break off, and embolize to the brain. Since the cerebrovascular system receives 20% of the cardiac output, there is at least a 1 in 5 chance of a single embolus reaching the cerebral vessels.

Artery-to-Artery Embolus. When embolization occurs from more proximal vessels it is called artery-to-artery embolization. For example, if thrombus or atheromatous material becomes dislodged from a carotid plaque, it may embolize to a cerebral artery.

Clinical Presentation of Ischemic Cerebrovascular Disease

Whether thrombotic or embolic, the classic presentation of ischemic cerebrovascular disease is that of sudden onset of a neurologic defect which conforms to a specific arterial distribution. Refer to Table 68-1 for a summary of these clinical correlations. Ischemic cerebrovascular syndromes are defined by the duration of the resulting neurologic deficit. This approach predicts the disability that will be incurred by the patient and directs the appropriate diagnostic and therapeutic response.

Transient Ischemic Attack (TIA)

By definition, a TIA is a brief impairment of neurologic function secondary to an interruption of regional cerebral blood flow which may last only several seconds or up to 24 hours in duration. The signs and symptoms of a TIA will depend upon the region of brain denied its blood flow. To educate the public of the importance of these events, current trends are geared towards calling these episodes "brain attacks." This will hopefully emphasize the importance of these events in heralding potentially more serious problems, much like the initial "heart attack" (angina) may be the harbinger of a myocardial infarction.

Reversible Ischemic Neurologic Deficit (RIND)

A neurologic deficit lasting more than 24 hours, but which resolves before 3 weeks, is referred to as a RIND. The temporal length of this event implies greater ischemia or a subclinical infarct. Frequently, neuro-imaging with such modalities as MRI can delineate a subclinical infarct.

Cerebral Infarction

A continuum of cerebrovascular disease exists with the TIA being the least severe and the cerebral infarction at the other end of the spectrum. Irreversible damage to the brain occurs during an infarct due to neuronal cell death from inadequate blood supply. The clinical hallmark is a persistent neurologic deficit.

Evaluating Cerebrovascular Disease

The history and physical exam are the most important diagnostic tools a clinician possesses to localize the site and source of a cerebrovascular lesion. The pattern of neurologic dysfunction can give important clues as to the arterial distribution affected. A patient that is suffering TIAs in both hemispheres will very likely have a cardiogenic source, whereas unilateral stereotypical TIAs suggest a more distal arterial source. A patient may complain of episodic monocular blindness (amaurosis fugax), described like the aperture of a lens closing or a window shade being drawn over the eye. Amaurosis fugax localizes to the ophthalmic artery distribution and is most commonly from microembolization from a carotid plaque ulceration. By physical exam, a bruit may be auscultated by the bell of the stethoscope over the course of the carotid, indicating stenosis. It is important to note however that one-third of lesions with significant stenosis have no audible bruits. Diagnosis of carotid artery disease is enhanced by duplex ultrasound. This noninvasive procedure allows the clinician to examine the lumen size and flow characteristics of affected vessels and it is the study of choice for an asymptomatic bruit. Combined with magnetic resonance arteriography, these modalities can be quite sensitive. Conventional arteriography, however, remains as the gold standard for visualizing the carotid, vertebral, and cerebral vessels. This is achieved by placing a small catheter in the femoral artery and directing it into the carotid or vertebral circulation. Radiographic contrast material is infused at the same time that rapid successive x-rays are exposed. This technique defines the anatomy while also delineating the flow characteristics intracranially. For example, the patency of the anastomotic circle of Willis can be determined by injecting radiopaque dye into a carotid artery while carefully applying pressure to the contralateral artery.

Treatment of Ischemic Cerebrovascular Disease

Treatment is dependent upon the source of the ischemic event and includes antiplatelet drugs, anticoagulation, and, in some cases, surgical therapies. Prevention, however, through management of risk factors for atherosclerosis is also an important aspect of therapy.

Hemorrhagic Cerebrovascular Disease

Hemorrhage can either be intra-axial (parenchymal) or extra-axial (subarachnoid, subdural, epidural). An intracranial cerebral hemorrhage, whether intra- or extra-axial, causes the sudden onset of headache. Patients may describe a headache with an onset similar to that of a "thunder clap" or "gun blast" going off near their head. It is important to realize that an intra-axial hemorrhage may expand into the subarachnoid space and vice versa.

Subarachnoid Hemorrhage

A fine lace network of arachnoid is attached to vessels and pia and creates the subarachnoid space in which cerebrospinal fluid circulates. Trauma is the most common cause of hemorrhage into the subarachnoid space. Spontaneous subarachnoid hemorrhage (SAH) is caused primarily by cerebral aneurysm or arteriovenous malformation (AVM) ruptures. Intracerebral, intraventricular, and subdural hemorrhages frequently occur in association with SAH and increase the already high morbidity and mortality. Blood in the subarachnoid space is very irritative and causes most of its deleterious effects by producing vasospasm of the cerebral vessels or communicating hydrocephalus from obstruction of CSF absorption.

Mechanism of Vasospasm from SAH

Vasospasm is a complication of subarachnoid hemorrhage that has an incidence of 20–30% and is associated with significant mortality and morbidity due to cerebral ischemia and infarction. Constriction of the cerebral vessels is primarily induced by the components of subarachnoid blood. The smooth muscle contraction is probably caused by a combination of hemoglobin, prostaglandins, catecholamines, calcium influx, free radicals, and mechanical injury. The onset of vasospasm is typically at least 3 days after the initial bleed.

Aneurysms

An abnormal dilation of the vascular lumen is termed a cerebral aneurysm. The autopsy prevalence of cerebral aneurysms is 0.2–7.9%. Morphologically, aneurysms can be saccular (berry) 95%, fusiform 4%, or dissecting 1%. Saccular aneurysms result from a congenital loss or absence of the internal elastic membrane along with a defect in the muscularis layer of the media (Fig. 68-5).

Aneurysms are rarely seen before the first decade of life and rupture most frequently in the fifth and sixth decades. The most common locations of saccular aneurysms are at the (1) bifurcation of the anterior cerebral and anterior communicating arteries (30–40%), (2) bifurcation of the posterior communicating with the internal carotid, and the (3) first major bifurcation of middle cerebral artery. The risk of rerupture is 19% during the first 2 weeks after

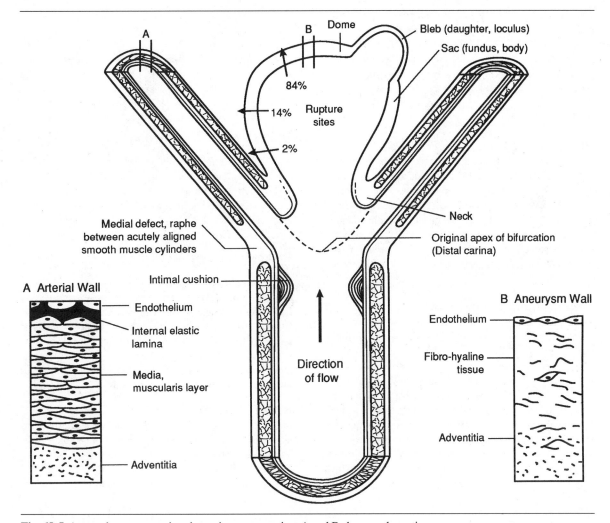

Fig. 68-5. A saccular aneurysm in schematic representation. A and B show a schematic cross-section of normal arterial wall and aneurysm wall respectively. (Used with permission from: Compton MR. The pathogenesis of cerebral aneurysm. *Brain* 89:805, l966. By permission of Oxford University Press.)

the original event. Rebleeding will most likely recur in the first 24 hours. Factors influencing risk of rupture include hypertension and the size, location, and aneurysm type. The average size of cerebral aneurysms at the time of rupture is 8 mm. Bacterial infections of a vessel wall in the cerebral circulation can cause weakness of the artery, causing a mycotic or infectious aneurysm. These are generally treatable with antibiotics but may require surgery.

Clinical Presentation

By far the most common symptom of a SAH from a cerebral aneurysm or AVM rupture is the sudden onset of a severe headache (generally the worst ever in the patient's life). Most patients will have accompanying nausea and vomiting. A decreased level of consciousness may occur at the time of rupture or shortly thereafter. Several hours later, meningeal signs will usually occur secondary to the irritative effect of blood on the meningeal linings. Aneurysmal rupture can create an intraparenchymal hemorrhage from blood forced into the brain substance at the time of rupture. The Hunt and Hess classification system (Table 68-2) is the most commonly used scale to grade the severity of subarachnoid hemorrhage from aneurysm rupture. This classification closely correlates with survival from such an event.

Diagnosis of SAH

It is generally carried out initially by computerized tomography (CT) of the head. Subarachnoid blood and intraparenchymal hemorrhage can be readily seen in the acute stage; however, some patients with aneurysmal subarachnoid hemorrhage will have a negative CT scan and require a lumbar puncture to confirm the diagnosis. Occasionally, the aneurysm can be seen on the contrast infused CT scan but the definitive diagnosis is generally made with cerebral arteriography.

Treatment of Cerebral Aneurysm

Treatment is usually surgical. Saccular aneurysms are the most amenable to surgery. They will have an anatomic neck, across which a spring-loaded clip can be placed. This will prevent further risk from rupture. Much investigation has been geared towards managing the unfavorable effects of vasospasm. Treatment is aimed at providing adequate blood supply through the area of constriction and decreasing the amount of vasospasm, while at the same time preventing ICP from increasing. Inducing moderate hypertension by hypervolemia or by chemotherapeutic means provides greater pressure at the area of constriction, which may allow an adequate perfusion pressure of the artery af-

fected. This global increase in pressure however may detrimentally increase ICP in an already compromised brain. Volume expansion with normal saline and colloid solutions will decrease the viscosity of blood, increasing perfusion past the point of restriction. Calcium channel blocking agents, such as Nicardipine, may be used to decrease the smooth muscle tone, thus decreasing vasospasm.

Intracerebral Hemorrhage

Spontaneous intraparenchymal hemorrhage accounts for 6.3–12% of all new cerebrovascular accidents in the United States each year. Intracerebral hemorrhages present with the acute onset of headache and focal neurologic signs. Hemorrhages can be lobar or involve deep cerebral structures. Hypertension is the cause in 70–90% of the cases.

Pathophysiologic Mechanisms

Hypertension.   Hypertension is associated with hyalinization of the vessel walls as well as microaneurysm formation at the apex of bifurcations. These are known as Charcot-Bouchard aneurysms or miliary aneurysms. The mortality from intracerebral hemorrhage approaches 50%, with serious morbidity in the majority of survivors. Hypertensive intracerebral hemorrhages most frequently occur in the basal ganglia, thalamus, and pons.

Arteriovenous Malformations (AVM).   Congenital malformations of blood vessels occur when arteries connect directly into veins without interposed capillary beds. Trauma may predispose the brain to some types of AVMs. They are approximately one-tenth as common as aneurysms and can occur anywhere in the neuraxis. AVMs produce

Table 68-2. Hunt and Hess Classification of Clinical Features of Subarachnoid Hemorrhage

Grade	Description
0	Unruptured aneurysm
1	Asymptomatic, or mild H/A and slight nuchal rigidity
1a	No acute meningeal/brain reaction, but with fixed neurologic deficit
2	Cranial nerve palsy, moderate to severe H/A, nuchal rigidity
3	Mild focal deficit, lethargy to confusion
4	Stupor, moderate to severe hemiparesis, early decerebrate rigidity
5	Deep coma, decerebrate rigidity, moribund appearance

Add one grade for serious systemic disease (e.g., HTN, DM, severe atherosclerosis, COPD, or severe vasospasm on arteriography).

Used with permission from: Greenberg MS. *Handbook of Neurosurgery* (3rd ed.). Lakeland, Fla: Greenberg Graphics, 1994, p. 714.

symptoms by either hemorrhage with destruction of parenchyma or by mass effect and compression of parenchyma. AVMs may occur near the surface; their rupture may present as a subarachnoid hemorrhage. The annual rate of hemorrhage is approximately 2–3%.

Bleeding Dyscrasias. They can be congenital, acquired, or iatrogenically induced. The hemophilias rarely induce spontaneous intracerebral hemorrhage but may do so after trauma so insignificant as to not be remembered. Acquired deficiencies of clotting factors can be caused from severe alcoholic liver disease. Thrombocytopenia of 25,000 platelets or less, from any cause, will increase the risk of intracerebral bleeding. Administration of heparin or warfarin may subject the patient to dangerous bleeding tendencies if not closely monitored.

Amyloid Angiopathy. Amyloidosis of the cerebral vessels is characterized by the deposition of proteinaceous amyloid in the wall of blood vessels and is frequently the cause of intracerebral hemorrhage in the elderly. Amyloidosis rarely affects the deep cortical structures such as occurs with hypertensive hemorrhages. The only accurate means of diagnosis is by brain biopsy, but there is no known treatment for this entity thus far.

Tumor. Intracerebral hemorrhages from tumors are generally from the malignant primary brain tumor, glioblastoma multiform, or from metastatic tumors. The most common metastatic tumors to bleed are the melanoma, bronchogenic carcinoma, renal cell carcinoma, and choriocarcinoma.

Sympathomimetic Drugs and Ethanol. Cocaine and methamphetamines, along with various derivatives, may cause hemorrhage by several means. These agents increase sympathetic outflow and thus blood pressure which will predispose the cerebral vessels to increased pressures. Due to the usually unsterile method of drug administration, there is also increased incidence in mycotic aneurysms. Chronic ethanol consumption may affect coagulation factors and may also incite systemic hypertension. Both conditions will increase the chances of intracerebral hemorrhage.

Clinical Presentation of Intracerebral Hemorrhage

Hemorrhage of the cerebral lobes (lobar hematoma) will cause symptoms by destruction or mass effect of the adjacent parenchyma. A left frontal hemorrhage in a right-handed patient (thus left-brain dominant), is likely to cause an expressive aphasia and possible paresis or plegia of the right upper extremity and face. Lesions of the deeper structures generally cause more widespread effects when compared with those of comparable size in the outer cortex. The most common sites include the lenticular nuclei, the thalamus, and the pons. A basal ganglia or thalamic hematoma will commonly involve the descending corticospinal system and the ascending somatosensory system, resulting in a contralateral hemiplegia and hemisensory deficit. A pontine hematoma may involve the descending corticospinal system along with lateral gaze centers, resulting in a quadriplegia and ophthalmoplegia. Larger hemorrhages can cause coma or death by brainstem compression.

Diagnosis

The history and physical exam can elucidate the location and cause of most hemorrhages. The history is usually obtained from the patient's family or witnesses of the event. Vascular events tend to be rapid in onset with symptoms occurring within seconds, yet they may progress if the intracerebral hemorrhage continues to expand.

It is difficult to tell from the physical exam alone whether a cerebrovascular accident is from an acute occlusion or from hemorrhage. If the patient has a history of poorly controlled hypertension or bleeding dyscrasia, the process is presumably hemorrhagic whereas occlusive disease would be expected in a patient with atherosclerosis. A CT scan of the head will show the degree and location of an intracerebral hemorrhage. If the cause of hemorrhage is unknown, an arteriogram may be useful to rule out an occult aneurysm or AVM.

Treatment

Treatment is generally conservative with supportive care in an intensive care situation. Hypertension should be diligently managed if present; replacement of absent or dysfunctional clotting factors should be performed. Anticoagulants should be reversed. If the hemorrhage is close to the cortical surface with significant mass effect, surgical debridement may offer palliation and may be a life-saving procedure.

Clinical Examples

1. A 42-year-old woman presented with the "worst headache of her life" which occurred suddenly over the frontal region. She reported no syncope or preceding trauma. She denied any prior history of headaches. A routine medical examination performed one month ago revealed no health problems and her past medical history was unremarkable, as was the family and social history.

She was oriented to person, place, and date but unsure of the time. She answered questions appropriately and she understood the events going on around her. The physical exam was remarkable for a fixed and dilated right pupil with the eye deviated down and out. The left pupil was reactive with normal extraocular movement. She had a mildly positive Brudzinski's sign. Motor and sensory exam were normal.

Discussion.   Her presenting complaint is headache which has negligible localizing features. The suddenness of the event directs the diagnosis towards a vascular event such as an intracerebral or subarachnoid hemorrhage. Her neck stiffness is an indicator of meningeal irritation which is probably from subarachnoid blood. The right third nerve palsy suggests a lesion along the course of the oculomotor nerve which exits the midbrain and traverses between the posterior cerebral and the superior cerebellar arteries. Aneurysms of the posterior communicating artery will cause a total or partial palsy of CNIII in 30–40% of patients. At this point, the most likely diagnoses would be cerebral aneurysm or least likely arteriovenous malformation rupture. She has a Hunt and Hess grade 2 SAH.

A CT scan of the brain should reveal hemorrhage. Blood in the cisterns would be compatible with a SAH versus intracerebral blood which may be more indicative of an AVM. A contrast-infused CT may even show the aneurysm or AVM. If no hemorrhage is seen and there is no contraindication, such as a mass lesion, a lumbar puncture should be performed. Subarachnoid hemorrhage is diagnosed if blood and xanthochromia (yellow color of supernatant of centrifuged bloody spinal fluid) is seen. The time window of blood demonstrated by CT after SAH is approximately one week, whereas xanthochromia in the CSF may be present for 2 weeks. A cerebral arteriogram should help identify the location of an aneurysm or AVM.

2. A 58-year-old, right-hand dominant man presented to the emergency room with a 6-month history of intermittent right-sided weakness and occasional speech difficulty. The episodes occurred two to three times per week and each episode was between 30 minutes to 4 hours in duration. His wife was concerned because he was unable to follow commands and "his speech was not quite right." He has frequently had trouble with his left eye in that he described visual blurring like "a window shade being brought down over my eye." He smoked 2 packs of cigarettes per day and was found to have borderline hypertension 7 years ago, the last time he had his blood pressure checked. He denied any history of syncope, cardiac palpitations, cardiac angina, headaches, or left-sided weakness.

His father and younger brother both died of acute myocardial infarctions.

Physical exam revealed a blood pressure of 185/105. Examination of the neck revealed no carotid bruits. The heart sounds were normal and there were no murmurs. He was alert and oriented with fluent conversation. There was good strength and sensation throughout. His cranial nerve exam was normal. The remainder of the physical exam was within normal limits.

Discussion.   The patient had transient episodes of left monocular blindness (amaurosis fugax) and transient right-sided weakness, and numbness, and aphasia. These symptoms localize to the left optic nerve and the left frontal-parietal lobe. These structures are supplied by the left carotid artery. His symptoms are those of carotid occlusive disease with embolization. He has no symptoms on the contralateral side, which makes cardiogenic embolization less likely. The family history of cardiac disease suggests a genetic predisposition for atherosclerotic disease in our patient. The presence of a carotid bruit would strongly favor a flow-limiting lesion; however, the absence of such is not helpful. An atheromatous plaque with ulceration may provide genesis for embolization without significant flow limitation.

A carotid duplex survey of the carotid artery may reveal flow-limiting lesions or an ulcerating plaque. The patient has such a classic presentation however that his workup should proceed with the gold standard of examining the carotid arteries: a carotid arteriogram. The right carotid should also be inspected because both carotids may be affected. In this case, an arteriogram revealed a 90% stenosis at the origination of the left internal carotid with an ulcerating plaque. A carotid endarterectomy of the left carotid at the site of the lesion will effectively remove the stenotic area and ulceration. Medical management should then be employed to prevent recurrence of disease on this and the contralateral side.

3. A 9-year-old child was brought to the emergency room by her mother. After playing in the park for several hours in the heat of the summer, the child complained of a severe headache. She was then observed to be confused and agitated. There was no history of trauma. The child had been in excellent health and has no relevant past medical or family history.

The child's temperature was 100.2°C. She was moderately paretic in both legs. Her cranial nerve exam was grossly normal with pupils of 4 mm size and 3+ reactive to light. During the exam, she was observed to have a tonic-clonic seizure.

Discussion. The decreased mentation, paraparesis, and seizure implies that the medial frontal lobes are the site of the problem. The suddenness of onset suggests a vascular etiology. Cerebrovascular disease is very rare in children, however. The history suggests possible dehydration with the child being active in the heat for several hours and the mild elevation of the body temperature. This scenario suggests dehydration-induced thrombosis of a cerebral sinus which is treated by anticoagulation and meticulous fluid management. However, any condition which results in increased viscosity or hypercoagulability (such as polycythemia, hyperthermia, antiphospholipid antibodies, sickle cell disease, paraneoplastic conditions, protein C or protein S deficiency, and antithrombin III deficiency) should be considered.

Bibliography

Adams AP and Biller J. Hemorrhagic intracranial vascular disease. In Joynt RJ (ed.). *Clinical Neurology*. Philadelphia: Lippincott, 1994. *An up-to-date review.*

Bhagwati SN and Deshpande HG. Study of Circle of Willis in 1021 consecutive autopsies: Incidence of aneurysms, anatomical variations and atherosclerosis. *Ann Acad Med Singapore* 22(3 Suppl.):443–446, 1993. *This article outlines statistics and common anomalies of the Circle of Willis.*

Carter LP and Spetzler R. *Neurovascular Surgery*. New York: McGraw-Hill, 1995. *This recently published text covers all facets of cerebrovascular disease.*

Crompton MR. Pathogenesis of cerebral aneurysms. *Brain* 89:797–814, 1966. *This historic article demonstrates the microanatomy and pathophysiology of cerebral aneurysms.*

Hopkins LN and Budney JL. Fibromuscular dysplasia. In Wilkins RH, Rengachary (eds.). *Neurosurgery* Vol. 2, pp. 1293–1296. *The incidence, etiology, and pathophysiology of fibromuscular dysplasia is described in detail in this chapter.*

Robinson MK and Toole JF. Ischemic cerebrovascular disease. In Joynt RJ (ed.). *Clinical Neurology*. Philadelphia: Lippincott, 1994. *A review of the pathogenesis and clinical features of ischemic cerebrovascular disease.*

Weinfeld FD (ed.). The National Survey of Stroke. *Stroke* 12 (Suppl. 1):1–91, 1981. *Spontaneous hemorrhage as a cause of cerebral vascular accident is detailed.*

69 Infections of the Central Nervous System

Richard W. Leech and Roger A. Brumback

Objectives

After completing this chapter, you should be able to

Define and distinguish between the terms meningitis, cerebritis, encephalitis, abscess, meningoencephalitis, pachymeningitis, empyema, cerebral vasculitis, granulomas, and aseptic meningitis

Understand how organisms gain access to the central nervous system and how they evade body defenses

Understand the clinical characteristics of infections: viral, fungal, bacterial, parasitic, and spirochetal

Develop concepts about the mode of onset, course, and clinical characteristics of infections which involve the nervous system

Understand the types of central nervous system infections associated with immune suppression

Virtually any microorganism that can infect the human body can involve the nervous system and its many components (Table 69-1). However, certain microorganisms have a predilection for specific nervous system structures (meninges or parenchyma) and sites (cerebral hemispheres, brainstem, cerebellum, or spinal cord). These considerations combined with the universal symptoms and signs of infection (fever, malaise, anorexia, and pain) can enhance the clinician's ability to diagnose infection as a cause of nervous system disease. Microorganisms that infect the nervous system generally present with symptoms and signs which imply either diffuse involvement (meningitis or encephalitis) or localized involvement (empyema or abscess).

Anatomy of the Meninges

The brain and spinal cord are supported and protected by several membranous layers — the dura mater (pachymeninges) and the leptomeninges (pia mater and arachnoid). In general usage, the term "meninges" is usually used to refer only to the leptomeninges. The dura mater is a thick fibrous membrane enveloping the brain and spinal cord. Within the skull the dura mater is firmly adherent to the periosteum. However, at the foramen magnum, the dura mater separates from the intracranial periosteum, and within the spinal canal the two layers are separated by the epidural space containing fat and blood vessels. The dura protects the nervous system from injury or contiguous spread of infection from the bone, sinuses, and soft tissues surrounding the brain and spinal cord. The leptomeninges are delicate membranes which cover the brain and lie under the dura. There is a potential space between the arachnoid membrane and the dura mater. The pia is closely adherent to the brain and spinal cord. The space between the arachnoid membrane and the pia mater is termed the subarachnoid space and is filled with cerebrospinal fluid.

Table 69-1. Definitions and Clinical Characteristics of CNS Infection

Type	Site of Involvement	Predominant Microorganism	Neurologic Features
DIFFUSE			
Meningitis	Inflammation of meninges	Bacterial Fungal Mycobacterial Spirochete Viral	Headache and nuchal rigidity
Encephalitis	Inflammation of parenchyma	Viral	Headache, confusion, and seizures
Meningoencephalitis	Inflammation of meninges and parenchyma	Viral	Headache, confusion, and nuchal rigidity
FOCAL			
Cerebritis	Focal inflammation of parenchyma	Bacterial	Focal signs and seizures
Abscess	Liquefactive necrosis with capsulation localized area for parenchyma	Bacterial	Focal signs, seizure, and mass effect
Empyema	Localization of pus within epidural or subdural space	Bacterial	Focal signs, seizure, and mass effect
Granuloma	Localized areas of chronic inflammation	Fungal Mycobacterial Spirochete	Focal signs and seizures
Vasculitis	Inflammation and arteritis	Bacterial Fungal Spirochetal	Focal signs localized to arterial distribution
Phlebitis	Inflammation of veins	Bacterial	Focal signs localized to venous distribution

Infections that Primarily Involve the Meninges

Meningitis is an inflammatory reaction of the meninges as the result of invasion of microorganisms, chemicals, blood, or neoplastic cells. The characteristic features of meningitis are headache and meningeal irritation (nuchal rigidity). Nuchal rigidity is reflex extension of the neck when tension is put on inflamed structures (meninges and nerve roots) by passive pressure on the head. When the neck is passively flexed and there is not only resistance to neck flexion but also simultaneous flexion of the hips, it is known as Brudzinski's sign. When the legs are flexed at the hips and there is resistance to leg extension, it is known as Kernig's sign. Both signs in addition to the nuchal rigidity suggest inflammation of the meninges.

Meningitis can be caused by a variety of organisms (bacterial, viral, spirochete, fungal, or protozoan). The clinical features and CSF findings can be used to differentiate between acute (bacterial or viral) and chronic (fungal, tuberculous) forms of meningitis. Table 69-2 outlines the course, CSF findings, and notable features in the different forms of meningitis.

Acute Bacterial Meningitis

Pathogens can gain access to the leptomeninges and cerebrospinal fluid by a variety of mechanisms, including trauma, surgical procedures, parameningeal foci (such as sinusitis or mastoiditis), congenital defects, retrograde venous flow, paravertebral lymphatics, axons, and Schwann cells. However, bacteria within the blood stream must

Table 69-2. Typical Cerebrospinal Abnormalities in Meningitis

Type of Meningitis	Course	Number of Cells per ml	Cell Type	Protein Concentration, in mg/100ml	Glucose	Other
Acute bacterial	Acute	500–20,000	polymorphonuclear	100–1000	decreased	35% have concurrent pyogenic process
Partially treated bacterial	Subacute	increased	mononuclear	increased	normal or increased	
Viral	Subacute	30–350	mononuclear	40–80	normal	serology and/or culture positive
Mycobacterial	Subacute or chronic	50–700	mononuclear	60–700	decreased	
Fungal	Chronic	50–600	mononuclear	50–600	decreased	serology positive in some
Spirochete	Subacute	300–600	mononuclear	50–400	normal	positive serology

breach the blood-brain barrier. For example, blood-borne infections initially colonize the upper respiratory tract and invade the blood before they breach the blood-brain barrier and produce inflammation of the meninges with complications such as brain edema and endarteritis. Many organisms elaborate capsular and cell wall substances that aid in evading host recognition and clearance or possess specialized appendages that bind to surface receptors on the nasopharyngeal mucosa (Table 69-3). The blood-brain barrier depends on cerebrovascular endothelial cells which have tight junctions between cells and a paucity of cytoplasmic pinocytotic vesicles. Specializations of the cell walls of pathogenic bacteria facilitate binding of the pathogen to the endothelial cell with consequent disruption of the tight junctions and resultant breakdown of the blood-brain barrier. An increase in endothelial cell vesicles coincides with this breakdown of the blood-brain barrier.

Once within the cerebrospinal fluid space, pathogens encounter an immunologic void. Humoral immune defenses (including complement and immunoglobulins) are in low concentration, opsonin activity is low, and targeting of bacteria by leukocytes is slow. In this setting, bacterial cell constituents (such as the endotoxin of gram-negative organisms and the teichoic acid and peptidoglycans of gram-positive organisms) stimulate release of cytokines (mediators of inflammation) by endothelial cells, central nervous system macrophages, and astrocytes. These cytokines, including tumor necrosis factor (TNF), interleukins, arachidonic acid metabolites, platelet activating factor, and interferons, induce leukocyte margination (ad-

Table 69-3. Pathophysiology of Bacterial Infections

MUCOSAL SURVIVAL

Binding adhesins (e.g., *N. meningitidis*)
Secretion of IgA proteases (e.g., *S. pneumoniae*, *H. influenzae*, and *N. meningitidis*)
Direct mucosal injury (e.g., *N. meningitidis*, *H. influenzae*)

BLOOD STREAM SURVIVAL (EVASION OF COMPLEMENT SYSTEM)

Antiphagocytosis lipopolysaccharide (e.g., *S. pneumoniae*, *H. meningitidis*)
K1 antigen of *E. coli*, group B streptococcus

BREECHING OF THE BLOOD BRAIN BARRIER

Release of inflammatory cell cytokines induce adhesion and then ingress of leukocytes into CSF
Tight junctions disrupted followed by ingress of protein
Increased pinocytosis

SURVIVAL OF LEUKOCYTES IN CSF FACILITATED BY IMMUNOLOGIC VOID

Low complement and immunoglobulins
Decreased opsonin activity
Slow targeting of leukocytes

CEREBRAL MICROVASCULATURE INJURY

Enhanced by release of inflammatory cytokines from endothelium, cerebral macrophages and astrocytes
Loss of vascular autoregulation

END RESULT OF VASCULAR INJURY

Cytotoxic cerebral edema
Increased intracranial pressure
Altered cerebral blood flow
Herniation, hypoxic-ischemic brain injury, etc.

hesion of leukocytes to endothelium) and ingress into the CSF compartments.

Increased permeability of the blood-brain barrier results in an elevated protein content in the cerebrospinal fluid and vasogenic edema of the brain. Leukocyte generation of oxygen radicals, proteases, and other toxins results in cytotoxic edema. Increased intracranial pressure from brain edema and interference with the normal flow of cerebrospinal fluid can compromise cerebral blood flow, further damaging an already dysfunctional central nervous system. Additional complications of the inflammation include vasculitis and vascular thrombosis from stimulation of the coagulation cascade.

Epidemiology

Approximately 15,000 cases of meningitis occur each year, with 70% being diagnosed in children under age 5 years. Most are found in infants under age 12 months. In children, *Haemophilus influenzae* type B accounts for most cases, whereas in neonates under age one month group B *Streptococcus* is more commonly identified. The most common pathogens causing meningitis in the United States continue to be *H. influenzae, Neisseria meningitidis* (meningococcus), and *Streptococcus pneumoniae* (pneumococcus), accounting respectively for 45%, 18%, and 14% of cases. Gram-negative bacillary meningitis is more common in neonates, the elderly, and the debilitated. Fortunately, since the introduction of specific vaccines, the incidence of *H. influenzae* meningitis has decreased. Unfortunately, the mortality rate for meningitis in adults has not changed over the past three decades, with an overall case-fatality rate of 25%. However, in children mortality rates are approximately 5–10% for meningococcal and *Haemophilus* infections and 25–30% for pneumococcal infections.

Predisposing and Prognostic Factors

Meningitis is a disease of the young and elderly. It is slightly more common in males, and clusters of meningococcal infections occur in day care centers or among recruits in military camps. Predisposing conditions for meningitis include infections at other body sites, head injury, diabetes mellitus, alcoholism, recent neurosurgery or presence of neurosurgical devices (such as a shunt or catheter), malignancy, chemotherapy, and immunosuppression.

Prognosis is affected adversely by age greater than 60 years, stupor or coma at the time of hospital admission, and onset of seizures within 24 hours of hospital admission. Other factors indicating a poor prognosis include the presence of a predisposing or associated illness, absence of

nuchal rigidity, markedly elevated CSF protein, organisms identifiable on a CSF smear, positive CSF culture, and presence of bacteremia.

Diagnosis

The diagnosis of bacterial meningitis is dependent upon finding of pleocytosis, elevated protein and reduced glucose in the CSF along with identification of the microorganisms on cultures. Detection of capsular antigens can be helpful in the diagnosis of *streptococcus pneumoniae, H. influenza, N. meningitides,* and group B *Streptococci.*

Complications

Complications of meningitis result from raised intracranial pressure and edema, cerebral ischemia, and the actions of mediators of inflammation. Although the case fatality rate of meningitis has dropped over the past few decades, morbidity remains very high. More than one-third of children demonstrate neurologic abnormalities one month after recovery, and more than one-fourth have permanent deficits at one year. Sensorineural hearing loss (10%) and seizures (7%) are the most common neurologic problems with mental retardation and motor system lesions less common. Fifty percent of adults suffer complications, including both neurologic and systemic problems. Systemic complications include septic shock, adult respiratory distress syndrome, and disseminated intravascular coagulation. Neurologic complications include brain edema, hydrocephalus, and intracerebral hemorrhage.

Management

Therapy includes antimicrobial chemotherapy along with management of sepsis, shock, pulmonary complications, cerebral edema, coagulopathy, metabolic imbalances, and seizures. Drug accessibility to the CSF in sufficiently high concentrations and drug resistance of some organisms are major problems. Prophylaxis must be considered for all individuals contacting a patient with the highly contagious *N. meningitidis* infection.

Chronic Meningitis

The onset of chronic meningitis is insidious over days or weeks. Neurologic complications are common and include: involvement of cranial nerves from meningeal inflammation or endarteritis, evidence of parenchymal damage secondary to arteritis, and hydrocephalus secondary to interference with normal CSF circulation. CSF studies are usually nonspecific, identification of the causative organism is frequently difficult, and delay in diagnosis is often long. The most common and important infectious causes of chronic meningitis include tuberculosis, fungi, spirochetes, and toxoplasmosis. Noninfectious etiologies include carcinomatous meningitis and granulomatous diseases such as sarcoidosis.

Tuberculosis

Although the prevalence of pulmonary and other forms of tuberculosis declined dramatically from the 1950s to 1984, there has been an almost 20% increase since 1985 with an even greater increase in children. Drug-resistant tuberculosis is becoming more common, with many cases now showing resistance to isoniazid or rifampin or both. Factors contributing to this resurgence in tuberculosis include its frequent association with human immunodeficiency virus (HIV) infection or other immunocompromised states, immigration from countries with high tuberculosis prevalence, substance abuse, homelessness, poverty, and deterioration in the public health infrastructure.

Tuberculous meningitis is the most life-threatening form of tuberculosis. It is characterized by a caseating granulomatous inflammation of the leptomeninges anywhere in the CSF space, but generally most severe at the base of the brain. Involvement of the base of the brain is responsible for the clinical finding of cranial neuropathies and hydrocephalus. Infection begins as a granuloma in the leptomeninges, with later spread of bacilli throughout the subarachnoid space. Large granulomas (tuberculomas) act as intracranial mass lesions. Tuberculous arteritis results in multiple infarcts.

Spirochetes

Syphilis.   The spirochete *Treponema pallidum* can produce several forms of central nervous system disease (tertiary neurosyphilis) to include meningovascular syphilis and later onset parenchymal neurosyphilis which is characterized by dementia (general paresis) or a constellation of sensory ataxia, areflexia, and lightening pains (tabes dorsalis). Since the introduction of penicillin, the parenchymal forms are rare. However, cases of chronic meningitis and stroke related to endarteritis in meningovascular syphilis are now increasing in incidence. This is a consequence of the spread of acquired immunodeficiency syndrome (AIDS), which results in increased susceptibility and virulence of *T. pallidum* infections.

Lyme Disease.   The agent of Lyme disease is the spirochete *Borrelia burgdorferi*. Like syphilis, Lyme disease has three stages. The early stage is characterized by arthralgias and rash. This is followed by meningoencephalitis, cranial neuritis (particularly facial palsy), and/or polyradiculopathy or mononeuritis. This stage can be quite protracted in duration. Late complications include encephalopathy and focal neurologic signs related to demyelination. Lyme disease is most prevalent in New England, along the Atlantic seaboard, in the upper Midwest, in southern United States, and in California. This distribution coincides with the distribution of its major tick vectors, *Ixodes dammini* and *I. pacificus*. It occurs predominantly in epidemics in individuals exposed through outdoor recreation. During 1992, Lyme disease accounted for more than 90% of all vector-borne illnesses in the United States.

Fungal Infections

Fungi produce all forms of primary central nervous system infections, including meningitis, abscess, granuloma, meningoencephalitis, and arteritis. Molds are the filamentous forms of fungi, producing septate and nonseptate hyphae, whereas yeasts are unicellular organisms. Dimorphic or diphasic fungi have a filamentous form when grown on artificial media and yeast form in tissue. Fungi typically produce a subacute or chronic meningitis that is often clinically indistinguishable from tuberculous meningitis. *Cryptococcus* is the most common fungus producing sporadic disease in apparently healthy people. *Candida, Cryptococcus, Rhizopus, Aspergillus, Blastomyces,* and *Histoplasma* often produce infections in patients with cancer or immunocompromise.

Cryptococcal Infection.   *Cryptococcus neoformans* is a yeast found worldwide in fruit, soil, and excreta of certain birds. The usual clinical disease is a basilar meningitis. The organism incites a granulomatous inflammation, but the inflammatory reaction may be scant in immunocompromised patients. Organisms can be identified both free and within multinucleated macrophages in the subarachnoid space and extending along the Virchow-Robin space. Clinical presentation is similar to that of tuberculous meningitis, and diagnosis requires visualization of the organism by culture or detection of antigen in CSF which is the most rapid and sensitive diagnostic technique. The mortality rate, as in tuberculous meningitis, is high (approximately 30%).

Candidal Infection.   *Candida* species is a ubiquitous, worldwide opportunistic fungus that produces infection most often involving skin and mucous membranes. Invasive or disseminated candidiasis is a disease of immunocompromised patients (such as those with malignancies, particularly lymphoma, or AIDS), in whom overwhelming infection of the oral cavity and gastrointestinal tract leads to blood vessel invasion and subsequent hematogenous dissemination of the organism. Within the central nervous system, there may be meningitis, abscesses, granulomas, and infarcts secondary to vascular thrombosis.

Mucormycosis. Species of the genera *Mucor, Rhizopus,* and *Absidia* of the order of Mucorales produce mucormycosis (phycomycosis or zygomycosis), with the lungs or nasal mucosa being the most common sites of entry of the organism. As with candida, these organisms invade blood vessels and are hematogenously disseminated. Rhinocerebral mucormycosis involves the nose, sinuses, adjacent orbits, and then spreads through the circulation to the intracranial compartment to produce infarcts and purulent meningitis. Granulomas are uncommon.

Infections That Involve the Parenchyma (Encephalitis)

Encephalitis is characterized by symptoms and signs which suggest diffuse involvement of the parenchyma (headache, confusion, and seizures). While any microorganism can display neurotropism (a predilection for nerve cells), thus producing encephalitis, viruses are the most common agent.

Viral Infections

Viruses enter the body through various routes and, as with bacteria, must elude both humoral and cellular immune responses. For example, enteric viruses enter primarily through the gastrointestinal tract and, after surviving the local environment, penetrate the intestinal epithelium, utilizing a variety of cell-to-cell mechanisms, including unique surface antigens or membrane alterations. The host inflammatory response produces diarrhea. Meanwhile organisms that gain access to the regional lymphatics proliferate within macrophages and lymphocytes or attach to surface receptors of such cells, which then carry the virus to distant sites. Viruses that escape the host's immune responses gain access to the CNS by penetrating the blood-brain barrier or by traveling along the axon from a peripheral site (retrograde axoplasmic transport).

Viruses selectively attack specific CNS regions and cells. This neurotropism is in part related to attraction to specific cell surface antigens and in part related to route of entry. Enteric viruses, such as the poliovirus, attack spinal cord motor neurons, but can also affect other areas. Rabies virus selectively attacks the brainstem, cytomegalovirus

prefers endothelial cells and ependymal cells, and papova viruses localize to oligodendrocytes. Viruses persist by using a variety of mechanisms, including preservation of viral DNA in the host cell, integration with host cell genes, and by antigenic mutation. In intrauterine and neonatal infections, viruses attack rapidly proliferating cells. Destruction of such precursor cells does not necessarily give rise to an encephalitis, but may simply result in a paucity of mature cells. Viral infection can also induce cell transformation and neoplasia, such as occurs in AIDS or HTLV-1 infections.

The histologic reaction of the CNS to virus infection is variable and includes acute encephalitis, glial nodules, or foci of lymphocytes. Dying and dead neurons are ingested by macrophages; such neuronophagic nodules are typically seen in poliomyelitis. Many viruses produce inclusions. The Cowdry type A intranuclear inclusion (eosinophilic inclusion surrounded by a clear halo) is seen in herpes simplex encephalitis, measles encephalitis, progressive multifocal leukoencephalopathy, and cytomegalovirus infection (Plate 9). Rabies produces an intracytoplasmic inclusion (Negri body).

Herpes Virus Infection

Herpes Simplex Infection. Herpes simplex encephalitis is the most common sporadic viral infection with serious neurologic consequences (over 70% mortality and morbidity with an untreated CNS infection), although herpes simplex type 1 virus is the cause of illness in less than 10% of patients presenting with an acute encephalitic picture. At least 25% of patients with herpes simplex encephalitis have a history of a previous contact with the virus, such as infections of the lips, mouth, and eyes. Latent or persistent infection of the trigeminal nerve ganglion is common and CNS infection represents spread from that latent site. Typically a severe necrotizing encephalitis begins in the medial temporal and basal frontal regions which is clinically characterized by change in behavior, confusion, and seizures often partial complex in type. Herpes simplex encephalitis is rapidly progressive, often fatal, and leaves severe neurologic deficits in survivors (amnestic state, personality disorder, and epilepsy). Imaging studies might suggest predominant frontal and temporal involvement (MRI, nuclear brain scan) and the EEG typically demonstrates periodic discharges. This finding, combined with the clinical picture, is often sufficient for the diagnosis. While brain biopsy is diagnostic, there are risks of hemorrhage and infection. Mortality is low when antiviral therapy (acyclovir) is initiated before loss of consciousness.

Neonatal herpes encephalitis is typically due to the herpes simplex type 2 virus acquired during vaginal delivery or through ruptured amniotic membranes from a mother with a genital herpes infection. Neonatal herpes encephalitis produces a widespread necrosis, and, as with the adult form of the disease, mortality is high if untreated (80%) and neurologic deficits in survivors are common (greater than 90%).

Cytomegalovirus Infection. Cytomegalovirus (CMV) is a member of the herpesvirus family and produces many different symptoms and signs related to retinitis, encephalitis, myelitis, and radiculitis. It commonly occurs in immunosuppressed patients or as a congenital infection. In patients with AIDS, CMV infection is commonly seen in the lungs, adrenal glands, and brain, where it infects endothelial cells, producing a vasculitis with consequent foci of encephalomalacia or infarcts. CMV also infects ependymal cells, resulting in a characteristic syndrome of cranial nerve deficits, nystagmus, CSF pleocytosis, decreased glucose levels, and progressive ventriculomegaly. Encouraging results have been obtained with antiviral agents.

Congenital infections produce both systemic and CNS disease with resultant congenital malformations, meningoencephalitis, and widespread calcifications. Clinically silent or asymptomatic CMV infection produces a sensorineural hearing loss in up to 15% of children.

Arborvirus Infection

The arborviruses (acronym for <u>ar</u>thropod-<u>bo</u>rne viruses) are the most common cause of epidemic outbreaks of encephalitis in the U.S., particularly California encephalitis and St. Louis encephalitis. The virus infects neurons and therefore histologic evidence of inflammation is in gray matter, often in basal ganglia and brainstem. Meningeal inflammation can also be present.

Rabies

Rabies is worldwide in distribution, but human infection is seldom seen in developed countries although the organism is present in many wild animals. On the North American continent, rabies is frequently found in skunks, raccoons, bats, and foxes. Transmitted by the bite of an infected animal, the virus multiplies locally in muscle fibers, and then spreads to the peripheral nerve, traveling in axons to enter the CNS via the nerve root. The rabies virus has a predilection for the brainstem, but is found elsewhere. The pathologic features are typical of encephalitis with focal mononuclear cell infiltrates. Negri bodies are usually identified in Purkinje cells and pyramidal neurons of the hippocampus.

Measles Infections

Measles produces three distinct pathologic and clinical entities.

Subacute Measles Encephalitis. This is seen in immunocompromised children with onset 5 weeks to 6 months after an initial illness. Death occurs within a few weeks. Pathologically there are giant cells, intranuclear neuronal inclusions, slight gliosis, and variable inflammation.

Subacute Sclerosing Panencephalitis. SSPE usually presents in children aged 6–12 years. The mutant measles virus lacks the gene necessary for coding of the matrix (M) protein necessary for viral release. Thus the organism persists within neural cells and escapes immune recognition. There is an intense gliosis of the white and gray matter with only minimal inflammation. Viral inclusion bodies are found in oligodendrocytes, astrocytes, endothelial cells, and neurons. The disease is characterized by insidious behavioral change and intellectual deterioration, followed by myoclonic jerks which are often provoked by stimuli. As the disease progresses, the child loses motor skills and manifests involuntary movement, poor coordination, and upper motor neuron weakness. The final stages of the disease are characterized by dementia and quadriparesis. Associated symptoms include seizures and visual impairments related to chorioretinitis, optic atrophy, and occipital lobe involvement. The EEG may show high-amplitude, slow-wave bursts and 2–3 Hz. Demonstration of measles antibody in the serum and CSF is diagnostic. Antiviral agents (isoprinosine) have been demonstrated to slow the course of SSPE.

Post-infectious Encephalomyelitis. This follows measles (although it can also occur after rubella, smallpox, varicella, herpes zoster, and infectious mononucleosis). Mortality is approximately 25% and neurologic sequelae are seen in 30%. Pathologically there is widespread perivenous demyelination, presumably from an autoimmune reaction.

Progressive Multifocal Leukoencephalitis

In immunocompromised patients, JC virus (a member of the papovavirus group) produces a disease characterized by progressive dementia and motor system dysfunction which is invariably fatal. The histopathology includes areas of necrotizing demyelination, usually in the parieto-occipital regions, with large, bizarre, almost neoplastic-appearing, astrocytes and oligodendrocytes containing homogeneous intranuclear inclusions (Fig. 69-1).

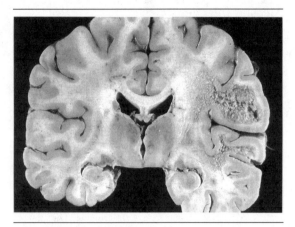

Fig. 69-1. Coronal section of cerebral hemispheres at level of arterial lateral geniculate nuclei showing granular discoloration and destruction of white matter most strikingly in the area of right frontal operculum characteristic of progressive multifocal leukoencephalopathy.

HIV Infection

HIV infection produces CNS disease in three ways: (1) by producing a primary infection, (2) by setting the stage for an opportunistic infection, and (3) by inducing CNS neoplasia (such as primary CNS lymphomas). Alterations in the brains of AIDS patients are common (as many as 80% showing alterations in the brain at autopsy).

The human immunodeficiency virus (a retrovirus) does not infect neurons directly, although significant neuronal loss occurs. The virus does infect and activate the microglial cell, producing a cascade of events to explain the loss of neurons which correlates with the clinical observation of progressive dementia. Activated microglia produce the cytokine interleukin-1alpha that promotes proliferation of astrocytes which express another cytokine S100β. These two cytokines increase expression of beta-amyloid precursor protein, elevate intracellular calcium levels, and promote excessive growth of abnormal (dystrophic) neurites. The end result is neuronal death. Other abnormalities occur within the white matter, resulting in a leukodystrophy with a pathogenesis similar to that for neuronal loss. The mildest white matter change is pallor associated with collections of microglial nodules and scattered multinucleated giant cells. Myelin and oligodendroglial cell loss is cytokine mediated. Activated microglial cells stimulate astrocytes and both cells then produce tissue necrosis factor,

which is myelinotoxic. Astrocytes also produce nitric oxide and microglia produce quinolinic acid, both substances being neurotoxic.

HIV infection can be associated with an acute infection which reflects seroconversion to HIV-1 and is characterized by meningoencephalitis, myelopathy, or polyneuropathy. While overt AIDS is characterized by the development of opportunistic infections and neoplasia, CNS manifestations of the HIV virus which occur during the immunocompromised stage include AIDS-dementia complex (insidious and progressive dementia), myelopathy (progressive paraparesis), atypical Guillain-Barré syndrome (CSF pleocytosis associated with areflexic paralysis), sensorimotor polyneuropathy, and myopathy.

Infections Producing Mass Lesions

Mass-producing infections (empyema, abscess, granuloma) produce localized symptoms and signs. Symptoms and signs of infection may be subtle or in fact absent, particularly when there is encapsulation of the infectious mass.

Subdural Empyema

A subdural empyema incites edema of the underlying brain such that in early stages the degree of displacement of brain parenchyma is out of proportion to the size of the empyema. Subsequently, the increased size of the empyema can itself act as a mass lesion. Causative organisms include those producing meningitis, as well as coagulase-negative staphylococci and anaerobic bacteria which gain access to the subdural space through contiguous spread from sinuses (ethmoids, sphenoids in particular).

Epidural Abscess (Empyema)

Cranial epidural abscess (empyema) is much less common than subdural empyema; however spinal epidural abscess is important because the diagnosis is difficult to establish, morbidity and mortality are high, and emergency neurosurgic drainage is indicated. A distant focus of infection is present in many of the patients, although discitis, vertebral osteomyelitis, paraspinal abscess, and recent back surgery are other predisposing conditions. The occurrence of localized pain and symptoms or signs of spinal cord compression in the face of predisposing factors should suggest an epidural abscess. Staphylococci are the causative agent in nearly two-thirds of cases.

Brain Abscess

A brain abscess begins as a focus of cerebritis, followed by increasing accumulation of leukocytes, destruction of brain parenchyma, edema, hyperemia, and finally development of a pocket of pus. The brain reacts with only limited production of fibrous scarring at the margins, with encapsulation taking place after 2–3 weeks. Because the capsule is thin, extension of the cerebritis outward into the surrounding brain is common. Unimpeded progression of an abscess results in the complications associated with a mass lesion, including displacement of adjacent brain, herniation, and death.

The most common sites of brain abscess are the frontal and temporal lobes. Males are affected twice as often as females, most occur between ages 30 to 40 years, and mortality is high (up to 20%). Brain abscesses are associated with head trauma (in 5% of cases), spread of contiguous foci of infection (uncommon with current medical therapy), and hematogenous dissemination of infection from the lungs or in association with congenital heart disease or immune compromise. The causative organism is generally related to the underlying disease process. Streptococci and staphylococci are most frequent, but anaerobes are also common. Brain abscesses in children and infants often occur in the setting of septicemia associated with pulmonary disease, congenital heart disease, or with neonatal meningitis.

Granulomas and Cysts

Fungal Infections

Aspergillosis. *Aspergillus* species are ubiquitous fungi, found in soil and decaying vegetation. The organism typically produces a cavitating pulmonary infection and CNS infection in immunosuppressed patients. The invasive form of the organism (the mycelium with branching septate hyphae) spreads via the circulation, producing an arteritis with infarcts and abscesses. Parenchymal granulomas can be found throughout the CNS, but meningitis is uncommon.

Parasitic Infections

Cerebral Cysticercosis. Cysticercosis is the most common parasitic infestation of the CNS in the world and is often seen in immigrants to the United States. Most cases occur in western United States among immigrants from areas with endemic cysticercosis, such as Mexico.

The disease is produced by the tissue-invading larval stage (cysticerci) of the pork tapeworm, *Taenia solium*. The mechanism by which these larval forms enter the body is by ingestion of tapeworm eggs shed in *human feces* (not by ingesting pork). The larvae migrate throughout the body, but clinical problems are most severe when the CNS is invaded. Cerebral forms of cysticercosis include arachnoiditis (50% of cases), hydrocephalus, and parenchymal cysts. Parenchymal calcifications indicate inactive disease.

Toxoplasmosis. *Toxoplasma gondii* is a common protozoan which is an obligate intracellular parasite that is able to remain alive in the host as encysted organisms. The major clinical forms of disease include lymphadenopathy, encephalitis, disseminated infection, and congenital infection. Disseminated infection is most often seen in the immunocompromised patient, with CNS, heart, and lung involvement in more than 70% of cases. Toxoplasmosis is commonly suspected in AIDS patients and probably is the most common cause of focal brain lesions, but its demonstration can be difficult (Plate 10). Diagnosis is made with serologic tests or by finding the organism in biopsies. The brain lesions are typically widespread, small, and include variable numbers of chronic inflammatory cells, encysted tachyzoites, or proliferative free tachyzoite (see Plate 10).

Congenital toxoplasmosis is a devastatingly destructive disease giving rise to microcephaly, hydrocephalus, microphthalmia, seizures, psychomotor retardation, cerebral calcifications, and chorioretinitis.

Clinical Example

1. A 30-year-old man presented with unilateral blindness, confusion and personality change, and weakness of the legs progressive over 2 weeks. He had been seropositive to HIV-1 for 3 years with a past history of genital herpes infection and syphilis. Within the past year he was formally diagnosed with AIDS when he developed *Pneumocytis carinii* pneumonia. On examination, the patient was confused. His vision was no light perception in the left eye and 20/100 in the right eye. Retinitis was observed on funduscopic examination. He was plegic in the legs with areflexia. He could not appreciate pain and temperature sensation on the lower extremities. CT scan was normal. CSF revealed a lymphocytic pleocytosis with a modestly elevated protein and normal glucose.

Discussion.   The problems demonstrated in this patient suggest extensive involvement of the neuraxis. The visual loss suggests a problem involving the visual pathways, which in this case is localized to the retina by the documentation of retinitis. The confusion suggests a problem involving the reticular activating system and its connections with the cerebral cortex. The paraplegia suggests a problem with the motor system which specifically localizes to the lower motor neuron by the demonstration of areflexia. This combined with the abnormalities in sensation localize to multiple nerve roots (polyradiculopathy) or peripheral nerve (polyneuropathy) .

With the prior documentation of seroconversion to HIV-1, the patient is at risk for development of disorders linked to HIV-1 (AIDS dementia complex, progressive myelopathy, neuropathy, myopathy) and disorders secondary to HIV-1 induced immunosuppression (infections and neoplasia). The extensive pattern of involvement (retina, ARAS system, and polyradiculopathy or polyneuropathy) and the rapid progression of symptoms would suggest the diagnosis of a diffuse infection which is supported by the absence of focal lesions on the CT and a CSF suggesting an inflammatory process involving the meninges or parenchyma. Most common infections to consider in this setting include viral (herpes simplex, cytomegalovirus, varicella zoster), fungal meningitis (cryptococcal, histoplasmosis), tuberculous meningitis, and toxoplasmosis. Although specific diagnosis is dependent upon identification of the microorganism by culture or serologic methods, the occurrence of retinitis, encephalitis, and polyradiculitis during the immunocompromised stage of AIDS would most likely suggest cytomegalovirus.

Bibliography

Bradley JS. Meningitis. *Hosp Pract* 28:15–19, 1993. *A practical and concise review.*

Quagliarello VJ and Scheld WM. New perspectives on bacterial meningitis. *Clin Infect Dis* 17:603–610, 1993. *A thorough review of the topic in general.*

Stanley LC, Mrak RE, Woody RC, et al. Glial cytokines as neuropathologic factors in HIV infection: Pathogenic similarities to Alzheimer's disease. *J Neuropathol Exp Neurol* 53:231–238, 1994. *Current hypothesis relating cytokines to neuronal abnormalities.*

Vinken PJ, Bruyn GW, Klawans HL, and Harris AA (eds.). Microbial Disease. In Vinken PJ, Bruyn GW, and Klawans HL (eds.), *Handbook of Clinical Neurology,* Vol 52. New York: Elsevier Science Pub. Co., 1988. *This volume contains a thorough review of bacterial, fungal and parasitic infections of the central nervous system.*

Vinken PJ, Bruyn GW, Klawans HL, and McKendall RR (eds.). Viral Disease. In Vinken PJ, Bruyn GW, and Klawans HL (eds.), *Handbook of Clinical Neurology,* Vol. 56. New York: Elsevier Science Pub. Co., 1989. *This volume contains a thorough review of the various viral disorders that can affect the central nervous system.*

Part VIII Questions: Neurologic Diseases and Special Senses

1. The acute onset of expressive aphasia and right-arm weakness is most likely the result of which of the following:
   A. Infarction in left middle cerebral artery distribution
   B. Hyponatremia
   C. Glioma in the left frontal lobe
   D. Meningitis
   E. Lead poisoning

2. A 45-year-old man developed muscular weakness and aching and dysphagia that progressed gradually over a 4-month period. Examination shows intact cranial nerve function, nonfluctuating weakness of proximal muscles in all extremities, and normal muscle stretch reflexes. The most likely diagnosis is
   A. myasthenia gravis.
   B. chronic inflammatory polyradiculoneuropathy.
   C. polymyositis.
   D. myotonic dystrophy.
   E. motor neuron disease.

3. A 50-year-old woman presents with numbness of her feet and hands, weakness of distal muscle groups of the feet and hands, and areflexia of the ankles. The type and pattern of abnormalities suggest which of the following:
   A. Mononeuropathy
   B. Radiculopathy
   C. Polyneuropathy
   D. Central cord syndrome
   E. Spinal cord transection

4. The key anatomic feature of Huntington's disease is
   A. depigmentation of the substantia nigra.
   B. atrophy of the caudate nuclei.
   C. sclerosis of the hippocampus.
   D. atrophy of subthalamic nucleus.

5. A "homeless" 50-year-old man is admitted for treatment of pneumonia. Neurologic examination reveals that he has a wide-based unsteady gait, ataxia of both lower limbs, mild distal and symmetric lower extremity weakness, loss of muscle stretch reflexes in the lower extremities, and a stocking-glove pattern of sensory loss to pain and temperature only. The most likely diagnosis to explain the ataxia is
   A. Guillain-Barré syndrome.
   B. myasthenia gravis.
   C. cerebellar degeneration secondary to alcoholism.
   D. cerebellar astrocytoma.

6. A 35-year-old painter has fallen from a ladder onto the back of his head on a concrete floor. He complains of vertigo, hearing loss, and facial weakness. Computed tomography of his skull reveals a left transverse temporal bone fracture involving his horizontal vestibular canal and cochlea. His facial nerve has been severed by the fracture. In which direction would the patient's nystagmus be?
   A. Clockwise rotatory nystagmus in both eyes
   B. Vertical left nystagmus with slow component to the right and fast component to the left in both eyes
   C. Vertical right nystagmus with slow component to the left and fast component to the right in both eyes
   D. Horizontal right nystagmus with slow component to the right and fast component to the left in both eyes
   E. Horizontal right nystagmus with slow component to the left and fast component to the right in both eyes

7. A 10-year-old boy with headaches is found on CT scan to have a tumor filling the aqueduct of Sylvius. This patient is not likely to have which of the following:
   A. Communicating hydrocephalus
   B. Noncommunicating hydrocephalus
   C. Increased intracranial pressure
   D. Decreased brain compliance
   E. Hydrostatic edema

8. A four-year-old white female was taken to her pediatrician by her mother, who noted that the little girl had
been day-dreaming a lot more than usual. Mother
hadn't thought too much of it until she noticed that
her child did it several times during Sesame Street,
her favorite television show. Her daughter would stare
straight ahead for 10–15 seconds, would occasionally
smack her lips a few times if it lasted longer than that,
and then immediately resumed what she had been
doing. The doctor prescribed carbamazepine three
times per day and scheduled her for an EEG. Ten days
later, the mother called, stating that the spells had
doubled in frequency.

What type of seizure is the most likely based on the
description given by mom?
A. Atonic seizure
B. Absence seizure
C. Myoclonic seizure
D. Focal seizure
E. Generalized tonic-clonic seizure

9. A 26-year-old man has the recent onset of persistent
and progressive pain around the right eye. The periorbital area is tender to palpation. There is reduced sensation over the right forehead. The vision is reduced
in the right eye. He cannot adduct, abduct, or elevate
the right eye and the pupil is larger on the right and
slower to respond than the left.

The headache described in this case represents
which of the following types of headache?
A. Migraine headache
B. Cluster headache
C. Tension headache
D. Headache from involvement of extracranial pain
sensitive structures
E. Trigeminal neuralgia

10. Intracerebral hemorrhage is *least* likely to be associ-
ated with
A. fibromuscular dysplasia.
B. hypertension.
C. arteriovenous malformations.
D. sympathomimetic drugs.
E. amyloid angiopathy.

11. The pathogenesis of neuronal and oligodendroglial
cell loss in AIDS dementia is related to all of the fol-
lowing except
A. activated microglia.
B. astrocytic production of cytokines.
C. direct neuronal or oligodendroglial cell invasion
by the human immunodeficiency virus.
D. direct infection of the microglial cell.

Answers

Part I: Cardiovascular Diseases

1. B. Interruption of the His bundle would sever the only electrical connection between the AV node and the ventricles, leading to complete heart block. Fibrosis of the sinus node might cause bradycardia due to pacemaker failure, but all the emitted sinus node impulses would be transmitted to the ventricle. Interruption of either the left or the right bundle would not prevent the impulse from being conducted to the ventricle through the other bundle. Interruption of both the left and the right bundle would result in complete heart block. Interruption of an accessory pathway would have no effect on conduction through the normal conduction system.

2. A. The systolic function of the myocardium is contraction; when contraction is impaired, systolic dysfunction results.

3. E. Valvular insufficiency produces diastolic volume loading of the chamber or chambers involved. The increased volume is accompanied by an increase in diastolic pressure since volume and pressure during diastole are related by the diastolic compliance curve. The increased diastolic volume results in an increase in stroke volume only a portion of which is reflected in forward flow (cardiac output). A reflex increase in heart rate may occur but bradycardia would not be expected.

4. A. Obstruction to pulmonary blood flow typically causes severe hypoxemia resulting in cyanosis. In left heart obstructive lesions the ductus is necessary to provide systemic (not pulmonary) blood flow. Hypercyanotic spells are caused by a lowering of systemic resistance and increased pulmonary vascular resistance. Children with large septal defects often do not have symptoms of CHF if their pulmonary vascular resistance remains elevated. The foramen ovale provides an important site of mixing of poorly and well oxygenated blood after birth in several types of congenital lesions.

5. E. Patient's symptoms of prolonged chest pain and

signs of CHF are suggestive of acute myocardial infarction. Anginal pain is similar but usually lasts less than 15–20 minutes.

6. B. In restrictive cardiomyopathy the ventricular cavities are usually normal in size. Amyloidosis is the prototype for restrictive cardiomyopathy, with the other causes for restrictive cardiomyopathy being sarcoidosis and hemochromatosis. Most patients with restrictive cardiomyopathy have predominantly diastolic dysfunction due to the restrictive process. Systolic dysfunction is uncommon and a rather late clinical feature. The differential diagnosis of restrictive cardiomyopathy is constrictive pericarditis and not pericardial effusion. Constrictive pericarditis is a condition characterized by thick pericardium which restricts diastolic filling, thereby sharing several clinical features with restrictive cardiomyopathy. The cardiomyopathy that occurs in the postpartum period is dilated cardiomyopathy and not restrictive cardiomyopathy.

7. E. RV hypertrophy or dilatation is required for the diagnosis of cor pulmonale but may be seen in other forms of heart disease such as mitral stenosis, pulmonic stenosis, or atrial septal defect. Similarly, an increase in the intensity of the pulmonic component of the second heart sound will accompany pulmonary hypertension of any cause. Shortness of breath on exertion is a common symptom and may be secondary to left ventricular systolic or diastolic dysfunction, for example. Chronic hypoxemia often leads to cor pulmonale, but acute hypoxemia may be seen without evidence of cor pulmonale.

8. E. Pericardial effusion is not a feature of constrictive pericarditis.

9. D. Vegetations may rarely be noninfectious. Echocardiograms may be negative. In greater than 95% of cases, continuous bacteremia or fungemia is the diagnostic hallmark of infective endocarditis.

10. D. Arteriovenous shunting may occur in distributive shock and result in inadequate oxygen delivery and utilization even in the presence of increased car-

diac output. Cardiac output is frequently high but may be in the normal range or depressed in distributive shock, especially in later stages of shock. The decrease in cardiac pump function may be due to cardiac ischemia or the postulated circulating "myocardial depressant factors." Creatine kinase MB fractions are used to diagnose acute myocardial infarction, which does not necessarily imply cardiogenic shock. In acute myocardial infarction, both a CVP and PAOP are required to assess the adequacy of filling of both ventricles. Pericardial effusion impairs filling, or flow into, rather than out of, the ventricles.

11. C. In mitral stenosis, left atrial pressure is elevated due to obstruction of blood flow from the left atrium to the left ventricle. This subsequently results in elevation of pulmonary capillary and pulmonary arterial pressure. Due to diminished blood flow into the left ventricle, this chamber is usually small and has lower than normal pressure. Thus in mitral stenosis failure is not due to left ventricular failure. Flow through the mitral valve is favored by longer diastole associated with a slower heart rate. Dyspnea is due to pulmonary venous congestion.

12. D. Hypercalcemia may cause hypertension, primarily through its direct effect on peripheral vascular resistance. All of the other conditions have predominant volume-dependent factors generating the hypertension.

13. C. Loss of integrity of the one-way valve in the communicating veins allows high-pressure flow from the deep veins to be transmitted to the superficial system; this flaw defines chronic venous insufficiency and it usually initiates a chain of pathophysiologic events which may lead to the postphlebitic syndrome. Valves are usually lost after a significant DVT episode, but identical valvular damage occurs occasionally in the absence of DVT. Patients with chronic venous insufficiency may have **recurrent** DVT with resultant PE but venous insufficiency alone isn't the cause of PE. Graduated compression hose is adequate treatment for most patients with venous insufficiency. Inflammation may be seen from time to time as part of the postphlebitic syndrome, but does not play a role in the pathogenesis of chronic venous insufficiency.

14. E. Taking in a greater proportion of saturated fat (animal fat) compared to the unsaturated variety (olive oil, etc.) is the only dietary change listed which would raise LDL levels.

Part II: Digestive Diseases and Nutrition

1. E. Esophageal motility disorders equally affect solid and liquid bolus transport, causing dysphagia for both. Mechanical obstructions to flow in the esophagus preferentially cause solid dysphagia, either progressive with esophageal cancer and stricture or intermittent with Schatzki ring. Globus sensation and water brash are symptoms characteristic of GERD.

2. E. Numerous pathogenic mechanisms have been suggested for duodenal ulcers. Whether these abnormalities are primary or secondary has not been established. Many abnormalities will probably prove to be secondary to *H. pylori* infection.

3. D. The intestinal phase of pancreatic secretion accounts for approximately 65% of enzyme release. During this phase, cholecystokinin, as well as secretin, both act upon the pancreas to cause an increase in secretion.

4. E. The inferior vena cava is not included in the portal circulation. Portal hypertension can arise from obstruction to portal venous blood flow at presinusoidal, sinusoidal, and postsinusoidal sites. Splenic vein and portal vein thrombosis are examples of presinusoidal obstruction to portal blood flow. Hepatic vein thrombosis illustrates a postsinusoidal obstruction to flow, and cirrhosis with regenerative nodule formation is a cause of sinusoidal obstruction to portal venous blood flow.

5. A. Bile salts are essential for fat and NOT carbohydrate absorption. Diseases of the pancreas cause decreased secretion of lipase and colipase required for lipolysis. Small bowel resection results in reduced surface area available for absorption. Vitamin B_{12} is primarily absorbed in the ileum, which is also a frequent site of involvement of Crohn's disease. The duodenum is the primary site of iron absorption.

6. D. Bleeding caused by diverticular disease is brisk and acute. It is usually self-limited but, if recurrent, may need surgery. It usually originates from the right colon. Colon cancer, on the other hand, is a common cause of iron deficiency anemia due to slow, chronic bleeding.

7. E. Deficiency of any of the B complex vitamins can lead to a beefy red tongue, known as glossitis. Vitamin C deficiency causes petechiae at the base of hair follicles. Essential fatty acid deficiency causes

an evanescent flaky rash over the truncal areas of the body. Vitamin D deficiency impairs calcium and phosphorus metabolism. Vitamin E deficiency does not lead to characteristic physical changes.

Part III: Endocrine and Metabolic Disorders

1. C. Both peptide and steroid hormones affect transcription in target cells, so this is not a distinguishing characteristic and is the correct answer. Only steroids are derived from cholesterol and must have a nuclear location for activity. Only peptide hormones use cAMP as a second messenger. Peptide hormone receptors are on the cell surface while steroid receptors are cytosolic or nuclear.

2. D. The absence of mineralocorticoids results in sodium loss with resulting decreased plasma volume and hypotension. Although diabetes mellitus might coexist with Addison's disease, hypoglycemia is characteristic of adrenal insufficiency. Hyperkalemia is characteristic of Addison's disease since, in the absence of aldosterone, reduced activity of the Na-K pump of the renal tubule impairs potassium excretion in the urine. Weight loss and not weight gain is characteristic of Addison's disease.

3. A. DKA and normal fasting are qualitatively similar in several respects. In DKA, however, insulin concentrations are significantly lower with respect to circulating glucose levels. In a normal overnight fast, free fatty acids and ketones are present and counter-regulatory hormones are mildly elevated. As the duration of the fast increases, counter-regulatory hormones, fatty acids and ketones all increase, but the prevailing insulin concentration controls lipolysis, glycogenolysis, and protein breakdown. The glucose produced in the liver via gluconeogenesis is sufficient for the brain's requirements but does not produce hyperglycemia. The ketones are taken up under the influence of the available insulin and used in non-neural tissue as an alternative energy source. The elevation of counter-regulatory hormones is not as extreme during fasting as in DKA because of the dehydration associated with the latter condition. Although fasting elevation of such counter-regulatory hormones as cortisol, GH, and epinephrine partially inhibit uptake of glucose by muscle and other non-neural tissues in fasting, greater inhibition is observed in DKA and this is associated with massive hepatic overproduction of glucose (gluconeogenesis) that overwhelms the peripheral utilization of glucose and leads to polyuria and electrolyte abnormalities. In DKA, the ketones are massively increased and are not utilized completely as energy substrate and therefore are excreted by the kidney as their salt, leading to systemic acidosis. These differences between fasting and DKA are due to the presence of "adequate" levels of insulin in the fasting state and lower or absent insulin activity in DKA.

4. C. Kleinefelter's syndrome has a 47,XXY karyotype. Typically these patients have gynecomastia and small, hard testes. Although they are somewhat eunuchoid, they often have normal sexual relationships. Mild mental retardation can be associated with this syndrome.

5. A. Prolactin is the only anterior pituitary hormone which is under tonic inhibition. Therefore, disruption of the tonic inhibition by hypothalamic dopamine would result in an increased secretion of prolactin. Since the secretion of all other anterior pituitary hormones is dependent upon stimulation by hypothalamic factors, disruption of the connection between the hypothalamus and anterior pituitary would result in decreased secretion of these hormones.

6. D. Graves' disease is a result of thyroid-stimulating immunoglobulins (TSIs) that bind the TSH receptor. Hyperthyroidism may result from autoimmune destruction of the thyroid, autonomous nodules, and rarely by decreased T4 suppression of pituitary TSH release; but the eponym Graves' is reserved for diffuse toxic goiter associated with TSH receptor activation.

7. D. Hypocalcemia (not hypercalcemia) contributes to renal osteodystrophy. It is a result of decreased renal production of calcitriol. Hyperphosphatemia — due to decreased renal phosphate clearance — also plays a major role. Aluminum, which is present in some phosphate-binding antacids, inhibits mineralization, causing osteomalacia, which can be seen in renal osteodystrophy.

Part IV: Hematologic and Neoplastic Disorders

1. B. Ineffective erythropoiesis results from defective maturation of erythroid precursors, and the erythroid marrow is hypercellular due to increased erythropoietin production in response to the ane-

mia. The blood reticulocyte count is low because a large proportion of the defective precursors does not develop to the reticulocyte stage.

2. C. Greater than 30% blast cells in the marrow aspirate is diagnostic of acute leukemia.

3. B. The finding of numerous mature lymphocytes and smudge cells with adenopathy and splenomegaly in an elderly patient virtually makes the diagnosis of chronic lymphocytic leukemia. Acute leukemia cells do not appear mature. Some lymphomas, particularly low-grade non-Hodgkin's lymphoma, may present in this fashion, but that disease is usually dominated by the lymphadenopathy. Hodgkin's disease and myeloma very rarely present in leukemic phase and infectious mononucleosis is very uncommon in the elderly.

4. A. A gene that is lost recurrently in tumors provides evidence for a tumor suppressor, not an oncogene, since gene deletion implies a loss of function. The common mechanisms to activate oncogenes in human tumors are amplification, translocation, and point mutation. Animal models involving RNA tumor viruses have often served to identify oncogenes.

5. D. Tumors which are curable with chemotherapy may be cured when they are quite large. Size is not as important prognostically in these tumors as it is in the slow-growing types that respond poorly to chemotherapy.

6. B. In patients with mild thrombocytopenia due to increased splenic pooling, measured platelet survivals are normal. All other statements about this clinical situation are true. The thrombocytopenia is simply the result of pooling much more than the normal one-third of circulating platelets within the congested sinusoids of the spleen. In some patients, as many as 90% of total body platelets may be contained within the spleen, so they are in slow equilibrium with the circulating blood.

Part V: Rheumatologic and Immunologic Disorders

1. E. Deficiency of early components of the classical pathway predispose to SLE. Deficiency of late components predispose to infection, particularly by *Neisseria* species. An association of complement component deficiency and lymphoma has not been established.

2. E. The late phase of immediate hypersensitivity is caused by inflammatory cells chemotactically attracted by mast cell products. It is seen 3–8 hours after allergen challenge in 50% of those who have an early-phase response. It is seen in asthma, allergic rhinitis, skin testing, and anaphylaxis. Fibrosis is not a common consequence.

3. B. IgE and allergy are not necessarily involved in asthma, although they often are. Mediator release, eosinophilia, potential reversibility, and bronchial hyperreactivity are all defining aspects of asthmatic disease, and are used to differentiate asthma from other bronchopulmonary disorders.

4. C. The autoantibody most closely associated with lupus nephritis is anti-native DNA.

5. i. D. Deficiencies of several late components of the complement system predispose to *Neisseria* infection.

   ii. C. The spleen has an important role in the phagocytosis of circulating microorganisms which might explain why fulminant bacteremia, especially pneumoccal occurs in children after splenectomy.

   iii. A. Recurrent infections with encapsulated bacteria, such as the *Pneumococcus,* is characteristic of patients with defective humoral immunity.

   iv. E. The host defense against *staphylococcus* depends upon intact granulocyte function.

   v. B. Defects in cellular immunity are characterized by infections with viruses and fungi including *Candida* species.

6. A. OA is not a disease where degeneration is the cardinal feature; it is a dynamic process reflecting cartilage injury with subsequent repair.

7. E. Joint instability results from distention of the joint capsule from swelling and synovial hypertrophy. Ligaments are damaged by inflammatory mediators and chronic distention. The muscular support is lost as muscles become weak and atrophy from joint immobilization secondary to pain. Joint denervation is not a feature of RA. Neuropeptides released from nerve endings actually contribute to joint destruction by stimulating degradative enzyme production. The importance of these neuropeptides to the inflammatory response is clinically demonstrated in RA patients who suffer strokes with unilateral paralysis; active joint disease often resolves on the paralyzed side.

8. E. A high-purine diet may contribute to hyperuricemia, but there is no evidence of increased absorption with a normal diet.

Part VI: Pulmonary Diseases

1. D. Answering this question requires calculating the oxygen content in each of these situations. Since oxygen is highly insoluble in plasma water, one can ignore the calculation for the dissolved oxygen and simply calculate oxyhemoglobin. Using the oxyhemoglobin dissociation curve, one can see that at a PaO_2 of 60 mm Hg, hemoglobin is approximately 90% saturated, at a PaO_2 of 50 mm Hg, 85% saturated, and at a PaO_2 of 40 mm Hg, 75% saturated. In the first option, the oxyhemoglobin level increased from approximately 8.75 to 12.5 ml/dl for an increase of approximately 3.75 ml/dl. In the second example the increase was from 8.75 to 9.4 ml/dl for an increase of approximately 0.65 ml/dl. In the third example the oxyhemoglobin level went from 7.3 to 8.95 ml/dl, an increase of 1.65 ml/dl. In the fourth example the oxyhemoglobin went from 7.3 to 11.4 ml/dl, an increase of 4.1 ml/dl, and in the last example the oxyhemoglobin went from 15.65 to 18.75 ml/dl, an increase of 3.1 ml/dl. Therefore, the greatest increase was in option D.

2. A. A restrictive defect has a decreased TLC by definition. The FEV_1/FVC ratio may be normal or increased in a restrictive defect. If the restrictive process increases lung elastic recoil and the driving pressure for expiratory flow, the FEV_1/FVC ratio may be increased. Reduced TLC and FEV_1/FVC ratio would be characteristic of a mixed obstructive and restrictive defect. A normal FVC and decreased FEV_1/FVC ratio would indicate a pure obstructive defect. An increase in FEV_1 following an inhaled bronchodilator is characteristic of an obstructive defect and is not found in a pure restrictive defect. A normal FVC and FEV_1 and decreased FEF_{25-75} would indicate an obstructive defect.

3. B. First, the PaO_2 is not low enough to produce dyspnea. A measurable increase in respiratory drive, at rest, does not occur with hypoxia until PO_2 falls below 50 mm Hg, and even then it is not sufficient to produce more than a few mm Hg reduction in PCO_2. Second, if you calculate the A – a gradient you will see that it is increased, $0.21 \times (747 - 47) - 25/.8 - 60 = 55.75$, which is above normal (10–25 mm Hg). This is good evidence of lung disease in this patient.

4. C. Patients with α_1-antitrypsin deficiency classically show lower lobe involvement with equal destruction of all parts of the acinus, hence the name "panacinar emphysema." Centrilobular is the most common form of emphysema and usually is associated with cigarette smoking. B, D, and E are different names for the limited peripheral disease seen in adults with spontaneous pneumothorax.

5. B. Poorly ventilated alveoli with good blood flow is the major cause of hypoxemia in interstitial disease. Impaired diffusion contributes to hypoxemia mainly with exercise. Shunt is increased but has less of an effect than low $\dot{V}/\dot{Q}$ as demonstrated by the marked improvement in PaO_2 by administration of oxygen to most patients with interstitial disease. Dead space is increased, but this contributes little to hypoxemia. There are more high $\dot{V}/\dot{Q}$ areas in interstitial lung disease but they do not contribute to hypoxemia.

6. C. Under normal conditions, when P_{CAP} is 10 mm Hg, π_{CAP} is 24 mm Hg and σ is close to one (0.9), the balance of intravascular forces should promote fluid absorption from the interstitial space, but this is not what is observed. Instead there is a continuous flow of lymph from the lung, indicating continuous filtration. The importance of the interstitial forces is demonstrated by the fact that the balance of intravascular *and* interstitial forces in fact favors filtration of fluid from the capillary into the interstitial space where it is picked up and removed by the lymphatics.

7. E. The visceral pleura is not innervated, so the presence of pleuritic pain indicates irritation of receptors in the parietal pleura. Lung compression produces both V/Q mismatching and reflex cough stimulation. Outward displacement of the chest wall causes the inspiratory muscles to work at a mechanical disadvantage and is a major factor contributing to dyspnea.

8. C. All statements concerning VTE are correct except for C. Autopsy studies indicate the incidence of VTE may be rising despite the use of prophylactic measures. The reasons are unclear. The aging populations of developed nations may be to blame, as risk of VTE rises exponentially with increasing age.

Part VII: Renal and Electrolyte Disorders

1. C. Hyponatremia can be associated with a normal or increased as well as decreased total body sodium.

Since sodium is lost exclusively from the extracellular space, the size of the intracellular compartment would change only if the osmolality of body fluids also changed. The sodium content is the major determinant of the volume of the extracellular space. Therefore, a decrease in extracellular volume exists whenever sodium depletion occurs. Sodium excess, not sodium depletion, would be associated with expansion of the extracellular space.

2. D. Normally, all the potassium presented to the glomerulus is freely filtered and that situation does not change in potassium depletion. All the potassium appearing in urine is *secreted* from the collecting duct. In chronic potassium depletion, potassium secretion in the collecting duct is decreased. This is mediated in part by reduction in plasma aldosterone level.

3. i. B. The low pH and increased AG indicate the presence of a metabolic acidosis. The $PaCO_2$, being greater than expected in the face of the metabolic disturbance, indicates that a concomitant respiratory acidosis is present as well.

    ii. A. The pH, pCO_2, and HCO_3^- are normal. However, the anion gap of 25 mEq/liter is markedly elevated. The increased anion gap suggests the presence of a metabolic acidosis. Since the pH is normal, an alkalosis must also be present. The normal pCO_2 indicates that the alkalosis can not be respiratory. Thus the only combination acid-base disturbance which can explain this combination of data is a metabolic acidosis and a coexisting metabolic alkalosis.

    iii. F. The presence of an alkalemia and a low pCO_2 indicates respiratory alkalosis. The slightly elevated plasma HCO_3^- indicates the presence of a concomitant metabolic alkalosis since HCO_3^- should be normal to low in isolated respiratory alkalosis.

    iv. E. The markedly depressed plasma bicarbonate indicates the presence of metabolic acidosis, since even the most severe and prolonged respiratory alkalosis is not associated with a plasma bicarbonate level less than 12–14 mEq/liter. The modest elevation of the anion gap suggests that both a normal anion gap and a high anion gap type of metabolic acidosis may be present. The respiratory response is appropriate. This can be confirmed by consulting Fig. 53-2. A good rule of thumb is that the $PaCO_2$ should match the last two digits of the arterial pH if compensation for metabolic acidosis is appropriate.

    v. D. The slightly increased pH indicates an alkalosis but the $[HCO_3^-]$ is too low and the anion gap is too high to be explained by respiratory alkalosis alone. These findings indicate that metabolic acidosis is also present.

    vi. C. The $PaCO_2$ of 58 mm Hg indicates respiratory acidosis ($PaCO_2$ rarely exceeds 55 mm Hg as a compensatory response to metabolic alkalosis). The presence of a normal arterial pH indicates that metabolic alkalosis is also present since renal compensation alone would not be expected to completely correct the acidemia (i.e., arterial pH is always low in uncomplicated respiratory acidosis).

4. D. By inhibiting Mg reabsorption in the thick ascending limb of Henle's loop, which is the major site of Mg reabsorption in the nephron, bumetanide (one of the loop-acting diuretics) increases urinary Mg excretion.

5. D. Nephrotic syndrome associated with membranous nephropathy has a high risk of thromboembolic complications, especially renal vein thrombosis. Although total serum calcium is often depressed, because of the low serum proteins available for binding, ionized calcium usually remains within the normal range. Most of these patients have normal blood volume; therefore congestive heart failure is unlikely, unless coexisting cardiac disease is present. Rapidly deteriorating renal functions is not a feature of membranous nephropathy. Total serum T_4 may be depressed due to low serum proteins, but free T_4 and TSH levels are usually normal.

6. D. Severe congestive heart failure often causes prerenal azotemia, which is characterized by a fractional excretion of sodium less than 1% (typically 0.1–0.2%). The other features listed are typical findings in prerenal azotemia.

7. E. Buffering of the protons created by the oxidative metabolism of sulfur and phosphorus containing amino and nucleic acids, respectively, lowers the serum bicarbonate concentration. Alveolar hyperventilation will ensue, thereby lowering arterial PCO_2. The serum chloride concentration under these circumstances will rise to maintain electroneutrality of the extracellular fluid as bicarbonate falls. Decreased renal ammonia production occurs

in chronic renal insufficiency because of reduced proximal tubular mass. Although the amount of acid excreted by the kidneys in chronic renal insufficiency is markedly reduced, the ability of the functioning nephrons to generate a urine-to-plasma pH difference is not.

8. A. Tubular damage impairs the ability to acidify the urine, often resulting in metabolic acidosis with a normal anion gap. Often severe damage of tubules and interstitium leads to fibrosis and destruction of the entire nephron. Therefore glomerular filtration rate decreases. Fractional excretion of sodium is invariably increased in patients with a decreased glomerular filtration rate. This occurs as a functional adaptation to the decrease in GFR in order to maintain sodium balance. Decreased ability to concentrate urine is a common finding in patients with tubulointerstitial nephropathy, especially when the medulla is affected. Medullary damage impairs the counter-current multiplier system and the medullary interstitium cannot maintain the desired hypertonicity. Tubular disease may produce proteinuria but it is usually less than 1–2 g in 24 hours.

Part VIII: Neurologic Diseases and Special Senses

1. A. Expressive aphasia and right monoparesis are localized to the left frontal lobe (response cortex). Since only the arm is involved, the lesion is more specifically localized to the lateral aspect of the frontal lobe which conforms to the frontal branches of the left middle cerebral artery. As the onset was acute, the lesion is most likely vascular such as infarction involving the left middle cerebral artery.

2. C. Polymyositis is often insidious in onset, causing progressive non-fluctuating weakness of proximal muscles. The disease is usually painless, but 15% of the patients will complain of muscle aching.

3. C. Distal greater than proximal sensory loss, weakness and areflexia are typical findings of a polyneuropathy. Radiculopathies produce dermatomal distribution of radiating pain or anesthesia and segmental weakness. Mononeuropathies produce sensory and motor abnormalities which conform to one nerve. A spinal cord transection would involve a sensory level which conformed to one dermatome, and corticospinal tract signs. A central cord syndrome would

produce dissociation of sensory modalities with a "suspended band" sensory deficit and segmental lower motor neuron signs.

4. B. The pathology of Huntington's disease demonstrates large lateral ventricles due to the atrophy of the caudate nuclei and to a lesser extent the putamen. On neuroimaging studies, this is often described as "box-car" ventricles, due to the large and somewhat rectangular appearance the anterior horns of the lateral ventricles assume. Pathologic cerebral atrophy can also be seen on neuroimaging studies. Depigmentation of the substantia nigra occurs in Parkinson's disease and hippocampal sclerosis is seen in certain types of epilepsy.

5. C. The gait ataxia and lower limb ataxia localizes to the vermis and anterior lobe of the cerebellum while distal weakness, sensory loss, and hyporeflexia suggest peripheral nerve damage. A combined toxic effect of ethanol and thiamine deficiency would explain the cerebellar dysfunction and the polyneuropathy, both of which are contributing to the ataxia.

6. D. With a left peripheral vestibular injury the tonic activity from the left labyrinth to move the eyes to the right (away) is lost and the intact right side then causes a slow deviation of the eyes to the left. The reticular formation rapidly moves the eyes back to the right again. Therefore, the patient will have a right beating horizontal nystagmus since the fast component defines the direction of the nystagmus.

7. A. This patient suffered headaches which were likely the result of increased intracranial pressure. The cause of this patient's increased intracranial pressure is the noncommunicating hydrocephalus as a result of the tumor blocking the aqueduct, thus obstructing flow of CSF from the lateral and 3rd ventricles. This noncommunicating hydrocephalus causes an increase in intracranial pressure with concomitant decreased brain compliance or a high brain elastance. The water content of the brain increases in this condition and this particular type of edema is termed hydrostatic or hydrocephalic edema.

8. B. The description is typical for absence seizures which are characterized by brief episodes of altered consciousness. In this case, partial complex seizures are also considered as she had associated lip smacking which can occur in either type.

9. D. The occurrence of a recent onset of localized pain which is reproducible would suggest involvement

of pain sensitive structure of the head. In this case, involvement of ethmoid or frontal sinus or orbital structures is suggested by the location of pain. While a cluster headache may be localized to the periorbital region, the pain typically occurs in clusters. Neither migraine nor cluster or tension headaches are associated with focal neurologic signs. Trigeminal neuralgia may involve the ophthalmic division of the trigeminal but is characterized by brief episodes of lancinating pain.

10. A. Fibromuscular dysplasia is associated with stenosis and thrombosis but does not directly cause intracranial hemorrhage.

11. C. Neuronal cell death is very likely cytokine mediated, through activation of the microglial cell. Activated microglia produce cell-damaging cytokines and stimulate the astrocyte to do likewise. The human immunodeficiency virus does not directly infect either neuron or oligodendroglia cell.

Index

Note: Numbers followed by the letter *f* indicate figures; numbers followed by the letter *t* indicate tables.